WHAT THE EXPERTS ARE SAYING ABOUT
THE PDR® POCKET GUIDE TO PRESCRIPTION DRUGS™

"An easy-to-read guide to medications, side effects, and efficacy... Now one can get understandable medical information that can help keep health costs down, yet give patients a fine comfort level with the medicines they take."

> —Leon G. Smith, MD
> Chairman of Medicine
> St. Michael's Medical Center
> Newark, NJ

"A must for every household where there are concerns about the safe use of medications. It is an ideal way to clarify and supplement the information provided by your healthcare provider."

> —Jack M. Rosenberg, PharmD, PhD
> Professor of Pharmacy Practice and Pharmacology
> Arnold & Marie Schwartz College of Pharmacy
> Long Island University—Brooklyn Campus
> Brooklyn, NY

W9-BNW-503

THE ⬛ PDR®

PDR®
FAMILY
GUIDES

POCKET GUIDE

TO PRESCRIPTION DRUGS™

7TH EDITION
FULLY REVISED AND UPDATED

Based on *Physicians' Desk Reference*®,
the Nation's Leading Drug Handbook

POCKET BOOKS
New York   London   Toronto   Sydney

PHYSICIANS' DESK REFERENCE®, PDR®, Pocket PDR®, The PDR® Family Guide to Prescription Drugs®, The PDR® Family Guide to Women's Health and Prescription Drugs®, and The PDR® Family Guide to Nutrition and Health® are registered trademarks used herein under license. PDR® for Ophthalmic Medicines, PDR® for Nonprescription Drugs and Dietary Supplements, PDR® Companion Guide, PDR® Pharmacopoeia Pocket Dosing Guide, PDR® Monthly Prescribing Guide™, PDR® for Herbal Medicines, PDR® for Nutritional Supplements, PDR® Medical Dictionary, PDR® Nurse's Drug Handbook™, PDR® Nurse's Dictionary, The PDR® Family Guide Encyclopedia of Medical Care, The PDR® Family Guide to Natural Medicines and Healing Therapies, The PDR® Family Guide to Common Ailments, The PDR® Family Guide to Over-the-Counter Drugs, The PDR® Family Guide to Nutritional Supplements, and PDR® Electronic Library are trademarks used herein under license.

Officers of Thomson Healthcare, Inc.: *President and Chief Executive Officer:* Kevin King; *Chief Financial Officer:* Paul Hilger; *Chief Technology Officer:* Frank Licata; *Executive Vice President, Medical Education:* Jeff MacDonald; *Executive Vice President, Medstat:* Carol Diephuis; *Executive Vice President, Micromedex:* Jeff Reihl; *Senior Vice President, Marketing:* Timothy Murray; *Vice President, Finance:* Joseph Scarfone; *Vice President, Human Resources:* Pamela M. Bilash

POCKET BOOKS, a division of Simon & Schuster, Inc.
1230 Avenue of the Americas, New York, NY 10020

Copyright © 1996, 1997, 1999, 2000, 2002, 2003, 2005 by Thomson PDR

Published by arrangement with Thomson PDR

ISBN-13: 978-1-4165-1085-7
ISBN-10: 1-4165-1085-0
ISBN-13: 978-1-4165-2331-4
ISBN-10: 1-4165-2331-6

This Pocket Books paperback edition December 2005

10 9 8 7 6 5 4 3 2 1

POCKET and colophon are registered trademarks of Simon & Schuster, Inc.

Cover design by John Vairo Jr.
Front cover photo © Davis & Starr/Getty Images

Manufactured in the United States of America

For information regarding special discounts for bulk purchases,
please contact Simon & Schuster Special Sales
at 1-800-456-6798 or business@simonandschuster.com.

Publisher's Note

The drug information contained in this book is based on product labeling published in the 2005 edition of *Physicians' Desk Reference®*, supplemented with facts from other sources the publisher believes reliable. While diligent efforts have been made to ensure the accuracy of this information, the book does not list every possible action, adverse reaction, interaction, and precaution; and all information is presented without guarantees by the authors, consultants, and publisher, who disclaim all liability in connection with its use.

This book is intended only as a reference for use in an ongoing partnership between doctor and patient in the management of the patient's health. It is not a substitute for a doctor's professional judgment, and serves only as a reminder of concerns that may need discussion. All readers are urged to consult with a physician before beginning or discontinuing use of any prescription drug or undertaking any form of self-treatment. Brand names listed in this book are intended to represent only the more commonly used products. Inclusion of a brand name does not signify endorsement of the product; absence of a name does not imply a criticism or rejection of the product. The publisher is not advocating the use of any product described in this book, does not warrant or guarantee any of these products, and has not performed any independent analysis in connection with the product information contained herein.

Contents

Contents

The PDR® Pocket Guide to Prescription Drugs™, based on the 2005 edition of PDR®

Editor-in-Chief: Bette LaGow

Director, Clinical Content: Thomas Fleming, PharmD

Senior Editor: Lori Murray

Production Editor: Gwynned Kelly

Drug Information Specialist: Gregory Tallis, RPh

Writers: Nancy K. Bannon; Rebecca Bowers; Janette Carlucci; Neil Chesanow; Mary Lou Hurley; Eileen McCaffrey; Leah E. Perry; Kathleen Rodgers, RPh; Marissa J. Ventura

Editorial Production: *Vice President, PDR Services:* Brian Holland; *Director, Operations:* Robert Klein; *Production Specialist:* Christina Klinger; *Digital Imaging Manager:* Christopher Husted; *Digital Imaging Coordinator:* Michael Labruyere; *Production Design Supervisor:* Adeline Rich; *Senior Electronic Publishing Designer:* Livio Udina

Thomson PDR

Senior Vice President, Sales & Marketing: Dikran M. Barsamian

Senior Director, Brand & Product Management: Valerie E. Berger

Director, Brand & Product Management: Carmen Mazzatta

Senior Director, Publishing Sales & Marketing: Michael Bennett

Director, Trade Sales: Bill Gaffney

Gardiner Morse, MS
Editor, Harvard Health Publications, Boston, MA

Louis V. Napolitano, MD
Family Practice
Hackensack University Medical Center, Hackensack, NJ

Mark D. Ravenscraft, MD
Creve Coeur, MO

Martin I. Resnick, MD
Professor and Chairman, Department of Urology
Case Western Reserve University, Cleveland, OH

Frank Simo, MD
St. Louis, MO

Karl Singer, MD
Exeter Family Medicine Associates, Exeter, NH

Eugene W. Sweeney, MD
Department of Dermatology
Columbia Presbyterian Medical Center
New York, NY

Foreword

The PDR® Pocket Guide to Prescription Drugs™ strives to make the many benefits of modern pharmaceuticals—as well as their undeniable risks—as clear and simple as can be. *The PDR Pocket Guide* spells out exactly why each drug is prescribed and the most important fact to remember about it, then discloses its most common side effects. As a safeguard against error, it also provides you with information on standard dosage recommendations. It tells exactly what to do when you miss a dose of your medication, while alerting you to the warning signs of an overdose. And to help you find all these facts as quickly as possible, it lists each medication under its familiar brand name—with a cross-reference in case the drug is dispensed generically.

Still, despite the depth and detail of the information you'll find here, *The PDR Pocket Guide* is not a replacement for your doctor's advice. Rather, it serves as a reminder of the basic instructions and caveats that may be forgotten by the time you leave your doctor's office, as well as providing you with a checklist of the problems and conditions that you must be certain the doctor knows about—facts that might call for a change in your prescription.

In this way, the book is designed to serve as an aid in an ongoing dialogue between you and your doctor—a collaboration necessary for any treatment to work. Just as the doctor must tell you how and why to use a particular drug, you must tell the doctor how it affects you, reporting any reactions or drug interactions you suspect you may have. And while it's up to the doctor to devise your treatment strategy, it's up to you to make sure that the right doses are administered at the right times, and that the prescribed course of therapy is completed as planned.

Physicians' Desk Reference® has been providing doctors with the information needed for safe, effective drug therapy for 60 years. Designed especially for healthcare professionals, it presents the facts in a detailed, technical format approved by the Food and Drug Administration (FDA). To make the key facts buried in this wealth of data accessible to everyone, *The PDR Pocket Guide* strips away the medical shorthand and technical terminology, and presents the core of this information in a simple, standard format designed for maximum convenience and ease of use by the consumer. Almost all the information you'll find in *The PDR Pocket Guide*'s consumer drug profiles has been extracted from *PDR* itself. When necessary, however, selected facts have been added from other authoritative sources—in particular, the databases maintained by Thomson Micromedex, another company within the Thomson Healthcare group of respected, authoritative healthcare, medical, and pharmacological content specialists.

Modern drug therapy is a vast and complicated field—so complicated that, for many questions about medicines, the answer varies with each patient. *The PDR Pocket Guide to Prescription Drugs* gives you general guidelines for safe drug use. But only your doctor, evaluating the unique details of your case, can give you the exact instructions best suited for you. The goal of this book is simply to alert you to the most pertinent questions to ask, and to help clarify your doctor's answers—in short, to give you the tools you need to supervise your own medical care as effectively as possible.

We wish you good health.

Robert W. Hogan, MD
Chair, Board of Medical Consultants

How to Use This Book

Although doctors today can often work miracles with advanced technology and sophisticated medicines, it's vital for you to take an active role in managing your health. Any medicine can prove worthless if taken improperly. Likewise, you must let your doctor know if you react badly to a drug or have a condition that makes taking it dangerous. While no book is a substitute for a visit to the doctor, this guide is designed to help you use your medications safely and effectively, and to help you determine things that deserve further discussion with your doctor.

The book is divided into two major parts. In the first, you'll find profiles of the more frequently prescribed medications. The second section has helpful references and an index of common diseases and disorders.

THE DRUG PROFILES

The profiles provide detailed information on the most frequently prescribed prescription drugs, plus a few widely used over-the-counter medications. Though the section covers more than 1,000 products, don't be alarmed if you don't find a profile for a prescription you've received. There are a number of specialized yet valuable drugs that have been omitted here due to lack of space.

The products described here are listed alphabetically by the manufacturer's brand name or the generic name. Full-profile headers appear in all uppercase letters; cross-references are either boldface upper- and lowercase (for brand names) or boldface upper- and lowercase italic (for generics). If there is more than one brand of a drug, you'll usually find the profile cross-referenced to the name most frequently prescribed.

The drug profiles begin with correct pronunciation of the name, followed by the generic name for the drug and, if applicable, the other brand names. The information that follows these names is divided into 10 sections. Here's what you'll find in each.

Why is this drug prescribed?
This is an overview of the major conditions for which the drug is generally prescribed.

Most important fact about this drug
Highlighted here is one key point about a drug that is especially worthwhile to know. We've placed it here for the sake of emphasis. Never regard this section as a definitive summary of the drug.

How should you take this medication?

This section details special instructions, including how and when to take the drug, and any dietary restrictions that may apply. Also found here is advice on what to do if you forget a dose, as well as any special storage requirements that apply.

What side effects may occur?

Shown here are only the most common side effects listed by the manufacturer in the drug's FDA-approved product labeling. Any drug will occasionally cause an unwanted reaction. Even the most common side effects are seen in only a small percentage of patients. Not included are side effects that can be detected only by a physician or laboratory. If you have any questions about side effects—or if you have any new or continuing symptoms—talk to your doctor

Why should this drug not be prescribed?

A few drugs are harmful under certain conditions, which are detailed here. The most common contraindication is a hypersensitivity to the drug itself. If you think one of these restrictions applies to you, alert your doctor immediately.

Special warnings about this medication

If you recognize any problems or conditions that your doctor may be unaware of, be sure to bring them to his or her attention. Do not change your dosage or discontinue the drug without first consulting your doctor, however. Such a change might well do more harm than good.

Possible food and drug interactions when taking this medication

This section lists specific drugs, classes of drugs, and foods that have been known to interact with the medicine being profiled. The examples are not all-inclusive. If you're not certain whether a medication you're taking falls into one of these categories, be sure to check with your doctor or pharmacist. But never stop taking any drug without first consulting your doctor.

Special information if you are pregnant or breastfeeding

This section will tell you whether a drug has been confirmed safe for use during pregnancy or breastfeeding, is known to be dangerous, or is part of that large group about which scientists are not really sure. With many of these drugs, the small theoretical risk they pose may be overshadowed by your need for treatment.

Recommended dosage

Shown here are excerpts of the dosage guidelines your doctor uses. The information is presented as a convenient double check in case you suspect a misunderstanding or a typographical error on your prescription label. Don't use it to determine an exact dosage yourself.

Overdosage

As another safety measure this section lists, when available, the signs of an overdose. If the symptoms listed in this section lead you to suspect an overdose, seek emergency medical attention immediately.

OTHER FEATURES

Drug Identification Guide

This full-color guide includes actual-sized photographs of the leading products discussed in the book, arranged alphabetically by brand name. Manufacturers occasionally change the color and shape of a product, so if a prescription does not match the photo shown here, check with your pharmacist before assuming there's been a mistake.

The Disease and Disorder Index

This index helps you quickly identify drugs available for a particular medical condition. Arranged alphabetically by ailment, it lists all the medications profiled in the book.

The Appendices

This section provides you with two important safeguards that every home should always have handy: Appendix 1 is a brief guide to safe medication use and Appendix 2 is a directory of poison control centers nationwide. Appendix 3, a new addition, lists the 200 drugs most commonly prescribed in the United States.

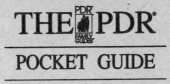

THE PDR PDR

POCKET GUIDE

TO PRESCRIPTION DRUGS™

Drug Profiles

Abacavir See Ziagen, page 1633.

Abacavir, Lamivudine, and Zidovudine See Trizivir, page 1505.

ABILIFY
Pronounced: a-BILL-i-fie
Generic name: Aripiprazole

Why is this drug prescribed?

Abilify is used in the treatment of schizophrenia, the psychological disorder that causes its victims to lose touch with reality, often triggering hallucinations, delusions (false beliefs), and disorganized thinking. It's also used to help control the manic phase of bipolar disorder, including the prevention of future episodes. The drug is thought to work by modifying sensitivity to two of the brain's chief chemical messengers, serotonin and dopamine.

Most important fact about this drug

Abilify can cause tardive dyskinesia, a condition marked by involuntary movements in the face and body. This condition may be permanent and appears to be most common among older adults, especially women. Ask your doctor for more information about this possible risk.

Drugs such as Abilify may increase the risk of death in elderly people with dementia-related psychosis. Abilify is not approved for use in such patients.

How should you take this medication?

Abilify should be taken once a day. It may be taken with food or on an empty stomach. The drug is available in tablet and oral solution forms.

■ *If you miss a dose…*
Take the forgotten dose as soon as you remember. However, if it is almost time for your next dose, skip the one you missed and return to your regular schedule. Do not take 2 doses at once.

■ *Storage instructions…*
Store the tablets at room temperature. Keep bottles of the oral solution in the refrigerator and use within 6 months after opening.

What side effects may occur?

Side effects cannot be anticipated. If any develop or change in intensity, tell your doctor as soon as possible. Only your doctor can determine if it is safe to continue using Abilify.

■ *Side effects may include:*
Anxiety, blurred vision, constipation, cough, headache, insomnia, light-headedness, nausea, rash, restlessness, runny nose, sleepiness, tremors, vomiting, weakness, weight gain

Why should this drug not be prescribed?
If Abilify causes an allergic reaction, you'll be unable to use it.

Special warnings about this medication
The risk of tardive dyskinesia (see *Most important fact about this drug*) increases with the total amount of Abilify that you've taken. To reduce the risk, the doctor will prescribe the lowest effective dose and resort to long-term therapy only if necessary. If you develop symptoms of tardive dyskinesia, see your doctor immediately. Therapy with Abilify may have to be discontinued.

In rare cases, Abilify has been known to cause a potentially fatal condition called Neuroleptic Malignant Syndrome (NMS). Symptoms include high fever, rigid muscles, irregular pulse or blood pressure, rapid heartbeat, excessive perspiration, altered mental status, and changes in heart rhythm. If you develop these symptoms, contact your doctor immediately. Abilify should be discontinued.

Certain antipsychotic drugs, including Abilify, are associated with an increased risk of developing high blood sugar, which on rare occasions has led to coma or death. See your doctor right away if you develop signs of high blood sugar, including dry mouth, unusual thirst, increased urination, and tiredness. If you have diabetes or have a high risk of developing it, see your doctor regularly for blood sugar testing. Also be aware that the oral solution contains 400 milligrams of sucrose and 200 milligrams of fructose per milliliter.

Because Abilify tends to make some people sleepy, you should be cautious about operating hazardous machinery such as cars until you are certain the drug will not impair your ability.

In a few people, Abilify can cause an abrupt drop in blood pressure when they stand up, leading to light-headedness or even fainting. Use Abilify with caution if you have any kind of heart or circulatory problem, take blood pressure medication, or tend to become dehydrated.

Abilify has triggered seizures in a very small number of patients, and can also interfere with the swallowing mechanism. The risk of either problem is greater among older adults. If you've ever had a seizure, be sure to tell the doctor. Abilify should be used with caution.

Drugs such as Abilify can cause the body to overheat. Be cautious in hot weather and when exercising strenuously, and be sure to get plenty of liquids.

Abilify has not been tested in children or teenagers. The drug should be used cautiously by older adults, especially those who have dementia-related psychosis.

Possible food and drug interactions when taking this medication

The doctor will need to reduce the dosage of Abilify when you take the following additional drugs:

Fluoxetine (Prozac)
Ketoconazole (Nizoral)
Paroxetine (Paxil)
Quinidine (Quinidex)

On the other hand, the dosage of Abilify should be increased when you take carbamazepine (Tegretol).

Be cautious when taking Abilify with blood pressure medications classified as alpha-adrenergic blockers, including Hytrin and Cardura. Caution is also advised when combining Abilify with drugs that act on the brain, including tranquilizers, antidepressants, sleeping pills, narcotic painkillers, and other schizophrenia medications.

Although Abilify does not interact with alcohol, the manufacturer recommends avoiding the combination.

Special information if you are pregnant or breastfeeding

The effects of Abilify during pregnancy have not been adequately studied. The drug is recommended only if its benefits are thought to outweigh the potential risk to the baby. If you are pregnant or planning to become pregnant, inform your doctor immediately.

Breastfeeding is not recommended during Abilify therapy.

Recommended dosage

ADULTS

Schizophrenia
The usual dose is 10 or 15 milligrams taken once a day. The doctor will wait at least 2 weeks before prescribing an increased dosage.

Bipolar Disorder
The usual starting dose is 30 milligrams once a day. If you experience side effects, the doctor may decrease your dose to 15 milligrams once a day.

Overdosage

Any medication taken in excess can have serious consequences. If you suspect an overdose, seek medical attention immediately.

■ *Symptoms of Abilify overdose may include:*
Sleepiness, vomiting

Acamprosate *See Campral, page 234.*

Acarbose *See Precose, page 1126.*

ACCOLATE
Pronounced: ACK-o-late
Generic name: Zafirlukast

Why is this drug prescribed?
Accolate helps prevent asthma attacks. It is prescribed for long-term treatment.

Most important fact about this drug
Accolate will not stop an asthma attack once it starts. You will still need to use an airway-opening medication when an attack occurs.

How should you take this medication?
Accolate should be taken twice every day, whether or not you have had any recent asthma attacks. Do not take the medication with food. Allow at least 1 hour to pass before eating, or wait for 2 hours after a meal. You can continue to take Accolate while using another medication to stop an attack.

- *If you miss a dose...*
  Take it as soon as you remember. If it is almost time for your next dose, skip the one you missed and go back to your regular schedule. Do not take 2 doses at once.
- *Storage instructions...*
  Store at room temperature in a dark, dry place.

What side effects may occur?
Side effects cannot be anticipated. If any develop or change in intensity, inform your doctor as soon as possible. Only your doctor can determine if it is safe for you to continue taking Accolate.

- *Side effects may include:*
  Headache, infection, nausea

Why should this drug not be prescribed?
If you have had an allergic reaction to Accolate or to any of its ingredients, avoid this drug.

Special warnings about this medication
While taking Accolate, you should not stop—or even cut down on—any other asthma medication you are using unless your doctor recommends it. Remember that Accolate is not an airway-opening medication. You will still need an inhaler to stop an attack.

If you have been taking an oral steroid drug and your doctor does decide to cut back the dosage, there is a remote chance that complications will follow. Inform your doctor of any new symptoms.

Also call your doctor if you develop any of the following: pain in the upper right abdomen, nausea, fatigue, lethargy, loss of appetite, itching, flu-like symptoms, or jaundice (yellowing of the skin and eyes). These are signs of a liver problem—a rare side effect of Accolate that tends to develop more often in women. If tests show the problem to be serious, you'll have to stop using the drug. The symptoms will disappear once you stop.

Possible food and drug interactions when taking this medication

A full stomach can reduce Accolate's effectiveness. Do not take with meals.

If Accolate is taken with certain other drugs, the effects of either could be increased, decreased, or altered. It is especially important to check with your doctor before combining Accolate with the following:

Aspirin (Ecotrin, Genuine Bayer, others)
Astemizole (Hismanal)
Blood-thinning drugs such as Coumadin
Carbamazepine (Tegretol)
Cyclosporine (Sandimmune, Neoral)
Erythromycin (E.E.S., E-Mycin, others)
Heart and blood pressure medications called calcium channel blockers, including Calan, Cardizem, and Procardia
Phenytoin (Dilantin)
Terfenadine (Seldane)
Theophylline (Theo-Dur, others)
Tolbutamide (Orinase)

Special information if you are pregnant or breastfeeding

Accolate should be taken during pregnancy only if clearly needed. If you are pregnant or plan to become pregnant, inform your doctor immediately.

Accolate does find its way into breast milk and should not be taken by nursing mothers.

Recommended dosage

ADULTS

The usual dose for adults and children 12 years of age and over is 20 milligrams twice a day.

CHILDREN

The usual dose for children 5 to 11 years of age is 10 milligrams twice a day. Safety and effectiveness in children under 5 years of age have not been established.

Overdosage

Any medication taken in excess can have serious consequences. If you suspect an overdose, seek medical attention immediately.

■ *Symptoms of Accolate overdose may include:*
Rash, upset stomach

AccuNeb *See Proventil, page 1185.*

ACCUPRIL

Pronounced: AK-you-prill
Generic name: Quinapril hydrochloride

Why is this drug prescribed?

Accupril is used in the treatment of high blood pressure. It can be taken alone or in combination with a thiazide type of water pill such as HydroDIURIL. Accupril is in a family of drugs known as *ACE inhibitors.* It works by preventing a chemical in your blood called angiotensin I from converting into a more potent form that increases salt and water retention in your body. Accupril also enhances blood flow throughout your blood vessels. Along with other drugs, Accupril is also prescribed in the treatment of congestive heart failure.

Most important fact about this drug

You must take Accupril regularly for it to be effective. Since blood pressure declines gradually, it may be several weeks before you get the full benefit of Accupril; and you must continue taking it even if you are feeling well. Accupril does not cure high blood pressure; it merely keeps it under control.

How should you take this medication?

You can take Accupril with or without meals.

Alcohol may increase the effect of Accupril, and could cause dizziness or fainting. Avoid alcoholic beverages until you have checked with your doctor.

Take Accupril exactly as prescribed, and see your doctor regularly to make sure the drug is working properly, without unwanted side effects. Do not stop taking this drug without first consulting your doctor.

■ *If you miss a dose...*
Take the forgotten dose as soon as you remember. However, if it is almost time for your next dose, skip the one you missed and go back to your regular schedule. Never try to catch up by doubling the dose.
■ *Storage instructions...*
Accupril can be stored at room temperature. Protect from light.

What side effects may occur?

Side effects cannot be anticipated. If any develop or change in intensity, inform your doctor as soon as possible. Only your doctor can determine if it is safe for you to continue taking Accupril.

■ *Side effects may include:*
Dizziness, headache

Why should this drug not be prescribed?

If you are sensitive to or have ever had an allergic reaction to Accupril or similar drugs, such as Capoten and Vasotec, you should not take this medication. Make sure your doctor is aware of any drug reactions you have experienced.

Special warnings about this medication

If you develop swelling of the face, lips, tongue, or throat, or of your arms and legs, or have difficulty swallowing or breathing, you should contact your doctor immediately. You may need emergency treatment.

If you develop abdominal pain with or without nausea and vomiting, contact your doctor. ACE inhibitors such as Accupril have been known to cause intestinal swelling.

You may feel light-headed, especially during the first few days of Accupril therapy. If this occurs, notify your doctor. If you actually faint, stop taking the medication until you have consulted with your doctor.

Vomiting, diarrhea, and heavy perspiration can all deplete your body fluid; and dehydration can cause your blood pressure to drop. If this leads to light-headedness or fainting, you should check with your doctor.

Inform your doctor or dentist that you are taking Accupril before undergoing surgery or anesthesia.

Do not use potassium supplements or salt substitutes containing potassium without consulting your doctor.

If you develop a sore throat, fever, or any other sign of infection, contact your doctor immediately. It could indicate a more serious illness.

If you are taking Accupril, your doctor will do a complete assessment of your kidney function and will watch it closely as long as you are taking this drug.

If you notice a yellow tinge to your skin and the whites of your eyes, stop taking the drug and notify your doctor immediately. This could be a sign of liver damage.

The safety and effectiveness of Accupril in children have not been established.

Possible food and drug interactions when taking this medication

If Accupril is taken with certain other drugs, the effects of either could be increased, decreased, or altered. It is especially important to check with your doctor before combining Accupril with the following:

Diuretics such as Lasix
Lithium (Eskalith, Lithobid)
Magnesium
Potassium-sparing diuretics such as Aldactone, Dyazide, and
  Moduretic
Potassium supplements such as Slow-K and K-Dur
Salt substitutes containing potassium
Tetracycline (Sumycin)

Special information if you are pregnant or breastfeeding

ACE inhibitors such as Accupril have been shown to cause injury and even death to the unborn child when used in pregnancy during the second and third trimesters. If you are pregnant, your doctor should discontinue Accupril as soon as possible. If you plan to become pregnant, make sure your doctor knows you are taking this medication. Accupril appears in breast milk and could affect a nursing infant. If this medication is essential to your health, your doctor may advise you to discontinue breastfeeding until your treatment is finished.

Recommended dosage

High Blood Pressure

The usual starting dose is 10 or 20 milligrams taken once a day. If you have any problems with your kidneys or if you are also taking a diuretic, your starting dose may be lower. For adults over age 65, the usual starting dose is 10 milligrams. Depending on how your blood pressure responds, your doctor may increase your dose up to a total of 80 milligrams a day taken once a day or divided into 2 doses.

Congestive Heart Failure

The usual starting dose is 5 milligrams taken twice a day. Your doctor may increase the dose from week to week, up to as much as 20 to 40 milligrams daily, divided into 2 equal doses. If you have kidney problems, the dosage will be lower.

Overdosage

Any medication taken in excess can have serious consequences. If you suspect an overdose, seek medical attention immediately.

A severe drop in blood pressure is the primary sign of an Accupril overdose.

ACCURETIC

Pronounced: AK-you-REH-tik
Generic ingredients: Quinapril hydrochloride,
Hydrochlorothiazide

Why is this drug prescribed?

Accuretic combines two types of blood pressure medication. The first, quinapril hydrochloride, is an ACE (angiotensin-converting enzyme) inhibitor. It works by preventing a chemical in your blood called angiotensin I from converting into a more potent form (angiotensin II) that increases salt and water retention in the body and causes the blood vessels to constrict—two actions that tend to increase blood pressure.

To aid in clearing excess water from the body, Accuretic also contains hydrochlorothiazide, a diuretic that promotes production of urine. Diuretics often wash too much potassium out of the body along with the water. However, the ACE inhibitor part of Accuretic tends to keep potassium in the body, thereby canceling this unwanted effect.

Accuretic is not used for the initial treatment of high blood pressure. It is saved for later use, when a single blood pressure medication is not sufficient for the job. In addition, some doctors are using Accuretic along with other drugs to treat congestive heart failure.

Most important fact about this drug

You must take Accuretic regularly for it to be effective. Since blood pressure declines gradually, it may be several weeks before you get the full benefit of Accuretic; and you must continue taking it even if you are feeling well. Accuretic does not cure high blood pressure; it merely keeps it under control.

How should you take this medication?

You can take Accuretic with or without meals.

Take Accuretic exactly as prescribed, and see your doctor regularly to make sure the drug is working properly, without unwanted side effects. Do not stop taking this drug without first consulting your doctor.

■ *If you miss a dose...*
  Take it as soon as you remember. If it is almost time for your next dose, skip the one you missed and go back to your regular schedule. Never take 2 doses at the same time.
■ *Storage instructions...*
  Store at room temperature in a tightly closed container. Protect from moisture and light.

What side effects may occur?

Side effects cannot be anticipated. If any develop or change in intensity, inform your doctor as soon as possible. Only your doctor can determine if it is safe for you to continue taking Accuretic.

■ *Side effects may include:*
Cough, dizziness, headache

Why should this drug not be prescribed?

If you are unable to urinate, avoid this medication.

You should not take this medication if you are sensitive to or have ever had an allergic reaction to any of the following: Accupril, thiazide diuretics such as HydroDIURIL and Esidrix, ACE inhibitors such as Capoten and Vasotec, or sulfa or other sulfonamide-derived drugs such as Bactrim and Septra. If you have a history of allergies, you may be at greater risk for an allergic reaction to this medication. Make sure your doctor is aware of any drug reactions you have experienced.

Special warnings about this medication

If you develop swelling of the face, lips, tongue, or throat, or of your arms and legs, or have difficulty swallowing or breathing, stop taking the medication and contact your doctor immediately. You may need emergency treatment.

If you develop abdominal pain with or without nausea and vomiting, contact your doctor. ACE inhibitors such as Accuretic have been known to cause intestinal swelling.

You may feel light-headed, especially during the first few days of Accuretic therapy. If this occurs, notify your doctor. If you actually faint, stop taking the medication until you have consulted with your doctor.

Dehydration, excessive sweating, vomiting, or diarrhea can all deplete your body's fluids and cause your blood pressure to drop. If this leads to light-headedness or fainting, you should check with your doctor.

Inform your doctor or dentist that you are taking Accuretic before undergoing surgery or anesthesia.

Do not use potassium supplements or salt substitutes containing potassium without consulting your doctor.

If you develop any type of infection such as a sore throat or fever, contact your doctor immediately. It could indicate a more serious illness.

If you are taking Accuretic, your doctor will do a complete assessment of your kidney function and will watch it closely as long as you are taking this drug. If you have kidney disease, Accuretic should be used with caution.

Caution is warranted, too, if you have liver disease. If you notice a yellow tinge to your skin and the whites of your eyes, stop taking the drug and notify your doctor. This could be a sign of liver damage.

Accuretic may increase your blood sugar levels if you have diabetes. It can also trigger gout or the connective tissue disease lupus erythematosus. Use Accuretic cautiously if you have any of these problems.

The safety and effectiveness of Accuretic in children have not been established.

Possible food and drug interactions when taking this medication

If Accuretic is taken with certain other drugs, the effects of either could be increased, decreased, or altered. It is especially important to check with your doctor before combining Accuretic with the following:

Barbiturates such as phenobarbital
Cholestyramine (Questran)
Colestipol (Colestid)
Corticosteroids such as prednisone and ACTH
Diabetes medications such as insulin and Micronase
Digoxin (Lanoxin)
Diuretics such as HydroDIURIL and Lasix
Lithium (Eskalith, Lithobid)
Narcotics such as Percocet
Nonsteroidal anti-inflammatory drugs such as Naprosyn
Norepinephrine (Levophed)
Other high blood pressure medications such as Aldomet
Potassium-sparing diuretics such as Aldactone, Dyazide, and
    Moduretic
Potassium supplements such as Slow-K and K-Dur
Salt substitutes containing potassium
Tetracycline (Achromycin V, Sumycin)

Alcohol may increase the effect of Accuretic, and could cause dizziness or fainting. Check with your doctor before drinking alcoholic beverages.

Special information if you are pregnant or breastfeeding

ACE inhibitors such as the one in Accuretic have been shown to cause injury and even death to the unborn child when used in pregnancy during the second and third trimesters. If you are pregnant, your doctor should discontinue this medication as soon as possible. If you plan to become pregnant, make sure your doctor knows you are taking this medication. The diuretic component of Accuretic, when taken during pregnancy, can cause jaundice (yellowing of the skin and whites of the eyes) and abnormal bruising and bleeding in newborns.

Accuretic appears in breast milk and could affect a nursing infant. Because of potential harm to the baby, you'll need to choose between breastfeeding and continuing your treatment with Accuretic.

Recommended dosage

ADULTS

Accuretic is usually taken once a day. Your doctor will adjust the dosage depending on how your blood pressure responds. Daily doses of up to 80 milligrams of quinapril and 50 milligrams of hydrochlorothiazide may be prescribed, but doctors aim for the smallest dose that proves effective.

Overdosage

Any medication taken in excess can have serious consequences. If you suspect an overdose, seek medical attention immediately.

■ *Symptoms of Accuretic overdose may include:*
A severe drop in blood pressure, dry mouth, excessive thirst, muscle pain or cramps, nausea and vomiting, weak or irregular heartbeat, weakness and dizziness

ACCUTANE

Pronounced: ACC-u-tane
Generic name: Isotretinoin
Other brand name: Amnesteem

Why is this drug prescribed?

Accutane, a chemical cousin of vitamin A, is prescribed for the treatment of severe, disfiguring cystic acne that has not cleared up in response to milder medications such as antibiotics. It works on the oil glands within the skin, shrinking them and diminishing their output. You take Accutane by mouth every day for several months, then stop. The antiacne effect can last even after you have finished your course of medication.

Most important fact about this drug

Because Accutane can cause severe birth defects, including mental retardation and physical malformations, a woman *must not* become pregnant while taking it. Before starting Accutane therapy, women of childbearing age will be asked to read a pamphlet, watch a video, and sign a detailed consent form regarding the danger of birth defects. You must have two negative pregnancy tests before beginning Accutane therapy, and must take monthly pregnancy tests while using this drug.

In addition, you must use 2 forms of birth control during Accutane therapy, and for 1 month before and after. Each prescription for Accutane must bear a yellow qualification sticker signifying that you meet these requirements. Scientists have not ruled out the possibility that hormone-based contraceptives (birth control pills and implants) may be less reliable when taken with Accutane, so a second form of birth control should always be used while taking this drug. If you accidentally become pregnant while taking Accutane, you should immediately consult your doctor.

How should you take this medication?

Take Accutane two times a day with a meal, unless your doctor tells you otherwise. Swallow the capsule. Don't suck or chew it. Take it with a full glass of water, milk, or other nonalcoholic liquid. Follow your doctor's instructions carefully.

Depending on your reaction to Accutane, your doctor may need to adjust the dosage upward or downward. If you respond quickly and very well, your doctor may take you off Accutane even before the 15 or 20 weeks are up.

After you finish taking Accutane, there should be at least a 2-month "rest period" during which you are off the drug. This is because your acne may continue to get better even though you are no longer taking the medication. Once the 2 months are up, if your acne is still severe, your doctor may want to give you a second course of Accutane. If you are still growing, your doctor may recommend a longer *rest period*.

Avoid consumption of alcoholic beverages.

Read the patient information leaflet available with the product.

Do not crush the capsules.

Do not share Accutane with anyone because of the risk of birth defects and other serious side effects.

■ *If you miss a dose...*
Take the forgotten dose as soon as you remember. If it is almost time for your next dose, skip the one you missed and go back to your regular schedule. Do not take 2 doses at the same time.

■ *Storage instructions...*
Store at room temperature, away from light.

What side effects may occur?

Side effects cannot be anticipated. If any develop or change in intensity, inform your doctor as soon as possible. Only your doctor can determine if it is safe for you to continue taking Accutane.

■ *Side effects may include:*
Abnormal hair growth or loss, allergic reaction, bleeding gums, blood in urine, bowel inflammation and pain, bruising, changes in blood sugar or cholesterol levels, changes in skin pigmentation, chest pain, decreased night vision, decreased tolerance to contact lenses, delay in wound healing, depression, difficulty sleeping, dizziness, drowsiness, dry or fragile skin, dry or cracked lips, dry mouth, dry nose, fatigue, flushing, headache, hearing problems, heartbeat irregularities, herpes, inflammation or sores in the esophagus, itching, joint pain, liver disorders, menstrual changes, muscle wasting, nail disorders, nausea, nervousness, nosebleeds, peeling palms or soles, pinkeye, rash, skin infections, stomach and intestinal discomfort, stroke, sudden drop in blood pressure (causing unconsciousness), sunburn-sensitive skin, suppression of growth, sweating, swelling due to fluid retention, ten-

don and ligament problems, urinary discomfort, vision problems, vomiting, weakness, weight loss

Why should this drug not be prescribed?

If Accutane gives you an allergic reaction, you will not be able to use it.

If you are a woman of childbearing age, you should not take Accutane if you are pregnant, if you think there is a possibility you might get pregnant during the treatment, or if you are unable to keep coming back to the doctor for monthly checkups, including pregnancy testing.

Special warnings about this medication

Stop taking Accutane and notify your doctor immediately at the first sign of a skin rash or any other allergic reaction. Although they are rare, serious and even fatal allergic reactions have been known to occur.

When you first start taking Accutane, it is possible that your acne will get worse before it starts to get better.

Accutane may cause depression or other mental problems. In rare cases, it has prompted thoughts of suicide. If you begin to feel depressed or become troubled by suicidal thoughts, contact your doctor immediately.

Before starting Accutane therapy, all patients must sign a consent form noting that they are aware of the possibility of mental side effects, the danger of birth defects, and the need for certain other precautions.

If you are a woman of childbearing age and you are considering taking Accutane, you will be given both spoken and written warnings about the importance of avoiding pregnancy during the treatment. You will also be asked to sign a second consent form noting that:

- You must not take Accutane if you are pregnant or may become pregnant during treatment;
- If you get pregnant while taking Accutane, your baby will be at high risk for birth defects;
- If you take Accutane, you must use 2 effective forms of birth control from 1 month before the start of treatment through 1 month after the end of treatment;
- You must have 2 negative pregnancy tests (one just before starting Accutane therapy), and must be tested every month during therapy;
- You may participate in a program that includes an initial free pregnancy test and birth control counseling session;
- If you become pregnant, you must immediately stop taking Accutane and see your doctor;
- You have read and understood the Accutane patient brochure and asked your doctor any questions you had;
- You have been invited to participate in a survey of women being treated with Accutane.

Some people taking Accutane, including some who simultaneously took tetracycline, have experienced headache, nausea, and visual disturbances caused by increased pressure within the skull. Avoid taking tetracycline while using Accutane. See a doctor immediately if you have these symptoms; if the doctor finds swelling of the optic nerve at the back of your eye, you must stop taking Accutane at once and see a neurologist for further care.

Be careful driving at night. Some people have experienced a sudden decrease in night vision.

Accutane affects the body's processing of fats and sugars. It should be used cautiously by people with diabetes, excess weight, high triglyceride or cholesterol levels, or a tendency to drink too much alcohol. If you have any of these conditions, your doctor will monitor you closely during Accutane therapy.

You may not be able to tolerate your contact lenses during and after your therapy with Accutane.

You should stop taking Accutane immediately if you have abdominal pain, bleeding from the rectum, or severe diarrhea. You may have an inflammatory disease of the bowel.

You should not donate blood during your therapy with Accutane and for a month after you stop taking it.

You may become more sensitive to light while taking this drug. Try to stay out of the sun as much as possible.

You should not use wax hair removal treatments or skin resurfacing procedures (dermabrasion, laser treatments) while taking Accutane or for 6 months after completing therapy.

Some people taking Accutane develop vision or hearing problems. If you notice changes in your vision or hearing, stop taking this drug and contact your doctor.

Possible food and drug interactions when taking this medication

While taking Accutane, do not take vitamin supplements containing vitamin A. Accutane and vitamin A are chemically related; taking them together is like taking an overdose of vitamin A.

Remember, too, that Accutane should not be combined with tetracycline antibiotics such as Doryx, Minocin, and Vibramycin.

Special information if you are pregnant or breastfeeding

Accutane causes birth defects; do not use it while pregnant. Nursing mothers should not take Accutane because of the possibility of passing the drug on to the baby via breast milk.

Recommended dosage

The recommended dosage range for Accutane is 0.5 to 1 milligram per 2.2 pounds of body weight, divided into 2 doses daily, for 15 to 20 weeks. For very severe cases, the doctor may increase the daily dose to as much as 2 milligrams per 2.2 pounds.

If after a period of 2 months or more off therapy, severe cystic acne persists, your doctor may prescribe a second course of therapy.

Overdosage

Any medication taken in excess can have serious consequences. If you suspect an overdose of Accutane, seek medical attention immediately.

■ *Overdosage of Accutane, like overdosage of vitamin A, can cause:*
Abdominal pain, dizziness, dry or cracked lips, facial flushing, incoordination and clumsiness, headache, vomiting

Acebutolol *See Sectral, page 1292.*

ACEON

Pronounced: A-see-on
Generic name: Perindopril erbumine

Why is this drug prescribed?

Aceon is used in the treatment of high blood pressure. It can be taken alone or in combination with thiazide diuretics that help rid the body of excess water. Aceon belongs to a family of drugs called angiotensin-converting enzyme (ACE) inhibitors. It works by preventing a chemical in your blood called angiotensin I from converting into a more potent form that increases salt and water retention in your body. Aceon also improves the flow of blood through the circulatory system.

Most important fact about this drug

You must take Aceon regularly for it to be effective. Since blood pressure declines gradually, it may be several weeks before you get the full benefit of the drug; and you must continue taking it even if you are feeling well. Aceon does not cure blood pressure; it merely keeps it under control.

How should you take this medication?

Aceon can be taken with or without food.

■ *If you miss a dose...*
Take the forgotten dose as soon as you remember. If it is almost time for your next dose, skip the one you missed and go back to your regular schedule. Never take 2 doses at the same time.
■ *Storage instructions...*
Store at room temperature, protected from moisture.

What side effects may occur?

If any side effects develop, they are usually mild and are likely to disappear as therapy continues. However, if any do appear, inform your doctor as soon as possible. Only your doctor can determine if it is safe for you to continue taking Aceon.

■ *Side effects may include:*
Cough, dizziness, headache, leg pain, light-headedness, nasal inflammation, sore throat, upper respiratory infection, weakness

Why should this drug not be prescribed?
If Aceon gives you an allergic reaction, or if you've had an allergic reaction to other ACE inhibitors, you should not take this medication.

Special warnings about this medication
If you develop signs of an allergic reaction (swelling of your face, lips, tongue, or throat; swollen arms and legs; difficulty swallowing or breathing), stop taking Aceon and contact your doctor immediately. You may need emergency treatment.

Contact your doctor if you develop abdominal pain with or without nausea and vomiting. ACE inhibitors such as Aceon have been known to cause intestinal swelling.

Aceon occasionally makes people dizzy, light-headed, or faint, especially during the first few days of therapy. If these symptoms occur, contact your doctor. Do not drive, operate dangerous machinery, or participate in any hazardous activity that requires full mental alertness until you know how Aceon affects you. If you actually faint, stop taking the drug and call your doctor immediately.

Aceon can cause excessively low blood pressure, especially if your body is short of fluid. This problem is more likely if you are also taking a diuretic or suffer from diarrhea, vomiting, or excessive sweating. Call your doctor if you develop such signs of fluid depletion as dry mouth, weakness or fatigue, unusual thirst, restlessness or confusion, or reduced urination.

In rare instances, Aceon can damage the kidneys. When prescribing Aceon, your doctor will perform a complete assessment of your kidney function and will continue to monitor it. If you have kidney disease, the drug should be used with caution. The doctor will also take extra care if you have congestive heart failure or circulatory problems.

Aceon occasionally causes an unwanted increase in the body's potassium level. Do not use potassium supplements or salt substitutes containing potassium without your doctor's okay.

Contact your doctor promptly if you develop any sign of infection, such as a sore throat or fever. Also be sure to let the doctor know if you develop a persistent, dry cough. It could be a side effect that will disappear if the doctor switches you to another medication.

There have been rare cases of liver damage linked to Aceon. If you develop signs of liver problems such as yellowish skin and eyes, stop taking the medication and contact your doctor.

If you are receiving bee or wasp venom to prevent an allergic reaction to stings, taking Aceon at the same time may cause a severe allergic reaction. Make sure the allergist knows you are taking Aceon. In fact, before any type of procedure, notify your doctor or dentist that you are taking this drug.

Possible food and drug interactions when taking this medication

If Aceon is taken with certain other drugs, the effects of either could be increased, decreased, or altered. It is especially important to check with your doctor before combining Aceon with the following:

Cyclosporine (Neoral, Sandimmune)
Digoxin (Lanoxin)
Diuretics such as Aldactone, Diuril, Dyazide, Lasix, and Moduretic
Gentamicin (Garamycin)
Indomethacin (Indocin)
Lithium (Eskalith, Lithobid, Lithonate)
Potassium supplements such as K-Lyte, K-Tab, and Slow-K

Special information if you are pregnant or breastfeeding

Aceon can cause injury or death to the developing baby when used during the last 6 months of pregnancy. Aceon should be stopped as soon as you know that you're pregnant; contact your doctor immediately.

Aceon may appear in breast milk and could affect a nursing infant. It should be used with caution if you are breastfeeding.

Recommended dosage

ADULTS

The usual starting dosage is 4 milligrams daily, taken as a single dose or divided into 2 smaller doses. Your doctor may increase the dosage until your blood pressure is under control, up to a maximum of 16 milligrams per day. A dose of 4 to 8 milligrams a day is usually sufficient.

If you have been taking a diuretic, your doctor may tell you to stop taking it 2 or 3 days before you start taking Aceon. If you need to continue the diuretic without interruption, the doctor may start you on Aceon at a reduced dose of 2 to 4 milligrams daily, then gradually increase the dosage if necessary.

If your blood pressure is not adequately controlled with Aceon alone, the doctor may add a diuretic to your regimen.

Aceon has not been tested in people with severe kidney disease. If you have mild kidney problems, the usual starting dosage is 2 milligrams or less per day. The dosage may be increased gradually to not more than 8 milligrams per day.

CHILDREN

Aceon has not been tested in children.

OLDER ADULTS

Higher doses (above 8 milligrams a day) are prescribed for older adults only with extra caution.

Overdosage

The most likely warning signs of an Aceon overdose are symptoms of excessively low blood pressure, including dizziness and light-headedness. If you suspect an overdose, seek medical attention immediately.

Acetaminophen *See Tylenol, page 1513.*

Acetaminophen with Codeine *See Tylenol with Codeine, page 1516.*

Acetaminophen with Oxycodone *See Percocet, page 1073.*

Acetazolamide *See Diamox, page 435.*

Achromycin V *See Tetracycline, page 1422.*

ACIPHEX

Pronounced: ASS-ih-fex
Generic name: Rabeprazole sodium

Why is this drug prescribed?

AcipHex blocks acid production in the stomach. It is prescribed for the short-term (4 to 8 weeks) treatment of sores and inflammation in the upper digestive canal (esophagus). This condition, known as gastroesophageal reflux disease (GERD), is caused by the backflow of stomach acid into the esophagus over a prolonged period of time. Because GERD can be chronic, your doctor may continue to prescribe AcipHex to prevent a relapse after your initial course of treatment and to relieve symptoms of GERD such as heartburn.

AcipHex can also be prescribed for the short-term (up to 4 weeks) treatment of duodenal ulcers (ulcers that form just outside the stomach at the top of the small intestine), and for Zollinger-Ellison syndrome, a disease which causes the stomach to produce too much acid. The drug is classified as a proton pump inhibitor. It works by blocking a specific enzyme essential to the production of stomach acid. It begins reducing acid within an hour of administration.

AcipHex is sometimes combined with the antibiotics amoxicillin and clarithromycin to treat infections caused by *H. pylori*, a type of bacteria that lives in the digestive tract and is often associated with recurrent ulcers.

Most important fact about this drug

AcipHex will work even if your symptoms are caused by a serious condition such as stomach cancer. For that reason, doctors are warned to rule out cancer whenever prescribing this drug.

How should you take this medication?

Take AcipHex once a day, with or without food. Swallow the tablet whole; it should not be crushed, chewed, or split. You can continue taking antacids during AcipHex therapy.

If you're using AcipHex along with amoxicillin and clarithromycin, take all three drugs at the same time twice a day, once in the morning and again in the evening. This three-drug regimen should be taken with meals.

■ *If you miss a dose...*
Take it as soon as you remember. If it is almost time for your next dose, skip the one you missed and go back to your regular schedule. Do not take 2 doses at once.

■ *Storage instructions...*
AcipHex should be stored at room temperature and protected from moisture.

What side effects may occur?

Side effects cannot be anticipated. If any develop or change in intensity, tell your doctor as soon as possible. Only your doctor can determine if it is safe for you to continue taking AcipHex. Headache is the most common side effect of AcipHex, occurring in 2 people out of 100.

Why should this drug not be prescribed?

If AcipHex gives you an allergic reaction, you will not be able to use it.

Special warnings about this medication

If you have stomach ulcers caused by the *H. pylori* bacteria, AcipHex could make the condition slightly worse. The doctor may order a test for *H. pylori* before prescribing this drug. If you test positive, the doctor may prescribe antibiotics along with AcipHex.

AcipHex has not been tested in children under 18 years of age.

Possible food and drug interactions when taking this medication

If AcipHex is taken with certain other drugs, the effects of either could be increase, decreased, or altered. It is especially important to check with your doctor before combining AcipHex with the following:

Cyclosporine (Neoral, Sandimmune)
Digoxin (Lanoxin)
Ketoconazole (Nizoral)
Warfarin (Coumadin)

Special information if you are pregnant or breastfeeding

The effects of AcipHex during pregnancy have not been adequately studied. If you are pregnant or plan to become pregnant, inform your doctor immediately. The drug may appear in breast milk and should not be taken while you're breastfeeding.

Recommended dosage

ADULTS

Gastroesophageal Reflux Disease (GERD)
The usual dose is 20 milligrams once a day for 4 to 8 weeks. For patients who have not healed after 8 weeks, the doctor may prescribe an additional 8-week course of AcipHex therapy.

To Relieve Symptoms or Prevent a Relapse of GERD
The usual dose is 20 milligrams once a day.

Duodenal Ulcer
The usual dose is 20 milligrams taken once daily after the morning meal for a period of up to 4 weeks. Some people may require an additional 4 weeks of treatment.

Combination Drug Treatment to Eliminate H. Pylori
The recommended combination is 20 milligrams of AcipHex, 1,000 milligrams of amoxicillin, and 500 milligrams of clarithromycin taken twice a day for 7 days. It's important to take all three drugs for the entire 7 days. Cutting the treatment short could fail to eliminate the infection and possibly lead to antibiotic resistance.

Zollinger-Ellison Syndrome
The usual starting dose is 60 milligrams once a day, although your doctor may adjust the dose based on your individual need. Doses of up to 100 milligrams once a day or 60 milligrams twice a day are sometimes prescribed.

Overdosage

Little is known about AcipHex overdose. However, any medication taken in excess can have serious consequences. If you suspect an overdose, seek medical attention immediately.

Acitretin *See Soriatane, page 1326.*

ACLOVATE

Pronounced: AK-low-vait
Generic name: Alclometasone dipropionate

Why is this drug prescribed?

Aclovate, a synthetic steroid medication of the cortisone family, is spread on the skin to relieve certain types of itchy rashes, including psoriasis.

Most important fact about this drug

When you use Aclovate, you inevitably absorb some of the medication through your skin and into the bloodstream. Too much absorption can lead to unwanted side effects elsewhere in the body. To keep this problem to a minimum, avoid using large amounts of Aclovate over large areas, and do not cover it with airtight dressings such as plastic wrap or adhesive bandages unless specifically told to by your doctor.

How should you use this medication?

Use Aclovate exactly as prescribed by your doctor and only to treat the condition for which your doctor prescribed it. The usual procedure is to spread a thin film of Aclovate cream or ointment over the rash and massage gently until the medication disappears. Do this 2 or 3 times a day.

For areas of deep-seated, persistent rash, your doctor may recommend a thick layer of Aclovate cream or ointment topped with waterproof bandaging, to be left in place for 1 to 4 days. If necessary, this procedure may be repeated 3 or 4 times. Do not use bandaging at all, however, unless your doctor so advises.

Aclovate is for use only on the skin. Be careful to keep it out of your eyes.

■ *If you miss a dose...*
Apply it as soon as you remember. If it is almost time for the next dose, skip the one you missed and go back to your regular schedule.

■ *Storage instructions...*
Store at room temperature.

What side effects may occur?

Side effects cannot be anticipated. If any develop or change in intensity, inform your doctor as soon as possible. Only your doctor can determine if it is safe for you to continue taking Aclovate.

■ *Side effects may include:*
Acne-like pimples, allergic rash/inflammation, burning, dryness, infection, irritation, itching, pale spots, prickly heat, rash, redness, stretch marks on skin

Why should this drug not be prescribed?

Do not use Aclovate if it has ever given you an allergic reaction.

Special warnings about this medication

Aclovate is for external use only. Do not let the cream or ointment get into your eyes. Avoid using the product on your face, underarms, or groin, unless the doctor tells you to.

Do not use Aclovate to treat diaper rash or apply it in the diaper area; waterproof diapers or plastic pants can increase unwanted absorption of Aclovate.

If your skin is inflamed or you have some other skin condition, tell your doctor. You may absorb more drug than usual.

If you use Aclovate over large areas of skin for prolonged periods of time, the amount of hormone absorbed into your bloodstream may eventually lead to Cushing's syndrome: a moon-faced appearance, fattened neck and trunk, and purplish streaks on the skin. Children, because of their relatively larger ratio of skin surface to body weight, are particularly susceptible to overabsorption of hormone from Aclovate. The drug should not be used on children under 1 year of age or for more than 3 weeks in children older than 1 year.

Possible food and drug interactions when taking this medication

Check with your doctor before combining Aclovate with other more potent steroids, since this could lead to undesirably large amounts of hormone circulating in your bloodstream.

Special information if you are pregnant or breastfeeding

Drug absorbed from Aclovate cream or ointment into the bloodstream may find its way into an unborn child's blood, or may seep into breast milk. To avoid any possible harm to your child, use Aclovate very sparingly—and only with your doctor's permission—if you are pregnant or nursing a baby.

Recommended dosage

Apply a thin film of Aclovate cream or ointment to the affected skin areas 2 or 3 times daily; massage gently until the medication disappears.

Bandages that block out air may be used to control psoriasis and other severe skin rashes, if your doctor recommends them. Apply as follows:

1. Cover the affected area with a thick layer of Aclovate cream or ointment and a light gauze dressing, then cover the area with a pliable plastic film.
2. Seal the edges to the normal skin by adhesive tape or other means.
3. Leave the dressing in place 1 to 4 days and repeat the procedure 3 or 4 times as needed.

With this method of treatment, marked improvement is often seen in a few days. If an infection develops, the use of airtight bandages should be discontinued. Your doctor will recommend an alternative treatment.

Once your condition is under control, you should stop using Aclovate. If you don't see any improvement within 2 weeks, check with your doctor.

Overdosage

Any medication taken in excess can have serious consequences. If you suspect an overdose, seek medical attention immediately.

In a child, an overdose of Aclovate may cause increased pressure within the skull leading to bulging soft spots (in an infant's head) or headache. If this happens, see a doctor without delay.

Over the long term, overuse of Aclovate can interfere with a child's normal growth and development.

Acrivastine with Pseudoephedrine See Semprex-D, *page 1295.*

ACTIGALL
Pronounced: AK-ti-gawl
Generic name: Ursodiol
Other brand name: Urso 250

Why is this drug prescribed?

Actigall is used to help dissolve certain kinds of gallstones. If you suffer from gallstones but do not want to undergo surgery to remove them, or if age, infirmity, or a poor reaction to anesthesia makes you a poor candidate for surgery, Actigall treatment may be a good alternative.

Actigall is also used to prevent gallstones in people on rapid-weight-loss diets. And under the brand name Urso 250, its active ingredient is prescribed to treat liver disease caused by hardening and blockage of the bile ducts (primary biliary cirrhosis).

Most important fact about this drug

Actigall is not a quick remedy. It takes months of Actigall therapy to dissolve gallstones; and there is a possibility of incomplete dissolution and recurrence of stones. Your doctor will weigh Actigall against alternative treatments and recommend the best one for you.

Actigall is most effective if your gallstones are small or "floatable" (high in cholesterol). In addition, your gallbladder must still be functioning properly.

How should you take this medication?

Take Actigall exactly as prescribed; otherwise the gallstones may dissolve too slowly or not dissolve at all. During treatment, your doctor will do periodic ultrasound exams to see if your stones are dissolving.

Urso should be taken 4 times a day with food.

■ *If you miss a dose...*
Take it as soon as you remember, or at the same time as the next dose.
■ *Storage instructions...*
Store at room temperature in a tightly closed container.

What side effects may occur?
Side effects cannot be anticipated. If any develop or change in intensity, inform your doctor as soon as possible. Only your doctor can determine if it is safe for you to continue taking Actigall.

■ *Side effects may include:*
Abdominal pain, allergy, arthritis, back pain, bronchitis, chest pain, constipation, cough, diarrhea, dizziness, fatigue, flu-like symptoms, gas, hair loss, headache, high blood sugar, indigestion, insomnia, joint pain, menstrual pain, muscle and bone pain, nasal inflammation, nausea, sinus inflammation, skin rash, sore throat, stomach or intestinal disorder, stomach ulcer, upper respiratory tract infection, urinary tract infection, viral infection, vomiting

Why should this drug not be prescribed?
Do not take these medications if you are sensitive to or have ever had an allergic reaction to ursodiol or to other bile acids.

Actigall will not dissolve certain types of gallstones. If your doctor tells you that your gallstones are calcified cholesterol stones, radio-opaque stones, or radiolucent bile pigment stones, you are not a candidate for treatment with Actigall.

Also, if you have biliary tract (liver, gallbladder, bile duct) problems or certain liver and pancreas diseases, your doctor may not be able to prescribe Actigall for you.

Special warnings about this medication
Although Actigall is not known to cause liver damage, it is theoretically possible in some people. Your doctor may run blood tests for liver function before you start to take Actigall and again while you are taking it.

Possible food and drug interactions when taking this medication
If Actigall or Urso is taken with certain other drugs, the effects of either could be increased, decreased, or altered. It is especially important to check with your doctor before combining Actigall or Urso with the following:

Aluminum-based antacid medications (Alu-Cap, Alu-Tab, Rolaids, others)
Cholesterol-lowering medications such as Atromid-S, Lopid, Mevacor, Questran, and Colestid
Estrogens such as Premarin
Oral contraceptives

Special information if you are pregnant or breastfeeding

If you are pregnant or plan to become pregnant, inform your doctor immediately. So far, there is no evidence that ursodiol can harm an unborn baby; but to be safe, the medication is not recommended during pregnancy. Caution is needed during breastfeeding; it is not known whether ursodiol taken by a nursing mother passes into her breast milk.

Recommended dosage

ACTIGALL

Dissolving Gallstones
The recommended daily dosage is 8 to 10 milligrams per 2.2 pounds of body weight, divided into 2 or 3 doses.

Preventing Gallstones
The usual dose in people losing weight rapidly is 300 milligrams twice a day.

URSO 250

Primary Biliary Cirrhosis
The recommended adult dosage is 13 to 15 milligrams per 2.2 pounds of body weight per day, divided into 4 small doses taken with food.

Overdosage

Although there have been no reports of overdose with Actigall, the most likely symptom of severe overdose would be diarrhea. Since any medication taken in excess can have serious consequences, you should seek medical attention immediately if you suspect an Actigall overdose.

ACTIVELLA AND FEMHRT

Generic ingredients: Estrogen, Progestin
Other brand name: Prefest

Why is this drug prescribed?

These medications are designed for use in hormone replacement therapy. Both combine a form of estrogen with a substance that acts like progesterone. Both relieve the symptoms of menopause, and both are prescribed to prevent osteoporosis in postmenopausal women. (Activella is also used for vaginal atrophy.)

Estrogen, when taken by itself, poses an increased risk of uterine cancer. The progestin in these products largely counteracts this effect.

Most important fact about this drug

Because of the risk of uterine cancer, be sure to alert your doctor if you experience any abnormal vaginal bleeding. There is little, if any, increase in risk during the first year of treatment, but the odds rise substantially after 5 to 10 years.

How should you take this medication?

Take 1 tablet at the same time each day, with or without food. If you are taking the medication to relieve menopausal symptoms, your doctor will reevaluate your need for medication every 3 to 6 months. If you are taking the product to prevent osteoporosis, you will probably continue for years.

■ *If you miss a dose...*
Take it as soon as you remember. If it is almost time for your next dose, skip the one you missed and go back to your regular schedule. Never take 2 doses at the same time.

■ *Storage instructions...*
Store at room temperature. Keep Activella in a tightly closed container away from moisture and light.

What side effects may occur?

Side effects cannot be anticipated. If any develop or change in intensity, inform your doctor as soon as possible. Only your doctor can determine if it is safe for you to continue taking this type of product.

■ *Side effects may include:*
Abdominal pain, breast tenderness and enlargement, depression, enlargement of uterine fibroids, headache, nausea, nervousness, skin reddening, urinary tract infection, vaginal inflammation, vomiting

Why should this drug not be prescribed?

Do not take these products if you have:

■ Known or suspected breast cancer, any other cancer stimulated by estrogen, or a past history of breast cancer associated with estrogen use
■ Unexplained genital bleeding
■ A history of blood clots or phlebitis
■ Sensitivity to estrogen or progesterone
■ Any reason to believe that you are pregnant

If you've had your uterus removed, you don't need the progestin in these products, and should take a different type of hormone replacement therapy. You should also avoid Activella if you have a liver condition.

Special warnings about this medication

In addition to increasing the chances of uterine cancer, estrogen replacement therapy may also raise the odds of breast cancer if taken at high doses or for long periods of time. Be sure to do a monthly self-exam of your breasts, and get regular mammograms.

Estrogen replacement therapy typically doubles the chances of gallbladder disease. Notify your doctor if you experience pain, tenderness, or swelling in your abdomen.

Estrogen replacement increases the risk of blood clots in the veins, especially during the first year of therapy. Call your doctor immediately if you experience any of the following warning signs: bulging eyes, changes in vision or speech, coughing up blood, dizziness, double vision, faintness, migraine, pains in the calves or chest, severe headache or vomiting, sudden shortness of breath, sudden vision loss, weakness or numbness of an arm or leg.

Estrogen therapy sometimes causes high blood pressure, so be sure to get periodic checkups. In women prone to high blood lipid levels, estrogen can also cause a sharp spike in triglycerides, possibly leading to pancreatitis. Fluid retention is another possibility. If it develops, it can aggravate conditions such as asthma, epilepsy, heart disease, kidney disease, and migraine.

Make sure your doctor knows if you have ever been diagnosed with depression. Treatment with the products should be discontinued if depression recurs.

If you have diabetes, watch your blood sugar levels especially carefully. There's a chance that estrogen/progestin products may make diabetes worse.

Possible food and drug interactions when taking this medication
If estrogen is taken with certain other drugs, the effects of either could be increased, decreased, or altered. It is especially important to check with your doctor before combining estrogen with the following:

Acetaminophen (Tylenol)
Aspirin
Clofibrate (Atromid-S)
Cyclosporine (Neoral)
Morphine
Seizure medications such as Dilantin, phenobarbital, and Tegretol
Steroid medications such as prednisone (Deltasone)
Rifampin (Rifadin)
Temazepam (Restoril)
Theophylline (Theo-Dur)

Special information if you are pregnant or breastfeeding
Although these medications are intended only for women who are no longer in their childbearing years, it's important to note that they should never be taken during pregnancy, since they can harm the developing baby. Additionally, estrogen decreases the quantity and quality of breast milk, and progesterone finds its way into the milk.

Recommended dosage

ADULTS

The recommended dose is 1 tablet daily.

Overdosage

Any medication taken in excess can have serious consequences. If you suspect an overdose, seek medical attention immediately.

■ *Symptoms of overdose may include:*
Nausea, vomiting, vaginal bleeding

ACTONEL

Pronounced: AK-ton-ell
Generic name: Risedronate

Why is this drug prescribed?

Although our bones seem solid and stable, they actually undergo constant renewal. Specialized cells called *osteoclasts* draw used calcium out of the bones while other cells called *osteoblasts* replace it.

Especially after menopause, this process can get out of balance. Calcium starts to leach out of the bones faster than it can be replaced, leading to the brittle bone disease called osteoporosis.

Actonel combats this problem by reducing the activity of the osteoclasts and slowing the loss of calcium from the bones. It is prescribed for postmenopausal women, both to prevent osteoporosis and to strengthen the bones once the disease has begun. It is also used to prevent or treat osteoporosis resulting from therapy with steroid medications, and it is used in the treatment of Paget's disease, a condition in which patches of bone become softened and enlarged.

Both Actonel and a similar drug called Fosamax are members of the family of drugs called bisphosphonates.

Most important fact about this drug

Actonel not only stops the bone loss of osteoporosis, but actually reverses the disease and increases bone mineral density. As the bones grow stronger, your chances of sustaining a fracture decline.

How should you take this medication?

Three types of Actonel are available: 5-milligram and 30-milligram tablets that can be taken daily, and a 35-milligram tablet that's taken once a week. The tablets should be taken at least 30 minutes before the first food or drink of the day other than water. Take the pill while standing or sitting in an upright position and wash it down with a full 6 to 8 ounce glass of plain water (do not use coffee, tea, juice, milk, or other dairy products).

Swallow the tablet whole, do not chew or suck on it. Do not lie down for 30 minutes after taking the medication.

Other treatment measures typically include weight-bearing exercise, reduction of excessive smoking and drinking, and supplemental calcium and vitamin D if you don't get enough in your diet. If you require calcium supplements or use any medications containing calcium, aluminum, or magnesium, avoid taking them at the same time of day as Actonel.

■ *If you miss a dose...*
If you realize that you missed a daily dose and have not yet had anything to eat or drink, it's okay to take your medication. If you have already eaten, skip the dose for that day and take your regular dose the following morning.

If you forget to take a weekly dose, take 1 tablet on the morning after you remember, then return to taking 1 tablet a week as originally scheduled on the chosen day. Never take 2 tablets on the same day.
■ *Storage instructions...*
Store at room temperature.

What side effects may occur?

Side effects cannot be anticipated. If any develop or change in intensity, inform your doctor as soon as possible. Only your doctor can determine if it is safe for you to continue taking Actonel.

■ *Side effects may include:*
Abdominal pain, anxiety, back pain, belching, bladder irritation, bone disorders and pain, bronchitis, bursitis, cataracts, chest pain, colitis, constipation, depression, diarrhea, difficulty breathing, dizziness, dry eyes, eye infection, flu-like symptoms, gas, headache, high blood pressure, infection, insomnia, itching, joint disorders and pain, leg cramps, muscle pain, muscle weakness, nausea, neck pain, nerve pain, pain, pneumonia, rash, ringing in ears, sinus problems, sore throat, stomach bleeding, stuffy or runny nose, swelling, tendon problems, tumor, ulcers, urinary tract infection, vertigo, vision problems, weakness

Why should this drug not be prescribed?

Your doctor will not prescribe Actonel if you have low calcium levels in your blood or the drug gives you an allergic reaction. You also cannot take Actonel if you are unable to stand or sit upright for at least 30 minutes after taking the drug. In addition, the drug is not recommended for people with severe kidney disease.

Special warnings about this medication

The drugs in Actonel's family have been known to cause problems in the canal between the mouth and the stomach (the esophagus). Among the disorders that have been reported are esophageal irritation, difficulty swallowing, esophageal ulcers, and gastric ulcers.

You can guard against such problems by taking the medication with plenty of water, swallowing the pill while standing or sitting upright, and remaining upright for 30 minutes afterwards. If you experience difficulty or pain on swallowing, chest pain, or heartburn that is severe or worse than usual, stop taking Actonel and check with your doctor immediately.

Possible food and drug interactions when taking this medication

If Actonel is taken with certain other drugs, the effects of either could be increased, decreased, or altered. It is especially important to check with your doctor before combining Actonel with the following:

Antacids
Calcium supplements
Laxatives such as milk of magnesia

Special information if you are pregnant or breastfeeding

Actonel has caused harm when tested on pregnant animals. It is not recommended during human pregnancy unless its benefits are judged to outweigh the potential risks. If you are pregnant or plan to become pregnant, notify your doctor immediately.

If you are nursing a baby, you'll need to choose between discontinuing nursing and discontinuing the drug.

Recommended dosage

ADULTS

Osteoporosis
For the prevention and treatment of osteoporosis, the recommended dose is one 5-milligram tablet once daily or one 35-milligram tablet once a week.

Steroid-Induced Osteoporosis
For treatment or prevention of steroid-induced osteoporosis, the recommended dose is one 5-milligram tablet once a day.

Paget's Disease
The recommended dose for Paget's disease is 30 milligrams once a day for 2 months. A second 2-month course of therapy may be required in certain individuals.

Overdosage

A large overdose of Actonel can dramatically reduce calcium levels in the blood. Warning signs include a tingling sensation and spasms. If you suspect an overdose, seek medical attention immediately.

ACTOS

Pronounced: ACK-toes
Generic name: Pioglitazone hydrochloride

Why is this drug prescribed?

Actos is used to control high blood sugar in type 2 diabetes. This form of the illness usually stems from the body's inability to make good use of insulin, the natural hormone that helps to transfer sugar out of the blood and into the cells, where it's converted to energy. Actos works by improving the body's response to its natural supply of insulin, rather than increasing its insulin output. Actos also reduces the production of unneeded sugar in the liver.

Actos (and the similar drug Avandia) can be used alone or in combination with insulin injections or other oral diabetes medications such as DiaBeta, Micronase, Glucotrol, or Glucophage.

Most important fact about this drug

Always remember that Actos is an aid to, not a substitute for, good diet and exercise. Failure to follow a sound diet and exercise plan can lead to serious complications, such as dangerously high or low blood sugar levels. Remember, too, that Actos is not an oral form of insulin, and cannot be used in place of insulin.

How should you take this medication?

Actos should be taken once a day with or without meals.

■ *If you miss a dose...*
Take it as soon as you remember. If you miss a dose on one day, skip it and go back to your regular schedule. Do not double your dose the following day.
■ *Storage instructions...*
Store at room temperature in a tight container, away from moisture and humidity.

What side effects may occur?

Side effects cannot be anticipated. If any develop or change in intensity, inform your doctor as soon as possible. Only your doctor can determine if it is safe for you to continue taking Actos.

■ *More common side effects may include:*
Headache, hypoglycemia, muscle aches, respiratory tract infection, sinus inflammation, sore throat, swelling, tooth disorder

Why should this drug not be prescribed?

If Actos gives you an allergic reaction, you should not take this drug.

Special warnings about this medication

In very rare cases, a drug similar to Actos has proven toxic to the liver. The manufacturer therefore recommends that your doctor check your liver function before you begin taking Actos and periodically thereafter. If you experience symptoms of liver problems such as jaundice (yellowing of the skin and eyes), nausea, vomiting, abdominal pain, fatigue, loss of appetite, or dark urine, report them to your doctor immediately. You will probably have to stop using Actos.

Because Actos works by improving the body's response to its own supply of insulin, it is not for type 1 diabetics, who are unable to produce any insulin at all. For the same reason, Actos can't be used to treat the condition known as diabetic ketoacidosis (excessively high sugar levels due to the lack of insulin).

In rare instances, Actos causes swelling and fluid retention that can lead to congestive heart failure. If you already have this problem, you should avoid Actos. If you develop symptoms that signal the problem—such as shortness of breath, fatigue, or weight gain—you should check with your doctor immediately; the drug will probably have to be discontinued. The problem is more likely when Actos is taken in combination with insulin.

Actos, by itself, will not cause excessively low blood sugar (hypoglycemia). However, when you combine it with insulin injections or some other oral diabetes drugs, the chance of hypoglycemia increases. If you begin to feel symptoms of hypoglycemia—shaking, sweating, agitation, clammy skin, or blurred vision—take some fast-acting sugar, such as 4 to 6 ounces of fruit juice. Let your doctor know about the incident; you may need a lower dose of insulin or oral medication.

To make sure that your blood sugar levels stay within the normal range, get regular tests of your blood sugar and glycosylated hemoglobin (a long-term measurement of blood sugar). Contact your doctor during periods of stress due to fever, infection, injury, surgery, and the like. The dosage of your diabetes medicines may need to be changed.

Possible food and drug interactions when taking this medication

It is possible that Actos may reduce the effectiveness of birth control pills containing ethinyl estradiol and norethindrone. To guard against an unwanted pregnancy, be sure to use some other form of contraception.

If Actos is taken with certain other drugs, the effects of either could be increased, decreased, or altered. It is especially important to check with your doctor before combining Actos with the following:

Ketoconazole (Nizoral)
Midazolam (Versed)

Special information if you are pregnant or breastfeeding

The effects of Actos during pregnancy have not been adequately studied. If you are pregnant or plan to become pregnant, tell your doctor immediately. He may switch you to insulin during your pregnancy, since normal blood sugar levels are very important for the developing baby.

It is not known whether Actos appears in breast milk. For safety's sake, do not use this drug while breastfeeding.

Recommended dosage

ADULTS

The recommended starting dose of Actos is 15 to 30 milligrams once a day.

If this fails to bring your blood sugar under control, the dose can be increased to a maximum of 45 milligrams a day. If your blood sugar still remains high, the doctor may add a second medication.

When Actos is added to other diabetes medications, your doctor may need to lower their dosage if you develop low blood sugar. If you are taking insulin, the dose should be lowered when blood sugar readings fall below 100.

Overdosage

The effects of a massive Actos overdose are unknown, but any medication taken in excess can have serious consequences. If you suspect an overdose with Actos, seek medical attention immediately.

Actron *See Orudis, page 1016.*

ACULAR

Pronounced: AK-yew-lar
Generic name: Ketorolac tromethamine

Why is this drug prescribed?

Acular relieves the itchy eyes brought on by seasonal allergies. Doctors also prescribe it to reduce inflammation after cataracts have been removed from the eyes. A preservative-free formulation (Acular PF) is used to reduce pain and light-sensitivity following operations to correct vision. Acular belongs to the class of medications called nonsteroidal anti-inflammatory drugs.

Most important fact about this drug

Acular sometimes causes an inflammation of the cornea (the clear tissue over the pupil of the eye). This can lead to a sight-threatening breakdown of the cornea. Warning signs may include sensitivity to light and a sensation like a foreign body in the eye. If you develop these problems, see your doctor immediately. Acular may have to be discontinued.

How should you take this medication?

Do not administer Acular while wearing contact lenses. If you are using Acular PF, open a new single-use vial for each dose and discard any unused contents after administering the drop. To prevent contamination and possible infections, avoid touching the eyedropper or single-use vial to the eye or any other surface.

■ *If you miss a dose...*
Apply the forgotten dose as soon as you remember. However, if it is almost time for your next dose, skip the one you missed and return to your regular schedule. Do not apply 2 doses at once.

■ *Storage instructions...*
Store at room temperature. Protect from light.

What side effects may occur?

Side effects cannot be anticipated. If any develop or change in intensity, tell your doctor as soon as possible. Only your doctor can determine if it is safe to continue using Acular.

■ *Side effects may include:*
Temporary stinging and burning when the drops are applied.

Why should this drug not be prescribed?

If you've ever had an allergic reaction to the active ingredient ketorolac (found in the painkiller Toradol), you should not use Acular.

Special warnings about this medication

A history of reactions to other nonsteroidal anti-inflammatory drugs, including aspirin, makes a reaction to Acular more likely. Tell the doctor about any drug reactions you've experienced.

Drugs such as Acular may make the blood slower to clot, leading to increased bleeding after eye surgery. Use Acular with caution if you tend to bleed easily or are taking a blood-thinning medication. Acular may also delay healing.

Problems in the cornea are more likely after complicated or repeated eye operations, or if you use Acular for more than 1 day prior to surgery or more than 14 days afterwards. The risk of such problems is also greater if you have diabetes, arthritis, dry eyes, or pre-existing corneal defects.

Acular is not recommended for children under 3 years of age.

Possible food and drug interactions when using this medication

No interactions with Acular have been reported.

Special information if you are pregnant or breastfeeding

Avoid Acular late in pregnancy; the drug could have harmful effects on the developing baby. If you are pregnant or plan to become pregnant, inform your doctor immediately.

Use Acular with caution while nursing a baby.

Recommended dosage

ACULAR

Itchy Eyes
The usual dose is 1 drop 4 times a day.

After Cataract Surgery
The usual dose is 1 drop 4 times a day, beginning 24 hours after the operation and continuing for the first 2 weeks postsurgery.

ACULAR PF

After Corrective Surgery
The usual dose is 1 drop 4 times a day for up to 3 days after the operation.

Overdosage

There is no information on Acular overdose. However, any medication taken in excess can have serious consequences. If you suspect an overdose, seek medical attention immediately.

Acyclovir *See Zovirax, page 1656.*

Adalat *See Procardia, page 1162.*

Adapalene *See Differin, page 438.*

ADDERALL

Pronounced: ADD-ur-all
Generic ingredients: Amphetamines

Why is this drug prescribed?

Adderall is prescribed in the treatment of Attention Deficit Hyperactivity Disorder (ADHD), the condition in which a child exhibits a short attention span and becomes easily distracted, overly emotional, excessively active, and highly impulsive. It should be used as part of a broader treatment plan that includes psychological, educational, and social measures. An extended-release form of the drug, called Adderall XR, is available for once-daily treatment of ADHD.

The regular form of Adderall is also prescribed for narcolepsy (uncontrollable attacks of sleep).

Most important fact about this drug

Adderall, like all amphetamines, has a high potential for abuse. If used in large doses over long periods of time, it can cause dependence and addiction. Be careful to take Adderall only as prescribed.

How should you take this medication?

Never take more Adderall than your doctor has prescribed. Do not take it for a longer time or for any other purpose than prescribed.

Take the first dose upon awakening. If additional doses are prescribed, take them at intervals of 4 to 6 hours. Avoid late evening doses, which can interfere with sleep.

Adderall XR capsules can be taken whole, or the contents can be sprinkled on applesauce. The applesauce should be eaten immediately, without chewing. Be sure to use the entire contents of the capsule.

■ *If you miss a dose...*
If you are taking 1 dose a day, and at least 6 hours remain before bedtime, take the dose as soon as you remember. If you don't remember until the next day, skip the dose and go back to your regular schedule. Do not take a double dose.

If you are taking more than 1 dose a day, and you remember within an hour or so of the scheduled time, take the missed dose immediately. Otherwise, skip the dose and go back to your regular schedule. Never take 2 doses at once.

■ *Storage instructions...*
Store at room temperature in a tight, light-resistant container.

What side effects may occur?

Side effects cannot be anticipated. If any develop or change in intensity, tell your doctor as soon as possible. Only your doctor can determine if it is safe for you or your child to continue taking Adderall.

■ *Side effects of Adderall may include:*
Dry mouth, high blood pressure, hives, impotence, overstimulation, rapid or pounding heartbeat, stomach and intestinal disturbances, weight loss

■ *Side effects of Adderall XR may include:*
Abdominal pain, diarrhea, dizziness, fever, infection (including viral), insomnia, loss of appetite, mood swings, nausea, nervousness, vomiting, weakness, weight loss

Why should this drug not be prescribed?

Do not use Adderall if you have any of the following conditions:

Hardening of the arteries
Heart disease
High blood pressure
High pressure in the eye (glaucoma)
Overactive thyroid gland

Never take Adderall within 14 days of taking an antidepressant classified as an MAO inhibitor, including Nardil and Parnate. A potentially life-threatening spike in blood pressure could result.

Your doctor will not prescribe Adderall if you have ever had a reaction to similar stimulant drugs. The doctor will also avoid prescribing Adderall if you appear agitated or are prone to substance abuse.

Special warnings about this medication

If you have even a mild case of high blood pressure, take Adderall with caution. Be careful, too, about driving or operating machinery until you know how this drug affects you. It may impair judgment and coordination.

Adderall can make tics and twitches worse. If you or a family member has this problem (or the condition called Tourette's syndrome), make sure the doctor is aware of it. Amphetamines such as Adderall have also been known to aggravate symptoms in seriously disturbed (psychotic) individuals.

If the problem is attention deficit disorder, the doctor will do a complete history and evaluation before prescribing Adderall, taking particular account of the severity of the symptoms and the age of your child. If the problem is a temporary reaction to a stressful situation, Adderall is probably not called for.

At present, there has been no experience with long-term Adderall therapy in children. However, other amphetamine-based medications have been known to stunt growth, so your doctor will need to watch the child carefully.

Possible food and drug interactions when taking this medication

If Adderall is taken with certain other drugs, the effects of either could be increased, decreased, or altered. It is especially important to check with your doctor before combining Adderall with the following:

Acetazolamide (Diamox)
Antihistamines such as Benadryl and Chlor-Trimeton
Drugs classified as MAO inhibitors, including the antidepressants
  Nardil and Parnate
Drugs that make the urine more acid, such as Uroquid-Acid No. 2
Glutamic acid (an amino acid related to MSG)
High blood pressure medications such as Calan, guanethidine,
  HydroDIURIL, Hytrin, Procardia, and reserpine
Lithium (Eskalith, Lithobid)
Major tranquilizers such as Haldol and Thorazine
Meperidine (Demerol)
Methenamine (Urised)
Norepinephrine (Levophed)
Propoxyphene (Darvon)
Seizure medications such as Dilantin, phenobarbital, and Zarontin
Tricyclic antidepressants such as Norpramin, Tofranil, and Vivactil
Vitamin C

Special information if you are pregnant or breastfeeding

Heavy use of amphetamines during pregnancy can lead to premature birth or low birth weight. Avoid taking Adderall unless absolutely necessary. Amphetamines do find their way into breast milk, so you should not take Adderall while breastfeeding.

Recommended dosage

Whether the problem is attention deficit disorder or narcolepsy, the doctor will keep the dosage as low as possible.

ADDERALL

Attention Deficit Hyperactivity Disorder

Children 3 to 5 years of age: The usual starting dose is 2.5 milligrams daily. Each week, the doctor will raise the daily dosage by 2.5 milligrams until the condition is under control.

Children 6 years of age and older: The usual starting dose is 5 milligrams once or twice a day. Each week, the daily dosage may be increased by 5 milligrams. Only in rare cases will a child need more than 40 milligrams per day.

The doctor may interrupt therapy occasionally to see if the drug is still needed.

Narcolepsy

Adults: The usual total daily dose ranges from 5 to 60 milligrams, taken as 2 or more smaller doses.

Children under 12 years of age: The usual starting dose is 5 milligrams daily. Each week, the doctor will raise the daily dose by 5 milligrams until the condition is under control.

Children 12 years of age and older: The usual starting dose is 10 milligrams daily, with weekly increases of 10 milligrams daily until the drug takes effect.

ADDERALL XR

Attention Deficit Hyperactivity Disorder

Children 6 years of age and older: The usual starting dose for children taking Adderall for the first time is 10 milligrams once daily in the morning. At weekly intervals, the doctor may increase the daily dosage by 5 or 10 milligrams, up to a maximum of 30 milligrams a day.

Children already taking regular Adderall are prescribed a single dose of Adderall XR equal to their previous daily total.

Adderall XR has not been tested on children under 6.

Overdosage

A large overdose of Adderall can be fatal. Warning signs of a massive overdose include convulsions and coma.

■ *Symptoms of Adderall overdose may include:*
Abdominal cramps, assaultiveness, changes in blood pressure, confusion, diarrhea, hallucinations, heightened reflexes, high fever, irregular heartbeat, nausea, panic, rapid breathing, restlessness, tremor, vomiting

If you suspect an overdose, seek emergency treatment immediately.

ADIPEX-P

Pronounced: ADD-i-pecks
Generic name: Phentermine hydrochloride
Other brand name: Ionamin

Why is this drug prescribed?

Adipex-P, an appetite suppressant, is prescribed for short-term use (a few weeks) as part of an overall weight reduction program that also includes dieting, exercise, and counseling. The drug is for use only by excessively overweight individuals who have a condition—such as diabetes, high blood pressure, or high cholesterol—that could lead to serious medical problems.

Most important fact about this drug

Be sure to use this drug only as directed. It will lose its effect after a few weeks, and should be discontinued when this happens. If you try to boost its effectiveness by increasing the dose, you will run the risk of serious side effects and dependence on the drug.

How should you take this medication?

Take Adipex-P before breakfast or up to 2 hours after breakfast. Tablets can be broken in half, if necessary.

Take Ionamin before breakfast or 10 to 14 hours before you go to bed. Ionamin capsules should be swallowed whole.

■ *If you miss a dose...*
Skip the missed dose completely; then take the next dose at the regularly scheduled time.
■ *Storage instructions...*
Store at room temperature.

What side effects may occur?

Side effects cannot be anticipated. If any develop or change in intensity, inform your doctor as soon as possible. Only your doctor can determine if it is safe for you to continue taking this medication.

■ *Side effects may include:*
Changes in sex drive, constipation, diarrhea, dizziness, dry mouth, exaggerated feelings of depression or elation, headache, high blood pressure, hives, impotence, inability to fall or stay asleep, increased heart rate, overstimulation, restlessness, stomach or intestinal problems, throbbing heartbeat, tremors, unpleasant taste

Why should this drug not be prescribed?

If you are sensitive to or have ever had an allergic reaction to phentermine hydrochloride or other drugs that stimulate the nervous system, you should not take this medication. Make sure your doctor is aware of any drug reactions you have experienced.

Do not take this drug if you have hardening of the arteries, symptoms of heart or blood vessel disease, an overactive thyroid gland, the eye condition known as glaucoma, or high blood pressure. Also avoid this drug if you are agitated, have ever abused drugs, or have taken an MAO inhibitor, including antidepressant drugs such as Nardil and Parnate, within the last 14 days.

Special warnings about this medication

This drug can cause a rare but potentially fatal condition called primary pulmonary hypertension. Call your doctor immediately if you develop such warning signs as chest pain, shortness of breath, fainting spells, or swollen ankles.

This drug may affect your ability to perform potentially hazardous activities. Therefore, you should be extremely careful if you have to drive a car or operate machinery.

You can become psychologically dependent on this drug. Consult your doctor if you rely on this drug to maintain a state of well-being.

If you stop taking this drug suddenly after you have taken high doses for a long time, you may find you are extremely fatigued or depressed, or that you have trouble sleeping.

If you continually take too much of any appetite suppressant, it can cause severe skin disorders, a pronounced inability to fall or stay asleep, irritability, hyperactivity, and personality changes.

Even if your blood pressure is only mildly high, be careful taking this drug.

Possible food and drug interactions when taking this medication

Remember that this drug should never be combined with the weight loss drug fenfluramine (Pondimin); very dangerous side effects could result. This drug may also react badly with alcohol. Avoid alcoholic beverages while you are taking it.

If Adipex-P is taken with certain other drugs, the effects of either can be increased, decreased, or altered. It is especially important that you check with your doctor before combining this drug with the following:

Diabetes medications such as insulin and Micronase
Drugs that boost serotonin levels, such as the antidepressants Luvox, Paxil, Prozac, and Zoloft
Drugs classified as MAO inhibitors, including the antidepressants Nardil and Parnate
High blood pressure medications such as guanethidine (Ismelin)

Special information if you are pregnant or breastfeeding

The effects of this drug during pregnancy have not been adequately studied. If you are pregnant, plan to become pregnant, or are breastfeeding, notify your doctor immediately.

Recommended dosage

ADULTS

Adipex-P
The usual dose is 1 capsule or tablet a day, taken before breakfast or up to 2 hours after breakfast. Some people need only half a tablet each day. Others may find it more effective to take half a tablet twice daily.

Ionamin
The usual dose is 1 capsule a day, taken before breakfast or 10 to 14 hours before bedtime.

CHILDREN

This drug is not recommended for use in children under 16 years of age.

Overdosage

Any medication taken in excess can have serious consequences. An overdose of this drug can be fatal. If you suspect an overdose, seek emergency medical treatment immediately.

■ *Symptoms of Adipex-P overdose may include:*
Abdominal cramps, aggressiveness, confusion, diarrhea, exaggerated reflexes, hallucinations, high or low blood pressure, irregular heartbeat, nausea, panic states, rapid breathing, restlessness, tremors, vomiting

Fatigue and depression may follow the stimulant effects of this drug.

In cases of fatal poisoning, convulsions and coma usually precede death.

ADVAIR DISKUS

Pronounced: AD-vare
Generic ingredients: Fluticasone propionate, Salmeterol

Why is this drug prescribed?

Advair Diskus is used to control asthma and chronic obstructive pulmonary disease (COPD) associated with chronic bronchitis. It is an oral inhaler that contains two types of medication. One is fluticasone propionate, a steroid that reduces inflammation in the lungs. The other, salmeterol, is a long-acting bronchodilator that opens up the airways. Together, the two ingredients provide better symptom control than either does individually.

Most important fact about this drug

Advair Diskus is used for long-term control of asthma and short-term control of COPD associated with bronchitis. The drug won't end a sudden attack. For relief of acute asthma or bronchial symptoms, your doctor will prescribe a short-acting inhaler such as Proventil or Ventolin.

How should you take this medication?

Advair Diskus should be used twice a day, once in the morning and once in the evening. You may be able to taste or feel your dose of Advair Diskus. Do not be concerned, however, if you can't detect anything. You're getting the proper dose whether you can taste the medication or not. Never exceed the recommended dose of one inhalation twice daily.

Follow the detailed directions that came with the inhaler. If you have any questions, ask your doctor or pharmacist. Some important points to keep in mind:

- Do not use a spacer with this medication.
- Never exhale into the diskus.
- Do not try to take the diskus apart.
- Always activate and use the diskus in a level, horizontal position.
- It is important to keep the diskus dry—do not wash any part of the mouthpiece or any part of the diskus.
- To reduce the risk of developing an infection in your mouth, rinse your mouth with water after each inhalation without swallowing.

When first using this medication, you may notice some improvement within 30 minutes, but its maximum benefits may take a week or more to appear.

- *If you miss a dose...*
  Take it as soon as you remember. If it is almost time for your next dose, skip the one you missed and go back to your regular schedule.

■ *Storage instructions…*
Store the diskus at room temperature, away from heat, sunlight, and moisture. Discard the diskus one month after removing it from its moisture-protective foil overwrap pouch or after all blisters have been used, whichever comes first.

What side effects may occur?
Side effects cannot be anticipated. If any develop or change in intensity, inform your doctor as soon as possible. Only your doctor can determine if it is safe for you to continue taking Advair Diskus.

■ *Side effects may include:*
Bronchitis, cough, diarrhea, difficulty speaking, fungal infection of the mouth, gastrointestinal discomfort and pain, headaches, hoarseness, muscle pain, nausea, sinus problems, sore throat, upper respiratory infection or inflammation, vomiting

Why should this drug not be prescribed?
Advair cannot be used for acute episodes of asthma that require intensive therapy. You'll also have to avoid it if it gives you an allergic reaction.

Special warnings about this medication
Call your doctor immediately if you develop hives, rash, or swelling, or if you have shortness of breath that does not respond to your usual medication. Advair Diskus has been known to cause allergic reactions and acute attacks of asthma or bronchial spasms.

A safety study found that one of the ingredients in Advair Diskus, salmeterol, may be associated with rare cases of serious asthma attacks or asthma-related death. If you're concerned, talk with the doctor about your options. Do not, however, stop using Advair Diskus without first consulting your doctor.

Very rarely, Advair Diskus can cause a severe allergic reaction in people who are highly allergic to milk protein.

Be sure to keep track of how often you have to use your short-acting inhaler for relief of acute asthma symptoms. Your doctor will use this information to help determine how well Advair Diskus is working. Notify your doctor if you do not get relief from your short-acting inhaler or if you need more inhalations than usual to get relief. Keep track of your peak flow readings, too. Call your doctor if you notice a drop in this measurement of lung capacity.

Do not use Advair Diskus more often than your doctor has prescribed. Excessive use can cause heart irregularities. Use Advair Diskus with caution if you have any kind of heart disorder or high blood pressure. Alert your doctor immediately if you develop chest pain, heart palpitations, nervousness, or tremor.

Long-term use of the medications in Advair Diskus could exacerbate certain conditions. Your doctor will monitor you closely if you have any of the following: infections caused by a virus, fungus, or bacteria (including tuberculosis); blood sugar problems; overactive thyroid; seizures; eye problems (such as cataracts or glaucoma); blood disorders; and osteoporosis or an increased risk of losing bone mineral density.

Steroids taken by mouth or injection have been shown to slow or stop growth in children and cause reduced adrenal gland function. If enough medication is absorbed following inhalation, it's possible that Advair Diskus could also cause these effects. The doctor will prescribe the lowest possible dose to lessen the chance of an effect on growth or adrenal gland function.—It is important that children taking this medication visit their doctors regularly so that their growth rates may be monitored.— Before this medicine is given to a child, you and your doctor should talk about the benefits as well as the risks of using it.

People taking this medicine may be more susceptible to infections. Try to avoid contact with people who have measles or chickenpox, and notify your doctor if you or your child is exposed. The steroid component of Advair Diskus tends to lower immunity and could make these infections worse.

Do not use Serevent (salmeterol), Foradil (formoterol), or other long-acting inhalers while using Advair Diskus. They contain the same type of active ingredient, and will provide no extra benefit.

Possible food and drug interactions when taking this medication

If Advair Diskus is used with certain other drugs, the effects of either could be increased, decreased, or altered. It is especially important to check with your doctor before combining this medication with the following:

Antidepressants categorized as tricyclics, such as Elavil and Tofranil
Antidepressants called monoamine oxidase inhibitors, such as Nardil and Parnate
Beta-blockers (drugs such as Inderal and Tenormin that are used to control blood pressure and treat various heart conditions)
Ketoconazole (Nizoral)
Long-acting inhalers such as Foradil and Serevent
Ritonavir (Norvir)
Water pills (diuretics) such as HydroDIURIL and Lasix

Special information if you are pregnant or breastfeeding

The possibility of harm to a developing baby has not been ruled out. Advair Diskus should be used during pregnancy only if the potential benefit justifies the risk.

It is possible that the ingredients of Advair Diskus may appear in breast milk, so you'll need to choose between nursing the baby and continuing your therapy.

Recommended dosage

ADULTS

The recommended dosage of Advair Diskus is one inhalation twice daily. Take the inhalations morning and evening, 12 hours apart.

The product comes in three strengths. Your doctor will select the best strength for you based on your current therapy. If this selection fails to improve your symptoms after 2 weeks, the doctor may prescribe a higher strength.

CHILDREN

Advair Diskus can be used by adolescents 12 years of age and older. The dosage is the same as for adults.

Advair Diskus can sometimes be used to control asthma in children 4 to 11 years of age. For these children, only the lowest strength of medication is given.

Advair Diskus should not be used by children under 4 years of age.

Overdosage

Any medication taken in excess can have serious consequences. If you suspect an overdose, seek medical attention immediately.

■ *Symptoms of acute Advair Diskus overdose may include:*
Fast or irregular heartbeat, headache, muscle cramps, tremor

Advanced Natalcare *See Prenatal Vitamins, page 1141.*

ADVICOR
Pronounced: AD-vih-core
Generic ingredients: Lovastatin, Niacin

Why is this drug prescribed?

Advicor is a cholesterol-lowering drug. Excess cholesterol in the bloodstream can lead to hardening of the arteries and heart disease. Advicor lowers total cholesterol and LDL ("bad") cholesterol, while raising the amount of HDL ("good") cholesterol.

Advicor is a combination of two cholesterol-fighting ingredients: extended-release niacin and lovastatin (Mevacor). It is prescribed only when other drugs and a program of diet, exercise, and weight reduction have been unsuccessful in lowering cholesterol levels.

Most important fact about this drug

Although you cannot feel any symptoms of high cholesterol, it is important to take Advicor every day. The drug will be more effective if it is taken as part of a program of diet, exercise, and weight loss. All these efforts keep your cholesterol levels normal and lower your risk of heart disease.

How should you take this medication?

Advicor should be taken at bedtime, with a low-fat snack. Do not take this medication on an empty stomach.

Advicor is an extended-release medication. Swallow the tablets whole. Do not break, chew, or crush the tablets.

If you stop taking Advicor for more than a week, check with your doctor; you may need to gradually build up your dosage again.

■ *If you miss a dose...*
Take it as soon as you remember. If it is almost time for your next dose, skip the one you missed and go back to your regular schedule. Do not take 2 doses at once.
■ *Storage instructions...*
Store at room temperature.

What side effects may occur?

Side effects cannot be anticipated. If any develop or change in intensity, inform your doctor as soon as possible. Only your doctor can determine if it is safe for you to continue taking Advicor.

■ *Side effects may include:*
Abdominal pain, back pain, diarrhea, flu-like symptoms, flushing, headache, high blood sugar, indigestion, infection, itching, muscle pain, nausea, pain, rash, vomiting, weakness

Why should this drug not be prescribed?

If you are allergic to niacin or lovastatin, you cannot take Advicor. You should also avoid Advicor if you have liver disease, an ulcer, or arterial bleeding. Never take Advicor during pregnancy or while you are breast-feeding.

Special warnings about this medication

Advicor can cause liver problems. Your doctor will test your liver function before you start taking this medication, then every 6 to 12 weeks for the first 6 months after you begin therapy, and every 6 months thereafter. If the tests reveal a problem, you may have to stop taking Advicor. Individuals who regularly drink alcohol or have a history of liver disease should use this drug with caution. Avoid Advicor completely if you currently have liver disease.

The extended-release niacin in Advicor is not interchangeable with immediate-release niacin. Substituting doses of extended-release niacin for immediate-release niacin can cause severe liver damage.

Drugs like Advicor may trigger a muscle-wasting condition that also can affect the kidneys. The risk is increased if Advicor is taken with certain drugs or grapefruit juice. Contact your doctor immediately if you experience unexplained muscle pain, tenderness, or weakness. You may have to stop taking Advicor. Use Advicor with caution if you have kidney disease, gout, or the chest pain of angina.

Advicor may cause flushing. This side effect usually goes away after taking the medication for several weeks. Flushing can be accompanied by dizziness, fainting, heartbeat irregularities, chills, shortness of breath, or swelling. Notify your doctor if you experience dizziness. If you awaken because of flushing, rise slowly to avoid dizziness and fainting. Taking aspirin or ibuprofen before taking Advicor may help decrease the flushing. Avoid drinking alcohol or hot drinks near the time you take Advicor; these can increase flushing.

If you have diabetes, Advicor may affect your blood sugar levels. Tell your doctor if you note any changes.

Advicor can cause abnormalities in the blood. If you are scheduled for surgery, your doctor will have you stop taking Advicor a few days before the operation.

Tell your doctor if you are taking any nutritional supplements that contain niacin.

Advicor is not recommended for children.

Possible food and drug interactions when taking this medication
Avoid drinking large amounts of grapefruit juice (more than a quart a day) while on Advicor therapy. It can increase the risk of muscle wasting.

If Advicor is taken with certain other drugs, the effects of either could be increased, decreased, or altered. It is especially important to check with your doctor before combining Advicor with any of the following:

Antifungal drugs such as Nizoral and Sporanox
Blood pressure medications such as Inderal, Lopressor, and
    Tenormin
Calcium channel blockers such as Norvasc, Plendil, and Procardia
Cholesterol-lowering drugs called fibrates such as Atromid and
    Lopid
Cimetidine (Tagamet)
Clarithromycin (Biaxin)
Cyclosporine (Sandimmune)
Erythromycin (E.E.S., Erythrocin)
HIV protease inhibitors such as Norvir and Viracept
Nefazodone (Serzone)
Nitroglycerin (Nitro-Bid, Nitro-Dur, Nitrostat)
Nutritional supplements containing niacin or nicotinamide
Spironolactone (Aldactone)
Warfarin (Coumadin)

Special information if you are pregnant or breastfeeding

Developing babies need plenty of cholesterol, so cholesterol-lowering drugs should never be used during pregnancy or while breastfeeding. Advicor should be taken by women of childbearing age only if it is very unlikely that they will become pregnant. If you do become pregnant while taking Advicor, stop taking the medication immediately and contact your doctor.

Recommended dosage

ADULTS

The usual starting dose of Advicor is one tablet containing 500 milligrams of extended-release niacin and 20 milligrams of lovastatin, taken at bedtime with a low-fat snack. After four weeks, your doctor may increase the dosage if the initial dose has not been effective. The maximum recommended dosage is 2,000 milligrams of extended-release niacin and 40 milligrams of lovastatin.

Overdosage

Any medication taken in excess can have dangerous consequences. If you suspect an overdose, seek medical attention immediately.

■ *Symptoms of Advicor overdose may include:*
Diarrhea, dizziness, fainting, heartbeat irregularities, indigestion, nausea, severe flushing, vomiting

Advil *See Motrin, page 895.*

AEROBID
Pronounced: AIR-oh-bid
Generic name: Flunisolide
Other brand names: AeroBid-M, Nasalide

Why is this drug prescribed?

AeroBid is prescribed for people who need long-term treatment to control and prevent the symptoms of asthma. It contains an anti-inflammatory steroid type of medication and may reduce or eliminate your need for other corticosteroids. A nasal-spray form of the drug (Nasalide) is available for relief of hay fever.

Most important fact about this drug

AeroBid helps to reduce the likelihood of an asthma attack, but will not relieve one that has already started. To be effective as a preventive measure, it must be taken every day at regularly spaced intervals. It may be several weeks before you receive its full benefit.

How should you take this medication?

Take this medication at regular intervals, exactly as prescribed by your doctor.

Administration technique:

1. Place the metal cartridge inside the plastic container.
2. Remove the cap; inspect the mouthpiece for foreign objects.
3. Shake the inhaler thoroughly.
4. Tilt your head slightly and breathe out as completely as possible.
5. Hold the inhaler upright and put the plastic mouthpiece in your mouth; close your lips tightly around it.
6. Press down on the metal cartridge. At the same time, take a slow, deep breath through your mouth.
7. Hold your breath as long as you can. While holding your breath, stop pressing down on the cartridge and remove the mouthpiece from your mouth.
8. Allow at least 1 minute between inhalations.

To help reduce hoarseness, throat irritation, and mouth infection, rinse out with water after each use. If your mouth is sore or has a rash, tell your doctor.

Illustrated instructions for use are available with the product.

◼ *If you miss a dose...*
Use it as soon as you remember. If it is almost time for your next dose, skip the one you missed and go back to your regular schedule. Do not take 2 doses at the same time.

◼ *Storage instructions...*
Store away from heat or cold and light. Keep away from open flames.

What side effects may occur?

Side effects cannot be anticipated. If any develop or change in intensity, inform your doctor as soon as possible. Only your doctor can determine if it is safe for you to continue taking AeroBid.

◼ *Side effects may include:*
Cold symptoms, diarrhea, flu, headache, infection of the upper respiratory tract, nasal congestion, nausea, sore throat, unpleasant taste, upset stomach, vomiting

Why should this drug not be prescribed?

This medication is not for treatment of prolonged, severe asthma attacks where more intensive measures are required.

If you are allergic or sensitive to AeroBid or other steroid drugs, advise your doctor. This medication may not be right for you.

Special warnings about this medication

Your asthma should be reasonably stable before treatment with AeroBid Inhaler is started. AeroBid should be started in combination with your usual dose of an oral steroid medication. After approximately 1 week, your doctor will start to withdraw gradually the oral steroid by reducing the daily or alternate daily dose. A slow rate of reduction is very important, as some people have experienced withdrawal symptoms such as joint and/or muscular pain, fatigue, and depression. Tell your doctor if you lose weight or feel light-headed. You may need to take more oral corticosteroid temporarily.

This medication is not useful when you need rapid relief of asthma symptoms.

Transferring from steroid tablet therapy to AeroBid Inhaler may produce allergic conditions that were previously controlled by the steroid tablet therapy. These include rhinitis (inflammation of the mucous membrane of the nose), conjunctivitis (pinkeye), and eczema.

Contact your doctor immediately if you have an asthma attack that isn't controlled by a bronchodilator while you are being treated with AeroBid. You may need an oral steroid drug.

While you are being treated with AeroBid, particularly at higher doses, your doctor will carefully observe you for any evidence of side effects such as the suppression of glandular function and diminished bone growth in children. If you have just had surgery or are under extreme stress, your doctor will also closely monitor you.

The use of AeroBid may cause a yeast-like fungal infection of the mouth, pharynx (throat), or larynx (voice box). If you suspect a fungal infection, notify your doctor. Treatment with antifungal medication may be necessary.

Since the contents of this inhalant are under pressure, do not puncture the container and do not use or store the medication near heat or an open flame. Exposure to temperatures above 120 degrees Fahrenheit may cause the container to explode.

People taking drugs such as AeroBid that suppress the immune system are more open to infection. Take extra care to avoid exposure to measles and chickenpox if you've never had them or never had shots. Such diseases can be serious or even fatal when your immune system is below par. If you are exposed, tell your doctor immediately.

Also, if you have tuberculosis, a herpes infection of the eye, or any other kind of infection, make sure the doctor knows about it. You probably should not use AeroBid.

Possible food and drug interactions when taking this medication
No interactions have been reported.

Special information if you are pregnant or breastfeeding
The effects of AeroBid during pregnancy have not been adequately studied. If you are pregnant or plan to become pregnant, inform your doctor immediately. It is not known whether AeroBid appears in breast milk. If this medication is essential to your health, your doctor may advise you to

discontinue breastfeeding your baby until your treatment with this medication is finished.

Recommended dosage

The AeroBid Inhaler system is for oral inhalation only.

ADULTS

The recommended starting dose is 2 inhalations twice daily, in the morning and evening, for a total daily dose of 1 milligram. The daily dose should not exceed 4 inhalations twice a day, for a total daily dose of 2 milligrams.

CHILDREN

For children 6 to 15 years of age, 2 inhalations may be used twice daily, for a total daily dose of 1 milligram.

The safety and effectiveness of AeroBid have not been established in children under 6 years of age.

Overdosage

Any medication taken in excess can have serious consequences. If you suspect an overdose, seek emergency medical treatment immediately.

AGENERASE

Pronounced: ah-JEN-eh-race
Generic name: Amprenavir

Why is this drug prescribed?

Agenerase is one of the many drugs now used to combat human immunodeficiency virus (HIV) infection. HIV undermines the immune system, reducing the body's ability to fight off other infections and eventually leading to the deadly condition known as acquired immune deficiency syndrome (AIDS).

Agenerase slows the progress of HIV by interfering with an important step in the virus's reproductive cycle. The drug is a member of the group of protease inhibitors, famous for having successfully halted the advance of the virus in many HIV-positive individuals. Agenerase is prescribed only as part of a drug regimen that attacks the virus on several fronts. It is not used alone.

Most important fact about this drug

Agenerase is not a cure for HIV infection or AIDS. It does not completely eliminate HIV from the body or totally restore the immune system. There is still a danger of developing serious opportunistic infections (infections that develop when the immune system falters). It's important, therefore, to continue seeing your doctor for regular blood counts and tests. And notify your doctor immediately of any changes in your general health.

How should you take this medication?

With the exception of high-fat meals, Agenerase may be taken with or without food. (Excessive fat decreases the amount of medicine that gets into the bloodstream.)

It is important to keep adequate levels of the drug in your bloodstream at all times, so be sure to take Agenerase exactly as prescribed, even when you're feeling better. Do not substitute Agenerase oral solution for the capsules. The two are not interchangeable.

If you are also taking antacids or the HIV drug didanosine (Videx), be sure to allow at least 1 hour between a dose of either medicine and a dose of Agenerase.

■ *If you miss a dose...*
Take it as soon as you remember. If it is almost time for your next dose, skip the one you missed and go back to your regular schedule. Do not take 2 doses at once.

■ *Storage instructions...*
Both the capsules and the oral solution can be stored at room temperature. Do not refrigerate the oral solution.

What side effects may occur?

Side effects cannot be anticipated. If any develop or change in intensity, inform your doctor as soon as possible. Only your doctor can determine if it is safe for you to continue taking Agenerase.

■ *Side effects may include:*
Abdominal discomfort or pain, diarrhea, fatigue, gas, headache, nausea, skin rash, vomiting, mouth tingling

Why should this drug not be prescribed?

If Agenerase gives you an allergic reaction, you will not be able to use it. Agenerase oral solution should be taken only when the capsule form is not an option. The oral solution contains an ingredient, propylene glycol, that some people have difficulty processing. It should not be taken by children under age 4, pregnant women, people with kidney or liver failure, or anyone who is also taking disulfiram (Antabuse) or metronidazole (Flagyl). It should be used with caution by women and individuals who have an Asian, Eskimo, or Native American ethnic background. Possible reactions to the propylene glycol in Agenerase oral solution include seizures, drowsiness, and fast heartbeat.

Special warnings about this medication

Remember that Agenerase does not completely eliminate HIV, and that it is still possible to pass the virus to others through sexual contact or blood contamination. Continue to practice safe sex while using Agenerase.

Agenerase can interfere with oral contraceptives. Use a backup form of birth control (such as condoms) to avoid an unwanted pregnancy.

Agenerase must be used with caution if you have kidney or liver problems. If you have such a disorder, make sure your doctor is aware of it.

Do not take vitamin E supplements with this drug. Agenerase is already fortified with vitamin E.

One serious potential side effect of Agenerase is a rash that occasionally becomes so severe as to be life-threatening. If you notice any signs of rash, inform your doctor immediately. If the rash gets worse or is accompanied by fever, blisters, mouth sores, red eyes, swelling, or flu-like symptoms, stop taking the drug and call your doctor.

Agenerase may trigger diabetes or make it worse. If this occurs, you may have to start taking insulin or oral diabetes drugs, or have your dosage of these medications adjusted. Agenerase can also increase cholesterol levels, possibly resulting in the need for treatment.

Like other protease inhibitors, Agenerase may also lead to a redistribution of body fat, with an increase in weight around the middle and on the upper back, and a loss of fat in the arms and legs. The long-term health effects of this change are still unknown.

Agenerase belongs to the sulfonamide family of drugs. If you have an allergy to other sulfa drugs, such as Bactrim or Septra, be sure to tell your doctor.

Possible food and drug interactions when taking this medication
Be sure to check with your doctor about the medicines and herbal remedies that should NOT be taken with this drug. Due to the danger of life-threatening side effects, Agenerase should never be combined with dihydroergotamine (Migranal), ergonovine (Ergotrate), ergotamine (Ergostat), methylergonovine (Methergine), pimozide (Orap), midazolam (Versed), or triazolam (Halcion). Serious or life-threatening side effects can also occur when Agenerase is taken with amiodarone (Cordarone), lidocaine, lovastatin (Mevacor), quinidine (Quinidex), simvastatin (Zocor), or tricyclic antidepressants such as Elavil and Tofranil. If you are taking both Agenerase and the HIV drug ritonavir (Norvir), you must be careful to avoid the heart medications flecainide (Tambocor) and propafenone (Rythmol).

Rifampin (Rifadin, Rifamate, Rifater) and St. John's wort should be avoided because they combat the antiviral effects of Agenerase. Combining Agenerase oral solution with Norvir oral solution is not recommended. And while taking Agenerase oral solution, it's best to avoid drinking alcohol.

Be cautious, too, about combining Agenerase and Viagra. The combination increases the risk of Viagra-related side effects such as low blood pressure, changes in vision, and persistent painful erection.

A variety of other drugs may also interact with Agenerase. Here is a list of the major possibilities.

Abacavir (Ziagen)
Amiodarone (Cordarone)
Antacids such as Maalox and Mylanta
Antidepressants classified as tricyclics, such as Elavil, Pamelor, and
    Tofranil
Benzodiazepine drugs used to treat anxiety, including Dalmane,
    Tranxene, Valium, and Xanax
Calcium channel blockers (used for high blood pressure and angina),
    including Adalat, Calan, Cardene, Cardizem, Dilacor, DynaCirc,
    Nimotop, Norvasc, Plendil, Procardia, Sular, and Vascor
Carbamazepine (Tegretol)
Cholesterol-lowering agents such as Lipitor, Mevacor, and Zocor
Cimetidine (Tagamet)
Clarithromycin (Biaxin)
Clozapine (Clozaril)
Cyclosporine (Sandimmune, Neoral)
Dapsone
Delavirdine (Rescriptor)
Dexamethasone (Decadron)
Didanosine (Videx)
Dihydroergotamine (D.H.E. 45 Injection, Migranal Nasal Spray)
Disulfiram (Antabuse)
Efavirenz (Sustiva)
Ergonovine (Ergotrate)
Ergotamine (Ergostat)
Erythromycin (Eryc, Ery-Tab)
Indinavir (Crixivan)
Itraconazole (Sporanox)
Ketoconazole (Nizoral)
Lidocaine
Lopinavir/ritonavir (Kaletra)
Loratadine (Claritin)
Methadone
Methylergonovine (Methergine)
Metronidazole (Flagyl)
Midazolam (Versed)
Nelfinavir (Viracept)
Nevirapine (Viramune)
Oral contraceptives
Phenobarbital
Phenytoin (Dilantin)
Pimozide (Orap)
Quinidine (Quinaglute, Quinidex)
Rapamycin (Rapamune)
Rifabutin (Mycobutin)

Rifampin (Rifadin, Rimactane)
Ritonavir (Norvir)
Saquinavir (Invirase)
Sildenafil (Viagra)
St. John's wort
Tacrolimus (Prograf)
Triazolam (Halcion)
Warfarin (Coumadin)
Zidovudine (Retrovir)

Special information if you are pregnant or breastfeeding

The effects of Agenerase during pregnancy have not been adequately studied. If you are pregnant or plan to become pregnant, tell your doctor immediately. Do not take the oral solution while pregnant.

Since HIV infection can be passed to your baby through breast milk, you should avoid breastfeeding.

Recommended dosage

ADULTS

Capsules
The usual dosage for adults and adolescents 13 years of age and over is 1,200 milligrams (eight 150-milligram capsules) twice a day in combination with other anti-HIV medications. When combined with Norvir, the recommended dosage is 1,200 milligrams of Agenerase and 200 milligrams of Norvir once a day, or half that amount twice a day.

Oral Solution
The usual dose for adults and children 13 years of age and over is 1,400 milligrams twice a day in combination with other anti-HIV medications.

CHILDREN

The recommended dosage for children between 4 and 12 years old (and those over 13 who weigh 110 pounds or less) is as follows.

Capsules
20 milligrams per 2.2 pounds of body weight twice a day or 15 milligrams per 2.2 pounds of body weight 3 times daily in combination with other anti-HIV medications.

Oral Solution
22.5 milligrams per 2.2 pounds of body weight twice a day or 17.5 milligrams per 2.2 pounds of body weight 3 times daily in combination with other anti-HIV medications.

Dosage should never exceed 2,400 milligrams daily in capsule form or 2,800 milligrams daily of oral solution.

THOSE WITH REDUCED LIVER FUNCTION

The doctor will prescribe a reduced dosage ranging from 300 milligrams twice a day to 450 milligrams twice a day depending on the amount of liver damage you've suffered.

Overdosage

Little is known about the symptoms of Agenerase overdose. However, any medication taken in excess can have serious consequences. If you suspect an overdose, seek medical attention immediately.

AGGRENOX

Pronounced: AG-reh-noks
Generic ingredients: Aspirin, Extended-release dipyridamole

Why is this drug prescribed?

Aggrenox is prescribed to stave off a stroke in people who have had a mini-stroke (transient ischemic attack) or a full-scale stroke due to a blood clot blocking an artery in the brain.

   Both the ingredients in Aggrenox prevent the formation of clots by interfering with the tendency of blood platelets to clump together. However, the two ingredients together are more effective at preventing strokes than either ingredient taken alone. Aggrenox doesn't eliminate the possibility of a stroke; but it does reduce the odds by almost six percentage points during the first 2 years of treatment.

Most important fact about this drug

Because of the aspirin in Aggrenox, this product cannot be used by people who have an allergy to aspirin and other nonsteroidal anti-inflammatory drugs such as Advil, Motrin, and Naprosyn, or by people who suffer asthma attacks after taking aspirin.

How should you take this medication?

Aggrenox should be taken once in the morning and once in the evening. The capsule should be swallowed whole without chewing. This drug may be taken with or without food.

■ *If you miss a dose...*
   Take it as soon as you remember. If it is almost time for your next dose, skip the one you missed and go back to your regular schedule. Never take 2 doses at the same time.
■ *Storage instructions...*
   Store at room temperature and protect from excessive moisture.

What side effects may occur?

Side effects cannot be anticipated. If any develop or change in intensity, inform your doctor as soon as possible. Only your doctor can determine if it is safe for you to continue taking Aggrenox.

■ *Side effects may include:*

Abdominal pain, back pain, bleeding, diarrhea, dizziness, fatigue, headache, indigestion, joint pain, nausea, pain, vomiting

Why should this drug not be prescribed?

You should not take Aggrenox if you have ever had an allergic reaction to aspirin, dipyridamole, or nonsteroidal anti-inflammatory drugs. You should also avoid this drug if you have asthma, a persistent runny nose, or nasal polyps, or if you have severe liver or kidney disease.

Aspirin can cause a dangerous brain disorder called Reye's syndrome in children and teenagers who have a viral illness. Since Aggrenox contains aspirin, it is not recommended for children or teenagers.

Special warnings about this medication

The aspirin in Aggrenox can cause stomach bleeding. You should avoid this drug if you have a stomach ulcer, and should use it with care if you have liver disease or any kind of bleeding disorder. (Regular heavy drinking increases the danger of bleeding problems.) Also, be sure to tell the doctor that you are taking Aggrenox if you have a medical emergency or plan to have surgery or dental work.

The dipyridamole in Aggrenox causes blood vessels to expand and should be used cautiously by people with heart disease, especially those with chest pain (unstable angina) or a recent heart attack. It can make chest pain worse and trigger episodes of very low blood pressure.

Possible food and drug interactions when taking this medication

If Aggrenox is taken with certain other drugs, the effects of either could be increased, decreased, or altered. It is especially important to check with your doctor before combining Aggrenox with the following:

ACE inhibitors (heart and blood pressure medications such as Capoten and Vasotec)
Acetazolamide (Diamox)
Blood pressure medications classified as beta-blockers, including Inderal, Sectral, and Tenormin
Blood-thinning drugs such as Coumadin
Gout medications such as Benemid and Anturane
Methotrexate (Rheumatrex)
Nonsteroidal anti-inflammatory drugs such as Advil, Motrin, and Indocin
Oral diabetes drugs such as Diabinese and Micronase

Seizure medications such as Depakene and Dilantin
Water pills (diuretics) such as HydroDiuril and Lasix

If you suffer from the muscle disease myasthenia gravis, treatment with Aggrenox may interfere with your drug therapy.

Special information if you are pregnant or breastfeeding

Aggrenox can seriously harm a developing baby, leading to low birth weight, bleeding in the brain, birth defects, and even death. Aggrenox should not be used during the final 3 months of pregnancy, and should be taken during the first 6 months only if its benefits outweigh the possibility of harm to the developing baby. Notify your doctor immediately if you are pregnant or plan to become pregnant.

Use Aggrenox with caution if you are breastfeeding a baby, since this drug appears in breast milk.

Recommended dosage

ADULTS

The recommended dosage of Aggrenox is one capsule twice a day, in the morning and evening.

Overdosage

Any medication taken in excess can have serious consequences. If you suspect an overdose, seek medical attention immediately.

■ *Symptoms of Aggrenox overdose may include:*
  Dizziness, flushes, irregular heartbeat, restlessness, ringing in the ears, sweating, warm feeling, weakness

Aktob *See Tobrex, page 1446.*

ALAMAST
Pronounced: allah-mast
Generic name: Pemirolast

Why is this drug prescribed?

Alamast is taken to prevent the itchy eyes caused by allergies such as hay fever.

Most important fact about this drug

Alamast does not provide immediate relief. It may take a few days or as much as 4 weeks for the medication to start working.

How should you take this medication?

Use Alamast solution only in the eyes; never swallow it. Be careful to keep the dropper tip from touching the eyelid or surrounding areas when administering this medication.

If you wear soft contact lenses, remove them before administering the eye drops and wait 10 minutes before re-inserting them.

■ *If you miss a dose...*
Take it as soon as you remember. If it is almost time for your next dose, skip the one you missed and go back to your regular schedule. Never take 2 doses at the same time.
■ *Storage instructions...*
Store at room temperature. Keep the bottle tightly closed.

What side effects may occur?

Side effects cannot be anticipated. If any develop or change in intensity, inform your doctor as soon as possible. Only your doctor can determine if it is safe for you to continue taking Alamast.

■ *Side effects may include:*
Allergy, back pain, bronchitis, burning eyes, cough, dry eyes, eye discomfort, fever, flu-like symptoms, headache, menstrual pain, nasal congestion, sinus inflammation, sneezing, stuffy or runny nose

Why should this drug not be prescribed?

Do not take Alamast if you have ever had an allergic reaction to it.

Special warnings about this medication

Do not use Alamast if your eye irritation is caused by your contact lenses. Do not wear a lens if the eye is red.

Possible food and drug interactions when taking this medication

No interactions have been reported.

Special information if you are pregnant or breastfeeding

The possibility of harm to the developing baby has not been completely ruled out. Before using Alamast, let your doctor know if you are pregnant or are planning to become pregnant.

It is not known whether Alamast appears in breast milk. If you plan to breastfeed, discuss your medication options with your doctor.

Recommended dosage

ADULTS AND CHILDREN OVER 3

The recommended dosage is 1 or 2 drops in each affected eye 4 times a day. Alamast has not been evaluated in children under the age of 3.

Overdosage
There has been no experience with Alamast overdose. However, any medication taken in excess can have serious consequences. If you suspect an overdose, seek medical attention immediately.

Albuterol See Proventil, page 1185.

Alclometasone See Aclovate, page 22.

ALDACTAZIDE
Pronounced: al-DAK-tah-zide
Generic ingredients: Spironolactone, Hydrochlorothiazide

Why is this drug prescribed?
Aldactazide is used in the treatment of high blood pressure and other conditions that require the elimination of excess fluid from the body. These conditions include congestive heart failure, cirrhosis of the liver, and kidney disease. Aldactazide combines two diuretic drugs that help your body produce and eliminate more urine. Spironolactone, one of the ingredients, helps to minimize the potassium loss that can be caused by the hydrochlorothiazide component.

Most important fact about this drug
If you have high blood pressure, you must take Aldactazide regularly for it to be effective. Since blood pressure declines gradually, it may be several weeks before you get the full benefit of Aldactazide; and you must continue taking it even if you are feeling well. Aldactazide does not cure high blood pressure; it merely keeps it under control.

How should you take this medication?
Take Aldactazide exactly as prescribed. Stopping Aldactazide suddenly could cause your condition to worsen.

■ *If you miss a dose...*
Take it as soon as you remember. If it is almost time for your next dose, skip the one you missed and go back to your regular schedule. Never take 2 doses at the same time.

■ *Storage instructions...*
Store at room temperature.

What side effects may occur?
Side effects cannot be anticipated. If any develop or change in intensity, inform your doctor as soon as possible. Only your doctor can determine if it is safe for you to continue taking Aldactazide.

■ *Side effects may include:*
Abdominal cramps, breast development in males, change in potassium levels (leading to such symptoms as dry mouth, excessive thirst, weak or irregular heartbeat, and muscle pain or cramps), deepening of the voice, diarrhea, dizziness, dizziness on rising, drowsiness, excessive hairiness, fever, headache, hives, inflammation of blood vessels or lymph vessels, inflammation of the pancreas, irregular menstruation, kidney problems, lack of coordination, liver problems, loss of appetite, mental confusion, muscle spasms, nausea, postmenopausal-bleeding, rash, red or purple spots on skin, restlessness, sensitivity to light, severe allergic reaction, sexual dysfunction, sluggishness, stomach bleeding, stomach inflammation, stomach ulcers, tingling or pins and needles, vertigo, vomiting, weakness, yellow eyes and skin, yellow vision

Why should this drug not be prescribed?

Aldactazide should not be used if you have acute kidney disease or liver failure, have difficulty urinating or are unable to urinate, or have high potassium levels in your blood.

If you are sensitive to or have ever had an allergic reaction to spironolactone, hydrochlorothiazide, or similar drugs, or if you are sensitive to sulfa drugs, you should not take this medication. Make sure your doctor is aware of any drug reactions you may have experienced.

Special warnings about this medication

This medication should be used only if your doctor has determined that the precise amount of each ingredient in Aldactazide meets your specific needs.

Drugs such as the hydrochlorothiazide component of Aldactazide have been known to trigger gout and allergic reactions. They can also raise your blood sugar levels.

Potassium supplements (including salt substitutes) or diuretics that leave high levels of potassium in your body should not be used while taking Aldactazide, unless specifically recommended by your doctor. Symptoms of excess potassium include tingling sensations, fatigue, muscle weakness or paralysis, and a slow heartbeat. If you develop these problems, call your doctor immediately.

If you are taking an ACE inhibitor type of blood pressure medication such as Vasotec, this drug should be used with extreme caution.

If you have liver or kidney disease or lupus erythematosus (a disease that causes skin eruptions), Aldactazide should be used with caution.

Excessive sweating, severe diarrhea, or vomiting could cause you to lose too much water and cause your blood pressure to become too low. Signs of dehydration include thirst, dry mouth, weakness, drowsiness, muscle fatigue, muscle cramps, restlessness, reduced urination, and a rapid heartbeat. Be sure to drink plenty of fluids whenever dehydration threatens, and be careful when exercising in hot weather.

Notify your doctor or dentist that you are taking Aldactazide if you have a medical emergency, and before you have surgery or dental treatment.

Possible food and drug interactions when taking this medication

If Aldactazide is taken with certain other drugs, the effects of either could be increased, decreased, or altered. It is especially important to check with your doctor before combining Aldactazide with the following:

ACE inhibitor blood pressure drugs such as Vasotec
Alcohol
Antigout medications such as Zyloprim
Barbiturates such as phenobarbital and Seconal
Digoxin (Lanoxin)
Diuretics such as Lasix and Midamor
Insulin or oral antidiabetic drugs such as Micronase
Lithium (Lithonate)
Narcotic drugs such as those containing codeine
Nonsteroidal anti-inflammatory drugs (NSAIDs) such as Advil, Aleve, and Motrin
Norepinephrine (Levophed)
Potassium supplements such as Slow-K
Steroids such as prednisone

Special information if you are pregnant or breastfeeding

The effects of Aldactazide during pregnancy have not been adequately studied. If you are pregnant or plan to become pregnant, inform your doctor immediately. Aldactazide appears in breast milk and could affect a nursing infant. If this medication is essential to your health, your doctor may advise you to discontinue breastfeeding until your treatment is finished.

Recommended dosage

ADULTS

Congestive Heart Failure, Cirrhosis, Nephrotic Syndrome (Kidney Disorder)
The usual dosage is 100 milligrams each of spironolactone and hydrochlorothiazide daily, taken as a single dose or in divided doses. Dosage may range from 25 to 200 milligrams of each ingredient daily, depending on your individual needs.

High Blood Pressure
The usual dose is 50 to 100 milligrams each of spironolactone and hydrochlorothiazide daily, in a single dose or divided into smaller doses.

CHILDREN

The usual dose of Aldactazide should provide 0.75 to 1.5 milligrams of spironolactone per pound of body weight.

Overdosage

Any medication taken in excess can have serious consequences. If you suspect an overdose, seek medical attention immediately.

■ *Symptoms of Aldactazide overdose may include:*
Confusion, diarrhea, dizziness, drowsiness, nausea, patchy raised skin rash, vomiting

ALDACTONE

Pronounced: al-DAK-tone
Generic name: Spironolactone

Why is this drug prescribed?

Aldactone flushes excess salt and water from the body and controls high blood pressure. It is used in the diagnosis and treatment of hyperaldosteronism, a condition in which the adrenal gland secretes too much aldosterone (a hormone that regulates the body's salt and potassium levels). It is also used in treating other conditions that require the elimination of excess fluid from the body. These conditions include congestive heart failure, high blood pressure, cirrhosis of the liver, kidney disease, and unusually low potassium levels in the blood. When used for high blood pressure, Aldactone can be taken alone or with other high blood pressure medications.

Most important fact about this drug

If you have high blood pressure, you must take Aldactone regularly for it to be effective. Since blood pressure declines gradually, it may be several weeks before you get the full benefit of Aldactone; and you must continue taking it even if you are feeling well. Aldactone does not cure high blood pressure; it merely keeps it under control.

How should you take this medication?

Take Aldactone exactly as prescribed by your doctor. Stopping Aldactone suddenly could cause your condition to worsen.

■ *If you miss a dose...*
Take it as soon as you remember. If it is almost time for your next dose, skip the one you missed and go back to your regular schedule. Never take 2 doses at the same time.
■ *Storage instructions...*
Store at room temperature.

What side effects may occur?

Side effects cannot be anticipated. If any develop or change in intensity, inform your doctor as soon as possible. Only your doctor can determine if it is safe for you to continue taking Aldactone.

■ *Side effects may include:*

Abdominal cramps, breast development in males, change in potassium levels (leading to such symptoms as dry mouth, excessive thirst, weak or irregular heartbeat, and muscle pain or cramps), deepening of the voice, diarrhea, drowsiness, excessive hairiness, fever, headache, hives, irregular menstruation, kidney problems, lack of coordination, lethargy, liver problems, mental confusion, postmenopausal bleeding, severe allergic reaction, sexual dysfunction, skin eruptions, stomach bleeding, stomach inflammation, ulcers, vomiting

Why should this drug not be prescribed?

You should not take Aldactone if you have kidney disease, an inability to urinate, difficulty urinating, or high potassium levels in your blood.

Special warnings about this medication

Potassium supplements or other diuretics that leave your potassium levels high, such as Maxzide, should not be used while taking Aldactone, unless specifically indicated by your doctor. Symptoms of excess potassium include tingling sensations, fatigue, muscle weakness or paralysis, and a slow heartbeat. If you develop these problems, call your doctor immediately.

ACE inhibitors (Vasotec, Capoten), used for blood pressure and heart failure, should not be taken while using Aldactone.

If you are taking Aldactone, your kidney function should be given a complete assessment and should continue to be monitored.

If you have liver disease, your doctor will be cautious about using this medication.

Excessive sweating, severe diarrhea, or vomiting could cause you to lose too much water and cause your blood pressure to become too low. Signs of dehydration include thirst, dry mouth, weakness, drowsiness, muscle fatigue, muscle cramps, restlessness, reduced urination, and a rapid heartbeat. Be sure to drink plenty of fluids whenever dehydration threatens, and be careful when exercising in hot weather.

Notify your doctor or dentist that you are taking Aldactone if you have a medical emergency, and before you have surgery or dental treatment.

Possible food and drug interactions when taking this medication

If Aldactone is taken with certain other drugs, the effects of either could be increased, decreased, or altered. It is especially important to check with your doctor before combining Aldactone with the following:

ACE inhibitors such as Capoten and Vasotec

Alcohol

Barbiturates such as phenobarbital and Seconal

Digoxin (Lanoxin)

Indomethacin (Indocin)

Lithium (Lithonate)

Narcotic drugs such as those containing codeine

Nonsteroidal anti-inflammatory drugs (NSAIDs) such as Advil, Aleve, and Motrin

Norepinephrine (Levophed)

Other high blood pressure medications such as Aldomet and Procardia XL

Other water pills such as HydroDIURIL and Lasix

Steroids such as prednisone

Special information if you are pregnant or breastfeeding

The effects of Aldactone during pregnancy have not been adequately studied. If you are pregnant or plan to become pregnant, inform your doctor immediately. Aldactone appears in breast milk and could affect a nursing infant. If this medication is essential to your health, your doctor may advise you to discontinue breastfeeding until your treatment with this medication is finished.

Recommended dosage

ADULTS

Primary Hyperaldosteronism

Initial dosages of this medication are used to determine the presence of primary hyperaldosteronism (too much secretion of the adrenal hormone aldosterone). People can be tested with this medication over either a long or a short period of time.

In the long test, you take 400 milligrams per day for 3 to 4 weeks. If your potassium levels and blood pressure are corrected with this dosage in this time period, your physician may assume you have this condition.

In the short test, you receive 400 milligrams per day for 4 days. A laboratory test compares potassium levels while you are on Aldactone and after the medication is stopped. Your doctor may then make a diagnosis.

After the diagnosis of primary hyperaldosteronism is made and confirmed by more tests, the usual dose is 100 to 400 milligrams per day, prior to surgery. In those who are not good candidates for surgery, this drug is given over the long term at the lowest effective dose.

Fluid Retention (Congestive Heart Failure, Cirrhosis of the Liver, or Kidney Disorders)

The usual starting dosage is 100 milligrams daily either in a single dose or divided into smaller doses. However, your doctor may have you take daily doses as low as 25 milligrams or as high as 200 milligrams.

Your doctor may choose to adjust your dosage after an initial 5-day trial period or add another diuretic medication to this one.

Essential Hypertension (High Blood Pressure)

The usual starting dosage is 50 to 100 milligrams daily in a single dose or divided into smaller doses. This medication may be given with another diuretic or with other high blood pressure medications.

It may be up to 2 weeks before the full effect of this medication is seen. Your doctor can then adjust the dosage according to your response.

Hypokalemia (Potassium Loss)

Your doctor may have you take daily dosages of 25 to 100 milligrams when potassium loss caused by the effects of a diuretic cannot be treated by a potassium supplement.

Overdosage

Any medication taken in excess can have serious consequences. If you suspect an overdose, seek medical attention immediately.

■ *Symptoms of Aldactone overdose may include:*
Confusion, diarrhea, dizziness, drowsiness, nausea, patchy raised skin rash, vomiting

ALDOMET

Pronounced: AL-doe-met
Generic name: Methyldopa

Why is this drug prescribed?

Aldomet is used to treat high blood pressure. It is effective when used alone or with other high blood pressure medications.

Most important fact about this drug

You must take Aldomet regularly for it to be effective. Since blood pressure declines gradually, it may be several weeks before you get the full benefit of Aldomet; and you must continue taking it even if you are feeling well. Aldomet does not cure high blood pressure; it merely keeps it under control.

How should you take this medication?

Take this medication exactly as prescribed. Try not to miss any doses. Do not stop taking the drug without your doctor's knowledge.

Drowsiness may occur when the dosage is increased. If your doctor increases the amount of Aldomet you take, start the new dosage in the evening.

■ *If you miss a dose...*
Take it as soon as you remember. If it is almost time for your next dose, skip the one you missed and go back to your regular schedule. Never take 2 doses at the same time.

■ *Storage instructions...*
Keep Aldomet in the container it came in, tightly closed. Store Aldomet tablets at room temperature. Protect from light.

What side effects may occur?
Side effects cannot be anticipated. If any develop or change in intensity, inform your doctor as soon as possible. Only your doctor can determine if it is safe for you to continue taking Aldomet.

■ *Side effects may include:*
Drowsiness during the first few weeks of therapy, fluid retention or weight gain, headache, weakness

Why should this drug not be prescribed?
If you have liver disease or cirrhosis, or if you have taken Aldomet before and developed liver disease, do not take this medication.

If you are sensitive to or have ever had an allergic reaction to Aldomet, or if you have been prescribed the oral suspension form of Aldomet and have ever had an allergic reaction to sulfites, you should not take this medication.

If you are taking drugs known as monoamine oxidase (MAO) inhibitors, you should not take Aldomet.

Special warnings about this medication
Before you begin taking Aldomet, your doctor should perform a complete study of your liver function, and it should be monitored periodically thereafter.

Aldomet can cause liver disorders. You may develop a fever, jaundice (yellow eyes and skin), or both, usually within the first 2 to 3 months of therapy. If either of these symptoms occurs, stop taking Aldomet and contact your doctor immediately. If the fever and/or jaundice were caused by the medication, your liver function should gradually return to normal.

If you have a history of liver disease, this medication should be used with caution.

Hemolytic anemia, a blood disorder in which red blood cells are destroyed, can develop with long-term use of Aldomet; your doctor will do periodic blood counts to check for this problem.

Aldomet can cause water retention or weight gain in some people. A diuretic will usually relieve these symptoms.

If you are on dialysis and are taking Aldomet for high blood pressure, your blood pressure may rise after your dialysis treatments.

Aldomet can cause you to become drowsy or less alert, especially during the first few weeks of therapy or when dosage levels are increased. If it affects you this way, driving or operating heavy machinery or participating in any hazardous activity that requires full mental alertness is not recommended.

Notify your doctor or dentist that you are taking Aldomet if you have a medical emergency and before you have surgery or dental treatment.

Possible food and drug interactions when taking this medication

If Aldomet is taken with certain other drugs, the effects of either could be increased, decreased, or altered. It is especially important to check with your doctor before combining Aldomet with the following:

Antidepressants known as MAO inhibitors, including Nardil and Parnate
Dextroamphetamine (Dexedrine)
Imipramine (Tofranil)
Iron-containing products such as ferrous sulfate (Feosol) and ferrous gluconate (Fergon)
Lithium (Lithonate)
Other blood pressure medications such as Catapres and Calan
Phenylpropanolamine (a decongestant used in common cold remedies such as Dimetapp, Entex LA, and others)
Propranolol (Inderal)
Tolbutamide (Orinase)

Special information if you are pregnant or breastfeeding

The use of Aldomet during pregnancy appears to be relatively safe. However, if you are pregnant or plan to become pregnant, inform your doctor immediately. Aldomet appears in breast milk and could affect a nursing infant. If this medication is essential to your health, your doctor may advise you to discontinue breastfeeding until your treatment is finished.

Recommended dosage

ADULTS

The usual starting dose is 250 milligrams, 2 or 3 times per day, in the first 48 hours of treatment. Your doctor may increase or decrease your dose over the next few days to achieve the correct blood pressure.

To reduce the effect of any sedation the medication may cause, dosage increases will usually be given in the evening.

The usual maintenance dosage is 500 milligrams to 2 grams per day, divided into 2 to 4 doses. The maximum dose is usually 3 grams.

Your doctor will also adjust your dosage of Aldomet when it is taken in combination with certain other high blood pressure drugs.

If you take Aldomet with a non-thiazide high blood pressure medicine, your doctor will limit the initial dosage to 500 milligrams daily divided into small doses.

Dosages will be adjusted, and other high blood pressure drugs may be added, during the first few months of treatment with Aldomet. Those with reduced kidney function may require smaller doses. Older people who are prone to fainting spells due to arterial disease may also require smaller doses.

CHILDREN

The usual starting dose is 10 milligrams per 2.2 pounds of body weight daily, divided into 2 to 4 doses. Doses will be adjusted until blood pressure is normal. The maximum daily dose is usually 65 milligrams per 2.2 pounds of body weight or 3 grams, whichever is less.

OLDER ADULTS

Dosages of this drug are adjusted to each individual's needs. Lower doses may be prescribed by your doctor.

Overdosage

Any medication taken in excess can have serious consequences. If you suspect an overdose, seek medical attention immediately.

■ *Symptoms of Aldomet overdose may include:*
Bloating, constipation, diarrhea, dizziness, extreme drowsiness, gas, light-headedness, nausea, severely low blood pressure, slow heartbeat, vomiting, weakness

Alendronate *See Fosamax, page 607.*

Alesse *See Oral Contraceptives, page 1000.*

Aleve *See Anaprox, page 105.*

Alfuzosin *See Uroxatral, page 1536.*

ALINIA
Pronounced: ah-LIN-ee-ah
Generic name: Nitazoxanide

Why is this drug prescribed?

Alinia is used to treat children with infectious diarrhea caused by the organisms *Cryptosporidium parvum* or *Giardia lamblia.*

It is prescribed for children 1 year old and older.

For infectious diarrhea caused by the organism *Cryptosporidium parvum,* only the oral suspension form of Alinia should be used to treat children 1 to 11 years old.

Infectious diarrhea is marked by abnormal bowel habits, including increased stool frequency, as well as watery stools. It is normally caused by contaminated food or water.

Most important fact about this drug

The safety and effectiveness of Alinia have not been studied in children less than 12 months old. The tablets contain a greater amount of the drug than the oral suspension and should not be used in children under 11 years old. The drug has also not been studied in adults or people with weakened immune systems, including those with HIV or AIDS.

How should you take this medication?

Be sure to give this medication with food. Shake the oral suspension vigorously before you give each dose. The oral suspension will keep for 7 days. After this time any unused solution must be thrown away.

■ *If your child misses a dose...*
  Give the forgotten dose with food as soon as you remember. However, if it is almost time for your child's next dose, skip the missed dose and return to the regular schedule. Do not give 2 doses at once.

■ *Storage instructions...*
  Store the tablets or oral suspension at room temperature. Keep the bottles tightly closed.

What side effects may occur?

Side effects cannot be anticipated. If any develop or change in intensity, tell your doctor as soon as possible. Only your doctor can determine if it is safe for your child to continue using Alinia.

■ *Side effects may include:*
  Abdominal pain, diarrhea, headache, nausea

Why should this drug not be prescribed?

Alinia should not be given to children who have an allergic reaction to the drug. It should also not be taken by children less than 12 months old or greater than 11 years old. In addition, Alinia should not be used by adults or people with kidney or liver problems or with weakened immune systems, including those with HIV or AIDS.

Special warnings about this medication

If your child has diabetes, you should be aware that Alinia contains about 1 teaspoon of sugar per dose.

Possible food and drug interactions when taking this medication

If Alinia is taken with certain other drugs, the effects of either could be increased, decreased, or altered. It is important to check with your doctor before combining Alinia with other drugs your child is taking.

Special information if you are pregnant or breastfeeding

Alinia has not been adequately studied in pregnant or breastfeeding women.

Recommended dosage

CHILDREN

Giardia Lamblia
Ages 1 to 3 years: The recommended dosage of oral suspension is 1 teaspoon every 12 hours for 3 days.

Ages 4 to 11 years: The recommended dosage of oral suspension is 2 teaspoons every 12 hours for 3 days.

Ages 12 years and older: The recommended dosage is 5 teaspoons of oral suspension or one 500-milligram tablet every 12 hours for 3 days.

Cryptosporidium Parvum
Ages 1 to 3 years: The recommended dosage of oral suspension is 1 teaspoon every 12 hours for 3 days.

Ages 4 to 11 years: The recommended dosage of oral suspension is 2 teaspoons every 12 hours for 3 days.

This drug's safety and effectiveness have not been studied for treating diarrhea caused by *Cryptosporidium parvum* in children 12 years and older or in adults.

Overdosage

Any medication taken in excess can have serious consequences. If you suspect an overdose, seek medical help immediately.

ALLEGRA

Pronounced: ah-LEG-rah
Generic name: Fexofenadine hydrochloride
Other brand name: Allegra-D

Why is this drug prescribed?

Allegra relieves the itchy, runny nose, sneezing, and itchy, red, watery eyes that come with hay fever. It is also used to relieve the itching and welts of hives. Allegra is a type of antihistamine that rarely causes drowsiness.

In addition to the antihistamine in Allegra, Allegra-D also contains the nasal decongestant pseudoephedrine.

Most important fact about this drug
Seldane, an antihistamine related to Allegra, has been implicated in dangerous interactions with the common antibiotic erythromycin, the antifungal medication ketoconazole (Nizoral), and several similar drugs. Allegra poses no such risks. It is also safe for people with liver disease.

How should you take this medication?
Take Allegra-D on an empty stomach with water. You can take regular Allegra with or without food.

■ *If you miss a dose...*
Take it as soon as you remember. If it is almost time for your next dose, skip the one you missed and go back to your regular schedule. Do not take 2 doses at once.

■ *Storage instructions...*
Store at room temperature. Protect blister packs from moisture.

What side effects may occur?
Side effects cannot be anticipated. If any develop or change in intensity, tell your doctor as soon as possible. Only your doctor can determine if it is safe for you to continue taking Allegra.

■ *Side effects of Allegra may include:*
Colds or flu, coughing, drowsiness, fatigue, fever, headache, indigestion, menstrual problems, nausea, pain including back or ear pain
■ *Side effects of Allegra-D may include:*
Abdominal pain, agitation, anxiety, back pain, dizziness, dry mouth, headache, heart palpitations, indigestion, insomnia, nausea, nervousness, respiratory tract infection, throat irritation

Why should this drug not be prescribed?
If Allegra or Allegra-D gives you an allergic reaction, avoid it in the future. Do not give either product to children under 6 years of age.

Do not take Allegra-D if you have glaucoma, urination problems, or severe high blood pressure or heart disease. Also avoid taking Allegra-D within 2 weeks of using an MAO inhibitor drug such as Marplan, Nardil, or Parnate.

Special warnings about this medication
Use Allegra-D with caution if you have high blood pressure, diabetes, heart disease, increased pressure in the eyes, prostate problems, or

hyperthyroidism. Stop using it and check with your doctor if it causes nervousness, dizziness, or sleeplessness.

Possible food and drug interactions when taking this medication
Check with your doctor before combining Allegra with erythromycin (E.E.S., Ery-Tab, PCE) or ketoconazole (Nizoral). These drugs may increase Allegra's effects.

Allow a little time between a dose of Allegra and antacids such as Maalox that contain aluminum and magnesium. This type of antacid can decrease Allegra's effects.

Allegra-D should never be taken within 2 weeks of using an MAO inhibitor drug such as the antidepressants Marplan, Nardil, and Parnate. Also check with your doctor before combining it with the following:

Mecamylamine (Inversine)
Methyldopa (Aldomet)
Reserpine (Diupress, Hydropres)

You should also avoid Allegra-D if you have a pacemaker and take digoxin (Lanoxin). And you should not combine it with over-the-counter antihistamines and decongestants.

Special information if you are pregnant or breastfeeding
The effects of this drug during pregnancy have not been adequately studied. If you are pregnant or plan to become pregnant, inform your doctor immediately. It is not known whether Allegra appears in breast milk. If the drug is essential to your health, your doctor may advise you to stop nursing until your treatment is finished.

Recommended dosage

ALLEGRA

Adults and Children 12 Years and Older
For hay fever, the usual dosage is 60 milligrams twice a day or 180 milligrams once a day. For hives, it's 60 milligrams twice a day. If you have kidney problems, your doctor may have you take only one 60-milligram dose daily.

Children 6 Through 11 Years Old
For hay fever or hives, the usual dosage is 30 milligrams twice a day. Children with kidney problems may be prescribed only one 30-milligram dose each day.

ALLEGRA-D

Adults and Children 12 Years and Older
12-Hour Tablets: Take 1 tablet twice a day. People with kidney problems should take only 1 tablet daily.

24-Hour Tablets: Take 1 tablet once a day. Allegra-D 24-hour tablets should generally not be taken by people with kidney problems.

Allegra-D is not recommended for children less than 12 years old.

Overdosage
An excessive dose of any medicine can have serious consequences. Seek medical attention whenever an overdose is suspected.

■ *Symptoms of Allegra overdose may include:*
Dizziness, drowsiness, dry mouth

Allopurinol See Zyloprim, page 1665.

Almotriptan See Axert, page 171.

Alora See Estrogen Patches, page 538.

ALPHAGAN P
Pronounced: AL-fuh-gan
Generic name: Brimonidine tartrate

Why is this drug prescribed?
Alphagan P lowers high pressure in the eye, a problem typically caused by the condition known as open-angle glaucoma. Alphagan P works in two ways: it reduces production of the liquid that fills the eyeball, and it promotes drainage of this liquid. This drug is free of the preservative benzalkonium chloride.

Most important fact about this drug
Alphagan P may have a slight effect on blood pressure. If you have severe heart disease, make sure the doctor is aware of it. Caution is warranted.

How should you take this medication?
Alphagan P is administered with an eyedropper. If you are using other eyedrops or ointments, allow at least 5 minutes between doses of each product.

■ *If you miss a dose...*
Take the forgotten dose as soon as you remember. However, if it is almost time for your next dose, skip the one you missed and return to your regular schedule. Do not take 2 doses at once.

■ *Storage instructions...*
Store at room temperature.

What side effects may occur?
Side effects cannot be anticipated. If any develop or change in intensity, tell your doctor as soon as possible. Only your doctor can determine if it is safe to continue using Alphagan P.

■ *Side effects may include:*
Abnormal vision, allergic reaction, blurred vision, burning and stinging, dizziness, drowsiness, dry eyes, dry mouth, eye pain or irritation, fatigue, feeling of foreign body in the eye, headache, inflamed or swollen eyelids, itchy eyes, loss of tissue or staining of the cornea, muscle pain, red or swollen eyes, sensitivity to light, stomach problems, tearing, upper respiratory symptoms, watery eyes, weakness

Why should this drug not be prescribed?
You'll need to avoid Alphagan P if it gives you an allergic reaction, or if you're taking a medication classified as an MAO inhibitor, such as the antidepressants Nardil and Parnate.

Special warnings about this medication
Use Alphagan P with caution if you have circulation problems, low blood pressure, or depression. Caution is also warranted if you have liver or kidney problems, since the effects of Alphagan P under these conditions have not been studied.

The effect of Alphagan P may diminish over time. The doctor should check your eye pressure periodically.

Alphagan P makes some people drowsy. Do not engage in hazardous activities such as driving until you know how this drug affects you.

Alphagan P has not been studied in children under 2 years of age.

Possible food and drug interactions when using this medication
If Alphagan P is taken with certain other drugs, the effects of either could be increased, decreased, or altered. It is especially important to check with your doctor before combining Alphagan P with the following:

Alcohol
Barbiturates such as phenobarbital and Seconal
Drugs classified as beta-blockers, such as the high blood pressure
    medications Inderal, Sectral, and Tenormin
Heart drugs such as Isordil, Lanoxin, and Nitro-Dur
Narcotic painkillers such as Darvon, Percodan, and Vicodin
Other high blood pressure drugs
Other sleep medications such as Ambien and Sonata
Tricyclic antidepressant drugs such as Sinequan, Surmontil, and
    Vivactil

Special information if you are pregnant or breastfeeding

Although there is no evidence that Alphagan P can cause harm, the effects of the drug during pregnancy have not been adequately studied. If you are pregnant or plan to become pregnant, inform your doctor immediately.

It is not known whether Alphagan P appears in breast milk. If you are nursing, its use is not recommended.

Recommended dosage

The usual dose is 1 drop in the affected eye(s) 3 times daily, approximately 8 hours apart.

Overdosage

No information is available on Alphagan P overdose. However, any medication taken in excess can have serious consequences. If you suspect an overdose, seek medical attention immediately.

Alprazolam See Xanax, page 1594.

Alprostadil See Caverject, page 257.

ALTACE

Pronounced: AL-tayce
Generic name: Ramipril

Why is this drug prescribed?

Altace is used in the treatment of high blood pressure. It is effective when used alone or in combination with other high blood pressure medications, especially thiazide-type water pills (diuretics). Altace works by preventing the conversion of a chemical in your blood called angiotensin I into a more potent substance that increases salt and water retention in your body. It also enhances blood flow in your circulatory system. It is a member of the group of drugs called ACE inhibitors.

Altace is also prescribed to reduce the chances of heart attack, stroke, and heart-related death in people 55 years or older who are in danger of such an event. Typical candidates include those who suffer from coronary artery disease, poor circulation, stroke, or diabetes and have at least one other risk factor, such as high blood pressure, high cholesterol levels, low HDL ("good") cholesterol, or cigarette smoking.

If you do suffer a heart attack and develop heart failure, Altace can be prescribed to prevent the condition from getting worse.

Most important fact about this drug

If you are taking Altace for high blood pressure, you must take the drug regularly for it to be effective. Since blood pressure declines gradually, it may be several weeks before you get the full benefit of Altace; and you must continue taking it even if you are feeling well. Altace does not cure high blood pressure; it merely keeps it under control.

How should you take this medication?

Take this medication exactly as prescribed by your doctor. If you have difficulty swallowing the capsule, you can sprinkle the contents on a small amount (about 4 ounces) of applesauce, or mix the contents with 4 ounces of water or apple juice. Be sure to eat or drink the entire mixture so that you get the full dose of the drug. You can prepare the mixture ahead of time; it will keep for 24 hours at room temperature or 48 hours in the refrigerator.

■ *If you miss a dose...*
If you forget to take a dose, take it as soon as you remember. If it is almost time for your next dose, skip the one you missed and go back to your regular schedule. Never take 2 doses at the same time.
■ *Storage instructions...*
Store Altace at room temperature in a tightly closed container.

What side effects may occur?

Side effects cannot be anticipated. If any develop or change in intensity, inform your doctor as soon as possible. Only your doctor can determine if it is safe for you to continue taking Altace.

■ *Side effects may include:*
Chest pain, cough (in people with high blood pressure), dizziness, low blood pressure (in people with congestive heart failure)
People prescribed the drug after a heart attack may also experience light-headedness when standing; more severe heart failure is also a possibility.

Why should this drug not be prescribed?

If you are sensitive to or have ever had an allergic reaction to Altace, or if you have a history of swelling of the face, tongue, or throat while taking similar drugs such as Capoten, Vasotec, and Zestril, you should not take this medication. Make sure that your doctor is aware of any drug reactions that you have experienced.

Special warnings about this medication

If you develop swelling of the face around your lips, tongue, or throat or difficulty swallowing, difficulty breathing, swelling of arms and legs, or infection, sore throat, and fever, you should contact your doctor immediately. You may have a serious side effect of the drug and need emergency treatment.

If you develop abdominal pain with or without nausea and vomiting, contact your doctor. ACE inhibitors such as Altace have been known to cause intestinal swelling.

If you are taking Altace, your kidney function should be given a complete assessment and should continue to be monitored.

If you notice your skin or the whites of your eyes turning yellow, notify your doctor. Your liver may be affected, and you may have to stop taking Altace. Your doctor should routinely test your liver function while you are on this drug.

Altace should be used with caution if you have impaired kidney function, since rare cases of kidney failure have been reported. Also use caution if you have impaired liver function, or if you have a connective tissue disease such as lupus erythematosis or scleroderma.

If you are taking diuretics and Altace, or have congestive heart failure, you may develop excessively low blood pressure.

Do not use salt substitutes containing potassium or potassium supplements without consulting your doctor. Altace can cause increased potassium levels in your blood, especially if you have diabetes and kidney problems.

Light-headedness can occur when taking Altace, especially during the first days of therapy, and should be reported to your doctor. If fainting occurs, stop taking the medication and notify your doctor immediately.

Dehydration, excessive sweating, severe diarrhea, or vomiting could deplete your body's fluids, causing your blood pressure to drop dangerously.

Altace may reduce the number of infection-fighting white blood cells in your bloodstream, especially if you have a kidney problem or a connective tissue disorder such as lupus. Contact your doctor immediately if you develop a sore throat or fever, which could be a sign of this condition.

ACE inhibitors such as Altace have been known to cause severe allergic reactions in people undergoing desensitization therapy with bee or wasp venom. These drugs have also caused severe reactions in kidney dialysis patients.

Possible food and drug interactions when taking this medication

If Altace is taken with certain other drugs, the effects of either could be increased, decreased, or altered. It is especially important to check with your doctor before combining Altace with the following:

Alcohol
Diuretics such as hydrochlorothiazide (found in many blood
    pressure medicines)
Diuretics that don't wash out potassium, such as spironolactone
    (Aldactone) and the diuretic component in Dyazide, Maxzide,
    Moduretic, and others
Lithium (Eskalith, Lithobid)

Nonsteroidal anti-inflammatory drugs such as Motrin, Naprosyn, and
   Orudis
Oral diabetes drugs such as DiaBeta, Glucotrol, Micronase, and
   Orinase
Potassium-containing salt substitutes
Potassium supplements such as K-lyte and K-Tab

Special information if you are pregnant or breastfeeding

When used during the second and third trimesters, Altace can lead to
birth defects, prematurity, and death in developing and newborn babies.
If you are pregnant or plan to become pregnant and are taking Altace, it
should be discontinued as soon as possible. Contact your doctor immediately. Altace may appear in breast milk and could affect a nursing infant.
If this medication is essential to your health, your doctor may advise you
to avoid breastfeeding.

Recommended dosage

ADULTS

As a precaution, your doctor may have you take the first dose of Altace in
his office. To reduce the risk of a severe drop in blood pressure, the
dosage of any diuretic you're taking should be reduced or, if possible,
eliminated.

High Blood Pressure

For patients not on diuretics, the usual starting dose is 2.5 milligrams,
taken once daily. After blood pressure is under control, the dosage will
range from 2.5 to 20 milligrams a day in a single dose or divided into
2 equal doses. If Altace proves insufficient, the doctor may then add a
diuretic.

Heart Attack and Stroke Prevention

Patients usually receive 2.5 milligrams once a day for the first week. The
dose is then increased to 5 milligrams once a day for the next 3 weeks,
and to as much as 10 milligrams daily for the long term. The doctor may
recommend dividing each dose into 2 smaller ones if you have high blood
pressure or are recovering from a recent heart attack.

Heart Failure After a Heart Attack

The usual starting dose is 2.5 milligrams taken twice a day. If your blood
pressure drops severely, your doctor will reduce the dose to 1.25 milligrams, then slowly increase it back to the starting dose, aiming for a
maintenance dose of 5 milligrams twice a day.

If you have kidney problems, your doctor may prescribe a lower than
normal dose.

CHILDREN

The safety and effectiveness of Altace in children have not been established.

Overdosage

Any medication taken in excess can have serious consequences. If you suspect an overdose, seek medical attention immediately.

Symptoms of low blood pressure are likely to be the primary warning of an Altace overdose.

ALTOCOR

Pronounced: AL-tow-core
Generic name: Lovastatin

Why is this drug prescribed?

Altocor is an extended-release form of the cholesterol-lowering drug lovastatin. By releasing small amounts of the drug throughout the day, Altocor maintains a relatively steady level of lovastatin in the bloodstream.

In many people, high cholesterol levels contribute to the development of clogged arteries and heart disease. Altocor is prescribed to slow the clogging process in people who already have heart disease, and to fend off clogged arteries in people at risk of developing the disease.

Like other drugs in its class, Altocor reduces the level of "bad" LDL cholesterol and raises the level of "good" HDL cholesterol. For people at high risk of heart disease, current guidelines suggest drug therapy when the LDL level reaches 130. For people at lower risk, the cutoff is 160. For those at little or no risk, it's 190.

Most important fact about this drug

Altocor is usually prescribed only if diet, exercise, and weight loss fail to bring your cholesterol level under control. It is important to remember that Altocor is a supplement to—not a substitute for—those other measures. To get the full benefit of the medication, you need to stick to the diet and exercise program prescribed by your doctor.

How should you take this medication?

Altocor is taken once a day at bedtime. Swallow Altocor whole. Do not break, chew, crush, or cut the tablets.

■ *If you miss a dose...*
   Take it as soon as you remember. If it is almost time for your next dose, skip the dose you missed and go back to your regular schedule. Never take 2 doses at once.

■ *Storage instructions...*
   Store at room temperature. Protect from heat and humidity.

What side effects may occur?

The side effects of Altocor generally are mild and temporary. Nevertheless, if any develop or change in intensity, tell your doctor as soon as possible. Only your doctor can determine whether it is safe for you to continue taking Altocor.

■ *Side effects may include:*
 Back pain, diarrhea, flu-like symptoms, headache, infection, injury, joint pain, muscle pain, sinus inflammation, unspecified pain, weakness

Why should this drug not be prescribed?

Cholesterol is essential for developing babies, so Altocor must never be taken during pregnancy or when nursing an infant. You'll also need to avoid Altocor if you have active liver disease or the drug gives you an allergic reaction.

Special warnings about this medication

In rare cases, drugs such as Altocor cause rhabdomyolysis, a potentially fatal condition that destroys muscle cells and sometimes causes kidney failure. Alert your doctor immediately if you experience any unexplained muscle tenderness, weakness, or pain, especially if you also have a fever or feel sick. You'll probably need to give up Altocor therapy.

Because Altocor may affect the liver, your doctor may order blood tests to check your liver function. Blood tests will probably be done before you start taking this medication, at 6 weeks and 12 weeks after you start taking the drug, when your dosage is increased, and periodically after that (semi-annually). If the tests detect a significant problem, Altocor therapy will have to be stopped. You'll be monitored especially closely if you have a history of liver disease or drink substantial quantities of alcohol.

If you have surgery or a major illness, you'll be told to stop taking Altocor until you get better.

Altocor is not recommended for individuals below age 20.

Possible food and drug interactions when taking this medication

If you take Altocor with certain other drugs, the effects of either could be increased, decreased, or altered. It is especially important to check with your doctor before combining Altocor with any of the following:

Antipyrine
Blood-thinning drugs such as Coumadin and Dicumarol
Cimetidine (Tagamet)
Clarithromycin (Biaxin)
Cyclosporine (Neoral, Sandimmune)
Erythromycin (E.E.S., PCE, and others)
Gemfibrozil (Lopid)
HIV protease inhibitors such as Agenerase, Norvir, and Viracept

Itraconazole (Sporanox)
Ketoconazole (Nizoral)
Spironolactone (Aldactone)
Nefazodone (Serzone)
Nicotinic acid or niacin (Niacor, Niaspan)
Verapamil (Calan, Verelan)

Do not take Altocor with large amounts of grapefruit juice.

Special information if you are pregnant or breastfeeding

Because of potential harm to the developing baby, Altocor should never be taken during pregnancy or by anyone who may become pregnant. If you become pregnant while taking Altocor, stop taking this medication immediately and notify your doctor.

Because of the potential for harm to the nursing infant, do not breast-feed while taking Altocor.

Recommended dosage

You will have to follow a standard cholesterol-lowering diet before starting treatment with Altocor, and continue this diet while using Altocor. Your dose may be adjusted to meet your individual needs.

ADULTS

The usual starting dose is 20 to 60 milligrams, taken once a day at bedtime. Dosage adjustments may be made every 4 weeks, and dose levels may be reduced as cholesterol levels come down.

The usual starting dose is 10 milligrams for people who are taking cyclosporine and Altocor. The dosage should not be increased to more than 20 milligrams a day.

The usual starting dose is 20 milligrams or less for people with kidney disease or people who are taking gemfibrozil, niacin, or other cholesterol-lowering drugs.

Overdosage

Although there is no specific information available about Altocor overdose, any medication taken in excess can have serious consequences. If you suspect an overdose of Altocor, seek medical attention immediately.

ALUPENT

Pronounced: AL-yew-pent
Generic name: Metaproterenol sulfate

Why is this drug prescribed?

Alupent is a bronchodilator prescribed for the prevention and relief of bronchial asthma and bronchial spasms (wheezing) associated with bronchitis and emphysema. Alupent Inhalation Solution is also used to treat acute asthmatic attacks in children 6 years of age and older.

Most important fact about this drug

Alupent's effects last up to 6 hours. It should not be used more frequently than your doctor recommends.

Increasing the number of doses can be dangerous and may actually make symptoms of asthma worse. Fatalities have occurred with excessive use of this medication.

If the dose your doctor recommends does not provide relief of your symptoms, if your symptoms become worse, or if side effects occur, seek medical attention immediately.

How should you take this medication?

Take this medication exactly as prescribed by your doctor.

■ *If you miss a dose...*
Take the dose as soon as you remember. Take any remaining doses for the day at equal intervals thereafter. Do not increase the total for the day or take 2 doses at the same time.

■ *Storage instructions...*
Store at room temperature. Protect from light and excessive humidity. Keep out of reach of children.

What side effects may occur?

Side effects cannot be anticipated. If any develop or change in intensity, inform your doctor as soon as possible. Only your doctor can determine if it is safe for you to continue taking Alupent.

■ *Side effects may include:*
Bad taste in the mouth, cough, dizziness, headache, high blood pressure, nausea, nervousness, rapid or throbbing heartbeat, stomach and intestinal upset, throat irritation, tremors, vomiting, worsening or aggravation of asthma

Side effects can occur when a new aerosol container is used, even though you have had no trouble with the medication in the past. Replacing the container may solve the problem.

Why should this drug not be prescribed?

If you are sensitive to or have ever had an allergic reaction to Alupent or similar drugs, such as Proventil, you should not take this medication. Make sure your doctor is aware of any drug reactions you have experienced.

Unless you are directed to do so by your doctor, do not take this medication if you have an irregular, rapid heart rate.

Special warnings about this medication

When taking Alupent, you should not use other inhaled medications (called sympathomimetics) before checking with your doctor. Only your doctor can determine the sufficient amount of time between inhaled medications.

A single dose of nebulized Alupent used to treat an acute attack of asthma may temporarily relieve symptoms but not completely stop the attack.

Consult your doctor before using this medication if you have a heart condition, a convulsive disorder such as epilepsy, high blood pressure, hyperthyroidism, or diabetes mellitus. Alupent can cause significant changes in blood pressure.

Possible food and drug interactions when taking this medication

If Alupent is taken with certain other drugs, the effects of either could be increased, decreased, or altered. It is especially important to check with your doctor before combining Alupent with the following:

MAO inhibitors (antidepressant drugs such as Nardil and Parnate)
Bronchodilators such as Ventolin and Proventil inhalers
Tricyclic antidepressants such as Elavil and Tofranil

Special information if you are pregnant or breastfeeding

The effects of Alupent during pregnancy have not been adequately studied. If you are pregnant or plan to become pregnant, inform your doctor immediately. It is not known whether Alupent appears in breast milk. If this medication is essential to your health, your doctor may advise you to stop nursing your baby until your treatment is finished.

Recommended dosage

ADULTS

Inhalation Aerosol

The usual single dose is 2 to 3 inhalations. Inhalation should usually not be repeated more often than about every 3 to 4 hours. Total dosage per day should not exceed 12 inhalations.

Inhalation Solution 5%

Treatment usually need not be repeated more often than every 4 hours to relieve acute attacks of bronchospasm.

As part of a total treatment program for chronic breathing disorders, the inhalation solution may be taken 3 to 4 times per day, as determined by your doctor.

Inhalation solution is given by oral inhalation with the aid of a nebulizer or an intermittent positive pressure breathing (IPPB) apparatus.

The usual single dose with the nebulizer is 10 inhalations. However, a single dose of 5 to 15 inhalations can be taken, as determined by your doctor. The usual single daily dose with the IPPB is 0.3 milliliter diluted in approximately 2.5 milliliters of saline solution. The dosage range is 0.2 to 0.3 milliliter, as determined by your doctor.

Inhalation Solution 0.4% and 0.6% Unit-Dose Vials
The inhalation solution unit-dose vial is administered by oral inhalation using an intermittent positive pressure breathing (IPPB) apparatus. The usual adult dose is 1 vial per treatment. You usually should not need to repeat the treatment more often than every 4 hours for severe attacks of wheezing. You can use the unit-dose vials 3 to 4 times a day.

CHILDREN

Inhalation Aerosol
Alupent Inhalation Aerosol is not recommended for use in children under 12 years of age.

Inhalation Solution 5%
For children aged 6 to 12 years, the usual single dose is 0.1 milliliter, given by oral inhalation with a nebulizer. Dosage can be increased to 0.2 milliliter 3 to 4 times a day.

The unit-dose vial is not recommended for children under 12 years of age.

Overdosage
Any medication taken in excess can have serious consequences. If you suspect an overdose, seek medical attention immediately.

■ *Symptoms of Alupent overdose may include:*
Dizziness, dry mouth, fatigue, general feeling of bodily discomfort, headache, high or low blood pressure, inability to fall or stay asleep, irregular heartbeat, nausea, nervousness, rapid, fluttery heartbeat, severe, suffocating chest pain, tremors

AMARYL
Pronounced: AM-a-ril
Generic name: Glimepiride

Why is this drug prescribed?
Amaryl is an oral medication used to treat type 2 (non-insulin-dependent) diabetes when diet and exercise alone fail to control abnormally high levels of blood sugar. Like other diabetes drugs classified as sulfonylureas, Amaryl lowers blood sugar by stimulating the pancreas to produce more insulin. Amaryl is often prescribed along with the insulin-boosting drug Glucophage. It may also be used in conjunction with insulin and other diabetes drugs.

Most important fact about this drug

Always remember that Amaryl is an aid to, not a substitute for, good diet and exercise. Failure to follow a sound diet and exercise plan may diminish the results of Amaryl and can lead to serious complications such as dangerously high or low blood sugar levels. Remember, too, that Amaryl is not an oral form of insulin, and cannot be used in place of insulin.

How should you take this medication?

Do not take more or less of this medication than directed by your doctor. Amaryl should be taken with breakfast or the first main meal.

■ *If you miss a dose...*
Take it as soon as you remember. If it is almost time for the next dose, skip the one you missed and go back to your regular schedule. Do not take 2 doses at the same time.

■ *Storage instructions...*
Amaryl should be stored at room temperature in a well-closed container.

What side effects may occur?

Side effects cannot be anticipated. If any develop or change in intensity, tell your doctor as soon as possible. Only your doctor can determine if it is safe for you to continue taking Amaryl.

■ *Side effects may include:*
Anemia and other blood disorders, blurred vision, diarrhea, dizziness, headache, itching, liver problems and jaundice, muscle weakness, nausea, sensitivity to light, skin rash and eruptions, stomach and intestinal pain, vomiting

Amaryl, like all oral antidiabetics, can result in hypoglycemia (low blood sugar). The risk of hypoglycemia can be increased by missed meals, alcohol, fever, injury, infection, surgery, excessive exercise, and the addition of other medications such as Glucophage or insulin. To avoid hypoglycemia, closely follow the dietary and exercise regimen suggested by your doctor.

■ *Symptoms of mild low blood sugar may include:*
Blurred vision, cold sweats, dizziness, fast heartbeat, fatigue, headache, hunger, light-headedness, nausea, nervousness

■ *Symptoms of more severe low blood sugar may include:*
Coma, disorientation, pale skin, seizures, shallow breathing

Ask your doctor what steps you should take if you experience mild hypoglycemia. If symptoms of severe low blood sugar occur, contact your doctor immediately; severe hypoglycemia is a medical emergency.

Why should this drug not be prescribed?

Avoid Amaryl if you have ever had an allergic reaction to it.

Do not take Amaryl to correct diabetic ketoacidosis (a life-threatening medical emergency caused by insufficient insulin and marked by excessive thirst, nausea, fatigue, and fruity breath). This condition should be treated with insulin.

Special warnings about this medication

It's possible that drugs such as Amaryl may lead to more heart problems than diet treatment alone, or treatment with diet and insulin. If you have a heart condition, you may want to discuss this with your doctor.

When taking Amaryl, you should check your blood and urine regularly for abnormally high sugar (glucose) levels. The effectiveness of any oral antidiabetic, including Amaryl, may decrease with time. This may occur because of either a diminished responsiveness to the medication or a worsening of the diabetes.

Even people with well-controlled diabetes may find that stress such as injury, infection, surgery, or fever triggers a loss of control. If this happens, your doctor may recommend that you add insulin to your treatment with Amaryl or that you temporarily stop taking Amaryl and use insulin instead.

Possible food and drug interactions when taking this medication

If Amaryl is taken with certain other drugs, the effects of either could be increased, decreased, or altered. It is especially important to check with your doctor before combining Amaryl with the following:

Airway-opening drugs such as Proventil and Ventolin
Aspirin and other salicylate medications
Chloramphenicol (Chloromycetin)
Corticosteroids such as prednisone (Deltasone)
Diuretics such as hydrochlorothiazide (HydroDIURIL) and
    chlorothiazide (Diuril)
Estrogens such as Premarin
Heart and blood pressure medications called beta-blockers,
    including Tenormin, Inderal, and Lopressor
Isoniazid (Nydrazid)
Major tranquilizers such as Mellaril and Thorazine
MAO inhibitors (antidepressants such as Nardil and Parnate)
Miconazole (Monistat)
Nicotinic acid (Nicobid)
Nonsteroidal anti-inflammatory drugs such as Advil, Motrin,
    Naprosyn, Nuprin, Ponstel, and Voltaren
Oral contraceptives
Phenytoin (Dilantin)
Probenecid (Benemid)
Sulfa drugs such as Bactrim DS and Septra DS
Thyroid medications such as Synthroid
Warfarin (Coumadin)

Use alcohol with care; excessive alcohol intake can cause low blood sugar.

Special information if you are pregnant or breastfeeding

Do not take Amaryl while pregnant. Since studies suggest the importance of maintaining normal blood sugar levels during pregnancy, your doctor may prescribe injected insulin instead. Drugs similar to Amaryl do appear in breast milk and may cause low blood sugar in nursing infants. You should not take Amaryl while nursing. If diet alone does not control your sugar levels, your doctor may prescribe injected insulin.

Recommended dosage

ADULTS

The usual starting dose is 1 to 2 milligrams taken once daily with breakfast or the first main meal. The maximum starting dose is 2 milligrams.

If necessary, your doctor will gradually increase the dose 1 or 2 milligrams at a time every 1 or 2 weeks. Your diabetes will probably be controlled on 1 to 4 milligrams a day; the most you should take in a day is 8 milligrams. If the maximum dose fails to do the job, your doctor may add Glucophage to your regimen.

Weakened or malnourished people and those with adrenal, pituitary, kidney, or liver disorders are particularly sensitive to hypoglycemic drugs such as Amaryl and should start at 1 milligram once daily. Your doctor will increase your medication based on your response to the drug.

CHILDREN

Safety and effectiveness in children have not been established.

Overdosage

An overdose of Amaryl can cause low blood sugar (see *What side effects may occur?* for symptoms).

Eating sugar or a sugar-based product will often correct mild hypoglycemia. For severe hypoglycemia, seek medical attention immediately.

AMBIEN

Pronounced: AM-bee-en
Generic name: Zolpidem tartrate

Why is this drug prescribed?

Ambien is used for short-term treatment of insomnia (difficulty falling asleep or staying asleep, or early awakening). A relatively new drug, it is chemically different from other common sleep medications such as Halcion and Dalmane.

Most important fact about this drug

Sleep problems are usually temporary and require medication for a week or two at most. Insomnia that lasts longer could be a sign of another medical problem. If you find that you need this medicine for more than 7 to 10 days, be sure to check with your doctor.

How should you take this medication?

Ambien works very quickly. Take it just before going to bed. Take only the prescribed dose, exactly as instructed by your doctor.

■ *If you miss a dose...*
Take Ambien only as needed. Never double the dose.
■ *Storage instructions...*
Store at room temperature. Protect from extreme heat.

What side effects may occur?

Side effects cannot be anticipated. If any develop or change in intensity, tell your doctor immediately. Only your doctor can determine whether it is safe to continue taking Ambien.

■ *Side effects may include:*
Allergy, daytime drowsiness, dizziness, drugged feeling, headache, indigestion, nausea

Why should this drug not be prescribed?

There are no known situations in which Ambien cannot be used.

Special warnings about this medication

When sleep medications are used every night for more than a few weeks, some may lose their effectiveness. Remember, too, that you can become dependent on some sleep medications if you use them for a long time or at high doses.

Some people using Ambien—especially those taking serotonin-boosting antidepressants—have experienced unusual changes in their thinking and/or behavior. Alert your doctor if you notice a change.

Ambien and other sleep medicines can cause a special type of memory loss. It should not be taken on an overnight airplane flight of less than 7 to 8 hours, since traveler's amnesia may occur.

When you first start taking Ambien, until you know whether the medication will have any *carryover* effect the next day, use extreme care while doing anything that requires complete alertness, such as driving a car or operating machinery. Older adults, in particular, should be aware that they may be more apt to fall.

Use Ambien cautiously if you have liver problems. It will take longer for its effects to wear off.

If you take Ambien for more than 1 or 2 weeks, consult your doctor before stopping. Sudden discontinuation of a sleep medicine can bring on withdrawal symptoms ranging from unpleasant feelings to vomiting and cramps.

When taking Ambien, do *not* drink alcohol. It can increase the drug's side effects.

If you have breathing problems, they may become worse when you use Ambien.

Possible food and drug interactions when taking this medication

If Ambien is used with certain other drugs, the effects of either drug could be increased, decreased, or altered. It is especially important to check with your doctor before combining Ambien with the following:

Drugs that depress the central nervous system, including Valium, Percocet, and Benadryl
Serotonin-boosting antidepressants such as Paxil, Prozac, and Zoloft
The antidepressant drug imipramine (Tofranil)
The antipsychotic drug chlorpromazine

Special information if you are pregnant or breastfeeding

If you are pregnant or plan to become pregnant, inform your doctor immediately. Babies whose mothers take some sedative/hypnotic drugs may have withdrawal symptoms after birth and may seem limp and flaccid. Ambien is not recommended for use by nursing mothers.

Recommended dosage

ADULTS

The recommended dosage for adults is 10 milligrams right before bedtime. Your doctor will prescribe a smaller dose if you are likely to be sensitive to the drug or have a liver problem. Never take more than 10 milligrams of Ambien per day.

CHILDREN

The safety and effectiveness of Ambien have not been established in children below the age of 18.

OLDER ADULTS

Because older people and those in a weakened condition may be more sensitive to Ambien's effects, the recommended starting dosage is 5 milligrams just before bedtime.

Overdosage

People who take too much Ambien may become excessively sleepy or even go into a light coma. The symptoms of overdose are more severe if the person is also taking other drugs that depress the central nervous system. Some cases of multiple overdose have been fatal.

If you suspect an overdose, seek medical attention immediately.

Amcinonide *See Cyclocort, page 370.*

AMERGE

Pronounced: *ah-MERJ*
Generic name: *Naratriptan hydrochloride*

Why is this drug prescribed?

Amerge is used for relief of classic migraine headaches. It's helpful whether or not the headache is preceded by an aura (visual disturbances, usually sensations of halos or flickering lights). The drug works only during an actual attack. It will not reduce the number of headaches that develop.

Most important fact about this drug

Amerge should be used only for acute, classic migraine attacks. It should not be taken for other types of headache, including cluster headache and certain unusual types of migraine.

How should you take this medication?

Amerge may be taken any time after the headache starts. Swallow the tablet whole, with liquid. If you have no response, a partial response, or return of your headache after the first tablet, consult your doctor. You may take a second tablet, but should wait at least 4 hours after the first dose. Do not take more than 2 doses within 24 hours.

■ *If you miss a dose...*
Amerge is not for regular use. Take it only during an attack.
■ *Storage instructions...*
    Store Amerge tablets at room temperature, away from heat and light. If your medication has expired (the expiration date is printed on the treatment pack), throw it away. If your doctor decides to stop your treatment, do not keep any leftover medicine unless your doctor recommends it.

What side effects may occur?

Side effects cannot be anticipated. If any develop or change in intensity, inform your doctor as soon as possible. Only your doctor can determine if it is safe for you to continue taking Amerge.

■ *Side effects may include:*
Nausea, sensation of pain and pressure, strange sensations

Why should this drug not be prescribed?

You should avoid Amerge if you are prone to any type of impaired circulation, including angina (crushing chest pain), heart attack, stroke, or ischemic bowel disease. Also avoid Amerge if you have severe kidney or liver disease, or suffer from uncontrolled high blood pressure.

Do not use Amerge within 24 hours of another medication in the same drug class, such as Imitrex or Zomig, or an ergotamine-based medication such as Cafergot, D.H.E. 45 Injection, Migranal Nasal Spray, or Sansert.

If Amerge gives you an allergic reaction, stop using it and notify your doctor.

Special warnings about this medication

People with a heart or circulatory condition have been known to suffer a heart attack or stroke after taking Amerge. If you have heart disease, or know of any factors that make undetected heart disease a possibility, be sure to tell the doctor. Risk factors include high blood pressure, high cholesterol, diabetes, excess weight, smoking, a history of heart disease in your family, and menopause.

If there's any chance of a heart problem, your doctor may administer the first dose of Amerge in the office and monitor your response. After later doses, call your doctor immediately if you experience chest discomfort (including, pain, heaviness, tightness), sudden or severe stomach pain, numbness or tingling, heat sensations, or facial flushing after taking Amerge.

Amerge is only for classic migraine headache. If the first dose fails to relieve your symptoms, your doctor should reevaluate you. Your problem may not be migraine.

If a headache feels different from any you've had previously, check with your doctor. It could be a warning of a problem unrelated to migraine.

If you have kidney or liver problems, or if you have any trouble with your eyes, inform your doctor.

Although very rare, severe and even fatal allergic reactions have occurred in people taking Amerge. Call your doctor immediately if you have shortness of breath; wheezing; palpitations; swelling of the eyelids, face, or lips; or a skin rash, lumps, or hives. Such reactions are more likely in people who have multiple allergies.

Amerge has not been tested in children or adults over age 65.

Possible food and drug interactions when taking this medication

If Amerge is taken with certain other drugs, the effects of either may be increased, decreased, or altered. Do not combine Amerge with the following:

Antidepressants that boost serotonin levels, including Luvox, Paxil, Prozac, and Zoloft.

Ergot-containing drugs such as Cafergot and Ergostat
Sumatriptan (Imitrex)
Zolmitriptan (Zomig)

Special information if you are pregnant or breastfeeding

The effects of Amerge during pregnancy have not been adequately studied. If you are pregnant or plan to become pregnant, inform your doctor immediately. Amerge may appear in breast milk and could affect a nursing infant. If this medication is essential to your health, your doctor may advise you to discontinue breastfeeding while using Amerge.

Recommended dosage

ADULTS

Amerge comes in 1- and 2.5-milligram tablets. The most you should take at one time is 2.5 milligrams, and the maximum for each 24 hours is 5 milligrams. Doses should be spaced at least 4 hours apart.

If you have kidney or liver problems, the recommended dose is 1 milligram, with a 24-hour maximum of 2.5 milligrams.

Overdosage

Any medication taken in excess can have serious consequences. If you suspect an overdose, seek medical attention immediately.

■ *Symptoms of Amerge overdose may include:*
Light-headedness, loss of coordination, tension in the neck, tiredness

Amiloride with Hydrochlorothiazide *See Moduretic, page 882.*

Amitriptyline *See Elavil, page 499.*

Amitriptyline with Perphenazine *See Triavil, page 1478.*

Amlodipine *See Norvasc, page 976.*

Amlodipine and Atorvastatin *See Caduet, page 223.*

Amlodipine with Benazepril *See Lotrel, page 790.*

Ammonium lactate *See Lac-Hydrin, page 716.*

Amnesteem *See Accutane, page 12.*

Amoxicillin *See Amoxil, page 95.*

Amoxicillin, Clarithromycin, and Lansoprazole *See Prevpac, page 1153.*

Amoxicillin with Clavulanate *See Augmentin, page 150.*

AMOXIL

Pronounced: a-MOX-il
Generic name: Amoxicillin
Other brand name: Trimox

Why is this drug prescribed?

Amoxil, an antibiotic, is used to treat a wide variety of infections, including: gonorrhea, middle ear infections, skin infections, upper and lower respiratory tract infections, and infections of the genital and urinary tract. In combination with other drugs such as Prilosec, Prevacid, and/or Biaxin, it is also used to treat duodenal ulcers caused by *H. pylori* bacteria (ulcers in the wall of the small intestine near the exit from the stomach).

Most important fact about this drug

If you are allergic to either penicillin or cephalosporin antibiotics in any form, consult your doctor before taking Amoxil. There is a possibility that you are allergic to both types of medication; and if a reaction occurs, it could be extremely severe. If you take the drug and feel signs of a reaction, seek medical attention immediately.

How should you take this medication?

Amoxil can be taken with or without food. If you are using Amoxil suspension, shake it well before using.

Your doctor will prescribe only Amoxil to treat a bacterial infection. Amoxil will not cure a viral infection such as the common cold. It's important to take all of your medication as instructed by your doctor, even if you're feeling better in a few days. Not finishing the complete dosage of Amoxil may decrease the drug's effectiveness and increase the chances for bacterial resistance to Amoxil and similar antibiotics.

■ *If you miss a dose...*
Take it as soon as you remember. If it is almost time for the next dose, and you take 2 doses a day, take the one you missed and the next dose 5 to 6 hours later. If you take 3 or more doses a day, take the one you missed and the next dose 2 to 4 hours later. Then go back to your regular schedule.

■ *Storage instructions...*
Amoxil suspension and pediatric drops should be stored in a tightly closed bottle. Discard any unused medication after 14 days. Refrigeration is preferable.

Store capsules at or below 68 degrees Fahrenheit. Store chewable tablets and tablets at or below 77 degrees Fahrenheit in a tightly closed container.

What side effects may occur?

Side effects cannot be anticipated. If any develop or change in intensity, inform your doctor as soon as possible. Only your doctor can determine if it is safe for you to continue taking Amoxil.

■ *Side effects may include:*

Agitation, anemia, anxiety, changes in behavior, colitis, confusion, convulsions, diarrhea, dizziness, hives, hyperactivity, insomnia, liver problems and jaundice, nausea, peeling skin, rash, tooth discoloration in children, vomiting.

When used in combination with Prilosec, Prevacid, and/or Biaxin for the treatment of ulcers, the most common side effects are changes in taste sensation, diarrhea, and headache.

Why should this drug not be prescribed?

You should not use Amoxil if you are allergic to penicillin, or cephalosporin antibiotics (for example, Ceclor).

Special warnings about this medication

If you have ever had asthma, hives, hay fever, or other allergies, consult with your doctor before taking Amoxil.

You should stop using Amoxil if you experience reactions such as bruising, fever, skin rash, itching, joint pain, swollen lymph nodes, and/or sores on the genitals. If these reactions occur, stop taking Amoxil unless your doctor advises you to continue.

For infections such as strep throat, it is important to take Amoxil for the entire amount of time your doctor has prescribed. Even if you feel better, you need to continue taking Amoxil. If you stop taking Amoxil before your treatment time is complete, you may get other infections, such as glomerulonephritis (a kidney infection) or rheumatic fever.

If you are diabetic, be aware that Amoxil may cause a false positive Clinitest (urine glucose test) result to occur. You should consult with your doctor about using different tests while taking Amoxil.

Before taking Amoxil, tell your doctor if you have ever had asthma, colitis (inflammatory bowel disease), diabetes, or kidney or liver disease.

The chewable tablet form of Amoxil contains phenylalanine. If you or your child has the hereditary disease phenylketonuria, this form of Amoxil should not be used.

Possible food and drug interactions when taking this medication

If Amoxil is taken with certain other drugs, the effects of either could be increased, decreased, or altered. It is especially important to check with your doctor before combining Amoxil with the following:

Chloramphenicol (Chloromycetin)
Erythromycin (E.E.S., PCE, others)
Oral contraceptives

Probenecid
Tetracycline (Achromycin V, others)

Special information if you are pregnant or breastfeeding

Amoxil should be used during pregnancy only when clearly needed. If you are pregnant or plan to become pregnant, inform your doctor immediately. Since Amoxil may appear in breast milk, you should consult your doctor if you plan to breastfeed your baby.

Recommended dosage

Dosages will be determined by the type of infection being treated.

ADULTS

Ear, Nose, Throat, Skin, Genital, and Urinary Tract Infections
For mild or moderate infections, the usual dose is 250 milligrams every 8 hours, or 500 milligrams every 12 hours. For severe infections, the usual dose is 500 milligrams every 8 hours, or 875 milligrams every 12 hours.

Lower Respiratory Tract Infections
For mild, moderate, or severe infections, the usual dose is 500 milligrams every 8 hours, or 875 milligrams every 12 hours.

*Gonorrhea, Acute, Uncomplicated Anogenital and
Urethral Infections*
The usual dosage is 3 grams in a single oral dose.

Ulcers
For ulcer treatment, Amoxil is combined with Biaxin, Prevacid, or Prilosec. There are several dosage regimens available. For more information, refer to the *Recommended dosage* section under Biaxin, Prevacid, or Prilosec.

If your kidneys are severely impaired or you are undergoing hemodialysis, your doctor may have to adjust your dosage accordingly.

CHILDREN OLDER THAN 3 MONTHS

Children weighing 88 pounds and over should follow the recommended adult dose schedule.

Children weighing under 88 pounds will have their dosage determined by their weight.

Ear, Nose, Throat, Genital, and Urinary Tract Infections
For mild or moderate infections, the usual dose is 25 milligrams per 2.2 pounds of body weight, divided into two daily doses and taken every 12 hours; or 20 milligrams per 2.2 pounds of body weight, divided into three daily doses and taken every 8 hours.

For severe infections, the usual dose is 45 milligrams per 2.2 pounds of body weight, divided into two daily doses and taken every 12 hours; or

40 milligrams per 2.2 pounds of body weight, divided into three daily doses and taken every 8 hours.

Lower Respiratory Tract Infections

For mild, moderate, or severe infections, the usual dose is 45 milligrams per 2.2 pounds of body weight, divided into two daily doses and taken every 12 hours; or 40 milligrams per 2.2 pounds of body weight, divided into three daily doses and taken every 8 hours.

For infants 3 months or younger the maximum daily dose is 30 milligrams per 2.2 pounds of body weight, divided into two daily doses and taken every 12 hours.

The required amount of liquid medication should be placed directly on the child's tongue for swallowing. It can also be added to formula, milk, fruit juice, water, ginger ale, or cold drinks. The preparation should be taken immediately. To be certain the child is getting the full dose of medication, make sure he or she drinks the entire preparation.

If your child is taking the pediatric drops, use the dropper provided to measure the dosage.

Overdosage

Any medication taken in excess can have serious consequences. If you suspect an overdose, seek medical attention immediately.

■ *Symptoms of Amoxil overdose may include:*
Diarrhea, nausea, stomach cramps, vomiting

Amphetamines See Adderall, page 36.

AMPICILLIN
Pronounced: AM-pi-sill-in
Brand name: Principen

Why is this drug prescribed?

Ampicillin is a penicillin-like antibiotic prescribed for a wide variety of infections, including gonorrhea and other genital and urinary infections, respiratory infections, and gastrointestinal infections, as well as meningitis (inflamed membranes of the spinal cord or brain).

Most important fact about this drug

If you are allergic to either penicillin or cephalosporin antibiotics in any form, consult your doctor *before taking ampicillin*. There is a possibility that you are allergic to both types of medication; and if a reaction occurs, it could be extremely severe. If you take the drug and develop a skin reaction, diarrhea, shortness of breath, wheezing, sore throat, or fever, seek medical attention immediately.

How should you use this medication?

Take ampicillin capsules with a full glass of water, a half hour before or 2 hours after a meal.

The oral suspension should be shaken well before using.

Take this medication exactly as prescribed. It works best when there is a constant amount in the body. Take your doses at evenly spaced times around the clock, and try not to miss a dose.

■ *If you miss a dose...*

Take it as soon as you remember. If it is almost time for the next dose, and you take 2 doses a day, take the one you missed and the next dose 5 to 6 hours later. If you take 3 or more doses a day, take the one you missed and the next dose 2 to 4 hours later. Then go back to your regular schedule. Do not take 2 doses at once.

■ *Storage instructions...*

Store capsules at room temperature in a tightly closed container.

Keep the oral suspension in the refrigerator, in a tightly closed container. Discard the unused portion after 14 days.

What side effects may occur?

Side effects cannot be anticipated. If any develop or change in intensity, inform your doctor as soon as possible. Only your doctor can determine whether it is safe for you to continue taking this drug.

■ *Side effects may include:*

Colitis (inflammation of the bowel), diarrhea, fever, itching, nausea, rash or other skin problems, sore tongue or mouth, vomiting

Why should this drug not be prescribed?

You should not take ampicillin if you are allergic to penicillin or cephalosporin antibiotics.

Special warnings about this medication

If you have an allergic reaction, stop taking this drug and contact your doctor immediately.

After you have taken ampicillin for a long time, you may get a new infection (called a superinfection) due to an organism this medication cannot treat. Consult your doctor if your symptoms do not improve or seem to get worse.

Ampicillin sometimes causes diarrhea. Some diarrhea medications can make the diarrhea worse. Check with your doctor before taking any diarrhea remedy.

Oral contraceptives may not work properly while you are taking ampicillin. For greater certainty, use other measures while taking this drug.

If you are diabetic, be aware that ampicillin may cause a false positive in certain urine glucose tests. You should talk to your doctor about the right tests to use while you are taking ampicillin.

For infections such as strep throat, it is important to take ampicillin for the entire amount of time your doctor has prescribed. Even if you feel better, you need to continue taking the medication.

Possible food and drug interactions when taking this medication

If ampicillin is taken with certain other drugs, the effects of either could be increased, decreased, or altered. It is especially important to check with your doctor before combining ampicillin with any of the following:

Allopurinol (Zyloprim)
Atenolol (Tenormin)
Chloroquine (Aralen)
Mefloquine (Lariam)
Oral contraceptives

Special information if you are pregnant or breastfeeding

The effects of ampicillin during pregnancy have not been adequately studied. If you are pregnant or plan to become pregnant, inform your doctor immediately. Ampicillin should be used during pregnancy only if the potential benefit justifies the potential risk to the developing baby.

Ampicillin appears in breast milk and could affect a nursing infant. If this medication is essential to your health, your doctor may advise you to stop breastfeeding until your treatment is finished.

Recommended dosage

Unless you are being treated for gonorrhea, your doctor will have you continue to take ampicillin for 2 to 3 days after your symptoms have disappeared. Dosages are for capsules and oral suspension.

ADULTS

Infections of the Genital, Urinary, or Gastrointestinal Tracts
The usual dose is 500 milligrams, taken every 6 hours.

Gonorrhea
The usual dose is 3.5 grams in a single oral dose along with 1 gram of probenecid.

Respiratory Tract Infections
The usual dose is 250 milligrams, taken every 6 hours.

CHILDREN

Children weighing over 44 pounds should follow the adult dose schedule.

Children weighing 44 pounds or less should have their dosage determined by their weight.

Infections of the Genital, Urinary, or Gastrointestinal Tracts
The usual dose is 100 milligrams for each 2.2 pounds of body weight daily, divided into 4 doses for the capsules, and 3 to 4 doses for the suspension.

Respiratory Tract Infections
The usual dose is 50 milligrams for each 2.2 pounds of body weight daily, divided into 3 to 4 doses.

Overdosage

Although no specific symptoms have been reported, any medication taken in excess can have serious consequences. If you suspect an overdose of ampicillin, seek medical attention immediately.

Amprenavir *See Agenerase, page 52.*

ANAFRANIL
Pronounced: an-AF-ran-il
Generic name: Clomipramine hydrochloride

Why is this drug prescribed?

Anafranil, a chemical cousin of tricyclic antidepressant medications such as Tofranil and Elavil, is used to treat people who suffer from obsessions and compulsions.

An obsession is a persistent, disturbing idea, image, or urge that keeps coming to mind despite the person's efforts to ignore or forget it—for example, a preoccupation with avoiding contamination.

A compulsion is an irrational action that the person knows is senseless but feels driven to repeat again and again—for example, hand-washing perhaps dozens or even scores of times throughout the day.

Most important fact about this drug

Serious, even fatal, reactions have been known to occur when drugs such as Anafranil are taken along with drugs known as MAO inhibitors. Drugs in this category include the antidepressants Nardil and Parnate. Never take Anafranil with one of these drugs.

How should you take this medication?

Take Anafranil with meals, at first, to avoid stomach upset. After your regular dosage has been established, you can take 1 dose at bedtime to avoid sleepiness during the day. Always take it exactly as prescribed.

This medicine may cause dry mouth. Hard candy, chewing gum, or bits of ice may relieve this problem.

■ *If you miss a dose...*
If you take 1 dose at bedtime, consult your doctor. Do not take the missed dose in the morning. If you take 2 or more doses a day, take the missed dose as soon as you remember. If it is almost time for your next dose, skip the one you missed and go back to your regular schedule. Do not take 2 doses at the same time.

■ *Storage instructions...*
Store at room temperature in a tightly closed container, away from moisture.

What side effects may occur?

Side effects cannot be anticipated. If any develop or change in intensity, inform your doctor as soon as possible. Only your doctor can determine if it is safe for you to continue taking Anafranil.

The most significant risk is that of seizures (convulsions). Headache, fatigue, and nausea can be a problem. Men are likely to experience problems with sexual function. Unwanted weight gain is a potential problem for many people who take Anafranil, although a small number actually lose weight.

■ *Side effects may include:*
Constipation, dizziness, dry mouth, impotence, increased appetite, increased sweating, indigestion, libido changes, nausea, nervousness, sleepiness, tremor, twitching, visual changes, weight gain, weight loss

Why should this drug not be prescribed?

Do not take this medication if you are sensitive to or have ever had an allergic reaction to a tricyclic antidepressant such as Tofranil, Elavil, or Tegretol.

Be sure to avoid Anafranil if you are taking, or have taken within the past 14 days, an MAO inhibitor such as the antidepressants Parnate or Nardil. Combining Anafranil with one of these medications could lead to fever, seizures, coma, and even death.

Do not take Anafranil if you have recently had a heart attack.

Special warnings about this medication

This drug should be used with caution in children with depression. In clinical studies, antidepressants increased the risk of suicidal thinking and behavior in children and adolescents with depression and other psychiatric disorders. Anyone considering the use of Anafranil or any other antidepressant in a child or adolescent must balance this risk with the clinical need. In children, Anafranil is approved only to treat obsessive-compulsive disorder.

Additionally, the progression of major depression is associated with a worsening of symptoms and/or the emergence of suicidal thinking or behavior in both adults and children, whether or not they are taking antidepressants. Individuals being treated with Anafranil and their caregivers should watch for any change in symptoms or any new symptoms that appear suddenly—especially agitation, anxiety, hostility, panic, restlessness, extreme hyperactivity, and suicidal thinking or behavior—and report them to the doctor immediately. Be especially observant at the beginning of treatment or whenever there is a change in dose.

If you have narrow-angle glaucoma (increased pressure in the eye) or are having difficulty urinating, Anafranil could make these conditions worse. Use Anafranil with caution if your kidney function is not normal.

If you have a tumor of the adrenal gland, this medication could cause your blood pressure to rise suddenly and dangerously.

Because Anafranil poses a possible risk of seizures, and because it may impair mental or physical ability to perform complicated tasks, your doctor will probably warn you to take special precautions if you need to drive a car, operate complicated machinery, or take part in activities such as swimming or climbing, in which suddenly losing consciousness could be dangerous. Note that your risk of seizures is increased:

If you have ever had a seizure

If you have a history of brain damage or alcoholism

If you are taking another medication that might predispose you to seizures

As with Tofranil, Elavil, and other tricyclic antidepressants, an overdose of Anafranil can be fatal. Do not be surprised if your doctor prescribes only a small quantity of Anafranil at a time. This is standard procedure to minimize the risk of overdose.

Anafranil may cause your skin to become more sensitive to sunlight. Avoid prolonged exposure to sunlight.

Before having any kind of surgery involving the use of general anesthesia, tell your doctor or dentist that you are taking Anafranil. You may be advised to discontinue the drug temporarily.

When it is time to stop taking Anafranil, do not stop abruptly. Your doctor will have you taper off gradually to avoid withdrawal symptoms such as dizziness, fever, general feeling of illness, headache, high fever, irritability or worsening emotional or mental problems, nausea, sleep problems, vomiting.

Possible food and drug interactions when taking this medication
Avoid alcoholic beverages while taking Anafranil.

If Anafranil is taken with certain other drugs, the effects of either could be increased, decreased, or altered. It is especially important to check with your doctor before combining Anafranil with the following:

Antipsychotic drugs such as chlorpromazine and Haldol

Barbiturates such as phenobarbital

Certain blood pressure drugs such as Catapres-TTS and Ismelin

Cimetidine (Tagamet)

Digoxin (Lanoxin)

Drugs that ease spasms, such as Bentyl, Cogentin, and Donnatal

Flecainide (Tambocor)

MAO inhibitors such as Nardil and Parnate

Methylphenidate (Ritalin)

Phenytoin (Dilantin)

Propafenone (Rythmol)

Quinidine (Quinidex)

Serotonin-boosting drugs such as the antidepressants Luvox, Paxil, Prozac, and Zoloft

Thyroid medications such as Synthroid

Tranquilizers such as Valium and Xanax

Warfarin (Coumadin)

Special information if you are pregnant or breastfeeding

If you are pregnant or plan to become pregnant, inform your doctor immediately. Anafranil should not be used during pregnancy unless absolutely necessary; some babies born to women who took Anafranil have had withdrawal symptoms such as jitteriness, tremors, and seizures. Anafranil appears in breast milk. Your doctor may advise you to stop breastfeeding while you are taking Anafranil.

Recommended dosage

ADULTS

The usual recommended initial dose is 25 milligrams daily. Your doctor may gradually increase this dosage to 100 milligrams during the first 2 weeks. During this period you will be asked to take this drug, divided into smaller doses, with meals. The maximum daily dosage is 250 milligrams. After the dose has been determined, your doctor may direct you to take a single dose at bedtime, to avoid sleepiness during the day.

CHILDREN

The usual recommended initial dose is 25 milligrams daily, divided into smaller doses and taken with meals. Your doctor may gradually increase the dose to a maximum of 100 milligrams or 3 milligrams per 2.2 pounds of body weight per day, whichever is smaller. The maximum dose is 200 milligrams or 3 milligrams per 2.2 pounds of body weight, whichever is smaller. Once the dose has been determined, the child can take it in a single dose at bedtime.

Overdosage

An overdose of Anafranil can be fatal. If you suspect an overdose, seek medical attention immediately.

- *Critical signs and symptoms of Anafranil overdose may include:*
  Impaired brain activity (including coma), irregular heartbeat, seizures, severely low blood pressure
- *Other signs and symptoms of overdosage may include:*
  Agitation, bluish skin color, breathing difficulty, delirium, dilated pupils, drowsiness, high fever, incoordination, little or no urine output, muscle rigidity, overactive reflexes, rapid heartbeat, restlessness, severe perspiration, shock, stupor, twitching or twisting movements, vomiting

There is a danger of heart malfunction and even, in rare cases, cardiac arrest.

Anakinra *See Kineret, page 711.*

ANAPROX

Pronounced: AN-uh-procks
Generic name: Naproxen sodium
Other brand names: Aleve, Anaprox DS, Naprelan

Why is this drug prescribed?

Anaprox and Naprelan are nonsteroidal anti-inflammatory drugs used to relieve mild to moderate pain and menstrual cramps. They are also prescribed for relief of the inflammation, swelling, stiffness, and joint pain associated with rheumatoid arthritis and osteoarthritis (the most common form of arthritis), and for ankylosing spondylitis (spinal arthritis), tendinitis, bursitis, acute gout, and other conditions. Anaprox also may be prescribed for juvenile arthritis.

The over-the-counter form of naproxen sodium, Aleve, is used for temporary relief of minor aches and pains, and to reduce fever.

Most important fact about this drug

You should have frequent checkups with your doctor if you take Anaprox regularly. Ulcers or internal bleeding can occur without warning.

How should you take this medication?

Your doctor may ask you to take Anaprox with food or an antacid to avoid stomach upset. Take Aleve with a full glass of water.

Take this medication exactly as prescribed by your doctor.

If you are using Anaprox for arthritis, it should be taken regularly.

- *If you miss a dose...*
  Anaprox: Take the forgotten dose as soon as you remember. If it is almost time for your next dose, skip the one you missed and go back to your regular schedule. Never take 2 doses at the same time.

Naprelan: Take the forgotten dose only if you remember within 2 hours after the appointed time. Otherwise, skip the dose and go back to your regular schedule.

■ *Storage instructions...*
Store at room temperature in a tightly closed container.

What side effects may occur?
Side effects cannot be anticipated. If any develop or change in intensity, inform your doctor as soon as possible. Only your doctor can determine if it is safe for you to continue taking Anaprox.

■ *Side effects of Anaprox may include:*
Abdominal pain, bruising, constipation, diarrhea, difficult or labored breathing, dizziness, drowsiness, headache, hearing disturbances, heartburn, indigestion, inflammation of the mouth, itching, light-headedness, nausea, rapid, fluttery heartbeat, red or purple spots on the skin, ringing in the ears, skin eruptions, sweating, swelling due to fluid retention, thirst, vertigo, vision changes

Naprelan shares some of the above side effects, but also has some of its own:

■ *Side effects of Naprelan may include:*
Back pain, flu symptoms, infection, nasal inflammation, sinus inflammation, sore throat, urinary infection

Why should this drug not be prescribed?
If you are sensitive to or have ever had an allergic reaction to Anaprox, aspirin, or similar drugs such as Motrin, if you have had asthma attacks caused by aspirin or other drugs of this type, or if you have ever retained fluid or had hives or nasal tumors, you should not take this medication. Make sure your doctor is aware of any drug reactions you have experienced.

Special warnings about this medication
Remember that peptic ulcers and bleeding can occur without warning.

This drug should be used with caution if you have kidney or liver disease. It can cause liver inflammation in some people.

Do not take aspirin or any other anti-inflammatory medications while taking Anaprox, unless your doctor tells you to do so.

Anaprox and Naprelan contain sodium. If you are on a low-sodium diet, discuss this with your doctor.

Use with caution if you have heart disease or high blood pressure. This drug can increase water retention. It also may cause vision problems. If you experience any changes in your vision, inform your doctor.

This drug makes some people drowsy or less alert. Avoid driving, operating dangerous machinery, and participating in any hazardous activity that requires full mental alertness if you find that the drug has this effect on you.

Do not take Aleve for more than 10 days for pain or 3 days for fever. Contact your doctor if pain or fever persists or gets worse, if the painful area becomes red or swollen, or if you develop more than a mild digestive upset.

Possible food and drug interactions when taking this medication

If Anaprox is taken with certain other drugs, the effects of either could be increased, decreased, or altered. It is especially important to check with your doctor before combining Anaprox with the following:

ACE inhibitors such as the blood pressure medication Capoten
Antiseizure drugs such as Dilantin
Aspirin
Beta-blockers, including blood pressure drugs such as Inderal
Blood thinners such as Coumadin
Certain water pills (diuretics) such as Lasix
Lithium (Lithonate)
Methotrexate
Naproxen in other forms, such as Naprosyn
Oral diabetes drugs such as Micronase
Other pain relievers such as aspirin, acetaminophen (Tylenol),
    and ibuprofen (Motrin)
Probenecid (Benemid)

If you have more than 3 alcoholic drinks per day, check with your doctor before using painkillers.

Special information if you are pregnant or breastfeeding

The effects of Anaprox during pregnancy have not been adequately studied. If you are pregnant or plan to become pregnant, inform your doctor immediately. Avoid Anaprox, Naprelan, and Aleve during the last 3 months of pregnancy. Anaprox appears in breast milk and could affect a nursing infant. If this medication is essential to your health, your doctor may advise you to discontinue breastfeeding until your treatment with this medication is finished.

Recommended dosage

ADULTS

Mild to Moderate Pain, Menstrual Cramps, Acute Tendinitis and Bursitis
The starting dose is 550 milligrams, followed by 275 milligrams every 6 to 8 hours or 550 milligrams every 12 hours. You should not take more than 1,375 milligrams a day to start, or 1,100 milligrams a day thereafter.

Rheumatoid Arthritis, Osteoarthritis,
and Ankylosing Spondylitis
The starting dose is 275 milligrams or 550 milligrams 2 times a day (morning and evening). Your physician can adjust the doses for maximum benefit. Symptoms should improve within 2 to 4 weeks.

Acute Gout
The starting dose is 825 milligrams, followed by 275 milligrams every 8 hours, until symptoms subside.

CHILDREN

Juvenile Arthritis
The usual daily dosage is a total of 10 milligrams per 2.2 pounds of body weight, divided into 2 doses. Dosage should not exceed 15 milligrams per 2.2 pounds per day.

The safety and effectiveness of Anaprox have not been established in children under 2 years of age.

OLDER ADULTS

Your doctor will determine the dosage based on your particular needs. Adjustments in the normal adult dosage may be needed.

NAPRELAN

Rheumatoid Arthritis, Osteoarthritis,
and Ankylosing Spondylitis
The usual dose is two 375- or 500-milligram tablets taken once a day. Your doctor will adjust your dose. You should not take more than three 500-milligram tablets daily.

Pain, Menstrual Cramps, Acute Tendinitis and Bursitis
The starting dose is two 500-milligram tablets taken once a day. For a short time, the doctor may increase the dose to three 500-milligram tablets daily.

Acute Gout
The usual dose is two to three 500-milligram tablets taken together on the first day, then two 500-milligram tablets once daily until the attack subsides.

It is not known whether Naprelan is safe for children.

ALEVE

1 tablet or caplet every 8 to 12 hours, to a maximum of 3 per day. For those over age 65, no more than 1 tablet or caplet every 12 hours. Not recommended for children under 12.

Overdosage

Any medication taken in excess can cause symptoms of overdose. If you suspect an overdose of Anaprox, seek medical attention immediately.

■ *Symptoms of Anaprox overdose may include:*
Drowsiness
heartburn
indigestion
nausea
vomiting

Anaspaz *See Levsin, page 742.*

Anastrozole *See Arimidex, page 125.*

Androderm *See Testosterone Patches, page 1420.*

ANDROGEL

Pronounced: AN-droe-jel
Generic name: Testosterone gel
Other brand name: Testim

Why is this drug prescribed?

AndroGel is a hormone replacement product for men suffering from hypogonadism, a low level of the male hormone testosterone. This condition is marked by symptoms such as impotence and decreased interest in sex, lowered mood, fatigue, and decreases in bone density and lean body mass. Testosterone replacement therapy helps correct these problems. AndroGel, applied daily to the skin, provides an especially convenient way of taking the hormone, which was previously administered only by injection or skin patch.

Most important fact about this drug

Men using AndroGel must be careful to prevent contact between gel-covered areas and other people's skin. The drug can be transferred by skin-to-skin contact and can have harmful effects on women, especially pregnant women and their unborn babies. Women who touch AndroGel should wash with soap and water as soon as possible. Female partners of men who use AndroGel should contact a physician if they develop signs that the hormone is being transferred, such as acne, increased body hair, or other male sexual characteristics.

How should you take this medication?

Apply AndroGel once daily in the morning to clean, dry skin. Empty the entire contents of the package into a clean hand and apply to the shoulders and upper arms and/or the abdomen. Wash hands thoroughly with soap and water. Allow the application site to dry before dressing, then be sure to cover the treated area with clothing. Avoid bathing, showering, or swimming for 5 to 6 hours after application. Do not apply AndroGel to the genitals.

Gels are flammable. Be sure to avoid fire, an open flame, and smoking while using AndroGel.

■ *If you miss a dose...*
Apply it as soon as you remember. If it is almost time for your next application, skip the missed dose and go back to your regular schedule.
■ *Storage instructions...*
Store at room temperature.

What side effects may occur?

Side effects cannot be anticipated. If any develop or change in intensity, inform your doctor as soon as possible. Only your doctor can determine if it is safe for you to continue using topical AndroGel.

■ *Side effects may include:*
Acne, application site reaction, breast enlargement, emotional instability, headache, high blood pressure, prostate disorder

Why should this drug not be prescribed?

Women must not use AndroGel, and men with prostate cancer or cancer of the breast should also avoid it. Do not use the product if it gives you an allergic reaction.

Special warnings about this medication

AndroGel is flammable when wet. You should avoid fire, flames, and smoking until the gel has dried.

Before using AndroGel, you should be aware that prolonged, high-dose therapy with male hormones is associated with liver disease and, in some cases, liver cancer. Breast enlargement is also a common problem.

Remember, too, that older men who take male hormones are at higher risk for developing prostate disease or prostate cancer. Your doctor should check you carefully before prescribing AndroGel if you have a medical profile that increases your risk for prostate cancer.

Testosterone replacement therapy also tends to worsen sleep apnea, a condition that causes breathing to stop temporarily during sleep. Obese men and those with chronic lung disease are especially at risk.

If you have a history of heart, kidney, or liver disease and develop swelling in the hands, feet, or ankles, stop using AndroGel and alert your doctor immediately. Also contact your doctor if you develop too frequent or persistent erections, nausea, vomiting, or changes in breathing or skin color.

This drug has not been tested in males under 18 years of age.

Possible food and drug interactions when taking this medication
Combining AndroGel with adrenocorticotropic hormone (Cortrosyn), or steroid drugs such as hydrocortisone (Hytone), prednisolone (Pediapred), and betamethasone (Diprolene) may increase fluid retention and swelling, especially in people with heart or kidney disease.

If AndroGel is taken with certain other drugs, the effects of either could be increased, decreased, or altered. It is especially important to check with your doctor before combining AndroGel with the following:

Insulin (Humulin, Novolin)
Oxyphenbutazone
Propranolol (Inderal)

Special information if you are pregnant or breastfeeding
Maternal contact with AndroGel can harm a developing baby. The product must be avoided by pregnant and breastfeeding women. If you are exposed to AndroGel while pregnant, notify your doctor immediately.

Recommended dosage

ADULTS

The recommended adult male starting dose of AndroGel is one 5-gram packet (or for Testim, one 5-gram tube), applied once daily, which delivers 50 milligrams of testosterone. Your doctor should take a blood test to measure your testosterone level about 2 weeks after you start treatment, and may adjust the dose accordingly. The maximum recommended dose is 2 packets or tubes daily.

Overdosage
One reported overdose of injectable testosterone is believed to have caused a stroke. If you suspect an overdose of AndroGel, seek medical attention immediately.

Anexsia *See Vicodin, page 1557.*

Anisindione *See Miradon, page 870.*

Anolor 300 *See Fioricet, page 565.*

ANSAID
Pronounced: AN-sed
Generic name: Flurbiprofen

Why is this drug prescribed?
Ansaid, a nonsteroidal anti-inflammatory drug, is used to relieve the inflammation, swelling, stiffness, and joint pain associated with rheumatoid arthritis and osteoarthritis (the most common form of arthritis).

Most important fact about this drug

You should have frequent checkups with your doctor if you take Ansaid regularly. Ulcers or internal bleeding can occur without warning.

How should you take this medication?

Your doctor may ask you to take Ansaid with food or an antacid.

Take this medication exactly as prescribed by your doctor.

If you are using Ansaid for arthritis, it should be taken regularly.

■ *If you miss a dose...*

Take the forgotten dose as soon as you remember. If it is almost time for your next dose, skip the one you missed and go back to your regular schedule. Never take 2 doses at the same time.

■ *Storage instructions...*

Store at room temperature.

What side effects may occur?

Side effects cannot be anticipated. If any develop or change in intensity, inform your doctor as soon as possible. Only your doctor can determine if it is safe for you to continue taking Ansaid.

■ *Side effects may include:*

Abdominal pain, diarrhea, general feeling of illness, headache, indigestion, nausea, swelling due to fluid retention, urinary tract infection

Why should this drug not be prescribed?

If you are sensitive to or have ever had an allergic reaction to Ansaid, aspirin, or similar drugs such as Motrin, or if you have had asthma attacks caused by aspirin or other drugs of this type, you should not take this medication. Fatal attacks have occurred in people allergic to this drug. Make sure your doctor is aware of any drug reactions you have experienced.

Special warnings about this medication

This drug should be used with caution if you have kidney or liver disease. Kidney problems are most likely to develop in such people, as well as in those with heart failure, those taking water pills, and older adults.

If you have asthma, take Ansaid with extra caution. Do not take aspirin or similar drugs while taking Ansaid, unless your doctor tells you to do so.

Ansaid can cause vision problems. If you experience a change in your vision, inform your doctor. Blurred and/or decreased vision has occurred while taking this medication.

Ansaid slows the clotting process. If you are taking blood-thinning medication, this drug should be taken with caution.

This drug can increase water retention. If you have heart disease or high blood pressure, use with caution.

If you want to take Ansaid for pain less serious than that of arthritis, be sure to discuss the risks of using this drug with your doctor.

Possible food and drug interactions when taking this medication

If Ansaid is taken with certain other drugs, the effects of either could be increased, decreased, or altered. It is especially important to check with your doctor before combining Ansaid with the following:

Antacids
Aspirin
Beta-blockers such as the blood pressure medications Inderal and Tenormin
Blood thinners such as Coumadin
Cimetidine (Tagamet)
Methotrexate (Rheumatrex)
Oral diabetes drugs such as Micronase
Ranitidine (Zantac)
Water pills such as Lasix and Bumex

Special information if you are pregnant or breastfeeding

The effects of Ansaid during pregnancy have not been adequately studied. If you are pregnant or plan to become pregnant, inform your doctor immediately. In particular, you should not use Ansaid in late pregnancy, as it can affect the developing baby's circulatory system. Ansaid appears in breast milk and could affect a nursing infant. If this medication is essential to your health, your doctor may advise you to discontinue breastfeeding until your treatment is finished.

Recommended dosage

ADULTS

Rheumatoid Arthritis or Osteoarthritis
The usual starting dosage is a total of 200 to 300 milligrams a day, divided into 2, 3, or 4 smaller doses (usually 3 or 4 for rheumatoid arthritis). Your doctor will tailor the dose to suit your needs, but you should not take more than 100 milligrams at any one time or more than 300 milligrams in a day.

CHILDREN

The safety and effectiveness of Ansaid have not been established in children.

OLDER ADULTS

Older people are among those most apt to develop kidney problems while taking this drug.
Your doctor will determine the dosage according to your needs.

Overdosage

Any medication taken in excess can cause symptoms of overdose. If you suspect an overdose of Ansaid, seek medical attention immediately.

■ *The symptoms of Ansaid overdose may include:*
Agitation, change in pupil size, coma, disorientation, dizziness, double vision, drowsiness, headache, nausea, semiconsciousness, shallow breathing, stomach pain

ANTACIDS

Brand names: Gaviscon, Maalox, Mylanta, Rolaids, Tums

Why is this drug prescribed?

Available under a number of brand names, antacids are used to relieve the uncomfortable symptoms of acid indigestion, heartburn, gas, and sour stomach.

Most important fact about this drug

Do not take antacids for longer than 2 weeks or in larger than recommended doses unless directed by your doctor. If your symptoms persist, contact your doctor. Antacids should be used only for occasional relief of stomach upset.

How should you take this medication?

If you take a chewable antacid tablet, chew thoroughly before swallowing so that the medicine can work faster and be more effective. Allow Mylanta Soothing Lozenges to completely dissolve in your mouth. Shake liquids well before using.

■ *If you miss a dose...*
Take this medication only as needed or as instructed by your doctor.
■ *Storage instructions...*
Store at room temperature. Keep liquids tightly closed and protect from freezing.

What side effects may occur?

When taken as recommended, antacids are relatively free of side effects. Occasionally, one of the following symptoms may develop.

■ *Side effects may include:*
Chalky taste, constipation, diarrhea, increased thirst, stomach cramps

Why should this drug not be prescribed?

Do not take antacids if you have signs of appendicitis or an inflamed bowel; symptoms include stomach or lower abdominal pain, cramping, bloating, soreness, nausea, or vomiting.

If you are sensitive to or have ever had an allergic reaction to aluminum, calcium, magnesium, or simethicone, do not take an antacid containing these ingredients. If you are elderly and have bone problems or if you are taking care of an elderly person with Alzheimer's disease, do not use an antacid containing aluminum.

Special warnings about this medication

If you are taking any prescription drug, check with your doctor before you take an antacid. Also, tell your doctor or pharmacist about any drug allergies or medical conditions you have.

If you have kidney disease, do not take an antacid containing aluminum or magnesium. If you are on a sodium-restricted diet, do not take Gaviscon without checking first with your doctor or pharmacist.

Possible food and drug interactions when taking this medication

If antacids are taken with certain other medications, the effects of either could be increased, decreased, or altered. It is especially important to check with your doctor before combining antacids with the following:

Cellulose sodium phosphate (Calcibind)
Isoniazid (Rifamate)
Ketoconazole (Nizoral)
Mecamylamine (Inversine)
Methenamine (Mandelamine)
Sodium polystyrene sulfonate resin (Kayexalate)
Tetracycline antibiotics (Achromycin, Minocin)

Special information if you are pregnant or breastfeeding

As with all medications, ask your doctor or health care professional whether it is safe for you to use antacids while you are pregnant or breastfeeding.

Recommended dosage

ADULTS

Take antacids according to the following schedules, or as directed by your doctor.

Gaviscon and Gaviscon Extra Strength Relief Formula Chewable Tablets

Chew 2 to 4 tablets 4 times a day after meals and at bedtime or as needed. Follow with half a glass of water or other liquid. Do not swallow the tablets whole.

Gaviscon Extra Strength Relief Formula Liquid

Take 2 to 4 teaspoonfuls 4 times a day after meals and at bedtime. Follow with half a glass of water or other liquid.

Gaviscon Liquid
Take 1 or 2 tablespoonfuls 4 times a day after meals and at bedtime. Follow with half a glass of water.

Maalox Antacid Caplets
Take 1 caplet as needed. Swallow the tablets whole; do not chew them.

Maalox Heartburn Relief Chewable Tablets
Chew 2 to 4 tablets after meals and at bedtime. Follow with half a glass of water or other liquid.

Maalox Heartburn Relief Suspension, Maalox Magnesia and Alumina Oral Suspension, and Extra Strength Maalox Antacid Plus Anti-Gas Suspension
Take 2 to 4 teaspoonfuls 4 times a day, 20 minutes to 1 hour after meals and at bedtime.

Maalox Plus Chewable Tablets
Chew 1 to 4 tablets 4 times a day, 20 minutes to 1 hour after meals and at bedtime.

Extra Strength Maalox Antacid Plus Anti-Gas
Chewable Tablets
Chew 1 to 3 tablets 20 minutes to 1 hour after meals and at bedtime.

Mylanta and Mylanta Double Strength Liquid and Chewable Tablets Antacid/Anti-Gas
Take 2 to 4 teaspoonfuls of liquid or chew 2 to 4 tablets between meals and at bedtime.

Mylanta Gelcaps
Take 2 to 4 gelcaps as needed.

Mylanta Soothing Lozenges
Dissolve 1 lozenge in your mouth. If needed, follow with a second. Repeat as needed.

Rolaids, Calcium-Rich/Sodium Free Rolaids, and
Extra Strength Rolaids
Chew 1 or 2 tablets as symptoms occur. Repeat hourly if symptoms return.

Tums, Tums E-X, and Tums Anti-Gas Formula
Chew 1 or 2 tablets as symptoms occur. Repeat hourly if symptoms return. You may also hold the tablet between your gum and cheek and let it dissolve gradually.

CHILDREN

Do not give to children under 6 years of age, unless directed by your doctor.

Overdosage

Any medication taken in excess can have serious consequences. If you suspect an overdose, seek medical attention immediately.

■ *For aluminum-containing antacids (Gaviscon, Maalox, Mylanta):*
Bone pain, constipation (severe and continuing), feeling of discomfort (continuing), loss of appetite (continuing), mood or mental changes, muscle weakness, swelling of wrists or ankles, weight loss (unusual)

■ *For calcium-containing antacids (Mylanta, Rolaids, Tums):*
Constipation (severe and continuing), difficult or painful urination, frequent urge to urinate, headache (continuing), loss of appetite (continuing), mood or mental changes, muscle pain or twitching, nausea or vomiting, nervousness or restlessness, slow breathing, unpleasant taste, unusual tiredness or weakness

■ *For magnesium-containing antacids (Gaviscon, Maalox, Mylanta):*
Difficult or painful urination, dizziness or light-headedness, irregular heartbeat, mood or mental changes, unusual tiredness or weakness

ANTIPYRINE AND BENZOCAINE

Pronounced: AN-tee-pie-rheen and BEN-zoh-cane

Why is this drug prescribed?

This medication is prescribed to reduce the inflammation and congestion and relieve the pain and discomfort of severe middle ear infections. This drug may be used in combination with an antibiotic for curing the infection.

This medication is also used to remove excessive or impacted earwax.

Most important fact about this drug

Discard this product 6 months after the dropper is first placed in the drug solution.

How should you use this medication?

Use this medication exactly as prescribed. Administer as follows:

1. Warm the drops to body temperature by holding the bottle in your hand for a few minutes.
2. Shake the bottle.
3. Lie on your side or tilt the affected ear up.
4. Gently pull the earlobe up.
5. Administer the prescribed number of drops.
6. Avoid touching the dropper to the ear.
7. Keep the ear tilted up for about 5 to 7 minutes.

Do not rinse the dropper; replace it in the bottle after each use. Hold the dropper assembly by the screw cap and, without squeezing the rubber bulb, insert the dropper into the bottle and screw down tightly.

■ *If you miss a dose...*
Use it as soon as you remember. If it is almost time for your next dose, skip the one you missed and go back to your regular schedule.
■ *Storage instructions...*
Store at room temperature.

What side effects may occur?

Side effects cannot be anticipated. If any develop or change in intensity, inform your doctor as soon as possible. No specific side effects have been reported for this medication.

Why should this drug not be prescribed?

Do not take Antipyrine and Benzocaine if you are sensitive or allergic to any ingredients in this medication or similar drugs. Make sure your doctor is aware of any drug reactions you have experienced.

Unless directed to do so by your doctor, do not use this medication if you have a punctured eardrum.

Special warnings about this medication

Notify your doctor if irritation occurs or if you develop an allergic reaction to this medication.

Possible food and drug interactions when taking this medication

No food or drug interactions have been reported.

Special information if you are pregnant or breastfeeding

The effects of this medication during pregnancy have not been adequately studied. If you are pregnant or plan to become pregnant, notify your doctor immediately. It is not known whether this medication appears in breast milk. If it is essential to your health, your doctor may advise you to discontinue breastfeeding until your treatment is finished.

Recommended dosage

ADULTS AND CHILDREN

Acute Otitis Media (Severe Middle Ear Infection)
Apply the medication drop by drop into the ear, permitting the solution to run along the wall of the ear canal until it is filled. Avoid touching the ear with the dropper. Then moisten a piece of cotton dressing material, such as gauze, with the medication and insert it into the opening of the ear. Repeat every 1 to 2 hours until pain and congestion are relieved.

Removal of Earwax.
Apply the medication drop by drop into the ear 3 times daily for 2 or 3 days to help detach and remove earwax from the wall of the ear canal.

After the wax has been removed, the medication is useful for drying out the canal or relieving discomfort.

Before and after the removal of earwax, cotton dressing material such as gauze should be moistened with the medication and inserted into the opening of the ear.

Overdosage
No information on overdosage with this medication is available.

ANTIVERT
Pronounced: AN-tee-vert
Generic name: Meclizine hydrochloride
Other brand names: Bonine

Why is this drug prescribed?
Antivert, an antihistamine, is prescribed for the management of nausea, vomiting, and dizziness associated with motion sickness.

Antivert may also be prescribed for the management of vertigo (a spinning sensation or a feeling that the ground is tilted) due to diseases affecting the vestibular system (the bony labyrinth of the ear, which contains the sensors that control your balance).

Most important fact about this drug
Antivert may cause you to become drowsy or less alert; therefore, driving a car or operating dangerous machinery is not recommended.

How should you take this medication?
Take this medication exactly as prescribed by your doctor.

■ *If you miss a dose...*
Take it as soon as you remember. If it is almost time for your next dose, skip the one you missed and go back to your regular schedule. Do not take 2 doses at the same time.

■ *Storage instructions...*
Store away from heat, light, and moisture.

What side effects may occur?
Side effects cannot be anticipated. If any develop or change in intensity, inform your doctor as soon as possible. Only your doctor can determine if it is safe for you to continue taking Antivert.

■ *Side effects may include:*
Drowsiness, dry mouth

Why should this drug not be prescribed?

If you are sensitive to or have ever had an allergic reaction to Antivert or similar drugs, do not take this drug. Make sure that your doctor is aware of any drug reactions you have experienced.

Special warnings about this medication

If you have asthma, glaucoma, or an enlarged prostate gland, check with your doctor before using Antivert.

Possible food and drug interactions when taking this medication

Antivert may intensify the effects of alcohol. Do not drink alcohol while taking this medication.

Special information if you are pregnant or breastfeeding

Studies regarding the use of Antivert in pregnant women do not indicate that this drug increases the risk of abnormalities. However, if you are pregnant or plan to become pregnant, inform your doctor before using Antivert. Check with him, too, if you are breastfeeding your baby.

Recommended dosage

ADULTS AND CHILDREN 12 AND OVER

Motion Sickness
For protection against motion sickness, take 25 to 50 milligrams 1 hour before traveling. You may repeat the dose every 24 hours for the duration of the journey.

Vertigo
The recommended dosage is 25 to 100 milligrams per day, divided into equal, smaller doses as determined by your doctor.

CHILDREN

The safety and effectiveness of Antivert have not been established in children under 12 years of age.

Overdosage

Any medication taken in excess can have serious consequences. If you suspect an overdose of Antivert, seek emergency medical treatment immediately.

Apidra *See Insulin, page 689.*

Apri *See Oral Contraceptives, page 1000.*

ARAVA

Pronounced: ah-RAV-ah
Generic name: Leflunomide

Why is this drug prescribed?

Arava is used in the treatment of rheumatoid arthritis. It reduces the pain, stiffness, inflammation, and swelling associated with this disease, improves physical function, and staves off the joint damage that ultimately results.

Most important fact about this drug

You MUST NOT take Arava if you are pregnant; it can harm the developing baby. If you are still in your childbearing years, your doctor will want to see negative results from a pregnancy test before starting you on Arava. You'll also need to use reliable contraceptive measures as long as you take the drug.

If you become pregnant while taking Arava, your doctor will stop the drug immediately and prescribe a regimen of cholestyramine (Questran) in 8-gram doses 3 times a day for 11 days. Questran helps to clear Arava from the bloodstream, possibly preventing harm to the unborn child.

How should you take this medication?

Your dosage of Arava will be decreased after the first 3 days. Never take more than your doctor prescribes.

- *If you miss a dose...*
  Take it as soon as you remember. If it is almost time for your next dose, skip the one you missed and go back to your regular schedule. Do not take 2 doses at the same time.
- *Storage instructions...*
  Store at room temperature away from light.

What side effects may occur?

Side effects cannot be anticipated. If any develop or change in intensity, inform your doctor as soon as possible. Only your doctor can determine if it is safe for you to continue taking Arava.

- *Side effects may include:*
  Abdominal pain, back pain, bronchitis, cough, diarrhea, dizziness, hair loss, headache, high blood pressure, indigestion, itching, joint disorders, loss of appetite, mouth ulcers, nausea, rash, respiratory infection, sore throat, stomach inflammation, tendon inflammation, urinary tract infection, vomiting, weakness, weight loss

Why should this drug not be prescribed?

Remember that you must not take Arava if you are pregnant or plan to become pregnant. You'll also need to avoid this drug if it gives you an allergic reaction.

Special warnings about this medication

Arava is potentially damaging to the liver. Your doctor will test your liver function before starting Arava therapy. If you have significant liver disease, including hepatitis, you'll be unable to take Arava. If you develop liver problems while taking the drug, your dose will have to be reduced or eliminated.

Theoretically, Arava may interfere with your body's ability to fight off infection. The drug is therefore not recommended for people with cancer, bone marrow problems, severe infections, AIDS, or any other immune system problems. You should also avoid immunization with live vaccines while taking Arava.

Since there is a possibility that Arava could damage your liver or cause blood problems (such as a loss of white blood cells used to fight infection or a loss of cells that help your blood clot), it is essential that your doctor conduct a monthly blood test for the first 6 months of therapy, then every 6 to 8 weeks thereafter. If you are taking Arava and the cancer drug methotrexate together, you may be even more susceptible to these problems. Your doctor will need to test your blood every month. Notify your doctor promptly if any signs of a blood problem appear. Warnings include easy bruising, frequent infections, unusual fatigue, and paleness.

Arava has been known to cause rare but serious skin reactions. If you develop a skin rash or eruption, stop taking Arava and contact your doctor. Arava can also reduce your blood cell count.

Your doctor will prescribe the drug cautiously if you have kidney problems, since poor kidney function can increase the amount of Arava in your system.

Arava does not appear to cause fetal harm when taken by the father prior to conception. Nevertheless, if you plan to father a child, your doctor will instruct you to stop taking Arava and will prescribe a regimen of cholestyramine to clear Arava from your system.

Possible food and drug interactions when taking this medication

If Arava is taken with certain other drugs, the effects of either could be increased, decreased, or altered. It is especially important to check with your doctor before combining Arava with the following:

Cholestyramine (Prevalite, Questran)
Methotrexate (Rheumatrex)
Nonsteroidal anti-inflammatory drugs such as Advil, Aleve, Motrin, and Naprosyn
Rifampin (Rifadin, Rifamate, Rifater)
Tolbutamide (Orinase)

Special information if you are pregnant or breastfeeding

Do not take Arava while pregnant or breastfeeding. Taken during pregnancy, the drug can cause birth defects. And although it is not known whether Arava appears in breast milk, there is good reason to suspect that it will cause serious side effects in nursing infants.

Recommended dosage

ADULTS

The recommended starting dose is one 100-milligram tablet daily for the first 3 days. If you have an increased risk for blood disorders or liver problems, your doctor may choose to eliminate the 100-milligram starting dose to reduce the risk of serious side effects.

After the first 3 days, the doctor will reduce the dose to 20 milligrams a day. If side effects appear, the dose may be further decreased to 10 milligrams a day.

CHILDREN

Arava is not recommended for children less than 18 years old.

Overdosage

Any medication taken in excess can have serious consequences. If you suspect an overdose of Arava, seek medical treatment immediately.

■ *Symptoms of Arava overdose may include:*
Abdominal pain, anemia, blood disorders, diarrhea, liver problems

ARICEPT

Pronounced: AIR-ih-sept
Generic name: Donepezil hydrochloride

Why is this drug prescribed?

Aricept is one of the few drugs that can provide some relief from the symptoms of early Alzheimer's disease. (Cognex, Exelon, and Razadyne are others.) Alzheimer's disease causes physical changes in the brain that disrupt the flow of information and interfere with memory, thinking, and behavior. Aricept can temporarily improve brain function in some Alzheimer's sufferers, although it does not halt the progress of the underlying disease.

Most important fact about this drug

To maintain any improvement, Aricept must be taken regularly. If the drug is stopped, its benefits will soon be lost. Patience is in order when starting the drug. It can take up to 3 weeks for any positive effects to appear.

How should you take this medication?

Aricept should be taken once a day just before bedtime. Be sure it's taken every day. If Aricept is not taken regularly, it won't work. It can be taken with or without food.

■ *If you miss a dose...*
Make it up as soon as you remember. If it is almost time for the next dose, skip the one that was missed and go back to the regular schedule. Never double the dose.

■ *Storage instructions...*
Store at room temperature.

What side effects may occur?

Side effects cannot be anticipated. If any develop or change in intensity, tell the doctor as soon as possible. Only the doctor can determine if it is safe to continue Aricept.

Side effects are more likely with higher doses. The most common are diarrhea, fatigue, insomnia, loss of appetite, muscle cramps, nausea, and vomiting. When one of these effects occurs, it is usually mild and gets better as treatment continues.

■ *Other side effects may include:*
Abnormal dreams, arthritis, bruising, depression, dizziness, fainting, frequent urination, headache, pain, sleepiness, weight loss

Why should this drug not be prescribed?

There are two reasons to avoid Aricept: an allergic reaction to the drug itself, or an allergy to the group of antihistamines that includes Claritin, Allegra, Atarax, Periactin, and Optimine.

Special warnings about this medication

Aricept can aggravate asthma and other breathing problems, and can increase the risk of seizures. It can also slow the heartbeat, cause heartbeat irregularities, and lead to fainting episodes. Contact your doctor if any of these problems occurs.

In patients who have had stomach ulcers, and those who take a non-steroidal anti-inflammatory drug such as Advil, Nuprin, or Aleve, Aricept can make stomach side effects worse. Be cautious when using Aricept and report all side effects to your doctor.

Possible food and drug interactions when taking this medication

Aricept will increase the effects of certain anesthetics. Make sure the doctor is aware of Aricept therapy prior to any surgery.

If Aricept is taken with certain other drugs, the effects of either could be increased, decreased, or altered. It is especially important to check with your doctor before combining Aricept with the following:

Antispasmodic drugs such as Bentyl, Cogentin, and Pro-Banthine
Bethanechol chloride (Urecholine)
Carbamazepine (Tegretol)
Dexamethasone (Decadron)
Ketoconazole (Nizoral)
Phenobarbital
Phenytoin (Dilantin)
Quinidine (Quinidex)
Rifampin (Rifadin, Rifamate)

Special information if you are pregnant or breastfeeding

Since it is not intended for women of childbearing age, Aricept's effects during pregnancy have not been studied, and it is not known whether it appears in breast milk.

Recommended dosage

ADULTS

The usual starting dose is 5 milligrams once a day at bedtime for at least 4 to 6 weeks. Do not increase the dose during this period unless directed. The doctor may then change the dosage to 10 milligrams once a day if response to the drug warrants it.

CHILDREN

The safety and effectiveness of Aricept have not been established in children.

Overdosage

Any medication taken in excess can have serious consequences. If you suspect an overdose, seek medical attention immediately.

■ *Symptoms of Aricept overdose include:*
   Collapse, convulsions, extreme muscle weakness (possibly ending in death if breathing muscles are affected), low blood pressure, nausea, salivation, slowed heart rate, sweating, vomiting

ARIMIDEX

Pronounced: AR-i-mi-deks
Generic name: Anastrozole

Why is this drug prescribed?

Arimidex is a first-line treatment of breast cancer in postmenopausal women. It slows the growth of advanced cancer within the breast and cancer that has spread to other parts of the body. Arimidex is also used to treat advanced breast cancer in postmenopausal women whose disease has spread to other parts of the body following treatment with tamoxifen (Nolvadex), another anticancer drug. Arimidex can also be prescribed along with other drugs to treat the early stages of breast cancer in postmenopausal women.

Arimidex combats the kind of breast cancer that thrives on estrogen. One of the hormones produced by the adrenal gland is converted to a form of estrogen by an enzyme called aromatase. Arimidex suppresses this enzyme and thereby reduces the level of estrogen circulating in the body.

Most important fact about this drug
Arimidex, like many other anticancer medications, may prolong survival and improve quality of life. To keep this medication working properly, it's important to continue taking it even when you don't feel well. If you develop bothersome side effects, call your doctor. He or she can recommend ways to reduce your discomfort.

How should you take this medication?
Take Arimidex exactly as directed.

■ *If you miss a dose...*
Take the forgotten dose if you remember within 12 hours. If it is almost time for your next dose, skip the one you missed and go back to your regular schedule. Never take 2 doses at once.

■ *Storage instructions...*
Store at room temperature.

What side effects may occur?
Side effects cannot be anticipated. If any develop or change in intensity, tell your doctor as soon as possible. Only your doctor can determine if it is safe for you to continue taking Arimidex.

■ *Side effects may include:*
Abdominal pain, accidental injury, anxiety, arthritis, back pain, bone pain, breast pain, cataracts, chest pain, constipation, cough, depression, diarrhea, dizziness, dry mouth, flu-like symptoms, fractures, headache, heart disease, high blood pressure or cholesterol, hot flashes, infection, insomnia, joint disease or pain, loss of appetite, nausea, osteoporosis, pain, pelvic pain and stiffness, pins and needles sensation, rash, shortness of breath, sore throat, stomach and intestinal upset, sweating, swelling of arms and legs, urinary tract infection, vaginal discharge or inflammation, vomiting, weakness, weight gain

Why should this drug not be prescribed?
Do not take Arimidex if you are pregnant or if you have an allergic reaction to the drug.

Special warnings about this medication

Because Arimidex may raise the level of cholesterol in your blood, your doctor may periodically do blood tests to check.

Possible food and drug interactions when taking this medication

Certain drugs may decrease the effectiveness of Arimidex, including tamoxifen (Nolvadex) and estrogen-containing drugs. Be sure to tell your doctor about any medication you are taking.

Special information if you are pregnant or breastfeeding

If you are pregnant or plan to become pregnant, do not take Arimidex. In animal studies, this medication has caused severe birth defects, including incomplete bone formation and low birth weight; it could be poisonous to your unborn child. Arimidex also increases your chances of having a miscarriage or a stillborn baby. If you should accidentally become pregnant, tell your doctor immediately.

Because of the possibility of Arimidex passing through your breast milk to your baby, you should probably avoid breastfeeding.

Recommended dosage

ADULTS

The usual dose is a 1-milligram tablet taken once a day. If Arimidex is being used as an initial treatment for advanced breast cancer, you will continue taking the medication until it no longer works against the tumor. The optimal duration of therapy for early breast cancer has not been determined.

Overdosage

Although there have been no reports of Arimidex overdose, any medication taken in excess can have serious consequences. If you suspect an overdose, seek medical attention immediately.

Aripiprazole See Abilify, page 1.

ARMOUR THYROID

Pronounced: ARE-more THIGH-roid
Generic name: Natural thyroid hormones TC and TD

Why is this drug prescribed?

Armour Thyroid is prescribed when your thyroid gland is unable to produce enough hormone. It is also used to treat or prevent goiter (enlargement of the thyroid gland), and is given in a suppression test to diagnose an overactive thyroid.

Most important fact about this drug

Although Armour Thyroid will speed up your metabolism, it is not effective as a weight-loss drug and should not be used for that purpose. Too much Armour Thyroid may cause severe side effects, especially if you are also taking appetite suppressants.

How should you take this medication?

Take Armour Thyroid exactly as prescribed by your doctor. There is no *typical* dosage; the amount you need to take will depend on how much thyroid hormone your body is able to produce. Take no more or less than the amount your doctor prescribes. Take your dose at the same time every day for consistent effect.

Do not change brands of medication without consulting your doctor.

If you are taking Armour Thyroid to compensate for an underactive thyroid gland, you will probably need to take the medication indefinitely.

■ *If you miss a dose...*
Take it as soon as you remember. If it is almost time for your next dose, skip the one you missed and go back to your regular schedule. Do not take 2 doses at the same time. If you miss 2 or more doses in a row, consult your doctor.

■ *Storage instructions...*
Store at room temperature in a tightly closed container.

What side effects may occur?

Side effects are rare when Armour Thyroid is taken at the correct dosage. However, taking too much medication or increasing the dosage too quickly may lead to overstimulation of the thyroid gland.

■ *Symptoms of overstimulation may include:*
Changes in appetite, diarrhea, fever, headache, increased heart rate, irritability, nausea, nervousness, sleeplessness, sweating, weight loss

Although children treated with Armour Thyroid may initially lose some hair, the hair loss is temporary.

Why should this drug not be prescribed?

You should not take Armour Thyroid if you have ever had an allergic reaction to this drug; your thyroid gland is overactive; or your adrenal glands are not making enough corticosteroid hormone.

Special warnings about this medication

If you are elderly, particularly if you suffer from angina (chest pain due to a heart condition), you should take Armour Thyroid at a lower dosage, and your doctor should schedule frequent checkups.

Armour Thyroid tends to aggravate symptoms of diabetes and underactive adrenal glands. If you take medication to treat one of these disorders, your dosage of that medication will probably need to be adjusted once you start taking Armour Thyroid.

Possible food and drug interactions when taking this medication
If you take Armour Thyroid with certain other drugs, the effect of either drug could be increased, decreased, or altered. It is especially important to check with your doctor before combining Armour Thyroid with the following:

Asthma medications such as Theo-Dur
Blood thinners such as Coumadin
Cholestyramine (Questran)
Colestipol (Colestid)
Estrogen preparations (including some birth control pills such as Ortho-Novum and Premarin)
Insulin
Oral diabetes drugs such as Diabinese and Glucotrol)

Special information if you are pregnant or breastfeeding
If you need to take Armour Thyroid because of a thyroid hormone deficiency, you may continue using the medication during pregnancy, but your doctor will test you regularly and may change your dosage. Once your baby is born, you may breastfeed while continuing treatment with Armour Thyroid.

Recommended dosage

ADULTS

Your doctor will tailor the dosage of Armour Thyroid to meet your individual requirements, taking into consideration the status of your thyroid gland and any other medical conditions you may have.

Overdosage
An overdose of Armour Thyroid will speed up all of the body's vital processes, causing physical and mental hyperactivity, increased appetite, excessive sweating, chest pain, increased pulse rate, palpitations, nervousness, intolerance to heat, and possibly tremors or a rapid heartbeat.

ARTHROTEC
Pronounced: ARE-throw-teck
Generic ingredients: Diclofenac sodium, Misoprostol

Why is this drug prescribed?
Arthrotec is designed to relieve the symptoms of arthritis in people who are also prone to ulcers. It contains diclofenac, a nonsteroidal anti-

inflammatory drug (NSAID) for control of the inflammation, swelling, stiffness, and joint pain associated with rheumatoid arthritis and osteoarthritis. However, since NSAIDs can cause stomach ulcers in susceptible people, Arthrotec also contains misoprostol, a synthetic prostaglandin that serves to reduce the production of stomach acid, protect the stomach lining, and thus prevent ulcers.

Most important fact about this drug

Be certain to avoid taking Arthrotec during pregnancy. It can cause a miscarriage with potentially dangerous bleeding, sometimes leading to hospitalization, surgery, infertility, and even death. Arthrotec can also deform or kill the developing baby. If you haven't passed menopause, your doctor should do a pregnancy test less than 2 weeks before your therapy begins. Once you've started taking the drug, it is vitally important that you also use reliable contraceptive measures. If you do become pregnant, stop taking Arthrotec and contact your doctor immediately.

How should you take this medication?

To minimize diarrhea and related side effects, take Arthrotec with meals, exactly as prescribed. Antacids containing magnesium can make Arthrotec-induced diarrhea worse. If you need an antacid, use one containing aluminum or calcium instead. Arthrotec tablets should be swallowed whole and not chewed, crushed, or dissolved.

■ *If you miss a dose...*
If you are following a regular schedule, take the dose as soon as you remember. If it is almost time for the next one, skip the dose you missed and go back to your regular schedule. Do not take 2 doses at once.

■ *Storage instructions...*
Store at room temperature in a dry place.

What side effects may occur?

Side effects cannot be anticipated. If any develop or change in intensity, inform your doctor as soon as possible. Only your doctor can determine if it is safe for you to continue taking Arthrotec.

■ *Side effects may include:*
Abdominal pain, acid indigestion, diarrhea, gas, nausea

Why should this drug not be prescribed?

Remember that it is essential to avoid Arthrotec during pregnancy. You should also avoid this medication if you've ever had an allergic reaction to either of its components (diclofenac and misoprostol). Avoid it, too, if you've had a reaction to any other prostaglandin medication, or to any NSAID, including aspirin. Make sure the doctor is aware of any drug reactions you've experienced.

Special warnings about this medication

Although Arthrotec is designed to protect against stomach ulcers and bleeding, they remain a possibility. Contact your doctor immediately if you notice signs of bleeding such as black tarry stools. Also call the doctor if you develop severe diarrhea, cramping, or nausea, or if milder symptoms persist for more than 7 days.

This drug should be used with caution if you have kidney problems or liver disease. Your doctor will do a blood test to monitor your liver within 4 to 8 weeks after starting Arthrotec therapy and periodically thereafter. If you develop signs of a liver problem, such as nausea, fatigue, tiredness, itching, yellowed eyes and skin, tenderness in the upper right area of your stomach, or flu-like symptoms, stop taking Arthrotec and notify your doctor at once.

Use Arthrotec cautiously if you have systemic lupus or a similar connective tissue disease. Certain rare side effects are more likely to occur. Be cautious, too, if you have heart disease or high blood pressure. Arthrotec can increase water retention. Also exercise caution if you have asthma. In some people, Arthrotec could trigger an attack.

Do not take Arthrotec if you're dehydrated (a possibility after severe vomiting or diarrhea). You should also avoid Arthrotec if you have a condition known as porphyria.

Arthrotec is not an ordinary pain reliever. It is a potent medication, and poses extreme danger during pregnancy. Never share it with anyone else.

Possible food and drug interactions when taking this medication

If Arthrotec is taken with certain other drugs, the effects of either could be increased, decreased, or altered. It is especially important to check with your doctor before combining Arthrotec with the following:

Aspirin
Blood pressure medications such as Cardizem, Inderal, Procardia, and Vasotec
Cyclosporine (Neoral, Sandimmune)
Digoxin (Lanoxin)
Diuretics (HydroDIURIL, Lasix)
Glipizide (Glucotrol, Glucotrol XL)
Glyburide (Diabeta, Micronase)
Insulin
Lithium (Lithobid, Lithonate)
Magnesium-containing antacids such as Maalox and Mylanta
Methotrexate (Rheumatrex)
Phenobarbital
Prednisolone (Delta-Cortef, Pediapred, Prelone)
Warfarin (Coumadin)

Special information if you are pregnant or breastfeeding

Arthrotec must be strictly avoided during pregnancy. If you are in your childbearing years, your doctor will have you take your first dose on the second or third day of your menstrual period to be sure you're not pregnant. Use reliable contraception for the duration of your treatment.

Because Arthrotec appears in breast milk, your doctor may have you stop breastfeeding until your treatment is finished.

Recommended dosage

ADULTS

Osteoarthritis
The recommended dose is 50 milligrams 3 times daily.

Rheumatoid Arthritis
The recommended dose is 50 milligrams 3 or 4 times daily.

If you cannot tolerate the recommended dosage, your doctor can prescribe a dose of 50 or 75 milligrams twice daily. However, such lower dosages are less effective at preventing ulcers.

Your doctor may prescribe misoprostol (Cytotec) in addition to Arthrotec for better ulcer protection.

CHILDREN

The safety and effectiveness of Arthrotec have not been established in children below the age of 18.

Overdosage

If you suspect an overdose of Arthrotec, seek medical attention immediately.

■ *Symptoms of Arthrotec overdose may include:*
Abdominal pain, confusion, diarrhea, difficulty breathing, digestive discomfort, drowsiness, fever, lack of muscle tone, low blood pressure, tremors, seizures, slow heartbeat, throbbing heartbeat, vomiting

Asacol *See Rowasa, page 1280.*

ASPIRIN

Pronounced: ASS-per-in
Brand names: Empirin, Ecotrin, Genuine Bayer, Halfprin

Why is this drug prescribed?

Aspirin is an anti-inflammatory pain medication (analgesic) that is used to relieve headaches, toothaches, and minor aches and pains, and to reduce fever. It also temporarily relieves the minor aches and pains of arthritis, muscle aches, colds, flu, and menstrual discomfort. In some patients, a small daily dose of aspirin may be used to ensure sufficient blood flow to the brain and prevent stroke. Aspirin may also be taken to decrease recurrence of a heart attack or other heart problems.

Most important fact about this drug

Aspirin should not be used during the last 3 months of pregnancy unless specifically prescribed by a doctor. It may cause problems in the unborn child or complications during delivery.

How should you take this medication?

Do not take more than the recommended dose.

Do not use aspirin if it has a strong, vinegar-like odor.

If aspirin upsets your stomach, use of a coated or buffered brand may reduce the problem.

Do not chew or crush sustained-release brands, such as Bayer time-release aspirin, or pills coated to delay breakdown of the drug, such as Ecotrin. To make them easier to swallow, take them with a full glass of water.

■ *If you miss a dose...*
Take it as soon as you remember. If it is almost time for your next dose, skip the one you missed and go back to your regular schedule. Never take 2 doses at the same time.

■ *Storage instructions...*
Store at room temperature.

What side effects may occur?

Side effects cannot be anticipated. If any develop or change in intensity, inform your doctor as soon as possible. Only your doctor can determine if it is safe for you to continue using aspirin.

■ *Side effects may include:*
Heartburn, nausea and/or vomiting, possible involvement in formation of stomach ulcers and bleeding, small amounts of blood in stool, stomach pain, stomach upset

Why should this drug not be prescribed?

Do not take aspirin if you are allergic to it, if you have asthma, ulcers or ulcer symptoms, or if you are taking a medication that affects the clotting of your blood, unless specifically told to do so by your doctor.

Special warnings about this medication

Aspirin should not be given to children or teenagers for flu symptoms or chickenpox. Aspirin has been associated with the development of Reye's syndrome, a dangerous disorder characterized by disorientation and lethargy leading to coma.

If you have a continuous or high fever, or a severe or persistent sore throat, especially with a high fever, vomiting, and nausea, consult your doctor. It could indicate a more serious illness.

If pain persists for more than 10 days or if redness or swelling appears at the site of inflammation, consult your doctor immediately.

If you experience ringing in the ears, hearing loss, upset stomach, or dizziness, consult your doctor before taking more aspirin.

Check with your doctor before giving aspirin for arthritis or rheumatism to a child under 12.

Possible food and drug interactions when taking this medication

If aspirin is taken with certain other drugs, the effects of either could be increased, decreased, or altered. It is especially important to check with your doctor before combining aspirin with the following:

Acetazolamide (Diamox)
ACE-inhibitor-type blood pressure medications such as Capoten
Antigout medications such as Zyloprim
Arthritis medications such as Motrin and Indocin
Blood thinners such as Coumadin
Certain diuretics such as Lasix
Diabetes medications such as DiaBeta and Micronase
Diltiazem (Cardizem)
Dipyridamole (Persantine)
Insulin
Seizure medications such as Depakene
Steroids such as prednisone

Special information if you are pregnant or breastfeeding

The use of aspirin during pregnancy should be discussed with your doctor. Aspirin should not be used during the last 3 months of pregnancy unless specifically indicated by your doctor. It may cause problems in the fetus and complications during delivery. Aspirin may appear in breast milk and could affect a nursing infant. Ask your doctor whether it is safe to take aspirin while you are breastfeeding.

Recommended dosage

ADULTS

Treatment of Minor Pain and Fever
The usual dose is 1 or 2 tablets every 3 to 4 hours up to 6 times a day.

Prevention of Stroke
The usual dose is 1 tablet 4 times daily or 2 tablets 2 times a day.

Prevention of Heart Attack
The usual dose is 1 tablet daily. Your physician may suggest that you take
a larger dose, however. If you use Halfprin low-strength tablets (162 milligrams), adjust the dosage accordingly.

CHILDREN

Consult your doctor.

Overdosage

Any medication used in excess can have serious consequences. If you
suspect symptoms of an aspirin overdose, seek medical treatment immediately.

Aspirin Free Anacin *See Tylenol, page 1513.*

Aspirin with Extended-release dipyridamole
    See Aggrenox, page 57.

ASTELIN

Pronounced: AST-eh-linn
Generic name: Azelastine hydrochloride

Why is this drug prescribed?

Astelin is an antihistamine nasal spray. It is prescribed for the relief of hay
fever symptoms such as itchy, runny nose and sneezing, and can also be
used to relieve cases of congested, runny nose and postnasal drip unrelated to allergies.

Most important fact about this drug

Astelin can cause drowsiness. Do not drive a car, operate machinery, or
undertake any other activity that requires mental alertness until you know
how the drug affects you. Avoid combining Astelin with alcohol, antihistamines, and other drugs that slow the central nervous system; worse
drowsiness could result.

How should you take this medication?

Use Astelin nasal spray only as prescribed. Avoid spraying into the eyes.

Before initial use, prime the pump by depressing it 4 times, or until
a fine mist appears. When 3 or more days have elapsed since the last
use, you should reprime the pump with 2 strokes, or until a fine mist
appears.

Relief of symptoms usually occurs within 3 hours and lasts up to 12
hours.

■ *If you miss a dose...*
Take the forgotten dose as soon as you remember. If it is almost time for your next dose, skip the one you missed and go back to your regular schedule. Never double your dose.

■ *Storage instructions...*
Store the bottle in an upright position at room temperature with the nasal pump tightly closed. Do not freeze.

What side effects may occur?

Side effects cannot be anticipated. If any develop or change in intensity, inform your doctor as soon as possible. Only your doctor can determine if it is safe for you to continue taking Astelin.

■ *Side effects may include:*
Bitter taste, drowsiness, headache, loss of sensation, nasal, burning, sneezing, sore throat

Why should this drug not be prescribed?

If you are sensitive to or have ever had an allergic reaction to Astelin or any of its ingredients, you should not take this medication.

Special warnings about this medication

Remember that Astelin makes some people drowsy. See *Most important fact about this drug* for precautions to take.

If you have a kidney condition, make sure your doctor is aware of it. Your dosage of Astelin may have to be reduced.

Possible food and drug interactions when taking this medication

If Astelin is taken with certain other drugs, the effects of either could be increased, decreased, or altered. It is especially important to check with your doctor before combining Astelin with the following:

Alcohol
Cimetidine (Tagamet)
Drugs that slow the nervous system, including codeine, phenobarbital, and Restoril
Ketoconazole (Nizoral)
Other antihistamines such as Benadryl and Claritin

Special information if you are pregnant or breastfeeding

The effects of Astelin during pregnancy have not been adequately studied. If you are pregnant or plan to become pregnant, inform your doctor immediately. Because of the possibility of harming the developing baby, you may need to give up the medication. It is not known whether Astelin appears in breast milk. Your doctor may want you to stop breastfeeding while using this drug.

Recommended dosage

ADULTS

The usual dose for adults and children 12 years of age and older is 2 sprays into each nostril twice a day.

CHILDREN

To relieve hay fever in children between 5 and 12 years of age, the usual dose is 1 spray into each nostril twice a day. Astelin is not recommended for other types of congestion in this age group. Safety and effectiveness in children under 5 have not been established.

Overdosage

A severe overdose is unlikely, and would probably cause no other symptoms than extreme drowsiness. However, if you suspect an overdose, it's still wise to seek medical attention immediately.

ATACAND
Pronounced: AT-uh-kand
Generic name: Candesartan cilexetil

Why is this drug prescribed?

Atacand controls high blood pressure. It works by blocking the effect of a hormone called angiotensin II. Unopposed, this substance prompts the blood vessels to contract, an action that tends to raise blood pressure. Atacand relaxes and expands the blood vessels, allowing pressure to drop. The drug may be prescribed alone or with other blood pressure medications.

Most important fact about this drug

You must take Atacand regularly for it to be effective. Since blood pressure declines gradually, it may be a couple of weeks before you get significant benefits from Atacand, and you must continue taking it even though you feel well. Atacand does not cure high blood pressure; it merely keeps it under control.

How should you take this medication?

So you won't forget, make a habit of taking your dose of Atacand around the same time every day. This medication can be taken with or without food.

■ *If you miss a dose...*
Take it as soon as you remember. If it's almost time for your next dose, skip the one you missed and go back to your regular schedule. Do not take 2 doses at the same time.

■ *Storage instructions…*
Store at room temperature in a tightly sealed container.

What side effects may occur?
Side effects cannot be anticipated. If any develop or change in intensity, inform your doctor as soon as possible. Only your doctor can determine if it is safe for you to continue taking Atacand.

■ *Side effects may include:*
Back pain, dizziness, respiratory tract infection

Why should this drug not be prescribed?
If Atacand gives you an allergic reaction, you cannot continue using it.

Special warnings about this medication
Atacand can cause a severe drop in blood pressure, especially when you first start taking the drug. The problem is more likely to occur if your body's supply of water has been depleted by diuretics (water pills). Symptoms include light-headedness, dizziness, and faintness. Call your doctor if they occur. You may need to have your dose adjusted.

If you have kidney or liver disease, or congestive heart failure, Atacand must be used with caution.

Possible food and drug interactions when taking this medication
The chances of a drug interaction with Atacand are low. Check with your doctor, however, before combining it with lithium (Eskalith).

Special information if you are pregnant or breastfeeding
Atacand can cause injury or even death to an unborn child when used during the last 6 months of pregnancy. As soon as you learn that you are pregnant, stop taking Atacand and call your doctor.

It is not known whether Atacand appears in breast milk, but because of the potential risks to the nursing infant, it's considered best to avoid the drug while breastfeeding. You should decide whether to give up nursing or discontinue Atacand.

Recommended dosage

ADULTS

Atacand can be taken once or twice a day in doses totaling 8 to 32 milligrams per day. However, the recommended starting dose is 16 milligrams taken once daily. If you are taking a diuretic (water pill) or if you have kidney or liver problems, your doctor will start you on a lower dose.

Overdosage
There have been few reports of overdose with Atacand. However, the most likely results are low blood pressure, dizziness, and an abnormally

slow or rapid heartbeat. If you suspect an overdose, seek medical attention immediately.

ATACAND HCT

Pronounced: AT-uh-kand HCT
Generic name: Candesartan cilexetil, Hydrochlorothiazide

Why is this drug prescribed?

Atacand HCT is a combination medication used in the treatment of high blood pressure. One component, candesartan, belongs to a class of blood pressure medications that work by preventing the hormone angiotensin II from constricting the blood vessels. This allows the blood to flow more freely and helps keep blood pressure down. The other component, hydrochlorothiazide, is a diuretic that increases the output of urine. This removes excess fluid from the body and helps lower blood pressure. Doctors usually prescribe Atacand HCT in place of its individual components. It can also be prescribed along with other blood pressure medications.

Most important fact about this drug

You must take Atacand HCT regularly for it to be effective. Since blood pressure declines gradually, it may be several weeks before you get the full benefit of Atacand HCT, and you must continue taking it even though you feel well. Atacand HCT does not cure high blood pressure; it merely keeps it under control.

How should you take this medication?

Atacand HCT may be taken with or without food. Take Atacand HCT exactly as directed. Try to take it at the same time each day so that it is easier to remember.

■ *If you miss a dose...*
Take it as soon as you remember. If it is almost time for your next dose, skip the one you missed and go back to your regular schedule. Do not take 2 doses at once.

■ *Storage instructions...*
Keep in a tightly closed container at room temperature.

What side effects may occur?

Side effects cannot be anticipated. If any develop or change in intensity, inform your doctor as soon as possible. Only your doctor can determine if it is safe for you to continue taking Atacand HCT.

■ *Side effects may include:*
Back pain, dizziness, flu-like symptoms, headache, upper respiratory infection

Why should this drug not be prescribed?
Do not take Atacand HCT if you have ever had an allergic reaction to candesartan, hydrochlorothiazide, or any sulfa drugs. You should also avoid this drug if you are unable to urinate.

Special warnings about this medication
Atacand HCT can cause low blood pressure, especially if you are also taking another diuretic. This may make you feel light-headed or faint, especially during the first days of therapy. If these symptoms occur, contact your doctor. Your dosage may need to be adjusted. If you actually faint, stop taking this medication until you have talked to your doctor.

If you have congestive heart failure, liver or kidney disease, lupus, gout, or diabetes, Atacand HCT should be used with caution. This drug may bring out hidden diabetes. If you are already taking insulin or oral diabetes drugs, your medication may have to be adjusted. The hydrochlorothiazide component of Atacand HCT also has a tendency to increase cholesterol levels.

If you have bronchial asthma or a history of allergies, you may be at greater risk for an allergic reaction to this medication.

The diuretic in Atacand HCT can cause a chemical imbalance in the body, especially if dehydration has depleted your fluids. Your doctor will perform blood tests periodically to check for this imbalance. Signs include dry mouth, thirst, weakness, sluggishness, drowsiness, restlessness, confusion, seizures, muscle pain or cramps, muscle fatigue, low blood pressure, decreased urination, rapid heartbeat, nausea, and vomiting. Call your doctor if you experience any of these symptoms.

Diuretics also can cause your body to lose too much potassium. Signs of an excessively low potassium level include muscle weakness and rapid or irregular heartbeat. To boost your potassium level, your doctor may recommend eating potassium-rich foods or taking a potassium supplement. If you think you need a supplement, check with your doctor; do not start taking one on your own. Likewise, check with your doctor before using a potassium-containing salt substitute.

Excessive sweating, severe diarrhea, or vomiting could deplete your body's fluids and cause your blood pressure to become too low. Be careful when exercising and during hot weather.

Atacand HCT has not been evaluated for use in children.

Possible food and drug interactions when taking this medication
If Atacand HCT is taken with certain other drugs, the effects of either could be increased, decreased, or altered. It is especially important to check with your doctor before combining Atacand HCT with the following:

Alcohol
Barbiturates such as phenobarbital and Seconal
Cholestyramine (Questran)

Colestipol (Colestid)
Insulin
Lithium (Eskalith)
Muscle relaxants such as tubocurarine
Narcotic painkillers such as Percocet
Nonsteroidal anti-inflammatory drugs such as Advil, Motrin,
 and Naprosyn
Norepinephrine (Levophed)
Oral diabetes drugs such as Diabinese, Diabeta, and Glucotrol
Other blood pressure–lowering drugs
Steroid medications such as prednisone

Special information if you are pregnant or breastfeeding

Atacand HCT can cause injury or even death to an unborn child when
used during the last 6 months of pregnancy. As soon as you learn that
you are pregnant, stop taking Atacand HCT and call your doctor. Atacand
HCT appears in breast milk and can affect the nursing infant. You'll need
to choose between breastfeeding and using Atacand HCT.

Recommended dosage

ADULTS

Atacand HCT is available in tablets containing either 16 or 32 milligrams
of candesartan and 12.5 milligrams of hydrochlorothiazide. The usual
starting dose is one 16/12.5 tablet or one 32/12.5 tablet per day, depending on the medicine that you have been taking before starting Atacand
HCT. If the starting dose is not effective in lowering your blood pressure,
after four weeks your doctor may increase your dosage.

Your doctor may need to adjust your dose of Atacand HCT if you have
liver or kidney problems. If your kidney problems are severe, you will not
be able to take Atacand HCT.

Overdosage

Any medication taken in excess can have serious consequences. If you
suspect an overdose, seek medical help immediately.

■ *Symptoms of Atacand HCT overdose may include:*
 Dehydration, dizziness, low blood pressure, slow or irregular heartbeat

ATARAX

Pronounced: AT-a-raks
Generic name: Hydroxyzine hydrochloride
Other brand name: Vistaril

Why is this drug prescribed?

Atarax is an antihistamine used to relieve the symptoms of common anxiety and tension and, in combination with other medications, to treat anxiety that results from physical illness. It also relieves itching from allergic reactions and can be used as a sedative before and after general anesthesia. Antihistamines work by decreasing the effects of histamine, a chemical the body releases that narrows air passages in the lungs and contributes to inflammation. Antihistamines reduce itching and swelling and dry up secretions from the nose, eyes, and throat.

Most important fact about this drug

Atarax is not intended for long-term use (more than 4 months). Your doctor should re-evaluate the prescription periodically.

How should you take this medication?

Take this medication exactly as prescribed by your doctor.

■ *If you miss a dose...*
  Take it as soon as you remember. If it is almost time for your next dose, skip the one you missed and go back to your regular schedule. Do not take 2 doses at once.

■ *Storage instructions...*
  Store tablets and syrup away from heat, light, and moisture. Keep the syrup from freezing.

What side effects may occur?

Side effects cannot be anticipated. If any develop or change in intensity, inform your doctor as soon as possible. Only your doctor can determine if it is safe for you to continue taking Atarax.

Drowsiness, the most common side effect of Atarax, is usually temporary and may disappear in a few days or when dosage is reduced. Other side effects include dry mouth, twitches, tremors, and convulsions. The last two usually occur with higher than recommended doses of Atarax.

Why should this drug not be prescribed?

Atarax should not be taken in early pregnancy or if you are sensitive to or have ever had an allergic reaction to it. Make sure your doctor is aware of any drug reactions you have experienced.

Special warnings about this medication
Atarax increases the effects of drugs that depress the activity of the central nervous system. If you are taking narcotics, non-narcotic analgesics, or barbiturates in combination with Atarax, their dosage should be reduced.

This medication can cause drowsiness. Driving or operating dangerous machinery or participating in any hazardous activity that requires full mental alertness is not recommended until you know how you react to Atarax.

Possible food and drug interactions when taking this medication
Atarax may increase the effects of alcohol. Avoid alcohol while taking this medication.

If Atarax is taken with certain other drugs, the effects of either could be increased, decreased, or altered. It is especially important to check with your doctor before combining Atarax with the following:

Barbiturates such as Phenobarbital and Seconal
Narcotics such as Demerol and Percocet
Non-narcotic analgesics such as Motrin and Tylenol

Special information if you are pregnant or breastfeeding
Although the effects of Atarax during pregnancy have not been adequately studied in humans, birth defects have appeared in animal studies with this medication. You should not take Atarax in early pregnancy. If you are pregnant or plan to become pregnant, inform your doctor immediately. Atarax may appear in breast milk and could affect a nursing infant. If this medication is essential to your health, your doctor may advise you to discontinue breastfeeding until your treatment is finished.

Recommended dosage
When treatment begins with injections, it can be continued in tablet form.

Your doctor will adjust your dosage based on your response to the drug. Due to an increased risk of drowsiness, older adults usually start at the low end of the dosage range.

FOR ANXIETY AND TENSION

Adults: The usual dose is 50 to 100 milligrams 4 times per day.

Children under age 6: The total dose is 50 milligrams daily, divided into several smaller doses.

Children over age 6: The total dose is 50 to 100 milligrams daily, divided into several smaller doses.

FOR ITCHING DUE TO ALLERGIC CONDITIONS

Adults: The usual dose is 25 milligrams 3 or 4 times a day.

Children under age 6: The total dose is 50 milligrams daily, divided into several smaller doses.

Children over age 6: The total dose is 50 to 100 milligrams daily, divided into several smaller doses.

BEFORE AND AFTER GENERAL ANESTHESIA

Adults: The usual dose is 50 to 100 milligrams.

Children: The usual dose is 0.6 milligram per 2.2 pounds of body weight.

Overdosage

Any medication taken in excess can have serious consequences. If you suspect an overdose of Atarax, seek medical attention immediately.

The most common symptom of Atarax overdose is excessive calm; your blood pressure may drop, although it is not likely.

Atazanavir *See Reyataz, page 1251.*

Atenolol *See Tenormin, page 1405.*

Atenolol with Chlorthalidone *See Tenoretic, page 1402.*

ATIVAN
Pronounced: AT-i-van
Generic name: Lorazepam

Why is this drug prescribed?

Ativan is used in the treatment of anxiety disorders and for short-term (up to 4 months) relief of the symptoms of anxiety. It belongs to a class of drugs known as benzodiazepines.

Most important fact about this drug

Tolerance and dependence can develop with the use of Ativan. You may experience withdrawal symptoms if you stop using it abruptly. Only your doctor should advise you to discontinue or change your dose.

How should you take this drug?

Take this medication exactly as prescribed by your doctor.

- *If you miss a dose...*
  If it is within an hour or so of the scheduled time, take the forgotten dose as soon as you remember. Otherwise, skip the dose and go back to your regular schedule. Do not take 2 doses at once.

■ *Storage instructions…*
Store at room temperature in a tightly closed container, away from light.

What side effects may occur?
Side effects cannot be anticipated. If any develop or change in intensity, inform your doctor as soon as possible. Only your doctor can determine if it is safe for you to continue taking Ativan.

If you experience any side effects, it will usually be at the beginning of your treatment; they will probably disappear as you continue to take the drug, or if your dosage is reduced.

■ *Side effects may include:*
Dizziness, memory problems, sedation, transient amnesia, unsteadiness, weakness
■ *Side effects due to a rapid decrease in dose or abrupt withdrawal from Ativan:*
Abdominal and muscle cramps, convulsions, depressed mood, inability to fall or stay asleep, sweating, tremors, vomiting

Why should this drug not be prescribed?
If you are sensitive to or have ever had an allergic reaction to Ativan or similar drugs such as Valium, you should not take this medication.

Also avoid Ativan if you have the eye disease acute narrow-angle glaucoma.

Anxiety or tension related to everyday stress usually does not require treatment with Ativan. Discuss your symptoms thoroughly with your doctor.

Special warnings about this medication
Ativan may cause you to become drowsy or less alert; therefore, driving or operating dangerous machinery or participating in any hazardous activity that requires full mental alertness is not recommended.

If you are severely depressed or have suffered from severe depression, consult with your doctor before taking this medication.

If you have decreased kidney or liver function, use of this drug should be discussed with your doctor.

If you are an older person or if you have been using Ativan for a prolonged period of time, your doctor will watch you closely for stomach and upper intestinal problems.

Possible food and drug interactions when taking this medication
Ativan may intensify the effects of alcohol. Avoid alcohol while taking this medication.

If Ativan is taken with certain other drugs, the effects of either could be increased, decreased, or altered. It is especially important to check with your doctor before combining Ativan with barbiturates (phenobarbital, Seconal, Amytal) or sedative-type medications such as Valium and Halcion.

Special information if you are pregnant or breastfeeding

Do not take Ativan if you are pregnant or planning to become pregnant. There is an increased risk of birth defects. It is not known whether Ativan appears in breast milk. If this medication is essential to your health, your doctor may advise you to discontinue breastfeeding until your treatment is finished.

Recommended dosage

ADULTS

The usual recommended dosage is a total of 2 to 6 milligrams per day divided into smaller doses. The largest dose should be taken at bedtime. The daily dose may vary from 1 to 10 milligrams.

Anxiety
The usual starting dose is a total of 2 to 3 milligrams per day taken in 2 or 3 smaller doses.

Insomnia Due to Anxiety
A single daily dose of 2 to 4 milligrams may be taken, usually at bedtime.

CHILDREN

The safety and effectiveness of Ativan have not been established in children under 12 years of age.

OLDER ADULTS

The usual starting dosage for older adults and those in a weakened condition should not exceed a total of 1 to 2 milligrams per day, divided into smaller doses, to avoid oversedation. This dose can be adjusted by your doctor as needed.

Overdosage

Any medication taken in excess can have serious consequences. An overdose of Ativan can be fatal, though this is rare. If you suspect an overdose, seek medical attention immediately.

■ *The symptoms of Ativan overdose may include:*
Coma, confusion, drowsiness, hypnotic state, lack of coordination, low blood pressure, sluggishness

Atomoxetine See Strattera, page 1348.

Atorvastatin See Lipitor, page 764.

ATROVENT

Pronounced: AT-row-vent
Generic name: Ipratropium bromide

Why is this drug prescribed?

Atrovent inhalation aerosol and solution are prescribed for long-term treatment of bronchial spasms (wheezing) associated with chronic obstructive pulmonary disease, including chronic bronchitis and emphysema. When inhaled, Atrovent opens the air passages, allowing more oxygen to reach the lungs.

Atrovent nasal spray relieves runny nose. The 0.03% spray is used for year-round runny nose due to allergies and other causes. The 0.06% spray is prescribed for hay fever and for runny nose due to colds. The spray does not relieve nasal congestion or sneezing.

Most important fact about this drug

Atrovent inhalation aerosol and solution are not for initial use in acute attacks of bronchial spasm when fast action is needed.

How should you take this medication?

Atrovent inhalation aerosol and solution are not intended for occasional use. To get the most benefit from this drug, you must use it consistently throughout your course of treatment, as prescribed by your doctor.

To take the inhalation aerosol, insert the metal canister in the special Atrovent mouthpiece and shake well. Holding the canister upside down, exhale deeply through the mouth, enclose the mouthpiece with your lips, and inhale slowly through the mouth while firmly pressing once on the base of the upended canister. Hold your breath for 10 seconds then exhale. Wait 15 seconds and repeat. Test-spray the canister 3 times whenever it has not been used for 24 hours. Be careful to avoid spraying in the eyes.

The nasal spray pump must be primed; your doctor will show you how.

■ *If you miss a dose...*
 Take it as soon as you remember. If it is almost time for your next dose, skip the one you missed and go back to your regular schedule. Do not take 2 doses at once.

■ *Storage instructions...*
 All forms of Atrovent may be stored at room temperature. Do not freeze.

 Keep the inhalation aerosol away from heat and flame; the canister could burst. Discard after 200 sprays. Keep the nasal spray tightly closed.

What side effects may occur?

Side effects cannot be anticipated. If any develop or change in intensity, inform your doctor as soon as possible. Only your doctor can determine if it is safe for you to continue taking Atrovent.

INHALATION AEROSOL AND SOLUTION

■ *Side effects may include:*
Blurred vision, breathlessness, bronchitis, cough, dizziness, dry mouth, headache, irritation from aerosol, nausea, nervousness, rash, stomach and intestinal upset, wheezing, worsening of symptoms

NASAL SPRAY

■ *Side effects may include:*
Blurred vision, change in taste, conjunctivitis (pinkeye), cough, diarrhea, dizziness, dry mouth/throat, eye irritation, headache, hoarseness, increased runny nose or nasal inflammation, inflamed nasal ulcers, nasal congestion, nasal dryness, nasal irritation/itching/burning, nasal tumors, nausea, nosebleed, pain, posterior nasal drip, pounding heartbeat, ringing in the ears, sinus inflammation, skin rash, sneezing, sore throat, swollen nose, thirst, upper respiratory infection

Why should this drug not be prescribed?

If you are sensitive to or have ever had an allergic reaction to Atrovent or any of its ingredients, or to soybeans, soy lecithin, or peanuts, you should not take this medication.

You should also avoid Atrovent if you are allergic to drugs based on atropine. Make sure your doctor is aware of any drug reactions you have experienced.

Special warnings about this medication

An immediate allergic reaction (hives, swelling, rash, wheezing) is possible when you first use this drug.

Unless you are directed to do so by your doctor, do not take this medication if you have the eye condition called narrow-angle glaucoma (high pressure inside the eye), an enlarged prostate, or obstruction in the neck of the bladder.

Keep Atrovent away from your eyes. It can cause blurred vision, visual halos and colors, red eyes, pain, or even narrow-angle glaucoma. If any of these symptoms develop, see your doctor immediately.

If you develop eye pain, blurred vision, very dry nose, or nosebleeds after using the nasal spray, call your doctor.

Do not increase your use of Atrovent without your doctor's approval. If the drug begins to lose its effect, check with your doctor immediately.

Possible food and drug interactions when taking this medication

When using the aerosol or solution, do not take other inhaled medications unless your doctor approves. Check with your doctor before combining Atrovent with spasm-quelling medications such as Donnatal and Levsin.

Special information if you are pregnant or breastfeeding

The effects of Atrovent during pregnancy have not been adequately studied. If you are pregnant or plan to become pregnant, inform your doctor immediately. It is not known whether Atrovent appears in breast milk. If this drug is essential to your health, your doctor may advise you to stop nursing your baby until your treatment is finished.

Recommended dosage

AEROSOL OR SOLUTION

The usual starting dose is 2 inhalations, 4 times per day. Additional inhalations may be taken, but the total should not exceed 12 in 24 hours. Not for use in children under 12.

NASAL SPRAY 0.03%

The usual dose is 2 sprays in each nostril 2 or 3 times a day. Not for use in children under 6.

NASAL SPRAY 0.06%

Runny Nose Due to Colds
The usual adult dose is 2 sprays in each nostril 3 or 4 times a day. The recommended dose for children ages 5 to 11 is 2 sprays in each nostril 3 times a day. Do not use for more than 4 days and do not give it to children under 5.

Runny Nose Due to Hay Fever
The usual dose for adults and children 5 and over is 2 sprays in each nostril 4 times a day. Can be used safely for hay fever for up to 3 weeks.

Overdosage

There is no information on specific symptoms of Atrovent overdose. However, any drug taken in excess can have serious consequences. If you suspect an overdose of Atrovent, seek medical attention immediately.

A/T/S *See Erythromycin, Topical, page 524.*

AUGMENTIN

Pronounced: awg-MENT-in
Generic ingredients: Amoxicillin, Clavulanate potassium
Other brand name: Augmentin XR

Why is this drug prescribed?

Augmentin is used in the treatment of lower respiratory, middle ear, sinus, skin, and urinary tract infections that are caused by certain specific bacteria. These bacteria produce a chemical enzyme called beta lactamase that makes some infections particularly difficult to treat.

Augmentin ES-600, a stronger, oral-suspension form of the drug, is prescribed for certain stubborn ear infections that previous treatment has failed to clear up in children two and under, or those attending day care.

Augmentin XR is an extended-release form of the drug used to treat pneumonia and sinus infections.

Most important fact about this drug

If you are allergic to either penicillin or cephalosporin antibiotics in any form, consult your doctor *before taking Augmentin.* You may be allergic to it, and if a reaction occurs, it could be extremely severe. If you take the drug and feel signs of a reaction, seek medical attention immediately.

How should you take this medication?

Augmentin should be taken every 8 or 12 hours, depending on the dosage strength. It may be taken with or without food, but taking it with meals or snacks will help prevent stomach upset. However, the extended-release form, Augmentin XR, should always be taken with food to improve absorption.

Your doctor will prescribe Augmentin only to treat a bacterial infection; it will not cure a viral infection, such as the common cold. It's important to take the full dosage schedule of Augmentin, even if you're feeling better in a few days. Not completing the full dosage schedule may decrease the drug's effectiveness and increase the chances that the bacteria may become resistant to Augmentin and similar antibiotics.

Shake the suspension well. Use a dosing spoon or medicine dropper to give a child the medication; rinse the spoon or dropper after each use.

■ *If you miss a dose...*
Take it as soon as you remember. If it is almost time for the next dose, and you take 2 doses a day, take the one you missed and the next dose 5 to 6 hours later. If you take 3 doses a day, take the one you missed and the next dose 2 to 4 hours later. Then go back to your regular schedule.

■ *Storage instructions…*
Store the suspension under refrigeration and discard after 10 days.
Store tablets away from heat, light, and moisture.

What side effects may occur?
Side effects cannot be anticipated. If any develop or change in intensity, inform your doctor as soon as possible. Only your doctor can determine if it is safe for you to continue taking Augmentin.

■ *Side effects may include:*
Diarrhea/loose stools, nausea, skin rashes and hives

Why should this drug not be prescribed?
If you are sensitive to or have ever had an allergic reaction to any penicillin medication, do not take this drug.

Also avoid taking Augmentin if it has ever given you liver problems or yellowing of the skin and eyes. Additionally, do not take Augmentin XR if you have severe kidney problems or need dialysis.

Special warnings about this medication
Augmentin and other penicillin-like medicines are generally safe; however, anyone with liver, kidney, or blood disorders is at increased risk when using this drug. Alternative choices may be available to your doctor.

If you have diabetes and test your urine for the presence of sugar, you should ask your doctor or pharmacist if this medication will interfere with the type of test you use.

Allergic reactions to this medication can be serious and possibly fatal. Let your doctor know about previous allergic reactions to medicines, food, or other substances before using Augmentin. If you experience a reaction, report it to your doctor immediately and seek medical treatment.

If you develop diarrhea while taking Augmentin, inform your doctor. It could be a sign of a potentially dangerous form of bowel inflammation.

Some formulations of Augmentin contain phenylalanine. If you have the hereditary disease phenylketonuria, check with your doctor or pharmacist before taking this drug.

Possible food and drug interactions when taking this medication
Augmentin may react with the antigout medication Benemid, resulting in changes in blood levels. A reaction with another antigout drug, Zyloprim, may cause a rash. Notify your doctor if you are taking either of these drugs.

Like many antibiotics, Augmentin may reduce the effectiveness of birth control pills. You may want to take additional measures while taking Augmentin.

Special information if you are pregnant or breastfeeding

The effects of Augmentin during pregnancy have not been adequately studied. Because there may be risk to the developing baby, doctors usually recommend Augmentin to pregnant women only when the benefits of therapy outweigh any potential danger. Augmentin appears in breast milk and could affect a nursing infant. If Augmentin is essential to your health, your doctor may advise you to stop breastfeeding until your treatment with this drug is finished.

Recommended dosage

ADULTS

The usual adult dose is one 500-milligram tablet every 12 hours or one 250-milligram tablet every 8 hours. For more severe infections and infections of the respiratory tract, the dose should be one 875-milligram tablet every 12 hours or one 500-milligram tablet every 8 hours. It is essential that you take this medicine according to your doctor's directions.

The total daily dose of Augmentin XR is 4,000 milligrams of amoxicillin and 250 milligrams of clavulanate potassium, given in divided doses every 12 hours for 10 days (for sinus infections) or for 7 to 10 days (for pneumonia).

CHILDREN

Older than 3 Months

For middle ear infections, sinus inflammation, lower respiratory tract infections, and more severe infections, the usual dose of the 200- or 400-milligram suspension is 45 milligrams per 2.2 pounds per day, in 2 doses, every 12 hours, and of the 125- or 250-milligram suspension, 40 milligrams per 2.2 pounds per day, in 3 doses, every 8 hours.

For less severe infections, the usual dose is 25 milligrams of the 200- or 400-milligram suspension for each 2.2 pounds of weight per day, divided into 2 doses, every 12 hours, or 20 milligrams of the 125- or 250-milligram suspension per 2.2 pounds per day, divided into 3 doses, every 8 hours.

The usual dosage of Augmentin ES-600 oral suspension is 90 milligrams per 2.2 pounds of body weight per day, divided into 2 doses taken every 12 hours. Treatment lasts 10 days.

Children weighing 88 pounds or more will take the adult dosage of standard Augmentin.

Less than 3 Months

Children in this age group take 30 milligrams per 2.2 pounds of body weight per day, divided into 2 doses and taken every 12 hours.

Augmentin XR has not been studied in children younger than 16 years old and should not be used in this group.

Overdosage

Augmentin is generally safe; however, large amounts may cause overdose symptoms. Suspected overdoses of Augmentin must be treated immediately; contact your physician or an emergency room.

■ *Symptoms of Augmentin overdose may include:*
Diarrhea, drowsiness, kidney problems, overactivity, rash, stomach and abdominal pain, vomiting

Auranofin See Ridaura, page 1261.

AVALIDE

Pronounced: AV-a-lide
Generic name: Irbesartan, Hydrochlorothiazide

Why is this drug prescribed?

Avalide is a combination medication used to treat high blood pressure. One component, irbesartan, belongs to a class of blood pressure medications that prevents the hormone angiotensin II from constricting the blood vessels, thereby allowing blood to flow more freely and keeping blood pressure down. The other component, hydrochlorothiazide, is a diuretic that increases the output of urine, removing excess fluid from the body and thus lowering blood pressure.

Combinations such as Avalide are usually prescribed only when treatment with a single medication fails to lower blood pressure sufficiently. Avalide can be combined with yet other blood pressure medicines if your pressure remains too high.

Most important fact about this drug

If you have high blood pressure, you must take Avalide regularly for it to be effective. Since blood pressure declines gradually, it may be several weeks before you get the full benefit of Avalide and you must continue taking it even if you are feeling well. Avalide does not cure high blood pressure; it merely keeps it under control.

How should you take this medication?

Avalide can be taken with or without food.

■ *If you miss a dose...*
Take it as soon as you remember. If it is almost time for your next dose, skip the one you missed and go back to your regular schedule. Never take 2 doses at the same time.

■ *Storage instructions...*
Store Avalide at room temperature.

What side effects may occur?

Avalide is unlikely to produce side effects, and if any do occur they are usually mild and temporary. Nevertheless, be sure to report all side effects to your doctor as soon as possible. Only your doctor can determine if it is safe for you to continue taking Avalide.

■ *Side effects may include:*
Dizziness, fatigue, influenza, muscle and bone pain, nausea, swelling due to water retention, vomiting

Why should this drug not be prescribed?

If Avalide gives you an allergic reaction, you'll be unable to use it. You should also avoid it if you have an allergy to sulfa drugs or if you're unable to urinate.

Special warnings about this medication

Avalide can cause low blood pressure, especially if your body is short of fluid. This can happen due to excessive sweating, inadequate fluid intake, diarrhea, or vomiting, as well as dialysis or use of another diuretic. Be sure to drink plenty of fluids, and call your doctor if your mouth becomes dry, you feel weak or tired or sluggish, you are unusually thirsty, you feel restless or confused, you ache all over, you find you are urinating less frequently, your heart starts beating faster, or you become nauseous.

If your blood pressure drops excessively, you may feel light-headed or faint, especially during the first few days of therapy. If these symptoms occur, contact your doctor. Your dosage may need adjustment. If you actually faint, stop taking the medication until you have talked with your doctor.

If you have liver or kidney disease, diabetes, gout, or lupus erythematosus, use Avalide with caution. This drug may bring out hidden diabetes. If you are already taking insulin or oral diabetes drugs, your dosage may have to be adjusted. If you have bronchial asthma or a history of allergies, you may be at greater risk for an allergic reaction to this medication.

This drug has not been tested in children.

Possible food and drug interactions when taking this medication

Alcohol may increase the effects of Avalide. Use it with caution.

If Avalide is taken with certain other drugs, the effects of either could be increased, decreased, or altered. It is especially important to check with your doctor before combining Avalide with the following:

Adrenocorticotropic hormone (ACTH)
Barbiturates such as phenobarbital and Seconal
Cholestyramine (Questran)
Colestipol (Colestid)
Insulin
Lithium (Eskalith, Lithobid)
Narcotic painkillers such as Demerol, Tylenol with Codeine, and Percocet

Nonsteroidal anti-inflammatory drugs such as Aleve, Anaprox, and Motrin

Other blood pressure medications such as Procardia XL and Tenormin

Oral diabetes drugs such as Diabinese, DiaBeta, and Glucotrol

Steroids such as prednisone

Special information if you are pregnant or breastfeeding

When used in the second and third trimesters of pregnancy, Avalide can cause injury and even death to the unborn child. Stop taking Avalide as soon as you know you are pregnant. If you know you are pregnant or plan to become pregnant, tell your doctor immediately.

Avalide appears in breast milk and can affect the nursing infant. If this medication is essential to your health, your doctor may advise you to stop breastfeeding while you are taking Avalide.

Recommended dosage

Avalide tablets come in two strengths:

150 milligrams irbesartan with 12.5 milligrams hydrochlorothiazide
300 milligrams irbesartan with 12.5 milligrams hydrochlorothiazide

ADULTS

The usual starting dose of Avalide is 1 lower-strength tablet daily.

It will take 2 to 4 weeks for Avalide to reach its maximum effectiveness. If your blood pressure does not respond to the initial dosage, your doctor may increase the dosage to 1 higher-strength tablet or 2 lower-strength tablets taken once a day.

Overdosage

Any medication taken in excess can have serious consequences. Information on Avalide overdosage is limited, but extremely low blood pressure and an unusually rapid or slow heartbeat are likely signs of an overdose. Other signs may include dry mouth, excessive thirst, muscle cramps, weakness, restlessness, confusion, and nausea. If you suspect an overdose, seek medical attention immediately.

AVANDAMET

Pronounced: ah-VAN-duh-met
Generic ingredients: Rosiglitazone maleate, Metformin hydrochloride

Why is this drug prescribed?

Avandamet is an oral medication used to control blood sugar levels in people with type 2 (non-insulin-dependent) diabetes. It contains two drugs commonly used to lower blood sugar, rosiglitazone (Avandia) and metformin (Glucophage). Avandamet replaces the need to take these two drugs separately. It is also used when treatment with Glucophage alone doesn't work. Avandamet is not, however, meant to take the place of weight loss or diet and exercise. You should continue to follow the regimen your doctor recommends.

Blood sugar levels are ordinarily controlled by the body's natural supply of insulin, which helps sugar move out of the bloodstream and into the cells to be used for energy. People who have type 2 diabetes do not make enough insulin or do not respond normally to the insulin their bodies make, causing a buildup of unused sugar in the bloodstream. Avandamet helps remedy this problem in two ways: by decreasing your body's production of sugar and making your body more sensitive to its own insulin supply. Avandamet does not increase the body's production of insulin.

Most important fact about this drug

Avandamet could cause a very rare—but potentially fatal—side effect known as lactic acidosis. It is caused by a buildup of lactic acid in the blood. The problem is most likely to occur in people whose liver or kidneys are not working well, and in those who have multiple medical problems, take several medications, or have congestive heart failure. The risk also is higher if you are an older adult or drink alcohol. Lactic acidosis is a medical emergency that must be treated in a hospital. Notify your doctor immediately if you experience any of the following.

■ *Symptoms of lactic acidosis may include:*
Dizziness, extreme weakness or tiredness, light-headedness, low body temperature, slow or irregular heartbeat, rapid breathing or trouble breathing, sleepiness, unexpected or unusual stomach discomfort (especially after you have been taking Avandamet for a while), unusual muscle pain

How should you take this medication?

Do not take more or less of this medication than directed by your doctor. Avandamet should be taken in divided doses with meals to reduce the possibility of nausea or diarrhea, especially during the first few weeks of therapy. Avandamet may start to work within the first week or two after you begin taking it, but it can take up to 3 months before the drug's full effects are seen. Be sure to check your blood sugar as your doctor recommends.

■ *If you miss a dose...*
Take the forgotten dose as soon as you remember. However, if it is almost time for your next dose, skip the one you missed and return to your regular schedule. Do not take two doses at once.

■ *Storage instructions...*
Store at room temperature in a tight, light-resistant container.

What side effects may occur?
Side effects cannot be anticipated. If any develop or change in intensity, tell your doctor as soon as possible. Only your doctor can determine if it is safe for you to continue using Avandamet.

■ *Side effects may include:*
Accidental injury, anemia, back pain, diarrhea, fatigue, headache, joint pain, nausea, sinus inflammation, swelling, upper respiratory infection, upset stomach, viral infection

Why should this drug not be prescribed?
Avandamet is processed primarily by the kidneys, and can build up to excessive levels in the body if the kidneys aren't working properly. It should be avoided if you have kidney disease or your kidney function has been impaired by a condition such as shock, blood poisoning, or a heart attack.

You should not use Avandamet if you need to take medicine for congestive heart failure.

Do not take Avandamet if you have ever had an allergic reaction to rosiglitazone or metformin.

Do not take Avandamet if you have metabolic or diabetic ketoacidosis (a life-threatening medical emergency caused by insufficient insulin and marked by excessive thirst, nausea, fatigue, pain below the breastbone, and fruity breath).

You should not use Avandamet if you have type 1 (insulin-dependent) diabetes, or if you are already taking insulin.

Special warnings about this medication
Use Avandamet with caution if you have a problem with fluid retention or swelling. The drug has been known to cause this problem, which in turn can lead to heart failure. Also use caution if you're at risk for heart failure. Call the doctor immediately if you develop symptoms of heart failure such as a sudden weight change, fatigue, shortness of breath, or swelling of the ankles or legs.

Before you start therapy with Avandamet, and at least once a year thereafter, your doctor will do a complete assessment of your kidney function. If you develop kidney problems while on Avandamet, your doctor will discontinue this medication. If you are an older person, you will need to have your kidney function monitored more frequently, and your doctor may want to start you at a lower dosage.

Poor liver function could increase the risk of lactic acidosis. Therefore, your doctor will check to make sure your liver function is normal before prescribing Avandamet, then recheck it every 2 months for the first 12 months and periodically thereafter. Warning signs of liver damage include nausea, vomiting, abdominal pain, fatigue, loss of appetite, dark urine, and yellowing of the skin or whites of the eyes. If you develop any of these symptoms, tell your doctor immediately. You may need to discontinue treatment with Avandamet.

You should not take Avandamet for 2 days before and after having an X-ray procedure (such as an angiogram) that uses an injectable dye. Also, if you are going to have surgery, except minor surgery, you should stop taking Avandamet. Once you have resumed normal food and fluid intake, your doctor will tell you when you can start drug therapy again.

Avoid drinking too much alcohol while taking Avandamet. Heavy drinking increases the danger of lactic acidosis and can also trigger an attack of low blood sugar.

Avandamet occasionally causes a mild deficiency of vitamin B_{12}. Your doctor will check for this with yearly blood tests and may prescribe a supplement if necessary.

While taking Avandamet, you should check your blood or urine periodically for abnormal sugar levels. If you notice sudden changes after you've been stabilized for a while, tell your doctor immediately. It could be a sign you're developing lactic acidosis or ketoacidosis.

Avandamet does not usually cause hypoglycemia (low blood sugar). However, it remains a possibility, especially in older, weak, and undernourished people and those with kidney, liver, adrenal, or pituitary gland problems. The risk of low blood sugar increases when Avandamet is combined with other diabetes medications. The risk is also boosted by missed meals, alcohol, and excessive exercise. To avoid low blood sugar, you should closely follow the diet and exercise plan suggested by your doctor.

If your blood sugar becomes unstable due to the stress of a fever, injury, infection, or surgery, your doctor may temporarily take you off Avandamet and ask you to take insulin instead.

You should stop taking Avandamet if you become seriously dehydrated, since this increases the likelihood of developing lactic acidosis. Tell your doctor if you lose a significant amount of fluid due to vomiting, diarrhea, fever, or some other condition.

Avandamet could trigger ovulation in premenopausal women who have stopped ovulating. It is important for all women who do not wish to get pregnant to use adequate birth control while taking this drug.

Possible food and drug interactions when taking this medication

If Avandamet is taken with certain other drugs, the effects of either could be increased, decreased, or altered. It is especially important to check with your doctor before combining Avandamet with the following:

Amiloride (Moduretic)
Calcium channel blockers (heart medications) such as Calan, Isoptin, and Procardia
Cimetidine (Tagamet)
Decongestant, airway-opening drugs such as Sudafed and Ventolin

Digoxin (Lanoxin)
Estrogens such as Premarin
Furosemide (Lasix)
Isoniazid (Rifamate), a drug used for tuberculosis
Morphine
Niacin (Niaspan)
Nifedipine (Adalat, Procardia)
Oral contraceptives
Phenytoin (Dilantin)
Procainamide (Procanbid, Pronestyl)
Quinidine (Quinidex)
Quinine
Ranitidine (Zantac)
Steroids such as prednisone (Deltasone)
Thyroid hormones such as Synthroid
Tranquilizers such as Thorazine
Triamterene (Dyazide, Dyrenium)
Trimethoprim (Bactrim, Septra)
Vancomycin (Vancocin)
Water pills (diuretics) such as HydroDIURIL, Dyazide, and Moduretic

Do not drink too much alcohol, since excessive alcohol consumption can cause low blood sugar and increase the risk of developing lactic acidosis.

Special information if you are pregnant or breastfeeding

If you are pregnant or plan to become pregnant, tell your doctor immediately. Avandamet has not been adequately studied in pregnant women and should not be taken during pregnancy unless the potential benefit outweighs the potential risk. Since studies suggest the importance of maintaining normal blood sugar levels during pregnancy, your doctor may prescribe insulin injections instead.

It is not known whether Avandamet appears in human breast milk. Therefore, you should discuss with your doctor whether to discontinue the medication or to stop breastfeeding. If the medication is discontinued and if diet alone does not control your blood sugar levels, your doctor may prescribe insulin injections.

Recommended dosage

ADULTS

Your doctor will start therapy at a low dose and increase it until your blood sugar levels are under control.

For Patients Who Are Inadequately Controlled on Metformin Therapy Alone
The recommended daily starting dose is 4 milligrams of rosiglitazone plus the dose of metformin you are already taking.

*For Patients Who Are Inadequately Controlled on
Rosiglitazone Therapy Alone*
The recommended daily starting dose is 1,000 milligrams of metformin
plus the dose of rosiglitazone you are already taking.

*For Patients on Combination Therapy Taking Separate Doses
of Rosiglitazone and Metformin*
The usual starting dose of Avandamet is based on your current doses of
rosiglitazone and metformin.

*For Patients Who Need to Increase Their Current Dose
of Avandamet*
The daily dose of Avandamet may be increased by increments of 4 milligrams of rosiglitazone and/or 500 milligrams of metformin, up to a maximum daily dose of 8 milligrams of rosiglitazone and 2,000 milligrams of
metformin.

CHILDREN

Children should not take Avandamet, since the safety and effectiveness of
the drug have not been studied in this group.

Overdosage

An overdose of Avandamet can cause lactic acidosis (see *Most important
fact about this drug*). If you suspect an overdose, seek emergency treatment immediately.

AVANDIA

Pronounced: AH-van-DEE-ah
Generic name: Rosiglitazone maleate

Why is this drug prescribed?

Avandia is used to hold down blood sugar levels in people with type 2
diabetes (also known as *non-insulin-dependent* or *adult onset* diabetes).
   Blood sugar levels are ordinarily controlled by the body's natural supply of insulin, which helps sugar move out of the bloodstream and into
the cells. In type 2 diabetes, the buildup of sugar in the blood is often due
not to a lack of insulin, but to the body's inability to make proper use of it.
Avandia works first by decreasing sugar production, then by helping the
body make more efficient use of whatever insulin is available. It does not
increase the actual amount of insulin in circulation.
   Avandia is a new type of diabetes medication. It can be used alone or
in conjunction with insulin, metformin (Glucophage), or a member of the
sulfonylurea class of diabetes drugs (Diabinese, Micronase, Orinase). It
takes effect slowly. You may not see a reduction in blood sugar levels for
the first 2 weeks of therapy, and it may take 2 to 3 months for the medication to deliver maximum results.

Most important fact about this drug

Always remember that Avandia is an aid to, not a substitute for, good diet, weight loss, and exercise. Failure to follow a sound diet and exercise plan can lead to serious complications, such as dangerously high or low blood sugar levels. Remember, too, that Avandia is not an oral form of insulin, and cannot be used in place of insulin.

How should you take this medication?

Your dose of Avandia may be taken once a day in the morning or divided in half and taken in the morning and evening, with or without food.

■ *If you miss a dose...*
Take it as soon as you remember. If it is almost time for the next dose, skip the one you missed and go back to your regular schedule. Do not take 2 doses at once.

■ *Storage instructions...*
Store at room temperature in a tight, light-resistant container.

What side effects may occur?

Side effects cannot be anticipated. If any develop or change in intensity, inform your doctor as soon as possible. Only your doctor can determine if it is safe for you to continue taking Avandia.

■ *Side effects may include:*
Back pain, fatigue, headache, high blood sugar, low blood sugar, respiratory tract infections, sinus inflammation, swelling

Why should this drug not be prescribed?

Do not take Avandia if it has ever given you an allergic reaction.

Special warnings about this medication

If you have liver disease, you should not take Avandia. Your doctor will check to make sure your liver function is normal before prescribing Avandia, then recheck it every 2 months for the first 12 months and periodically thereafter. Warning signs of liver damage include nausea, vomiting, abdominal pain, fatigue, loss of appetite, and dark urine. If you develop any of these symptoms, tell your doctor immediately. You may need to discontinue treatment with Avandia.

People taking Avandia in combination with insulin or other diabetes drugs sometimes develop *low* blood sugar. If this happens, check with your doctor. The dosage of the other diabetes drug may have to be reduced.

People with kidney problems can take Avandia, but should not take Glucophage. If you have poor kidney function, you'll be unable to take advantage of this combination.

Avandia can increase the chances of conception. Be sure to use some form of birth control if you don't want a pregnancy.

Avandia won't help type 1 diabetics, who are unable to produce any insulin at all. Insulin shots are a necessity for this form of the illness. Nor can Avandia relieve diabetic ketoacidosis (excessively high sugar levels due to lack of insulin).

Use Avandia with caution if you have a problem with fluid retention or swelling. The drug has been known to cause this problem, which in turn can lead to heart failure or other heart problems. Avandia should be avoided by anyone who has been diagnosed with heart failure, and it should be discontinued by anyone who develops it. Make sure your doctor is aware of any heart problems you may have. Alert him immediately if you develop symptoms of heart failure such as fatigue and shortness of breath.

If you are being treated with Avandia and insulin, you will need to be monitored for heart problems. Notify your doctor if you develop any unusual swelling or a rapid weight increase.

You should be aware that people taking Avandia tend to gain a little weight, typically around 5 to 10 pounds. The cause is thought to be a combination of fluid retention and fat accumulation.

Avandia is not recommended for children under 18.

Possible food and drug interactions when taking this medication

No drug interactions with Avandia have been reported at this time.

Special information if you are pregnant or breastfeeding

It's important to maintain normal blood sugar levels while pregnant, but the safety of Avandia during pregnancy remains unproven. Since insulin shots are known to be safe, your doctor may switch you from Avandia to insulin until the baby is born.

It is not known whether Avandia appears in breast milk. Because many drugs do find their way into breast milk, however, the safest bet is to avoid taking Avandia while nursing.

Recommended dosage

ADULTS

The usual starting dose of Avandia either alone or in combination with insulin or another diabetes drug is 4 milligrams once a day or 2 milligrams twice a day. If your sugar levels remain too high after 12 weeks of treatment, the doctor may increase your dose to 8 milligrams once a day or 4 milligrams twice a day. However, the maximum recommended dose of Avandia in combination with insulin or a sulfonylurea diabetes drug is 4 milligrams per day. If you do develop low blood sugar, your insulin or sulfonylurea drug dosage will need to be decreased by your doctor.

Overdosage

Although there is no information on the potential results of Avandia overdose, any medication taken in excess can have serious consequences. If you suspect an overdose, seek medical attention immediately.

AVAPRO

Pronounced: AVE-ah-pro
Generic name: Irbesartan

Why is this drug prescribed?

Avapro is used to treat high blood pressure. A member of the new family of drugs called angiotensin II receptor antagonists, it works by preventing the hormone angiotensin II from narrowing the blood vessels, an action that tends to raise blood pressure. Avapro may be prescribed alone or with other blood pressure medications.

In people with type 2 diabetes and high blood pressure, Avapro is also prescribed to stave off damage to the kidneys, often delaying the need for dialysis and a kidney transplant.

Most important fact about this drug

You must take Avapro regularly for it to be effective. Since blood pressure declines gradually, it may be a couple of weeks before you get the full benefit of Avapro, and you must continue taking it even if you are feeling well. Avapro does not cure high blood pressure; it merely keeps it under control.

How should you take this medication?

Take your dose of Avapro around the same time every day, with or without food.

■ *If you miss a dose...*
Take it as soon as you remember. If it is almost time for your next dose, skip the one you missed and go back to your regular schedule. Do not take 2 doses at the same time.

■ *Storage instructions...*
Store at room temperature.

What side effects may occur?

Side effects cannot be anticipated. If any develop or change in intensity, tell your doctor as soon as possible. Only your doctor can determine if it is safe for you to continue taking Avapro.

■ *Side effects may include:*
Diarrhea, fatigue, respiratory tract infection
In people taking Avapro for diabetic kidney disease, the most common side effects are dizziness, dizziness when standing up, or low blood pressure when standing up.

Why should this drug not be prescribed?

If Avapro gives you an allergic reaction, you will not be able to use this drug.

Special warnings about this medication

In rare cases, Avapro can cause a severe drop in blood pressure. The problem is more likely if your body's supply of water has been depleted by dialysis treatments or high doses of diuretics. Symptoms include light-headedness, dizziness, and faintness, and are more likely when you first start taking the drug. Call your doctor if they occur. You may need to have your dose adjusted.

If you have kidney disease, Avapro must be used with caution.

Possible food and drug interactions when taking this medication

The chances of an interaction with Avapro are low. Check with your doctor, however, before combining it with tolbutamide (Orinase).

Special information if you are pregnant or breastfeeding

Avapro can cause injury or even death to the unborn child when used during the last 6 months of pregnancy. As soon as you learn you're pregnant, stop taking Avapro and call your doctor.

It is not known whether Avapro appears in breast milk, but because of potential risks to the newborn, it's considered best to avoid using the drug while breastfeeding. You and your doctor should decide whether you should give up breastfeeding or discontinue Avapro.

Recommended dosage

ADULTS

High Blood Pressure
The recommended starting dose of Avapro is 150 milligrams once a day. If your blood pressure remains elevated, your dose will be gradually increased to 300 milligrams once a day.

If you are being treated with hemodialysis or high doses of diuretics, you'll be started at a lower dose of 75 milligrams once a day.

Kidney Damage from Type 2 Diabetes
The usual dose is 300 milligrams once a day.

CHILDREN

For children under 6, safety and effectiveness have not been established. For children 6 to 12 years old, the typical starting dose is 75 milligrams once a day. If blood pressure is still too high, the dose may be increased to 150 milligrams once a day. Children 13 to 16 years old are usually given the adult dosage.

Overdosage

There has been little experience with overdosage of drugs such as Avapro. However, the most likely results would be low blood pressure and an abnormally slow or rapid heartbeat. If you suspect an overdose, seek medical attention immediately.

AVAR

Pronounced: AY-var
Generic ingredients: Sulfacetamide sodium and Sulfur

Why is this drug prescribed?

Avar is a gel used to treat the inflammation and skin eruptions associated with acne and rosacea. Avar Green is a tinted version of the gel that helps tone down redness. Avar can also be used to treat the dry, scaly skin known as seborrheic dermatitis.

Avar is intended for use on a daily basis. It may take several weeks to see an improvement in the skin.

Most important fact about this drug

Avar contains an ingredient similar to sulfa drugs such as Bactrim and Septra. On rare occasions these medications have caused severe allergic reactions. If you are allergic to any sulfa drug, you may also be allergic to Avar. In addition, if you have taken one of these medications in the past, you may have developed a hidden allergy to sulfa drugs that might show up when you use Avar. Notify your doctor immediately at the first sign of a severe reaction such as skin rash, sore throat, fever, joint pain, cough, shortness of breath, abnormal skin paleness, reddish or purplish skin spots, or yellowing of the skin or whites of the eyes.

How should you take this medication?

Apply a thin film to the skin, being careful to avoid the eyes. Wash your hands after each application.

If you have rosacea, be sure to avoid things that make your face turn red or flush. Typical offenders include hot or spicy foods, hot drinks such as tea or coffee, and alcohol. You should also avoid using cleansers and other facial products that contain alcohol or astringents.

■ *If you miss a dose...*
Take it as soon as you remember. If it is almost time for the next dose, skip the one you missed and go back to your regular schedule.
■ *Storage instructions...*
Store at room temperature. Do not allow the gel to freeze.

What side effects may occur?

Side effects cannot be anticipated. If any develop or change in intensity, inform your doctor as soon as possible. Only your doctor can determine if it is safe for you to continue using Avar.

■ *Side effects may include:*
Reddening of the skin, scaling skin, skin irritation

Why should this drug not be prescribed?

Do not use Avar if you are allergic to sulfa drugs (see *Most important fact about this drug*) or if you have kidney disease.

Special warnings about this medication

Inform your doctor if your skin becomes excessively red or irritated while using Avar.

Possible food and drug interactions when taking this medication

No interactions have been reported.

Special information if you are pregnant or breastfeeding

The effects of this medication during pregnancy and breastfeeding have not been adequately studied. If you are pregnant or plan to become pregnant, notify your doctor immediately. Small amounts of the drug could appear in breast milk. If you are nursing, use this medication with caution.

Recommended dosage

Apply a thin film of Avar gel to the affected areas 1 to 3 times daily, or as directed by your doctor.

Overdosage

An overdose is unlikely. However, if your skin becomes severely irritated, you should stop applying the medication and call your doctor.

AVELOX

Pronounced: AV-eh-locks
Generic name: Moxifloxacin hydrochloride

Why is this drug prescribed?

Avelox, an antibiotic, is prescribed to treat sinus and lung infections. It kills bacteria that can cause sinusitis, pneumonia, and secondary infections in chronic bronchitis. It also fights skin infections caused by staph or strep.

Avelox is a member of the quinolone family of antibiotics. Like all antibiotics, Avelox works only against bacteria. It will not cure an infection caused by a virus.

Most important fact about this drug

In rare cases, antibiotics can cause a serious allergic reaction. Stop taking Avelox and call your doctor immediately if you develop any of the following warning signs: skin rash, tingling, hives, shortness of breath, swelling of the face or throat, or difficulty swallowing.

How should you take this medication?

Avelox may be taken with or without food. Your doctor will prescribe Avelox only to treat a bacterial infection; it will not cure a viral infection, such as the common cold. It's important to take the full dosage schedule of Avelox, even if you're feeling better in a few days. Not completing the full dosage schedule may decrease the drug's effectiveness and increase the chances that the bacteria may become resistant to Avelox and similar antibiotics.

Be sure to drink plenty of fluids while taking Avelox.

■ *If you miss a dose...*
Take it as soon as you remember. If it is almost time for your next dose, skip the one you missed and go back to your regular schedule. Do not take a double dose in an effort to catch up.

■ *Storage instructions...*
Store Avelox at room temperature. Avoid high humidity.

What side effects may occur?

Most people taking Avelox do not experience side effects; and when reactions do occur, they are usually mild. If you do develop a side effect, however, inform your doctor as soon as possible. Only your doctor can determine if it is safe for you to continue taking Avelox.

■ *Side effects may include:*
Nausea, diarrhea, dizziness

Why should this drug not be prescribed?

If you have ever had an allergic reaction to any other quinolone antibiotic, such as Cipro, Floxin, Levaquin, Maxaquin, Noroxin, or Penetrex, you should not take Avelox.

Special warnings about this medication

Avelox may make you dizzy or light-headed. Do not drive a car, operate machinery, or engage in activities requiring mental alertness or coordination until you know how the drug affects you.

Avelox can cause certain heart irregularities in people already prone to the problem. If you are being treated for an abnormal heartbeat, make sure your doctor is aware of it. You may have to avoid Avelox. Also tell your doctor if you or anyone in your family has a history of heart problems. If you develop palpitations or fainting spells while taking Avelox, contact your doctor immediately.

Before you take Avelox, you should tell your doctor if you have a history of convulsions or blockage of the arteries in the brain. Quinolone-type antibiotics like Avelox have been known to cause convulsions and other problems with the nervous system, including symptoms such as agitation, anxiety, dizziness, confusion, depression, hallucinations, nervousness, nightmares, tremors, and suicidal thoughts. Contact your doctor immediately if you experience any of these reactions.

Avelox may cause Achilles and other tendon ruptures, especially in older adults and those taking steroids. If you experience pain or inflammation in a tendon, contact your doctor. Like other antibiotics, it can also cause serious intestinal inflammation. If you develop diarrhea, let your doctor know immediately.

Rare cases of peripheral neuropathy (changes or disturbances of the nervous system) have been reported with this type of antibiotic. Contact your doctor if you experience muscle weakness, paralysis, pain or numbness, a burning sensation, or a pins and needles sensation.

Avelox can make your skin more sensitive to light, so you should avoid excess sunlight and tanning beds.

You should avoid Avelox if you have a low level of potassium in your blood. Low potassium can be caused by the water pills (diuretics) often prescribed for high blood pressure. If you are taking a diuretic, make sure the doctor knows about it before you begin treatment with Avelox.

A case of diarrhea during Avelox therapy could signal development of a potentially dangerous bowel inflammation. Call your doctor for treatment at the first sign of a problem.

Avelox has not been tested in children under 18.

Possible food and drug interactions when taking this medication

Multivitamins containing iron or zinc; antacids containing magnesium, calcium, or aluminum; Carafate (sucralfate); and Videx (didanosine) reduce the effectiveness of Avelox. Take it at least 4 hours before or 8 hours after any of these products.

Do not take Avelox with nonsteroidal anti-inflammatory drugs (NSAIDs) such as Advil, Motrin, and Naprosyn because it may increase the risk of nerve stimulation and convulsions.

Other drugs to use cautiously while taking Avelox include:

Amiodarone (Cordarone)
Antipsychotic drugs such as Haldol, Stelazine, and Thorazine
Erythromycin (E-Mycin, Erythrocin)
Procainamide (Procan SR)
Quinidine (Quinidex)
Sotalol (Betapace)
Tricyclic antidepressants such as Elavil, Norpramin, and Triavil
Warfarin (Coumadin)

You also should avoid Avelox if the amount of potassium in your blood is low. Low potassium can sometimes be caused by diuretic medications such as Lasix. If you are taking a diuretic medicine, tell your doctor before taking Avelox. In fact, inform your doctor of all medications you are taking, including over-the-counter remedies.

Special information if you are pregnant or breastfeeding

The effects of Avelox during pregnancy have not been studied. It should be used during pregnancy only if the benefits outweigh the possible risk to the unborn baby. If you are expecting, make sure the doctor is aware of it before you start taking this drug.

Avelox may appear in breast milk and could affect a nursing infant. If this medication is essential to your health, your doctor may advise you to discontinue breastfeeding until your treatment is finished.

Recommended dosage

ADULTS

Acute Bacterial Sinusitis
The usual dose is one 400-milligram tablet daily for 7 to 14 days.

Acute Bacterial Infection with Chronic Bronchitis
The usual dose is one 400-milligram tablet daily for 5 days.

Pneumonia
The usual dose is one 400-milligram tablet daily for 7 to 14 days.

Skin Infections
The usual dose is one 400-milligram tablet daily for 7 days.

Overdosage

Any medication taken in excess can have serious consequences. If you suspect an overdose, seek medical attention immediately.

■ *Symptoms of Avelox overdose may include:*
Convulsions, decreased activity, diarrhea, sleepiness, tremors, vomiting

Aventyl *See Pamelor, page 1026.*

Avita *See Retin-A and Renova, page 1242.*

AVODART

Pronounced: AVE-oh-dart
Generic name: Dutasteride

Why is this drug prescribed?

Avodart is used to treat prostate enlargement, a condition that is medically known as benign prostatic hyperplasia, or BPH.

The prostate is a chestnut-shaped gland that is part of the male reproductive system. It produces a liquid that forms part of the semen. This gland completely encloses the upper part of the urethra, the tube through which urine flows out of the bladder. Many men over age 50 suffer from a benign (noncancerous) enlargement of the prostate. The enlarged gland squeezes the urethra, obstructing the normal flow of urine. Resulting problems may include difficulty in starting urination, weak flow of urine, and the need to urinate urgently or more frequently. Sometimes surgical removal of the prostate is necessary.

By shrinking the enlarged prostate, Avodart may alleviate the various urinary symptoms, making surgery unnecessary. You will need to see your doctor for periodic examinations to assess your response to treatment. It may take several months before you notice an improvement in symptoms.

Most important fact about this drug

Avodart can be absorbed through the skin. Because the drug could affect a developing baby, pregnant women, women who may become pregnant, and breastfeeding women should strictly avoid skin contact with the drug.

How should you take this medication?

Take 1 capsule once a day. The capsule should be swallowed whole and can be taken with or without meals.

■ *If you miss a dose...*
  If you miss a dose, take it as soon as you remember. If it is almost time for your next dose, skip the one you missed and go back to your regular schedule. Do not take 2 doses at once.
■ *Storage instructions...*
  Store at room temperature.

What side effects may occur?

Side effects cannot be anticipated. If any develop or change in intensity, inform your doctor as soon as possible. Only your doctor can determine if it is safe for you to continue taking Avodart.

■ *Side effects may include:*
  Breast tenderness, decreased sex drive, ejaculation problems, enlarged breasts in males, impotence

Why should this drug not be prescribed?

You should not take Avodart if you have ever had an allergic reaction to it or to similar drugs such as finasteride (Proscar).
  Women and children should not use Avodart.

Special warnings about this medication

If a pregnant or breastfeeding woman is exposed to Avodart, the drug may harm the developing baby (see *Special information if you are pregnant or breastfeeding*).

You should not donate blood while taking Avodart or for 6 months after stopping treatment to avoid exposing pregnant or breastfeeding women to blood that contains the drug.

Possible food and drug interactions when taking this medication

If Avodart is taken with certain other drugs, the effects of either could be increased, decreased, or altered. Check with your doctor before combining Avodart with other medication.

Use Avodart cautiously if you're taking HIV drugs such as ritonavir (Norvir), since there is a theoretical chance of an interaction.

Special information if you are pregnant or breastfeeding

Because Avodart can be absorbed through the skin, pregnant women, women who may become pregnant, and breastfeeding women should strictly avoid skin contact with the drug. If Avodart is accidentally absorbed by a pregnant woman who is carrying a male fetus, the drug could cause abnormal development of the baby's genital organs. Because it's not known if Avodart appears in breast milk, breastfeeding women must also avoid handling the drug.

Recommended dosage

ADULT MEN

Take one 0.5-milligram capsule once a day. The capsule should be swallowed whole.

Avodart has not been evaluated for use in children under 18.

Overdosage

Any medication taken in excess can have serious consequences. If you suspect an overdose, seek medical attention immediately.

AXERT

Pronounced: AKS-ert
Generic name: Almotriptan

Why is this drug prescribed?

Axert is a migraine treatment. It relieves the type of migraine that's accompanied by an aura (a set of symptoms that includes visual disturbances, speech difficulties, tingling, numbness, and weakness), as well as the kind that lacks an aura.

Axert is a member of a family of drugs called selective serotonin receptor agonists. These medications are thought to work by stopping abnormal dilation of blood vessels in the head, fighting inflammation, and reducing pain transmissions along certain nerve pathways near the brain.

Axert relieves migraines already in progress, but it won't prevent them from starting. It has not been tested for other types of headache, such as cluster headache, and should be used only for migraine attacks.

Most important fact about this drug

In people with heart disease, this type of drug has been known to trigger irregular heartbeat and heart attacks, sometimes leading to death. Do not take this medication if you have angina, a history of heart attack, or any other serious heart problem.

How should you take this medication?

Take one Axert tablet when a migraine begins. If the headache comes back, consult your doctor. You may be able to take a second dose 2 hours after the first one. Do not take more than 2 tablets in 24 hours.

■ *If you miss a dose...*
Axert should be used only when needed. Do not take it on a regular basis.
■ *Storage instructions...*
Axert should be stored at room temperature.

What side effects may occur?

Side effects cannot be anticipated. If any develop or change in intensity, inform your doctor as soon as possible. Only your doctor can determine if it is safe for you to continue taking Axert.

■ *Side effects may include:*
Dry mouth, headache, nausea, sleepiness, tingling or burning feeling

Why should this drug not be prescribed?

Do not take Axert if you have a history of heart attack, chest pain (angina), or any other condition that diminishes the supply of blood to the muscle of the heart. Axert could cause the coronary arteries to constrict, triggering an attack.

Do not use Axert if you have uncontrolled high blood pressure. The drug could cause your pressure to rise.

Do not use Axert within 24 hours of taking another serotonin agonist drug such as naratriptan (Amerge), rizatriptan (Maxalt), sumatriptan (Imitrex), or zolmitriptan (Zomig).

Also avoid Axert within 24 hours of taking an ergot-based drug such as ergotamine (Cafergot, Ergomar, Wigraine), dihydroergotamine (D.H.E. 45, Migranal), or methylsergide (Sansert).

Ask your doctor what kind of migraine headache you have. If it is categorized as hemiplegic or basilar migraine, you should not take Axert.

If Axert gives you an allergic reaction, you will not be able to use this drug.

Special warnings about this medication

Some patients taking serotonin agonists have suffered strokes, though it's unclear whether the drug was at fault. If you've ever had a stroke or mini-stroke, make sure the doctor is aware of it.

Symptoms such as tightness, pain, pressure, or a heavy feeling in the chest, throat, neck, or jaw may occur after taking Axert. If you develop any of these symptoms, or develop circulatory problems such as pale or blue fingers, notify your doctor. You will probably need to have a complete cardiac exam.

Let your doctor know if you have liver or kidney problems. Axert should be used with caution.

Axert is not for children under 18 years of age.

Possible food and drug interactions when taking this medication

Remember that Axert must never be used within 24 hours of taking another drug in its class, including Amerge, Maxalt, Imitrex, and Zomig. You should also avoid taking Axert within 24 hours of an ergot-based migraine remedy such as Cafergot, D.H.E. 45, Ergomar, Migranal, Sansert, or Wigraine.

If Axert is taken with certain other drugs, the effects of either could be increased, decreased, or altered. It is especially important to check with your doctor before combining Axert with any of the following:

Antidepressants that boost serotonin levels, including Luvox, Paxil, Prozac, and Zoloft
Erythromycin (E.E.S, E-Mycin, Ery-Tab, PCE)
Itraconazole (Sporanox)
Ketoconazole (Nizoral)
Ritonavir (Norvir)

Special information if you are pregnant or breastfeeding

Axert has not been studied in pregnant women. Consult your doctor if you are pregnant or plan to become pregnant. It is not known whether Axert appears in breast milk. If you are breastfeeding, caution is advised.

Recommended dosage

ADULTS

Take one tablet (either 6.25 or 12.5 milligrams) at the onset of the headache. If the headache returns, a second dose can be taken 2 hours later with your doctor's approval. Do not take more than 2 doses in 24 hours.

Inform your doctor if you experience more than 4 headaches in a 1-month period.

If you have liver or kidney problems, you should use the 6.25-milligram tablets and should not exceed 12.5 milligrams per day.

Overdosage

Little is known about Axert overdose, but the most likely results would be a rise in blood pressure and other heart and circulatory problems. If you suspect an overdose, seek medical attention immediately.

AXID

Pronounced: AK-sid
Generic name: Nizatidine

Why is this drug prescribed?

Axid is prescribed for the treatment of duodenal ulcers and noncancerous stomach ulcers. Full-dose therapy for these problems lasts no longer than 8 weeks. However, your doctor may prescribe Axid at a reduced dosage after a duodenal ulcer has healed. The drug is also prescribed for the heartburn and the inflammation that result when acid stomach contents flow backward into the esophagus. Axid belongs to a class of drugs known as histamine H_2 blockers.

Most important fact about this drug

Although Axid can be used for up to 8 to 12 weeks, most ulcers are healed within 4 weeks of therapy.

How should you take this medication?

Take this medication exactly as prescribed by your doctor.

■ *If you miss a dose...*
Take it as soon as you remember. If it is almost time for your next dose, skip the one you missed and go back to your regular schedule. Do not take 2 doses at once.
■ *Storage instructions...*
Store at room temperature.

What side effects may occur?

Side effects cannot be anticipated. If any develop or change in intensity, inform your doctor as soon as possible. Only your doctor can determine if it is safe for you to continue taking Axid.

■ *Side effects may include:*
Abdominal pain, diarrhea, dizziness, gas, headache, indigestion, inflammation of the nose, nausea, pain, sore throat, vomiting, weakness

Why should this drug not be prescribed?

If you are sensitive to or have ever had an allergic reaction to Axid or similar drugs such as Zantac, you should not take this medication. Make sure your doctor is aware of any drug reactions you have experienced.

Special warnings about this medication

Axid could mask a stomach malignancy. If you continue to have any problems, notify your doctor.

If you have moderate to severe kidney disease, your doctor will reduce your dosage.

Possible food and drug interactions when taking this medication

If Axid is taken with certain other drugs, the effects of either could be increased, decreased, or altered. It is especially important to check with your doctor before combining Axid with aspirin, especially in high doses.

Special information if you are pregnant or breastfeeding

The effects of Axid during pregnancy have not been adequately studied. If you are pregnant or plan to become pregnant, inform your doctor immediately. Axid appears in breast milk and could affect a nursing infant. If this medication is essential to your health, your doctor may advise you to discontinue breastfeeding until your treatment with this medication is finished.

Recommended dosage

ADULTS

Active Duodenal Ulcer
The usual dose is 300 milligrams once a day at bedtime, but your doctor may have you take 150 milligrams twice a day.

Active Noncancerous Stomach Ulcer
The usual dose is 150 milligrams twice a day or 300 milligrams once a day at bedtime.

Maintenance of a Healed Duodenal Ulcer
The usual dose is 150 milligrams once a day at bedtime.

If you have moderate to severe kidney disease, your doctor will prescribe a lower dose.

CHILDREN

The safety and effectiveness of Axid have not been established in children.

Overdosage

No specific information on Axid overdose is available. However, any medication taken in excess can have serious consequences. If you suspect an overdose of Axid, seek medical attention immediately.

AYGESTIN

Pronounced: Eye-JES-tin
Generic name: Norethindrone acetate

Why is this drug prescribed?

Aygestin contains a type of hormone known as progesterone. It is used to restore menstruation in women who have stopped having menstrual cycles (also called amenorrhea). Aygestin can also help treat endometriosis, a condition where the endometrium (the lining of the uterus) doesn't shed properly and attaches to the outside of the uterus or other areas such as the ovaries or bowels. Aygestin also helps control unusual and heavy bleeding of the uterus caused by hormonal imbalance. However, the drug is not used to control bleeding caused by fibroids or cancer.

Most important fact about this drug

Aygestin increases the risk of blood clots, which can lead to phlebitis, breathing problems, vision problems, or stroke. If you experience any symptoms that might suggest the onset of a clot-related disorder—pain with swelling, warmth and redness in a leg vein, coughing or shortness of breath, loss of vision or double vision, migraine, or weakness or numbness in an arm or leg—stop taking Aygestin and see your doctor immediately.

How should you take this medication?

Take Aygestin as directed by your doctor.

- *If you miss a dose...*
  Take it as soon as you remember. If it is almost time for your next dose, skip the one you missed and go back to your regular schedule. Never take 2 doses at the same time.
- *Storage instructions...*
  Store at room temperature in a tightly closed container.

What side effects may occur?

All progesterone drugs are associated with certain side effects, none of which can be anticipated. If any side effects develop or change in intensity, inform your doctor as soon as possible. Only your doctor can determine whether it is safe for you to continue taking Aygestin. bulging eye, depression, double vision, cervical changes or secretions, change in menstrual flow, headache, hives, inflammation of the optic nerve, insomnia, menstrual spotting, migraine, mood swings, nausea, rash with or without itchy spots, skin discoloration, stopping of menstrual flow, swelling, vision loss, weight increase or decrease, yellowing of the skin or eyes

■ *Side effects caused by progesterone drugs may include:*
Acne, allergic reaction, blood clots in the arteries, veins, eyes, or lungs, breakthrough menstrual bleeding, breast enlargement or tenderness, bulging eye, depression, double vision, cervical changes or secretions, change in menstrual flow, headache, hives, inflammation of the optic nerve, insomnia, menstrual spotting, migraine, mood swings, nausea, rash with or without itchy spots, skin discoloration, stopping of menstrual flow, swelling, vision loss, weight increase or decrease, yellowing of the skin or eyes

■ *Side effects caused by estrogen/progesterone combinations may include:*
Appetite changes, backache, blood pressure increase, bull's-eye rash, changes in appetite, changes in sex drive, dizziness, fatigue, hair growth or loss, headache, inflammation of the urinary tract, itching, nervousness, red or tender skin nodules, skin bruising, symptoms similar to premenstrual syndrome

Why should this drug not be prescribed?

Do not take Aygestin if you have ever had an allergic reaction to it.

Do not take Aygestin if you are pregnant or have had an incomplete miscarriage. Avoid it if you have ever had a blood clotting disorder or a stroke. Do not take this drug if you have breast cancer, unexplained vaginal bleeding, or severe liver disease.

Aygestin should not be used to test for pregnancy.

Special warnings about this medication

Remember that Aygestin can cause clot-related disorders. Check with your doctor immediately if you experience any of the warning signs listed in *Most important fact about this drug.*

To rule out cancer and other problems before you start taking Aygestin, your doctor will give you a complete physical exam, including examination of your breasts and pelvic organs. You also should have a Pap test (cervical smear).

Aygestin may cause some degree of fluid retention. If you have a medical condition that could be made worse by fluid retention—such as epilepsy, migraine, asthma, or a heart or kidney problem—make sure your doctor knows about it.

Be sure to tell your doctor if you experience any irregular or unexplained vaginal bleeding while taking this medication.

Aygestin makes some women depressed. If you've suffered from serious depression in the past, alert your doctor if you think you're having a relapse. You will probably need to stop taking Aygestin.

The long-term effects of drugs such as Aygestin on the function of certain organs—including the pituitary, ovaries, adrenal glands, liver, and uterus—are unknown.

Aygestin may affect cholesterol and blood sugar levels. If you have diabetes or high cholesterol, your doctor will want to watch you closely while you are taking this drug.

Aygestin may mask the onset of menopause. However, women who are of menopausal age are still eligible to take the drug.

If you're being screened for cancer, make sure the doctor or lab technician knows you are taking Aygestin.

Possible food and drug interactions when taking this medication

If Aygestin is taken with certain other drugs, the effects of either could be increased, decreased, or altered. Make sure your doctor knows about all the prescription and over-the-counter drugs you are taking.

In general, when you are taking a progesterone drug such as Aygestin, it is especially important to check with your doctor before taking the following:

Aminoglutethimide (Cytadren)
Carbamazepine (Tegretol)
Phenobarbital
Phenytoin (Dilantin)
Rifabutin (Mycobutin)
Rifampin (Rifadin, Rimactane)

Special information if you are pregnant or breastfeeding

Do not take Aygestin if you are pregnant or trying to become pregnant, since the drug may cause harm to a developing baby.

Aygestin appears in breast milk. Because the effect of Aygestin on a nursing infant is unknown, it is best to avoid the drug while breastfeeding unless it's clearly necessary.

Recommended dosage

To Prevent Abnormal Uterine Bleeding Due to Hormonal Imbalance or to Restore Menstrual Periods

The usual dose is 2.5 to 10 milligrams a day taken for 5 to 10 days during the second half of a 28-day cycle. Your period should start 3 to 7 days after you stop taking Aygestin.

To Treat Endometriosis

The recommended starting dose is 5 milligrams a day for 2 weeks. The doctor may increase your dose by 2.5 milligrams a day every 2 weeks up to a maximum of 15 milligrams a day. Treatment may continue for 6 to 9 months or until intolerable breakthrough bleeding occurs.

Overdosage

Although no specific information is available on Aygestin overdose, any medication taken in excess can have serious consequences. If you suspect an overdose, seek medical attention immediately.

Azatadine with Pseudoephedrine See *Trinalin, page 1502*.

Azelaic acid for acne See *Azelex, below*.

Azelaic acid for rosacea See *Finacea, page 564*.

Azelastine eyedrops See *Optivar, page 999*.

Azelastine nasal spray See *Astelin, page 135*.

AZELEX

Pronounced: AY-zuh-lecks
Generic name: Azelaic acid
Other brand names: Finevin

Why is this drug prescribed?

Azelex is a cream used to help clear up mild to moderate acne. The skin eruptions and inflammation of acne typically begin during puberty, when oily secretions undergo an increase.

Most important fact about this drug

You should keep using Azelex regularly, even if you see no immediate improvement. It takes up to 4 weeks for Azelex to show results.

How should you use this medication?

Use Azelex once in the morning and again in the evening. Wash the areas to be treated and pat dry. Apply a thin film of the medication and gently but thoroughly massage it into the skin. Wash your hands afterwards.

Do not put bandages or dressings over the treated areas. Avoid getting the medication into the eyes, mouth, or nose. If any of it does get into your eyes, wash it out with large amounts of water. Call your doctor if your eyes remain irritated.

■ *If you miss a dose...*
Apply it as soon as you remember. If it is almost time for the next dose, skip the one you missed and go back to your regular schedule.

■ *Storage instructions...*
Store at room temperature. Protect the cream from freezing.

What side effects may occur?

Side effects cannot be anticipated. If any develop or change in intensity, inform your doctor as soon as possible. Only your doctor can determine if it is safe for you to continue using this medication.

■ *Side effects may include:*
Burning, itching, stinging, tingling

Why should this drug not be prescribed?

Do not use this medication if it causes an allergic reaction.

Special warnings about this medication

Azelex may cause some itching, burning, or stinging when you first begin treatment. You can expect this to stop as treatment continues. If it doesn't, you should check with your doctor. You may have to cut back to a single application daily, or even temporarily stop using this medication.

Azelex has been known to occasionally have a bleaching effect on the skin. Report any abnormal changes in skin color to your doctor.

Possible food and drug interactions when using this medication

No interactions have been reported.

Special information if you are pregnant or breastfeeding

The effects of Azelex during pregnancy and breastfeeding have not been adequately studied. If you are pregnant or plan to become pregnant, notify your doctor immediately. Small amounts of Azelex could appear in breast milk. If you are nursing, use this medication with caution.

Recommended dosage

The usual dose is a thin film of Azelex applied twice a day.

Overdosage

An overdose is unlikely. However, if your skin becomes severely irritated, you should stop applying the medication and call your doctor.

Azithromycin See Zithromax, page 1635.

AZMACORT

Pronounced: AZ-ma-court
Generic name: Triamcinolone acetonide
Other brand names: Nasacort, Nasacort AQ

Why is this drug prescribed?

Azmacort and Nasacort are metered-dose inhalers containing the anti-inflammatory steroid medication triamcinolone acetonide; Nasacort AQ is a metered-dose pump spray. Azmacort is used as long-term therapy to control bronchial asthma attacks. Nasacort and Nasacort AQ are prescribed to relieve the symptoms of hay fever and other nasal allergies. Nasacort is also used in the treatment of nasal polyps (projecting masses of tissue in the nose).

Most important fact about this drug
Azmacort does not provide rapid relief in an asthma attack. Instead, it reduces the frequency and severity of attacks when taken on a regular basis. For quick relief, you must still use airway-opening medications.

How should you take this medication?
Take these drugs on a regular daily basis, exactly as prescribed. With Azmacort and Nasacort, you should begin to see improvement after a week, although it may take 2 weeks or more to achieve the greatest benefit. Nasacort AQ should begin to produce results on the first day, but will take a week to yield maximum benefit.

Shake the canister or bottle before each use. The Azmacort inhaler must be primed with 2 activations whenever it has been unused for more than 3 days. Do not use an Azmacort inhaler more than 240 times. Discard the Nasacort canister after 100 inhalations and the Nasacort AQ bottle after 120 actuations.

If the drug irritates your throat, gargling and rinsing your mouth with water after each dose can help to relieve the problem.

If you are using a bronchodilator inhalant, it should be used before the Azmacort inhalant to derive the best effects from this drug. Use of the two inhalers should be separated by several minutes.

Do not spray Nasacort directly onto the bone that separates the nostrils. Avoid spraying either medication in your eyes.

Illustrated instructions for use are available with the product.

■ *If you miss a dose...*
Use it as soon as you remember. If it is almost time for your next dose, skip the one you missed and go back to your regular schedule. Do not take 2 doses at once.

■ *Storage instructions...*
Store at room temperature. Since the contents of the aerosol inhalant are under pressure, do not puncture the container and do not use or store the medication near heat or open flame. Exposure to temperatures above 120 degrees Fahrenheit may cause the container to explode.

What side effects may occur?
Side effects cannot be anticipated. If any develop or change in intensity, inform your doctor as soon as possible. Only your doctor can determine if it is safe for you to continue taking these medications.

AZMACORT

■ *Side effects of Azmacort may include:*
Back pain, flu symptoms, headache, sinus inflammation, sore throat

NASACORT

- ■ *Side effects of Nasacort may include:*
  Headache
- ■ *Side effects of Nasacort in children aged 6 to 11 may include:*
  Cough, ear inflammation, fever, indigestion, nausea, nosebleed, throat discomfort

NASACORT AQ

- ■ *Side effects of Nasacort AQ may include:*
  Headache, nosebleed, stuffy nose
- ■ *Side effects of Nasacort AQ in children aged 6 to 11 may include:*
  Asthma, headache, infection, earache, sinus problems, vomiting

Why should this drug not be prescribed?
Do not use any of these medications if you are allergic to or sensitive to any of the ingredients. Do not use Azmacort if:

- ■ Your asthma can be controlled with airway openers and other non-steroid medications.
- ■ You require only occasional steroid treatment for asthma. (Azmacort is not for treatment of prolonged, severe asthma attacks where fast-acting measures are required.)
- ■ You have bronchitis not associated with asthma.

Special warnings about this medication
Your doctor will see that your asthma is reasonably under control before starting you on Azmacort. For about a week, he or she will have you take Azmacort along with your usual dose of oral steroid. After that, you will gradually take less and less of the oral drug. If you develop joint or muscular pain, weariness, and depression, contact your doctor immediately. If you feel light-headed or find that you are losing weight, also tell your doctor.

If you are using Azmacort and your airway-opening medication is not effective during an asthma attack, contact your doctor immediately. Also get medical help immediately if your wheezing gets worse after a dose of Azmacort.

The use of triamcinolone acetonide may cause a yeast-like fungal infection in the mouth and throat (Azmacort) or nose and throat (Nasacort and Nasacort AQ). If you suspect a fungal infection, notify your doctor. Treatment with antifungal medication may be necessary.

People using steroid medications such as these are more susceptible to infection. Chickenpox and measles, for example, can be far more serious for children and for adults who have not had them. Try to avoid exposure, but if you are exposed, inform your doctor. Medication may be needed.

Switching from steroid tablet therapy to Azmacort Inhaler may allow allergic conditions to surface that were previously controlled by the tablets. These include rhinitis (inflammation of the inside of the nose), conjunctivitis (pinkeye), and eczema.

If your child is using any of these medications, your doctor will watch to be sure he or she is growing properly. If you have just had an operation, or if you are experiencing extreme stress, your doctor will watch you closely.

Use these medications with extreme caution if you have tuberculosis, an untreated infection, or a herpes infection of the eye.

If your symptoms do not improve after 3 weeks, or if they get worse, contact your doctor. If you are using Nasacort or Nasacort AQ, also notify your doctor if you develop nosebleeds or notice nasal irritation, burning, or stinging after using the medication.

Use Nasacort or Nasacort AQ with caution if you have not fully healed from nasal ulcers, or an injury to your nose. Steroids can slow wound healing, and there have been rare cases of perforation inside the nose caused by inhaled steroids.

Possible food and drug interactions while taking this medication

Inhaled steroids such as Azmacort, Nasacort, and Nasacort AQ are not recommended for long-term use while you are taking prednisone (Deltasone).

Special information if you are pregnant or breastfeeding

The effects of triamcinolone acetonide during pregnancy have not been adequately studied. If you are pregnant or plan to become pregnant, inform your doctor immediately. It is not known whether triamcinolone acetonide appears in breast milk. If this medication is essential to your health, your doctor may advise you to discontinue breastfeeding until your treatment with this medication is finished.

Recommended dosage

AZMACORT

The Azmacort Inhaler unit is for oral inhalation only.

Adults
The usual dose is 2 inhalations (about 200 micrograms), taken 3 or 4 times a day or 4 inhalations taken twice a day. The daily dose should not exceed 16 inhalations.

Children 6 to 12 Years of Age
The usual dose is 1 or 2 inhalations (100 to 200 micrograms), taken 3 or 4 times a day or 2 to 4 inhalations taken twice a day. The daily dose should not exceed 12 inhalations.

Children Under 6 Years of Age
The safety and effectiveness of Azmacort have not been established in children under 6 years of age.

NASACORT

Adults and Children Aged 12 and Older
The usual starting dose is 220 micrograms a day, taken as 2 sprays in each nostril once a day. (One spray is 55 micrograms.) If necessary, your doctor may increase the dose up to 440 micrograms a day, taken all at once, twice a day, or 4 times a day. Once Nasacort has started to work, your doctor may decrease the dose to 110 micrograms a day.

Children 6 to 11 Years of Age
The usual starting dose is 2 sprays in each nostril once a day, for a total of 220 micrograms a day. Your doctor will adjust the dose to best suit the child.

Children Under 6 Years of Age
The safety and effectiveness of Nasacort in children under 6 years of age have not been established.

NASACORT AQ

Adults and Children Aged 12 and Older
The usual starting dose is 220 micrograms, taken as 2 sprays in each nostril once a day. Once your symptoms are under control, your doctor may reduce the dose to 110 micrograms a day.

Children 6 to 12 Years of Age
The recommended starting dose is 110 micrograms per day, taken as 1 spray in each nostril once a day. The maximum dose is 220 micrograms per day taken as 2 sprays in each nostril once a day.

Children Under 6 Years of Age
The safety and effectiveness of Nasacort AQ have not been established in children under 6 years of age.

Overdosage
Any medication taken in excess can have serious consequences. If you suspect an overdose, seek emergency medical treatment immediately.

An overdose is likely to be signaled by an increase in side effects. Accidental contact with the contents of the canister would most likely irritate your nose and give you a headache.

Overuse of Nasacort AQ may upset your stomach and intestines.

Continual overuse of Azmacort inhalation aerosol could lower your resistance; cause weakness; wasting, or swelling; and interfere with healing.

AZULFIDINE

Pronounced: A-ZUL-fi-deen
Generic name: Sulfasalazine

Why is this drug prescribed?

Azulfidine, an anti-inflammatory medicine, is prescribed for the treatment of mild to moderate ulcerative colitis (a long-term, progressive bowel disease) and as an added treatment in severe ulcerative colitis (chronic inflammation and ulceration of the lining of large bowel and rectum, the main symptom of which is bloody diarrhea). This medication is also prescribed to decrease severe attacks of ulcerative colitis.

Azulfidine EN-tabs are prescribed for people with ulcerative colitis who cannot take the regular Azulfidine tablet because of symptoms of stomach and intestinal irritation such as nausea and vomiting when taking the first few doses of the drug, or for those in whom a reduction in dosage does not lessen the stomach or intestinal side effects. The EN-tabs are also prescribed for adults and children with rheumatoid arthritis who fail to get relief from salicylates (such as aspirin) or other nonsteroidal anti-inflammatory drugs (such as ibuprofen).

Most important fact about this drug

Although ulcerative colitis rarely disappears completely, the risk of recurrence can be substantially reduced by the continued use of this drug.

How should you take this medication?

Take this medication in evenly spaced, equal doses, as determined by your doctor, preferably after meals or with food to avoid stomach upset. Swallow Azulfidine EN-tabs whole.

It is important that you drink plenty of fluids while taking this medication to avoid kidney stones.

If you are taking Azulfidine EN-tabs for rheumatoid arthritis, it may take up to 12 weeks for relief to occur.

■ *If you miss a dose...*
Take it as soon as you remember. If it is almost time for your next dose, skip the one you missed and go back to your regular schedule. Do not take 2 doses at once.
■ *Storage instructions...*
Store at room temperature.

What side effects may occur?

Side effects cannot be anticipated. If any develop or change in intensity, inform your doctor as soon as possible. Only your doctor can determine if it is safe for you to continue taking Azulfidine.

■ *Side effects may include:*
Abdominal pain, anemia, bluish skin, fever, headache, hives, inflammation of the mouth, itching, lack of appetite, nausea, rash, stomach distress, vomiting

Why should this drug not be prescribed?

If you are sensitive to or have ever had an allergic reaction to Azulfidine, salicylates (aspirin), or other sulfa drugs, you should not take this medication. Make sure your doctor is aware of any drug reactions you have experienced.

Unless you are directed to do so by your doctor, do not take Azulfidine if you have an intestinal or urinary obstruction or if you have porphyria (an inherited disorder involving the substance that gives color to the skin and iris of the eyes).

Special warnings about this medication

If you have kidney or liver damage or any blood disease, your doctor will check you very carefully before prescribing Azulfidine. Deaths have been reported from allergic reactions, blood diseases, kidney or liver damage, changes in nerve and muscle impulses, and fibrosing alveolitis (inflammation of the lungs due to a thickening or scarring of tissue). Signs such as sore throat, fever, abnormal paleness of the skin, purple or red spots on the skin, or jaundice (yellowing of the skin) may be an indication of a serious blood disorder. Your doctor will do frequent blood counts and urine tests. Use caution taking Azulfidine if you have a severe allergy or bronchial asthma.

If you develop loss of appetite, nausea, or vomiting, report it immediately. The doctor may need to adjust your dosage or change the prescription.

If Azulfidine EN-tabs are eliminated undisintegrated, stop taking the drug and notify your doctor immediately. (You may lack the intestinal enzymes necessary to dissolve this medication.)

Men taking Azulfidine may experience temporary infertility and a low sperm count.

Skin and urine may become yellow-orange in color while you are taking Azulfidine.

In addition, prolonged exposure to the sun should be avoided.

This drug is generally not prescribed for children under 6. Azulfidine EN-tabs are not recommended for children with the type of juvenile rheumatoid arthritis that affects the whole system, only for children with the type that stays in the joints.

Possible food and drug interactions when taking this medication

If Azulfidine is taken with certain other drugs, the effects of either could be increased, decreased, or altered. It is especially important to check with your doctor before combining Azulfidine with the following:

Digoxin (Lanoxin)
Folic acid (a B-complex vitamin)
Methotrexate (Rheumatrex)

Special information if you are pregnant or breastfeeding

The effects of Azulfidine during pregnancy have not been adequately studied. If you are pregnant or plan to become pregnant, inform your doctor immediately. Azulfidine is secreted in breast milk and could affect a nursing infant. If this medication is essential to your health, your doctor may advise you to discontinue breastfeeding until your treatment is finished.

Recommended dosage

Your doctor will carefully individualize your dosage and monitor your response periodically.

ULCERATIVE COLITIS

Adults

The usual recommended initial dose of Azulfidine and Azulfidine EN-tabs is 3 to 4 grams daily, divided into smaller doses (intervals between nighttime doses should not exceed 8 hours). In some cases the initial dosage is set at 1 to 2 grams daily to lessen side effects. As therapy continues, the dose is usually reduced to 2 grams daily.

Children Aged 6 and Older

The usual recommended initial dose is 40 to 60 milligrams per 2.2 pounds of body weight in each 24-hour period, divided into 3 to 6 doses. For the longer term, the dose is usually reduced to 30 milligrams per 2.2 pounds of body weight in each 24-hour period, divided into 4 doses.

RHEUMATOID ARTHRITIS

Adults

The usual dose of Azulfidine EN-tabs is 2 grams a day, divided into smaller doses. Your doctor may have you start with a lower dose, then raise the dosage to 3 grams after 12 weeks.

Children Aged 6 and Older

The typical recommended daily dosage is 30 to 50 milligrams per 2.2 pounds of body weight, up to a maximum of 2 grams, taken in 2 equally divided doses. To reduce the chance of digestive side effects and other reactions, the doctor will probably start with a fraction of the typical dose and build up to it over a period of weeks.

Overdosage

Any medication taken in excess can have serious consequences. If you suspect an Azulfidine overdose, seek emergency medical attention immediately.

■ *Symptoms of Azulfidine overdose may include:*
Abdominal pain, convulsions, drowsiness, nausea, stomach upset, vomiting

BACTRIM

Pronounced: BAC-trim
Generic ingredients: Trimethoprim, Sulfamethoxazole
Other brand name: Septra

Why is this drug prescribed?

Bactrim, an antibacterial combination drug, is prescribed for the treatment of certain urinary tract infections, severe middle ear infections in children, long-lasting or frequently recurring bronchitis in adults that has increased in seriousness, inflammation of the intestine due to a severe bacterial infection, and travelers' diarrhea in adults. Bactrim is also prescribed for the treatment of *Pneumocystis carinii* pneumonia, and for prevention of this type of pneumonia in people with weakened immune systems.

Most important fact about this drug

Sulfamethoxazole, an ingredient in Bactrim, is one of a group of drugs called sulfonamides, which prevent the growth of bacteria in the body. Rare but sometimes fatal reactions have occurred with use of sulfonamides. These reactions include Stevens-Johnson syndrome (severe eruptions around the mouth, anus, or eyes), progressive disintegration of the outer layer of the skin, sudden and severe liver damage, a severe blood disorder (agranulocytosis), and a lack of red and white blood cells because of a bone marrow disorder.

Notify your doctor at the first sign of an adverse reaction such as skin rash, sore throat, fever, joint pain, cough, shortness of breath, abnormal skin paleness, reddish or purplish skin spots, or yellowing of the skin or whites of the eyes.

Frequent blood counts by a doctor are recommended for patients taking sulfonamide drugs.

How should you take this medication?

It is important that you drink plenty of fluids while taking this medication in order to prevent sediment in the urine and the formation of stones.

Bactrim works best when there is a constant amount in the blood. Take Bactrim exactly as prescribed; try not to miss any doses. It is best to take doses at evenly spaced times day and night.

If you are taking Bactrim suspension, ask your pharmacist for a specially marked measuring spoon that delivers accurate doses.

■ *If you miss a dose...*
Take the forgotten dose as soon as you remember. If it is almost time for your next dose, skip the one you missed and go back to your regular schedule. Do not take 2 doses at once.

■ *Storage instructions...*
Store tablets and suspension at room temperature and protect from light. Keep tablets in a dry place. Protect the suspension from freezing.

What side effects may occur?

Side effects cannot be anticipated. If any develop or change in intensity, inform your doctor as soon as possible. Only your doctor can determine if it is safe for you to continue taking Bactrim.

■ *Side effects may include:*
Hives, lack or loss of appetite, nausea, skin rash, vomiting

Why should this drug not be prescribed?

If you are sensitive to or have ever had an allergic reaction to trimethoprim, sulfamethoxazole, or other sulfa drugs, you should not take this medication. Make sure that your doctor is aware of any drug reactions that you have experienced.

Unless you are directed to do so by your doctor, do not take this medication if you have been diagnosed as having megaloblastic anemia, which is a blood disorder due to a deficiency of folic acid.

This drug should not be given to infants less than 2 months of age.

Bactrim is not recommended for preventative or prolonged use in middle ear infections and should not be used in the treatment of streptococcal pharyngitis (strep throat) or certain other strep infections.

You should not take Bactrim if you are pregnant or nursing a baby.

Special warnings about this medication

Make sure your doctor knows if you have impaired kidney or liver function, have a folic acid deficiency, are a chronic alcoholic, are taking anticonvulsants, have been diagnosed as having malabsorption syndrome (abnormal intestinal absorption), are in a state of poor nutrition, or have severe allergies or bronchial asthma. Bactrim should be used cautiously under these conditions.

If you develop severe diarrhea, call your doctor. This drug can cause a serious intestinal inflammation.

If you have AIDS (acquired immunodeficiency syndrome) and are taking Bactrim to treat or prevent *Pneumocystis carinii* pneumonia, you will experience more side effects than will someone without AIDS.

Possible food and drug interactions when taking this medication

If Bactrim is taken with certain other drugs, the effects of either could be increased, decreased, or altered. It is especially important to check with your doctor before combining Bactrim with the following:

Amantadine (Symmetrel)
Blood thinners such as Coumadin
Cyclosporine (Neoral, Sandimmune)
Digoxin (Lanoxin)
Indomethacin (Indocin)
Methotrexate (Rheumatrex)
Oral diabetes medications such as Micronase and Glucotrol
Pyrimethamine (Daraprim)
Seizure medications such as Dilantin
Tricyclic antidepressants such as Elavil, Norpramin, Sinequan,
    and Tofranil
Water pills (diuretics) such as HydroDIURIL

Special information if you are pregnant or breastfeeding

Bactrim should not be taken during pregnancy. If you are pregnant or plan
to become pregnant, notify your doctor immediately. Bactrim does appear in breast milk and could affect a nursing infant. It should not be
taken while breastfeeding.

Recommended dosage

ADULTS

Urinary Tract Infections and Intestinal Inflammation
The usual adult dosage in the treatment of urinary tract infection is
1 Bactrim DS (double strength tablet) or 2 Bactrim tablets, or 4 teaspoonfuls (20 milliliters) of Bactrim Pediatric Suspension every 12 hours
for 10 to 14 days. The dosage for inflammation of the intestine is the
same but is taken for 5 days.

Worsening of Chronic Bronchitis
The usual recommended dosage is 1 Bactrim DS (double strength tablet),
2 Bactrim tablets, or 4 teaspoonfuls (20 milliliters) of Bactrim Pediatric
Suspension every 12 hours for 14 days.

Treatment of Pneumocystis carinii *Pneumonia*
The recommended dosage is 15 to 20 milligrams of trimethoprim and 75
to 100 milligrams of sulfamethoxazole per 2.2 pounds of body weight per
24 hours divided into equal doses every 6 hours for 14 to 21 days.

Prevention of Pneumocystis carinii *Pneumonia*
The recommended dosage is 1 Bactrim DS (double strength tablet) once
daily.

Travelers' Diarrhea
The usual recommended dosage is 1 Bactrim DS (double strength tablet),
2 Bactrim tablets, or 4 teaspoonfuls (20 milliliters) of Bactrim Pediatric
Suspension every 12 hours for 5 days.

CHILDREN

Urinary Tract Infections or Middle Ear Infections
The recommended dosage for children 2 months of age or older, given every 12 hours for 10 days, is determined by weight. The following table is a guideline for this dosage:

22 pounds, 1 teaspoonful (5 milliliters)
44 pounds, 2 teaspoonfuls (10 milliliters) or 1 tablet
66 pounds, 3 teaspoonfuls (15 milliliters) or 1½ tablets
88 pounds, 4 teaspoonfuls (20 milliliters) or 2 tablets or 1 DS tablet

Intestinal Inflammation
The recommended dosage is identical to the dosage recommended for urinary tract and middle ear infections; however, it should be taken for 5 days.

Treatment of Pneumocystis carinii Pneumonia
The recommended dosage, taken every 6 hours for 14 to 21 days, is determined by weight. The following table is a guideline for this dosage:

18 pounds, 1 teaspoonful (5 milliliters)
35 pounds, 2 teaspoonfuls (10 milliliters) or 1 tablet
53 pounds, 3 teaspoonfuls (15 milliliters) or 1½ tablets
70 pounds, 4 teaspoonfuls (20 milliliters) or 2 tablets or 1 DS tablet

Prevention of Pneumocystis carinii Pneumonia
The recommended dosage, taken twice a day, on 3 consecutive days per week, is determined by body surface area. The total daily dose should not exceed 320 milligrams trimethoprim and 1,600 milligrams sulfamethoxazole.

The safety of repeated use of Bactrim in children under 2 years of age has not been established.

OLDER ADULTS

There may be an increased risk of severe side effects when Bactrim is taken by older people, especially in those who have impaired kidney and/or liver function or who are taking other medication. Consult with your doctor before taking Bactrim.

Overdosage
If you suspect an overdose of Bactrim, seek emergency medical attention immediately.

■ *Symptoms of an overdose of Bactrim include:*
Blood or sediment in the urine, colic, confusion, dizziness, drowsiness, fever, headache, lack or loss of appetite, mental depression, nausea, unconsciousness, vomiting, yellowed eyes and skin

BACTROBAN

Pronounced: BAC-tro-ban
Generic name: Mupirocin

Why is this drug prescribed?

Bactroban is prescribed for the treatment of impetigo, a bacterial infection of the skin.

Most important fact about this drug

If the use of Bactroban does not clear your skin infection within 3 to 5 days, or if the infection becomes worse, notify your doctor.

How should you use this medication?

Do not use Bactroban more often or for longer than prescribed. Avoid contact with eyes. This drug is for external use only.

■ *If you miss a dose...*
   Apply it as soon as you remember. If it is almost time for the next dose, skip the one you missed and go back to your regular schedule.
■ *Storage instructions...*
   Store at room temperature.

What side effects may occur?

Side effects cannot be anticipated. If any develop or change in intensity, inform your doctor as soon as possible. Only your doctor can determine if it is safe for you to continue using Bactroban.

■ *Side effects may include:*
   Burning, pain, stinging

Why should this drug not be prescribed?

If you are sensitive to or have ever had an allergic reaction to Bactroban or similar drugs, you should not use this medication. Make sure your doctor is aware of any drug reactions you have experienced.

Special warnings about this medication

Continued or prolonged use of Bactroban may result in the growth of bacteria that do not respond to this medication and can cause a secondary infection.

   This drug is not intended for use in the eyes.

   If your skin shows signs of an allergic reaction or irritation, stop using Bactroban and consult your doctor.

Possible food and drug interactions when taking this medication

There are no known interactions.

Special information if you are pregnant or breastfeeding

The effects of Bactroban during pregnancy have not been adequately studied. If you are pregnant or plan to become pregnant, inform your doctor immediately. It is not known whether Bactroban appears in breast milk. Your doctor may advise you to discontinue breastfeeding until your treatment with this medication is finished.

Recommended dosage

Apply a small amount of this medication to the affected area 3 times a day. Cover the treated area with gauze if you want.

Overdosage

There is no information available on overdosage.

Balsalazide See Colazal, page 319.

BECLOMETHASONE

Pronounced: BECK-low-METH-ah-sone
Brand names: Beclovent, Beconase AQ Nasal Spray, Beconase
Inhalation Aerosol, Qvar Inhalation Aerosol, Vancenase AQ
Nasal Spray and Double Strength Nasal Spray, Vancenase
Nasal Inhaler and PocketHaler Nasal Inhaler, Vanceril
Inhalation Aerosol and Double Strength Inhalation Aerosol,
Vanceril Inhaler

Why is this drug prescribed?

Beclomethasone is a type of steroid used for respiratory problems. Beclovent and Vanceril are prescribed for the prevention of recurring symptoms of bronchial asthma.

Beconase and Vancenase are used to relieve the symptoms of hay fever and to prevent regrowth of nasal polyps following surgical removal.

Most important fact about this drug

Beclomethasone is not a bronchodilator medication (it does not quickly open the airways), and it should not be used for relief of asthma when bronchodilators and other nonsteroid drugs prove effective. Do not expect immediate relief from beclomethasone, and do not take higher doses in an attempt to make it work. It is not intended for rapid relief, but it will help control symptoms when taken routinely.

How should you take this medication?

Beclomethasone is prescribed in an oral inhalant or a nasal-spray form. Use this medication only as preventive therapy, and take only the dose prescribed.

Although some people begin to notice improvement within a day or two, it may take 1 or 2 weeks for the full benefits to appear. If there's no improvement after 3 weeks, let your doctor know.

If you are already taking a steroid in tablet form for asthma, you'll need to make a gradual transition to the oral inhalant. During the first week, you'll probably take the usual number of tablets. After that, you'll be instructed to slowly reduce the number of tablets, replacing them with the inhalant.

Be sure to take the drug regularly, even if you have no symptoms. Many people will require additional drugs to control asthma symptoms fully, but this drug may allow other drugs to be used in smaller doses.

If you are also using a bronchodilator inhalant, take it before inhaling beclomethasone. This will improve the effect of the second drug. Take the 2 inhalations several minutes apart.

Spray the inhalation aerosol into the air twice before you use it for the first time and when you have not used it for more than 7 days. Use it within 6 months.

Before you use Vancenase AQ 84 microgram nasal spray, press the pump 6 times or until you see a fine spray. If you don't use it for more than 4 days, reprime the pump by spraying once or until a fine spray appears.

To use the inhaler:
1. Remove the cap and hold inhaler upright.
2. Shake the inhaler thoroughly.
3. Take a drink of water to moisten the throat.
4. Breathe out as fully as you comfortably can. Hold the inhaler upright and close your lips around the mouthpiece, keeping your tongue below it.
5. While pressing down on the can, inhale deeply. Hold your breath as long as you can.
6. Take your finger off the can, remove the inhaler, and breathe out gently.
7. Allow at least 1 minute between inhalations.

Gargling and rinsing your mouth with water after each dose may help prevent hoarseness and throat irritation. Do not swallow the water after you rinse.

Be careful to avoid spraying the medication into your eyes. This medication comes with directions. Read them carefully before using it.

■ *If you miss a dose...*
Take it as soon as you remember and take the remaining doses for that day at evenly spaced intervals. If it is time for your next dose, skip the one you missed. Never take 2 doses at the same time.

■ *Storage instructions...*
Store at room temperature in a dry place, away from heat and cold. Do not puncture the container, store it near open flame, or dispose of it in a fire or incinerator.

What side effects may occur?

Side effects cannot be anticipated. If any develop or change in intensity, inform your doctor as soon as possible. Only your doctor can determine if it is safe for you to continue taking this medication.

■ *Side effects may include:*

Acne, agitation, allergic reactions, breathing problems, bruising, cataracts, chest pain, cold sores, cough, depression, dizziness, dry mouth, ear infections, fever, fluid retention, flu-like symptoms, headache, hives, hoarseness, increased pressure within the eye (glaucoma), itching, joint pain, light-headedness, mental disturbances, moon face, mouth or throat infection, muscle pain, nasal and throat dryness and irritation, nasal burning, nausea, nose infection, nosebleed, pain, pinkeye, pins and needles sensation, ringing in the ears, runny nose, skin rash, skin wasting, sneezing, sore mouth or throat, stuffy nose, stunted growth, tearing eyes, unpleasant—or loss of—taste and smell, upset stomach, vomiting, weight gain, wheezing

Why should this drug not be prescribed?

Your doctor will prescribe beclomethasone only if your asthma cannot be controlled with bronchodilators and other nonsteroid medications.

Beclomethasone is not used for the treatment of non-asthmatic bronchitis, or for intermittent asthma therapy.

Do not use beclomethasone nasal products if you've recently had nasal ulcers, nose surgery, or an injury to the nose. They could interfere with the healing process.

If you are sensitive to or have ever had an allergic reaction to beclomethasone or other steroid drugs, you should not take this medication. Rare cases of immediate and delayed allergic reactions, such as hives, a rash, or wheezing, have occured. Make sure that your doctor is aware of any drug reactions that you have experienced.

Although unlikely, immediate allergic reactions to beclomethasone have been known to occur.

Special warnings about this medication

When steroid drugs are taken by mouth, they substitute for and decrease the body's normal ability to make its own steroids as well as its ability to respond to stress.

There is a risk of causing a serious condition called adrenal insufficiency when people change from steroid tablets taken by mouth to aerosol beclomethasone. Although the aerosol may provide adequate control of asthma during the changeover period, it does not provide the normal amount of steroid the body needs during acute stress situations, such as injury, surgery, and infection—particularly stomach flu. If you are being transferred from steroid tablets to beclomethasone and you experience a period of stress or a severe asthma attack, contact your doctor immediately. He may prescribe additional treatment with steroid tablets. You should also carry a warning card indicating that you may need steroid tablets during such incidents. As you continue taking beclomethasone, your doctor may conduct periodic tests to measure your adrenal function.

Transfer from steroid tablet therapy to beclomethasone aerosol may reactivate allergic conditions that were previously suppressed by the steroid tablet therapy, such as runny nose, inflamed eyelids, and eczema. Some people also experience withdrawal side effects when they switch from tablets to aerosol. Potential symptoms include joint or muscle pain, weakness, and depression. Inform your doctor if you experience any of these symptoms.

High doses of steroids can suppress your immune system. When beclomethasone is used nasally, your chances of developing nose and throat infections increase. Also, take extra care to avoid exposure to measles or chickenpox if you have never had them or never had shots. These infections can be serious or even fatal if your immune system is below par. If you are exposed, seek medical advice immediately.

Symptoms such as mental disturbances, increased bruising, weight gain, facial swelling (moon face), acne, menstrual irregularities, increased pressure in the eyes, and cataracts may occur with steroids. If you experience any of these symptoms, notify your doctor immediately. If you've ever had cataracts or increased eye pressure, your doctor will monitor you closely if you have any problems with your vision.

Long-term use of steroids can slow down growth in children. If your child seems to be growing more slowly than normal, call your doctor.

If bronchodilator medications seem less effective after you start taking beclomethasone, be sure to tell your doctor. Do not abruptly stop using beclomethasone on your own.

If you have tuberculosis, a herpes infection of the eye, or any untreated fungal, bacterial, viral, or parasitic infections, your doctor may not want you to use an inhaled steroid.

Special information if you are pregnant or breastfeeding

The effects of beclomethasone in pregnancy have not been adequately studied. If you are pregnant or are planning a pregnancy, let your doctor know. Steroids do appear in breast milk and could harm your baby. Your doctor may want you to avoid breastfeeding while you are using beclomethasone.

Recommended dosage

ADULTS

Beclomethasone Oral Inhalant
The usual recommended dose for adults and children 12 years of age and over is 2 inhalations, taken 3 to 4 times a day. Four inhalations taken twice

daily have been shown to be effective in some people. If you have severe asthma, your doctor may advise you to start with 12 to 16 inhalations a day. Daily intake should not exceed 20 inhalations.

For the double strength inhalation aerosol, the usual dose is 2 inhalations twice a day. If your asthma is severe, your doctor may have you start with 6 to 8 inhalations a day. The maximum daily dosage is 10 inhalations.

For Qvar, a CFC-free form of the drug, the recommended starting dose is 40 to 80 micrograms twice daily if you've been using bronchodilators alone, and 40 to 160 micrograms if you've been using other inhaled steroid products. Take no more than 320 micrograms twice a day.

Beclomethasone Nasal Inhalation

For adults and children 12 years of age and over, the dosage of Vancenase PocketHaler is 1 inhalation in each nostril 2 to 4 times a day. A 3-times-daily schedule is often sufficient.

Beclomethasone Nasal Spray

For adults and children 12 years of age and older, the usual dosage is 1 or 2 inhalations in each nostril 2 to 4 times a day, depending on the brand. For the double strength nasal spray, the dosage is 1 or 2 inhalations in each nostril once a day.

The usual dosage of Vancenase AQ 84 micrograms for adults and children 6 years and over is 1 or 2 inhalations in each nostril once a day.

CHILDREN

Beclomethasone Oral Inhalant

Children 6 to 12 years of age: The usual recommended dose is 1 or 2 inhalations 3 or 4 times a day. Four inhalations twice daily have been effective for some children. Daily intake should not exceed 10 inhalations.

For the double strength inhalation aerosol, the usual dose is 2 inhalations twice daily, with a maximum of 5 inhalations a day.

For the Qvar brand, the recommended starting dose for children 5 to 11 is 40 micrograms twice daily. The highest recommended dose is 80 micrograms twice daily.

Beclomethasone Nasal Inhalation

Children 6 to 12 years of age: The usual dose of Vancenase PocketHaler is 1 inhalation 3 times a day.

Beclomethasone Nasal Spray

Children 6 to 12 years of age: The usual dosage is 1 inhalation in each nostril 2 times a day. Some children may need 2 inhalations. However, once adequate control is achieved, the dose should be decreased to 1 inhalation in each nostril twice daily. The maximum daily dose should not exceed 2 inhalations in each nostril twice daily. The dosage for the double strength nasal spray is 1 or 2 inhalations in each nostril once a day.

Beclomethasone should not be given to children under the age of 6 unless advised by your doctor.

Overdosage
Any medication taken in excess can have serious consequences. The main risk in an overdose of beclomethasone is adrenal insufficiency. If you suspect an overdose, seek medical attention immediately.

Beclovent *See Beclomethasone, page 193.*

Beconase *See Beclomethasone, page 193.*

Bellatal *See Donnatal, page 469.*

Benazepril *See Lotensin, page 784.*

Benazepril with Hydrochlorothiazide *See Lotensin HCT, page 787.*

BENICAR
Pronounced: BEN-ick-ar
Generic name: Olmesartan medoxomil
Other brand name: Benicar HCT

Why is this drug prescribed?
Benicar controls high blood pressure. It works by blocking the effect of a hormone called angiotensin II. Unopposed, this substance prompts the blood vessels to contract, an action that tends to raise blood pressure. Benicar relaxes and expands the blood vessels, allowing pressure to drop. Benicar may be prescribed alone or with other blood pressure medications, such as diuretics that help the body get rid of excess water. Benicar HCT provides just such a combination. It contains Benicar plus hydrochlorothiazide, a common diuretic that increases the output of urine. This removes excess fluid from the body and helps lower blood pressure.

Most important fact about this drug
You must take Benicar or Benicar HCT regularly for it to be effective. Since blood pressure declines gradually, it may be a couple of weeks before you get significant benefits, and you must continue taking it even though you feel well. This drug does not cure high blood pressure; it merely keeps it under control.

How should you take this medication?
Benicar or Benicar HCT should be taken once a day, preferably at the same time each day. It can be taken with or without food.

■ *If you miss a dose...*
Take it as soon as you remember. If it's almost time for your next dose, skip the one you missed and go back to your regular schedule. Do not take two doses in the same day.

■ *Storage instructions...*
Store at room temperature.

What side effects may occur?

Side effects cannot be anticipated. If any develop or change in intensity, inform your doctor as soon as possible. Only your doctor can determine if it is safe for you to continue taking Benicar or Benicar HCT.

■ *Side effects may include:*
Dizziness, gout, nausea, upper respiratory infection

Why should this drug not be prescribed?

Do not take Benicar or Benicar HCT while pregnant. Avoid both drugs if they cause an allergic reaction, and do not take Benicar HCT if you have ever had an allergic reaction to a sulfa drug such as Bactrim or Septra. Also avoid Benicar HCT if you have trouble urinating.

Special warnings about this medication

Benicar or Benicar HCT can cause a severe drop in blood pressure, especially when you first start taking the drug. The problem is more likely to occur if your body's supply of water has been depleted by diuretics (water pills). If your blood pressure drops too low, you could also experience light-headedness, dizziness, and faintness (lying down may relieve these symptoms). If you develop any of these problems, contact your physician. You may need to have your dose adjusted.

Likewise, excessive sweating, severe diarrhea, or vomiting could deplete your body's fluids and cause your blood pressure to drop too low. If you feel severely dehydrated, contact your doctor. Be careful, too, about avoiding excessive fluid loss when exercising and during hot weather.

Use Benicar and Benicar HCT with caution if you have a history of allergy or bronchial asthma.

If you have congestive heart failure, liver or kidney disease, lupus, gout, or diabetes, Benicar and Benicar HCT should be used with caution. Both drugs have been known to impair kidney function or even lead to kidney failure. They could also bring out hidden diabetes. If you are already taking insulin or oral diabetes drugs, your medication may have to be adjusted. The hydrochlorothiazide component of Benicar HCT also has a tendency to increase cholesterol levels.

The diuretic in Benicar HCT can lower the levels of electrolytes (salts and other minerals) in the blood, especially if you become dehydrated. Signs include dry mouth, thirst, weakness, sluggishness, drowsiness, restlessness, confusion, seizures, muscle pain or cramps, muscle fatigue, low blood pressure, decreased urination, rapid heartbeat, nausea, and vomiting. Call your doctor immediately if you experience any of these problems.

Likewise, the diuretic in Benicar HCT can cause excessive potassium loss. Signs include muscle weakness and rapid or irregular heartbeat. To boost your potassium level, your doctor may recommend eating potassium-rich foods or taking a potassium supplement. If you think you need a supplement, check with your doctor; do not start taking one on your own. Also check with your doctor before using a potassium-containing salt substitute.

Possible food and drug interactions when taking this medication

No significant drug interactions have been reported with Benicar.

The hydrochlorothiazide in Benicar HCT may interact with a variety of drugs. Be sure to check with your doctor before combining Benicar HCT with the following:

Alcohol
Barbiturates such as phenobarbital and Seconal
Cholestyramine (Questran)
Colestipol (Colestid)
Corticosteroids such as hydrocortisone and prednisone
Digoxin (Lanoxin)
Insulin
Lithium (Lithobid, Lithonate)
Muscle relaxants such as Tubocurarine
Narcotic drugs such as morphine or codeine products (Percocet)
Nonsteroidal anti-inflammatory drugs such as Advil, Aleve, Motrin, and Naprosyn
Norepinephrine
Oral diabetes drugs such as Diabeta, Diabinese, Glucotrol, and Micronase
Other blood pressure medications such as Cardizem, Lopressor, and Procardia

Special information if you are pregnant or breastfeeding

Drugs such as Benicar and Benicar HCT can cause injury or even death to a developing baby when used during the last 6 months of pregnancy. If you discover you're pregnant, stop taking the drug immediately and call your doctor. Likewise, alert your doctor if you plan to become pregnant.

Hydrochlorothiazide appears in breast milk and could affect a nursing infant. If this medication is essential to your health, your doctor may advise you to avoid breastfeeding until your treatment is finished.

Recommended dosage

ADULTS

Benicar

The usual starting dose is 20 milligrams once daily. If your blood pressure hasn't dropped sufficiently after 2 weeks, the doctor may raise the dose to 40 milligrams once a day. If you are taking a diuretic, your starting dose may be smaller than usual.

Benicar HCT

The starting dose of Benicar HCT is one tablet containing 20 milligrams of olmesartan/12.5 milligrams of hydrochlorothiazide once daily. If needed, the doctor may increase the dose every 2 to 4 weeks until your blood pressure is under control. The maximum dose is 40 milligrams of olmesartan/25 milligrams of hydrochlorothiazide once daily.

Overdosage

Any medication taken in excess can have serious consequences. If you suspect an overdose, seek medical attention immediately.

- *Symptoms of Benicar overdose may include:*
  Dehydration (dry mouth, excessive thirst, muscle pain or cramps, nausea and vomiting, weakness), dizziness, low blood pressure, slow or irregular heartbeat

Benicar HCT *See Benicar, page 198.*

BENTYL
Pronounced: BEN-til
Generic name: Dicyclomine hydrochloride

Why is this drug prescribed?

Bentyl is prescribed for the treatment of functional bowel/irritable bowel syndrome (abdominal pain, accompanied by diarrhea and constipation associated with stress).

Most important fact about this drug

Heat prostration (fever and heat stroke due to decreased sweating) can occur with use of this drug in hot weather. If symptoms occur, stop taking the drug and notify your doctor immediately.

How should you take this medication?

Take this medication exactly as prescribed.

■ *If you miss a dose...*
Take it as soon as you remember. If it is almost time for your next dose, skip the one you missed and go back to your regular schedule. Do not take 2 doses at once.

■ *Storage instructions...*
Store at room temperature. Keep tablets out of direct sunlight. Keep syrup away from excessive heat.

What side effects may occur?

Side effects cannot be anticipated. If any develop or change in intensity, inform your doctor as soon as possible. Only your doctor can determine if it is safe for you to continue taking Bentyl.

■ *Side effects may include:*
Blurred vision, dizziness, drowsiness, dry mouth, light-headedness, nausea, nervousness, weakness

Not all of the following side effects have been reported with dicyclomine hydrochloride, but they have been reported for similar drugs with anti-spasmodic action; contact your doctor if they occur.

Abdominal pain, bloated feeling, constipation, decreased sweating, difficulty in urinating, double vision, enlargement of the pupil of the eye, eye paralysis, fainting, headache, hives, impotence, inability to urinate, increased pressure in the eyes, itching, labored, difficult breathing, lack of coordination, lack or loss of appetite, nasal stuffiness or congestion, numbness, rapid heartbeat, rash, severe allergic reaction, sluggishness, sneezing, suffocation, suppression of breast milk, taste loss, temporary cessation of breathing, throat congestion, tingling, vomiting

Why should this drug not be prescribed?

If you are sensitive to or have ever had an allergic reaction to Bentyl, you should not take this medication. Make sure your doctor is aware of any drug reactions you have experienced.

Unless you are directed to do so by your doctor, do not take this drug if you have a blockage of the urinary tract, stomach, or intestines; severe ulcerative colitis (inflammatory disease of the large intestine); reflux esophagitis (inflammation of the esophagus usually caused by the back-flow of acid stomach contents); glaucoma; or myasthenia gravis (a disease characterized by long-lasting fatigue and muscle weakness).

This drug should not be given to infants less than 6 months of age or used by women who are nursing an infant.

Special warnings about this medication

Bentyl may produce drowsiness or blurred vision. Therefore, driving a car, operating machinery, or participating in any activity that requires full mental alertness is not recommended.

Diarrhea may be an early symptom of a partial intestinal blockage, especially in people who have had bowel removal and an ileostomy or colostomy. If this occurs, notify your doctor immediately.

You should use this medication with caution if you have autonomic neuropathy (a nerve disorder); liver or kidney disease; hyperthyroidism; high blood pressure; coronary heart disease; congestive heart failure; rapid, irregular heartbeat; hiatal hernia (protrusion of part of the stomach through the diaphragm); or enlargement of the prostate gland.

Possible food and drug interactions when taking this medication

If Bentyl is taken with certain other drugs, the effects of either could be increased, decreased, or altered. It is especially important to check with your doctor before combining Bentyl with the following:

Airway-opening drugs such as Proventil and Ventolin
Amantadine (Symmetrel)
Antacids such as Maalox
Antiarrhythmics such as quinidine (Quinidex)
Antiglaucoma drugs such as Pilopine
Antihistamines such as Tavist
Benzodiazepines (tranquilizers) such as Valium and Xanax
Corticosteroids such as prednisone (Deltasone)
Digoxin (the heart failure medication Lanoxin)
Major tranquilizers such as Mellaril and Thorazine
MAO inhibitors (antidepressants such as Nardil and Parnate)
Metoclopramide (the gastrointestinal stimulant Reglan)
Narcotic analgesics (pain relievers such as Demerol)
Nitrates and nitrites (heart medications such as nitroglycerin)
Tricyclic antidepressant drugs such as Elavil and Tofranil

Special information if you are pregnant or breastfeeding

The effects of Bentyl during pregnancy have not been adequately studied. If you are pregnant or plan to become pregnant, notify your doctor. Bentyl does appear in breast milk and could affect a nursing infant. Do not use it when breastfeeding.

Recommended dosage

ADULTS

The usual dosage is 160 milligrams per day, divided into 4 equal doses. Since this dose is associated with a significant incidence of side effects, your doctor may recommend a starting dose of 80 milligrams per day, divided into 4 equal doses. If no side effects appear, the doctor will then increase the dose.

If this drug is not effective within 2 weeks or side effects require doses below 80 milligrams per day, your doctor may discontinue it.

Overdosage
Any medication taken in excess can have serious consequences. If you suspect an overdose, seek medical attention immediately.

■ *Symptoms of a Bentyl overdose include:*
Blurred vision, difficulty in swallowing, dilated pupils, dizziness, dryness of the mouth, headache, hot, dry skin, nausea, nerve blockage causing weakness and possible paralysis, vomiting

BENZACLIN
Pronounced: BEN-za-klin
Generic ingredients: Benzoyl peroxide, Clindamycin

Why is this drug prescribed?
BenzaClin is an acne treatment. Both its ingredients—the antibiotic clindamycin and the antibacterial agent benzoyl peroxide—attack the bacteria that help cause acne.

Most important fact about this drug
Although BenzaClin is applied only to the skin, some of this medication could be absorbed into the bloodstream. Once in the system, it has been known to cause severe colitis. Symptoms include severe or bloody diarrhea and abdominal cramps.

How should you use this medication?
Before applying BenzaClin, gently wash the affected skin and rinse with warm water. Pat the skin dry. Apply the medication to the entire area, not just the pimples. Do not use BenzaClin more often than recommended by your doctor. Excessive use can make your skin dry or irritated.

■ *If you miss a dose...*
Apply it as soon as you remember. If it is almost time for your next application, skip the one you missed and go back to your regular schedule.

■ *Storage instructions...*
Store BenzaClin in the refrigerator in a tightly closed container. Do not freeze. Discard any unused medication after two months.

What side effects may occur?
Side effects cannot be anticipated. If any develop or change in intensity, inform your doctor as soon as possible. Only your doctor can determine if it is safe for you to continue using BenzaClin.

■ *Side effects may include:*
Dry skin, skin irritation

Why should this drug not be prescribed?

Do not use BenzaClin if you are allergic to either of its ingredients, or to the antibiotic lincomycin. Also avoid BenzaClin if you have a history of colitis.

Special warnings about this medication

BenzaClin gel is for external use only. Avoid contact with your eyes, nose, mouth, and all mucous membranes.

BenzaClin can cause skin irritation, especially if it is used with other skin treatments that are abrasive or cause peeling. Do not combine BenzaClin with other treatments unless directed by your doctor. If your skin becomes severely irritated, stop using BenzaClin and call your doctor.

As you use this antibiotic, organisms that are resistant to it may start to grow. If this occurs, your doctor will have you stop using BenzaClin.

BenzaClin may bleach hair or colored fabric.

This product has not been tested in children under 12.

Possible food and drug interactions when taking this medication

Do not use BenzaClin with medications containing erythromycin (E.E.S., Eryc, PCE, others).

If you develop diarrhea while taking BenzaClin, check with your doctor before taking an antidiarrhea medication. Some can make your diarrhea worse. For instance, you should avoid the commonly used drugs that slow movement through the intestinal tract, such as Lomotil and products containing paregoric.

Special information if you are pregnant or breastfeeding

If you are pregnant or plan to become pregnant, inform your doctor immediately. The possibility that BenzaClin could harm the developing baby has not been ruled out.

Clindamycin can make its way into breast milk, where it could harm a nursing infant. You'll need to choose between breastfeeding and continuing your treatment with BenzaClin.

Recommended dosage

ADULTS

Apply to the affected areas twice daily, once in the morning and once in the evening.

Overdosage

A massive overdose of BenzaClin is unlikely. However, any medication taken in excess can have serious consequences. If you suspect an overdose, seek medical help immediately.

Benzac W *See Desquam-E, page 421.*

Benzagel *See Desquam-E, page 421.*

BENZAMYCIN

Pronounced: BEN-za-MI-sin
Generic ingredients: Erythromycin, Benzoyl peroxide

Why is this drug prescribed?
A combination of the antibiotic erythromycin and the antibacterial agent benzoyl peroxide, Benzamycin is effective in stopping the bacteria that cause acne and in reducing acne infection.

Most important fact about this drug
If you experience excessive irritation, stop using Benzamycin and notify your doctor.

How should you use this medication?
Use Benzamycin 2 times per day, once in the morning and once in the evening, or as directed by your doctor.

Before applying Benzamycin, thoroughly wash the affected area with soap and warm water, rinse well, and gently pat dry. Apply Benzamycin to the entire area, not just the pimples.

■ *If you miss a dose...*
Apply it as soon as you remember. If it is almost time for your next dose, skip the one you missed and go back to your regular schedule.

■ *Storage instructions...*
This medication should be stored in your refrigerator in a tightly closed container and discarded after 3 months. Do not freeze.

What side effects may occur?
Very few side effects have been reported with the use of Benzamycin. However, those reported include dryness and swelling. Occasionally, use of this medication has caused a burning sensation; eye irritation; inflammation of the face, eyes, and nose; itching; oiliness; reddened skin; skin discoloration; skin irritation and peeling; and skin tenderness.

If any side effects develop or change in intensity, inform your doctor as soon as possible. Only your doctor can determine if it is safe for you to continue using Benzamycin.

Why should this drug not be prescribed?
If you are sensitive to or have ever had an allergic reaction to erythromycin or benzoyl peroxide, or any other ingredients in Benzamycin, you should not use this medication. Make sure your doctor is aware of any drug reactions you have experienced.

Special warnings about this medication

Benzamycin Topical Gel is for external use only. Avoid contact with your eyes, nose, mouth, and all mucous membranes.

Benzamycin may bleach hair or colored fabric. Avoid contact with scalp and clothes.

As you use this antibiotic, organisms that are resistant to it may start to grow. Your doctor will have you stop using Benzamycin and will give you a medication to fight the new bacteria.

If you develop diarrhea after you start using Benzamycin, call your doctor. You may have an intestinal inflammation that could be serious.

Possible food and drug interactions when using this medication

If Benzamycin is used with other acne medications, the effects of either could be increased, decreased, or altered. Always check with your doctor before combining any other prescription or over-the-counter acne remedy with Benzamycin.

Special information if you are pregnant or breastfeeding

The effects of Benzamycin during pregnancy have not been adequately studied. If you are pregnant or plan to become pregnant, inform your doctor immediately. It is not known whether Benzamycin appears in breast milk, but erythromycin does if it is swallowed or injected. If this medication is essential to your health, your doctor may advise you to discontinue breastfeeding your baby until your treatment with this medication is finished.

Recommended dosage

ADULTS

Apply to affected areas twice daily, once in the morning and once in the evening.

CHILDREN

The safety and effectiveness of Benzamycin have not been established in children under 12 years of age.

Overdosage

There is no information available on overdosage.

Benzashave *See Desquam-E, page 421.*

Benzonatate *See Tessalon, page 1416.*

Benzoyl peroxide *See Desquam-E, page 421.*

BETAGAN

Pronounced: BAIT-ah-gan
Generic name: Levobunolol hydrochloride

Why is this drug prescribed?

Betagan eyedrops are given to treat chronic open-angle glaucoma (increased pressure inside the eye). This medication is in a class called beta-blockers. It works by lowering pressure within the eyeball.

Most important fact about this drug

Although Betagan eyedrops are applied to the eye, the medication is absorbed and may have effects in other parts of the body. If you have diabetes, asthma or other respiratory diseases, or decreased heart function, make sure your doctor is aware of the problem.

How should you use this medication?

Use Betagan eyedrops exactly as prescribed. Some people also need to use eyedrops that constrict their pupils.

Administer Betagan eyedrops as follows:
1. Wash your hands thoroughly.
2. Gently pull your lower eyelid down to form a pocket between your eye and eyelid.
3. Hold the bottle on the bridge of your nose or on your forehead.
4. Do not touch the applicator tip to any surface, including your eye.
5. Tilt your head back and squeeze the medication into your eye.
6. Close your eyes gently.
7. Keep your eyes closed for 1 to 2 minutes.
8. Wait 5 to 10 minutes before using any other eyedrops.
9. Do not rinse the dropper.

■ *If you miss a dose...*
If you take Betagan once a day, use it as soon as you remember. If you do not remember until the next day, skip the dose you missed and go back to your regular schedule. Do not take 2 doses at once. If you take Betagan 2 or more times a day, use it as soon as you remember. If it is almost time for your next dose, skip the one you missed and go back to your regular schedule. Do not take 2 doses at once.

■ *Storage instructions...*
Store at room temperature, away from light.

What side effects may occur?

Side effects from Betagan cannot be anticipated. If any develop or change in intensity, inform your doctor. Only your doctor can determine whether it is safe for you to continue using this medication. You may feel a momentary burning and stinging when you place the drops in your eyes. More rarely, you may develop an eye inflammation.

Beta-blockers may cause muscle weakness; weakened muscles around the eyes may cause double vision or drooping eyelids.

Why should this drug not be prescribed?

Do not use Betagan if you have ever had an allergic reaction to it or are sensitive to it.

You should not use Betagan if you have any of the following conditions:

Asthma
Cardiogenic shock (shock due to insufficient heart action)
Certain heart irregularities
Heart failure
Severe chronic obstructive lung disease
Slow heartbeat (sinus bradycardia)

Special warnings about this medication

Betagan contains a sulfite preservative. In a few people, sulfites can cause an allergic reaction, which may be life-threatening. If you suffer from asthma, you are at increased risk for sulfite allergy.

Betagan may be absorbed into your bloodstream. If too much of the drug is absorbed, this may worsen asthma or other lung diseases or lead to heart failure, which sometimes happens with oral beta-blocker medications.

Beta-blockers may increase the risks of anesthesia. If you are facing elective surgery, your doctor may want you to taper off Betagan prior to your operation.

Use Betagan cautiously if you have diminished lung function.

Since beta-blockers may mask some signs and symptoms of low blood sugar (hypoglycemia), you should use Betagan very carefully if you have low blood sugar, or if you have diabetes and are taking insulin or an oral antidiabetic medication.

If your body tends to produce too much thyroid hormone, you should taper off Betagan very gradually rather than stopping the drug all at once. Abrupt withdrawal of any beta-blocker may provoke a rush of thyroid hormone *(thyroid storm)*.

Do not use 2 or more beta-blocker eye medications at the same time.

Possible food and drug interactions when taking this medication

If Betagan is used with certain other drugs, the effects of either could be increased, decreased, or altered. It is especially important to check with your doctor before combining Betagan with the following:

Calcium-blocking blood pressure medications such as Calan and
    Cardizem

Digitalis (the heart medication Lanoxin)
Epinephrine (Epifrin)
Oral beta-blockers such as the blood pressure medications Inderal
   and Tenormin
Reserpine (Serpasil)

Special information if you are pregnant or breastfeeding

The use of Betagan in pregnancy has not been adequately studied. If you are pregnant or plan to become pregnant, notify your doctor immediately. Betagan eyedrops should be used during pregnancy only if the benefit justifies the potential risk to the unborn child. Since other beta-blocker medications are known to appear in breast milk, use Betagan eyedrops with caution if you are breastfeeding.

Recommended dosage

ADULTS

The recommended starting dose is 1 or 2 drops of Betagan 0.5% in the affected eye(s) once a day.

The typical dose of Betagan 0.25% is 1 or 2 drops twice daily.

For more severe glaucoma, your doctor may have you use Betagan 0.5% twice a day.

Overdosage

Overuse of Betagan eyedrops may produce symptoms of beta-blocker overdosage—slowed heartbeat, low blood pressure, breathing difficulty, and/or heart failure. Any medication taken in excess can have serious consequences. If you suspect an overdose of Betagan, seek medical attention immediately.

Betaine See Cystadane, page 375.

Betamethasone See Diprolene, page 455.

Betaxolol See Betoptic, below.

Betimol See Timoptic, page 1440.

BETOPTIC

Pronounced: bet-OP-tick
Generic name: Betaxolol hydrochloride

Why is this drug prescribed?

Betoptic Ophthalmic Solution and Betoptic S Ophthalmic Suspension contain a medication that lowers internal eye pressure and is used to treat open-angle glaucoma (high pressure of the fluid in the eye).

Most important fact about this drug

Although Betoptic, a type of drug called a beta-blocker, is applied directly to the eye, it may be absorbed into the bloodstream. Because it may have effects in other parts of the body, you should use Betoptic cautiously if you have diabetes, asthma or other respiratory diseases, or decreased heart function.

How should you use this medication?

Use this medication exactly as prescribed. You may need to use other medications at the same time.

Betoptic S Suspension should be shaken well before each dose.

Administer Betoptic as follows:

1. Wash your hands thoroughly.
2. Gently pull your lower eyelid down to form a pocket between your eye and eyelid.
3. Hold the bottle on the bridge of your nose or on your forehead.
4. Do not touch the applicator tip to any surface, including your eye.
5. Tilt your head back and squeeze the medication into your eye.
6. Close your eyes gently.
7. Keep your eyes closed for 1 to 2 minutes.
8. Wait for 5 to 10 minutes before using any other eyedrops.
9. Do not rinse the dropper.

■ *If you miss a dose...*
Use it as soon as you remember. If it is almost time for your next dose, skip the one you missed and go back to your regular schedule. Do not use 2 doses at once.

■ *Storage instructions...*
Store at room temperature.

What side effects may occur?

Side effects cannot be anticipated. If any develop or change in intensity, inform your doctor as soon as possible. Only your doctor can determine if it is safe for you to continue using Betoptic.

■ *Side effects may include:*
Temporary eye discomfort

Why should this drug not be prescribed?

Do not use Betoptic if you are sensitive to or have ever had an allergic reaction to it.

People with certain heart conditions should not use Betoptic.

Special warnings about this medication

Before you use Betoptic, tell your doctor if you have any of the following:

> Asthma
> Diabetes
> Heart disease
> Thyroid disease

If you are having surgery, your doctor may advise you to gradually stop using Betoptic before you undergo general anesthesia.

This drug may lose some of its effectiveness for glaucoma after you have been taking it a long time.

Possible food and drug interactions when using this medication

If Betoptic is used with certain other drugs, the effects of either could be increased, decreased, or altered. It is especially important to check with your doctor before combining Betoptic with the following:

> Drugs that alter mood, such as Nardil and Elavil
> Oral beta-blockers such as Inderal and Tenormin
> Reserpine (Serpasil)

Special information if you are pregnant or breastfeeding

The effects of Betoptic during pregnancy have not been adequately studied. If you are pregnant or plan to become pregnant, inform your doctor immediately. Betoptic may appear in breast milk and could affect a nursing infant. If this medication is essential to your health, your doctor may advise you to stop breastfeeding until your treatment with Betoptic is finished.

Recommended dosage

Your doctor may have you take another medication with Betoptic or Betoptic-S.

ADULTS

Betoptic
The usual recommended dose is 1 to 2 drops of Betoptic in the affected eye(s) twice daily.

Betoptic S
The usual recommended dose is 1 to 2 drops of Betoptic S in the affected eye(s) twice daily.

Overdosage

Any medication used in excess can have serious consequences. If you suspect an overdose of Betoptic, seek medical attention immediately.

■ *With an oral beta-blocker, symptoms of overdose might include:*
Heart failure, low blood pressure, slow heartbeat

BIAXIN

Pronounced: buy-AX-in
Generic name: Clarithromycin
Other brand name: Biaxin XL

Why is this drug prescribed?

Biaxin, an antibiotic chemically related to erythromycin, is used to treat certain bacterial infections of the respiratory tract, including:

Strep throat
Pneumonia
Sinusitis (inflamed sinuses)
Tonsillitis (inflamed tonsils)
Acute middle ear infections
Acute flare-ups of chronic bronchitis (inflamed airways)

Biaxin is also prescribed to treat infections of the skin. Combined with Prilosec or Prevacid and amoxicillin, it is used to cure ulcers near the exit from the stomach (duodenal ulcers) caused by *H. pylori* bacteria. It can also be prescribed to combat *Mycobacterium avium* infections in people with AIDS.

Biaxin is available in tablet and suspension form, and in extended-release tablets (Biaxin XL). The extended-release form is used only for sinus inflammation and flare-ups of bronchitis.

Most important fact about this drug

Biaxin, like any other antibiotic, works best when there is a constant amount of drug in the blood. To keep the amount constant, try not to miss any doses.

How should you take this medication?

You may take Biaxin suspension or tablets with or without food. Biaxin XL, however, should always be taken with food. Do not chew or crush Biaxin XL tablets. Shake Biaxin suspension before each dose and use it within 14 days.

Take the medication exactly as prescribed, and be sure to continue taking it for the full course of treatment.

■ *If you miss a dose...*
Take it as soon as you remember. If it is almost time for your next dose, take the one you missed and take the next one 5 to 6 hours later. Then go back to your regular schedule.

■ *Storage instructions...*
Store at room temperature in a tightly closed container, away from light. Do not refrigerate the suspension.

What side effects may occur?

Side effects cannot be anticipated. If any side effects develop or change in intensity, tell your doctor immediately. Only your doctor can determine whether it is safe for you to continue taking Biaxin.

■ *Side effects may include:*
Abdominal pain, abnormal taste, diarrhea, nausea, rash, vomiting

Side effects of Biaxin XL are generally milder than those of regular Biaxin. They may include diarrhea, abnormal taste, and nausea.

Why should this drug not be prescribed?

Do not take Biaxin if you have ever had an allergic reaction to it, or if you are sensitive to it or erythromycin, or similar antibiotics such as Tao and Zithromax. Also avoid Biaxin if you have a heart condition or an imbalance in the body's water and minerals; and do not take the drug while taking Orap, Propulsid, or Seldane.

Special warnings about this medication

If you have severe kidney disease, the doctor may need to prescribe a smaller dose of Biaxin. Make sure the doctor is aware of any kidney problems you may have.

Like other antibiotics, Biaxin may cause a potentially life-threatening form of diarrhea that signals a condition called pseudomembranous colitis (inflammation of the large intestine). Mild diarrhea, a fairly common Biaxin side effect, may disappear as your body gets used to the drug. However, if Biaxin gives you prolonged or severe diarrhea, stop taking the drug and call your doctor immediately.

Possible food and drug interactions when taking this medication

If Biaxin is taken with certain other drugs, the effects of either can be increased, decreased, or altered. It is especially important to check with your doctor before combining Biaxin with the following:

Alprazolam (Xanax)
Blood thinners such as Coumadin
Bromocriptine (Parlodel)
Carbamazepine (Tegretol)
Cholesterol-lowering drugs such as Mevacor and Zocor
Cilostazol (Pletal)
Cyclosporine (Sandimmune, Neoral)
Digoxin (Lanoxin)
Disopyramide (Norpace)
Ergot-based migraine drugs such as Cafergot, DHE, Sansert, and Wigraine
Fluconazole (Diflucan)
Hexobarbital
Methylprednisolone (Medrol)

Midazolam (Versed)
Phenytoin (Dilantin)
Pimozide (Orap)
Quinidine (Quinidex)
Rifabutin (Mycobutin)
Ritonavir (Norvir)
Sildenafil (Viagra)
Tacrolimus (Prograf)
Theophylline (Slo-Phyllin, Theo-Dur, others)
Triazolam (Halcion)
Valproate (Depakene, Depakote)
Zidovudine (Retrovir)

Special information if you are pregnant or breastfeeding

If you are pregnant or plan to become pregnant, notify your doctor immediately. Since Biaxin may have the potential to cause birth defects, it is prescribed during pregnancy only when there is no alternative. Caution is advised when using Biaxin while breastfeeding. Biaxin may appear in breast milk, as does its chemical cousin, erythromycin.

Recommended dosage

BIAXIN

Adults
Respiratory, ear, and skin infections: Your doctor will carefully tailor your individual dosage of Biaxin depending upon the type of infection and organism causing it.

The usual dose varies from 250 to 500 milligrams every 12 hours for 7 to 14 days.

Duodenal ulcers: You can expect one of the following treatment regimens:

500 milligrams of Biaxin, 30 milligrams of Prevacid, and 1 gram of amoxicillin every 12 hours for 10 or 14 days.

500 milligrams of Biaxin, 20 milligrams of Prilosec, and 1 gram of amoxicillin every 12 hours for 10 days. Some patients need to continue taking 20 milligrams of Prilosec on a once-daily basis for an additional 18 days.

500 milligrams of Biaxin every 8 hours plus 40 milligrams of Prilosec every morning for 14 days. Some patients need to continue taking Prilosec at a reduced dosage of 20 milligrams once a day for an additional 14 days.

500 milligrams of Biaxin every 8 or 12 hours plus 400 milligrams of Tritec every 12 hours for 14 days. Some patients need to continue taking 400 milligrams of Tritec every 12 hours for an additional 14 days.

Mycobacterium Avium infections: For prevention or treatment, the recommended dose is 500 milligrams twice a day.

Children

Biaxin is not recommended for children under 6 months of age.

The dose for children older than 6 months depends on how much the child weighs. Biaxin is usually given twice a day for 10 days.

BIAXIN XL

Adults

Sinusitis: The usual dosage is 1,000 milligrams once a day for 14 days.

Bronchitis or pneumonia: The usual dosage is 1,000 milligrams once a day for 7 days.

Children

Safety and effectiveness of Biaxin XL have not been established for children.

Overdosage

Any medication taken in excess can have serious consequences. If you suspect an overdose, seek medical attention immediately.

■ *Symptoms of Biaxin overdose may include:*
   Abdominal pain, diarrhea, nausea, vomiting

Bimatoprost *See Lumigan, page 798.*

Bismuth subsalicylate, Metronidazole, and Tetracycline
   See Helidac Therapy, page 649.

Bisoprolol *See Zebeta, page 1615.*

Bisoprolol with Hydrochlorothiazide *See Ziac, page 1629.*

Bleph-10 *See Sodium Sulamyd, page 1320.*

Bonine *See Antivert, page 119.*

BRETHINE
Pronounced: Breath-EEN
Generic name: Terbutaline sulfate

Why is this drug prescribed?

Brethine is a bronchodilator (a medication that opens the bronchial tubes), prescribed for the prevention and relief of bronchial spasms in asthma. This medication is also used for the relief of bronchial spasms associated with bronchitis and emphysema.

Most important fact about this drug

If you experience an immediate allergic reaction or a worsening of a bronchial spasm, notify your doctor immediately.

How should you take this medication?

Take this drug exactly as prescribed by your doctor.

The action of Brethine may last up to 8 hours. Do not use it more frequently than recommended.

- *If you miss a dose…*
  Take it as soon as you remember. Then take the rest of your medication for that day in evenly spaced doses. Do not take 2 doses at once.
- *Storage instructions…*
  Store at room temperature in a tightly closed container, away from light.

What side effects may occur?

Side effects cannot be anticipated. If any develop or change in intensity, inform your doctor as soon as possible. Only your doctor can determine if it is safe for you to continue taking Brethine.

- *Side effects may include:*
  Chest discomfort, difficulty in breathing, dizziness, drowsiness, fast, fluttery heartbeat, flushed feeling, headache, increased heart rate, nausea, nervousness, pain at injection site, rapid heartbeat, sweating, tremors, vomiting, weakness

Why should this drug not be prescribed?

If you are sensitive to or have ever had an allergic reaction to Brethine or similar drugs such as Ventolin, you should not take this medication. Make sure your doctor is aware of any drug reactions you have experienced.

Special warnings about this medication

When taking Brethine, you should not use other asthma medications before checking with your doctor. Only your doctor can determine what is a sufficient amount of time between doses. If you find that Brethine is not working, tell your doctor immediately.

Consult with your doctor before using this medication if you have diabetes, high blood pressure, or an overactive thyroid gland, or if you have had seizures at any time.

Unless you are directed to do so by your doctor, do not take this medication if you have heart disease, especially if you also have an irregular heart rate.

Possible food and drug interactions when taking this medication

If Brethine is taken with certain other drugs, the effects of either could be increased, decreased, or altered. It is especially important to check with your doctor before combining Brethine with the following:

Antidepressant drugs known as MAO inhibitors (Nardil, Parnate, others)

Beta-blockers (blood pressure medications such as Inderal and Tenormin)

Diuretics (water pills, such as Lasix or HydroDIURIL)

Other bronchodilators such as Proventil and Ventolin

Tricyclic antidepressant drugs such as Elavil and Tofranil

Special information if you are pregnant or breastfeeding

The effects of Brethine during pregnancy have not been adequately studied. If you are pregnant or plan to become pregnant, inform your doctor immediately. It is not known whether Brethine appears in breast milk. If this drug is essential to your health, your doctor may advise you to stop nursing your baby until your treatment is finished.

Recommended dosage

ADULTS

The usual tablet dose is 5 milligrams taken at approximately 6-hour intervals, 3 times per day during waking hours. If side effects are excessive, your doctor may reduce your dose to 2.5 milligrams, 3 times per day.

Do not take more than 15 milligrams in a 24-hour period.

CHILDREN

This medication is not recommended for use in children below 12 years of age.

For children 12 to 15 years of age, the usual dose is 2.5 milligrams, 3 times per day, not to exceed a total of 7.5 milligrams in a 24-hour period.

Overdosage

Any drug taken or used in excess can have serious consequences. Signs of a Brethine overdose are the same as the side effects. If you suspect an overdose, seek medical attention immediately.

Brevicon *See Oral Contraceptives, page 1000.*

Brimonidine *See Alphagan P, page 75.*

Bromocriptine *See Parlodel, page 1033.*

Brontex *See Tussi-Organidin NR, page 1510.*

Budesonide *See Rhinocort Aqua, page 1255.*

Budesonide inhalation powder *See Pulmicort Turbuhaler, page 1206.*

Budesonide inhalation suspension *See Pulmicort Respules, page 1202.*

Budesonide, oral *See Entocort EC, page 515.*

Bumetanide *See Bumex, below.*

BUMEX

Pronounced: BYOO-meks
Generic name: Bumetanide

Why is this drug prescribed?

Bumex is used to lower the amount of excess salt and water in your body by increasing the output of urine. It is prescribed in the treatment of edema, or fluid retention, associated with congestive heart failure and liver or kidney disease. It is also occasionally prescribed, along with other drugs, to treat high blood pressure.

Most important fact about this drug

Bumex is a powerful drug. If taken in excessive amounts, it can severely decrease the levels of water and minerals, especially potassium, your body needs to function. Therefore, your doctor should monitor your dose carefully.

How should you take this medication?

Bumex can increase the frequency of urination and may cause loss of sleep if taken at night. Therefore, if you are taking a single dose of Bumex daily, it should be taken in the morning after breakfast. If you take more than one dose a day, take the last dose no later than 6:00 PM.

■ *If you miss a dose…*
   Take the forgotten dose as soon as you remember. If it is almost time for your next dose, skip the one you missed and go back to your regular schedule. Never take 2 doses at the same time.
■ *Storage instructions…*
   Store at room temperature.

What side effects may occur?

Side effects cannot be anticipated. If any develop or change in intensity, inform your doctor as soon as possible. Only your doctor can determine if it is safe for you to continue taking Bumex.

■ *More common side effects may include:*
   Dizziness, headache, low blood pressure, muscle cramps, nausea
■ *Signs of too much potassium loss are:*
   Dry mouth, irregular heartbeat, muscle cramps or pains, unusual tiredness or weakness

Why should this drug not be prescribed?

Bumex should not be used if you are unable to urinate or if you are dehydrated.

If you are sensitive to or have ever had an allergic reaction to Bumex or similar drugs such as Lasix, you should not take this medication. Make sure your doctor is aware of any drug reactions you have experienced.

Special warnings about this medication

If you are allergic to sulfur-containing drugs such as sulfonamides (antibacterial drugs), check with your doctor before taking Bumex.

Bumex can decrease the number of platelets in your blood. Your doctor should monitor your blood status regularly.

Bumex can cause a loss of potassium from the body. Your doctor may recommend foods or fluids high in potassium or may want you to take a potassium supplement to help prevent this. Follow your doctor's recommendation carefully.

While taking this medication you may feel dizzy or light-headed or actually faint when getting up from a lying or sitting position. If getting up slowly does not help or if this problem continues, notify your doctor.

Possible food and drug interactions when taking this medication

If Bumex is taken with certain other drugs, the effects of either could be increased, decreased, or altered. It is especially important to check with your doctor before combining Bumex with the following:

Blood pressure medications such as Vasotec and Tenormin
Indomethacin (Indocin) and other nonsteroidal anti-inflammatory
    drugs
Probenecid (Benemid)

The combination of Bumex and certain antibiotics or cisplatin (Platinol) may increase the risk of hearing loss.

Because Bumex can lower potassium levels, the combination of Bumex and digitalis or digoxin (Lanoxin) may increase the risk of changes in heartbeat.

The combination of Bumex and lithium (Lithonate) may increase the levels of lithium in the body, causing it to become poisonous.

Special information if you are pregnant or breastfeeding

The effects of Bumex during pregnancy have not been adequately studied. If you are pregnant or plan to become pregnant, inform your doctor immediately. It is not known if this medication appears in breast milk. Your doctor may advise you to discontinue breastfeeding your baby until your treatment with Bumex is finished.

Recommended dosage

ADULTS

The usual total daily dose is 0.5 to 2.0 milligrams a day. For most people, this is taken as a single dose. However, if the initial dose is not adequate, your doctor may have you take a second and, possibly, a third dose at 4- to 5-hour intervals, up to a maximum daily dose of 10 milligrams.

For the continuing control of edema, your doctor may tell you to take Bumex on alternate days or for 3 to 4 days at a time with rest periods of 1 to 2 days in between.

If you have liver failure, your dose will be kept to a minimum and increased very carefully.

CHILDREN

The safety and effectiveness of Bumex have not been established in children below the age of 18.

Overdosage

An overdose of Bumex can lead to severe dehydration, reduction of blood volume, and severe problems with the circulatory system.

■ *The signs of an overdose include:*
Cramps, dizziness, lethargy (sluggishness), loss or lack of appetite, mental confusion, vomiting, weakness

If you suspect an overdose, get medical attention immediately.

Bupropion for depression *See Wellbutrin, page 1587.*

Bupropion for smoking *See Zyban, page 1659.*

BUSPAR

Pronounced: BYOO-spar
Generic name: Buspirone hydrochloride

Why is this drug prescribed?

BuSpar is used in the treatment of anxiety disorders and for short-term relief of the symptoms of anxiety.

Most important fact about this drug

BuSpar should not be used with antidepressant drugs known as monoamine oxidase (MAO) inhibitors. Brands include Nardil and Parnate.

How should you take this medication?

Take BuSpar exactly as prescribed. Do not be discouraged if you feel no immediate effect. The full benefit of this drug may not be seen for 1 to 2 weeks after you start to take it.

■ *If you miss a dose…*
Take the forgotten dose as soon as you remember. If it is almost time for your next dose, skip the one you missed and go back to your regular schedule. Never take 2 doses at the same time.

■ *Storage instructions…*
Store at room temperature in a tightly closed container, away from light.

What side effects may occur?
Side effects cannot be anticipated. If any develop or change in intensity, inform your doctor as soon as possible. Only your doctor can determine if it is safe for you to continue taking BuSpar.

■ *Side effects may include:*
Dizziness, dry mouth, fatigue, headache, light-headedness, nausea, nervousness, unusual excitement

Why should this drug not be prescribed?
If you are sensitive to or have ever had an allergic reaction to BuSpar or similar mood-altering drugs, you should not take this medication. Make sure your doctor is aware of any drug reactions you have experienced.

Anxiety or tension related to everyday stress usually does not require treatment with BuSpar. Discuss your symptoms thoroughly with your doctor.

The use of BuSpar is not recommended if you have severe kidney or liver damage.

Special warnings about this medication
The effects of BuSpar on the central nervous system (brain and spinal cord) are unpredictable. Therefore, you should not drive or operate dangerous machinery or participate in any hazardous activity that requires full mental alertness while you are taking BuSpar.

Possible food and drug interactions when taking this medication
Although BuSpar does not intensify the effects of alcohol, it is best to avoid alcohol while taking this medication.

If BuSpar is taken with certain other drugs, the effects of either can be increased, decreased, or altered. It is especially important to check with your doctor before combining BuSpar with the following:

Haloperidol (Haldol)
MAO inhibitors (antidepressant drugs such as Nardil and Parnate)
The blood-thinning drug Coumadin
Trazodone (Desyrel)

Special information if you are pregnant or breastfeeding
The effects of BuSpar during pregnancy have not been adequately studied. If you are pregnant or plan to become pregnant, inform your doctor

immediately. It is not known whether BuSpar appears in breast milk. If this medication is essential to your health, your doctor may advise you to discontinue breastfeeding until your treatment is finished.

Recommended dosage

ADULTS

The recommended starting dose is a total of 15 milligrams per day, divided into smaller doses, usually 5 milligrams 3 times a day. Every 2 to 3 days, your doctor may increase the dosage 5 milligrams per day as needed. The daily dose should not exceed 60 milligrams.

CHILDREN

The safety and effectiveness of BuSpar have not been established in children under 18 years of age.

Overdosage

Any medication taken in excess can have serious consequences. If you suspect an overdose of BuSpar, seek medical attention immediately.

■ *The symptoms of BuSpar overdose may include:*
Dizziness, drowsiness, nausea or vomiting, severe stomach upset, unusually small pupils

Buspirone *See BuSpar, page 221.*

Butalbital, Acetaminophen, and Caffeine *See Fioricet, page 565.*

Butalbital, Aspirin, and Caffeine *See Fiorinal, page 568.*

Butalbital, Codeine, Aspirin, and Caffeine *See Fiorinal with Codeine, page 571.*

Butoconazole *See Mycelex-3, page 903.*

CADUET

Pronounced: CA-due-et
Generic ingredients: Amlodipine and Atorvastatin

Why is this drug prescribed?

Caduet is a combination of two drugs, amlodipine (also known as Norvasc) and atorvastatin (also known as Lipitor). It is used for people who need both medications.

Amlodipine is used to treat high blood pressure and angina. Angina is characterized by episodes of crushing chest pain that usually results from a lack of oxygen in the heart muscle due to clogged arteries. Amlodipine is a calcium channel blocker, a type of drug that dilates blood vessels and slows the heart to reduce blood pressure and the pain of angina.

Atorvastatin is a cholesterol-lowering drug. Your doctor may prescribe it along with a special diet if your blood cholesterol or triglyceride level is high enough to put you in danger of heart disease, and you have been unable to lower your readings by diet alone. Atorvastatin works by helping to clear harmful low-density lipoprotein (LDL) cholesterol out of the blood and by limiting the body's ability to form new cholesterol.

Most important fact about this drug

You must take Caduet regularly for it to be effective. Caduet does not cure high blood pressure or high cholesterol; it merely helps keep them under control. To get the full benefits of the drug, you should follow any diet, exercise, and weight-loss program prescribed by your doctor.

How should you take this medication?

You should take Caduet exactly as prescribed, even if your symptoms improve. Your dosage will be tailored depending on how much of each individual component is needed. The doctor may also direct you to take atorvastatin or amlodipine separately while you're taking Caduet.

Caduet may be taken with or without food.

■ *If you miss a dose...*
Take the forgotten dose as soon as you remember. However, if it is almost time for your next dose, skip the one you missed and return to your regular schedule. Do not take two doses at once.
■ *Storage instructions...*
Store at room temperature.

What side effects may occur?

Side effects cannot be anticipated. If any develop or change in intensity, tell your doctor as soon as possible. Only your doctor can determine if it is safe to continue using Caduet. Clinical trials have shown no side effect specific to Caduet. Side effects are similar to those reported with amlodipine and atorvastatin.

■ *Side effects of amlodipine may include:*
Dizziness, fatigue, flushing, fluid retention and swelling, headache, palpitations (fluttery or throbbing heartbeat)
■ *Side effects of atorvastatin may include:*
Abdominal pain, constipation, gas, indigestion

Why should this drug not be prescribed?

Never take Caduet during pregnancy or while breastfeeding. Avoid Caduet if you have liver disease, or if the drug gives you an allergic reaction.

Special warnings about this medication

There is a slight chance of liver damage from the atorvastatin contained in Caduet. Your doctor may order a blood test to check your liver function before you start taking the drug, again at 12 weeks after you begin therapy or your dosage is increased, and periodically thereafter. If the tests reveal a problem, you may have to stop using the drug.

Drugs like atorvastatin, one of the ingredients in Caduet, have occasionally been known to damage muscle tissue. Be sure to tell your doctor immediately if you notice any unexplained muscle tenderness, weakness, or pain, especially if you also have a fever or feel sick. Your doctor may want to do a blood test to check for signs of muscle damage.

Check with your doctor before you stop taking Caduet. You may need to reduce the medication slowly.

Your doctor will prescribe Caduet with caution if you have certain heart conditions or liver disease. Make sure your doctor is aware of all your medical problems before you start therapy with Caduet. Although very rare, if you have severe heart disease, you may experience an increase in frequency and duration of angina attacks, or even have a heart attack, when you are starting on Caduet or when your dosage is increased.

Possible food and drug interactions when taking this medication

If you take Caduet with certain other drugs, the effects of either could be increased, decreased, or altered. It is especially important to check with your doctor before combining Caduet with any of the following:

Antacids such as Maalox TC Suspension
Cimetidine
Colestipol (Colestid)
Cyclosporine (Sandimmune, Neoral)
Digoxin (Lanoxin)
Erythromycin (E.E.S., Erythrocin, others)
Fluconazole (Diflucan)
Gemfibrozil (Lopid)
Itraconazole (Sporanox)
Ketoconazole (Nizoral)
Niacin (Niaspan, Niacor, Slo-Niacin)
Oral contraceptives
Spironolactone (Aldactone)

Special information if you are pregnant or breastfeeding

Cholesterol-lowering drugs such as Caduet should never be used during pregnancy, since developing babies need plenty of cholesterol. In fact, your doctor is unlikely to prescribe Caduet if there is even a chance that you may become pregnant. If you do conceive while taking this drug, notify your doctor right away. Caduet does make its way into breast milk, so you should not take this drug while breastfeeding your baby.

Recommended dosage

HIGH BLOOD PRESSURE

Adults

The usual starting dose of amlodipine is 5 milligrams once a day, up to a maximum of 10 milligrams once a day. Individuals who have liver problems and those who are small, fragile, or elderly may be started at 2.5 milligrams a day.

If needed, the doctor may increase your dosage of amlodipine gradually over 1 to 2 weeks depending on how your body responds.

Children 6 to 17 Years Old

The usual dose is 2.5 to 5 milligrams once a day. Doses higher than 5 milligrams daily have not been studied in children.

ANGINA

Adults

The usual dose of amlodipine is 5 to 10 milligrams once a day. The elderly and individuals with liver problems will usually be started at the 5-milligram dose.

HIGH CHOLESTEROL OR TRIGLYCERIDES

Adults

The recommended starting dose is 10 or 20 milligrams once a day. (The doctor may start with 40 milligrams daily if your LDL levels need to be reduced by more than 45 percent.) The doctor will check your cholesterol levels every 2 to 4 weeks and adjust the dose accordingly. The maximum recommended daily dose is 80 milligrams.

Children 10 to 17 Years Old

The recommended starting dose is 10 milligrams once a day. The dosage may be increased after 4 weeks, as determined by the doctor, up to a maximum of 20 milligrams a day. Girls must be having regular menstrual cycles before starting therapy with Lipitor.

The safety and effectiveness of Lipitor in children under 10 years old or in doses greater than 20 milligrams a day have not been studied.

Caduet tablets come in doses ranging from 2.5 milligrams amlodipine/10 milligrams atorvastatin up to 10 milligrams amlodipine/80 milligrams atorvastatin. However, a 2.5-milligram/80-milligram Caduet tablet is not available. If your doctor prescribes this dosage combination, you'll need to take each drug separately.

Overdosage

If you suspect an overdose, seek medical attention immediately. Although no specific information on Caduet overdose is available, any medication taken in excess can have serious consequences.

In addition, no specific information about atorvastatin overdose is available. Experience with amlodipine overdose is limited, but the most likely symptoms include a severe drop in blood pressure and a faster heartbeat.

CAFERGOT

Pronounced: KAF-er-got
Generic ingredients: Ergotamine tartrate, Caffeine

Why is this drug prescribed?

Cafergot is prescribed for the relief or prevention of vascular headaches—for example, migraine, migraine variants, or cluster headaches.

Most important fact about this drug

The excessive use of Cafergot can lead to ergot poisoning, resulting in symptoms such as headache, pain in the legs when walking, muscle pain, numbness, coldness, and abnormal paleness of the fingers and toes. If this condition is not treated, it can lead to gangrene (tissue death due to decreased blood supply).

How should you take this medication?

Cafergot is available in both tablet and suppository form. Be sure to take it exactly as prescribed, remaining within the limits of your recommended dosage.

Cafergot works best if you use it at the first sign of a migraine attack. If you get warning signals of a coming migraine, take the drug before the headache actually starts.

Lie down and relax in a quiet, dark room for at least a couple of hours or until you feel better.

Avoid exposure to cold.

To use the suppositories, follow these steps:

1. If the suppository feels too soft, leave it in the refrigerator for about 30 minutes or put it, still wrapped, in ice water until it hardens.
2. Remove the foil wrapper and dip the tip of the suppository in water.
3. Lie down on your side and with a finger insert the suppository into the rectum. Hold it in place for a few moments.

■ *If you miss a dose...*
Take this medication only when threatened with an attack.

■ *Storage instructions...*
Store at room temperature in a tightly closed container away from light. Keep suppositories away from heat.

What side effects may occur?

Side effects cannot be anticipated. If any develop or change in intensity, inform your doctor as soon as possible. Only your doctor can determine if it is safe for you to continue taking Cafergot.

■ *Side effects may include:*
Fluid retention, high blood pressure, itching, nausea, numbness, rapid heart rate, slow heartbeat, tingling or pins and needles, vertigo, vomiting, weakness

■ *Complications caused by constriction of the blood vessels can be serious. They include:*
Bluish tinge to the skin, chest pain, cold arms and legs, gangrene, muscle pains

Although these symptoms occur most commonly with long-term therapy at relatively high doses, they have been reported with short-term or normal doses. A few people on long-term therapy have developed heart valve problems.

Why should this drug not be prescribed?

If you are sensitive to or have ever had an allergic reaction to ergotamine tartrate, caffeine, or similar drugs, you should not take this medication. Make sure your doctor is aware of any drug reactions you have experienced.

Unless directed to do so by your doctor, do not take this medication if you have coronary heart disease, circulatory problems, high blood pressure, impaired liver or kidney function, or an infection, or if you are pregnant.

Special warnings about this medication

It is extremely important that you do not exceed your recommended dosage, especially when Cafergot is used over long periods. There have been reports of psychological dependence in people who have abused this drug over long periods of time. Discontinuance of the drug may produce withdrawal symptoms such as sudden, severe headaches.

If you experience excessive nausea and vomiting during attacks, making it impossible for you to retain oral medication, your doctor will probably tell you to use rectal suppositories.

This drug is effective only for migraine and migraine-type headaches. Do not use it for any other kind of headache.

Possible food and drug interactions when taking this medication

If Cafergot is taken with certain other drugs, the effects of either could be increased, decreased, or altered. It is especially important to check with your doctor before combining Cafergot with the following:

Beta-blocker drugs (blood pressure medications such as Inderal and Tenormin)

Drugs that constrict the blood vessels, such as EpiPen and the oral decongestant Sudafed

Macrolide antibiotics such as PCE, E.E.S., and Biaxin

Nicotine (Nicoderm, Habitrol, others)

Special information if you are pregnant or breastfeeding

Do not take Cafergot if you are pregnant. Cafergot appears in breast milk and may have serious effects in your baby. If this medication is essential for your health, your doctor may advise you to discontinue breastfeeding.

Recommended dosage

Dosage should start at the first sign of an attack.

ADULTS

Orally

The total dose for any single attack should not exceed 6 tablets.

Rectally

The maximum dose for an individual attack is 2 suppositories.

The total weekly dosage should not exceed 10 tablets or 5 suppositories.

A preventive, short-term dose may be given at bedtime to certain people, but only as prescribed by a doctor.

Overdosage

If you suspect an overdose of Cafergot, seek emergency medical treatment immediately.

■ *Symptoms of Cafergot overdose include:*
Coma, convulsions, diminished or absent pulses, drowsiness, high or low blood pressure, numbness, shock, stupor, tingling, pain and bluish discoloration of the limbs, unresponsiveness, vomiting

CALAN

Pronounced: CAL-an
Generic name: Verapamil hydrochloride
Other brand names: Calan SR, Covera-HS, Isoptin,
  Isoptin SR, Verelan, Verelan PM

Why is this drug prescribed?

Verapamil-based medications can be prescribed for several heart and blood pressure problems. The fast-acting brands (Calan and Isoptin) are taken for angina (chest pain due to clogged cardiac arteries), as well as irregular heartbeat and high blood pressure. The longer-acting brands (Calan SR, Isoptin SR, Verelan, and Verelan PM) are typically used only for high blood pressure. Covera-HS is prescribed for both high blood pressure and angina.

Verapamil is a type of medication called a calcium channel blocker. It eases the heart's workload by slowing down the passage of nerve impulses through it, and hence the contractions of the heart muscle. This improves blood flow through the heart and throughout the body, reduces blood pressure, corrects irregular heartbeat, and helps prevent angina pain.

Some doctors also prescribe verapamil to prevent migraine headache and asthma and to treat manic depression and panic attacks.

Most important fact about this drug

If you have high blood pressure, you must take verapamil regularly for it to be effective. Since blood pressure declines gradually, it may be several weeks before you get the full benefit of verapamil; and you must continue taking it even if you are feeling well. Verapamil does not cure high blood pressure; it merely keeps it under control.

How should you take this medication?

Calan, Isoptin, and Verelan can be taken with or without food. Calan SR and Isoptin SR should be taken with food.

Covera-HS, Calan SR, Isoptin SR, Verelan, and Verelan PM must be swallowed whole and should not be crushed, broken, or chewed.

You may open Verelan capsules and sprinkle the pellets on a spoonful of cool applesauce. Swallow all of the mixture immediately, and then drink a glass of cool water.

Take this medication exactly as prescribed, even if you are feeling well. Try not to miss any doses. If the drug is not taken regularly, your condition can get worse.

Check with your doctor before you stop taking this drug; a slow reduction in the dose may be required.

■ *If you miss a dose...*
Take it as soon as you remember. If it is almost time for your next dose, skip the one you missed and go back to your regular schedule. Never take 2 doses at the same time.
■ *Storage instructions...*
Store at room temperature, away from heat, light, and moisture.

What side effects may occur?

Side effects cannot be anticipated. If any develop or change in intensity, inform your doctor as soon as possible. Only your doctor can determine if it is safe for you to continue taking verapamil.

■ *Side effects may include:*
Congestive heart failure, constipation, dizziness, fatigue, fluid retention, headache, low blood pressure, nausea, rash, shortness of breath,
slow heartbeat, upper respiratory infection

Why should this drug not be prescribed?

If you have low blood pressure or certain types of heart disease or heartbeat irregularities, you should not take verapamil. Make sure your doctor
is aware of any cardiac problems you may have.

If you are sensitive to or have ever had an allergic reaction to Calan or
any other brands of verapamil, or other calcium channel blockers, do not
take this medication.

Special warnings about this medication

Verapamil can reduce or eliminate angina pain caused by exertion or
exercise. Be sure to discuss with your doctor how much exertion is safe
for you.

Verapamil may cause your blood pressure to become too low. If you
experience dizziness or light-headedness, notify your doctor.

Congestive heart failure and fluid in the lungs have occurred in people
taking verapamil together with other heart drugs known as beta-blockers.
Make sure your doctor is aware of all medications you are taking.

If you have a heart condition, liver disease, kidney disease, myasthenia
gravis, or Duchenne's dystrophy (the most common type of muscular
dystrophy), make certain your doctor knows about it. Verapamil should
be used with caution.

If you are taking Covera-HS and you have a narrowing in your stomach
or intestines, be sure your doctor is aware of it when the drug is prescribed.

The outer shell of Covera-HS does not dissolve; do not worry if you see
it in your stool.

Possible food and drug interactions when taking this medication

If verapamil is taken with certain other drugs, the effects of either could
be increased, decreased, or altered. It is especially important to check
with your doctor before combining verapamil with the following:

ACE inhibitor–type blood pressure drugs such as Capoten and
    Vasotec
Beta-blocker-type blood pressure drugs such as Lopressor,
    Tenormin, and Inderal
Vasodilator-type blood pressure drugs such as Loniten
Other high blood pressure drugs such as Minipress
Alcohol
Amiodarone (Cordarone)

Aspirin
Carbamazepine (Tegretol)
Chloroquine (Aralen)
Cimetidine (Tagamet)
Cyclosporine (Sandimmune, Neoral)
Dantrolene (Dantrium)
Digitalis (Lanoxin)
Disopyramide (Norpace)
Diuretics such as Lasix and HydroDIURIL
Erythromycin (E.E.S., Ery-Tab, PCE)
Flecainide (Tambocor)
Glipizide (Glucotrol)
Grapefruit juice
Imipramine (Tofranil)
Lithium (Lithonate)
Nitrates such as Transderm Nitro and Isordil
Phenobarbital
Phenytoin (Dilantin)
Quinidine (Quinidex)
Rifampin (Rifadin)
Ritonavir (Kaletra, Norvir)
Theophylline (Theo-Dur)

Special information if you are pregnant or breastfeeding

The effects of verapamil during pregnancy have not been adequately studied. If you are pregnant or plan to become pregnant, inform your doctor immediately. The drug appears in breast milk and could affect a nursing infant. If this medication is essential to your health, your doctor may advise you to discontinue breastfeeding until your treatment is finished.

Recommended dosage

CALAN AND ISOPTIN

Dosages of this medication must be adjusted to meet individual needs. In general, dosages of this medication should not exceed 480 milligrams per day. Your doctor will closely monitor your response to this drug, usually within 8 hours of the first dose.

Safety and effectiveness of this drug in children have not been established.

Angina

The usual initial dose is 80 to 120 milligrams, 3 times a day. Lower doses of 40 milligrams, 3 times a day, may be used by people who have a stronger response to this medication, such as the elderly or those with decreased liver function. The dosage may be increased by your doctor either daily or weekly until the desired response is seen.

Irregular Heartbeat

The usual dose in people who are also on digitalis ranges from 240 to 320 milligrams per day, divided into 3 or 4 doses.

In those not on digitalis, doses range from a total of 240 to 480 milligrams per day, divided into 3 or 4 doses.

Maximum effects of this drug should be seen in the first 48 hours of use.

High Blood Pressure

The effects of this drug on blood pressure should be seen within the first week of use. Any adjustment of this medication to a higher dose will be based on its effectiveness as determined by your doctor.

The usual dose of this drug, when used alone for high blood pressure, is 80 milligrams, 3 times per day. Total daily doses of 360 milligrams and 480 milligrams may be used. Smaller doses of 40 milligrams, 3 times per day, may be taken by smaller individuals and the elderly.

CALAN SR, ISOPTIN SR, AND VERELAN

Dosages for high blood pressure should be adjusted to meet each individual's needs.

Adults

The usual starting dose of Calan SR and Isoptin SR is 180 milligrams, taken in the morning. For Verelan, it is 240 milligrams. A lower starting dose of 120 milligrams may be taken if the person is smaller. Your doctor will monitor your response to this drug and may adjust it each week. In addition, your doctor may increase the dose and add evening doses to the morning dose, based on the effectiveness of the drug.

You should see results from the drug within a week.

Children

The safety and effectiveness of this drug in children under age 18 have not been established.

Older Adults

Your doctor may start you at a lower dose of 120 milligrams and then adjust it according to your response.

COVERA-HS AND VERELAN PM

Adults

For use only at bedtime, these delayed-action forms of verapamil are timed to deliver their peak benefits in the morning, when blood pressure tends to spike. The usual starting dose is 180 milligrams of Covera-HS or 200 milligrams of Verelan PM. Your doctor may raise the dose gradually if you need more.

Children
Safety and effectiveness in children under age 18 have not been established.

Older Adults
If you have poor kidneys, the dosage may need to be lowered.

Overdosage

Any medication taken in excess can have serious consequences. If you suspect an overdose, seek medical attention immediately.

An overdose of Calan can cause fluid buildup in the lungs, kidney problems, seizures, dangerously low blood pressure, and life-threatening heart problems such as a slow or irregular heartbeat.

After treatment for an overdose, you should remain under observation in the hospital for at least 48 hours, especially if you have taken the sustained-release form of the drug.

Calcipotriene *See Dovonex, page 478.*

Calcitonin-salmon *See Miacalcin, page 845.*

Calcitriol *See Rocaltrol, page 1276.*

CAMPRAL
Pronounced: CAM-prawl
Generic name: Acamprosate calcium

Why is this drug prescribed?

Campral is prescribed to treat alcohol dependence. It helps people who have already stopped drinking alcohol keep from starting again.

You must be alcohol-free before taking Campral for it to work. You must also be prepared to follow a complete alcohol treatment plan that includes mental and behavioral health counseling.

Campral is thought to work by restoring and regulating brain chemicals that have been disrupted by long-term exposure to alcohol. Campral is not used for any type of substance dependence other than alcohol.

Most important fact about this drug

Individuals being treated with Campral and their caregivers should be aware that alcohol dependence and mental health problems frequently occur together. Pay special attention to any worsening of depression or any new symptoms that occur while taking Campral—especially agitation, anxiety, hostility, and suicidal thoughts or behavior—and report them to your doctor immediately.

How should you take this medication?

Campral may be taken with food or on an empty stomach. However, taking it with meals may make it easier to keep on a regular schedule. Continue taking Campral regularly even if you experience a relapse.

■ *If you miss a dose...*
Take the forgotten dose as soon as you remember. However, if it is almost time for your next dose, skip the one you missed and return to your regular schedule. Do not take two doses at once.

■ *Storage instructions...*
Store at room temperature.

What side effects may occur?

Side effects cannot be anticipated. If any develop or change in intensity, tell your doctor as soon as possible. Only your doctor can determine if it is safe to continue using Campral.

■ *Side effects may include:*
Anxiety, body pain or weakness, chest pain, depression, diarrhea, dizziness, headache, heart failure, insomnia, irregular heartbeat, kidney failure, nausea, seizure, sudden death, and suicidal thinking or suicide attempt

Why should this drug not be prescribed?

You cannot use Campral if you have severe kidney disease. You must also avoid the drug if it causes an allergic reaction.

Special warnings about this medication

You must completely avoid alcohol while taking Campral. If you begin drinking again, keep taking Campral and call your doctor right away to discuss your relapse. Campral does not relieve the symptoms of alcohol withdrawal.

Use Campral with caution if you have kidney problems.

Because mental health problems and alcoholism frequently occur together, tell your doctor about any change in mood or behavior while using Campral (see *Most important fact about this drug*).

Campral could affect your judgment, thinking, or motor skills. Do not drive, operate dangerous machinery, or participate in hazardous activities until you know how this drug affects you.

Possible food and drug interactions when taking this medication

At this time, there are no documented drug interactions with Campral. However, you should always tell the doctor about any medicines you take, including over-the-counter drugs, vitamins, and herbal supplements.

Special information if you are pregnant or breastfeeding

Campral has not been studied in pregnant women and should be used only if the benefits outweigh the potential risks. Be sure to tell your doctor if you're pregnant or plan to become pregnant.

In lab studies Campral showed up in the milk of breastfeeding animals. It is not known whether Campral appears in human breast milk. Your doctor may advise you not to breastfeed while taking this drug.

Recommended dosage

ADULTS

The usual starting dose is 2 tablets (each tablet contains 333 milligrams) taken 3 times a day, for a total of 6 tablets a day. Your doctor may lower the dose as needed.

People with moderate kidney disease take half the regular dose— 1 tablet three times a day.

CHILDREN

The safety and effectiveness of Campral have not been studied in children.

Overdosage

Any medication taken in excess can have serious consequences. If you suspect an overdose, seek emergency treatment immediately.

■ *Symptoms of overdose may include:*
Diarrhea

Canasa *See Rowasa, page 1280.*

Candesartan *See Atacand, page 137.*

Candesartan with Hydrochlorothiazide *See Atacand HCT, page 139.*

CAPOTEN

Pronounced: KAP-o-ten
Generic name: Captopril

Why is this drug prescribed?

Capoten is used in the treatment of high blood pressure and congestive heart failure. When prescribed for high blood pressure, it is effective used alone or combined with diuretics. If it is prescribed for congestive heart failure, it is used in combination with digitalis and diuretics. Capoten is in a family of drugs known as ACE (angiotensin converting enzyme) inhibitors. It works by preventing a chemical in your blood called angiotensin I from converting into a more potent form that increases salt and water retention in your body. Capoten also enhances blood flow throughout your blood vessels.

In addition, Capoten is used to improve survival in certain people who have suffered heart attacks and to treat kidney disease in diabetics.

Some doctors also prescribe Capoten for angina pectoris (crushing chest pain), Raynaud's phenomenon (a disorder of the blood vessels that causes the fingers to turn white when exposed to cold), and rheumatoid arthritis.

Most important fact about this drug

If you have high blood pressure, you must take Capoten regularly for it to be effective. Since blood pressure declines gradually, it may be several weeks before you get the full benefit of Capoten; you must continue taking it even if you are feeling well. Capoten does not cure high blood pressure; it merely keeps it under control.

How should you take this medication?

Capoten should be taken 1 hour before meals. If you are taking an antacid such as Mylanta, take it 2 hours prior to Capoten.

Take this medication exactly as prescribed. Stopping Capoten suddenly could cause your blood pressure to increase.

■ *If you miss a dose...*
Take it as soon as you remember. If it is almost time for your next dose, skip the one you missed and go back to your regular schedule. Never take 2 doses at the same time.

■ *Storage instructions...*
Store Capoten at room temperature, away from moisture, in a tightly closed container.

What side effects may occur?

Side effects cannot be anticipated. If any develop or change in intensity, inform your doctor as soon as possible. Only your doctor can determine if it is safe for you to continue taking Capoten.

■ *Side effects may include:*
Itching, loss of taste, low blood pressure, rash

Why should this drug not be prescribed?

If you are sensitive to or have ever had an allergic reaction to Capoten or similar drugs such as Vasotec, you should not take this medication. Make sure that your doctor is aware of any drug reactions that you have experienced.

Special warnings about this medication

If you develop swelling of the face around your lips, tongue, or throat (or of your arms and legs) or have difficulty swallowing, you should stop taking Capoten and contact your doctor immediately. You may need emergency treatment.

If you are receiving bee or wasp venom to prevent an allergic reaction to stings, use of Capoten at the same time may cause a severe allergic reaction.

If you are taking Capoten, a complete assessment of your kidney function should be done, and your kidney function should continue to be monitored. If you have kidney disease, Capoten should be used only if you have taken other blood pressure medications and your doctor has determined that the results were unsatisfactory.

Some people taking Capoten have had a severe allergic reaction during kidney dialysis.

If you are taking Capoten for your heart, be careful not to increase physical activity too quickly. Check with your doctor as to how much exercise is safe for you.

If you are taking Capoten for congestive heart failure, your blood pressure may drop temporarily after the first few doses and you may feel light-headed for a time. Your doctor should monitor you closely when you start taking the medication or when your dosage is increased.

If you are taking high doses of diuretics and Capoten, you may develop excessively low blood pressure. Your doctor may reduce your diuretic dose so that your blood pressure doesn't drop too far.

If you notice a yellow coloring to your skin or the whites of your eyes, stop taking the drug and notify your doctor immediately. You could be developing a liver problem.

Capoten may cause you to become drowsy or less alert, especially if you are also taking a diuretic at the same time. If it has this effect on you, driving or participating in any potentially hazardous activity is not recommended.

Dehydration may cause a drop in blood pressure. If you experience symptoms such as excessive perspiration, vomiting, and/or diarrhea, notify your doctor immediately.

If you develop a sore throat or fever, you should contact your doctor immediately. It could indicate a more serious illness.

If you develop a persistent, dry cough, tell your doctor. It may be due to the medication and, if so, will disappear if you stop taking Capoten.

Possible food and drug interactions when taking this medication

If Capoten is taken with certain other drugs, the effects of either could be increased, decreased, or altered. It is especially important to check with your doctor before combining Capoten with the following:

Allopurinol (Zyloprim)
Aspirin
Blood pressure drugs known as beta-blockers, such as Inderal and Tenormin

Cyclosporine (Sandimmune)
Digoxin (Lanoxin)
Diuretics such as HydroDIURIL
Lithium (Lithonate)
Nitroglycerin and similar heart medicines (Nitro-Dur, Transderm-Nitro, others)
Nonsteroidal anti-inflammatory drugs such as Indocin and Feldene
Potassium preparations such as Micro-K and Slow-K
Potassium-sparing diuretics such as Aldactone and Midamor

Do not use potassium-containing salt substitutes while taking Capoten.

Special information if you are pregnant or breastfeeding

ACE inhibitors such as Capoten have been shown to cause injury and even death to the developing baby when used in pregnancy during the second and third trimesters. If you are pregnant or plan to become pregnant, contact your doctor immediately. Capoten appears in breast milk and could affect a nursing infant. If this medication is essential to your health, your doctor may advise you to discontinue breastfeeding until your treatment is finished.

Recommended dosage

ADULTS

High Blood Pressure
The usual starting dose is 25 milligrams, taken 2 or 3 times a day. If you have any problems with your kidneys or suffer from other major health problems, your starting dose may be lower. Depending on how your blood pressure responds, your doctor may increase your dose later, up to a total of 150 milligrams 2 or 3 times a day. The maximum recommended daily dose is 450 milligrams.

Heart Failure
For most people, the usual dose is 25 milligrams, taken 3 times a day. A daily dosage of 450 milligrams should not be exceeded.

After a Heart Attack
The usual starting dose is 6.25 milligrams, taken once, followed by 12.5 milligrams 3 times a day. Your doctor will increase the dose over the next several days to 25 milligrams, taken 3 times a day and then, over the next several weeks, to 50 milligrams 3 times a day.

Kidney Disease in Diabetes
The usual dose is 25 milligrams, taken 3 times a day.

CHILDREN

The safety and effectiveness of Capoten in children have not been established.

Overdosage

Any medication taken in excess can cause symptoms of overdose. If you suspect an overdose of Capoten, seek medical attention immediately.

Light-headedness or dizziness due to a sudden drop in blood pressure is the primary effect of a Capoten overdose.

CAPOZIDE

Pronounced: KAP-oh-zide
Generic ingredients: Captopril, Hydrochlorothiazide

Why is this drug prescribed?

Capozide is used in the treatment of high blood pressure. It combines an ACE inhibitor with a thiazide diuretic. Captopril, the ACE inhibitor, works by preventing a chemical in your blood called angiotensin I from converting into a more potent form that increases salt and water retention in your body. Captopril also enhances blood flow throughout your blood vessels. Hydrochlorothiazide, the diuretic, helps your body produce and eliminate more urine, which helps in lowering blood pressure.

Most important fact about this drug

You must take Capozide regularly for it to be effective. Since blood pressure declines gradually, it may be several weeks before you get the full benefit of Capozide; and you must continue taking it even if you are feeling well. Capozide does not cure high blood pressure; it merely keeps it under control.

How should you take this medication?

Capozide should be taken 1 hour before meals. Take it exactly as prescribed. Stopping Capozide suddenly could cause your blood pressure to increase.

- *If you miss a dose...*
  Take it as soon as you remember. If it is almost time for your next dose, skip the one you missed and go back to your regular schedule. Never take 2 doses at the same time.
- *Storage instructions...*
  Capozide should be stored at room temperature in a tightly closed container, away from moisture.

What side effects may occur?

Side effects cannot be anticipated. If any develop or change in intensity, inform your doctor as soon as possible. Only your doctor can determine if it is safe for you to continue taking Capozide.

■ *Side effects may include:*
Itching, loss of taste, low blood pressure, rash

Why should this drug not be prescribed?

If you are sensitive to or have ever had an allergic reaction to captopril, hydrochlorothiazide, other ACE inhibitors such as Vasotec, or other thiazide diuretics such as Diuril, or if you are sensitive to other sulfonamide-derived drugs, you should not take this medication. If you have a history of angioedema (swelling of face, extremities, and throat) or inability to urinate, you should not take this medication.

Special warnings about this medication

If you develop swelling of your face around your lips, tongue, or throat, or in your arms and legs, or if you begin to have difficulty swallowing, you should contact your doctor immediately. You may need emergency treatment.

If you develop a sore throat or fever, you should contact your doctor immediately. It could indicate a more serious illness.

If you are taking Capozide, your doctor will make a complete assessment of your kidney function and will continue to monitor it.

If you have impaired kidney function, Capozide should be used only if you have taken other blood pressure medications and your doctor has determined that the results were unsatisfactory.

If you have liver disease or a disease of the connective tissue called lupus erythematosus, Capozide should be used with caution. Tell your doctor immediately if you notice a yellowish color in your skin or the whites of your eyes.

If you have congestive heart failure, you should be carefully watched for low blood pressure. You should not increase your physical activity too quickly.

Excessive sweating, dehydration, severe diarrhea, or vomiting could deplete your fluids and cause your blood pressure to become too low. Be careful when exercising and in hot weather.

This drug should be used with caution if you are on dialysis. There have been reports of extreme allergic reactions during dialysis in people taking ACE-inhibitor medications such as Capozide. Your odds of an allergic reaction also increase if you are being desensitized with bee venom while you are taking Capozide.

While taking Capozide, do not use potassium-sparing diuretics (such as Moduretic), potassium supplements, or salt substitutes containing potassium without talking to your doctor first.

Possible food and drug interactions when taking this medication
Capozide may intensify the effects of alcohol. Do not drink alcohol while taking this medication.

If Capozide is taken with certain other drugs, the effects of either could be increased, decreased, or altered. It is especially important to check with your doctor before combining Capozide with the following:

Antigout drugs such as Zyloprim
Barbiturates such as phenobarbital or Seconal
Calcium
Cardiac glycosides such as Lanoxin
Cholestyramine (Questran)
Colestipol (Colestid)
Corticosteroids such as prednisone (Deltasone)
Diabetes medications such as Micronase and Insulin
Diazoxide (Proglycem)
Heart medications such as Lanoxin
Lithium (Lithonate)
MAO inhibitors (antidepressants such as Nardil)
Methenamine (Mandelamine)
Narcotics such as Percocet
Nitroglycerin or other nitrates such as Transderm-Nitro
Nonsteroidal anti-inflammatory drugs such as Naprosyn
Norepinephrine (Levophed)
Oral blood thinners such as Coumadin
Other blood pressure drugs such as Hytrin and Minipress
Potassium-sparing diuretics such as Moduretic
Potassium supplements such as Slow K
Probenecid (Benemid)
Salt substitutes containing potassium
Sulfinpyrazone (Anturane)

Special information if you are pregnant or breastfeeding
ACE inhibitors such as Capozide have been shown to cause injury and even death to the developing baby when used in pregnancy during the second or third trimesters. If you are pregnant, your doctor should discontinue your use of this medication as soon as possible. If you plan to become pregnant and are taking Capozide, contact your doctor immediately to discuss the potential hazard to your unborn child. Capozide appears in breast milk and could affect a nursing infant. If this medication is essential to your health, your doctor may advise you to discontinue breastfeeding until your treatment is finished.

Recommended dosage

ADULTS

Dosages of this drug are always individualized, and your doctor will determine what combination works best for you. This medication can be used in conjunction with other blood pressure medications such as beta-blockers. Dosages are also adjusted for people with decreased kidney function.

The initial dose is one 25-milligram/15-milligram tablet, once a day. If this is not effective, your doctor may adjust the dosage upward every 6 weeks. In general, the daily dose of captopril should not exceed 150 milligrams. The maximum recommended daily dose of hydrochlorothiazide is 50 milligrams.

CHILDREN

The safety and effectiveness of Capozide in children have not been established. Capozide should be used in children only if other measures for controlling blood pressure have not been effective.

OLDER ADULTS

Your doctor will determine the dosage according to your particular needs.

Overdosage

Any medication taken in excess can have serious consequences. If you suspect an overdose, seek medical attention immediately.

■ *The symptoms of Capozide overdose may include:*
Coma, lethargy, low blood pressure, sluggishness, stomach and intestinal irritation and hyperactivity

Captopril *See Capoten, page 236.*

Captopril with Hydrochlorothiazide *See Capozide, page 240.*

Carac *See Efudex, page 496.*

CARAFATE

Pronounced: CARE-uh-fate
Generic name: Sucralfate

Why is this drug prescribed?

Carafate Tablets and Suspension are used for the short-term treatment (up to 8 weeks) of an active duodenal ulcer; Carafate Tablets are also used for longer-term therapy at a reduced dosage after a duodenal ulcer has healed.

Carafate helps ulcers heal by forming a protective coating over them.

Some doctors also prescribe Carafate for ulcers in the mouth and esophagus that develop during cancer therapy, for digestive tract irritation caused by drugs, for long-term treatment of stomach ulcers, and to relieve pain following tonsil removal.

Most important fact about this drug
A duodenal ulcer is a recurring illness. While Carafate can cure an acute ulcer, it cannot prevent other ulcers from developing or lessen their severity.

How should you take this medication?
Carafate works best when taken on an empty stomach. If you take an antacid to relieve pain, avoid doing it within one-half hour before or after you take Carafate. Always take Carafate exactly as prescribed.

- *If you miss a dose...*
  Take it as soon as you remember. If it is almost time for your next dose, skip the one you missed and go back to your regular schedule. Never take 2 doses at the same time.
- *Storage instructions...*
  Store at room temperature. Protect the suspension from freezing.

What side effects may occur?
Side effects cannot be anticipated. If any develop or change in intensity, inform your doctor as soon as possible. Only your doctor can determine if it is safe for you to continue taking Carafate.

- *Side effects may include:*
  Constipation

Why should this drug not be prescribed?
There are no restrictions on the use of this drug.

Special warnings about this medication
If you have kidney failure or are on dialysis, the doctor will be cautious about prescribing this drug. Use of Carafate while taking aluminum-containing antacids may increase the possibility of aluminum poisoning in those with kidney failure.

Possible food and drug interactions when taking this medication
If Carafate is taken with certain other drugs, the effects of either could be increased, decreased, or altered. It is especially important to check with your doctor before combining Carafate with the following:

Antacids such as Mylanta and Maalox
Blood-thinning drugs such as Coumadin
Cimetidine (Tagamet)

Digoxin (Lanoxin)
Drugs for controlling spasms, such as Bentyl
Ketoconazole (Nizoral)
Levothyroxine (Synthroid)
Phenytoin (Dilantin)
Quinidine (Quinidex)
Quinolone antibiotics such as Cipro and Floxin
Ranitidine (Zantac)
Tetracycline (Sumycin)
Theophylline (Theo-Dur)

Special information if you are pregnant or breastfeeding

The effects of Carafate during pregnancy have not been adequately studied. If you are pregnant or plan to become pregnant, inform your doctor
immediately. Carafate may appear in breast milk and could affect a nursing infant. If this medication is essential to your health, your doctor may
advise you to discontinue breastfeeding until your treatment with this
medication is finished.

Recommended dosage

ADULTS

Active Duodenal Ulcer
The usual dose is 1 gram (1 tablet or 2 teaspoonfuls of suspension) 4
times a day on an empty stomach. Although your ulcer may heal during
the first 2 weeks of therapy, Carafate should be continued for 4 to 8
weeks.

Maintenance Therapy
The usual dose is 1 gram (1 tablet) 2 times a day.

CHILDREN

The safety and effectiveness of Carafate in children have not been established.

Overdosage

Although the risk of overdose with Carafate is low, any medication taken
in excess can have serious consequences. If you suspect an overdose,
seek medical attention immediately.

■ *Symptoms of overdose may include:*
Abdominal pain, indigestion, nausea, vomiting

Carbamazepine *See Tegretol, page 1395.*

Carbatrol *See Tegretol, page 1395.*

Carbidopa with Levodopa *See Sinemet CR, page 1309.*

Carbidopa, Levodopa, and Entacapone
See Stalevo, page 1342.

CARDENE
Pronounced: CAR-deen
Generic name: Nicardipine hydrochloride

Why is this drug prescribed?

Cardene, a type of medication called a calcium channel blocker, is prescribed for the treatment of chronic stable angina (chest pain usually caused by lack of oxygen to the heart resulting from clogged arteries, brought on by exertion) and for high blood pressure. When used to treat angina, Cardene is effective alone or in combination with beta-blocking medications such as Tenormin or Inderal. If it is used to treat high blood pressure, Cardene is effective alone or in combination with other high blood pressure medications. Calcium channel blockers ease the workload of the heart by slowing down its muscle contractions and the passage of nerve impulses through it. This improves blood flow through the heart and throughout the body, reducing blood pressure.

Cardene SR, a long-acting form of the drug, is prescribed only for high blood pressure.

Some doctors also prescribe Cardene to prevent migraine headache and to treat congestive heart failure. In combination with other drugs, such as Amicar, Cardene is also prescribed to manage neurological problems following certain kinds of stroke.

Most important fact about this drug

If you have high blood pressure, you must take Cardene regularly for it to be effective. Since blood pressure declines gradually, it may be several weeks before you get the full benefit of Cardene, and you must continue taking it even if you are feeling well. Cardene does not cure high blood pressure; it merely keeps it under control.

How should you take this medication?

Take this medication exactly as prescribed, even if your symptoms have disappeared.

If you are taking Cardene SR, swallow the capsule whole; do not chew, crush, or divide it.

Try not to miss any doses. If Cardene is not taken regularly, your condition may worsen.

■ *If you miss a dose…*
  Take it as soon as you remember. If it is almost time for the next dose, skip the one you missed and go back to your regular schedule. Do not take 2 doses at the same time.

■ *Storage instructions...*
Store at room temperature, away from light and moisture.

What side effects may occur?
Side effects cannot be anticipated. If any develop or change in intensity, inform your doctor as soon as possible. Only your doctor can determine if it is safe for you to continue taking Cardene.

■ *Side effects may include:*
Dizziness, flushing, headache, increased chest pain (angina), indigestion, nausea, pounding or rapid heartbeat, sleepiness, swelling of feet, weakness

Why should this drug not be prescribed?
If you have advanced aortic stenosis (a narrowing of the aorta that causes obstruction of blood flow from the heart to the body), you should not take this medication.

If you are sensitive to or have ever had an allergic reaction to Cardene, you should not take this medication. Make sure your doctor is aware of any drug reactions you may have experienced.

Special warnings about this medication
Cardene can reduce or eliminate chest (angina) pain caused by exertion or exercise. Be sure to discuss with your doctor how much exercise or exertion is safe for you.

If you experience increased chest pain when you start taking Cardene or when your dosage is increased, contact your doctor immediately.

Your doctor will monitor your progress especially carefully if you have congestive heart failure, particularly if you are also taking a beta-blocking medication such as Tenormin or Inderal.

Cardene can cause your blood pressure to become too low, making you feel light-headed or faint. Your doctor should check your blood pressure when you start taking Cardene and continue to monitor it while your dosage is being adjusted.

If you have liver disease or decreased liver function, use this drug with caution.

Possible food and drug interactions when taking this medication
If Cardene is taken with certain other drugs, the effects of either could be increased, decreased, or altered. It is especially important to check with your doctor before combining Cardene with the following:

Amiodarone (Cordarone)
Cimetidine (Tagamet)
Cyclosporine (Sandimmune)
Digoxin (Lanoxin)
Phenytoin (Dilantin)
Propranolol (Inderal)

Special information if you are pregnant or breastfeeding
The effects of Cardene during pregnancy have not been adequately studied. If you are pregnant or plan to become pregnant, inform your doctor immediately. Cardene may appear in breast milk and could affect a nursing infant. If this medication is essential to your health, your doctor may advise you to discontinue breastfeeding until your treatment with Cardene is finished.

Recommended dosage

ADULTS

Angina
Your doctor will adjust the dosage according to your needs, usually beginning with 20 milligrams 3 times a day. The usual regular dose is 20 to 40 milligrams 3 times a day. Your physician may monitor your condition for at least 3 days before adjusting your dose.

High Blood Pressure
Your doctor will adjust the dosage to suit your needs. The starting dose of Cardene is usually 20 milligrams 3 times a day. The regular dose ranges from 20 to 40 milligrams 3 times a day.

The starting dose of Cardene SR is usually 30 milligrams 2 times a day. The regular dose ranges from 30 to 60 milligrams 2 times a day.

Your doctor may monitor your response to this medication for a few hours after the first dose, and will check your condition for at least 3 days before adjusting your dose.

CHILDREN

The safety and effectiveness of this drug in children under age 18 have not been established.

Overdosage

■ *Symptoms of Cardene overdose may include:*
Confusion, drowsiness, severe low blood pressure, slow heartbeat, slurred speech

If you suspect an overdose, seek medical attention immediately.

CARDIZEM

Pronounced: CAR-di-zem
Generic name: Diltiazem hydrochloride
Other brand names: Cardizem CD, Cardizem LA,
   Cardizem SR, Dilacor XR, Tiazac

Why is this drug prescribed?

Cardizem and Cardizem CD (a controlled-release form of diltiazem) are used in the treatment of angina pectoris (chest pain usually caused by lack of oxygen to the heart due to clogged arteries). Cardizem, Cardizem CD, and Cardizem LA (an extended-release, once-a-day tablet form of diltiazem) are used to control chronic stable angina (caused by exertion). Cardizem CD and Cardizem LA are also used to treat high blood pressure. Another controlled-release form, Cardizem SR, is used only in the treatment of high blood pressure. Cardizem, a calcium channel blocker, dilates blood vessels and slows the heart to reduce blood pressure and the pain of angina.

Doctors sometimes prescribe Cardizem for loss of circulation in the fingers and toes (Raynaud's phenomenon), for involuntary movements (tardive dyskinesia), and to prevent heart attack.

Tiazac and Dilacor XR are used in the treatment of high blood pressure and chronic stable angina. They may be taken alone or combined with other blood pressure medications.

Most important fact about this drug

If you are taking Cardizem for high blood pressure, remember that it does not cure the problem; it merely controls it. You may need to take a blood pressure medication for the rest of your life.

If you are taking Cardizem for angina, do not stop suddenly. This can lead to an increase in your attacks.

How should you take this medication?

Cardizem should be taken before meals and at bedtime. Cardizem CD, Cardizem LA, Cardizem SR, and Dilacor XR should be swallowed whole; do not chew, crush, or divide. Tiazac capsules may be swallowed whole or opened and sprinkled on a spoonful of applesauce. Swallow the applesauce immediately, without chewing, and wash it down with a glass of cool water.

Take this medication exactly as prescribed by your doctor, even if your symptoms have disappeared.

■ *If you miss a dose...*
   If you forget to take a dose, take it as soon as you remember. If it's almost time for your next dose, skip the missed dose and go back to your regular schedule. Never take 2 doses at the same time.

■ *Storage instructions...*
Cardizem should be stored at room temperature; protect from moisture.

What side effects may occur?
Side effects cannot be anticipated. If any develop or change in intensity, inform your doctor as soon as possible. Only your doctor can determine if it is safe for you to continue taking Cardizem.

■ *Side effects may include:*
Abnormally slow heartbeat (more common with Cardizem SR, Cardizem LA, and Cardizem CD), dizziness, fatigue, fluid retention, flushing (more common with Cardizem SR, Cardizem LA, and Cardizem CD), headache, nausea, rash, weakness

Why should this drug not be prescribed?
If you suffer from *sick sinus* syndrome or second- or third-degree heart block (various types of irregular heartbeat), you should not take diltiazem unless you have a ventricular pacemaker. Also avoid diltiazem if you've just suffered a heart attack or have lung congestion.

Do not take diltiazem if you have low blood pressure or an allergy to the drug.

Special warnings about this medication
If you have congestive heart failure or suffer from kidney or liver disease, use Cardizem with caution.

This medication may cause your heart rate to become too slow. You should check your pulse regularly.

Possible food and drug interactions when taking this medication
If Cardizem is taken with certain other drugs, the effects of either could be increased, decreased, or altered. It is especially important to check with your doctor before combining Cardizem with the following:

Beta-blockers (heart and blood pressure drugs such as Tenormin
and Inderal)
Carbamazepine (Tegretol)
Cimetidine (Tagamet)
Cyclosporine (Sandimmune, Neoral)
Digoxin (Lanoxin)
Lovastatin (Mevacor)
Midazolam (Versed)
Rifampin (Rifadin)
Triazolam (Halcion)

Special information if you are pregnant or breastfeeding
The effects of Cardizem during pregnancy have not been adequately studied. If you are pregnant or plan to become pregnant, inform your doctor

immediately. Cardizem appears in breast milk and could affect a nursing infant. If this medication is essential to your health, your doctor may advise you to discontinue breastfeeding until your treatment with this medication is finished.

Recommended dosage

ADULTS

Dosage levels are determined by each individual's needs.

Cardizem
The average daily dosage is between 180 milligrams and 360 milligrams, divided into 3 or 4 smaller doses.

Cardizem SR
The recommended starting dosage is 60 to 120 milligrams 2 times a day, to be increased to 240 to 360 milligrams a day.

Cardizem CD
This is a once-a-day form of this drug. For high blood pressure, starting doses range from 180 to 240 milligrams; for angina, 120 to 180 milligrams.

Cardizem LA
This is also a once-a-day drug. For high blood pressure, when used alone, doses start at 180 to 240 milligrams and may be increased to as much as 540 milligrams once daily. For angina, the starting dose is 180 milligrams once daily with increases every 7 to 14 days if necessary.

Dilacor XR
This is another once-a-day drug. For high blood pressure, doses start at 180 to 240 milligrams and may be increased to as much as 540 milligrams. For angina, doses start at 120 milligrams and may be increased to 480 milligrams.

Tiazac
The usual starting dose for high blood pressure is 120 to 240 milligrams once a day. After the drug has taken effect—in about 2 weeks—the dose can range from 120 to 540 milligrams. For angina, once-daily doses start at 120 to 180 milligrams and may be increased to 540 milligrams if necessary.

CHILDREN

Safety and effectiveness in children have not been established.

Overdosage

Any medication taken in excess can have serious consequences. If you suspect an overdose of Cardizem, seek medical attention immediately.

■ *Symptoms of Cardizem overdose may include:*
Dizziness, fainting, heart failure, irregular pulse, low blood pressure, very slow heartbeat

CARDURA

Pronounced: car-DUHR-uh
Generic name: Doxazosin mesylate

Why is this drug prescribed?

Cardura is used in the treatment of benign prostatic hyperplasia, a condition in which the prostate gland grows larger, pressing on the urethra and threatening to block the flow of urine from the bladder. The drug relieves symptoms such as a weak stream, dribbling, incomplete emptying of the bladder, frequent urination, and burning during urination.

Cardura is also used in the treatment of high blood pressure. It is effective when used alone or in combination with other blood pressure medications, such as diuretics, beta-blocking medications, calcium channel blockers, or ACE inhibitors.

Doctors also prescribe Cardura, along with other drugs such as digitalis and diuretics, for treatment of congestive heart failure.

Most important fact about this drug

If you have high blood pressure, you must take Cardura regularly for it to be effective. Since blood pressure declines gradually, it may be several weeks before you get the full benefit of Cardura; and you must continue taking it even if you are feeling well. Cardura does not cure high blood pressure; it merely keeps it under control.

How should you take this medication?

This medication can be taken with or without food.

Cardura should be taken exactly as prescribed, even if your symptoms have disappeared. Try not to miss any doses. If this medication is not taken regularly, your condition may worsen.

If you have benign prostatic hyperplasia, you should see improvement in a week. Your blood pressure will fall in 2 to 6 hours.

■ *If you miss a dose...*
Take it as soon as you remember. If it is almost time for your next dose, skip the one you missed and go back to your regular schedule. Never take 2 doses at the same time.

■ *Storage instructions...*
Store at room temperature.

What side effects may occur?
Side effects cannot be anticipated. If any develop or change in intensity, inform your doctor as soon as possible. Only your doctor can determine if it is safe for you to continue taking Cardura.

■ *Side effects may include:*
Dizziness, drowsiness, fatigue, headache

Why should this drug not be prescribed?
Cardura should not be taken if you are sensitive to or have ever had an allergic reaction to Cardura or such drugs as Minipress or Hytrin. Make sure your doctor is aware of any drug reactions you may have experienced.

Special warnings about this medication
Cardura can cause low blood pressure, especially when you first start taking the medication and when dosage is increased. This can cause you to become faint, dizzy, or light-headed, particularly when first standing up. You should avoid driving or any hazardous tasks where injury could occur for 24 hours after taking the first dose, after your dose has been increased, or if Cardura has been stopped and then restarted.

In rare cases, men taking drugs such as Cardura have developed priapism—a painful, long-lasting erection that persists for hours. This condition can lead to impotence, so if it occurs, contact your doctor right away.

If you have liver disease or are taking other medications that alter liver function, your doctor will monitor you closely when you take Cardura.

Cardura may lower blood counts. Your doctor will most likely monitor your blood counts while you are taking this medication.

This medication may cause you to become drowsy or sleepy. For this reason, too, driving or operating dangerous machinery or participating in any hazardous activity that requires full mental alertness is not recommended.

Prostate cancer has some of the same symptoms as benign prostatic hyperplasia; your doctor will want to make sure you do not have cancer before starting you on Cardura.

Possible food and drug interactions when taking this medication
No significant interactions have been reported.

Special information if you are pregnant or breastfeeding
The effects of Cardura during pregnancy have not been adequately studied. If you are pregnant or plan to become pregnant, inform your doctor immediately. Cardura may appear in breast milk and could affect a nursing infant. If this medication is essential to your health, your doctor may advise you to discontinue breastfeeding until your treatment with this medication is finished.

Recommended dosage

ADULTS

Your doctor will adjust the dosage to fit your needs.

The usual starting dose is 1 milligram, taken once a day. To minimize the potential for dizziness or fainting associated with Cardura, which may occur between 2 and 6 hours after a dose, your doctor will monitor your blood pressure during this period and afterwards.

After the effects of the starting dose are measured, your doctor may increase the daily dose to 2 milligrams and then, if necessary, to 4 milligrams, 8 milligrams, or, in people with high blood pressure only, up to 16 milligrams. As the dose increases, the potential for side effects such as dizziness, vertigo, light-headedness, and fainting also increases.

CHILDREN

The safety and effectiveness of this drug in children have not been established.

Overdosage

Any medication taken in excess can have serious consequences. Although no specific information is available, low blood pressure is the most likely symptom of an overdose of Cardura.

If you suspect an overdose, seek medical attention immediately.

Carisoprodol See Soma, page 1322.

Carvedilol See Coreg, page 335.

Cataflam See Voltaren, page 1579.

CATAPRES

Pronounced: KAT-uh-press
Generic name: Clonidine hydrochloride

Why is this drug prescribed?

Catapres is prescribed for high blood pressure. It is effective when used alone or with other high blood pressure medications.

Doctors also prescribe Catapres for alcohol, nicotine, or benzodiazepine (tranquilizer) withdrawal; migraine headaches; smoking cessation programs; Tourette's syndrome (tics and uncontrollable utterances); narcotic/methadone detoxification; premenstrual tension; and diabetic diarrhea.

Most important fact about this drug

If you have high blood pressure, you must take Catapres regularly for it to be effective. Since blood pressure declines gradually, it may be several weeks before you get the full benefit of Catapres; and you must continue taking it even if you are feeling well. Catapres does not cure high blood pressure; it merely keeps it under control.

How should you take this medication?
Take this medication exactly as prescribed, even if you are feeling well. Try not to miss any doses. If Catapres is not taken regularly, your condition may get worse.

The Catapres-TTS patch should be put on a hairless, clean area of the outer upper arm or chest. Normally, a new one is applied every 7 days to a new area of the skin. If the patch becomes loose, use some adhesive tape or an adhesive bandage to keep it in place.

■ *If you miss a dose...*
Take it as soon as you remember, then go back to your regular schedule. If you forget to take the medication 2 or more times in a row, or if you forget to change the transdermal patch for 3 or more days, contact your doctor.

■ *Storage instructions...*
Store at room temperature in a tightly closed container, away from light.

What side effects may occur?
Side effects cannot be anticipated. If any develop or change in intensity, inform your doctor as soon as possible. Only your doctor can determine if it is safe for you to continue taking Catapres.

■ *Side effects may include:*
Agitation, constipation, dizziness, drowsiness, dry mouth, fatigue, impotence, loss of sex drive, nausea, nervousness, sedation (calm), vomiting, weakness

Why should this drug not be prescribed?
Do not take this medication if you have ever had an allergic reaction to Catapres or to any of the components of the transdermal patch.

Special warnings about this medication
Catapres should not be stopped suddenly. Headache, nervousness, agitation, tremor, confusion, and rapid rise in blood pressure can occur. Severe reactions such as disruption of brain functions, stroke, fluid in the lungs, and death have also been reported. Your doctor should gradually reduce your dosage over several days to avoid withdrawal symptoms.

If you see redness, blistering, or a rash near the transdermal patch, call your doctor. You may need to remove the patch. If you are troubled by mild irritation before completing 7 days of use, you may remove the patch and apply a new one at a different site.

If your doctor has switched you to oral Catapres (tablet) because you had an allergic reaction, such as a rash or hives, to the transdermal skin patch, be aware that you may have a similar reaction to the Catapres tablet.

If you have severe heart or kidney disease, are recovering from a heart attack, or have a disease of the blood vessels of the brain, your doctor will prescribe Catapres with caution.

If you are taking Catapres and a beta-blocker such as Inderal or Tenormin, and your doctor wants to stop your medication, the beta-blocker should be stopped several days before the gradual withdrawal of Catapres.

Catapres may cause drowsiness. If it has this effect on you, avoid driving, operating dangerous machinery, and participating in any hazardous activity that requires full mental alertness.

The used Catapres-TTS patch still contains enough drug to be harmful to children and pets. Fold the patch in half with the adhesive sides together and dispose of it out of the reach of children.

Possible food and drug interactions when taking this medication

Catapres may increase the effects of alcohol. Do not drink alcohol while taking this medication.

If Catapres is taken with certain other drugs, the effects of either could be increased, decreased, or altered. It is especially important to check with your doctor before combining Catapres with the following:

Barbiturates such as Nembutal and Seconal
Beta-blocker drugs such as the blood pressure medications Inderal and Lopressor
Calcium blockers such as the heart medications Calan and Cardizem
Digitalis
Sedatives such as Valium, Xanax, and Halcion
Tricyclic antidepressants such as Elavil and Tofranil

Special information if you are pregnant or breastfeeding

The effects of Catapres during pregnancy have not been adequately studied. If you are pregnant or plan to become pregnant, inform your doctor immediately. Catapres appears in breast milk and could affect a nursing infant. If this medication is essential to your health, your doctor may advise you to discontinue breastfeeding until your treatment with this medication is finished.

Recommended dosage

ADULTS

The dosage will be adjusted to your individual needs.

The usual starting dose is 0.1 milligram twice a day (usually in the morning and at bedtime).

The regular dose of Catapres is determined by increasing the daily dose by 0.1 milligram at weekly intervals until the desired response is achieved. A larger portion of the increased dose can be taken at bedtime to reduce the potential side effects of drowsiness and dry mouth that may appear when you begin taking this drug.

The most common effective dosages range from 0.2 milligram to 0.6 milligram per day, divided into smaller doses. The maximum effective dose is 2.4 milligrams per day; however, this dose is not usually prescribed.

Transdermal Patch
The patch comes in different strengths, and your doctor will determine which is best for you based on your blood pressure response.

People who are using another high blood pressure medication should not stop taking it abruptly when they begin using the patch, because the medication in the patch may take a few days to begin working. The other medication should be discontinued slowly as the patch begins to take effect.

CHILDREN

The safety and effectiveness of Catapres tablets and patches in children below the age of 12 have not been established.

OLDER ADULTS

Dosages are generally as above; however, the initial dosage for an older person may be lower than the regular starting dose.

Overdosage

■ *Symptoms of Catapres overdose may include:*
Constriction of pupils of the eye, drowsiness, high blood pressure followed by a drop in pressure, irritability, low body temperature, slowed breathing, slowed heartbeat, slowed reflexes, weakness

Large overdoses can cause changes in heart function or rhythm, coma, seizures, and temporary interruptions in breathing.

Getting a patch in the mouth or swallowing one can cause an overdose.

If you suspect symptoms of a Catapres overdose, seek medical attention immediately.

CAVERJECT
Pronounced: CA-vur-jekt
Generic name: Alprostadil
Other brand names: Edex, Muse

Why is this drug prescribed?
Caverject is used to treat male impotence. Your doctor also may use Caverject to help diagnose the exact nature of your impotence.

Caverject and the similar brand Edex are both taken by injection. A third brand, Muse, is taken as a small suppository inserted into the penis.

Most important fact about this drug

Caverject is known to have caused extremely long-lasting erections. Serious harm can occur from such a prolonged erection, so call your doctor or seek other professional help if an erection lasts more than 4 hours. Usually the erection should last about 1 hour.

How should you use this medication?

Caverject is injected into a specific area of the penis and produces an erection within 5 to 20 minutes. Do not use Caverject more than 3 times a week. Wait at least 24 hours between use.

The first injections are performed by your doctor in the doctor's office in order to determine the proper dosage. Afterwards, you can inject Caverject yourself as needed. Your doctor will train you in the proper technique for injecting Caverject, and you'll be given complete printed instructions. Follow these directions exactly, and do not change the dose your doctor has determined.

Do not use a Caverject solution that appears cloudy or colored or that contains particles. Do not shake the vial.

Wash your hands thoroughly and do not touch the needle. Carefully choose the injection site as instructed by your doctor, always avoiding visible veins. Cleanse the site with an alcohol swab. With each use, alternate the side of the penis and the site of the injection.

Use the needle/syringe and vial only once, then discard them properly. Do not share needles or allow anyone else to use your medication.

Caverject comes in both 10-microgram and 20-microgram strengths. Make sure you are using a vial with the correct strength.

After injecting Edex, put pressure on the injection site for 5 minutes, or until the bleeding stops.

If you have been prescribed Muse, your doctor will instruct you in the correct way to insert the suppository. An erection should occur within 5 to 10 minutes of insertion. Do not use more than 2 suppositories in 24 hours. Discard each applicator after a single use.

■ *Storage instructions...*

Store unused packs of Caverject at room temperature for up to 3 months. Protect from freezing or from overheating.

Once the Caverject solution is mixed, you must use it immediately or discard it.

When traveling, take care to prevent exposing Caverject to freezing or excessive heat. Do not store Caverject in checked luggage or leave it in a closed car.

Muse suppositories should be stored in the refrigerator, but may be left at room temperature for up to 14 days before use. Protect the suppositories from high temperatures and direct sunlight. Carry them in a portable cooler when traveling.

What side effects may occur?

Side effects cannot be anticipated. If any develop or change in intensity, inform your doctor as soon as possible. Only your doctor can determine if it is safe for you to continue using this drug.

CAVERJECT AND EDEX

The most common side effect is mild to moderate pain in the penis during and/or after injection, reported by about one-third of users. A small amount of bleeding may occur at the injection site. Notify your doctor if you have a condition or are taking a medication that interferes with blood clotting. As with any injection, the site can become infected. Call your doctor if you notice any redness, lumps, swelling, tenderness, or curving of the erect penis.

Your doctor should examine your penis regularly if you use Caverject. Use of Caverject may result in formation of fibrous (hardened) tissue in the penis or erections at an unusual angle. If those side effects occur, inform your doctor and stop using Caverject.

■ *Side effects may include:*
Blood-filled swelling at the site of injection, disorder of the penis (such as discoloration of the head, strange feeling, tearing of the skin), hardened tissue in the penis, pain in the penis, prolonged erection, upper respiratory infection

MUSE

■ *Side effects may include:*
Extremely low blood pressure, flu symptoms, headache, infection, pain, penis bleeding, penis burning or pain, testicular pain

In addition, Muse may cause vaginal burning and itching in your partner.

Why should this drug not be prescribed?

Do not use Caverject if you have a condition that might result in long-lasting erections, such as sickle-cell anemia, increased levels of white cells in your blood, and tumor of the bone marrow.

Men with penile implants or an unusually formed penis should not use Caverject. The drug is not for use in women, children, or men whose doctors have advised them not to have sex.

Do not use Caverject, Edex, or Muse if it causes an allergic reaction or if you have ever had a reaction to any prostaglandin drugs.

Do not use Muse for sexual intercourse with a pregnant woman unless you use a condom.

Special warnings about this medication

These drugs offer no protection from the transmission of sexually transmitted diseases, such as HIV, the virus that causes AIDS. Small amounts of bleeding at the injection or suppository site can increase the risk of transmission of blood-borne diseases such as HIV.

Remember that development of any unusual deformity of the penis while using Caverject is a signal to stop taking the injections and inform your doctor.

Because Muse has been known to cause low blood pressure and fainting, you should avoid driving and other hazardous activities after using it. When using Muse with a partner in her child-bearing years, contraception is recommended.

Possible food and drug interactions when using this medication

No interactions have been reported, but these products should not be used with other drugs that act on blood vessels, such as blood pressure medications.

You may have some bleeding at the site of injection or insertion. If you are taking anticoagulants such as heparin or Coumadin you may bleed more. Make sure that any doctor who prescribes an anticoagulant is aware that you are using one of these medications.

Recommended dosage

CAVERJECT AND EDEX

The correct dose of Caverject must be carefully determined by your doctor. Each man will need a different dose of Caverject, but the usual starting dosage is 1.25 or 2.5 micrograms, which is then increased gradually. Your doctor will adjust the dosage, particularly if it produces erections lasting longer than 1 hour. Doses should not exceed 60 micrograms.

The dosage range for Edex is 1 to 40 micrograms, given over 5 to 10 seconds.

Do not change your dosage without your doctor's approval. See your doctor every 3 months for a checkup.

MUSE

The suppositories come in four strengths, ranging from 125 to 1,000 micrograms. The 125- or 250-microgram strength is recommended at the start. Your doctor will prescribe a higher strength if necessary. Remember that you must not use more than 2 suppositories in each 24 hours.

Overdosage

No overdose of Caverject has been reported. However, any medication taken in excess can have serious consequences. The chief symptom of an overdose of this drug would be a prolonged erection. If you suspect an overdose, seek medical attention immediately.

CECLOR

Pronounced: SEE-klor
Generic name: Cefaclor

Why is this drug prescribed?

Ceclor, a cephalosporin antibiotic, is used in the treatment of ear, nose, throat, respiratory tract, urinary tract, and skin infections caused by specific bacteria, including staph, strep, and *E. coli.* Uses include treatment of sore or strep throat, pneumonia, and tonsillitis. Ceclor CD, an extended-release form of the drug, is also used for flare-ups of chronic bronchitis.

Most important fact about this drug

If you are allergic to either penicillin or cephalosporin antibiotics in any form, consult your doctor *before* taking Ceclor. There is a possibility that you are allergic to both types of medication; and if a reaction occurs, it could be extremely severe. If you take the drug and feel signs of a reaction, seek medical attention immediately.

How should you take this medication?

Your doctor will prescribe Ceclor only to treat a bacterial infection; it will not cure a viral infection, such as the common cold. It's important to take the full dosage schedule of Ceclor, even if you're feeling better in a few days. Not completing the full dosage schedule may decrease the drug's effectiveness and increase the chances that the bacteria may become resistant to Ceclor and similar antibiotics.

Ceclor works fastest when taken on an empty stomach. However, your doctor may ask you to take this drug with food to avoid stomach upset.

Ceclor CD should be taken with meals or at least within 1 hour of eating because it's better absorbed with food. Do not cut, crush, or chew the tablets.

Ceclor suspension should be shaken well before using.

■ *If you miss a dose…*
Take it as soon as you remember. If it is almost time for your next dose, skip the one you missed and go back to your regular schedule. Never take 2 doses at the same time.

■ *Storage instructions…*
Keep Ceclor capsules in the container they came in, tightly closed. Store at room temperature.

Refrigerate Ceclor suspension. Discard any unused portion after 14 days.

What side effects may occur?

Side effects cannot be anticipated. If any develop or change in intensity, inform your doctor as soon as possible. Only your doctor can determine if it is safe for you to continue taking Ceclor.

■ *Side effects of Ceclor may include:*
Diarrhea, hives, itching

■ *Side effects of Ceclor CD may include:*
Diarrhea, headache, nasal inflammation, nausea

Why should this drug not be prescribed?

If you are sensitive to or have ever had an allergic reaction to Ceclor or any other cephalosporin antibiotic, you should not take this medication. Make sure your doctor is aware of any drug reactions you have experienced.

Unless you are directed to do so by your doctor, do not take this medication if you have a history of gastrointestinal problems, particularly bowel inflammation (colitis). You may be at increased risk for side effects.

Special warnings about this medication

Ceclor may cause a false positive result with some urine sugar tests for diabetics. Your doctor can advise you of any adjustments you may need to make in your medication or diet.

Ceclor occasionally causes diarrhea. Some diarrhea medications can make this diarrhea worse. Check with your doctor before taking any diarrhea remedy.

Oral contraceptives may not work properly while you are taking Ceclor. For greater certainty, use other measures while taking Ceclor.

Possible food and drug interactions when taking this medication

If Ceclor is taken with certain other drugs, the effects of either could be increased, decreased, or altered. It is especially important to check with your doctor before combining Ceclor with the following:

Antacids containing magnesium or aluminum, including Gelusil,
  Maalox, and Mylanta (interact with Ceclor CD only)
Certain antibiotics such as Amikin
Certain potent diuretics such as Edecrin and Lasix
Probenecid (Benemid)
Warfarin (Coumadin)

Special information if you are pregnant or breastfeeding

The effects of Ceclor during pregnancy have not been adequately studied. If you are pregnant or plan to become pregnant, this drug should be used only under special circumstances. Ceclor appears in breast milk and could affect a nursing infant. If this medication is essential to your health, your doctor may advise you to stop nursing your baby until your treatment with Ceclor is finished.

Recommended dosage

CECLOR

Adults
The usual adult dose is 250 milligrams every 8 hours. For more severe infections (such as pneumonia), your doctor may increase the dosage.

Children
The usual daily dosage is 20 milligrams per 2.2 pounds of body weight per day, divided into smaller doses and taken every 8 or 12 hours. In more serious infections, such as middle ear infection, the usual dose is 40 milligrams per 2.2 pounds of body weight per day, divided into smaller doses. The total daily dose should not exceed 1 gram.

CECLOR CD

Adults: Bronchitis
The usual dose is 500 milligrams every 12 hours for 7 days.

Adults: Sore throat, Tonsillitis, and Skin Infections
The usual dose is 375 milligrams every 12 hours for 10 days (sore throat and tonsillitis) or 7 to 10 days (skin infections).

Children
The safety and effectiveness of Ceclor CD in children under age 16 have not been established.

Overdosage

■ *Symptoms of Ceclor overdose may include:*
  Diarrhea, nausea, stomach upset, vomiting

If other symptoms are present, they may be related to an allergic reaction or other underlying disease. In any case, you should contact your doctor or an emergency room immediately.

CEDAX
Pronounced: SEE-daks
Generic name: Ceftibuten

Why is this drug prescribed?
Cedax cures mild to moderate bacterial infections of the throat, ear, and respiratory tract. Among these infections are strep throat, tonsillitis, and acute otitis media (middle ear infection) in children and adults. Cedax is also prescribed for acute flare-ups of chronic bronchitis in adults. Cedax is a cephalosporin antibiotic.

Most important fact about this drug

If you are allergic to either penicillin or cephalosporin antibiotics in any form, double-check with your doctor *before* taking Cedax. There is a possibility that you are allergic to both types of medication and if a reaction occurs, it could be extremely severe. (Symptoms include swelling of the face, lips, tongue, and throat, making it difficult to breathe.) If you take the drug and feel any signs of this reaction, seek medical attention immediately.

How should you take this medication?

To make certain your infection is fully cleared up, take all the Cedax your doctor prescribes, even if you begin to feel better after the first few days.

If you are using the oral suspension, it must be taken at least 2 hours before a meal or 1 hour after. Shake well before using.

■ *If you miss a dose...*
Take it as soon as you remember. If it is almost time for your next dose, skip the one you missed and go back to your regular schedule. Never take 2 doses at the same time.

■ *Storage instructions...*
Keep the oral suspension in the refrigerator, and discard any unused portion after 14 days. Capsules may be stored at room temperature.

What side effects may occur?

Side effects cannot be anticipated. If any develop or change in intensity, notify your doctor as soon as possible. Only your doctor can determine whether it is safe for you to continue taking Cedax.

■ *Side effects in adults may include:*
Diarrhea, headache, nausea

■ *The most common side effect in children is:*
Diarrhea (especially in children age 2 and under)

Why should this drug not be prescribed?

If you are sensitive to or have ever had an allergic reaction to Cedax or other cephalosporins, such as Keflex, do not take this medication.

Make sure your doctor is aware of any drug reactions you have experienced. If you've ever had a reaction to penicillin, you're more likely to react to Cedax. If a reaction occurs, you'll have to stop taking Cedax.

Special warnings about this medication

If you have a history of gastrointestinal disease, particularly colitis, take Cedax with caution. If you develop diarrhea while taking Cedax, check with your doctor. The problem could be a sign of a serious condition.

Tell your doctor if you have kidney problems. Your dosage may have to be lowered. If you are diabetic, be sure to tell your doctor before starting therapy with Cedax; the oral suspension contains sugar.

If new infections (called superinfections) occur, talk to your doctor. You may need to be treated with a different antibiotic.

Do not give this medication to other people or use it for other infections before checking with your doctor. The drug is not effective against every type of germ.

Possible food and drug interactions when taking this medication

Zantac may boost the level of Cedax in your system. Check with your doctor before combining these drugs.

Special information if you are pregnant or breastfeeding

The effects of Cedax during pregnancy have not been adequately studied. If you are pregnant or plan to become pregnant, tell your doctor immediately. Cedax may appear in breast milk and could affect a nursing infant. If this medication is essential to your health, your doctor may advise you to stop breastfeeding until your treatment is finished.

Recommended dosage

ADULTS

The usual dose is a single 400-milligram capsule once a day. People with serious kidney problems are prescribed a smaller dose.

CHILDREN

Cedax oral suspension is taken once daily. The usual dose is determined by the child's weight.

22 pounds: 1 teaspoon
44 pounds: 2 teaspoons
88 pounds: 4 teaspoons

Children weighing over 100 pounds receive the adult dose. Cedax has not been tested for treatment of infants less than 6 months old.

Overdosage

Although no specific information is available, an overdose of cephalosporins has been known to cause convulsions. Any medication taken in excess can have serious consequences. If you suspect an overdose of Cedax, seek medical attention immediately.

Cefaclor See Ceclor, page 261.

Cefadroxil See Duricef, page 483.

Cefdinir See Omnicef, page 996.

Cefditoren See Spectracef, page 1332.

Cefixime *See Suprax, page 1356.*

Cefprozil *See Cefzil, page 269.*

Ceftibuten *See Cedax, page 263.*

CEFTIN
Pronounced: SEF-tin
Generic name: Cefuroxime axetil

Why is this drug prescribed?
Ceftin, a cephalosporin antibiotic, is prescribed for mild to moderately severe bacterial infections of the throat, lungs, ears, skin, sinuses, and urinary tract, and for gonorrhea. Ceftin tablets are also prescribed in the early stages of Lyme disease.

Most important fact about this drug
If you are allergic to either penicillin or cephalosporin antibiotics such as Ceclor, Cefzil, or Keflex, consult your doctor *before* taking Ceftin. There is a possibility that you are allergic to both types of medication; if a reaction occurs, it could be extremely severe. If you take the drug and develop shortness of breath, a pounding heartbeat, a skin rash, or hives, seek medical attention immediately.

How should you take this medication?
Ceftin tablets can be taken on a full or empty stomach. However, this drug enters the bloodstream and works faster when taken after meals. Ceftin oral suspension must be taken with food. Shake the suspension well before each use.

Take this medication exactly as prescribed: It is important that you finish taking all of this medication to obtain the maximum benefit.

The crushed tablet has a strong, persistent, bitter taste. Children who cannot swallow the tablet whole should take the oral suspension. Shake the oral suspension well before each use.

- *If you miss a dose...*
  Take it as soon as you remember. If it is almost time for your next dose skip the one you missed and go back to the regular schedule. Do not take 2 doses at once.
- *Storage instructions...*
  Store tablets at room temperature in a tightly closed container. Protect from moisture. The oral suspension may be stored either in the refrigerator or at room temperature. Replace the cap securely after each use. Discard any unused suspension after 10 days.

What side effects may occur?

Side effects cannot be anticipated. If any develop or change in intensity, inform your doctor as soon as possible. Only your doctor can determine if it is safe for you to continue taking Ceftin.

■ *Side effects may include:*
Diaper rash in infants, diarrhea, nausea, vomiting

Ceftin has also been reported to occasionally cause allergic reactions, blood disorders, colitis, jaundice (yellowing of the skin and eyes), kidney and liver problems, peeling skin, seizures, severe blisters in the mouth and eyes, and impaired blood clotting.

Why should this drug not be prescribed?

Ceftin should not be prescribed if you have a known allergy to cephalosporin antibiotics.

Special warnings about this medication

Inflammation of the bowel (colitis) has been reported with the use of Ceftin; therefore, if you develop diarrhea while taking this medication, notify your doctor.

Continued or prolonged use of Ceftin may result in an overgrowth of bacteria that do not respond to this medication and can cause a second infection. You should take this drug only when it is prescribed by your doctor, even if you have symptoms like those of a previous infection. Tell your doctor if you have any kidney problems. If you do, the drug must be used cautiously.

If you are allergic to penicillin, you may also be allergic to Ceftin. Make sure your doctor is aware of any allergies you have.

Cephalosporin antibiotics such as Ceftin sometimes trigger a tendency to bleed, especially in people with liver or kidney damage, individuals who are malnourished, those on long courses of antibiotic therapy, and people taking blood-thinning medications. If you fall into one of these categories, the doctor will monitor you carefully.

The safety and effectiveness of Ceftin have not been studied in people with kidney failure. If you have kidney problems, your doctor will need to monitor you carefully.

Possible food and drug interactions when taking this medication

It is important to consult your doctor before taking this drug with probenecid, a gout medication.

If diarrhea occurs while taking Ceftin, consult your doctor before taking an antidiarrhea medication. Certain drugs, such as Lomotil, may cause your diarrhea to become worse.

Be cautious if you are taking potent water pills (diuretics) such as Lasix while on Ceftin. The combination could affect your kidneys.

Special information if you are pregnant or breastfeeding

The effects of Ceftin during pregnancy have not been adequately studied. If you are pregnant or plan to become pregnant, inform your doctor immediately. Ceftin appears in breast milk and could affect a nursing infant. If this medication is essential to your health, your doctor may advise you to discontinue breastfeeding until your treatment with this medication is finished.

Recommended dosage

ADULTS

The usual dose for adults and children 13 years and older is 250 milligrams 2 times a day for up to 10 days. For more severe infections the dose may be increased to 500 milligrams 2 times a day.

Throat and Tonsil Infections
The usual dose is 250 milligrams 2 times a day for 10 days.

Sinus Infection
The usual dose is 250 milligrams 2 times a day for 10 days.

Bronchitis
The usual dose is 250 or 500 milligrams 2 times a day for 5 to 10 days.

Skin Infections
The usual dose is 250 or 500 milligrams 2 times a day for 10 days.

Urinary Tract Infection
The usual dose is 250 milligrams 2 times a day for 7 to 10 days.

Gonorrhea
The usual treatment is a single dose of 1 gram.

Early Lyme Disease
The usual dosage is 500 milligrams, taken twice a day for 20 days.

CHILDREN

Ceftin oral suspension may be given to children ranging in age from 3 months to 12 years.

Your doctor will determine the dosage based on your child's weight and the type of infection being treated. Ceftin oral suspension is given twice a day for 10 days. The maximum daily dose ranges from 500 to 1,000 milligrams.

For children who are able to swallow tablets whole, the usual dosage for ear infection or sinus infection is 250 milligrams 2 times a day for 10 days.

Overdosage

Any medication taken in excess can have serious consequences. Overdosage with cephalosporin antibiotics can cause brain irritation, leading to convulsions. If you suspect an overdose, seek medical attention immediately.

Cefuroxime *See Ceftin, page 266.*

CEFZIL

Pronounced: SEFF-zil
Generic name: Cefprozil

Why is this drug prescribed?

Cefzil, a cephalosporin antibiotic, is prescribed for mild to moderately severe bacterial infections of the throat, ear, sinuses, respiratory tract, and skin. Among these infections are strep throat, tonsillitis, bronchitis, and pneumonia.

Most important fact about this drug

If you are allergic to penicillin or cephalosporin antibiotics in any form, consult your doctor *before* taking Cefzil. An allergy to either type of medication may signal an allergy to Cefzil; and if a reaction occurs, it could be extremely severe. If you take the drug and feel signs of a reaction, seek medical attention immediately.

How should you use this medication?

Your doctor will prescribe Cefzil only to treat a bacterial infection; it will not cure a viral infection, such as the common cold. It's important to take the full dosage schedule of Cefzil, even if you're feeling better in a few days. Not completing the full dosage schedule may decrease the drug's effectiveness and increase the chances that the bacteria may become resistant to Cefzil and similar antibiotics.

Cefzil works fastest when taken on an empty stomach, but can be taken with food to avoid stomach upset.

Cefzil oral suspension should be shaken well before using.

■ *If you miss a dose…*
Take it as soon as you remember. If it is almost time for your next dose, skip the one you missed and go back to your regular schedule. Never take 2 doses at the same time.

■ *Storage instructions…*
Store Cefzil tablets at room temperature. Keep the oral suspension in the refrigerator; discard any unused portion after 14 days.

What side effects may occur?

Side effects cannot be anticipated. If any develop or change in intensity, notify your doctor as soon as possible. Only your doctor can determine whether it is safe for you to continue taking Cefzil.

The most common side effect is nausea.

■ *Other side effects may include:*
Abdominal pain, confusion, diaper rash, diarrhea, difficulty sleeping, dizziness, genital itching, headache, hives, hyperactivity, nervousness, rash, sleepiness, superinfection (additional infection), vaginal inflammation, vomiting, yellow eyes and skin

Although not reported for Cefzil, similar antibiotics have been known occasionally to have severe side effects such as anaphylaxis (a severe allergic reaction), skin rash with blisters, Stevens-Johnson syndrome (a rare skin condition characterized by severe blisters and bleeding in the lips, eyes, mouth, nose, and genitals), and "serum-sickness" (itchy rash, fever, and pain in the joints).

Why should this drug not be prescribed?
If you are sensitive to or have ever had an allergic reaction to Cefzil or other cephalosporin antibiotics, do not take this medication. Make sure your doctor is aware of any drug reactions you have experienced.

Special warnings about this medication
Cefzil occasionally causes colitis (inflammation of the bowel), leading to diarrhea. Some diarrhea medications can make this diarrhea worse. Check with your doctor before taking any diarrhea remedy.

Oral contraceptives may not work properly while you are taking Cefzil. For greater certainty, use other measures while taking Cefzil.

Your doctor will check your kidney function before and during your treatment with this medication.

Use Cefzil with caution if you are taking a strong diuretic, or if you have ever had stomach and intestinal disease, particularly colitis.

If new infections (called superinfections) occur, talk to your doctor. You may need to be treated with a different antibiotic.

Cefzil may alter the results of some urine sugar tests for diabetics. Your doctor can advise you of any adjustments you may need to make in your medication or diet.

Possible food and drug interactions when taking this medication
When Cefzil is taken with certain other drugs, the effects of either could be increased, decreased, or altered. It is especially important to check with your doctor before combining Cefzil with the following:

Certain other antibiotics such as Amikin
Certain potent diuretics such as Edecrin and Lasix
Oral contraceptives
Probenecid (Benemid)
Propantheline (Pro-Banthine)

Special information if you are pregnant or breastfeeding

The effects of Cefzil during pregnancy have not been adequately studied. If you are pregnant or plan to become pregnant, inform your doctor immediately. Cefzil does appear in breast milk and could affect a nursing infant. If this medication is essential to your health, your doctor may advise you to stop breastfeeding until your treatment with this medication is finished.

Recommended dosage

ADULTS

Throat and Respiratory Tract Infections
The usual dose is 500 milligrams, taken once or twice a day for 10 days.

Sinus Infection
The usual dose is 250 milligrams every 12 hours for 10 days; for severe infections, the dose is 500 milligrams.

Skin Infections
The dosage is usually either 250 milligrams, taken 2 times a day, or 500 milligrams taken once or twice a day for 10 days.

CHILDREN 2 TO 12 YEARS OLD

Throat Infections and Tonsillitis
The usual dose is 7.5 milligrams for each 2.2 pounds of body weight, taken 2 times a day for 10 days.

Skin Infections
The usual dose is 20 milligrams for each 2.2 pounds of body weight, taken once a day for 10 days.

INFANTS AND CHILDREN 6 MONTHS TO 12 YEARS OLD

Ear Infections
The usual dose is 15 milligrams for each 2.2 pounds of body weight, taken 2 times a day for 10 days.

Sinus Infection
The usual dose is 7.5 milligrams for each 2.2 pounds of body weight every 12 hours for 10 days. For severe infections, the amount may be doubled.

Overdosage

Although no specific information is available, any medication taken in excess can have serious consequences. If you suspect an overdose of Cefzil, seek medical attention immediately.

CELEBREX

Pronounced:.SELL-eh-breks
Generic name: Celecoxib

Why is this drug prescribed?

Celebrex is prescribed for acute pain, menstrual cramps, and the pain and inflammation of osteoarthritis and rheumatoid arthritis. It is a member of a new class of nonsteroidal anti-inflammatory drugs (NSAIDs) called COX-2 inhibitors. Like older NSAIDs such as Motrin and Naprosyn, Celebrex is believed to fight pain and inflammation by inhibiting the effect of a natural enzyme called COX-2. Unlike the older medications, however, it does not interfere with a similar substance, called COX-1, which exerts a protective effect on the lining of the stomach. Therefore, Celebrex may be less likely to cause the bleeding and ulcers that sometimes accompany sustained use of the older NSAIDs.

Celebrex has also been found to reduce the number of colorectal polyps (growths in the wall of the lower intestine and rectum) in people who suffer from the condition called familial adenomatous polyposis (FAP), an inherited tendency to develop large numbers of colorectal polyps that eventually become cancerous.

Most important fact about this drug

Like other NSAID medication, Celebrex could increase the chance of having a heart attack or stroke, possibly resulting in death. The risk is greater if you have heart disease or use NSAIDs for a long time. It's important to discuss the risks and benefits of using Celebrex with your doctor and to use the lowest effective dose for the shortest amount of time possible.

Although Celebrex is easy on the stomach, it still poses some degree of risk—especially if you've had a stomach ulcer or gastrointestinal bleeding in the past. All NSAIDs, including Celebrex, can cause serious—and even life-threatening—ulcers and bleeding in the stomach and intestines. These side effects can happen without symptoms and may occur at any time during treatment. If you've ever had ulcers or stomach bleeding, make sure the doctor is aware of it. And be sure to alert the doctor if you develop any digestive problems or notice a change in your bowel movement (such as blood in the stool or black, sticky stools).

How should you take this medication?

Take Celebrex exactly as prescribed. You can take it with or without food.

- *If you miss a dose…*
  Take it as soon as you remember. If it is almost time for your next dose, skip the one you missed and go back to your regular schedule. Do not take 2 doses at the same time.
- *Storage instructions…*
  Store at room temperature.

What side effects may occur?

Side effects cannot be anticipated. If any develop or change in intensity, inform your doctor as soon as possible. Only your doctor can determine if it is safe for you to continue taking Celebrex.

■ *Side effects may include:*
Abdominal pain, diarrhea, headache, indigestion, nausea, respiratory infection, sinus inflammation

Why should this drug not be prescribed?

Do not take Celebrex right before or after heart bypass surgery (also called coronary artery bypass graft, or CABG).

In addition, you should not use Celebrex if you are allergic to sulfonamide drugs such as sulfadiazine, sulfisoxazole, Gantanol, and Thiosulfil. Also avoid the drug if you've ever suffered an asthma attack, face and throat swelling, or skin eruptions after taking aspirin or other NSAIDs. If you find that you are allergic to Celebrex, you will not be able to use it.

Special warnings about this medication

Remember to tell your doctor about any stomach ulcers or bleeding you've had in the past. Also alert your doctor if you develop any digestive problems, swelling, or rash. The chance of developing a stomach ulcer or bleeding while taking Celebrex increases if you also take steroid drugs or blood thinners, smoke, drink alcohol, or use Celebrex or other NSAID medications for a long time. The risk is also greater if you're older or in poor health. Be sure the doctor is aware of your full medical history.

If you have asthma, use Celebrex with caution. It could trigger an attack, especially if you are also sensitive to aspirin.

If you are taking a steroid medication for your arthritis, do not discontinue it abruptly when you begin therapy with Celebrex. Celebrex is not a substitute for such drugs.

Celebrex has been known to cause kidney or liver problems, particularly in people with an existing condition. If you have such a disorder, take Celebrex with caution. If you develop symptoms of liver poisoning, stop taking the drug and see your doctor immediately. Warning signs include nausea, fatigue, itching, yellowish skin, pain in the right side of the stomach, and flu-like symptoms.

If you are prone to anemia (loss of red blood cells), make sure your doctor knows about it. Celebrex occasionally fosters this problem.

Celebrex sometimes causes water retention, which can aggravate swelling, high blood pressure, and heart failure. Use this drug with caution if you have any of these conditions.

There is no proof that Celebrex reduces the odds of cancer in people who take the drug for FAP. Although Celebrex can reduce the number of growths, you'll still need the other treatments and frequent checkups that this condition requires.

The safety and effectiveness of Celebrex have not been tested in children under 18.

Possible food and drug interactions when taking this medication

If Celebrex is taken with certain other drugs, the effects of either could be increased, decreased, or altered. It is especially important to check with your doctor before combining Celebrex with the following:

> ACE inhibitors (a type of blood pressure and heart medication, including such drugs as Capoten, Vasotec, and Prinivil)
> Blood-thinning agents such as Coumadin
> Fluconazole (Diflucan)
> Furosemide (Lasix)
> Lithium (Eskalith, Lithobid)
> Thiazide diuretics (water pills) such as hydrochlorothiazide and Dyazide

If you take low-dose aspirin to protect against heart attack, you can continue taking it with Celebrex. Using aspirin increases your risk of stomach ulcers or bleeding, but Celebrex does not have aspirin's protective effect on the heart.

Special information if you are pregnant or breastfeeding

Celebrex can harm a developing baby if taken during the third trimester, and its safety earlier in pregnancy has not been confirmed. Take it during pregnancy only if you feel the risk is justified.

It's possible that Celebrex makes its way into breast milk (limited data from one subject indicated that the drug was excreted in human milk), and it could cause serious reactions in a nursing infant. If this drug is essential to your health, your doctor may advise you to discontinue breastfeeding.

Recommended dosage

The following dosages are typically cut in half for people with moderate liver problems.

ADULTS

Osteoarthritis
The recommended daily dose is 200 milligrams, taken as a single dose or in 100-milligram doses twice a day.

Rheumatoid Arthritis
The recommended dose is 100 to 200 milligrams twice a day.

Acute Pain and Menstrual Cramps
The recommended starting dose is 400 milligrams, followed by an additional 200 milligrams if needed on the first day. On subsequent days, the recommended dosage is 200 milligrams twice a day.

Familial Adenomatous Polyposis
The recommended dose is 400 milligrams twice a day with food.

Overdosage
Any medication taken in excess can have serious consequences. If you suspect an overdose, seek medical attention immediately.

■ *Symptoms of Celebrex overdose may include:*
Breathing difficulties, coma, drowsiness, gastrointestinal bleeding, high blood pressure, kidney failure, nausea, sluggishness, stomach pain, vomiting

Celecoxib *See Celebrex, page 272.*

CELEXA
Pronounced: sell-EX-ah
Generic name: Citalopram hydrobromide

Why is this drug prescribed?
Celexa is used to treat major depression—a stubbornly low mood that persists nearly every day for at least 2 weeks and interferes with everyday living. Symptoms may include loss of interest in your usual activities, insomnia or excessive sleeping, a change in weight or appetite, constant fidgeting or a slowdown in movement, fatigue, feelings of worthlessness or guilt, difficulty thinking or concentrating, and repeated thoughts of suicide.

Like the antidepressant medications Paxil, Prozac, and Zoloft, Celexa is thought to work by boosting serotonin levels in the brain. Serotonin, one of the nervous system's primary chemical messengers, is known to elevate mood.

Most important fact about this drug
Be careful to avoid taking Celexa for 2 weeks before or after using an antidepressant known as an MAO inhibitor. Drugs in this category include Marplan, Nardil, and Parnate. Combining Celexa with one of these medications could lead to a serious—even fatal—reaction.

How should you take this medication?
Celexa is available in tablet and liquid forms. Take either formulation once a day, in the morning or evening, with or without food. Although your depression will begin to lift in 1 to 4 weeks, you should continue taking Celexa regularly. It takes several months for the medication to yield its full benefits.

■ *If you miss a dose…*
Take it as soon as you remember. If it is almost time for your next dose, skip the one you missed and go back to your regular schedule. Do not take 2 doses at the same time.

■ *Storage instructions…*
Store at room temperature.

What side effects may occur?

Side effects cannot be anticipated. If any develop or change in intensity, inform your doctor as soon as possible. Only your doctor can determine if it is safe for you to continue taking Celexa.

■ *Side effects may include:*
Abdominal pain, agitation, anxiety, diarrhea, drowsiness, dry mouth, ejaculation disorders, fatigue, impotence, indigestion, insomnia, loss of appetite, nausea, painful menstruation, respiratory tract infection, sinus or nasal inflammation, sweating, tremor, vomiting

Why should this drug not be prescribed?

If Celexa gives you an allergic reaction, you cannot continue using it. Also remember that Celexa must never be combined with an MAO inhibitor (see *Most important fact about this drug*).

Special warnings about this medication

In clinical studies, antidepressants increased the risk of suicidal thinking and behavior in children and adolescents with depression and other psychiatric disorders. Anyone considering the use of Celexa or any other antidepressant in a child or adolescent must balance this risk with the clinical need. Celexa has not been studied in children or adolescents and is not approved for treating anyone less than 18 years old.

Additionally, the progression of major depression is associated with a worsening of symptoms and/or the emergence of suicidal thinking or behavior in both adults and children, whether or not they are taking antidepressants. Individuals being treated with Celexa and their caregivers should watch for any change in symptoms or any new symptoms that appear suddenly—especially agitation, anxiety, hostility, panic, restlessness, extreme hyperactivity, and suicidal thinking or behavior—and report them to the doctor immediately. Be especially observant at the beginning of treatment or whenever there is a change in dose.

In recommended doses, Celexa does not seem to impair judgment or motor skills. However, a theoretical possibility of such problems remains, so you should use caution when driving or operating dangerous equipment until you are certain of Celexa's effect.

There is a slight chance that Celexa will trigger a manic episode. Use Celexa with caution if you suffer from manic-depression (bipolar disorder). Use caution, too, if you are over 60 years old, have liver or kidney problems, suffer from heart disease or high blood pressure, or have ever had seizures.

Possible food and drug interactions when taking this medication

Celexa does not increase the effects of alcohol. Nevertheless, it's considered unwise to combine Celexa with alcohol or any other drug that affects the brain. (Be particularly careful to avoid MAO inhibitors.)

If Celexa is taken with certain other drugs, the effects of either could be increased, decreased, or altered. Tell your doctor about any prescription or over-the-counter drugs you are planning to take, and be especially certain to check with him before combining Celexa with the following:

Carbamazepine (Tegretol)
Cimetidine (Tagamet)
Erythromycin (Eryc, Ery-Tab)
Fluconazole (Diflucan)
Itraconazole (Sporanox)
Ketoconazole (Nizoral)
Lithium (Lithobid, Lithonate)
Metoprolol (Lopressor)
Omeprazole (Prilosec)
Other antidepressants such as Elavil, Norpramin, Pamelor,
    and Tofranil
Sumatriptan (Imitrex)
Warfarin (Coumadin)

Special information if you are pregnant or breastfeeding

The effects of Celexa during pregnancy have not been adequately studied, and the potential for harm has not been ruled out. If you are pregnant or plan to become pregnant while on Celexa therapy, tell your doctor immediately.

Celexa appears in breast milk and will affect the nursing infant. You should consider discontinuing either breastfeeding or Celexa. Talk with your doctor about the pros and cons of each option.

Recommended dosage

ADULTS

The recommended starting dose of Celexa tablets or oral solution is 20 milligrams once a day. Dosage is usually increased to 40 milligrams once daily after at least a week has passed. Do not exceed 40 milligrams a day.

For older adults and those who have liver problems, the recommended dose is 20 milligrams once a day.

Overdosage

Any medication taken in excess can have serious consequences. If you suspect an overdose, seek medical attention immediately.

■ *Symptoms of Celexa overdose may include:*
Amnesia, bluish or purplish discoloration of the skin, coma, confusion, convulsions, dizziness, drowsiness, hyperventilation, nausea, rapid heartbeat, sweating, tremor, vomiting

Cenestin *See Premarin, page 1135.*

Centrum *See Multivitamins, page 901.*

Cephalexin *See Keflex, page 703.*

Cetacort *See Hydrocortisone Skin Preparations, page 656.*

Cetirizine *See Zyrtec, page 1673.*

Cetirizine with Pseudoephedrine *See Zyrtec-D, page 1676.*

Chlordiazepoxide *See Librium, page 759.*

Chlordiazepoxide with Clidinium *See Librax, page 756.*

Chlorhexidine *See Peridex, page 1080.*

Chlorothiazide *See Diuril, page 463.*

Chlorpheniramine with Pseudoephedrine *See Deconamine, page 397.*

CHLORPROMAZINE
Pronounced: klor-PROME-ah-zeen

Why is this drug prescribed?

Chlorpromazine is used for the treatment of schizophrenia (severe disruptions in thought and perception). It is also prescribed for the short-term treatment of severe behavioral disorders in children, including explosive hyperactivity and combativeness; and for the manic phase of bipolar disorder.

Chlorpromazine is also used to control nausea and vomiting, and to relieve restlessness and apprehension before surgery. It is used as an aid in the treatment of tetanus, and is prescribed for uncontrollable hiccups and acute intermittent porphyria (attacks of severe abdominal pain sometimes accompanied by psychiatric disturbances, cramps in the arms and legs, and muscle weakness).

Most important fact about this drug

Chlorpromazine may cause tardive dyskinesia—a condition marked by involuntary muscle spasms and twitches in the face and body. This condition may be permanent, and appears to be most common among the elderly, especially women. Ask your doctor for information about this possible risk.

How should you take this medication?

If taking chlorpromazine in a liquid concentrate form, you will need to dilute it with a liquid such as a carbonated beverage, coffee, fruit juice, milk, tea, tomato juice, or water. Puddings, soups, and other semisolid foods may also be used. Chlorpromazine will taste best if it is diluted immediately prior to use. You should not take chlorpromazine with alcohol.

Do not take antacids such as Gelusil at the same time as chlorpromazine. Leave at least 1 to 2 hours between doses of the two drugs.

■ *If you miss a dose...*
If you take chlorpromazine once a day, take the dose you missed as soon as you remember. If you do not remember until the next day, skip the dose, then go back to your regular schedule.

If you take more than 1 dose a day, take the one you missed as soon as you remember if it is within an hour or so of the scheduled time. If you do not remember until later, skip the dose, then go back to your regular schedule.

Never take 2 doses at once.

■ *Storage instructions...*
Store away from heat, light, and moisture. Do not freeze the liquid. Since the liquid concentrate form of chlorpromazine is light-sensitive, it should be stored in a dark place, but it does not need to be refrigerated.

What side effects may occur?

Side effects cannot be anticipated. If any develop or change in intensity, inform your doctor as soon as possible. Only your doctor can determine if it is safe for you to continue taking chlorpromazine.

■ *Side effects may include:*
Constipation, drowsiness, dry mouth, involuntary muscle spasms and twitches (tardive dyskinesia), jaundice, low blood pressure, low white blood cell count, movements similar to those of Parkinson's disease, neuroleptic malignant syndrome (see *Special warnings about this medication*), rapid heartbeat, restlessness, vision problems

Why should this drug not be prescribed?

You should not be using chlorpromazine if you are taking substances that slow down mental function such as alcohol, barbiturates, or narcotics.

You should not take chlorpromazine if you have ever had an allergic reaction to any major tranquilizer containing phenothiazine.

Special warnings about this medication

You should use chlorpromazine cautiously if you have ever had: asthma; a brain tumor; breast cancer; intestinal blockage; emphysema; the eye condition known as glaucoma; heart, kidney, or liver disease; respiratory infections; seizures; or an abnormal bone marrow or blood condition; or if you are exposed to pesticides or extreme heat. Be aware that chlorpromazine can mask symptoms of brain tumor, intestinal blockage, and the neurological condition called Reye's syndrome.

Stomach inflammation, dizziness, nausea, vomiting, and tremors may result if you suddenly stop taking chlorpromazine. Follow your doctor's instructions closely when discontinuing chlorpromazine.

Chlorpromazine can suppress the cough reflex; you may have trouble vomiting.

This drug may impair your ability to drive a car or operate potentially dangerous machinery. Do not participate in any activities that require full alertness if you are unsure about your ability.

This drug can increase your sensitivity to light. Avoid being out in the sun too long.

Chlorpromazine can cause a group of symptoms called Neuroleptic Malignant Syndrome, which can be fatal. Seek medical help immediately if you develop any of the following symptoms: extremely high body temperature, rigid muscles, mental changes, irregular pulse or blood pressure, rapid or irregular heartbeat, excessive sweating, and high fever.

If you are on chlorpromazine for prolonged therapy, you should see your doctor for regular evaluations, since side effects can get worse over time.

Possible food and drug interactions when taking this medication

If chlorpromazine is taken with certain other drugs, the effects of either could be increased, decreased, or altered. It is especially important to check with your doctor before combining chlorpromazine with the following:

Anesthetics
Antacids such as Gelusil
Antiseizure drugs such as Dilantin
Antispasmodic drugs such as Cogentin
Atropine (Donnatal)
Barbiturates such as phenobarbital
Blood-thinning drugs such as Coumadin
Captopril (Capoten)
Cimetidine (Tagamet)
Diuretics such as Dyazide
Epinephrine (EpiPen)
Guanethidine
Lithium (Lithobid, Eskalith)

    MAO inhibitors (antidepressants such as Nardil and Parnate)
    Narcotics such as Percocet
    Propranolol (Inderal)

Extreme drowsiness and other potentially serious effects can result if chlorpromazine is combined with alcohol and other mental depressants such as narcotic painkillers like Demerol.

Because chlorpromazine prevents vomiting, it can hide the signs and symptoms of overdose of other drugs.

Special information if you are pregnant or breastfeeding

The effects of chlorpromazine during pregnancy have not been adequately studied. If you are pregnant or plan to become pregnant, notify your doctor. Pregnant women should use chlorpromazine only if clearly needed.

Chlorpromazine appears in breast milk and may affect a nursing infant. If this medication is essential to your health, your doctor may advise you not to breastfeed until your treatment is finished.

Recommended dosage

Dosage recommendations shown here are for the oral and rectal forms of the drug. For certain problems, chlorpromazine is also given by injection.

ADULTS

Schizophrenia and Mania

Your doctor will gradually increase the dosage until symptoms are controlled. You may not see full improvement for weeks or even months.

Initial dosages may range from 30 to 75 milligrams daily. The amount is divided into equal doses and taken 3 or 4 times a day. If needed, your doctor may increase the dosage by 20 to 50 milligrams at semiweekly intervals.

Nausea and Vomiting

The usual tablet dosage is 10 to 25 milligrams, taken every 4 or 6 hours, as needed.

One 100-milligram suppository can be used every 6 to 8 hours.

Uncontrollable Hiccups

Dosages may range from 75 to 200 milligrams daily, divided into 3 or 4 equal doses.

Acute Intermittent Porphyria

Dosages may range from 75 to 200 milligrams daily, divided into 3 or 4 equal doses.

CHILDREN

Chlorpromazine is generally not prescribed for children younger than 6 months.

Severe Behavior Problems, Nausea, and Vomiting
Dosages are based on the child's weight.

Oral: The daily dose is one-quarter milligram for each pound of the child's weight, taken every 4 to 6 hours, as needed.

Rectal: The usual dose is one-half milligram per pound of body weight, taken every 6 to 8 hours, as necessary.

OLDER ADULTS

In general, older people take lower dosages of chlorpromazine, and any increase in dosage will be gradual. Because of a greater risk of low blood pressure, your doctor will watch you closely while you are taking chlorpromazine. Older people (especially older women) may be more susceptible to tardive dyskinesia—a possibly permanent condition characterized by involuntary muscle spasms and twitches in the face and body. Consult your doctor for information about these potential risks.

Overdosage

Any medication taken in excess can have serious consequences. An overdose of chlorpromazine can be fatal. If you suspect an overdose, seek medical help immediately.

■ *Symptoms of chlorpromazine overdose may include:*
Agitation, coma, convulsions, difficulty breathing, difficulty swallowing, dry mouth, extreme sleepiness, fever, intestinal blockage, irregular heart rate, low blood pressure, restlessness

Chlorpropamide *See Diabinese, page 431.*

Chlorthalidone *See Thalitone, page 1429.*

Chlorzoxazone *See Parafon Forte DSC, page 1032.*

Cholestyramine *See Questran, page 1211.*

Choline magnesium trisalicylate *See Trilisate, page 1499.*

CHRONULAC SYRUP

Pronounced: KRON-yoo-lak
Generic name: Lactulose

Why is this drug prescribed?

Chronulac treats constipation. In people who are chronically constipated, Chronulac increases the number and frequency of bowel movements.

Most important fact about this drug

It may take 24 to 48 hours to produce a normal bowel movement.

How should you take this medication?

Take this medication exactly as prescribed. If you find the taste of Chronulac unpleasant, it can be mixed with water, fruit juice, or milk.

■ *If you miss a dose...*
Take the forgotten dose as soon as you remember; but do not try to catch up by taking a double dose.

■ *Storage instructions...*
Store at room temperature. Avoid excessive heat or direct light. The liquid may darken in color, which is normal. Do not freeze.

What side effects may occur?

Side effects cannot be anticipated. If any develop or change in intensity, inform your doctor as soon as possible. Only your doctor can determine if it is safe for you to continue taking Chronulac.

■ *Side effects may include:*
Diarrhea, gas (temporary, at the beginning of use), intestinal cramps (temporary, at the beginning of use), nausea, potassium and fluid loss, vomiting

Why should this drug not be prescribed?

Chronulac contains galactose, a simple sugar. If you are on a low-galactose diet, do not take this medication.

Special warnings about this medication

Because of its sugar content, this medication should be used with caution if you have diabetes.

If unusual diarrhea occurs, contact your doctor.

Possible food and drug interactions when taking this medication

If Chronulac is taken with certain other drugs, the effects of either could be increased, decreased, or altered. It is especially important to check with your doctor before combining Chronulac with non-absorbable antacids such as Maalox and Mylanta.

Special information if you are pregnant or breastfeeding

The effects of Chronulac during pregnancy have not been adequately studied. If you are pregnant or plan to become pregnant, inform your doctor immediately. Chronulac may appear in breast milk and could affect a nursing infant. If this medication is essential to your health, your doctor may advise you to stop breastfeeding until your treatment is finished.

Recommended dosage

The usual dose is 1 to 2 tablespoonfuls (15 to 30 milliliters) daily. Your doctor may increase the dose to 60 milliliters a day, if necessary.

The safety and effectiveness for children have not been established.

Overdosage
Any medication taken in excess can have serious consequences. If you suspect an overdose, seek medical treatment immediately.

■ *Symptoms of Chronulac overdose may include:*
Abdominal cramps, diarrhea

CIALIS
Pronounced: See-AL-iss
Generic name: Tadalafil

Why is this drug prescribed?
Cialis is an oral drug for male impotence, also known as erectile dysfunction (ED). It works by dilating blood vessels in the penis, allowing the inflow of blood needed for an erection.

Most important fact about this drug
Cialis causes erections only during sexual excitement. It does not work in the absence of arousal and does not increase sexual desire.

How should you take this medication?
Take one Cialis tablet before sexual activity, with or without food. The best time to take Cialis depends on how and when the drug works for you, but some men are able to have an erection 30 minutes after taking it. Others are able to wait up to 36 hours after taking Cialis before engaging in sexual activity.

■ *If you miss a dose...*
Take Cialis only before sexual activity, but no more than once a day. Do not take 2 doses at once.
■ *Storage instructions...*
Store at room temperature.

What side effects may occur?
Side effects cannot be anticipated. If any develop or change in intensity, tell your doctor as soon as possible. Only your doctor can determine if it is safe to continue using Cialis.

■ *Side effects may include:*
Arm and leg pain, back pain, flushing, headache, indigestion, muscle aches, nasal congestion

This side effects list is not complete. If you have any questions about side effects, you should consult your doctor. Report any new or continuing symptoms to your doctor right away.

Why should this drug not be prescribed?

Do not take Cialis if you are taking any nitrate-based drug, including nitroglycerin patches (Nitro-Dur, Transderm-Nitro), nitroglycerin ointment (Nitro-Bid, Nitrol), nitroglycerin pills (Nitro-Bid, Nitrostat), and isosorbide pills (Dilatrate-SR, Isordil, Sorbitrate). This also includes street drugs known as "poppers," including amyl nitrate and butyl nitrate. Combining Cialis with any of these drugs can cause a dangerous drop in blood pressure.

Likewise, do not take Cialis with certain blood pressure and prostate drugs known as alpha-blockers, including Cardura (doxazosin), Hytrin (terazosin), Minipress (prazosin), and Uroxatral (alfuzosin). However, you can take the alpha-blocker Flomax (tamsulosin) at a dose of 0.4 milligram once a day.

If Cialis gives you an allergic reaction, do not use it again.

Special warnings about this medication

If you have heart problems severe enough to make sexual activity a danger, you should avoid using Cialis. If you take this drug and develop cardiac symptoms (for example, dizziness, nausea, and chest pain) during sexual activity, do not continue. Alert your doctor to the problem as soon as possible.

Because Cialis has not been studied in people with cardiovascular disease, it's best to avoid this drug if you've had a stroke or heart failure within the past 6 months, or a heart attack within the past 3 months. Be equally cautious if you have severe high or low blood pressure, heartbeat irregularities, or unstable angina (crushing heart pain that occurs at any time). If you develop angina after taking Cialis, seek medical attention immediately.

If you have severe kidney or liver problems, a bleeding disorder, stomach ulcer, or an inherited retinal disorder such as retinitis pigmentosa, use this medication with caution. Its safety under these circumstances has not yet been studied.

Rare cases of prolonged and sometimes painful erections (known as priapism) have been reported with drugs similar to Cialis. If you develop an erection that lasts more than 4 hours, seek medical treatment immediately. Otherwise, permanent damage and impotence could result.

If you have a condition that might result in long-lasting erections, such as sickle-cell anemia, multiple myeloma (a disease of the bone marrow), or leukemia, use Cialis with caution. Also use caution if you have a genital problem or deformity such as Peyronie's disease.

Remember that Cialis offers no protection from transmission of sexually transmitted diseases, such as HIV, the virus that causes AIDS.

Possible food and drug interactions when taking this medication

Be sure to check with your doctor about the medications that should never be taken with Cialis, including:

Alpha-blocking drugs prescribed for high blood pressure or prostate problems, including doxazosin (Cardura), terazosin (Hytrin), prazosin (Minipress), and alfuzosin (Uroxatral)

Nitrate-based drugs prescribed for chest pain, such as nitroglycerin patches (Nitro-Dur, Transderm-Nitro), nitroglycerin ointment (Nitro-Bid, Nitrol), nitroglycerin pills (Nitro-Bid, Nitrostat), and isosorbide pills (Dilatrate-SR, Isordil, Sorbitrate)

Street drugs known as poppers, including amyl nitrate and butyl nitrate

Cialis could intensify the effects of certain drugs used to lower blood pressure. Be sure to tell your doctor if you take any of the following:

Angiotensin II receptor blockers, such as candesartan (Atacand), eprosartan (Tevetan) and irbesartan (Avapro)
Bendrofluazide
Enalapril (Vasotec)
Metoprol (Lopressor)

If Cialis is taken with certain other drugs, the effects of either could be increased, decreased, or altered. It is especially important to check with your doctor before combining Cialis with the following:

Erythromycin (E-Mycin, Ery-Tab, PCE)
Grapefruit juice
Indinavir (Crixivan)
Itraconazole (Sporanox)
Ketoconazole (Nizoral)
Other impotence drugs, including alprostadil (Caverject), sildenafil (Viagra), and vardenafil (Levitra)
Rifampin (Rifadin, Rimactane)
Ritonavir (Norvir)

It's best not to drink too much alcohol while you're taking Cialis. Combining the two could lower your blood pressure and cause dizziness, especially upon standing. Drinking five or more servings of alcohol could intensify this effect and also cause headache and rapid heartbeat.

Special information about pregnancy and breastfeeding
Cialis should not be used by women. Its effects during pregnancy and breastfeeding have not been studied.

Recommended dosage

ADULT MALES

Doses range from 5 milligrams to 20 milligrams, depending on the drug's effect. The recommended starting dose is 10 milligrams.

Take Cialis only before sexual activity. The manufacturer recommends a maximum of 1 dose per day. If you're taking certain drugs that affect the liver, such as ritonavir (Norvir) or ketoconazole (Nizoral), the maximum recommended dose is 10 milligrams no more than once every 3 days.

If you have moderate kidney impairment, the recommended starting dose is 5 milligrams once a day, up to a maximum of 10 milligrams once every 2 days. If you have severe kidney impairment or need dialysis, the maximum recommended dose is 5 milligrams once a day. No dosage adjustment is required if you have mild kidney problems.

If you have mild or moderate liver impairment, your total daily dose should not exceed 10 milligrams once a day. If your liver is severely impaired, you will not be able to use Cialis.

Overdosage

Large doses of Cialis (up to 500 milligrams) have resulted in similar side effects as regular doses. However, any medication taken in excess can have serious consequences. If you suspect an overdose, seek medical attention immediately.

Ciclopirox See Loprox, page 779.

Ciclopirox nail lacquer See Penlac, page 1068.

CILOXAN

Pronounced: sill-OKS-an
Generic name: Ciprofloxacin hydrochloride

Why is this drug prescribed?

Ciloxan is an antibiotic used in the treatment of eye infections. The ointment form of the drug is prescribed for eye inflammations. The solution can also be used to treat ulcers or sores on the cornea (the transparent covering over the pupil). Ciprofloxacin, the active ingredient, is a member of the quinolone family of antibiotics.

Most important fact about this drug

Other forms of ciprofloxacin have been known to cause allergic reactions in a few patients. These reactions can be extremely serious, leading to loss of consciousness and cardiovascular collapse. Early warning signs include skin rash, hives, and itching. Other symptoms may include swelling of the face or throat, shortness of breath, and a tingling feeling. If you develop any of these symptoms, seek emergency help immediately.

How should you take this medication?

Ciloxan ointment should be applied in a ribbon on the inner eyelid. Ciloxan solution is administered with an eyedropper. Be careful to avoid touching the tip to the eye or any other surface. This could contaminate the solution.

■ *If you miss a dose...*
Take the forgotten dose as soon as you remember. However, if it is almost time for your next dose, skip the one you missed and return to your regular schedule. Do not take 2 doses at once.

■ *Storage instructions...*
Store at room temperature. Protect the solution from light.

What side effects may occur?

Side effects cannot be anticipated. If any develop or change in intensity, tell your doctor as soon as possible. Only your doctor can determine if it is safe to continue using Ciloxan.

■ *Side effects may include:*
Formation of crystals (with frequent application of solution only), local burning or discomfort

Why should this drug not be prescribed?

If you've ever had an allergic reaction to a quinolone antibiotic such as Cipro, Floxin, Levaquin, Noroxin, Avelox, or Tequin, you should not use this medication.

Special warnings about this medication

The manufacturer of Ciloxan warns against wearing contact lenses while suffering an eye infection.

When treating corneal ulcers with Ciloxan solution, you may notice a white buildup on the surface of the ulcer. This usually disappears within a week or two, and is no cause for concern.

Prolonged use of Ciloxan sometimes promotes the growth of germs that are unaffected by the medication. The doctor will examine your eyes for signs of this development.

The ointment form of Ciloxan may slow down healing of the cornea and cause blurred vision.

The safety and effectiveness have not been established in children under 2 years of age for Ciloxan ointment, or under 1 year of age for the solution.

Possible food and drug interactions when using this medication

There is no information on interactions with Ciloxan. When taken internally, however, ciprofloxacin is known to interact with the following:

Caffeine
Cyclosporine (Neoral, Sandimmune)
Theophylline (Theo-Dur)
Warfarin (Coumadin)

Special information if you are pregnant or breastfeeding

The effects of Ciloxan during pregnancy have not been adequately studied. If you are pregnant or plan to become pregnant, alert your doctor immediately.

Researchers do not know whether Ciloxan makes its way into breast milk; but when ciprofloxacin is taken internally, it definitely appears. Be cautious if using Ciloxan while nursing.

Recommended dosage

OINTMENT

Eye Inflammation
Apply a 1/2-inch ribbon on the inner eyelid 3 times a day for the first 2 days, then 2 times a day for the next 5 days.

SOLUTION

Eye Inflammation
Apply 1 or 2 drops every 2 hours for the first 2 days, then every 4 hours for the next 5 days.

Corneal Ulcers
Apply 2 drops in the affected eye every 15 minutes for the first 6 hours, then every 30 minutes for the rest of the first day. On the second day, apply 2 drops every hour. On the third through fourteenth days, apply 2 drops every 4 hours. Treatment can continue for more than 14 days if healing doesn't occur.

Overdosage

If you accidentally apply too many drops of solution, it can be flushed from the eye with warm water. The results of long-term overdosing are unknown. If you suspect a problem, check with your doctor.

Cimetidine See Tagamet, page 1378.

CIPRO

Pronounced: SIP-roh
Generic name: Ciprofloxacin hydrochloride
Other brand names: Cipro HC Otic, Cipro XR

Why is this drug prescribed?

Cipro is an antibiotic used to treat infections of the lower respiratory tract, the abdomen, the skin, the bones and joints, and the urinary tract, including cystitis (bladder inflammation) in women. It is also prescribed for severe sinus or bronchial infections, infectious diarrhea, typhoid fever, inhalational anthrax, infections of the prostate gland, and some sexually transmitted diseases such as gonorrhea. Additionally, some doctors prescribe Cipro for certain serious ear infections, tuberculosis, and some of the infections common in people with AIDS.

Cipro may also be prescribed for children with a urinary tract infection or kidney infection when other antibiotics are not effective.

Because Cipro is effective only for certain types of bacterial infections, before beginning treatment your doctor may perform tests to identify the specific organisms causing your infection.

Cipro is available as a tablet and an oral suspension (liquid). Cipro HC Otic is a suspension (ear drops) that also contains the anti-inflammatory drug hydrocortisone; it's used externally to treat ear infections.

Cipro XR, an extended-release form of the drug, is used to treat cystitis, urinary tract infection, and kidney infection.

Most important fact about this drug

Cipro kills a variety of bacteria, and is frequently used to treat infections in many parts of the body. However, be sure to stop taking Cipro and notify your doctor immediately at the first sign of a skin rash or any other allergic reaction. Although quite rare, serious and occasionally fatal allergic reactions—some following the first dose—have been reported in people receiving this type of antibacterial drug. Some reactions have been accompanied by collapse of the circulatory system, loss of consciousness, swelling of the face and throat, shortness of breath, tingling, itching, and hives. Fever and jaundice (yellowing of the skin and eyes) are other potential symptoms that should send you to the doctor immediately.

How should you take this medication?

Cipro can be taken with food or on an empty stomach. Cipro should *not* be taken with dairy products (such as milk or yogurt) or calcium-fortified juices alone; however, Cipro may be taken with a meal that contains these products. Drink plenty of fluids while taking this medication to prevent crystals from forming in your urine.

Like other antibiotics, Cipro work best when there is a constant amount in the blood and urine. To help keep the level constant, try not to miss any doses, and take them at approximately the same time every day.

Your doctor will only prescribe Cipro to treat a bacterial infection; it will not cure a viral infection, such as the common cold. It's important to take the full dosage schedule of Cipro, even if you're feeling better in a few days. Not completing the full dosage schedule may decrease the drug's effectiveness and increase the chances that the bacteria may become resistant to Cipro and similar antibiotics.

If you are taking the oral suspension, be sure to shake the bottle vigorously for 15 seconds before each dose. Swallow without chewing the microcapsules in the suspension. Reclose the bottle completely, following the instructions on the cap.

Do not use Cipro HC Otic suspension in your eyes, and avoid contaminating the dropper by letting it touch your ears, fingers, or other surfaces.

Administer the ear drops as follows:
1. Warm the otic suspension by holding the bottle in your hand for a minute or two; putting a cold suspension into the ear can cause dizziness.
2. Have the person lie down with the affected ear up.
3. Shake the bottle, then position the filled dropper above the entrance to the ear canal.
4. Squeeze 3 drops into the ear. The person should not get up for 30 to 60 seconds after the drops have been given.
5. Throw away any suspension that remains after treatment is finished.

■ *If you miss a dose…*
Take it as soon as you remember. If it is almost time for your next dose, skip the one you missed and go back to your regular schedule. Never take 2 doses at the same time.
■ *Storage instructions…*
Cipro tablets should be stored at room temperature. Cipro suspension may be stored at room temperature or in the refrigerator. The suspension is good for 14 days. Protect Cipro HC Otic suspension from light and avoid freezing.

What side effects may occur?
Side effects cannot be anticipated. If any develop or change in intensity, inform your doctor as soon as possible. Only your doctor can determine if it is safe for you to continue taking Cipro.

■ *Side effects may include:*
Abdominal pain/discomfort, diarrhea, headache, nausea, rash, restlessness, vomiting

Why should this drug not be prescribed?
If you are sensitive to or have ever had an allergic reaction to Cipro or certain other antibiotics of this type such as Floxin, Noroxin, and Trovan, you should not take this medication. Make sure that your doctor is aware of any drug reactions that you have experienced.

Cipro HC Otic suspension should not be used on anyone whose eardrum is perforated or who has a viral infection of the ear.

Special warnings about this medication
Cipro may cause you to become dizzy or light-headed; therefore, you should not drive a car, operate dangerous machinery, or participate in any

hazardous activity that requires full mental alertness until you know how the drug affects you.

Continued or prolonged use of this drug may result in a growth of bacteria that do not respond to this medication and can cause a secondary infection. Therefore, it is important that your doctor monitor your condition on a regular basis.

Cipro can cause increased pressure within the brain. Convulsions have been reported in people receiving the drug. If you experience a seizure or convulsion, notify your doctor immediately.

This medication may stimulate the central nervous system, which may lead to tremors, restlessness, light-headedness, confusion, depression, and hallucinations. If these reactions occur, consult your doctor at once. Other central nervous system reactions include nervousness, agitation, insomnia, anxiety, nightmares, and paranoia.

If you have a known or suspected central nervous system disorder such as epilepsy or hardening of the arteries in the brain, make sure your doctor knows about it when prescribing Cipro.

Remember to stop taking Cipro and see your doctor at the first hint of an allergic reaction (see *Most important fact about this drug*). Also call your doctor if you develop diarrhea. Antibiotics such as Cipro occasionally trigger a form of diarrhea that needs a doctor's attention.

Rare cases of peripheral neuropathy (changes or disturbances of the nervous system) have been reported with this type of antibiotic. Contact your doctor if you experience muscle weakness, paralysis, pain or numbness, a burning sensation, or a pins and needles sensation.

You may become more sensitive to light while taking this drug. Try to stay out of the sun as much as possible.

People taking Cipro have been known to suffer torn tendons. If you feel any pain or inflammation in a tendon area, stop taking the drug and call your doctor; you should rest and avoid exercise. You may need surgery to repair the tendon.

If you must take Cipro for an extended period of time, your doctor will probably order blood tests and tests for urine, kidney, and liver function. If you are taking Cipro to treat gonorrhea, the doctor should test you for syphilis after 3 months.

Possible food and drug interactions when taking this medication

Serious and fatal reactions have occurred when Cipro was taken in combination with theophylline (Theo-Dur). These reactions have included cardiac arrest, seizures, status epilepticus (continuous attacks of epilepsy with no periods of consciousness), and respiratory failure.

The following can interfere with the absorption of Cipro and should be taken no less than 6 hours before or 2 hours after a dose:

Antacids containing magnesium and aluminum
Carafate

Supplements and other products containing calcium, iron, or zinc
Videx chewable tablets and pediatric powder

You should also avoid taking Cipro with milk or yogurt alone, though calcium taken as part of a full meal has no significant effect on the drug.

Cipro may increase the effects of caffeine.

If Cipro is taken with certain other drugs, the effects of either could be increased, decreased, or altered. These drugs include:

Cyclophosphamide (Cytoxan)
Cyclosporine (Sandimmune, Neoral)
Glyburide (DiaBeta, Glynase, Micronase)
Methotrexate (Rheumatrex)
Metoclopramide (Reglan)
Metoprolol (Lopressor)
Phenytoin (Dilantin)
Probenecid
Warfarin (Coumadin)

Certain nonsteroidal anti-inflammatory drugs (NSAIDs), with the exception of aspirin, could cause convulsions when combined with high doses of this type of antibiotic.

Special information if you are pregnant or breastfeeding

Although there's reason to believe that Cipro poses little danger during pregnancy, its effects have not been adequately studied. If you are pregnant or plan to become pregnant, notify your doctor immediately. Cipro does appear in breast milk when it's taken internally, and could affect a nursing infant. If this medication is essential to your health, your doctor may advise you to discontinue breastfeeding your baby until your treatment is finished.

Recommended dosage

If you have kidney problems, your doctor may prescribe dosages lower than the ones listed below.

Note that if you're using the oral suspension, 1 teaspoonful of 5% suspension equals 250 milligrams and 1 teaspoonful of 10% suspension equals 500 milligrams.

ADULTS

Cipro
The usual adult dosage is 250 milligrams taken every 12 hours.

Complicated infections, as determined by your doctor, may require 500 milligrams taken every 12 hours. Treatment usually lasts 7 to 14 days.

Cystitis (Bladder Inflammation) in Women: The usual dosage is either 100 milligrams or 250 milligrams every 12 hours. Treatment usually lasts 3 days.

Lower Respiratory Tract, Skin, Bone, and Joint Infections: The usual recommended dosage is 500 milligrams taken every 12 hours. Complicated infections, as determined by your doctor, may require a dosage of 750 milligrams taken every 12 hours. Treatment usually lasts 7 to 14 days, except for bone and joint infections, which require 4 to 6 weeks.

Infectious Diarrhea; Typhoid Fever; Sinus, Prostate, and Abdominal Infections: The recommended dosage is 500 milligrams taken every 12 hours. Treatment lasts 5 to 7 days for diarrhea, 10 days for typhoid fever and sinus infections, 7 to 14 days for abdominal infections, and 28 days for prostate infections.

Inhalational Anthrax: For adults, the recommended dosage is 500 milligrams taken every 12 hours. Children's doses are calculated at a rate of 15 milligrams per 2.2 pounds of body weight up to a maximum of 500 milligrams per dose. Treatment continues for 60 days.

Gonorrhea in the Urethra or Cervix: For these sexually transmitted diseases, a single 250-milligram dose is the usual treatment.

Cipro HC Otic
Ear Infection: Instill 3 drops of suspension into the ear twice a day for 7 days.

Cipro
Cystitis (Bladder Inflammation) in Women: The usual dosage is 500 milligrams taken once daily for 3 days.

Urinary Tract and Kidney Infections: The usual dosage is 1,000 milligrams taken once daily for 7 to 14 days.

CHILDREN AGES 1 TO 17 YEARS OLD

Cipro
Urinary Tract and Kidney Infections: The usual dosage is based on your child's weight. It should be taken every 12 hours for 10 to 21 days.

Inhalational Anthrax: The usual dosage is based on your child's weight. It should be taken every 12 hours for 60 days.

Cipro HC Otic
The dosage is the same as for adults.

Cipro XR is not recommended for anyone less than 18 years old.

Overdosage
There is no information on the symptoms of Cipro overdose. However, any medication taken in excess can have serious consequences. If you suspect an overdose, seek medical attention immediately.

CIPRODEX

Pronounced: SIP-roh-decks
Generic name: Ciprofloxacin and Dexamethasone

Why is this drug prescribed?

Ciprodex is an ear drop medication used to treat middle ear infections in children ages 6 months or older who have tubes in their ears. It's also used to treat *swimmer's ear*—an inflammation, irritation, or infection of the outer ear and ear canal—in adults and children 6 months or older.

Ciprodex is a combination of two drugs. One is the antibiotic ciprofloxacin, which fights bacterial infections. The other is the steroid dexamethasone, which lessens inflammation.

Most important fact about this drug

Use Ciprodex for as long as the doctor has instructed, even if you begin to feel better. Otherwise, the infection could return.

Keep the infected ear clean and dry. Avoid getting it wet when bathing, and avoid swimming unless the doctor has instructed otherwise.

How should you take this medication?

Ciprodex drops should be used in the ear only; this drug is not approved for use in the eye.

Administer the drops as follows:

1. Wash hands with soap and water.
2. Clean the outer ear of any discharge.
3. Warm the bottle in your hand for 1 to 2 minutes before using. This will prevent a sense of dizziness that can result from putting a cold solution into the ear.
4. Have the person receiving the drops lie on his or her side with the affected ear up.
5. Shake the solution well and place 4 drops into the affected ear. Be careful not to let the tip of the bottle touch your fingers, the person's ear, or any other surface.
6. If a child receiving the medication has a tube in the ear, gently press on the small, thick flap that sticks out over the ear canal 5 times in a pumping motion. This allows the drops to pass through the tube into the eardrum and middle ear.
7. If the person receiving the medication has an outer ear infection (swimmer's ear), gently pull the ear upward and backward. This allows the drops to flow down into the ear canal.
8. The person should remain lying with the ear up for at least 1 minute. If both ears are affected, repeat the procedure on the other side.
9. Throw away any leftover medication.

■ *If you miss a dose...*
Take the forgotten dose as soon as you remember. However, if it is almost time for your next dose, skip the one you missed and go back to your regular schedule. Never take 2 doses at the same time.

■ *Storage instructions...*
Store at room temperature and protect from light.

What side effects may occur?

Side effects cannot be anticipated. If any develop or change in intensity, tell your doctor as soon as possible. Only your doctor can determine if it is safe to continue using Ciprodex.

■ *Side effects may include:*
Ear pain or discomfort, itching in the ear

Why should this drug not be prescribed?

You should not take Ciprodex if you have ever had an allergic reaction to Cipro or to any similar antibiotic, such as Floxin, Noroxin, or Trovan. You should also avoid Ciprodex if you have had an allergic reaction to dexamethasone or a similar steroid medication.

Special warnings about this medication

Stop using Ciprodex at the first sign of a skin rash or other allergic reaction.

Ciprodex may cause an overgrowth of other organisms, including yeast or fungus. If your symptoms are not better after a week of treatment, contact your doctor.

Possible food and drug interactions when taking this medication

There is no information on interactions between Ciprodex and other drugs.

Special information if you are pregnant or breastfeeding

The effects of Ciprodex during pregnancy have not been studied. Notify your doctor if you are pregnant or plan to become pregnant.

The drugs in Ciprodex—ciprofloxacin and dexamethasone—can show up in human breast milk if the drugs are swallowed. It is not known if the amount of medication absorbed through ear drops is enough to result in detectable amounts in breast milk. The doctor may advise you stop breastfeeding until your treating with Ciprodex is finished.

Recommended dosage

ADULTS AND CHILDREN 6 MONTHS AND OLDER

The recommended dose is 4 drops in the affected ear twice a day for 7 days. Try to use Ciprodex once in the morning and once at night, about 12 hours apart.

Overdosage
If you suspect an overdose, or if Ciprodex is swallowed, seek emergency treatment immediately.

Ciprofloxacin See Cipro, page 289.

Ciprofloxacin and Dexamethasone See Ciprodex, page 295.

Ciprofloxacin, ocular See Ciloxan, page 287.

Citalopram See Celexa, page 275.

CLARINEX
Pronounced: CLAR-in-ecks
Generic name: Desloratadine

Why is this drug prescribed?
Clarinex is an antihistamine used to relieve the symptoms of hay fever (seasonal and perennial allergic rhinitis).

Most important fact about this drug
If you have liver or kidney disease, your doctor should cut your starting dose in half.

How should you take this medication?
Clarinex can be taken with or without food. Take it exactly as directed.

Clarinex RediTabs should be placed on the tongue, where they dissolve quickly. Take the RediTabs immediately after removing them from the blister pack.

■ *If you miss a dose...*
Take it as soon as you remember. If it is almost time for your next dose, skip the one you missed and go back to your regular schedule. Never take 2 doses at the same time.
■ *Storage instructions...*
Store at room temperature. Protect from heat.

What side effects may occur?
Side effects cannot be anticipated. If any develop or change in intensity, inform your doctor as soon as possible. Only your doctor can determine if it is safe for you to continue taking Clarinex.

■ *Side effects may include:*
Dry mouth, fatigue, sleepiness, sore throat

Why should this drug not be prescribed?
If Clarinex or the similar drug Claritin gives you an allergic reaction, you'll be unable to use this drug.

Special warnings about this medication

Do not increase the dose of this drug or take it more than once a day. Higher doses have no additional effect on hay fever symptoms and may cause drowsiness.

The chewable tablet form of Clarinex contains phenylalanine. If you have the hereditary disease phenylketonuria, this form of Clarinex should not be used.

Clarinex is not approved for children under 12.

Possible food and drug interactions when taking this medication

No significant interactions have been reported.

Special information if you are pregnant or breastfeeding

The possibility that Clarinex could harm a developing baby has not been completely ruled out, and the drug should be used during pregnancy only if clearly needed.

Clarinex makes its way into breast milk. You'll need to choose between nursing and continuing to use the drug.

Recommended dosage

ADULTS AND CHILDREN 12 YEARS AND OLDER

For adults and children 12 and older, the usual dose is 5 milligrams (1 tablet or 2 teaspoonfuls of syrup) once a day. If you have kidney or liver disease, the recommended dose is 5 milligrams every other day.

CHILDREN 6 MONTHS TO 11 YEARS OLD

For children 6 years to 11 years old: The usual dose is 2.5 milligrams (1 teaspoonful of syrup) once a day.

For children 12 months to 5 years old: The usual dose is 1.25 milligrams (one-half teaspoonful) once a day. The dose should be given with a dropper that measures milliliters (one-half teaspoonful equals 2.5 milliliters).

For children 6 months to 11 months old: The usual dose is 1.0 milligram (2 milliliters) once a day. The dose should be given with a dropper that measures milliliters.

A recommended dose has not been established for children with kidney or liver disease.

Overdosage

Little is known about the effects of a Clarinex overdose. However, any medication taken in excess can have serious consequences. If you suspect an overdose, seek medical attention immediately.

■ *Symptoms of Clarinex overdose may include:*
   Rapid heartbeat, sleepiness

Clarithromycin *See Biaxin, page 213.*

CLARITIN

Pronounced: CLAR-i-tin
Generic name: Loratadine

Why is this drug prescribed?

Claritin is an antihistamine that relieves the sneezing, runny nose, stuffiness, itching, and tearing eyes caused by hay fever or other upper respiratory allergies. It also relieves the swollen, red, itchy patches of skin caused by hives. Claritin is also available as an over-the-counter product.

Most important fact about this drug

If you have liver or kidney disease, your doctor should prescribe a lower starting dose of Claritin.

How should you take this medication?

Claritin is available in syrup, regular tablets, and rapidly dissolving tablets called RediTabs. The RediTabs should be placed on the tongue rather than swallowed. They disintegrate rapidly and can be taken with or without water.

■ *If you miss a dose...*
Take the forgotten dose as soon as you remember. If it is almost time for your next dose, skip the one you missed. Never take two doses at the same time.

■ *Storage instructions...*
Claritin can be stored at room temperature. The Reditabs should be kept in a dry place. Use them within 6 months after opening the foil pouch in which they are packed. Take each tablet immediately after removing it from its individual blister.

What side effects may occur?

Side effects cannot be anticipated. If any develop or change in intensity, inform your doctor as soon as possible. Only your doctor can determine if it is safe for you to continue taking Claritin.

■ *Side effects may include:*
Dry mouth, fatigue, headache, sleepiness

Why should this drug not be prescribed?

Do not take Claritin if you are sensitive to or have ever had an allergic reaction to it. Make sure your doctor is aware of any drug reactions that you have experienced.

Special warnings about this medication

This medication may cause excessive sleepiness in people with liver or kidney disease, or older adults, and should be used with caution.

Possible food and drug interactions when taking this medication

Although no harmful interactions with Claritin have been reported, there is a theoretical possibility of an interaction with the following drugs:

Antibiotics such as erythromycin
Cimetidine (Tagamet)
Ketoconazole (Nizoral)

Special information if you are pregnant or breastfeeding

The effects of Claritin during pregnancy have not been adequately studied. If you are pregnant or plan to become pregnant, inform your doctor immediately. Claritin appears in breast milk and could affect a nursing infant. If this medication is essential to your health, your doctor may advise you to discontinue breastfeeding until your treatment with Claritin is finished.

Recommended dosage

ADULTS AND CHILDREN 6 YEARS AND OLDER

The usual dose is 10 milligrams once a day, taken as 1 tablet or 2 teaspoonfuls of syrup. In people with liver or kidney disease, the usual dose is 10 milligrams every other day.

CHILDREN 2 TO 5 YEARS OLD

The usual dose is 1 teaspoonful of syrup once a day. If the child has kidney or liver problems, give 1 teaspoonful every other day.

Overdosage

Any medication taken in excess can have serious consequences. If you suspect an overdose, seek medical attention immediately.

■ *Symptoms of Claritin overdose may include:*
Headache, rapid heartbeat, sleepiness

CLARITIN-D

Pronounced: CLAR-i-tin dee
Generic ingredients: Loratadine, Pseudoephedrine sulfate

Why is this drug prescribed?

Claritin-D is an antihistamine and decongestant that relieves the sneezing, runny nose, stuffiness, and itchy, tearing eyes caused by hay fever or other upper respiratory allergies. It also reduces swelling of the nasal passages, temporarily relieves sinus congestion and pressure, and temporarily restores freer breathing through the nose. Two versions are available: Claritin-D 12 Hour for twice-daily dosing and Claritin-D 24 Hour for once-a-day use. Claritin-D is also available as an over-the-counter product.

Most important fact about this drug
If you have liver disease, make sure the doctor is aware of it. Claritin-D is not recommended in this situation.

How should you take this medication?
Take Claritin-D exactly as prescribed by your doctor. Do not break or chew the tablet. Take the 24-hour variety with a glass of water.

■ *If you miss a dose...*
Take it as soon as you remember. If it is almost time for your next dose, skip the one you missed. Never take 2 doses at the same time.
■ *Storage instructions...*
Store at room temperature.

What side effects may occur?
Side effects cannot be anticipated. If any develop or change in intensity, inform your doctor as soon as possible. Only your doctor can determine if it is safe for you to continue taking Claritin-D.

■ *Side effects may include:*
Coughing, dizziness, dry mouth, fatigue, insomnia, nausea, nervousness, sleepiness, sore throat

Why should this drug not be prescribed?
Do not take Claritin-D if you have ever had an allergic reaction to any of its ingredients.

Avoid Claritin-D if you have the eye condition called narrow-angle glaucoma, very high blood pressure, or coronary artery disease; and do not take the drug if you have difficulty urinating. Also avoid taking Claritin-D within 14 days of taking any drug classified as an MAO inhibitor, including the antidepressants Nardil and Parnate.

Do not use Claritin-D 24 Hour if you have trouble swallowing or have been diagnosed with a narrowing of the food canal (esophagus) leading to your stomach.

Special warnings about this medication
If you are taking Claritin-D and experience insomnia, dizziness, weakness, tremor, or unusual heartbeats, tell your doctor; you may be having an allergic reaction.

You must be careful using Claritin-D if you have diabetes, heart dis-

ease, an overactive thyroid gland, kidney or liver problems, or an enlarged prostate gland.

Do not use Claritin-D with over-the-counter antihistamines and decongestants.

Claritin-D 24 Hour tablets have not been tested for safety in people
over 60, but it is known that side effects are more likely in this age group.

Possible food and drug interactions when taking this medication
Check with your doctor before combining Claritin-D with any of the following:

Blood pressure medications classified as beta-blockers, such as
    Inderal and Tenormin
Digoxin (Lanoxin)
MAO inhibitors, such as the antidepressants Nardil and Parnate
Mecamylamine (Inversine)
Methyldopa (Aldomet)
Reserpine

Special information if you are pregnant or breastfeeding
The effects of Claritin-D during pregnancy have not been adequately studied. If you are pregnant or plan to become pregnant, inform your doctor
immediately. Claritin-D may appear in breast milk. If this medication is
essential to your health, your doctor may advise you not to breastfeed
until your treatment is finished.

Recommended dosage

ADULTS AND CHILDREN 12 YEARS AND OLDER

The usual dose is 1 tablet every 12 hours for Claritin-D 12 Hour, 1 tablet
a day for Claritin-D 24 Hour. If you have kidney trouble, your doctor will
start you on 1 tablet a day (1 tablet every other day for Claritin-D 24
Hour).

Overdosage
Any medication taken in excess can have serious consequences. If you
suspect an overdose, seek medical attention immediately.

■ *Symptoms of Claritin-D overdose may include:*
    Anxiety, breathing difficulty, chest pain, coma, convulsions, delusions,
    difficulty urinating, fast, fluttery heartbeat, giddiness, hallucinations,
    headache, insomnia, irregular heartbeat, nausea, rapid heartbeat, rest-
    lessness, sleepiness, sweating, tension, thirst, vomiting, weakness

CLEOCIN T

Pronounced: KLEE-oh-sin tee
Generic name: Clindamycin phosphate

Why is this drug prescribed?

Cleocin T is an antibiotic used to treat acne.

Most important fact about this drug

Although applied only to the skin, some of this medication could be absorbed into the bloodstream; and it has been known to cause severe—sometimes even fatal—colitis (an inflammation of the lower bowel) when taken internally. Symptoms, which can occur a few days, weeks, or months after beginning treatment with this drug, include severe diarrhea, severe abdominal cramps, and the possibility of the passage of blood.

How should you take this medication?

Use this medication exactly as prescribed. Excessive use of Cleocin T can cause your skin to become too dry or irritated.

■ *If you miss a dose...*
Apply it as soon as you remember. If it is almost time for your next dose, skip the one you missed and go back to your regular schedule.
■ *Storage instructions...*
Store at room temperature. Keep from freezing. Store liquids in tightly closed containers.

What side effects may occur?

Side effects cannot be anticipated. If any develop or change in intensity, inform your doctor as soon as possible. Only your doctor can determine if it is safe for you to continue taking Cleocin T.

■ *Side effects may include:*
Burning, itching, peeling skin, reddened skin, skin dryness

Why should this drug not be prescribed?

If you are sensitive to or have ever had an allergic reaction to Cleocin T or similar drugs, such as Lincocin, you should not use this medication. Make sure your doctor is aware of any drug reactions you have experienced.

Unless you are directed to do so by your doctor, do not take this medication if you have ever had an intestinal inflammation, ulcerative colitis, or antibiotic-associated colitis.

Special warnings about this medication

Cleocin T contains an alcohol base, which can cause burning and irritation of the eyes. It also has an unpleasant taste. Use caution when applying this medication so as not to get it in the eyes, nose, mouth, or skin abrasions. In the event of accidental contact, rinse the affected area with cool water.

Use with caution if you have hay fever, asthma, or eczema.

Possible food and drug interactions when taking this medication

If you have diarrhea while taking Cleocin T, check with your doctor before taking an antidiarrhea medication, as certain drugs may cause your diarrhea to become worse.

The diarrhea should not be treated with the commonly used drugs that slow movement through the intestinal tract, such as Lomotil or products containing paregoric.

Special information if you are pregnant or breastfeeding

The effects of Cleocin T during pregnancy have not been adequately studied. If you are pregnant or plan to become pregnant, inform your doctor immediately. Cleocin T may appear in breast milk and could affect a nursing infant. If this medication is essential to your health, your doctor may advise you to discontinue breastfeeding your baby until your treatment with this medication is finished.

Recommended dosage

ADULTS

Apply a thin film of gel, solution, or lotion to the affected area 2 times a day, or use a solution pledget (application pad). Discard a pledget after you have used it once; you may use more than 1 pledget for a treatment. Do not remove the pledget from its foil container until you are ready to use it.

If you are using the lotion, shake it well immediately before using.

CHILDREN

The safety and effectiveness of Cleocin T have not been established in children under 12 years of age.

Overdosage

Cleocin T can be absorbed through the skin and produce side effects in the body. If you suspect an overdose, seek medical attention immediately.

Climara *See Estrogen Patches, page 538.*

Clinac BPO *See Desquam-E, page 421.*

Clindamycin *See Cleocin T, page 303.*

Clindamycin and Benzoyl peroxide *See BenzaClin, page 204.*

CLINORIL

Pronounced: CLIN-or-il
Generic name: Sulindac

Why is this drug prescribed?

Clinoril, a nonsteroidal anti-inflammatory drug, is used to relieve the inflammation, swelling, stiffness, and joint pain associated with rheumatoid arthritis, osteoarthritis (the most common form of arthritis), and ankylosing spondylitis (stiffness and progressive arthritis of the spine). It is also used to treat bursitis, tendinitis, acute gouty arthritis, and other types of pain.

The safety and effectiveness of this medication in the treatment of people with severe, incapacitating rheumatoid arthritis have not been established.

Most important fact about this drug

You should have frequent checkups with your doctor if you take Clinoril regularly. Ulcers or internal bleeding can occur without warning.

How should you take this medication?

Take this medication exactly as prescribed by your doctor.

If you are using Clinoril for arthritis, it should be taken regularly.

■ *If you miss a dose...*
Take it as soon as you remember. If it is almost time for your next dose, skip the one you missed and go back to your regular schedule. Never take two doses at the same time.

■ *Storage instructions...*
Do not store in damp places like the bathroom.

What side effects may occur?

Side effects cannot be anticipated. If any develop or change in intensity, inform your doctor as soon as possible. Only your doctor can determine if it is safe for you to continue taking Clinoril.

■ *Side effects may include:*
Abdominal pain, constipation, diarrhea, dizziness, gas, headache, indigestion, itching, loss of appetite, nausea, nervousness, rash, ringing in ears, stomach cramps, swelling due to fluid retention, vomiting

Why should this drug not be prescribed?

If you are sensitive to or have ever had an allergic reaction to Clinoril, aspirin, or similar drugs, or if you have had asthma attacks caused by aspirin or other drugs of this type, you should not take this medication. Make sure that your doctor is aware of any drug reactions that you have experienced.

Special warnings about this medication

Stomach ulcers and bleeding can occur without warning, especially if you are 65 or older. These and other side effects are also more likely if you have poor kidney function.

This drug should be used with caution if you have kidney or liver disease; it can cause liver inflammation in some people.

Do not take aspirin or any other anti-inflammatory medications while taking Clinoril, unless your doctor tells you to do so.

Nonsteroidal anti-inflammatory drugs such as Clinoril can hide the signs and symptoms of an infection. Be sure your doctor knows about any infection you may have.

Clinoril can cause vision problems. If you experience a change in your vision, inform your doctor.

If you have heart disease or high blood pressure, this drug can increase water retention. Use with caution.

If you develop pancreatitis (inflammation of the pancreas), Clinoril should be stopped immediately and not restarted.

Clinoril may cause you to become drowsy or less alert. If this happens, driving or operating dangerous machinery or participating in any hazardous activity that requires full mental alertness is not recommended.

Possible food and drug interactions when taking this medication

If Clinoril is taken with certain other drugs, the effects of either could be increased, decreased, or altered. It is especially important to check with your doctor before combining Clinoril with the following:

Aspirin
Blood thinners such as Coumadin
Cyclosporine (Sandimmune)
Diflunisal (Dolobid)
Dimethyl sulfoxide (DMSO)
Lithium
Loop diuretics such as Lasix
Methotrexate
Oral diabetes medications
Other nonsteroidal anti-inflammatory drugs (Aleve, Motrin, others)
The antigout medication Benemid

Special information if you are pregnant or breastfeeding

The effects of Clinoril during pregnancy have not been adequately studied; drugs of this class are known to cause birth defects. If you are pregnant or plan to become pregnant, inform your doctor immediately. Clinoril may appear in breast milk and could affect a nursing infant. If this medication is essential to your health, your doctor may advise you to discontinue breastfeeding until your treatment with Clinoril is finished.

Recommended dosage

ADULTS

Osteoarthritis, Rheumatoid Arthritis, Ankylosing Spondylitis
Starting dosage is 150 milligrams 2 times a day. Take with food. Doses should not exceed 400 milligrams per day.

Acute Gouty Arthritis or Arthritic Shoulder
and Joint Condition
400 milligrams daily taken in doses of 200 milligrams 2 times a day.
For acute painful shoulder, therapy lasting 7 to 14 days is usually adequate.
For acute gouty arthritis, therapy lasting 7 days is usually adequate.
The lowest dose that proves beneficial should be used.

CHILDREN

The safety and effectiveness of Clinoril have not been established in children.

Overdosage

Any medication taken in excess can cause symptoms of overdose. If you suspect an overdose, seek medical attention immediately.

■ *Symptoms of Clinoril overdose may include:*
Coma, low blood pressure, reduced output of urine, stupor

Clobetasol *See Temovate, page 1400.*

Clomid *See Clomiphene Citrate, below.*

CLOMIPHENE CITRATE

Pronounced: KLAHM-if-een SIT-rate
Brand names: Clomid, Serophene

Why is this drug prescribed?

Clomiphene is prescribed for the treatment of ovulatory failure in women who wish to become pregnant and whose husbands are fertile and potent.

Most important fact about this drug

Properly timed sexual intercourse is very important to increase the chances of conception. The likelihood of conception diminishes with each succeeding course of treatment. Your doctor will determine the need for continuing therapy after the first course. If you do not ovulate after 3 courses or do not become pregnant after 3 ovulations, your doctor will stop the therapy.

How should you take this medication?
Take this medication exactly as prescribed by your doctor.

■ *If you miss a dose...*
Take it as soon as you remember. If it is time for your next dose, take the 2 doses together and go back to your regular schedule. If you miss more than 1 dose, contact your doctor.

■ *Storage instructions...*
Store at room temperature in a tightly closed container, away from light, moisture, and excessive heat.

What side effects may occur?
Side effects occur infrequently and generally do not interfere with treatment at the recommended dosage of clomiphene. They tend to occur more frequently at higher doses and during long-term treatment.

■ *Side effects include:*
Abdominal discomfort, enlargement of the ovaries, hot flushes

Why should this drug not be prescribed?
If you are pregnant or think you may be, do not take this drug.

Unless directed to do so by your doctor, do not use this medication if you have an uncontrolled thyroid or adrenal gland disorder, an abnormality of the brain such as a pituitary gland tumor, a liver disease or a history of liver problems, abnormal uterine bleeding of undetermined origin, ovarian cysts, or enlargement of the ovaries not caused by polycystic ovarian syndrome (a hormonal disorder causing lack of ovulation).

Special warnings about this medication
Your doctor will evaluate you for normal liver function and normal estrogen levels before considering you for treatment with clomiphene.

Your doctor will also examine you for pregnancy, ovarian enlargement, and cyst formation prior to treatment with this drug and between each treatment cycle. He or she will do a complete pelvic examination before each course of this medication.

Clomiphene treatment increases the possibility of multiple births; also, birth defects have been reported following treatment to induce ovulation with clomiphene, although no direct effects of the drug on the unborn child have been established.

Because blurring and other visual symptoms may occur occasionally with clomiphene treatment, you should be cautious about driving a car or operating dangerous machinery, especially under conditions of variable lighting.

If you experience visual disturbances, notify your doctor immediately.

Symptoms of visual disturbance may include blurring, spots or flashes, double vision, intolerance to light, decreased visual sharpness, loss of peripheral vision, and distortion of space. Your doctor may recommend a complete evaluation by an eye specialist.

Ovarian hyperstimulation syndrome (or OHSS, enlargement of the ovary) has occurred in women receiving treatment with clomiphene. OHSS may progress rapidly and become serious. The early warning signs are severe pelvic pain, nausea, vomiting, and weight gain. Symptoms include abdominal pain, abdominal enlargement, nausea, vomiting, diarrhea, weight gain, difficult or labored breathing, and less urine production. If you experience any of these warning signs or symptoms, notify your doctor immediately.

To lessen the risks associated with abnormal ovarian enlargement during treatment with clomiphene, the lowest effective dose should be prescribed. Women with the hormonal disorder, polycystic ovarian syndrome may be unusually sensitive to certain hormones and may respond abnormally to usual doses of this drug. If you experience pelvic pain, notify your doctor. He may discontinue your use of clomiphene until the ovaries return to pretreatment size.

Because the safety of long-term treatment with clomiphene has not been established, your doctor will not prescribe more than about 6 courses of therapy. Prolonged use may increase the risk of a tumor in the ovaries.

Possible food and drug interactions when taking this medication
No food or drug interactions have been reported.

Special information if you are pregnant or breastfeeding
If you become pregnant, notify your doctor immediately. You should not be taking this drug while you are pregnant.

Recommended dosage
The recommended dosage for the first course of treatment is 50 milligrams (1 tablet) daily for 5 days. If ovulation does not appear to have occurred, your doctor may try up to 2 more times.

Overdosage
Taking any medication in excess can have serious consequences. If you suspect an overdose of clomiphene, contact your doctor immediately.

Clomipramine See Anafranil, page 101.

Clonazepam See Klonopin, page 713.

Clonidine See Catapres, page 254.

Clopidogrel See Plavix, page 1108.

Clorazepate See Tranxene, page 1470.

Clotrimazole *See Gyne-Lotrimin, page 640.*

Clotrimazole with Betamethasone *See Lotrisone, page 793.*

Clozapine *See Clozaril, below.*

CLOZARIL

Pronounced: KLOH-zah-ril
Generic name: Clozapine

Why is this drug prescribed?

Clozaril is given to help people with severe schizophrenia who have failed to respond to standard treatments. It is also used to help reduce the risk of suicidal behavior in people with schizophrenia. Clozaril is not a cure, but it can help some people return to more normal lives.

Most important fact about this drug

Even though it does not produce some of the disturbing side effects of other antipsychotic medications, Clozaril may cause agranulocytosis, a potentially lethal disorder of the white blood cells. Because of the risk of agranulocytosis, anyone who takes Clozaril is required to have a blood test once a week for the first 6 months. The drug is carefully controlled so that those taking it must get their weekly blood test before receiving the following week's supply of medication. If your blood counts have been acceptable for the 6-month period, you will need to have your blood tested only every other week thereafter. Anyone whose blood test results are abnormal will be taken off Clozaril either temporarily or permanently, depending on the results of an additional 4 weeks of testing.

How should you take this medication?

Take Clozaril exactly as directed by your doctor. Because of the significant risk of serious side effects associated with this drug, your doctor will periodically reassess the need for continued Clozaril therapy. Clozaril is distributed *only* through the Clozaril Patient Management System, which ensures regular white blood cell testing, monitoring, and pharmacy services prior to delivery of your next supply.

Clozaril may be taken with or without food.

■ *If you miss a dose...*
Take it as soon as you remember. If it is almost time for your next dose, skip the one you missed and go back to your regular schedule. Do not take 2 doses at once.

If you stop taking Clozaril for more than 2 days, do not start taking it again without consulting your physician.

■ *Storage instructions...*
Store at room temperature.

What side effects may occur?

Side effects cannot be anticipated. If any develop or change in intensity, inform your doctor as soon as possible. Only your doctor can determine if it is safe for you to continue taking Clozaril.

The most feared side effect is agranulocytosis, a dangerous drop in the number of a certain kind of white blood cell. Symptoms include fever, lethargy, sore throat, and weakness. If not caught in time, agranulocytosis can be fatal. That is why all people who take Clozaril must have a blood test every week. About 1 percent develop agranulocytosis and must stop taking the drug.

Seizures are another potential side effect, occurring in some 5 percent of people who take Clozaril. The higher the dosage, the greater the risk of seizures.

■ *Side effects may include:*
Abdominal discomfort, agitation, blood disorders, confusion, constipation, disturbed sleep, dizziness, drowsiness, dry mouth, fainting, fever, headache, heartburn, high blood pressure, inability to sit down, loss or slowness of muscle movement, low blood pressure, nausea, nightmares, rapid heartbeat and other heart conditions, restlessness, rigidity, salivation, sedation, sweating, tremors, vertigo, vision problems, vomiting, weight gain

Why should this drug not be prescribed?

Clozaril is considered a somewhat risky medication because of its potential to cause agranulocytosis and seizures. It should be taken only by people whose condition is serious, and who have not been helped by more traditional antipsychotic medications such as Haldol or Mellaril.

You should not take Clozaril if:

■ You have a bone marrow disease or disorder;
■ You have epilepsy that is not controlled;
■ You have ever developed an abnormal white blood cell count while taking Clozaril;
■ You are currently taking some other drug, such as Tegretol, that could cause a decrease in white blood cell count or a drug that could affect the bone marrow;
■ You have ever had an allergic reaction to any of its ingredients.

Special warnings about this medication

Clozaril can cause drowsiness, especially at the start of treatment. For this reason, and also because of the potential for seizures, you should not drive, swim, climb, or operate dangerous machinery while you are taking this medication, at least in the early stages of treatment.

Even though you will have blood tests weekly for the first 6 months of treatment and every other week after that, you should stay alert for early symptoms of agranulocytosis: weakness, lethargy, fever, sore throat, a general feeling of illness, a flu-like feeling, or ulcers of the lips, mouth, or other mucous membranes. If any such symptoms develop, tell your doctor immediately.

Especially during the first 3 weeks of treatment, you may develop a fever. If you do, notify your doctor.

While taking Clozaril, do not drink alcohol or use drugs of any kind, including over-the-counter medicines, without first checking with your doctor.

If you take Clozaril, you must be monitored especially closely if you have either the eye condition called narrow-angle glaucoma or an enlarged prostate; Clozaril could make these conditions worse.

On rare occasions, Clozaril can cause intestinal problems—constipation, impaction, or blockage—that can, in extreme cases, be fatal.

In very rare cases, Clozaril has been known to cause a potentially fatal inflammation of the heart. This problem is most likely to surface during the first month of treatment, but has also occurred later. Warning signs include unexplained fatigue, shortness of breath, fever, chest pain, and a rapid or pounding heartbeat. If you develop these symptoms, see your doctor immediately. Even a suspicion of heart inflammation warrants discontinuation of Clozaril.

Especially when you begin taking Clozaril, you may be troubled by a dramatic drop in blood pressure whenever you first stand up. This can lead to light-headedness, fainting, or even total collapse and cardiac arrest. Clozaril also tends to increase your heart rate. Both problems are more dangerous for someone with a heart problem. If you suffer from one, make sure your doctor knows about it.

Also, if you have kidney, liver, or lung disease, or a history of seizures or prostate problems, you should discuss these with your doctor before taking Clozaril. Nausea, vomiting, loss of appetite, and a yellow tinge to your skin and eyes are signs of liver trouble; call your doctor immediately if you develop these symptoms.

Drugs such as Clozaril can sometimes cause a set of symptoms called Neuroleptic Malignant Syndrome (NMS). Symptoms include high fever, muscle rigidity, irregular pulse or blood pressure, rapid heartbeat, excessive perspiration, and changes in heart rhythm. Your doctor will have you stop taking Clozaril while this condition is being treated.

There is also a risk of developing tardive dyskinesia, a condition of involuntary, slow, rhythmical movements. It happens more often in older adults, especially older women.

Clozaril has been known to occasionally raise blood sugar levels, causing unusual hunger, thirst, and weakness, along with excessive urination. If you develop these symptoms, alert your doctor. You may have to switch to a different medication.

In very rare instances, Clozaril may also cause a blood clot in the lungs. If you develop severe breathing problems or chest pain, call your doctor immediately.

Possible food and drug interactions when taking this medication

If Clozaril is taken with certain other drugs, the effects of either could be increased, decreased, or altered. It is especially important to check with your doctor before combining Clozaril with the following:

Alcohol
Antidepressants such as Paxil, Prozac, and Zoloft
Antipsychotic drugs such as chlorpromazine and Mellaril
Blood pressure medications such as Aldomet and Hytrin
Caffeine
Chemotherapy drugs
Cimetidine (Tagamet)
Digitoxin (Crystodigin)
Digoxin (Lanoxin)
Drugs that contain atropine such as Donnatal and Levsin
Drugs that depress the central nervous system, such as
    phenobarbital and Seconal
Epilepsy drugs such as Tegretol and Dilantin
Epinephrine (EpiPen)
Erythromycin (E-Mycin, Eryc, others)
Fluvoxamine
Heart rhythm stabilizers such as Rythmol, quinidine, and Tambocor
Nicotine
Rifampin (Rifadin, Rimactane)
Tranquilizers such as Valium and Xanax
Warfarin (Coumadin)

Special information if you are pregnant or breastfeeding

The effects of Clozaril during pregnancy have not been adequately studied. If you are pregnant or plan to become pregnant, inform your doctor immediately. Clozaril treatment should be continued during pregnancy only if absolutely necessary. You should not breastfeed if you are taking Clozaril, since the drug may appear in breast milk.

Recommended dosage

ADULTS

Your doctor will carefully individualize your dosage and monitor your response regularly.

The usual recommended initial dose is half of a 25-milligram tablet (12.5 milligrams) 1 or 2 times daily. Your doctor may increase the dosage in increments of 25 to 50 milligrams a day to achieve a daily dose of 300 to 450 milligrams by the end of 2 weeks. Dosage increases after that will be only once or twice a week and will be no more than 100 milligrams each time. Dosage is increased gradually because rapid increases and higher doses are more likely to cause seizures and changes in heart rhythm. The most you can take is 900 milligrams a day divided into 2 or 3 doses.

Your doctor will determine long-term dosage depending upon your response and results of the regular blood tests.

CHILDREN

Safety and efficacy have not been established for children up to 16 years of age.

Overdosage

Any medication taken in excess can have serious consequences. If you suspect an overdose, seek emergency medical attention immediately.

■ *Symptoms of overdose with Clozaril may include:*
Coma, delirium, drowsiness, excess salivation, low blood pressure, faintness, pneumonia, rapid heartbeat, seizures, shallow breathing or absence of breathing

Co-Gesic *See Vicodin, page 1557.*

COGNEX

Pronounced: COG-necks
Generic name: Tacrine hydrochloride

Why is this drug prescribed?

Cognex is used for the treatment of mild to moderate Alzheimer's disease. This progressive, degenerative disorder causes physical changes in the brain that disrupt the flow of information and affect memory, thinking, and behavior. As someone caring for a person with Alzheimer's, you should be aware that Cognex is not a cure, but has helped some people.

Most important fact about this drug

Do not abruptly stop Cognex treatment, or reduce the dosage, without consulting the doctor. A sudden reduction can cause the person you are caring for to become more disturbed and forgetful. Taking more Cognex than the doctor advises can also cause serious problems. Do not change the dosage of Cognex unless instructed by the doctor.

How should you take this medication?

This medication will work better if taken at regular intervals, usually 4 times a day. Cognex is best taken between meals; however, if it is irritating to the stomach, the doctor may advise taking it with meals. If Cognex is not taken regularly, as the doctor directs, the condition may get worse.

- *If you miss a dose...*
  Give the forgotten dose as soon as possible. If it is within 2 hours of the next dose, skip the missed dose and go back to the regular schedule. Do not double the doses.
- *Storage instructions...*
  Store at room temperature away from moisture.

What side effects may occur?

Side effects cannot be anticipated. If any develop or change in intensity, tell the doctor as soon as possible. Only the doctor can determine if it is safe to continue giving Cognex.

- *Side effects may include:*
  Abdominal pain, abnormal thinking, agitation, anxiety, chest pain, clumsiness or unsteadiness, confusion, constipation, coughing, depression, diarrhea, dizziness, fatigue, flushing, frequent urination, gas, headache, indigestion, inflamed nasal passages, insomnia, liver function disorders, loss of appetite, muscle pain, nausea, rash, sleepiness, upper respiratory infection, urinary tract infection, vomiting, weight loss

Be sure to report any symptoms that develop while on Cognex therapy. You should alert the doctor if the person you are caring for develops nausea, vomiting, loose stools, or diarrhea at the start of therapy or when the dosage is increased. Later in therapy, be on the lookout for rash or fever, yellowing of the eyes and skin, or changes in the color of the stool.

Why should this drug not be prescribed?

People who are sensitive to or have ever had an allergic reaction to Cognex (including symptoms such as rash or fever) should not take this medication. Before starting treatment with Cognex, it is important to discuss any medical problems with the doctor. If during previous Cognex therapy the person you are caring for developed jaundice (yellow skin and eyes), which signals that something is wrong with the liver, Cognex should not be used again.

Special warnings about this medication

Use Cognex with caution if the person you are caring for has a history of liver disease, certain heart disorders, stomach ulcers, or asthma.

Because of the risk of liver problems when taking Cognex, the doctor will schedule blood tests to monitor liver function every other week from at least the fourth week to the sixteenth week of treatment. After 16 weeks, blood tests will be given monthly for 2 months and every 3 months after that. If the person you are caring for develops any liver problems, the doctor may temporarily discontinue Cognex treatment until further testing shows that the liver has returned to normal. If the doctor resumes Cognex treatment, regular blood tests will be conducted again.

Before the person has any surgery, including dental surgery, tell the doctor that he or she is being treated with Cognex.

Cognex can cause seizures, and may cause difficulty urinating.

Possible food and drug interactions when taking this medication

If Cognex is taken with certain other drugs, the effects of either could be increased, decreased, or altered. It is especially important that you check with your doctor before combining Cognex with the following:

Antispasmodic drugs such as Bentyl and Levsin
Bethanechol chloride (Urecholine)
Cimetidine (Tagamet)
Fluvoxamine
Muscle stimulants such as Mestinon, Mytelase, and Prostigmin
Nonsteroidal anti-inflammatory drugs such as Aleve, Motrin, and
    Naprosyn
The Parkinson's medications Artane and Cogentin
Theophylline (Theo-24, Uniphyl)

Special information if you are pregnant or breastfeeding

The effects of Cognex during pregnancy have not been studied; and it is not known whether Cognex appears in breast milk.

Recommended dosage

ADULTS

The usual starting dose is 10 milligrams 4 times a day, for at least 4 weeks. Do not increase the dose during this 4-week period unless directed by your doctor.

Depending on the patient's tolerance of the drug, dosage may then be increased at 4-week intervals, first to 20 milligrams, then to 30 milligrams, and finally to 40 milligrams, always taken 4 times a day.

CHILDREN

The safety and effectiveness of Cognex have not been established in children.

Overdosage

Any medication taken in excess can have serious consequences. If you suspect an overdose, seek medical attention immediately.

■ *Symptoms of Cognex overdose include:*
Collapse, convulsions, extreme muscle weakness, possibly ending in death (if breathing muscles are affected), low blood pressure, nausea, salivation, slowed heart rate, sweating, vomiting

COLACE

Pronounced: KOH-lace
Generic name: Docusate
Other brand names: Ex-Lax Stool Softener,
  Phillips' Liqui-Gels, Surfak Liqui-Gels

Why is this drug prescribed?

Colace, a stool softener, promotes easy bowel movements without strain-ing. It softens the stool by mixing in fat and water.

Colace is helpful for people who have had recent rectal surgery, people with heart problems, high blood pressure, hemorrhoids, or hernias, and women who have just had babies.

Colace Microenema is used to relieve occasional constipation.

Most important fact about this drug

Colace is for short-term relief only, unless your doctor directs otherwise. It usually takes a day or two for the drug to achieve its laxative effect; some people may need to wait 4 or 5 days. Colace Microenema works in 2 to 15 minutes.

How should you take this medication?

To conceal the drug's bitter taste, take Colace liquid in half a glass of milk or fruit juice; it can be given in infant formula. The proper dosage of this medication may also be added to a retention or flushing enema.

To administer Colace Microenema:
1. Lubricate the tip by pushing out a drop of the medication.
2. Slowly insert the full length of the nozzle into the rectum. (Stop halfway for children 3 to 12 years of age.)
3. Squeeze out the contents of the tube.
4. Remove the nozzle before you release your grip on the tube.

■ *If you miss a dose...*
Take this medication only as needed.

■ *Storage instructions...*
Store at room temperature. Keep from freezing.

What side effects may occur?

Side effects are unlikely. The main ones reported are bitter taste, throat ir-ritation, and nausea (mainly associated with use of the syrup and liquid). Rash has occurred.

Why should this drug not be prescribed?

There are no known reasons this drug should not be prescribed.

Special warnings about this medication

Do not use this product if you have any abdominal pain, nausea, or vomiting, unless your doctor advises it. Do not take this product if you are taking mineral oil. If you have noticed a change in your bowel habits that has lasted for 2 weeks, ask your doctor before you use this product. If you bleed from the rectum or you do not have a bowel movement after using this product, stop using it and call your doctor; you may have a more serious condition. Do not use any laxative for more than a week without your doctor's approval.

Possible food and drug interactions when taking this medication

No interactions have been reported with Colace.

Special information if you are pregnant or breastfeeding

If you are pregnant, plan to become pregnant, or are breastfeeding your baby, notify your doctor before using this medication.

Recommended dosage

Your doctor will adjust the dosage according to your needs.

You will be using higher doses at the start of treatment with Colace. You should see an effect on stools 1 to 3 days after the first dose.

Colace Microenema should produce a bowel movement in 2 to 15 minutes.

ADULTS AND CHILDREN 12 AND OLDER

The suggested daily dosage of Colace is 50 to 200 milligrams.

In enemas, add 50 to 100 milligrams of Colace or 5 to 10 milliliters of Colace liquid to a retention or flushing enema, as prescribed by your doctor.

For Colace Microenema, use the entire contents of the tube.

CHILDREN UNDER 12 YEARS OLD

The suggested daily dosage of Colace for children 6 to 12 years of age is 40 to 120 milligrams; for children 3 to 6, it is 20 to 60 milligrams; for children under 3, it is 10 to 40 milligrams.

Colace Microenema should not be given to children under 3.

Overdosage

Overdose is unlikely with normal use of Colace. If you or your child should accidentally take too much, call your doctor or a Poison Control Center.

COLAZAL

Pronounced: KOHL-a-zahl
Generic name: Balsalazide disodium

Why is this drug prescribed?

Colazal is used in the treatment of mild to moderate ulcerative colitis (chronic inflammation and ulceration of the lower intestine). It is an anti-inflammatory medicine specially formulated to release the active ingredient, mesalamine, directly to the lining of the colon. Its ability to provide relief without the severe side effects found with similar drugs is believed to be due to this localized drug delivery mechanism.

Most important fact about this drug

Although there have been no reports of kidney damage from Colazal, other products containing mesalamine are known to have caused this problem. If you have kidney disease, your doctor will monitor your condition closely during treatment with Colazal. Report any problems or unusual symptoms immediately.

How should you take this medication?

Colazal can be taken with or without food.

■ *If you miss a dose...*
Take it as soon as possible. If it is within 2 hours of your next dose, skip the one you missed and go back to your regular schedule. Do not take 2 doses at once.

■ *Storage instructions...*
Store at room temperature.

What side effects may occur?

Side effects cannot be anticipated. If any develop or change in intensity, inform your doctor as soon as possible. Only your doctor can determine if it is safe for you to continue taking Colazal.

■ *Side effects may include:*
Abdominal pain, diarrhea, headache, joint pain, nausea, vomiting, respiratory infection

Why should this drug not be prescribed?

Do not take Colazal if you are allergic to mesalamine (Rowasa) or salicylates such as aspirin.

Special warnings about this medication

Some cases of fatal liver disease have been reported during treatment with Colazal. If you have a liver problem, make sure your doctor is aware of it before you start treatment.

If you have pyloric stenosis (narrowing of the stomach outlet), Colazal capsules may be slow to pass through the digestive tract.

Although many people get significant relief from Colazal, you should be aware that in rare cases it makes the symptoms worse.

This drug has not been tested in children.

Possible food and drug interactions when taking this medication

While drug interactions with Colazal have not yet been studied, it is possible that oral antibiotics could interfere with the release of this medication in the colon.

Special information if you are pregnant or breastfeeding

The effects of Colazal during pregnancy have not been adequately studied. If you are pregnant or plan to become pregnant, notify your doctor before taking this medication. It should be used during pregnancy only if clearly needed.

It is not known whether Colazal appears in breast milk. Because there's a chance that it may, caution is advised.

Recommended dosage

ADULTS

The usual dose of Colazal is three 750-milligram capsules taken 3 times daily for 8 to 12 weeks.

Overdosage

Little is known about Colazal overdose. However, any drug taken in excess can have serious consequences. If you suspect an overdose, seek emergency medical treatment immediately.

Colesevelam *See WelChol, page 1585.*

COLESTID
Pronounced: Koh-LESS-tid
Generic name: Colestipol hydrochloride

Why is this drug prescribed?

Colestid, in conjunction with diet, is used to help lower high levels of cholesterol in the blood. It is available in plain and orange-flavored granules and in tablet form.

Most important fact about this drug

Accidentally inhaling Colestid granules may cause serious effects. To avoid this, *NEVER* take them in their dry form. Colestid granules should always be mixed with water or other liquids *BEFORE* you take them.

How should you take this medication?

Colestid granules should be mixed with liquids such as:

Carbonated beverages (may cause stomach or intestinal discomfort)
Flavored drinks
Milk
Orange juice
Pineapple juice
Tomato juice
Water

Colestid may also be mixed with:

Milk used on breakfast cereals
Pulpy fruit (such as crushed peaches, pears, or pineapple) or fruit
cocktail
Soups with a high liquid content (such as chicken noodle or tomato)

To take Colestid granules with beverages:

1. Measure at least 3 ounces of liquid into a glass.
2. Add the prescribed dose of Colestid to the liquid.
3. Stir **until Colestid is completely mixed** (it will not dissolve) and then **drink the mixture.**
4. **Pour a small amount** of the beverage into the glass, swish it around, and drink it. This will help make sure you have taken all the medication.

Swallow Colestid tablets whole, one at a time. Although they are unusually large and may be hard to swallow, do not cut, chew, or crush them. Take the tablets with plenty of water or other liquid.

■ *If you miss a dose...*
Take the forgotten dose as soon as you remember. If it is almost time for the next dose, skip the one you missed and go back to your regular schedule. Never try to catch up by doubling the dose.

■ *Storage instructions...*
Store Colestid granules and tablets at room temperature.

What side effects may occur?

Side effects cannot be anticipated. If any develop or change in intensity, inform your doctor as soon as possible. Only your doctor can determine if it is safe for you to continue taking Colestid.

■ *Side effects may include:*
Constipation, worsening of hemorrhoids

Why should this drug not be prescribed?

You should not be using Colestid if you are allergic to it or any of its components.

Special warnings about this medication

Before starting treatment with Colestid, you should:

■ Be tested (and treated) for diseases that may contribute to increased blood cholesterol, such as an underactive thyroid gland, diabetes, nephrotic syndrome (a kidney disease), dysproteinemia (a blood disease), obstructive liver disease, and alcoholism.

■ Be on a diet plan (approved by your doctor) that stresses low-cholesterol foods and weight loss (if necessary).

Because certain medications may increase cholesterol, you should tell your doctor all of the medications you use.

Colestid may prevent the absorption of vitamins such as A, D, and K. Long-term use of Colestid may be connected to increased bleeding from a lack of vitamin K. Taking vitamin K$_1$ will help relieve this condition and prevent it in the future.

Your cholesterol and triglyceride levels should be checked regularly while you are taking Colestid.

Colestid may cause or worsen constipation. Dosages should be adjusted by your doctor. You may need to increase your intake of fiber and fluid. A stool softener also may be needed occasionally. People with coronary artery disease should be especially careful to avoid constipation. Hemorrhoids may be worsened by constipation related to Colestid.

If you have phenylketonuria (a hereditary disease caused by your body's inability to handle the amino acid phenylalanine), be aware that Flavored Colestid granules contain phenylalanine.

Possible food and drug interactions when taking this medication

Colestid may delay or reduce the absorption of other drugs. Allow as much time as possible between taking Colestid and taking other medications. Other drugs should be taken at least 1 hour before or 4 hours after taking Colestid.

If Colestid is taken with certain other drugs, the effects of either could be increased, decreased, or altered. It is especially important to check with your doctor before combining Colestid with the following:

Chlorothiazide (Diuril)
Digitalis (Lanoxin)
Folic acid and vitamins such as A, D, and K
Furosemide (Lasix)
Gemfibrozil (Lopid)
Hydrochlorothiazide (HydroDIURIL)
Hydrocortisone (Anusol-HC, Cortisporin, others)
Penicillin G, including brands such as Pentids
Phosphate supplements
Propranolol (Inderal)
Tetracycline drugs such as Sumycin

Special information if you are pregnant or breastfeeding

The effects of Colestid during pregnancy have not been adequately studied. If you are pregnant or planning to become pregnant, or plan to breastfeed, check with your doctor. Since Colestid interferes with the absorption of the fat-soluble vitamins A, D, and K, it may affect both the mother and the nursing infant.

Recommended dosage

ADULTS

One packet or 1 level scoopful of Flavored Colestid granules or one packet or 1 level teaspoon of unflavored granules contains 5 grams of Colestipol.

The usual starting dose is 1 packet or 1 level scoopful once or twice a day. Your doctor may increase this by 1 dose a day every month or every other month, up to 6 packets or 6 level scoopfuls taken once a day or divided into smaller doses.

If you are taking Colestid tablets, the usual starting dose is 2 grams (2 tablets) once or twice a day. Your doctor may increase the dose every month or every other month, to a maximum of 16 grams a day, taken once a day or divided into smaller doses.

CHILDREN

The safety and effectiveness of Colestid have not been established for children.

Overdosage

Overdoses of Colestid have not been reported. If an overdose occurs, the most likely harmful effect would be obstruction of the stomach and/or intestines. If you suspect an overdose, seek medical help immediately.

Colestipol See Colestid, page 320.

Colistin, Neomycin, Hydrocortisone, and Thonzonium
   See Cortisporin-TC Otic, page 343.

COMBIPATCH
Pronounced: KOM-bee-patch
Generic name: Estradiol and Norethindrone acetate

Why is this drug prescribed?

A remedy for the symptoms of menopause, CombiPatch combines the hormones estrogen (estradiol) and progestin (norethindrone acetate) in a slow-release patch that's applied to the skin. The product eases such symptoms of menopause as feelings of warmth in the face, neck, and chest, and the sudden intense episodes of heat and sweating known as hot flashes. It is also prescribed to relieve external vaginal irritation and internal vaginal dryness.

CombiPatch can also be used as an estrogen supplement by women unable to produce sufficient amounts of estrogen on their own. Problems prompting the need for supplementation include ovarian failure, hypogonadism (impaired hormone production), and surgical removal of the ovaries.

Most important fact about this drug

Using estrogen may increase your chances of getting heart attacks, strokes, blood clots, breast cancer, and endometrial cancer (cancer in the lining of the uterus). Because estrogen replacement therapy is not advisable if you are in any danger of developing cancer or blood clots, your doctor should take a complete medical and family history, and perform a complete physical exam, before prescribing CombiPatch. It is important to have regular checkups (at least once a year) and to report any unusual vaginal bleeding to your doctor immediately.

Hormone replacement therapy using estrogens, with or without progestin, should not be used to prevent heart disease. Recent studies have confirmed an increased rate of heart attack, stroke, and dangerous blood clots among women taking estrogen or estrogen combinations for 5 years. Blood clots can lead to phlebitis, stroke, heart attack, a loss of blood supply to the lungs, a blockage in the blood vessels serving the eye, and other serious disorders. Because of these risks, hormone replacement therapy should be given at the lowest effective dose for the shortest time. Your doctor will determine the dosage that is best for you.

How should you take this medication?

Apply the patch to a smooth, clean, dry area of the skin on your lower abdomen. Do not apply it on or near your breasts, at your waistline, or to oily, damaged, or irritated areas.

Rotate sites; the same area should not be used again for at least one week. Wear only one patch at a time.

Do not expose the patch to the sun for prolonged periods of time. If it falls off during bathing or other activities, reapply it to a different part of the lower abdomen. If necessary, use a new patch.

Remove the patch carefully to avoid skin irritation. If any adhesive remains, wait 15 minutes, then gently rub the area with a cream or lotion to remove the residue.

■ *If you miss a dose...*
If you forget to apply a new patch when you are supposed to, do it as soon as you remember. If it is almost time to change patches anyway, skip the one you missed and go back to your regular schedule. Do not apply more than one patch at a time unless directed by your doctor.

■ *Storage instructions…*
　Store the sealed foil patches at room temperature, away from extreme heat and cold, for up to 3 months.

What side effects may occur?
Side effects cannot be anticipated. If any develop or change in intensity, inform your doctor as soon as possible. Only your doctor can determine if it is safe for you to continue taking CombiPatch.

■ *Side effects may include:*
　Abdominal pain, back pain, breast pain, flu symptoms, menstrual problems, nausea, nervousness, painful menstruation, respiratory problems, skin reaction, sore throat, vaginal inflammation, weakness

Why should this drug not be prescribed?
The hormones in CombiPatch should not be used during pregnancy. You should also avoid this product if you have:

■ Unexplained vaginal bleeding
■ Known or suspected breast cancer
■ Any type of tumor stimulated by estrogen
■ Phlebitis, stroke, or any other clotting disorder
■ An allergy to any component of the patch

Special warnings about this medication
Estrogen, with or without progestins, has the potential of causing clot-related disorders, including heart attack and stroke, pulmonary embolism (a clot in the lungs), and thrombophlebitis (a clot in the veins). If you have a history of deep-vein thrombosis (a clot in the legs), or of thrombosis in your family, be sure to tell your doctor. The chance of developing a clot-related problem can be reduced by using the lowest dose of estrogen that still proves effective. If a problem develops, you'll have to stop using the patch. Likewise, you should discontinue the patch and call your doctor immediately if you suffer a loss of vision, any other eye problems, or a migraine headache.

Estrogen replacement therapy increases the risk of developing cancer of the lining of the uterus (endometrial cancer). The risk increases with longer use and higher doses. Combining estrogen and progestin reduces the risk of endometrial cancer caused by estrogen alone. However, this combination is not recommended for women who have had a hysterectomy (removal of the uterus), since they are not at risk for endometrial cancer.

Using estrogen may also increase your chances of breast cancer, ovarian cancer, and gallbladder disease.

Use estrogen with caution if you have severely low blood levels of calcium (hypocalcemia).

Tell your doctor if you've ever had liver problems, thyroid problems, or vision problems. Using estrogen could make these conditions worse. Other conditions that could worsen during estrogen therapy include asthma, diabetes, epilepsy, migraine, and the genetic disorder porphyria. Be sure your doctor is aware of any medical problems you have.

Hormone therapy occasionally causes a rise in blood pressure. If you have a blood pressure problem, use CombiPatch with caution and have your pressure checked regularly.

Hormones also tend to cause fluid retention. If you have a condition that could be aggravated by excess fluid, such as asthma, epilepsy, migraine headaches, heart disease, or kidney problems, use CombiPatch with caution.

If you suffer from endometriosis, a condition where the endometrium (the lining of the uterus) doesn't shed properly and attaches to the outside of the uterus or other areas such as the ovaries or bowels, hormone therapy may cause a worsening of this condition.

Because estrogen can increase triglyceride levels, you'll need to be closely monitored if your triglycerides tend to be high. If you have diabetes, CombiPatch may also affect your blood sugar levels.

Estrogen therapy occasionally causes abnormal uterine bleeding or breast pain. In view of concerns about cancer, you should have these symptoms checked by your doctor. In general, you should not take estrogen for more than 1 year without a follow-up physical exam. Ideally, you should have a checkup every 3 to 6 months.

Let your doctor know if you're going to have surgery or will be on bed rest; you may need to stop taking estrogens.

Possible food and drug interactions when taking this medication
The manufacturer has not reported interactions.

Special information if you are pregnant or breastfeeding
Estrogens such as the one in CombiPatch should not be used during pregnancy. They pose a danger of birth defects, particularly in the reproductive tract.

The hormones in CombiPatch do appear in breast milk and may affect its quantity and quality. You should avoid taking them while breastfeeding unless it's absolutely necessary.

Recommended dosage

ADULTS

Your doctor will determine the dosage that is right for you. Typically, hormone replacement therapy should be for the shortest duration to relieve your symptoms. You should be evaluated every three to six months.

The recommended starting dose is one patch containing 0.05 milligram estradiol and 0.14 milligram norethindrone acetate applied twice a week (every 3 to 4 days). Your doctor may increase your dose to a patch containing 0.05 milligram estradiol and 0.25 milligram norethindrone acetate if needed.

CombiPatch can also be used in conjunction with a 0.05-milligram estradiol-only patch such as the product brand-named Vivelle. The estradiol-only patch is applied twice a week for the first 14 days of a 28-day cycle, and CombiPatch is applied twice weekly for the remaining 14 days.

If you are currently taking another form of hormone replacement therapy, you should complete the current cycle before switching to Combi-Patch.

Irregular bleeding may occur, particularly in the first 6 months of therapy, but generally decreases with time and often stops completely.

Overdosage
Even a large overdose of the hormones in CombiPatch would pose little danger; and the patch form of delivery renders such a dose highly unlikely. Nevertheless, if you think there's a chance, seek medical attention immediately. Symptoms would include nausea and withdrawal bleeding.

COMBIVENT
Pronounced: COM-bi-vent
Generic name: Ipratropium bromide, Albuterol sulfate

Why is this drug prescribed?
Combivent is prescribed for people with chronic obstructive pulmonary disease (COPD) if they are already taking one airway-opening medication and need another. The product's two active ingredients act in distinctly different ways. Ipratropium quells airway-closing spasms in the bronchial walls. Albuterol relaxes the muscles in the walls, permitting them to expand. When used together, the two ingredients provide more relief than either can do alone.

Combivent is supplied in an aerosol canister for use only with the special Combivent mouthpiece.

Most important fact about this drug
Overuse of this product can be fatal. Do not increase the dose or frequency without your doctor's okay. If you find that Combivent is becoming less effective, that your symptoms are getting worse, or that you need the product more frequently than usual, see your doctor immediately.

How should you take this medication?
Remove the orange protective cap from the mouthpiece and shake the canister well. If you are starting a new canister, or if more than 24 hours have passed since your last dose, test-spray the canister 3 times. For best

results, make sure the canister is at room temperature. Do not use near an open flame.

1. Exhale deeply through your mouth, then close your lips around the mouthpiece. Keep your eyes closed to protect them against an accidental spray.
2. Inhale slowly through the mouth, and at the same time press down once on the canister's base.
3. Hold your breath for 10 seconds, then remove the mouthpiece from your lips and exhale slowly.
4. Wait 2 minutes, shake the canister again, and repeat.

The mouthpiece can be washed with soap and hot water. Rinse it and dry thoroughly. Keep the mouthpiece capped when not in use. Count the number of sprays and discard each canister after 200 sprays; canisters may fail to deliver the proper dose if used for more than that amount.

■ *If you miss a dose...*
Take the forgotten dose as soon as you remember. However, if it is almost time for your next dose, skip the one you missed and return to your regular schedule. Do not take 2 doses at once.

■ *Storage instructions...*
Store at room temperature. Protect from heat; a temperature of 120 degrees Fahrenheit can cause the canister to burst. Do not puncture the canister or discard it in an incinerator. Protect from high humidity.

What side effects may occur?
Side effects cannot be anticipated. If any develop or change in intensity, tell your doctor as soon as possible. Only your doctor can determine if it is safe to continue using Combivent.

■ *Side effects may include:*
Bronchitis, coughing, headache, shortness of breath, upper respiratory tract infection

Why should this drug not be prescribed?
You'll have to avoid Combivent if either of its ingredients has ever given you an allergic reaction. Avoid it, too, if you've had a reaction to atropine-containing drugs such as Donnatal, or if you are allergic to peanuts, soybeans, or soy lecithin.

Special warnings about this medication
Instead of opening the airways, Combivent sometimes causes them to close. This reaction—which can be life-threatening—is most likely to occur after the first use of a new canister. If you suffer severe breathing difficulties after a dose of Combivent, stop using it and see your doctor immediately.

The albuterol in Combivent has been known to raise heart rate and blood pressure. It can also cause changes in heart rhythm. If you have a weak heart, an irregular heartbeat, high blood pressure, or any other heart problem, you'll need to use Combivent with caution. If it triggers heart-related symptoms, check with your doctor at once. The product may have to be discontinued.

A severe allergic reaction can follow the first dose of Combivent. Possible symptoms include swelling of the face, mouth, or throat; hives, skin rash, breathing difficulties, or even collapse. Seek emergency care immediately if these symptoms occur.

The ipratropium in Combivent can aggravate glaucoma (high pressure in the eye), prostate enlargement, and urinary difficulties. The albuterol it contains can cause problems for people with epilepsy, diabetes, or an overactive thyroid. Use Combivent with caution if you have any of these conditions.

If the Combivent aerosol gets in your eyes, it can cause eye pain or discomfort, blurred vision, visual halos, colored images, or high pressure in the eye. Check with your doctor immediately if you develop any of these problems.

Possible food and drug interactions when using this medication

Combivent can be taken with other drugs for COPD, but you should use other inhaled medications only as directed by your doctor. If Combivent is taken with certain other drugs, the effects of either could be increased, decreased, or altered. It is especially important to check with your doctor before combining Combivent with the following:

Airway-opening drugs such as Advair, Alupent, Brethine, Proventil, Ventolin, and Xopenex

Drugs classified as beta-blockers, including Inderal, Sectral, and Tenormin

Drugs classified as monoamine oxidase inhibitors, such as the antidepressants Nardil and Parnate

Spasm-quelling medications such as Cogentin, Donnatal, and Levsin

Water pills (diuretics) such as Lasix and HydroDIURIL

Tricyclic antidepressants such as Etrafon, Norpramin, Sinequan, and Vivactil

Special information if you are pregnant or breastfeeding

The effects of Combivent during pregnancy have not been adequately studied. If you are pregnant or plan to become pregnant, tell your doctor immediately.

It's not known whether the components of Combivent appear in breast milk, but it's considered best to avoid use of the drug if you are breastfeeding.

Recommended dosage

ADULTS

The usual dosage is 2 inhalations 4 times a day. You can take additional inhalations as required up to a total of 12 inhalations each 24 hours.

Overdosage

An overdose of Combivent can be fatal. If you suspect an overdose, seek medical attention immediately.

■ *Symptoms of Combivent overdose may include:*
Cardiac arrest, chest pain (angina), high blood pressure, rapid heartbeat

COMBIVIR

Pronounced: KOM-bi-veer
Generic ingredients: Lamivudine, Zidovudine

Why is this drug prescribed?

Combivir is used to fight the human immunodeficiency virus (HIV), which causes AIDS. It is a combination product containing the two AIDS drugs lamivudine (Epivir) and zidovudine (Retrovir). It is intended for use with additional AIDS drugs.

HIV does its damage by slowly destroying the immune system, eventually leaving the body defenseless against infections. The drugs in Combivir interfere with the virus's ability to reproduce, thus staving off the decline of the immune system and preserving better health.

Most important fact about this drug

Combivir is not a cure for HIV infection or AIDS. It does not completely eliminate HIV from the body or totally restore the immune system. There is still a danger of serious infections, so you should be sure to see your doctor regularly for monitoring and tests.

How should you take this medication?

It's important to keep adequate levels of Combivir in your bloodstream at all times, so you need to take it regularly, exactly as prescribed, even when you're feeling better. Doses can be taken with or without food.

■ *If you miss a dose...*
Take it as soon as you remember. If it is almost time for your next dose, skip the one you missed and go back to your regular schedule. Do not take 2 doses at once.
■ *Storage instructions...*
Store at room temperature.

What side effects may occur?

Side effects cannot be anticipated. If any develop or change in intensity, inform your doctor as soon as possible. Only your doctor can determine if it is safe for you to continue taking Combivir.

■ *Side effects may include:*
Abdominal pain, abdominal cramps, allergic reactions, blisters, blood disorders, bone pain, breast enlargement, chills, cough, depression, diarrhea, dizziness, fat redistribution, fatigue, fever, flu-like symptoms, hair loss, headache, heart weakness, high blood sugar, indigestion, inflamed blood vessels, insomnia, joint pain, liver disorders, loss of appetite, mouth discoloration, mouth sores, muscle aches or weakness, nasal symptoms, nausea, nerve disorders, pancreatitis, seizures, skin rash, sleep disorders, vomiting, weakness, wheezing

Why should this drug not be prescribed?

You should not take Combivir if either component, Epivir or Retrovir, has ever given you an allergic reaction.

Special warnings about this medication

Remember that Combivir does not totally eliminate HIV from the body. The infection can still be passed on to others through sexual contact or blood contamination.

Combivir can upset the body's acid balance. It can also cause low blood cell counts (anemia), which can adversely affect your health. It should be used with extreme caution by anyone with an existing shortage of blood cells or a disease of the bone marrow (where blood cells are produced). It is very important to have your blood tested regularly, especially if you have an advanced case of HIV.

Combivir is known to occasionally cause serious liver problems.

If you have the chronic liver disease hepatitis B, the virus that causes it may become resistant to the Epivir component of Combivir. Your hepatitis may get worse when Combivir treatment is stopped.

Combivir can cause muscle pain and inflammation. Report these symptoms to your doctor.

If you weigh less than 110 pounds, you should not take Combivir. The Epivir component of Combivir is not recommended in people with low body weight.

Because Combivir contains fixed doses of Epivir and Retrovir, it cannot be used by people who might require a decrease or adjustment in the dosage of either drug, such as children and those with poor kidney or liver function.

Inflammation of the pancreas (pancreatitis) can be caused by the Epivir component of Combivir. If any signs of a pancreas problem develop, such as severe abdominal pain that goes on for days, accompanied by nausea and vomiting, stop taking Combivir and call your doctor immediately.

Another side effect seen in some people receiving drugs for HIV is a redistribution of body fat, leading to extra fat around the middle, a "buffalo hump" on the back, and wasting in the arms, legs, and face. Researchers don't know whether this represents a long-term health problem or not.

Possible food and drug interactions when taking this medication

If Combivir is taken with certain other drugs, the effects of either could be increased, decreased, or altered. It is especially important to check with your doctor before combining Combivir with the following:

Chemotherapy drugs
Doxorubicin (Doxil, Adriamycin)
Ganciclovir (Cytovene)
Interferon (Intron A, Roferon-A)
Ribavirin (Virazole)
Stavudine (Zerit)
Trimethoprim/Sulfamethoxazole (Bactrim, Septra)
Zalcitabine (Hivid)

Special information if you are pregnant or breastfeeding

The effects of Combivir during pregnancy have not been adequately studied. If you are pregnant or plan to become pregnant, notify your doctor immediately.

Since HIV infection can be passed to your baby through breast milk, you should not breastfeed your infant.

Recommended dosage

ADULTS

For adults and adolescents 12 and over, the recommended dose is one tablet (containing 150 milligrams of Epivir and 300 milligrams of Retrovir) twice a day.

CHILDREN

Combivir should not be taken by children under 12 years of age.

Overdosage

The symptoms of Combivir overdose are unknown at this time. However, any medication taken in excess can have serious consequences. If you suspect an overdose, seek medical attention immediately.

■ *Symptoms of overdose with the Retrovir component may include:*
Confusion, dizziness, drowsiness, headache, lack of energy, nausea, seizure, vomiting

COMTAN

Pronounced: COM-tan
Generic name: Entacapone

Why is this drug prescribed?

Comtan is used for Parkinson's disease. It is prescribed when doses of the combination drug levodopa/carbidopa (Sinemet) begin to wear off too soon. By extending the effect of each dose of Sinemet, it frees the patient from the stiffness and tremors of Parkinson's for a longer period of time.

Comtan works by inhibiting the effect of an enzyme that breaks down the levodopa in Sinemet. It has no effect on Parkinson's disease when used by itself.

Most important fact about this drug

Comtan's value lies in its ability to extend Sinemet's effectiveness when it begins to decline. It is helpful only when taken with the other drug, and has no benefit when used alone.

How should you take this medication?

Comtan should be taken with each dose of Sinemet. It can be taken up to 8 times per day, with or without food.

■ *If you miss a dose...*
Take it along with a dose of Sinemet as soon as you remember. If it is almost time for your next dose, skip the one you missed and go back to your regular schedule. Never take 2 doses at the same time.

■ *Storage instructions...*
Store at room temperature.

What side effects may occur?

Side effects cannot be anticipated. If any develop or change in intensity, inform your doctor as soon as possible. Only your doctor can determine if it is safe for you to continue taking Comtan.

■ *Side effects may include:*
Abdominal pain, back pain, constipation, diarrhea, discoloration of urine, dizziness, nausea, onset of new movement disorders, tired feeling, vomiting

Why should this drug not be prescribed?

If Comtan gives you an allergic reaction, you won't be able to use it. It is prescribed only with caution for people with liver disease.

Special warnings about this medication

Use of Comtan can cause low blood pressure, with symptoms such as dizziness, nausea, fainting, and sweating. Be careful when standing up after you have been sitting or lying down. See how the medication affects you before you drive a car or operate machinery.

Nausea and diarrhea are especially common side effects of Comtan, developing in more than 10 percent of those taking it. In rare cases, the problem is severe. Comtan may also cause hallucinations, and occasionally triggers new movement disorders. In about 10 percent of those taking it, it has the harmless side effect of turning the urine a brownish-orange color.

An abrupt discontinuation of Comtan can cause a reappearance of Parkinson's symptoms. If a decision is made to discontinue the drug, it should be withdrawn slowly, under a doctor's supervision.

This drug is not intended for use in children.

Possible food and drug interactions when taking this medication

If Comtan is taken with certain other drugs, the effects of either could be increased, decreased, or altered. It is especially important to check with your doctor before combining Comtan with the following:

Antidepressant drugs classified as MAO inhibitors, including Nardil and Parnate (Comtan can be used with a special type of MAO inhibitor called selegiline, which is used for treating Parkinson's disease)
Bitolterol (Tornalate)
Certain antibiotics, including ampicillin and erythromycin
Cholestyramine (Questran)
Methyldopa (Aldomet)
Isoproterenol (Isuprel)
Probenecid (Benemid)

Special information if you are pregnant or breastfeeding

The possibility of damage to a developing baby has not been ruled out. Tell your physician immediately if you are pregnant or plan to become pregnant. Comtan may appear in breast milk. It should be used with caution if you are nursing your baby.

Recommended dosage

ADULTS

The recommended dose is one 200-milligram tablet with each dose of Sinemet, up to a maximum of 8 doses per day. If you were taking more than 800 milligrams of levodopa per day before starting Comtan, you will probably need a reduction in your levodopa dose once you begin taking the drug.

Overdosage
Little is known about the result of Comtan overdose. However, the results could be serious, so if you suspect an overdose, seek medical attention immediately.

Concerta See Ritalin, page 1270.

Conjugated estrogens See Premarin, page 1135.

Copegus See Ribavirin, page 1258.

COREG
Pronounced: KOE-regg
Generic name: Carvedilol

Why is this drug prescribed?
Coreg lowers blood pressure and increases the output of the heart. It is prescribed for people with congestive heart failure to increase survival and reduce the need for hospitalization. Coreg may be prescribed if you have survived a heart attack and now suffer from left ventricular dysfunction, a condition where the left side of the heart no longer pumps properly. It is also used to control high blood pressure. It is often used with other drugs.

Most important fact about this drug
In some people, Coreg causes a drop in blood pressure when they first stand up, resulting in dizziness or even fainting. If this happens, sit or lie down and notify your doctor. Taking the drug with food reduces the chance of this problem. Even so, during the first month of therapy, or after a change in your dose, be careful about driving and operation of dangerous machinery.

How should you take this medication?
Take Coreg twice a day with food. If you are taking the drug for high blood pressure, there should be improvement within 7 to 14 days.

- ■ *If you miss a dose…*
  Take it as soon as you remember. If it is almost time for your next dose, skip the one you missed and go back to your regular schedule. Do not take 2 doses at once.
- ■ *Storage instructions…*
  Coreg should be stored at room temperature, away from light and moisture. Keep the container tightly closed.

What side effects may occur?

Side effects cannot be anticipated. If any develop or change in intensity, inform your doctor as soon as possible. Only your doctor can determine if it is safe for you to continue taking Coreg.

■ *Side effects may include:*

Anemia, back pain, bronchitis, cough, diarrhea, dizziness, fainting, fatigue, fluid in the lungs, headache, increased blood sugar levels, increased cholesterol, joint pain, low blood pressure, nausea, pain, shortness of breath, sinus problems, slow heartbeat, swelling, upper respiratory infection, vision changes, vomiting, weakness, weight gain, wheezing

Why should this drug not be prescribed?

Avoid Coreg if you have asthma, certain serious heart conditions, or liver disease. Do not take the drug if it causes an allergic reaction.

Special warnings about this medication

Coreg sometimes aggravates chronic bronchitis and emphysema. If you have either condition, make sure the doctor is aware of it. You'll need to use the drug cautiously. Report any weight gain or shortness of breath to your doctor immediately.

Liver damage is a rare side effect of the drug. Notify your doctor immediately if you develop these signs of liver disorder: appetite loss, dark urine, flu-like symptoms, itching, pain in your side, or yellowing of the skin. You will need to be switched from Coreg.

Make sure your doctor knows if you have diabetes or low blood sugar. Coreg can interfere with the effectiveness of diabetes drugs and can cover up the symptoms of low blood sugar. Monitor your blood sugar regularly, and report any changes to your doctor.

A few people starting Coreg therapy for heart failure suffer dizziness, light-headedness, or even fainting within an hour after taking each dose. The problem is most likely to occur during the first 30 days of treatment, and especially after a dosage increase. If Coreg has this effect on you, avoid driving or hazardous tasks for the hour following each dose.

When Coreg is taken for heart failure, there is also a slight chance that it will interfere with the kidneys. If this reaction seems likely, the doctor will monitor your kidney function and, if necessary, change your dosage—or take you off the drug. Your heart failure may continue to get worse during the first 3 months of treatment, possibly requiring a temporary reduction in the dose of Coreg. After that, Coreg's benefits should begin to appear.

If you have circulation problems in the arms and legs, Coreg may aggravate your symptoms. Use it with care and report any changes to your doctor.

Under no circumstances should you abruptly stop taking this drug on your own. Notify the doctor if you miss even a few doses of Coreg. Your symptoms could return with a vengeance; and if you have an overactive thyroid, those symptoms could be aggravated as well. If needed, the doctor will taper you off the drug gradually over a period of 1 to 2 weeks. During this time you should keep your physical activity to a minimum. If your angina worsens or heart problems occur, notify your doctor immediately; you may need to begin taking Coreg again, at least temporarily.

If you wear contact lenses, you should know that Coreg can dry your eyes.

Possible food and drug interactions when taking this medication

If Coreg is taken with certain other drugs, the effects of either could be increased, decreased, or altered. It is especially important to check with your doctor before combining Coreg with any of the following:

Calcium channel blockers (blood pressure and heart medications such as Calan, Cardizem, Isoptin, and Verelan)
Cimetidine (Tagamet)
Clonidine (Catapres)
Cyclosporine (Neoral, Sandimmune)
Diabetes pills such as Diabinese, Glucophage, and Rezulin
Drugs classified as MAO inhibitors, including the antidepressants Nardil and Parnate Digoxin (Lanoxin)
Fluoxetine (Prozac)
Insulin
Paroxetine (Paxil)
Propafenone (Rythmol)
Quinidine (Quinaglute)
Reserpine (Ser-Ap-Es)
Rifampin (Rifadin)

Special information if you are pregnant or breastfeeding

Coreg has not been adequately studied in pregnant women; and it is not known whether the drug appears in breast milk. If you are pregnant or plan to become pregnant, check with your doctor immediately.

Recommended dosage

ADULTS

Hypertension
The starting dose is 6.25 milligrams twice a day with food. Your doctor may raise the dosage every 1 or 2 weeks to a maximum of 50 milligrams a day.

Congestive Heart Failure
The starting dose is 3.125 milligrams twice a day with food. Your doctor may increase the dosage every 2 weeks. The maximum dosage, for people weighing over 187 pounds, is 100 milligrams a day.

Left Ventricular Dysfunction Following a Heart Attack
The starting dose ranges from 3.125 to 6.25 milligrams twice a day with food. Your doctor may increase the dosage after 3 to 10 days to 12.5 milligrams twice a day. Based on your response, the doctor may again increase the dose up to a maximum of 25 milligrams twice a day.

CHILDREN

The safety and effectiveness of Coreg have not been studied in children under 18.

Overdosage

Any medication taken in excess can have serious consequences. If you suspect an overdose, seek medical treatment immediately.

■ *Symptoms of Coreg overdose may include:*
  Breathing difficulties, heart problems, loss of consciousness, seizures, slow heartbeat, very low blood pressure, vomiting

CORGARD

Pronounced: CORE-guard
Generic name: Nadolol

Why is this drug prescribed?

Corgard is used in the treatment of angina pectoris (chest pain, usually caused by lack of oxygen to the heart due to clogged arteries) and to reduce high blood pressure.

When prescribed for high blood pressure, it is effective when used alone or in combination with other high blood pressure medications. Corgard is a type of drug known as a beta-blocker. It decreases the force and rate of heart contractions, reducing the heart's demand for oxygen and lowering blood pressure.

Most important fact about this drug

If you have high blood pressure, you must take Corgard regularly for it to be effective. Since blood pressure declines gradually, it may be several weeks before you get the full benefit of Corgard; and you must continue taking it even if you are feeling well. Corgard does not cure high blood pressure; it merely keeps it under control.

How should you take this medication?

Corgard can be taken with or without food. Take it exactly as prescribed even if your symptoms have disappeared.

Try not to miss any doses. Corgard is taken once a day. If it is not taken regularly, your condition may worsen.

■ *If you miss a dose...*
   Take it as soon as you remember. If it is within 8 hours of your next scheduled dose, skip the one you missed and go back to your regular schedule. Never take 2 doses at the same time.

■ *Storage instructions...*
   Store at room temperature, away from light and heat, in a tightly closed container.

What side effects may occur?

Side effects cannot be anticipated. If any develop or change in intensity, inform your doctor as soon as possible. Only your doctor can determine if it is safe for you to continue taking Corgard.

■ *Side effects may include:*
   Change in behavior, changes in heartbeat, dizziness or light-headedness, mild drowsiness, slow heartbeat, weakness or tiredness

Why should this drug not be prescribed?

If you have a slow heartbeat, bronchial asthma, certain types of heartbeat irregularity, cardiogenic shock (shock due to inadequate blood supply from the heart), or active heart failure, you should not take this medication.

Special warnings about this medication

If you have a history of congestive heart failure, your doctor will prescribe Corgard with caution.

Corgard should not be stopped suddenly. This can cause increased chest pain and even a heart attack. Dosage should be gradually reduced.

If you suffer from asthma, chronic bronchitis, emphysema, seasonal allergies or other bronchial conditions, or kidney or liver disease, this medication should be used with caution.

Ask your doctor if you should check your pulse while taking Corgard. It can cause your heartbeat to become too slow.

This medication may mask the symptoms of low blood sugar or alter blood sugar levels. If you are diabetic, discuss this with your doctor.

This medication may cause you to become drowsy or less alert; therefore, driving or operating dangerous machinery or participating in any hazardous activity that requires full mental alertness is not recommended until you know how you respond to this medication.

Notify your doctor or dentist that you are taking Corgard if you have a medical emergency or before you have surgery or dental treatment.

Possible food and drug interactions when taking this medication

If Corgard is taken with certain other drugs, the effects of either could be increased, decreased, or altered. It is especially important to check with your doctor before combining Corgard with the following:

Antidiabetic drugs, including insulin and oral drugs such as
  Micronase
Certain blood pressure drugs such as Diupres and Ser-Ap-Es
Epinephrine (EpiPen)

Special information if you are pregnant or breastfeeding

The effects of Corgard during pregnancy have not been adequately studied. If you are pregnant or plan to become pregnant, inform your doctor
immediately. Corgard appears in breast milk and could affect a nursing
infant. If this medication is essential to your health, your doctor may advise you to discontinue breastfeeding until your treatment with this medication is finished.

Recommended dosage

ADULTS

Dosage is tailored to each individual's needs.

Angina Pectoris
The usual starting dose is 40 milligrams once daily. The usual long-term
dose is 40 or 80 milligrams, once a day. Doses up to 160 or 240 milligrams, once a day, may be needed.

High Blood Pressure
The usual starting dose is 40 milligrams once daily.
  The usual long-term dose is 40 or 80 milligrams, once a day. Doses up
to 240 or 320 milligrams, once a day, may be needed.

CHILDREN

The safety and effectiveness of Corgard have not been established in
children.

Overdosage

Any medication taken in excess can have serious consequences. If you
suspect an overdose, seek medical attention immediately.

■ *Symptoms of Corgard overdose may include:*
  Difficulty breathing, heart failure, low blood pressure, slow heartbeat

Cormax *See Temovate, page 1400.*

CORTISPORIN OPHTHALMIC SUSPENSION

Pronounced: KORE-ti-SPORE-in
Generic ingredients:Polymyxin B sulfate, Neomycin sulfate,
  Hydrocortisone

Why is this drug prescribed?

Cortisporin Ophthalmic Suspension is a combination of the steroid drug hydrocortisone and two antibiotics. It is prescribed to relieve inflammatory conditions such as irritation, swelling, redness, and general eye discomfort, and to treat superficial bacterial infections of the eye.

Most important fact about this drug

Prolonged use of this medication may increase pressure within the eye, leading to potential damage to the optic nerve and visual problems. Prolonged use also may suppress your immune response and thus increase the hazard of secondary eye infections. Your doctor should measure your eye pressure periodically if you are using this product for 10 days or longer.

How should you use this medication?

To help clear up your infection completely, use this medication exactly as prescribed for the full time of treatment, even if your symptoms have disappeared.

Administer the eyedrops as follows:

1. Shake the dropper bottle well.
2. Wash your hands thoroughly.
3. Gently pull your lower eyelid down to form a pocket between your eye and eyelid.
4. Hold the bottle on the bridge of your nose or on your forehead.
5. Tilt your head back and squeeze the medication into your eye.
6. Do not touch the applicator tip to any surface, including your eye.
7. Close your eyes gently, and keep them closed for 1 to 2 minutes.
8. Do not rinse the dropper.
9. Wait 5 to 10 minutes before using any other eyedrops.

If you do not improve after 2 days, your doctor should re-evaluate your case.

Do not share this medication with anyone else; you may spread the infection.

■ *If you miss a dose...*
  Apply it as soon as you remember. If it is almost time for your next dose, skip the one you missed and go back to your regular schedule.

■ *Storage instructions...*
Store at room temperature. Keep tightly closed and protect from freezing.

What side effects may occur?

Side effects cannot be anticipated. If any develop or change in intensity, inform your doctor as soon as possible. Only your doctor can determine if it is safe for you to continue using Cortisporin.

■ *Side effects may include:*
Cataract formation (results in blurred vision), delayed wound healing, increased eye pressure (with possible development of glaucoma and, infrequently, optic nerve damage), irritation when drops are instilled, local allergic reactions (itching, swelling, redness), other infections (particularly fungal infections of the cornea and bacterial eye infections), severe allergic reactions

Why should this drug not be prescribed?

Cortisporin should not be used if you have certain viral or fungal diseases of the eye, including inflammation of the cornea caused by herpes simplex, chickenpox, or cowpox, or if you are sensitive to or have ever had an allergic reaction to any of its ingredients.

Special warnings about this medication

Remember that steroids such as hydrocortisone may hide the existence of an infection or worsen an existing one.

If you are using this medication for more than 10 days, your doctor should routinely check your eye pressure. If you already have high pressure within the eye (glaucoma), use this medication cautiously.

Neomycin, one of the ingredients in Cortisporin, may cause an allergic reaction—usually itching, redness, and swelling—or failure to heal. If you develop any of these signs, stop using Cortisporin; the symptoms should quickly subside. If the condition persists or gets worse, or if a rash or allergic reaction develops, call your doctor immediately. You are more likely to be sensitive to neomycin if you are sensitive to the following antibiotics: kanamycin, paromomycin, streptomycin, and possibly gentamicin.

The use of steroids in the eye can prolong and worsen many viral infections of the eye, including herpes simplex. Use this medication with extreme caution if you have this infection.

If you develop a sensitivity to Cortisporin, avoid other topical medications that contain neomycin.

Eye products that are not handled properly can become contaminated with bacteria that cause eye infections. If you use a contaminated product, you can seriously damage your eyes, even to the point of blindness.

Possible food and drug interactions when taking this medication
No interactions have been reported.

Special information if you are pregnant or breastfeeding
Although the effects of Cortisporin during pregnancy have not been adequately studied, steroids should be used during pregnancy only if the benefits outweigh the dangers to the fetus. If you are pregnant or plan to become pregnant, inform your doctor immediately. Hydrocortisone, when taken orally, appears in breast milk. Since medication may be absorbed into the bloodstream when it is applied to the eye, your doctor may advise you to stop breastfeeding until your treatment with Cortisporin is finished.

Recommended dosage

ADULTS

The usual recommended dose is 1 or 2 drops in the affected eye every 3 or 4 hours, depending on the severity of the condition. Cortisporin may be used more often if necessary.

Overdosage
Any medication used in excess can have serious consequences. If you suspect an overdose of Cortisporin Ophthalmic Suspension, seek medical treatment immediately.

CORTISPORIN-TC OTIC

Pronounced: KORE-ti-SPORE-in
Generic ingredients: Colistin sulfate, Neomycin sulfate,
* Hydrocortisone acetate, Thonzonium bromide*

Why is this drug prescribed?
Cortisporin-TC is a liquid suspension used to treat external ear infections. It may also be prescribed after ear surgery such as a mastoidectomy.

Colistin sulfate and neomycin sulfate are antibiotics used to treat the bacterial infection itself, while hydrocortisone acetate is a steroid that helps reduce the inflammation, swelling, itching, and other skin reactions associated with an ear infection; thonzonium bromide facilitates the drug's effects.

Most important fact about this drug
As with other antibiotics, long-term treatment may encourage other infections. Therefore, if your ear infection does not improve within a week, your physician may want to change your medication.

How should you use this medication?

Use this product for the full course of treatment (but no more than 10 days), even if you start to feel better in a few days.

Shake well before using. You can warm the suspension, but avoid heating it above body temperature. Excessive heat will reduce potency.

The external ear canal should be thoroughly cleaned and dried with a sterile cotton swab (applicator). The patient should lie with the infected ear facing up. Pull the earlobe down and back (for children) or up and back (for adults) to straighten the ear canal. Drop the suspension into the ear. The patient should lie in this position for 5 minutes to help the drops penetrate into the ear. If necessary, this procedure should be repeated for the other ear. To keep the medicine from leaking out, you can gently insert a sterile cotton plug.

If you prefer, a sterile cotton wick or plug may be inserted into the ear canal and then soaked with the suspension. This cotton wick should be moistened every 4 hours with more suspension and replaced at least once every 24 hours.

Avoid touching the dropper to the ear or other surfaces, and be careful to avoid getting the medication in your eyes.

■ *If you miss a dose...*
Apply it as soon as you remember. If it is almost time for your next dose, skip the one you missed and go back to your regular schedule.
■ *Storage instructions...*
Store at room temperature; avoid prolonged exposure to high temperatures. The medication expires after 18 months.

What side effects may occur?

No specific side effects have been reported; however, neomycin may be associated with an increased risk of allergic skin reaction.

Why should this drug not be prescribed?

You should not take this drug if you have had an allergic reaction to any of the ingredients, or if you suffer from herpes simplex, vaccinia (cowpox), or varicella (chickenpox).

Special warnings about this medication

Long-term use of Cortisporin-TC can lead to permanent hearing loss. Therefore, treatment should not continue for more than 10 days.

If an allergic reaction occurs, you should stop using the medication immediately. Your doctor may also recommend that future treatment with kanamycin, paromomycin, streptomycin, and possibly gentamicin be avoided, since you may also be allergic to these medications.

Use the medication with care if you have a perforated eardrum or chronic otitis media (inflammation and infection of the middle ear).

Possible food and drug interactions when using this medication
No interactions have been reported.

Special information if you are pregnant or breastfeeding
The effects of this product during pregnancy and nursing have not been adequately studied. If you are pregnant or plan to become pregnant, inform your doctor immediately.

Recommended dosage
This medication should not be used for longer than 10 days.

ADULTS

The usual dose is 5 drops (when using the supplied measured dropper) or 4 drops (when using the dropper-bottle container) in the affected ear, 3 or 4 times daily.

INFANTS AND CHILDREN

The usual dose is 4 drops (when using the supplied measured dropper) or 3 drops (when using the dropper-bottle container) in the affected ear 3 or 4 times daily.

Overdosage
Although no specific information is available, any medication taken in excess can have serious consequences. If you suspect an overdose, seek medical treatment immediately.

CORZIDE

Pronounced: CORE-zide
Generic ingredients: Nadolol, Bendroflumethiazide

Why is this drug prescribed?
Corzide is a combination drug used in the treatment of high blood pressure. It combines a beta-blocker and a thiazide diuretic. Nadolol, the beta-blocker, decreases the force and rate of heart contractions, thereby reducing blood pressure. Bendroflumethiazide, the diuretic, helps your body produce and eliminate more urine, which also helps in lowering blood pressure.

Most important fact about this drug
You must take Corzide regularly for it to be effective. Since blood pressure declines gradually, it may be several weeks before you get the full benefit of Corzide; and you must continue taking it even if you are feeling well. Corzide does not cure high blood pressure; it merely keeps it under control.

How should you take this medication?

Corzide may be taken with or without food. Take it exactly as prescribed, even if your symptoms have disappeared.

Try not to miss any doses. Corzide is taken once a day. If this medication is not taken regularly, your condition may worsen.

- ■ *If you miss a dose...*
  Take it as soon as you remember. If it's within 8 hours of your next scheduled dose, skip the one you missed and go back to your regular schedule. Never take 2 doses at the same time.
- ■ *Storage instructions...*
  Store at room temperature, away from heat, in a tightly closed container.

What side effects may occur?

Side effects cannot be anticipated. If any develop or change in intensity, inform your doctor as soon as possible. Only your doctor can determine if it is safe for you to continue taking Corzide.

- ■ *Side effects may include:*
  Asthma-like symptoms, changes in heart rhythm, cold hands and feet, dizziness, fatigue, low blood pressure, low potassium levels (symptoms include dry mouth, excessive thirst, weakness, drowsiness, restlessness, weak or irregular heartbeat, muscle pain or cramps, diminished urination, and digestive disturbances), slow heartbeat

Why should this drug not be prescribed?

If you have bronchial asthma, slow heartbeat, certain heartbeat irregularities (heart block), inadequate blood supply to the circulatory system (cardiogenic shock), active congestive heart failure, or inability to urinate, or if you are sensitive to or have ever had an allergic reaction to Corzide, its ingredients, or similar drugs, you should not take this medication.

Special warnings about this medication

If you have a history of congestive heart failure, your doctor will prescribe Corzide with caution.

Corzide should not be stopped suddenly. This can cause increased chest pain and even a heart attack. Dosage should be gradually reduced.

If you suffer from asthma, seasonal allergies, emphysema or other bronchial conditions, or kidney or liver disease, this medication should be used with caution.

Ask your doctor if you should check your pulse while taking Corzide. It can cause your heartbeat to become too slow.

Corzide may mask the symptoms of low blood sugar or alter blood sugar levels. If you are diabetic, discuss this with your doctor. The drug can also cause thyroid problems, and may aggravate the rash and joint pain of lupus erythematosus.

This medication can cause you to become drowsy or less alert; therefore, activity that requires full mental alertness is not recommended until you know how you respond to this medication.

Notify your doctor or dentist that you are taking Corzide if you have a medical emergency, or before you have surgery or dental treatment.

Possible food and drug interactions when taking this medication
Corzide may intensify the effects of alcohol. Do not drink alcohol while taking this medication.

If Corzide is taken with any other drug, the effects of either could be increased, decreased, or altered. It is especially important to check with your doctor before combining Corzide with the following:

Amphotericin B
Antidepressant drugs known as MAO inhibitors, such as Nardil and Parnate
Antidiabetic drugs, including insulin and oral drugs such as Micronase
Antigout drugs such as Benemid
Barbiturates such as phenobarbital
Blood thinners such as Coumadin
Calcium salt
Certain blood pressure drugs such as Diupres and Ser-Ap-Es
Cholestyramine (Questran)
Colestipol (Colestid)
Diazoxide (Proglycem)
Digitalis medications such as Lanoxin
Lithium (Lithonate)
Methenamine (Mandelamine)
Narcotics such as Percocet
Nonsteroidal anti-inflammatory drugs such as Motrin, Naprosyn, and Nuprin
Other antihypertensives such as Vasotec
Steroid medications such as prednisone
Sulfinpyrazone (Anturane)

Special information if you are pregnant or breastfeeding
The effects of Corzide during pregnancy have not been adequately studied. If you are pregnant or plan to become pregnant, inform your doctor immediately. Corzide appears in breast milk and could affect a nursing infant. If this medication is essential to your health, your doctor may advise you to discontinue breastfeeding until your treatment with Corzide is finished.

Recommended dosage

ADULTS

Dosages of this drug are always tailored to the individual's needs.

The usual dose is 1 Corzide 40/5-milligram tablet per day or, if necessary, 1 Corzide 80/5-milligram tablet per day. If you have kidney problems, you'll probably need Corzide less frequently. If this medication fails to bring your blood pressure under control, your doctor may gradually add another high blood pressure drug to your regimen.

CHILDREN

The safety and effectiveness of Corzide have not been established in children.

Overdosage

Any medication taken in excess can have serious consequences. If you suspect an overdose, seek medical attention immediately.

■ *Symptoms of Corzide overdose may include:*
Abdominal irritation, central nervous system depression, coma, extremely slow heartbeat, heart failure, lethargy, low blood pressure, wheezing

COSOPT

Pronounced: COH-sopt
Generic name: Dorzolamide hydrochloride, Timolol maleate

Why is this drug prescribed?

Cosopt lowers high pressure in the eye, a problem typically caused by the condition known as open-angle glaucoma. Cosopt works by reducing production of the liquid that fills the eyeball.

Most important fact about this drug

Although it often causes no symptoms at first, high pressure in the eye will eventually damage the optic nerve and lead to blindness. It's therefore very important to keep using this medicine even if your eyes seem okay.

How should you take this medication?

Cosopt is administered with an eyedropper bottle. If you are using other eyedrops or ointments, allow at least 10 minutes between doses of each product.

The benzalkonium chloride used as a preservative in Cosopt can be absorbed by soft contact lenses; wait 15 minutes after using the drug before you insert the lenses.

To apply the drops, first wash your hands, then tilt your head back and pull your lower eyelid down slightly to form a pocket between the lid and the eye. Turn the bottle upside down and press the "Finger Push Area" lightly with your thumb or index finger until one drop falls into the eye. Be careful to avoid touching the eyelids with the dropper tip. This could contaminate the solution.

■ *If you miss a dose...*
Take the forgotten dose as soon as you remember. However, if it is almost time for your next dose, skip the one you missed and return to your regular schedule. Do not take 2 doses at once.

■ *Storage instructions...*
Store at room temperature. Protect from light.

What side effects may occur?
Side effects cannot be anticipated. If any develop or change in intensity, tell your doctor as soon as possible. Only your doctor can determine if it is safe to continue using Cosopt.

■ *Side effects of Cosopt may include:*
Altered taste, blurred vision, burning or stinging eyes, inflamed cornea, itching eyes, red eyelids

Why should this drug not be prescribed?
You should not take Cosopt if you've ever had asthma, suffer from chronic obstructive pulmonary disease (COPD), or have heart failure or certain types of rhythm problems. The drug cannot be used if you are suffering from shock. You'll also need to avoid it if it causes an allergic reaction.

Special warnings about this medication
Although Cosopt is an eyedrop, the medications it contains affect the entire body. In rare cases, the timolol in Cosopt has caused fatal asthma attacks and heart failure. The dorzolamide it contains has been known to cause fatal allergic reactions. If you develop hives, blisters, swollen eyelids, inflamed eyes, or any other sign of an allergic reaction, stop using Cosopt and check with your doctor immediately.

If you are planning to have surgery, make sure the doctor knows you are using Cosopt. Your dose may be gradually lowered in preparation for the operation. Also alert the doctor immediately if you sustain an eye injury or infection.

Use Cosopt with caution if you have diabetes or a thyroid condition. It can mask some of the signs of these disorders. Caution is also warranted if you have myasthenia gravis; in rare cases, Cosopt may increase muscle weakness.

If you have severe kidney disease, make sure the doctor knows about it. Cosopt is not recommended under these circumstances.

Possible food and drug interactions when using this medication
If Cosopt is taken with certain other drugs, the effects of either could be increased, decreased, or altered. It is especially important to check with your doctor before combining Cosopt with the following:

Certain water pills (diuretics) such as Daranide
Clonidine (Catapres)
Digitalis (Lanoxin)
Drugs classified as beta-blockers, such as the high blood pressure medications Inderal, Sectral, and Tenormin
Drugs classified as calcium channel blockers, such as the heart medications Cardizem, Norvasc, and Procardia
Epinephrine (EpiPen)
Quinidine (Quinaglute, Quinidex)
Reserpine
Salicylate medications such as Disalcid and aspirin

Special information if you are pregnant or breastfeeding
The effects of Cosopt during pregnancy have not been adequately studied. If you are pregnant or plan to become pregnant, inform your doctor immediately. Cosopt should be used during pregnancy only if its benefits outweigh the potential risk to the developing baby.

The timolol component of Cosopt does appear in breast milk, and can cause serious reactions in nursing infants. If you are nursing, use of this drug is not recommended.

Recommended dosage
The usual dose is 1 drop in the affected eye(s) 2 times a day.

Overdosage
Any medication taken in excess can have serious consequences. If you suspect an overdose, seek medical attention immediately.

■ *Symptoms of Cosopt overdose may include:*
Cardiac arrest, dizziness, headache, shortness of breath, slow heartbeat, severe asthma

COUMADIN
Pronounced: COO-muh-din
Generic name: Warfarin sodium

Why is this drug prescribed?
Coumadin is an anticoagulant (blood thinner). It is prescribed to:
Prevent and/or treat a blood clot that has formed within a blood vessel or in the lungs.

Prevent and/or treat blood clots associated with certain heart conditions or replacement of a heart valve.

Aid in the prevention of blood clots that may form in blood vessels anywhere in the body after a heart attack.

Reduce the risk of death, another heart attack, or stroke after a heart attack.

Most important fact about this drug

The most serious risks associated with Coumadin treatment are hemorrhage (severe bleeding resulting in the loss of a large amount of blood) in any tissue or organ and, less frequently, the destruction of skin tissue cells (necrosis) or gangrene. The risk of hemorrhage usually depends on the dosage and length of treatment with this drug.

Hemorrhage and necrosis have been reported to result in death or permanent disability. Severe necrosis can lead to the removal of damaged tissue or amputation of a limb. Necrosis appears to be associated with blood clots located in the area of tissue damage and usually occurs within a few days of starting Coumadin treatment.

How should you take this medication?

The objective of treatment with a blood thinner is to control the blood-clotting process without causing severe bleeding, so that a clot does not form and cut off the blood supply necessary for normal body function. Therefore, it is very important that you take this medication exactly as prescribed by your doctor and that your doctor monitor your condition on a regular basis. Be especially careful to stick to the exact dosage schedule your doctor prescribes.

Effective treatment with minimal complications depends on your co-operation and communication with your doctor.

Do not take or discontinue any other medication unless directed to do so by your doctor. Avoid alcohol, salicylates such as aspirin, larger than usual amounts of foods rich in vitamin K (including liver, vegetable oil, egg yolks, and green leafy vegetables), which can counteract the effect of Coumadin, or any other drastic change in diet.

Note that Coumadin often turns urine reddish orange.

You should carry an identification card that indicates you are taking Coumadin.

■ *If you miss a dose...*
Take the forgotten dose as soon as you remember, then go back to your regular schedule. If you do not remember until the next day, skip the dose. Never try to catch up by doubling the dose. Keep a record for your doctor of any doses you miss.

■ *Storage instructions...*
Coumadin can be stored at room temperature. Close the container tightly and protect from light.

What side effects may occur?

Side effects cannot be anticipated. If any develop or change in intensity, inform your doctor as soon as possible. Only your doctor can determine if it is safe for you to continue taking Coumadin.

■ *Side effects may include:*

Hemorrhage: Signs of severe bleeding resulting in the loss of large amounts of blood depend upon the location and extent of bleeding. Symptoms include: chest, abdomen, joint, muscle, or other pain; difficulty breathing or swallowing; dizziness; headache; low blood pressure; numbness and tingling; paralysis; shortness of breath; unexplained shock; unexplained swelling; weakness

Why should this drug not be prescribed?

This drug should not be used for any condition where the danger of hemorrhage may be greater than the potential benefits of treatment. Unless directed to do so by your doctor, do not take this medication if one of the following conditions or situations applies to you:

A tendency to hemorrhage

Alcoholism

Allergy to any of the drug's ingredients

An abnormal blood condition

Aneurysm (balloon-like swelling of a blood vessel) in the brain or heart

Bleeding tendencies associated with ulceration or bleeding of the stomach, intestines, respiratory tract, or the genital or urinary system

Eclampsia (a rare and serious pregnancy disorder producing life-threatening convulsions) or preeclampsia (a toxic condition— including headache, high blood pressure, and swelling of the legs and feet—that can lead to eclampsia)

Excessive bleeding of brain blood vessels

Inflammation, due to bacterial infection, of the membrane that lines the inside of the heart

Inflammation of the sac that surrounds the heart or an escape of fluid from the heart sac

Malignant hypertension (extremely elevated blood pressure that damages the inner linings of blood vessels, the heart, spleen, kidneys, and brain)

Pregnancy

Recent or contemplated surgery of the central nervous system (brain and spinal cord) or eye

Spinal puncture or any procedure that can cause uncontrollable bleeding

Threatened miscarriage

Special warnings about this medication

Treatment with blood thinners may increase the risk that fatty plaque will break away from the wall of an artery and lodge at another point, causing the blockage of a blood vessel. If you notice any of the following symptoms, contact your doctor immediately:

Abdominal pain; abrupt and intense pain in the leg, foot, or toes; blood in the urine; bluish mottling of the skin of the legs and hands; foot ulcers; gangrene; high blood pressure; muscle pain; purple toes syndrome (see below); rash; or thigh or back pain.

If you have any of the following conditions, tell your doctor. He or she will have to weigh the risks against the benefits before giving you Coumadin.

A history of recurrent blood clot disorders in you or your family
An implanted catheter
An infectious disease or intestinal disorder
Dental procedures
Inflammation of a blood vessel
Moderate to severe high blood pressure
Moderate to severe kidney or liver dysfunction
Polycythemia vera (blood disorder)
Severe diabetes
Surgery or injury that leaves large raw surfaces
Trauma or injury that may result in internal bleeding

Purple toes syndrome can occur when taking Coumadin, usually 3 to 10 weeks after the start of anticoagulation therapy. Symptoms include a dark purplish or mottled color of the toes that turns white when pressure is applied and fades when you elevate your legs, pain and tenderness of the toes, and change in intensity of the color over a period of time. If any of these symptoms develops, notify your doctor immediately.

If you are taking Coumadin, your doctor should periodically check the time it takes for your blood to start the clotting process (prothrombin time). Numerous factors such as travel and changes in diet, environment, physical state, and medication may alter your response to treatment with an anticoagulant. Clotting time should also be monitored after your release from the hospital and whenever other medications are started, discontinued, or taken sporadically.

While taking Coumadin, avoid activities and sports that could cause an injury. Remain cautious after you stop taking Coumadin. It will continue to work for 2 to 5 days.

If you have congestive heart failure, you may become more sensitive to Coumadin and may need to have your dosage reduced. Your doctor will have you tested regularly.

Notify your doctor if any illness, such as diarrhea, infection, or fever develops; if any unusual symptoms, such as pain, swelling, or discomfort, appear; or if you see prolonged bleeding from cuts, increased menstrual flow, vaginal bleeding, nosebleeds, bleeding of gums from brushing, unusual bleeding or bruising, red or dark brown urine, red or tarry black stool, headache, dizziness, or weakness.

Possible food and drug interactions when taking this medication

Coumadin can interact with a very wide variety of drugs, both prescription and over the counter. Check with your doctor before taking ANY other medication or vitamin product.

Be extremely cautious, too, about taking any herbal remedies and supplements. A wide assortment of herbal products—including St. John's Wort, coenzyme Q10, bromelains, dan-shen, dong quai, garlic, and ginkgo biloba—are known to interact with Coumadin or otherwise affect coagulation.

Special information if you are pregnant or breastfeeding

Coumadin should not be taken by women who are or may become pregnant since the drug may cause fatal hemorrhage in the developing baby. There have also been reports of birth malformations, low birth weight, and retarded growth in children born to mothers treated with Coumadin during pregnancy. Spontaneous abortions and stillbirths are also known to occur. If you become pregnant while taking this drug, inform your doctor immediately.

Coumadin has not been found in the breast milk of mothers taking the drug. Nevertheless, the doctor may test the baby for coagulation abnormalities before recommending that you breastfeed while on Coumadin therapy.

Recommended dosage

ADULTS

The administration and dosage of Coumadin must be individualized by your doctor according to your sensitivity to the drug.

A common starting dosage of Coumadin tablets for adults is 2 to 5 milligrams per day. Individualized daily dosage adjustments are based on the results of tests that determine the amount of time it takes for the blood clotting process to begin.

A maintenance dose of 2 to 10 milligrams per day is satisfactory for most people. The duration of treatment will be determined by your physician.

CHILDREN

Although Coumadin has been widely used in children below the age of 18, its safety and effectiveness for this purpose have not been formally established.

OLDER ADULTS

Low starting and maintenance doses are recommended for older people, as the drug tends to have a greater effect.

Overdosage

Signs and symptoms of Coumadin overdose reflect abnormal bleeding.

■ *Symptoms of abnormal bleeding include:*
Black stools, blood in stools or urine, excessive menstrual bleeding, excessive bruising, persistent bleeding from superficial injuries, reddish or purplish spots on skin

If you suspect an overdose, seek emergency medical treatment immediately.

Covera-HS *See Calan, page 229.*

COZAAR

Pronounced: CO-zahr
Generic name: Losartan potassium

Why is this drug prescribed?

Cozaar is used in the treatment of high blood pressure. It is effective when used alone or with other high blood pressure medications, such as diuretics that help the body get rid of water.

Cozaar is also used to slow the progress of kidney disease caused by type 2 diabetes (the type of diabetes that doesn't require insulin shots). It is the first of a new class of blood pressure medications called angiotensin II receptor antagonists. Cozaar works, in part, by preventing the hormone angiotensin II from constricting the blood vessels, which tends to raise blood pressure.

Most important fact about this drug

You must take Cozaar regularly for it to be effective. Since blood pressure declines gradually, it may be several weeks before you get the full benefit of Cozaar, and you must continue taking it even if you are feeling well. Cozaar does not cure high blood pressure; it merely keeps it under control.

How should you take this medication?

Cozaar can be taken with or without food.

Take it at the same time each day. For example, if you take the medication every morning before or after breakfast, you will establish a regular routine and be less likely to forget your dose.

■ *If you miss a dose...*
Take it as soon as possible. If it is almost time for your next dose, skip the missed dose and go back to your regular schedule.
■ *Storage instructions...*
Store at room temperature. Keep in a tightly closed container, away from light.

What side effects may occur?
Side effects cannot be anticipated. If any develop or change in intensity, tell your doctor as soon as possible. Only your doctor can determine if it is safe for you to continue taking Cozaar.

■ *Side effects may include:*
Cough, dizziness, upper respiratory infection

Other side effects, such as weakness and chest pain, have been reported by people taking Cozaar for diabetic kidney disease. Severe allergic reactions, including swelling of the face and throat, are also a possibility.

Why should this drug not be prescribed?
Do not take Cozaar when you are pregnant. Avoid it if you have ever had an allergic reaction to it.

Special warnings about this medication
Cozaar can cause low blood pressure, especially if you are also taking a diuretic. You may feel light-headed or faint, especially during the first few days of therapy. If these symptoms occur, contact your doctor. Your dosage may need to be adjusted or discontinued. Be sure you know how you react to Cozaar before you drive or operate machinery.

Excessive sweating, dehydration, severe diarrhea, or vomiting could make you lose too much water, causing a severe drop in blood pressure. Call your doctor if you experience any of these symptoms.

Be sure to tell your doctor about any medical conditions you have, especially liver or kidney disease and congestive heart failure. In very rare cases, Cozaar has triggered fatal kidney problems in people with heart failure.

Cozaar tends to increase the level of potassium in the blood. Check with your doctor before taking potassium supplements or using a salt substitute.

Possible food and drug interactions when taking this medication
If Cozaar is taken with certain other drugs, the effects of either could be increased, decreased, or altered. It is especially important to check with your doctor before taking Cozaar with the following:

Diuretics that leave potassium in the body, such as Aldactone, triamterene, and amiloride

Indomethacin (Indocin)
Ketoconazole (Nizoral)
Troleandomycin (Tao)

Special information if you are pregnant or breastfeeding

Drugs such as Cozaar can cause injury or even death to the unborn child when used in the second or third trimester of pregnancy. Stop taking Cozaar as soon as you know you are pregnant. If you are pregnant or plan to become pregnant, tell your doctor before taking Cozaar. Cozaar may appear in breast milk and could affect the nursing infant. If this medication is essential to your health, your doctor may advise you to stop breastfeeding while you are taking Cozaar.

Recommended dosage

ADULTS

High blood pressure

The usual starting dose is 50 milligrams once daily. However, Cozaar can also be taken twice daily, with total daily doses ranging from 25 milligrams to 100 milligrams. If your blood pressure does not respond within 3 to 6 weeks, your doctor may increase your dose or add a low-dose diuretic to your regimen.

For people taking diuretics and people with liver problems, the usual starting dose is 25 milligrams daily. Your doctor may adjust your dosage according to your response.

Kidney disease caused by diabetes

The usual starting dose is 50 milligrams once daily. The doctor may increase the dose to 100 milligrams once a day if blood pressure remains too high.

CHILDREN

The safety and effectiveness of Cozaar in children have not been studied.

Overdosage

Any medication taken in excess can have serious consequences. If you suspect an overdose, seek medical attention immediately. Information concerning Cozaar overdosage is limited. However, hypotension (low blood pressure) and abnormally rapid or slow heartbeat may be signs of an overdose.

Creon *See Pancrease, page 1030.*

CRESTOR

Pronounced: CRES-tor
Generic name: Rosuvastatin calcium

Why is this drug prescribed?

Crestor is used to lower cholesterol levels when diet and exercise alone have failed to work. The drug can help lower the total cholesterol count as well as harmful levels of low-density lipoprotein (LDL) cholesterol. It can also lower triglycerides, a type of fat that is carried through the bloodstream and can end up being stored as body fat. Sometimes Crestor may be combined with another type of cholesterol-lowering drug such as Colestid, Questran, or WelChol.

In addition, Crestor can help increase the amount of "good" cholesterol known as high-density lipoprotein (HDL).

It's especially important to keep LDL cholesterol under control, since high levels are associated with heart disease. Federal guidelines recommend considering drug therapy when LDL levels reach 130 in people at high risk for heart disease. For people with a lower risk, the cutoff is 160. For those with little or no risk, it's 190.

Most important fact about this drug

Crestor is prescribed only if diet, exercise, and weight loss fail to lower your cholesterol levels. It's important to remember that Crestor is meant to supplement—not replace—these lifestyle changes. To get the full benefit of this medication, you need to stick to the diet and exercise program prescribed by your doctor. All of these efforts to keep your cholesterol levels normal are important because they may lower your risk of heart disease.

How should you take this medication?

Take Crestor once a day with or without food. You can take the drug at any time, but it's best to make a habit of taking it at the same time every day to prevent missed doses. Swallow each tablet whole with a glass of water.

If you need to take an antacid that contains aluminum and magnesium hydroxide, such as Maalox or Mylanta, be sure to take it at least 2 hours after you take Crestor.

■ *If you miss a dose…*
Take the forgotten dose as soon as you remember. However, if it is almost time for your next dose, skip the one you missed and go back to your regular schedule. Do not take 2 doses at the same time.

■ *Storage instructions…*
Store at room temperature and protect from moisture.

What side effects may occur?

Side effects cannot be anticipated. If any develop or change in intensity, tell your doctor as soon as possible. Only your doctor can determine if it is safe to continue using Crestor.

It's especially important to tell your doctor if you have unusual muscle pain, tenderness, or weakness that's accompanied by fever or a general feeling of illness and fatigue (see *Special warnings about this medication*).

■ *Side effects may include:*

Abdominal pain, constipation, diarrhea, headache, indigestion, nausea, sore throat

Why should this drug not be prescribed?

Do not take Crestor if you have liver disease, or if you've ever had an allergic reaction to the drug.

Also, never take Crestor during pregnancy or while breastfeeding.

Special warnings about this medication

Use Crestor with caution if you have a history of liver problems, if you have any symptoms associated with liver disease, or if you drink large amounts of alcohol. In rare cases, cholesterol-lowering drugs like Crestor have caused liver damage. To guard against such problems, your doctor will perform blood tests before you start taking the drug and again after 12 weeks. As therapy continues, you may have your blood tested periodically or whenever the doctor increases your dose.

There is a small chance that Crestor may cause damage to muscle tissue. Be especially cautious if you have any predisposing risk factors for muscle damage, including kidney problems or an underactive thyroid, or if you're past middle age. Promptly report to your doctor any unexplained muscle pain, tenderness, or weakness, especially if you also have a fever or you just generally do not feel well.

Use Crestor with caution if you have kidney problems. Studies have shown that the drug may affect kidney function, especially at higher doses. If your doctor finds evidence of this after routine testing, you may need to have your dosage lowered.

Be sure to tell the doctor if your ancestry is Japanese or Chinese, since these groups have been known to metabolize Crestor differently than others.

Crestor may be associated with abnormal lab test results, including tests for liver and thyroid function and blood sugar levels. If you're having any lab work done, be sure to let the doctor know you're taking Crestor.

The safety and effectiveness of Crestor have not been established in children.

Possible food and drug interactions when taking this medication
If you take Crestor with certain other drugs, the effects of either could be increased, decreased, or altered. It is especially important to check with your doctor before combining Crestor with any of the following:

Antacids such as Maalox or Mylanta
Cholesterol-lowering drugs such as clofibrate (Atromid-S) and fenofibrate (Tricor)
Cimetidine (Tagamet)
Cyclosporine (Sandimmune, Neoral)
Gemfibrozil (Lopid)
Ketoconazole (Nizoral)
Niacin (Niaspan, Niacor, Slo-Niacin)
Oral contraceptives
Spironolactone (Aldactone)
Warfarin (Coumadin)

Special information if you are pregnant or breastfeeding
Crestor should never be used during pregnancy because a developing baby needs plenty of cholesterol. Your doctor will prescribe Crestor only if you are highly unlikely to become pregnant while taking this drug. If you do become pregnant, tell your doctor immediately.

Likewise, Crestor should never be used while you're breastfeeding.

Recommended dosage

ADULTS

The usual starting dose is 10 milligrams once a day. However, your doctor may start you at 5 milligrams per day if your LDL cholesterol level doesn't require a high dose or if you have a predisposing risk factor for muscle damage (see *Special warnings about this medication*). If your LDL cholesterol level is above 190, the doctor may start you at 20 milligrams once a day. If this dose fails to lower your cholesterol, the doctor may increase your dose to 40 milligrams per day.

If you have a rare genetic disorder known as homozygous familial hypercholesterolemia, which causes unusually high cholesterol levels, the doctor will probably start you at 20 milligrams once a day. If needed, the doctor may raise the dose to a maximum of 40 milligrams a day.

If you have severe kidney problems, the recommended starting dose is 5 milligrams once a day, up to a maximum of 10 milligrams daily.

If you're taking cyclosporine, the doctor will limit your dose to 5 milligrams once a day. If you're taking the cholesterol-lowering drug gemfibrozil (Lopid), your dose must be limited to 10 milligrams once a day.

Your doctor will want to test your cholesterol levels within 2 to 4 weeks after you start taking Crestor and also after any dose adjustment.

Overdosage

Although no specific information is available, any medication taken in excess can have serious consequences. If you suspect an overdose of Crestor, seek medical attention immediately.

CRIXIVAN

Pronounced: CRIX-i-van
Generic name: Indinavir sulfate

Why is this drug prescribed?

Crixivan is used in the treatment of human immunodeficiency virus (HIV) infection. HIV causes the immune system to break down so that it can no longer fight off other infections. This leads to the fatal disease known as acquired immune deficiency syndrome (AIDS).

HIV thrives by taking over the immune system's vital CD4 cells (white blood cells) and using their inner workings to make additional copies of itself. Crixivan belongs to a class of HIV drugs called protease inhibitors, which work by interfering with an important step in the virus's reproductive cycle. Although Crixivan cannot eliminate HIV already present in the body, it can reduce the amount of virus available to infect other cells.

Crixivan can be taken alone or in combination with other HIV drugs such as Retrovir. Because Crixivan and Retrovir attack the virus in different ways, the combination is likely to be more effective than either drug alone.

Most important fact about this drug

It is important that you drink at least six 8-ounce glasses of liquid (preferably water) daily while taking Crixivan. If you do not get enough liquid, you may develop kidney stones and have to temporarily stop taking Crixivan or even discontinue it altogether.

How should you take this medication?

Take this medication exactly as prescribed by your doctor. Do not share this medication with anyone and do not take more than your recommended dosage.

To ensure maximum absorption, do not take Crixivan with food. Instead, take it with water 1 hour before or 2 hours after a meal. (Crixivan may also be taken with liquids such as skim milk, juice, coffee, or tea, or even with a light meal such as dry toast with jelly, juice, and coffee with skim milk and sugar, or corn flakes with skim milk and sugar.)

■ *If you miss a dose...*
Skip it and take the next dose at the regularly scheduled time. Do not double the dose.

■ *Storage instructions…*
Crixivan capsules are sensitive to moisture. Store Crixivan at room temperature in the original container and leave the drying agent in the bottle to keep the medication dry. Keep the container tightly closed.

What side effects may occur?
Side effects cannot be anticipated. If any develop or change in intensity, inform your doctor as soon as possible. Only your doctor can determine if it is safe for you to continue taking Crixivan.

■ *Side effects may include:*
Abdominal pain, acid regurgitation, back pain, bladder stones, changes in taste, diarrhea, dizziness, drowsiness, dry skin, fatigue, headache, itching, jaundice (yellowish skin or eyes, especially in children), kidney stones, liver problems, loss of appetite, nausea, pain in the side, rash, redistribution of body fat, sore throat or upper respiratory tract infection, vomiting, weakness

Why should this drug not be prescribed?
Certain drugs, when combined with Crixivan, may cause serious, even life-threatening reactions. The following drugs should not be taken if you are taking Crixivan:

Amiodarone (Pacerone)
Cisapride
Ergot-based drugs such as Cafergot, Methergine, and Migranal
Midazolam (Versed)
Pimozide (Orap)
Triazolam (Halcion)

If you suffer a severe allergic reaction to Crixivan or any of its ingredients, you should not take this medication.

Special warnings about this medication
Although Crixivan reduces the amount of HIV in the blood and increases the white blood cell count, its long-term effect on survival is still unknown. The virus remains in the body, and you will continue to face the possibility of complications, including opportunistic infections (rare infections that develop when the immune system falters), such as certain types of pneumonia, tuberculosis, and fungal infection. Therefore, it is important that you remain under the care of a doctor and keep all your follow-up appointments.

Crixivan is not a cure for HIV infection, and it does not reduce the risk of transmission of HIV to others through sexual contact or blood contamination. Therefore, you should continue to avoid practices that could spread HIV.

· Protease inhibitors such as Crixivan have been known to trigger diabetes (high blood sugar levels) or worsen existing diabetes. If you have diabetes, the dosages of your diabetes medications may have to be adjusted.

People taking HIV medications may also experience a redistribution of body fat, with wasting of the face, arms, and legs, and accumulation of fat around the middle, the upper back, and the breasts.

Cases of liver failure and death have occurred in patients treated with Crixivan and other medications. If you have a liver problem, particularly cirrhosis of the liver, make sure the doctor is aware of it. Kidney problems, including kidney and urinary stones, are also a possibility, so alert the doctor if you have any type of kidney disease.

Some patients have developed severe anemia (loss of red blood cells) while taking Crixivan. If this problem surfaces, you will have to stop taking the drug.

If you have hemophilia, you should also be aware that spontaneous bleeding has occurred in hemophilia victims taking protease inhibitors such as Crixivan.

Possible food and drug interactions when taking this medication

Avoid the following medications while taking Crixivan. The combination may cause serious or life-threatening effects.

Amiodarone (Pacerone)
Atazanavir (Reyataz)
Cisapride
Ergot-based drugs such as Cafergot, Methergine, and Migranal
Lovastatin (Mevacor)
Midazolam (Versed)
Pimozide (Orap)
Rifampin (Rifadin, Rifamate)
Simvastatin (Zocor)
St. John's wort
Triazolam (Halcion)

It's also best to avoid combining Crixivan with St. John's wort, which reduces Crixivan's effect.

Crixivan may interact with certain other drugs, and the effects of either could be increased, decreased, or altered. It is especially important to check with your doctor before combining Crixivan with the following:

Bepridil (Vascor)
Carbamazepine (Tegretol)
Cholesterol-lowering drugs such as Lescol, Lipitor, and Pravachol
Cimetidine (Tagamet)
Clarithromycin (Biaxin)
Cyclosporine (Neoral, Sandimmune)

Delavirdine (Rescriptor)
Didanosine (Videx)
Efavirenz (Sustiva)
Fluconazole (Diflucan)
Heart medications known as calcium channel blockers, including
   Cardene, Plendil, and Procardia
Isoniazid (Nydrazid)
Itraconazole (Sporanox)
Ketoconazole (Nizoral)
Lamivudine (Epivir)
Lidocaine (Lidoderm)
Methadone
Nelfinavir (Viracept)
Nevirapine (Viramune)
Ortho-Novum (ethinyl estradiol and norethindrone)
Phenobarbital
Phenytoin (Dilantin)
Quinidine (Quinidex)
Rifabutin (Mycobutin)
Rifampin (Rifadin)
Ritonavir (Norvir)
Saquinavir (Fortovase)
Sirolimus (Rapamune)
Stavudine (Zerit)
Sulfamethoxazole (Bactrim, Septra)
Tacrolimus (Prograf)
Theophylline (Theo-Dur)
Trimethoprim (Bactrim, Trimpex, Septra)
Zidovudine (Retrovir)

Check with your doctor before using any drug for erectile dysfunction (male impotence), such as Cialis, Levitra, or Viagra while on Crixivan. Combining an erectile dysfunction drug with Crixivan increases the risk of side effects, such as low blood pressure, vision problems, and a dangerously prolonged erection. If an erection lasts more than 4 hours, seek medical help immediately to avoid permanent damage to the penis.

Avoid drinking grapefruit juice while taking Crixivan. This kind of juice can reduce the drug's effectiveness.

Be sure to tell your doctor and pharmacist about all medications you are taking, both prescription and over the counter. Alert them, too, when you *stop* taking a medication.

Special information if you are pregnant or breastfeeding

The effects of Crixivan during pregnancy have not been adequately studied. If you are pregnant or plan to become pregnant, tell your doctor immediately. Do not breastfeed your baby. HIV appears in breast milk and can infect a nursing infant.

Recommended dosage

ADULTS

The recommended dose of Crixivan is 800 milligrams (usually two 400-milligram capsules) every 8 hours. Your doctor may lower the dose to 600 milligrams every 8 hours if you have mild to moderate liver problems due to cirrhosis. The dose will also need adjustment if you are taking Rescriptor, Mycobutin, Nizoral, Sporanox, or Videx.

CHILDREN

Crixivan is more likely to cause kidney stones in children than in adults. If the doctor finds it necessary to prescribe Crixivan anyway, dosage is calculated according to the weight of the child.

Overdosage

Any medication taken in excess can have serious consequences. If you suspect an overdose, seek emergency medical treatment immediately.

■ *Symptoms of Crixivan overdose may include:*
  Back pain, blood in urine, diarrhea, kidney stones, nausea, vomiting

CROLOM

Pronounced: CROW-lum
Generic name: Cromolyn sodium

Why is this drug prescribed?

Crolom is an eyedrop that relieves the itching, tearing, discharge, and redness caused by seasonal and chronic allergies. The drug works by preventing certain cells in the body from releasing histamine and other substances that can cause an allergic reaction. It may be prescribed alone or with a steroid medication.

Most important fact about this drug

In order for Crolom to work properly, you must continue to use it every day at regular intervals even if your symptoms have disappeared. It can take up to 6 weeks for your condition to clear up.

How should you use this medication?

Use Crolom exactly as directed by your doctor. Follow the instruction sheet that comes with the medication. Do not use more or less than required and apply it only when scheduled.

To administer Crolom, follow these steps:
1. Wash your hands thoroughly.
2. Tilt your head back.
3. Gently pull your lower eyelid down to form a pocket between your eye and the lid.
4. Drop the medicine into this pocket. Let go of the eyelid. Do not place Crolom directly over the pupil of the eye.
5. Blink a few times to make sure the eye is covered with medication.
6. Close the eye and with a tissue wipe away any excess medication.
7. Do not touch the applicator tip to your eye or any other surface. This could lead to infection.
8. Do not rinse the dropper.

■ *If you miss a dose...*
Use it as soon as possible. Then go back to your regular schedule.

■ *Storage instructions...*
Keep the container tightly closed and away from light. Store at room temperature.

What side effects may occur?
You may experience temporary burning or stinging in the eye after you apply Crolom.

■ *Side effects may include:*
Allergic reaction, dryness around the eye, eye irritation, inflammation of the eyelids, itchy eyes, puffy eyes, styes, watery eyes

Why should this drug not be prescribed?
If you have ever had an allergic reaction to cromolyn sodium, avoid this medication.

Special warnings about this medication
Crolom has been known to cause immediate, but rare, allergic reactions marked by breathlessness, swelling, or a rash. If you develop any of these symptoms, stop using this medication and contact your doctor immediately.

Do not wear contact lenses while suffering from allergy-induced eye irritation and while using Crolom.

If your symptoms do not begin to improve, alert your doctor.

Possible food and drug interactions when using this medication
No interactions have been reported.

Special information if you are pregnant or breastfeeding
There are no studies on use of Crolom with pregnant women. If you are pregnant or plan to become pregnant, tell your doctor. Crolom should be used during pregnancy only if clearly needed. It is not known whether

Crolom appears in human breast milk. If you are nursing and need to use Crolom, use it with caution.

Recommended dosage

ADULTS AND CHILDREN

Put 1 or 2 drops into each eye 4 to 6 times a day at evenly spaced intervals.

It is not known whether Crolom is safe and effective for children under 4 years.

Overdosage

Although there is no information on Crolom overdose, any medication taken in excess can have serious consequences. If you suspect an overdose, seek medical attention immediately.

Cromolyn, inhaled See *Intal, page 694*.

Cromolyn, ocular See *Crolom, page 365*.

CUTIVATE
Pronounced: KYOOT-i-vait
Generic name: Fluticasone propionate

Why is this drug prescribed?
Cutivate cream and ointment are prescribed for relief of inflamed, itchy rashes and other inflammatory skin conditions.

Most important fact about this drug
When you use Cutivate, you inevitably absorb some of the medication through your skin and into the bloodstream. Too much absorption can lead to unwanted side effects elsewhere in the body. To keep this problem to a minimum, avoid using large amounts of Cutivate over large areas, and do not cover it with airtight dressings such as plastic wrap or adhesive bandages unless specifically told to do so by your doctor.

How should you use this medication?
Cutivate is for use only on the skin. Be careful to keep it out of your eyes.

■ *If you miss a dose...*
Apply it as soon as you remember. If it is almost time for the next dose, skip the one you missed and go back to your regular schedule.

■ *Storage instructions...*
Store at room temperature.

What side effects may occur?
Side effects cannot be anticipated. If any develop or change in intensity, inform your doctor as soon as possible. Only your doctor can determine if it is safe for you to continue taking Cutivate.

■ *Side effects of Cutivate may include:*
Burning, dryness, infected or worsening eczema, itchy spots, rash, skin irritation, stinging

Side effects occur more frequently with the use of airtight bandages. In children, the more likely side effects may include a burning sensation, hives, inflammation, rash, and red blotches on the face and body.

Why should this drug not be prescribed?
If you are sensitive to or have ever had an allergic reaction to fluticasone propionate or other steroid medications, you should not use Cutivate. Make sure your doctor is aware of any drug reactions you have experienced.

Special warnings about this medication
Do not use this drug for any disorder other than the one for which it was prescribed.

Do not use Cutivate cream on the face, underarms, or groin areas unless your doctor tells you to do so. Do not apply Cutivate if you have an infection in the affected skin area. Tell your doctor if you have had any other problems in that area.

The treated skin area should not be bandaged, covered, or wrapped unless you have been directed to do so by your doctor.

Do not apply Cutivate cream to the diaper area because covering a treated area with waterproof diapers or plastic pants can increase unwanted absorption of Cutivate.

Do not use Cutivate to treat rosacea or skin inflammation near the mouth. Also avoid using Cutivate on thin, weakened skin that has lost its elasticity.

If an irritation or allergic reaction develops while using Cutivate, notify your doctor.

The drug can interfere with the thyroid, pituitary, and adrenal glands, causing a problem called Cushing's syndrome (weight gain, reddening of the face and neck, growth of excess facial hair, high blood pressure, and mental disturbances), hyperglycemia (excess glucose in the blood), and glucosuria (urinary excretion of glucose). Your doctor should monitor your condition and periodically check your glandular function if you are applying a large dose of any potent steroid preparation to a large area of your skin.

Steroid medications such as Cutivate are more likely to cause side effects in children. Problems can include Cushing's syndrome and other adrenal problems, stunted growth, and high pressure inside the head.

This excess pressure can lead to bulges in the skull, headaches, and eventually loss of vision.

Possible food and drug interactions when taking this medication
No interactions with food or other drugs have been reported.

Special information if you are pregnant or breastfeeding
The effects of Cutivate during pregnancy have not been adequately studied. If you are pregnant or plan to become pregnant, inform your doctor immediately. It is not known whether this medication appears in breast milk. If this drug is essential to your health, your doctor may advise you to discontinue breastfeeding until your treatment is finished.

Recommended dosage

ADULTS

Apply a thin film of Cutivate cream or ointment to the affected skin areas 1 or 2 times a day. Rub in gently. Contact your doctor if there is no improvement within 2 weeks.

Cutivate should not be used with tight, occlusive dressings or bandages.

CHILDREN

Cutivate cream may be used with caution to treat children over 3 months of age. Apply a thin film of Cutivate cream to the affected skin areas 1 or 2 times a day. Rub in gently. The safety of Cutivate cream to treat children for longer than 4 weeks has not been established.

Cutivate should not be used with tight, occlusive dressings or bandages.

The safety and effectiveness of Cutivate cream have not been established for treatments lasting more than 4 weeks in children or for infants below age 3 months.

Cutivate ointment is not recommended for use in children.

Overdosage
With extensive or long-term use of Cutivate, hormone absorbed into the bloodstream may cause a group of symptoms called Cushing's syndrome.

■ *Symptoms of Cushing's syndrome may include:*
Acne, depression, excessive hair growth, high blood pressure, humped upper back, insomnia, moon-faced appearance, obese trunk, paranoia, stretch marks, stunted growth (in children), susceptibility to bruising, fractures, and infections, wasted limbs

Cushing's syndrome may also trigger diabetes mellitus.

If it is left uncorrected, Cushing's syndrome may become serious. If you suspect your long-term use of Cutivate has led to this problem, seek medical attention immediately.

Cyclessa *See Oral Contraceptives, page 1000.*

Cyclobenzaprine *See Flexeril, page 577.*

CYCLOCORT
Pronounced: SIKE-low-court
Generic name: Amcinonide

Why is this drug prescribed?
Cyclocort is prescribed for the relief of the inflammatory and itchy symptoms of skin disorders that are responsive to corticosteroid treatment.

Most important fact about this drug
When you use Cyclocort, you inevitably absorb some of the medication through your skin and into the bloodstream. Too much absorption can lead to unwanted side effects elsewhere in the body. To keep this problem to a minimum, avoid using large amounts of Cyclocort over large areas, and do not cover it with airtight dressings such as plastic wrap or adhesive bandages unless specifically told to by your doctor.

How should you use this medication?
Use this medication exactly as prescribed by your doctor. It is for use only on the skin. Be careful to keep it out of your eyes.

Apply Cyclocort sparingly. Rub it in gently.

■ *If you miss a dose...*
Apply the forgotten dose as soon as you remember. Use the remaining doses for that day at evenly spaced intervals. Never try to catch up by doubling the amount applied.
■ *Storage instructions...*
Cyclocort can be stored at room temperature. Protect from freezing.

What side effects may occur?
Side effects cannot be anticipated. If any develop or change in intensity, inform your doctor as soon as possible. Only your doctor can determine if it is safe for you to continue taking Cyclocort.

■ *Side effects may include:*
Burning, itching, soreness, stinging

Why should this drug not be prescribed?

If you are sensitive to or have ever had an allergic reaction to amcinonide or other steroid medications, you should not use Cyclocort. Make sure your doctor is aware of any drug reactions you have experienced.

Special warnings about this medication

Do not use this drug for any disorder other than the one for which it was prescribed.

The use of tight-fitting diapers or plastic pants is not recommended for a child being treated in the diaper area. These garments may act as airtight dressings or bandages.

The treated skin area should not be bandaged, covered, or wrapped unless you have been directed to do so by your doctor.

If an irritation or allergic reaction develops while you are using Cyclocort, notify your doctor.

Possible food and drug interactions when taking this medication

No interactions with food or other drugs have been reported.

Special information if you are pregnant or breastfeeding

The effects of Cyclocort during pregnancy have not been adequately studied. If you are pregnant or plan to become pregnant, inform your doctor immediately. It is not known whether this medication appears in breast milk. If this drug is essential to your health, your doctor may advise you to discontinue breastfeeding until your treatment is finished.

Recommended dosage

ADULTS

Apply a thin film of Cyclocort to the affected area 2 or 3 times a day, depending on the severity of the condition.

Cyclocort lotion may be applied to the affected areas, particularly hairy areas, 2 times per day. The lotion should be rubbed in completely, and the area should not be washed and should be protected from clothing until the lotion has dried.

Your doctor may recommend airtight bandages or dressings if you are being treated for psoriasis (a skin disorder characterized by patches of red, dry, scale-covered skin) or other stubborn skin conditions. If an infection develops, stop bandaging the area.

CHILDREN

Topical use of Cyclocort on children should be limited to the smallest amount that is effective. Long-term treatment may interfere with children's growth and development.

Overdosage

A severe overdosage is unlikely with the use of Cyclocort; however, long-term or prolonged use can produce side effects throughout the body (see *Most important fact about this drug*).

Cyclophosphamide *See Cytoxan, page 380.*

Cyclosporine *See Sandimmune, page 1287.*

Cyclosporine eyedrops *See Restasis, page 1238.*

CYMBALTA

Pronounced: sim-BALL-ta
Generic name: Duloxetine hydrochloride

Why is this drug prescribed?

Cymbalta is used to treat major depression—a disorder marked by continuing, serious, and overwhelming feelings of depression that interfere with daily functioning. Symptoms may include major changes in appetite or sleep habits; lack of interest in social or work life; feelings of sadness, guilt, or worthlessness; fatigue; difficulty concentrating or making decisions; and suicidal thoughts or attempted suicide.

Cymbalta is also used to treat diabetic peripheral neuropathy, a painful nerve disorder associated with diabetes that affects the hands, legs, and feet.

Cymbalta is thought to work by correcting an imbalance of two brain chemicals known to influence mood—serotonin and norepinephrine. It belongs to a class of antidepressants called selective serotonin and norepinephrine reuptake inhibitors (SNRIs).

Most important fact about this drug

Serious, sometimes fatal reactions can occur if Cymbalta is taken with antidepressants known as MAO inhibitors, including Marplan, Nardil, and Parnate. Never combine Cymbalta with one of these drugs, and wait at least 14 days after stopping an MAO inhibitor before starting treatment with Cymbalta. Likewise, after stopping therapy with Cymbalta, allow at least 5 days before starting treatment with an MAO inhibitor.

How should you take this medication?

Take Cymbalta at about the same time each day. Swallow the capsule whole; do not chew it or break it open. Cymbalta may be taken with or without food.

It may take several weeks before the drug begins to work. Continue taking Cymbalta even if you begin to feel better. Do not stop taking this drug without your doctor's approval. Abruptly stopping treatment may cause severe side effects.

■ *If you miss a dose...*
Take the forgotten dose as soon as you remember. However, if it is almost time for your next dose, skip the one you missed and return to your regular schedule. Do not take 2 doses at once.

■ *Storage instructions...*
Store at room temperature.

What side effects may occur?

Side effects cannot be anticipated. If any develop or change in intensity, tell your doctor as soon as possible. Only your doctor can determine if it is safe to continue using Cymbalta.

■ *Side effects may include:*
Appetite changes, constipation, diarrhea, dizziness, dry mouth, fatigue, headache, insomnia, nausea, sexual difficulties, sleepiness, sweating, tremor, urinary difficulties, vomiting, weakness

Why should this drug not be prescribed?

You will not be able to use Cymbalta if it causes an allergic reaction. In addition, you should not take Cymbalta if you have uncontrolled narrow-angle glaucoma, a disease that causes increased pressure in the eyes.

Never combine Cymbalta with an MAO inhibitor such as Marplan, Nardil, or Parnate (see *Most important fact about this drug*).

Do not take the drug thioridazine (Mellaril) with Cymbalta, as it could cause fatal heartbeat irregularities.

Special warnings about this medication

In clinical studies, antidepressants increased the risk of suicidal thinking and behavior in children and adolescents with depression and other psychiatric disorders. Anyone considering the use of Cymbalta or any other antidepressant in a child or adolescent must balance this risk with the clinical need. Cymbalta has not been studied in children or adolescents and is not approved for treating anyone less than 18 years old.

Additionally, the progression of major depression is associated with a worsening of symptoms and/or the emergence of suicidal thinking or behavior in both adults and children, whether or not they're taking antidepressants. Individuals being treated with Cymbalta and their caregivers should watch for any change in symptoms or any new symptoms that come on suddenly or severely—especially agitation, anxiety, hostility, panic, restlessness, extreme hyperactivity, and suicidal thinking or behavior—and report them to the doctor immediately. Be especially observant at the beginning of treatment or whenever there is a change in dose.

Some medical conditions require careful monitoring during treatment with Cymbalta. Be sure to tell the doctor if you have diabetes, glaucoma, high blood pressure, or a seizure disorder. Cymbalta can cause episodes of mania (abnormally high feelings of excitement and energy), so be sure the doctor is aware if you have this condition.

Using Cymbalta is not recommended if you have liver problems or severe kidney disease.

Like other antidepressants, Cymbalta can cause drowsiness and affect judgment or motor skills. Use caution when driving, operating dangerous machinery, or participating in hazardous activities until you know how the drug affects you.

Possible food and drug interactions when taking this medication
Never take Cymbalta with MAO inhibitors (see *Most important fact about this drug*) or the drug thioridazine (Mellaril). Consult your doctor first before taking drugs that act on the central nervous system, such as antipsychotics, narcotic painkillers, sleep inducers, or tranquilizers.

Due to the possibility of liver damage, do not take Cymbalta if you use alcohol more than occasionally.

If Cymbalta is taken with certain other drugs, the effects of either could be increased, decreased, or altered. It is especially important to check with your doctor before combining Cymbalta with the following:

Antibiotics known as quinolones, such as Cipro, Floxin, and Trovan
Antidepressants known as tricyclics, including Elavil, Pamelor, and
   Tofranil
Antidepressants that raise serotonin levels, such as Effexor, Paxil,
   Prozac, and Zoloft
Antipsychotic medications known as phenothiazines, including
   Compazine, Prolixin, Serentil, Thorazine, and Trilafon
Flecainide (Tambocor)
Fluvoxamine
Propafenone (Rythmol)
Quinidine

Special information if you are pregnant or breastfeeding
Cymbalta had negative effects during pregnancy when given to animals. There have been no adequate studies in pregnant women. Cymbalta should be used during pregnancy only if the benefits outweigh the potential risks.

Cymbalta appears in the breast milk of animals. It is unknown whether the drug appears in human breast milk. Therefore, it's recommended that you avoid breastfeeding while taking Cymbalta.

Recommended dosage

ADULTS 18 YEARS AND OLDER

Major Depression
The total daily dose ranges from 40 milligrams (taken as one 20-milligram capsule twice a day) to 60 milligrams (taken as a 60-milligram capsule once a day or as a 30-milligram capsule twice a day).

Diabetic Peripheral Neuropathy
The recommended dose is 60 milligrams, taken once daily.

Overdosage

Any medication taken in excess can have serious consequences. If you suspect an overdose, seek emergency treatment immediately.

Cyproheptadine *See Periactin, page 1078.*

CYSTADANE

Pronounced: SIST-uh-dane
Generic name: Betaine anhydrous

Why is this drug prescribed?

Cystadane is prescribed to reduce dangerously high blood levels of the naturally occurring amino acid homocysteine. Excessive levels of homocysteine can lead to formation of clots within your blood vessels, brittle bones (osteoporosis), other bone abnormalities, and dislocation of the lens of the eye. Homocysteine is also linked with an increased risk of heart disease and heart attack.

When homocysteine levels are so high that the substance appears in the urine, the condition is called homocystinuria. The problem is usually the result of an inherited lack of the enzymes needed to process homocysteine and generally shows up within the first months or years of life. Early signs of homocystinuria include delays in development, failure to thrive, seizures, and sluggishness.

Most important fact about this drug

The active ingredient in Cystadane (betaine) is found in our bodies and in foods such as beets, cereals, seafood, and spinach. Your doctor may prescribe Cystadane along with vitamin B_6 (pyridoxine), vitamin B_{12} (cobalamin), and folate. All of these dietary substances aid in the proper processing of homocysteine.

How should you take this medication?

Take Cystadane exactly as directed. To avoid forgetting a dose, try to get into the habit of taking it at the same time each day.

Cystadane will start to work within a week, and should have your condition completely under control within a month. You can continue therapy indefinitely; people have taken betaine for years without a problem.

■ *If you miss a dose…*
Take the forgotten dose as soon as you remember. If it is almost time for your next dose, skip the one you missed and go back to your regular schedule.

■ *Storage instructions…*
Store Cystadane at room temperature and protect from moisture. Keep the bottle tightly closed.

What side effects may occur?
The side effects of Cystadane are minimal. If any develop or change in intensity, inform your doctor as soon as possible. Only your doctor can determine whether it is safe for you to continue taking Cystadane.

■ *Side effects may include:*
Diarrhea, nausea, odor, possible mental changes, stomach and intestinal problems

Why should this drug not be prescribed?
There are no known reasons for avoiding Cystadane.

Special warnings about this medication
Do not use the powder if it does not completely dissolve in water, or if it makes a colored solution.

Possible food and drug interactions when taking this medication
No interactions have been reported.

Special information if you are pregnant or breastfeeding
The effects of Cystadane during pregnancy have not been studied. If you are pregnant or plan to become pregnant, check with your doctor immediately. It is not known whether Cystadane appears in breast milk. If this medication is essential to your health, your doctor may advise you to avoid breastfeeding.

Recommended dosage
Shake the bottle of Cystadane before removing the cap. Measure the number of scoops your doctor has prescribed by using the scoop provided.

ADULTS

The usual dosage is 3 scoops (3 grams) mixed with 4 to 6 ounces of water twice a day (6 grams daily). Make sure the powder is completely dissolved before drinking. Drink immediately after mixing.

The doctor will gradually increase your dosage until your homocysteine levels are under control. Dosages of up to 20 grams daily are sometimes necessary.

CHILDREN

In children less than 3 years old, the usual starting dose is 100 milligrams per 2.2 pounds of body weight per day. Each week, the doctor will increase the daily dose by 100 milligrams per 2.2 pounds until homocysteine levels are normal.

Overdosage

There have been no reported cases of overdose with Cystadane. However, a massive overdose could be dangerous. If you suspect an overdose, seek medical attention immediately.

CYTOTEC

Pronounced: SITE-oh-tek
Generic name: Misoprostol

Why is this drug prescribed?

Cytotec, a synthetic prostaglandin (hormone-like substance), reduces the production of stomach acid and protects the stomach lining. People who take nonsteroidal anti-inflammatory drugs (NSAIDs) may be given Cytotec tablets to help prevent stomach ulcers.

Aspirin and other NSAIDs such as Motrin, Naprosyn, Feldene, and others, which are widely used to control the pain and inflammation of arthritis, are generally hard on the stomach. If you must take an NSAID for a prolonged period of time, and if you are elderly or have ever had a stomach ulcer, your doctor may want you to take Cytotec for as long as you take the NSAID.

Most important fact about this drug

You must not become pregnant while using Cytotec. This drug causes uterine contractions that could lead to a miscarriage. If you do have a miscarriage, there is a risk that it might be incomplete. This could lead to bleeding, hospitalization, surgery, infertility, or even death. It is vitally important to use reliable contraception while taking Cytotec.

How should you take this medication?

Take Cytotec with meals, exactly as prescribed.

Take Cytotec for the full course of NSAID treatment, even if you notice no stomach problems.

Take the final dosage at bedtime.

■ *If you miss a dose...*
Take it as soon as you remember. If it is almost time for your next dose, skip the one you missed and go back to your regular schedule. Do not take 2 doses at once.

■ *Storage instructions...*
Store at room temperature in a dry place.

What side effects may occur?

Cytotec may cause abdominal cramps, diarrhea, and/or nausea, especially during the first few weeks of treatment. These symptoms may disappear as your body gets used to the drug. Taking Cytotec with food can help minimize diarrhea. If you have prolonged difficulty (more than 8 days), or if you have severe diarrhea, cramping, or nausea, call your doctor.

■ *Other side effects may include:*
Constipation, gas, indigestion, headache, heavy menstrual bleeding, menstrual disorder, menstrual pain or cramps, paleness, spotting (light bleeding between menstrual periods), stomach or intestinal bleeding, vomiting

Cytotec may cause uterine bleeding even if you have gone through menopause. However, postmenopausal bleeding could be a sign of some other gynecological problem. If you experience any such bleeding while taking Cytotec, notify your doctor at once.

Why should this drug not be prescribed?

Do not take Cytotec if you are sensitive to or have ever had an allergic reaction to it or to another prostaglandin medication.

Do not take Cytotec if you are pregnant or might become pregnant while taking it.

Special warnings about this medication

Since Cytotec may cause diarrhea, you should use this drug very cautiously if you have inflammatory bowel disease or any other condition in which the loss of fluid caused by diarrhea would be particularly dangerous.

To reduce the risk of diarrhea, take Cytotec with food and avoid taking it with a magnesium-containing antacid, such as Di-Gel, Gelusil, Maalox, Mylanta, and others. Have frequent medical checkups.

Never give Cytotec to anyone else; the dosage might be wrong, and if the other person is pregnant, the drug might harm the unborn baby or cause a miscarriage.

If you have a history of heart disease, you may not be able to use Cytotec. Be sure to tell your doctor about any heart problems.

Possible food and drug interactions when taking this medication

Cytotec does not interfere with arthritis medications such as aspirin and ibuprofen.

Special information if you are pregnant or breastfeeding

If you are pregnant or plan to become pregnant, inform your doctor immediately. Because Cytotec can cause dangerous cases of miscarriage, sometimes leading to the mother's death, it should not be taken during pregnancy. If you are a woman of childbearing age, you should not take Cytotec unless you have thoroughly discussed the risks with your doctor and believe you are able to take effective contraceptive measures.

You will need to take a pregnancy test about 2 weeks before starting to take Cytotec. To be sure you are not pregnant at the start of Cytotec treatment, your doctor will have you take your first dose on the second or third day of your menstrual period.

Even the most scrupulous contraceptive measures sometimes fail. If you believe you may have become pregnant while taking Cytotec, stop taking the drug and contact your doctor immediately.

It is not known if Cytotec appears in breast milk. Because of the potential for severe diarrhea in a nursing infant, your doctor may have you stop breastfeeding until your treatment is finished.

Recommended dosage

ADULTS

The recommended oral dose of Cytotec for the prevention of NSAID-induced stomach ulcers is 200 micrograms 4 times daily with food. Take the last dose of the day at bedtime.

If you cannot tolerate this dosage, your doctor can prescribe a dose of 100 micrograms.

You should take Cytotec for the duration of NSAID therapy, as prescribed by your doctor.

For People with Kidney Impairment

You will not normally need an adjustment in the dosing schedule, but your doctor can reduce the dosage if you have trouble handling the usual dose.

Overdosage

Any medication taken in excess can have serious consequences. If you suspect symptoms of an overdose of Cytotec, seek medical attention immediately.

■ *Symptoms of Cytotec overdose may include:*
Abdominal pain, breathing difficulty, convulsions, diarrhea, fever, heart palpitations, low blood pressure, sedation (extreme drowsiness), slowed heartbeat, stomach or intestinal discomfort, tremors

CYTOXAN

Pronounced: sigh-TOKS-an
Generic name: Cyclophosphamide

Why is this drug prescribed?

Cytoxan, an anticancer drug, works by interfering with the growth of malignant cells. It may be used alone but is often given with other anticancer medications.

Cytoxan is used in the treatment of the following types of cancer:

Advanced mycosis fungoides (cancer of the skin and lymph nodes)
Breast cancer
Leukemias (cancers affecting the white blood cells)
Malignant lymphomas (Hodgkin's disease or cancer of the lymph nodes)
Multiple myeloma (a malignant condition or cancer of the plasma cells)
Neuroblastoma (a malignant tumor of the adrenal gland or sympathetic nervous system)
Ovarian cancer (adenocarcinoma)
Retinoblastoma (a malignant tumor of the retina)

In addition, Cytoxan may sometimes be given to children who have *minimal change* nephrotic syndrome (kidney damage resulting in loss of protein in the urine) and who have not responded well to treatment with steroid medications.

Most important fact about this drug

Cytoxan may cause bladder damage, probably from toxic by-products of the drug that are excreted in the urine. Potential problems include bladder infection with bleeding and fibrosis of the bladder.

While you are being treated with Cytoxan, drink 3 or 4 liters of fluid a day to help prevent bladder problems. The extra fluid will dilute your urine and make you urinate frequently, thus minimizing the Cytoxan by-products' contact with your bladder.

How should you take this medication?

Take Cytoxan exactly as prescribed. You will undergo frequent blood tests, and the doctor will adjust your dosage depending on your white blood cell count; a dosage reduction is necessary if the count drops below a certain level. You will also have frequent urine tests to check for blood in the urine, a sign of bladder damage.

Take Cytoxan on an empty stomach. If you have severe stomach upset, then you may take it with food.

If you are unable to swallow the tablet form, you may be given an oral solution made from the injectable form of Cytoxan and Aromatic Elixir. This solution should be used within 14 days.

■ *If you miss a dose...*
Do not take the dose you missed. Go back to your regular schedule and contact your doctor. Do not take 2 doses at once.

■ *Storage instructions...*
Store tablets at room temperature. Store the oral solution in the refrigerator.

What side effects may occur?
Side effects cannot be anticipated. If any develop or change in intensity, inform your doctor immediately. Only your doctor can determine if it is safe for you to continue using Cytoxan.

One possible Cytoxan side effect is the development of a secondary cancer, typically of the bladder, lymph nodes, or bone marrow. A secondary cancer may occur up to several years after the drug is given.

Cytoxan can lower the activity of your immune system, making you more vulnerable to infection.

Noncancerous bladder problems may occur during Cytoxan therapy (see *Most important fact about this drug,* above).

■ *Side effects may include:*
Loss of appetite, nausea and vomiting, temporary hair loss

Why should this drug not be prescribed?
Do not take this medication if you have ever had an allergic reaction to it.

Also, tell your doctor if you have ever had an allergic reaction to another anticancer drug such as Alkeran, CeeNU, Emcyt, Leukeran, Myleran, or Zanosar.

In adults, Cytoxan should not be given for "minimal change" nephrotic syndrome or any other kidney disease.

Also, Cytoxan should not be given to anyone who is unable to produce normal blood cells because the bone marrow—where blood cells are made—is not functioning well.

Special warnings about this medication
You are at increased risk for toxic side effects from Cytoxan if you have any of the following conditions:

Blood disorder (low white blood cell or platelet count)
Bone marrow tumors
Kidney disorder
Liver disorder
Past anticancer therapy
Past X-ray therapy .

Possible food and drug interactions when taking this medication

If Cytoxan is taken with certain other drugs, the effects of either could be increased, decreased, or altered. It is especially important to check with your doctor before combining Cytoxan with the following:

Anticancer drugs such as Adriamycin
Allopurinol (the gout medicine Zyloprim)
Phenobarbital

If you take adrenal steroid hormones because you have had your adrenal glands removed, you are at increased risk for toxic effects from Cytoxan; your dosage of both the steroids and Cytoxan may need to be modified.

Special information if you are pregnant or breastfeeding

If you are pregnant or plan to become pregnant, inform your doctor immediately. When taken during pregnancy, Cytoxan can cause defects in the unborn baby. Women taking Cytoxan should use effective contraception. Cytoxan does appear in breast milk. A new mother will need to choose between taking this drug and nursing her baby.

Recommended dosage

ADULTS AND CHILDREN

Malignant Diseases
Your doctor will tailor your dosage according to your condition and other drugs taken with Cytoxan.

The recommended oral dosage range is 1 to 5 milligrams per 2.2 pounds of body weight per day.

CHILDREN

"Minimal Change" Nephrotic Syndrome
The recommended oral dosage is 2.5 to 3 milligrams per 2.2 pounds of body weight per day for a period of 60 to 90 days.

Overdosage

Although there is no specific information on Cytoxan overdose, any medication taken in excess can have serious consequences. If you suspect an overdose of Cytoxan, seek medical attention immediately.

DALMANE

Pronounced: DAL-main
Generic name: Flurazepam hydrochloride

Why is this drug prescribed?

Dalmane is used for the relief of insomnia, defined as difficulty falling asleep, waking up frequently at night, or waking up early in the morning.

It can be used by people whose insomnia keeps coming back and in those who have poor sleeping habits. It belongs to a class of drugs known as benzodiazepines.

Most important fact about this drug

Tolerance and dependence can occur with the use of Dalmane. You may experience withdrawal symptoms if you stop using this drug abruptly. Discontinue or change your dose only in consultation with your doctor.

How should you take this medication?

Take this medication exactly as prescribed.

■ *If you miss a dose...*
Take the dose you missed as soon as you remember, if it is within an hour or so of the scheduled time. If you do not remember it until later, skip the dose you missed and go back to your regular schedule. Do not take 2 doses at once.
■ *Storage instructions...*
Store away from heat, light, and moisture.

What side effects may occur?

Side effects cannot be anticipated. If any develop or change in intensity, inform your doctor as soon as possible. Only your doctor can determine if it is safe for you to continue taking Dalmane.

■ *Side effects may include:*
Dizziness, drowsiness, falling, lack of muscular coordination, light-headedness, staggering
■ *Side effects due to a rapid decrease in dose or abrupt withdrawal from Dalmane:*
Abdominal and muscle cramps, convulsions, depressed mood, inability to fall asleep or stay asleep, sweating, tremors, vomiting

Why should this drug not be prescribed?

If you are sensitive to or have had an allergic reaction to Dalmane or similar drugs such as Valium, you should not take this medication. Make sure your doctor is aware of any drug reactions you have experienced.

Special warnings about this medication

Dalmane will cause you to become drowsy or less alert; therefore, you should not drive or operate dangerous machinery or participate in any hazardous activity that requires full mental alertness after taking Dalmane.

If you are severely depressed or have suffered from severe depression, consult with your doctor before taking this medication.

If you have decreased kidney or liver function or chronic respiratory or lung disease, discuss use of this drug with your doctor.

Possible food and drug interactions when taking this medication
Alcohol intensifies the effects of Dalmane. Do not drink alcohol while taking this medication.

If Dalmane is taken with certain other drugs, the effects of either could be increased, decreased, or altered. It is especially important to check with your doctor before combining Dalmane with the following:

Antidepressants such as Elavil and Tofranil
Antihistamines such as Benadryl and Tavist
Antipsychotic drugs such as Mellaril and chlorpromazine
Barbiturates such as Seconal and phenobarbital
Narcotic painkillers such as Demerol and Tylenol with Codeine
Sedatives such as Xanax and Halcion
Tranquilizers such as Librium and Valium

Special information if you are pregnant or breastfeeding
Do not take Dalmane if you are pregnant or planning to become pregnant. There is an increased risk of birth defects. This drug may appear in breast milk and could affect a nursing infant. If this medication is essential to your health, your doctor may advise you to discontinue breastfeeding until your treatment with Dalmane is finished.

Recommended dosage

ADULTS

The usual recommended dose is 30 milligrams at bedtime; however, 15 milligrams may be all that is necessary. Your doctor will adjust the dose to your needs.

CHILDREN

The safety and effectiveness of Dalmane have not been established in children under 15 years of age.

OLDER ADULTS

Your doctor will limit the dosage to the smallest effective amount to avoid oversedation, dizziness, confusion, and lack of muscle coordination. The usual starting dose is 15 milligrams.

Overdosage
Any medication taken in excess can cause symptoms of overdose. If you suspect an overdose of Dalmane, seek medical attention immediately.

■ *The symptoms of Dalmane overdose may include:*
Coma, confusion, low blood pressure, sleepiness

DARVOCET-N

Pronounced: DAR-voe-set en
Generic ingredients: Propoxyphene napsylate, Acetaminophen
Other brand names: Darvon-N (propoxyphene napsylate),
Darvon (propoxyphene hydrochloride), Darvon
Compound-65 (propoxyphene hydrochloride, aspirin,
and caffeine)

Why is this drug prescribed?

Darvocet-N and Darvon Compound-65 are mild narcotic analgesics prescribed for the relief of mild to moderate pain, with or without fever.

Darvon-N and Darvon are prescribed for the relief of mild to moderate pain.

Most important fact about this drug

You can build up tolerance to, and become dependent on, these drugs if you take them in higher than recommended doses over long periods of time.

How should you take this medication?

Take these drugs exactly as prescribed. Do not increase the amount you take without your doctor's approval. Do not take them for any reason other than those for which they are prescribed. Do not give them to others who may have similar symptoms.

■ *If you miss a dose...*
Take it as soon as you remember. If it is almost time for your next dose, skip the one you missed and go back to your regular schedule. Do not take 2 doses at once.
■ *Storage instructions...*
Store at room temperature.

What side effects may occur?

Side effects cannot be anticipated. If any develop or change in intensity, inform your doctor as soon as possible. Only your doctor can determine if it is safe for you to continue taking one of these medications.

■ *Side effects may include:*
Drowsiness, dizziness, nausea, sedation, vomiting

If these side effects occur, it may help if you lie down after taking the medication.

Why should this drug not be prescribed?

If you are sensitive to or have ever had an allergic reaction to propoxyphene, any of the other ingredients in these drugs, or other pain relievers of this type, you should not take this medication. Make sure your doctor is aware of any drug reactions you have experienced.

Special warnings about this medication

These medicines may cause you to become drowsy or less alert; therefore, you should not drive or operate dangerous machinery or participate in any hazardous activity that requires full mental alertness until you know how the drug affects you.

If you have a kidney or liver disorder, consult your doctor before taking Darvocet-N.

Darvon Compound-65 contains aspirin and caffeine. If you have an ulcer or a blood-clotting problem, consult your doctor before taking this medication. Aspirin may irritate the stomach lining and could cause bleeding.

Because there is a possible association between aspirin and the severe neurological disorder known as Reye's syndrome, children and teenagers with chickenpox or flu should not take Darvon Compound-65 unless prescribed by a doctor.

Aspirin may cause asthma attacks. If you have had an asthma attack while taking aspirin, consult your doctor before you take Darvon Compound-65.

Possible food and drug interactions when taking this medication

The propoxyphene in these drugs slows down the central nervous system and intensifies the effects of alcohol. Heavy use of alcohol with this drug may cause overdose symptoms. Therefore, limit or avoid use of alcohol while you are taking this medication.

If these medications are taken with certain other drugs, the effects of either could be increased, decreased, or altered. It is especially important to check with your doctor before combining them with the following:

Antidepressant drugs such as Elavil
Antihistamines such as Benadryl
Antiseizure medications such as Tegretol
Muscle relaxants such as Flexeril
Narcotic pain relievers such as Demerol
Sleep aids such as Halcion
Tranquilizers such as Xanax and Valium
Warfarin-like drugs such as Coumadin

The use of these drugs with propoxyphene can lead to potentially fatal overdose symptoms.

Severe neurologic disorders, including coma, have occurred with the use of propoxyphene in combination with Tegretol.

The use of anticoagulants (blood thinners such as Coumadin) in combination with Darvon Compound-65 may cause bleeding. If you are taking an anticoagulant, consult your doctor before taking this drug.

The use of aspirin with drugs for gout may alter the effects of the antigout medication. Consult your doctor before taking Darvon Compound-65.

Special information if you are pregnant or breastfeeding

Do not take these medications if you are pregnant or planning to become pregnant unless you are directed to do so by your doctor. Temporary drug dependence may occur in newborns when the mother has taken this drug consistently in the weeks before delivery. The use of Darvon Compound-65 (which contains aspirin) during pregnancy may cause problems in the developing baby or complications during delivery. Do not take it during the last 3 months of pregnancy. Darvocet-N does appear in breast milk. However, no adverse effects have been found in nursing infants.

Recommended dosage

ADULTS

These medicines may be taken every 4 hours as needed for pain. The usual doses are:

Darvocet-N 50: 2 tablets
Darvocet-N 100: 1 tablet
Darvon: 1 capsule
Darvon Compound-65: 1 capsule

Your doctor may lower the total daily dosage if you have kidney or liver problems.

The most you should take of Darvon or Darvon Compound-65 is 6 capsules a day.

CHILDREN

The safety and effectiveness of Darvocet-N have not been established in children.

OLDER ADULTS

Your doctor may lengthen the time between doses.

Overdosage

Any medication taken in excess can have serious consequences. If you suspect an overdose, seek medical attention immediately.

■ *Symptoms of a propoxyphene overdose may include:*
Bluish tinge to the skin, coma, convulsions, decreased or difficult breathing to the point of temporary stoppage, decreased heart function, extreme sleepiness, irregular heartbeat, low blood pressure, pinpoint pupils becoming dilated later, stupor

- *Additional symptoms of overdose with Darvocet-N:*
  Abdominal pain, excessive sweating, general feeling of illness, kidney failure, liver problems, loss of appetite, nausea, vomiting
- *Additional symptoms of overdose with Darvon Compound-65:*
  Confusion, deafness, excessive perspiration, headache, mental dullness, nausea, rapid breathing, rapid pulse, ringing in the ears, vertigo, vomiting

Extreme overdosage may lead to unconsciousness and death.

Darvon *See Darvocet-N, page 385.*

Darvon Compound-65 *See Darvocet-N, page 385.*

Darvon-N *See Darvocet-N, page 385.*

DAYPRO
Pronounced: DAY-pro
Generic name: Oxaprozin

Why is this drug prescribed?
Daypro is a nonsteroidal anti-inflammatory drug used to relieve the inflammation, swelling, stiffness, and joint pain associated with rheumatoid arthritis and osteoarthritis (the most common kind of arthritis).

Most important fact about this drug
You should have frequent check-ups with your doctor if you take Daypro regularly. Ulcers and internal bleeding can occur without warning.

How should you take this medication?
Take Daypro with a full glass of water. If the drug upsets your stomach, your doctor may recommend taking Daypro with food, milk, or an antacid, even though food may delay onset of relief.

It will also help to prevent irritation in your upper digestive tract if you avoid lying down for about 20 minutes after taking Daypro.

Take this medication exactly as prescribed.

- *If you miss a dose...*
  Try to take Daypro at the same time each day—for example, after breakfast. If you forget to take a dose and remember later in the day, you can still take it. If you completely forget to take your medication, do *not* double the dose the next day to make up for the missed dose. You should get back on your normal schedule as soon as possible.
- *Storage instructions...*
  Store at room temperature in a tightly closed container, away from light.

What side effects may occur?

Side effects cannot be anticipated. If any develop or change in intensity, tell your doctor as soon as possible. Only your doctor can decide if it is safe for you to continue taking Daypro.

■ *Side effects may include:*
Constipation, diarrhea, indigestion, nausea, rash

Why should this drug not be prescribed?

If you are sensitive to or have ever had an allergic reaction to Daypro, or if you have ever developed asthma, nasal tumors, or other allergic reactions due to aspirin or other nonsteroidal anti-inflammatory drugs, you should not take this medication. Make sure your doctor is aware of any drug reactions you have experienced.

Special warnings about this medication

Use Daypro with caution if you have kidney or liver disease.

Do not take aspirin or any other anti-inflammatory medications while taking Daypro, unless your doctor tells you to do so.

Daypro can increase water retention. Use with caution if you have heart disease or high blood pressure.

If you are taking Daypro for an extended period, your doctor should check your blood for anemia.

Daypro can prolong bleeding time. If you are taking a blood-thinning medication, use Daypro with caution.

Daypro may cause sensitivity to sunlight. Avoid prolonged exposure to the sun. Use sunscreens and wear protective clothing.

Do not use Daypro if you are planning to have surgery in the immediate future.

Possible food and drug interactions when taking this medication

If you take Daypro with certain other drugs, the effects of either medication could be increased, decreased, or altered. It is especially important to check with your doctor before combining Daypro with the following medications:

Aspirin
Beta-blocking blood pressure medications such as Inderal and
    Tenormin
Blood thinners such as Coumadin
Digitalis and digoxin (Lanoxin)
Diuretics such as Lasix and Midamor
Lithium (Lithonate)
Ulcer drugs such as Tagamet and Zantac

Avoid alcoholic beverages while taking Daypro.

Special information if you are pregnant or breastfeeding

The effects of Daypro during pregnancy have not been adequately studied. If you are pregnant or plan to become pregnant, tell your doctor immediately. Since the effects of Daypro on nursing infants are not known, tell your doctor if you are nursing or plan to nurse. If Daypro treatment is necessary for your health, your doctor may tell you to discontinue nursing until your treatment is finished.

Recommended dosage

ADULTS

Your doctor will adjust the dose based on your needs.

Rheumatoid Arthritis
The usual daily dose is 1,200 milligrams (two 600-milligram caplets) once a day.

Osteoarthritis
The usual starting dose for moderate to severe osteoarthritis is 1,200 milligrams (two 600-milligram caplets) once a day.

The most you should take in a day is 1,800 milligrams divided into smaller doses, or 26 milligrams per 2.2 pounds of body weight, whichever is lower.

CHILDREN

The safety and efficacy of Daypro in children have not been determined.

Overdosage

If you take too much of any medication, it can have serious consequences. If you suspect an overdose, seek medical attention immediately.

■ *Symptoms of Daypro overdose may include:*
Coma, drowsiness, fatigue, nausea, pain in the stomach, stomach and intestinal bleeding, vomiting

Acute kidney failure, high blood pressure, and a slowdown in breathing have occurred rarely.

DDAVP

Pronounced: dee-dee-ai-vee-pee
Generic name: Desmopressin acetate
Other brand name: Stimate

Why is this drug prescribed?

DDAVP nasal spray, nose drops, and tablets are given to prevent or control the frequent urination and loss of water associated with diabetes insipidus (a rare condition characterized by very large quantities of diluted urine and excessive thirst). They are also used to treat frequent passage of urine and increased thirst in people with certain brain injuries, and those who have undergone surgery in the pituitary region of the brain. DDAVP nasal spray and nose drops are also prescribed to help stop some types of bedwetting.

Stimate nasal spray is used to stop bleeding in certain types of hemophilia (failure of the blood to clot).

Most important fact about this drug

When taking DDAVP, elderly and young people in particular should limit their fluid intake to no more than what satisfies thirst. Although extremely rare, there is a possibility of water intoxication, in which reduced sodium levels in the blood can lead to seizures.

How should you use this medication?

Use DDAVP exactly as prescribed. The spray and drops are for nasal use only; never swallow the medication or allow the liquid to run into your mouth.

Your doctor may increase or decrease your dosage, depending on how you respond to DDAVP. Your response will be judged by how long you are able to sleep without having to get up to urinate and how much urine your kidneys produce.

The DDAVP nasal spray pump bottle accurately delivers 50 doses of the medication. After the 50th dose, the amount of medication that comes out with each spray will no longer be a full dose. When this happens, throw the bottle away even if it is not completely empty.

Stimate nasal spray delivers 25 doses; the same instructions apply. The Stimate nasal spray pump must be primed before you use it for the first time: Press down 4 times.

Since the DDAVP spray bottle delivers only a standard-sized dose, those who need more or less medication should use the nose drops instead of the spray.

If nasal congestion, scars, or swelling inside the nose make it difficult to absorb DDAVP, your doctor may temporarily stop the drug or give you tablets or an injectable form. If you are switched to tablets, you should start taking them 12 hours after you last used the nasal spray or nose drops.

■ *If you miss a dose...*
Take the forgotten dose as soon as you remember. If you take 1 dose a day and don't remember until the next day, skip the dose. If you take DDAVP more than once a day and it is almost time for the next dose, skip the one you missed and go back to your regular schedule. Never try to catch up by doubling the dose.

■ *Storage instructions...*
The drops should be stored in the refrigerator. If you are traveling, they will stay fresh at room temperature for up to 3 weeks.

The tablets and nasal spray can be kept at room temperature. Protect the tablets from heat and light.

What side effects may occur?
Too high a dosage of DDAVP nasal spray or drops may produce headache, nausea, mild abdominal cramps, stuffy nose, irritation of the nose, or flushing. These symptoms will probably disappear when the dosage is reduced. Some people have complained of nosebleed, sore throat, cough, or a cold or other upper respiratory infections after taking DDAVP nasal spray or drops.

- *Other potential side effects include:*
  Abdominal pain, chills, conjunctivitis (pinkeye), depression, dizziness, inability to produce tears, leg rash, nostril pain, rash, stomach or intestinal upset, swelling around the eyes, weakness
- *Side effects of Stimate nasal spray may include:*
  Agitation, chest pain, chills, dizziness, fluid retention and swelling, indigestion, inflammation of the penis, insomnia, itchy or light-sensitive eyes, pain, pounding heartbeat, rapid heartbeat, sleepiness, vomiting, warm feeling

Why should this drug not be prescribed?
Do not use DDAVP if you are sensitive to or have ever had an allergic reaction to any of its ingredients.

Special warnings about this medication
If you have cystic fibrosis or any other condition in which there is fluid and electrolyte imbalance, you should use DDAVP with extreme caution.

Because DDAVP may cause a rise in blood pressure, use this medication cautiously if you have high blood pressure and/or coronary artery disease. Your blood pressure could also fall temporarily. If you continue to experience bleeding after using Stimate nasal spray, contact your doctor.

Possible food and drug interactions when taking this medication
If DDAVP is taken with certain other drugs, the effects of either could be increased, decreased, or altered. It is especially important to check with your doctor before combining DDAVP with the following:

Any drug used to increase blood pressure
Clofibrate (Atromid-S)
Epinephrine (EpiPen)
Glyburide (Micronase)

Special information if you are pregnant or breastfeeding
If you are pregnant or plan to become pregnant, inform your doctor immediately. Although DDAVP is not known to cause birth defects, it should

be used with caution. DDAVP should be taken during pregnancy only if clearly needed. DDAVP is not believed to appear in breast milk. However, check with your doctor before using the drug while breastfeeding.

Recommended dosage

Your doctor will carefully tailor your dosage to meet your individual needs.

CENTRAL CRANIAL DIABETES INSIPIDUS

DDAVP Nasal Spray and Nose Drops

Adults: The usual recommended dosage range is 0.1 to 0.4 milliliter daily, either as a single dose or divided into 2 or 3 doses. Most adults require 0.2 milliliter per day divided into 2 doses.

Children: The usual dosage range for children aged 3 months to 12 years is 0.05 to 0.3 milliliter daily, either as a single dose or divided into 2 doses.

DDAVP Tablets

Adults and Children 4 Years and Older: The usual starting dose is half of a 0.1-milligram tablet twice a day. Your doctor will adjust the dose to suit you. You will eventually take 0.1 to 1.2 milligrams a day, divided into smaller doses.

PRIMARY NOCTURNAL ENURESIS (BEDWETTING)

DDAVP Nasal Spray/Nose Drops

Children 6 Years and Older: The usual recommended dose is 20 micrograms or 0.2 milliliter at bedtime. Dosage requirements range from 10 to 40 micrograms. One-half the dose should be taken in each nostril.

HEMOPHILIA

Stimate Nasal Spray

To stop bleeding, the usual dose is one 150-microgram spray in each nostril. If you use the spray more frequently than every 48 hours, you may not respond to the drug as well as you should.

Overdosage

An overdose of DDAVP may cause abdominal cramps, flushing, headache, or nausea. If you suspect an overdose of DDAVP, seek medical attention immediately.

DECADRON TABLETS

Pronounced: DECK-uh-drohn
Generic name: Dexamethasone

Why is this drug prescribed?

Decadron, a corticosteroid drug, is used to reduce inflammation and relieve symptoms in a variety of disorders, including rheumatoid arthritis and severe cases of asthma. It may be given to people to treat primary or secondary adrenal cortex insufficiency (lack of sufficient adrenal hormone). It is also given to help treat the following disorders:

Blood disorders such as various anemias
Certain cancers (along with other drugs)
Collagen (connective tissue) diseases such as systemic lupus
    erythematosus
Digestive tract disease such as ulcerative colitis
Eye diseases such as allergic conjunctivitis
Fluid retention due to nephrotic syndrome (a condition in which
    damage to the kidneys causes the body to lose protein in the
    urine)
High serum levels of calcium associated with cancer
Lung diseases such as tuberculosis (along with other drugs)
Severe allergic conditions such as drug-induced allergies
Skin diseases such as severe psoriasis

Most important fact about this drug

Decadron lowers your resistance to infections and can make them harder to treat. Decadron may also mask some of the signs of an infection, making it difficult for your doctor to diagnose the actual problem.

How should you take this medication?

Decadron should be taken exactly as prescribed by your doctor.

If you are taking large doses, your doctor may advise you to take Decadron with meals and to take antacids between meals, to prevent a peptic ulcer from developing.

Check with your doctor before stopping Decadron abruptly. If you have been taking the drug for a long time, you may need to reduce your dose gradually over a period of days or weeks.

The lowest possible dose should always be used, and as symptoms subside, dosage should be reduced gradually.

■ *If you miss a dose...*
Take the forgotten dose as soon as you remember. If it is almost time for the next dose, skip the one you missed and go back to your regular schedule. Never try to catch up by doubling the dose.

■ *Storage instructions...*
There are no special storage requirements.

What side effects may occur?

Side effects cannot be anticipated. If any develop or change in intensity, inform your doctor as soon as possible. Only your doctor can determine if it is safe for you to continue taking Decadron.

■ *Side effects may include:*
Abdominal distention, allergic reactions, blood clots, bone fractures and degeneration, bruises, cataracts, congestive heart failure, convulsions, cushingoid symptoms (moon face, weight gain, high blood pressure, emotional disturbances, growth of facial hair in women), excessive hairiness, fluid and salt retention, general feeling of illness, glaucoma, headache, hiccups, high blood pressure, high blood sugar, hives, increased appetite, increased eye pressure, increased pressure in head, increased sweating, increases in amounts of insulin or hypoglycemic medications needed in diabetes, inflammation of the esophagus, inflammation of the pancreas, irregular menstruation, loss of muscle mass, low potassium levels in blood (leading to symptoms such as dry mouth, excessive thirst, weak or irregular heartbeat, and muscle pain or cramps), muscle weakness, nausea, osteoporosis, peptic ulcer, perforated small and large bowel, poor healing of wounds, protruding eyeballs, suppression of growth in children, thin skin, tiny red or purplish spots on the skin, torn tendons, vertigo, weight gain

Why should this drug not be prescribed?

Decadron should not be used if you have a fungal infection, or if you are sensitive or allergic to any of its ingredients.

Special warnings about this medication

Decadron can alter the way your body responds to unusual stress. If you are injured, need surgery, or develop an acute illness, inform your doctor. Your dosage may need to be increased.

Corticosteroids such as Decadron can lower your resistance to infection. Diseases such as measles and chickenpox can be serious and even fatal in adults. Likewise, a simple case of threadworm can run rampant, producing life-threatening complications. If you are taking Decadron and are exposed to chickenpox or measles—or suspect a case of threadworm—notify your doctor immediately. Symptoms of threadworm include stomach pain, vomiting, and diarrhea.

Do not get a smallpox vaccination or any other immunizations while taking Decadron, especially in high doses. The vaccination might not take, and could do harm to the nervous system.

Decadron may reactivate a dormant case of tuberculosis. If you have inactive tuberculosis and must take Decadron for an extended period, your doctor will prescribe anti-TB medication as well.

When you stop taking Decadron after long-term therapy, you may develop withdrawal symptoms such as fever, muscle or joint pain, and a feeling of illness.

Long-term use of Decadron may cause cataracts, glaucoma, and eye infections.

If you have any of the following conditions, make sure your doctor knows about it:

Allergy to any cortisone-like drug
Cirrhosis
Diabetes
Diverticulitis
Eye infection (herpes simplex)
Glaucoma
High blood pressure
Impaired thyroid function
Kidney disease
Myasthenia gravis (a muscle disorder)
Osteoporosis (brittle bones)
Peptic ulcer
Recent heart attack
Tuberculosis
Ulcerative colitis

Steroids may alter male fertility.

This medication can aggravate existing emotional problems or cause emotional disturbances. Symptoms range from an exaggerated sense of well-being and difficulty sleeping to mood swings and psychotic episodes. If you experience any changes in mood, contact your doctor.

If you have recently been to the tropics or are suffering from diarrhea with no apparent cause, inform your doctor before taking Decadron.

Possible food and drug interactions when taking this medication
If Decadron is taken with certain other drugs, the effects of either could be increased, decreased, or altered. It is especially important to check with your doctor before combining Decadron with the following:

Aspirin
Blood-thinning medications such as Coumadin
Carbamazepine (Tegretol)
Ephedrine (a decongestant in drugs such as Rynatuss)
Erythromycin (E.E.S., Ery-Tab, PCE)
Indomethacin (Indocin)
Ketoconazole (Nizoral)
Phenobarbital

Phenytoin (Dilantin)
Rifampin (Rifadin, Rimactane)
Thalidomide (Thalomid)
Water pills that pull potassium out of the system, such as
     HydroDIURIL

Special information if you are pregnant or breastfeeding

The effects of Decadron during pregnancy have not been adequately studied. If you are pregnant or plan to become pregnant, inform your doctor immediately. Infants born to mothers who have taken substantial doses of corticosteroids during pregnancy should be carefully watched for adrenal problems. Corticosteroids appear in breast milk and can suppress growth in infants. If Decadron is essential to your health, your doctor may advise you to stop breastfeeding until your treatment with Decadron is finished.

Recommended dosage

ADULTS

Your doctor will tailor your individual dose to the condition being treated. Initial doses range from 0.75 milligram to 9 milligrams a day.

After the drug produces a satisfactory response, your doctor will gradually lower the dose to the minimum effective level.

Overdosage

Reports of overdose with this medication are rare. However, if you suspect an overdose, seek medical treatment immediately.

DECONAMINE

Pronounced: dee-CON-uh-meen
Generic ingredients: Chlorpheniramine maleate,
*   d-Pseudoephedrine hydrochloride*

Why is this drug prescribed?

Deconamine is an antihistamine and decongestant used for the temporary relief of persistent runny nose, sneezing, and nasal congestion caused by upper respiratory infections (the common cold), sinus inflammation, or hay fever. It is also used to help clear nasal passages and shrink swollen membranes and to drain the sinuses and relieve sinus pressure.

Most important fact about this drug

Deconamine may cause you to become drowsy or less alert. You should not drive or operate machinery or participate in any activity that requires full mental alertness until you know how you react to Deconamine.

How should you take this medication?

If Deconamine makes you nervous or restless, or you have trouble sleeping, take the last dose of the day a few hours before you go to bed. Take Deconamine exactly as prescribed.

Antihistamines can make your mouth and throat dry. It may help to suck on hard candy, chew gum, or melt bits of ice in your mouth.

■ *If you miss a dose...*
Take it as soon as you remember. If it is almost time for your next dose, skip the one you missed and go back to your regular schedule. Never take 2 doses at once.

■ *Storage instructions...*
Store at room temperature.

What side effects may occur?

Side effects cannot be anticipated. If any develop or change in intensity, inform your doctor as soon as possible. Only your doctor can determine if it is safe for you to continue taking Deconamine.

The most common side effect is mild to moderate drowsiness.

Why should this drug not be prescribed?

Do not use Deconamine if you have severe high blood pressure or severe heart disease, are taking an antidepressant drug known as an MAO inhibitor (Nardil, Parnate, others), or are sensitive to or have ever had an allergic reaction to antihistamines or decongestants.

Special warnings about this medication

Use Deconamine with extreme caution if you have the eye condition called glaucoma, peptic ulcer or stomach obstructions, an enlarged prostate, or difficulty urinating.

Also use caution if you have bronchial asthma, emphysema, chronic lung disease, high blood pressure, heart disease, diabetes, or an overactive thyroid.

Deconamine may cause excitability, especially in children.

Possible food and drug interactions when taking this medication

Alcohol increases the sedative effect of Deconamine. Avoid it while taking this medication.

If Deconamine is taken with certain other drugs, the effects of either may be increased, decreased, or altered. It is especially important to check with your doctor before combining Deconamine with the following:

Antidepressant drugs such as the MAO inhibitors Nardil and
  Parnate
Asthma medications such as Ventolin and Proventil
Bromocriptine (Parlodel)
Mecamylamine (Inversine)

Methyldopa (Aldomet)
Narcotic painkillers such as Demerol and Percocet
Phenytoin (Dilantin)
Reserpine (Ser-Ap-Es, others)
Sleep aids such as Halcion and Seconal
Tranquilizers such as Valium and Xanax

Special information if you are pregnant or breastfeeding

The effects of Deconamine during pregnancy have not been adequately studied. If you are pregnant or plan to become pregnant, notify your doctor immediately. Deconamine appears in breast milk and could affect a nursing infant. If this medication is essential to your health, your doctor may advise you to discontinue breastfeeding until your treatment with Deconamine is finished.

Recommended dosage

DECONAMINE TABLETS

Adults and Children over 12 Years: The usual dosage is 1 tablet 3 or 4 times daily.

Children Under 12 Years: Use Deconamine Syrup or Chewable Tablets instead of the tablets.

DECONAMINE SYRUP

Adults and Children over 12 Years: The usual dose is 1 to 2 teaspoonfuls (5 to 10 milliliters) 3 or 4 times daily.

Children 6 to 12 Years: The usual dose is one-half to 1 teaspoonful (2.5 to 5 milliliters) 3 or 4 times daily, not to exceed 4 teaspoonfuls in 24 hours.

Children 2 to 6 Years: The usual dose is one-half teaspoonful (2.5 milliliters) 3 or 4 times daily, not to exceed 2 teaspoonfuls in 24 hours.

Children Under 2 Years: Use as directed by your doctor.

DECONAMINE SR CAPSULES

Adults and Children over 12 Years: The usual dose is 1 capsule every 12 hours.

Children Under 12 Years: Use Deconamine Syrup or Chewable Tablets instead of the capsules.

DECONAMINE CHEWABLE TABLETS

Adults: The usual dose is 2 tablets 3 or 4 times a day.

Children 6 to 12 Years: The usual dose is 1 tablet 3 or 4 times a day.

Children 2 to 6 Years: The usual dose is half a tablet 3 or 4 times a day.

Overdosage

Any medication taken in excess can have serious consequences. If you suspect an overdose, seek medical attention immediately.

■ *Symptoms of Deconamine overdose include:*
Convulsions, diminished alertness, hallucinations, severe drowsiness, severe dryness of mouth, nose, and throat, shortness of breath/difficulty breathing, sleep problems, slow or rapid heartbeat, tremors

DEMADEX

Pronounced: DEH-muh-decks
Generic name: Torsemide

Why is this drug prescribed?

Demadex is a diuretic drug. It flushes excess water from the body by promoting the production of urine.

Demadex is prescribed to reduce the water retention and swelling that often accompany congestive heart failure, chronic kidney failure, and cirrhosis of the liver. It is also prescribed for high blood pressure, either alone or with other medications.

Most important fact about this drug

Demadex has been known to cause dehydration, chemical imbalances in the body, and a reduction in the volume of blood. Warning signs of these problems include dryness of the mouth, thirst, weakness, drowsiness, restlessness, muscle pain or fatigue, low blood pressure, diminished urination, rapid heartbeat, nausea, and vomiting. If any of these symptoms develop, see your doctor immediately. You'll probably need to stop taking Demadex temporarily, then resume at a lower dose.

How should you take this medication?

Demadex tablets can be taken with or without a meal. The diuretic effect begins within an hour and peaks during the first or second hour. Take Demadex exactly as prescribed.

■ *If you miss a dose...*
Take the forgotten dose as soon as you remember. However, if it is almost time for your next dose, skip the one you missed and return to your regular schedule. Do not take 2 doses at once.
■ *Storage instructions...*
Store at room temperature. Do not freeze.

What side effects may occur?

Side effects cannot be anticipated. If any develop or change in intensity, tell your doctor as soon as possible. Only your doctor can determine if it is safe to continue using Demadex.

■ *More common side effects may include:*
Excessive urination, dizziness, headache

Why should this drug not be prescribed?

You'll need to avoid Demadex if it gives you an allergic reaction. Avoid it, too, if you're allergic to sulfonylurea drugs such as the diabetes medications Amaryl, DiaBeta, Diabinese, and Glucotrol. Do not take Demadex if you are unable to urinate.

Special warnings about this medication

If you have cirrhosis, the doctor will use Demadex with great caution. The fluid and chemical imbalance that the drug can cause could send you into a coma.

Demadex may cause ringing in the ears and potential hearing loss, especially when large doses are given quickly.

In addition to potential imbalances in potassium, sodium, chloride, calcium, magnesium, and nitrogen, Demadex is known to cause a slight increase in blood sugar and cholesterol levels.

Possible food and drug interactions when using this medication

If Demadex is taken with certain other drugs, the effects of either could be increased, decreased, or altered. It is especially important to check with your doctor before combining Demadex with the following:

Aminoglycoside antibiotics such as Nebcin and streptomycin
Aspirin and other nonsteroidal anti-inflammatory drugs such as
Advil, Indocin, Motrin, and Naprosyn
Cholestyramine (Questran)
Ethacrynic acid (Edecrin)
Lithium (Eskalith, Lithobid)
Probenecid

Special information if you are pregnant or breastfeeding

The effects of Demadex during pregnancy have not been adequately studied. If you are pregnant or plan to become pregnant, inform your doctor immediately.

It is not known whether Demadex appears in breast milk. Use Demadex with caution if you are nursing a baby.

Recommended dosage

ADULTS

Congestive Heart Failure
The usual starting dose is 10 or 20 milligrams once a day. If this proves inadequate, the doctor will keep doubling the dose until the drug does its work. Doses of more than 200 milligrams are not recommended.

Chronic Kidney Failure

The usual starting dose is 20 milligrams once a day. If this proves inadequate, the doctor will keep doubling the dose until the drug does its work. Doses of more than 200 milligrams are not recommended.

Cirrhosis of the Liver

The usual starting dose is 5 or 10 milligrams once a day with other medications. If this proves inadequate, the doctor will keep doubling the dose until the drug does its work. Doses of more than 40 milligrams are not recommended.

High Blood Pressure

The usual starting dose is 5 milligrams once a day. If your blood pressure is still too high after 4 to 6 weeks, the doctor may increase the dose to 10 milligrams once a day. If that isn't sufficient, the doctor will add another drug to the regimen.

CHILDREN

The safety and effectiveness of Demadex in children have not been established.

Overdosage

An overdose of Demadex is likely to cause dehydration, chemical imbalances in the body, and a reduction in the volume of blood. Warning signs are those listed under *Most important fact about this drug*. If you suspect an overdose, seek medical attention immediately.

DEMEROL

Pronounced: DEM-er-awl
Generic name: Meperidine hydrochloride

Why is this drug prescribed?

Demerol, a narcotic analgesic, is prescribed for the relief of moderate to severe pain.

Most important fact about this drug

Do not take Demerol if you are currently taking drugs known as MAO inhibitors or have used them in the previous 2 weeks. Drugs in this category include the antidepressants Nardil and Parnate. When taken with Demerol, they can cause unpredictable, severe, and occasionally fatal reactions.

How should you take this medication?

Take Demerol exactly as prescribed. Do not increase the amount or length of time you take this drug without your doctor's approval. Likewise, do not abruptly stop taking Demerol, since this could increase the risk of withdrawal symptoms.

If you are using Demerol in syrup form, take each dose in a half glass of water.

■ *If you miss a dose...*
Take it as soon as you remember. If it is almost time for your next dose, skip the one you missed and go back to your regular schedule. Never take 2 doses at once.

■ *Storage instructions...*
Store at room temperature. Protect from heat.

What side effects may occur?

Side effects cannot be anticipated. If any develop or change in intensity, inform your doctor as soon as possible. Only your doctor can determine if it is safe for you to continue taking Demerol.

■ *Side effects of Demerol may include:*
Dizziness, light-headedness, nausea, sedation, sweating, vomiting

If any of these side effects occur, it may help if you lie down after taking the medication.

Why should this drug not be prescribed?

If you are sensitive to or have ever had an allergic reaction to Demerol or other narcotic painkillers, you should not use this medication. Make sure your doctor is aware of any drug reactions you have experienced.

Do not take Demerol with MAO inhibitors such as Nardil and Parnate.

Special warnings about this medication

Demerol may affect you both mentally and physically. You should not drive a car, operate machinery, or perform any other potentially hazardous activities until you know how the drug affects you.

You can build up tolerance to, and both mental and physical dependence on, Demerol if you take it repeatedly. Since it is possible that you could become addicted to Demerol, do not use it for any purpose other than what your doctor has prescribed it for. If you have ever had a problem with drug abuse, consult with your doctor before taking this drug.

Do not abruptly stop using Demerol, especially if you have been taking it for a while. Your doctor will have you gradually taper off this medication to reduce the risk of withdrawal symptoms, including restlessness, irritability, anxiety, insomnia, rapid heartbeat or breathing, increased blood pressure, or flu-like symptoms.

Use Demerol with caution if you have any of the following: a severe liver or kidney disorder, sickle-cell anemia, hypothyroidism (underactive thyroid gland), adrenal gland dysfunction or tumor, an enlarged prostate, a urethral stricture (narrowing of the tube leading from the bladder), a severe abdominal condition, an irregular heartbeat, a history of convulsions, or a history of alcoholism (including alcohol withdrawal marked by delirium tremens).

Be very careful taking this drug if you are having a severe asthma attack, if you have frequently recurring lung disease, if you are unable to inhale or exhale extra air when needed, or if you have any pre-existing breathing difficulties.

Use Demerol with caution if you have suffered any type of head injury. This medication may cause unusually slow or troubled breathing and may increase the pressure from fluid surrounding the brain and spinal cord. Demerol should be used by people with a head injury only if the doctor considers it absolutely necessary.

Demerol may make you feel light-headed or dizzy when you get up from lying down.

Before having surgery, make sure the doctor knows you are taking Demerol. Combining Demerol with a general anesthetic could cause serious side effects.

Possible food and drug interactions when taking this medication

It's very important not to combine Demerol with any sleep medications or tranquilizers, since this combination could cause serious injury or death.

Demerol slows brain activity and intensifies the effects of alcohol. Do not drink alcohol while taking this medication.

If Demerol is taken with certain other drugs, the effects of either could be increased, decreased, or altered. It is especially important to check with your doctor before combining Demerol with the following:

Acyclovir (Zovirax)
Antidepressant drugs such as Elavil or Tofranil
Buprenorphine
Butorphanol
Cimetidine (Tagamet)
General anesthetics such as Halothane or Versed
Major tranquilizers (phenothiazines) such as Mellaril and Thorazine
MAO inhibitors such as the antidepressant drugs Nardil and Parnate
Muscle relaxants such as Parafon Forte and Soma
Nalbuphine
Other narcotic painkillers such as Percocet and Tylenol with Codeine
Pentazocine
Phenytoin (Dilantin)
Ritonavir (Norvir)
Sedatives such as Halcion and Restoril
Sleep aids such as Ambien and Sonata
Tranquilizers such as Xanax and Valium

Special information if you are pregnant or breastfeeding

Do not take Demerol if you are pregnant or planning to become pregnant unless you are directed to do so by your doctor. Demerol appears in breast milk and could affect a nursing infant. If this medication is essential to your health, your doctor may advise you to discontinue breastfeeding your baby until your treatment is finished.

Recommended dosage

ADULTS

The usual dosage of Demerol is 50 milligrams to 150 milligrams every 3 or 4 hours, determined according to your response and the severity of the pain.

CHILDREN

The usual dosage is 1.1 milligrams to 1.8 milligrams per 2.2 pounds of body weight, taken every 3 or 4 hours, as determined by your doctor.

It's best to consult your doctor before giving Demerol to newborns or very young infants.

OLDER ADULTS

Your doctor may reduce the dosage.

Overdosage

■ *Symptoms of Demerol overdose include:*
Bluish discoloration of the skin, cold and clammy skin, coma or extreme sleepiness, limp, weak muscles, low blood pressure, slow heartbeat, troubled or slowed breathing

With severe overdose, a person may stop breathing, have a heart attack, and even die.

If you suspect an overdose, seek emergency medical treatment immediately.

Demulen *See Oral Contraceptives, page 1000.*

DENAVIR

Pronounced: DEN-a-veer
Generic name: Penciclovir

Why is this drug prescribed?

Denavir cream is used to treat recurrent cold sores on the lips and face. It works by interfering with the growth of the herpesvirus responsible for the sores.

Most important fact about this drug

You should begin applying Denavir at the first hint of a developing cold sore. The drug will not cure herpes, but it will reduce pain and may speed healing.

Check with your doctor if your cold sore does not improve or becomes worse. You could have an infection.

How should you use this medication?

Avoid using Denavir cream in or near the eyes; it can irritate them. Apply it only to sores on the lips and face.

■ *If you miss a dose...*
Apply it as soon as you remember. If it is almost time for your next dose, skip the one you missed and go back to your regular schedule.

■ *Storage instructions...*
Store at room temperature; avoid freezing.

What side effects may occur?

Reactions to Denavir are quite rare. If any develop or change in intensity, inform your doctor as soon as possible. Only your doctor can determine if it is safe for you to continue using this medication.

■ *Side effects may include:*
Headache, hives, itching, numbing of the skin, pain, rash, skin discoloration, skin reaction or swelling where the cream was applied, swelling in the mouth and throat, taste or smell alteration, tingling, worsened condition

Why should this drug not be prescribed?

If you have ever had an allergic reaction to any of the ingredients in Denavir, you should not use this medication.

Special warnings about this medication

It is not known whether Denavir is effective for people with weak immune systems.

Possible food and drug interactions when using this medication

No interactions with Denavir cream have been reported.

Special information if you are pregnant or breastfeeding

The effects of Denavir during pregnancy have not been adequately studied. If you are pregnant or plan to become pregnant, inform your doctor immediately. Researchers do not know whether this drug will appear in breast milk after external application. For safety's sake, your doctor may advise you to discontinue breastfeeding your baby until your treatment with Denavir is finished.

Recommended dosage

ADULTS AND CHILDREN 12 TO 17 YEARS OLD

Apply cream every 2 hours, while awake, for 4 days.

The safety and effectiveness of this drug in children less than 12 years old have not been established.

Overdosage

There have been no reported overdoses of this medication. Even if the cream is accidentally swallowed, it is unlikely to cause a harmful reaction.

DEPAKENE

Pronounced: DEP-uh-keen
Generic name: Valproic acid

Why is this drug prescribed?

Depakene, an epilepsy medicine, is used to treat certain types of seizures and convulsions. It may be prescribed alone or with other anticonvulsant medications.

Most important fact about this drug

Depakene can cause serious, even fatal, liver damage, especially during the first 6 months of treatment. Children under 2 years of age are the most vulnerable, especially if they are also taking other anticonvulsant medicines and have certain other disorders such as mental retardation. The risk of liver damage decreases with age; but you should always be alert for the following symptoms: loss of seizure control, weakness, dizziness, drowsiness, a general feeling of ill health, facial swelling, loss of appetite, vomiting, and yellowing of the skin and eyes. If you suspect a liver problem, call your doctor immediately.

Note too that Depakene has been known to cause rare cases of life-threatening damage to the pancreas. This problem can develop at any time, even after years of treatment. Call your doctor immediately if any of the following warning signs appear: abdominal pain, loss of appetite, nausea, and vomiting.

How should you take this medication?

If Depakene irritates your digestive system, take it with food. To avoid irritating your mouth and throat, swallow Depakene capsules whole; do not chew them.

■ *If you miss a dose…*
If you take 1 dose a day, take the dose you missed as soon as you remember. If you do not remember until the next day, skip the dose you missed and go back to your regular schedule.

If you take more than 1 dose a day and you remember the missed dose within 6 hours of the scheduled time, take it immediately. Take the rest of the doses for that day at equally spaced intervals. Never take 2 doses at once.

■ *Storage instructions...*
Store at room temperature.

What side effects may occur?

Side effects are more likely if you are taking more than one epilepsy medication, and when you are taking higher doses of Depakene. Indigestion, nausea, and vomiting are the most common side effects when you first start taking this drug.

If any side effects develop or change in intensity, inform your doctor as soon as possible. Only your doctor can determine if it is safe for you to continue taking Depakene.

■ *Side effects may include:*
Abdominal cramps, amnesia, breathing difficulty, depression, diarrhea, dimmed or blurred vision, drowsiness, hair loss, indigestion, infection, involuntary eye movements, loss of or increase in appetite, nausea, nervousness, ringing in the ears, sleeplessness, swelling of the arms and legs due to fluid retention, throat inflammation, tremors, vomiting

Why should this drug not be prescribed?

You should not take this drug if you have liver disease or your liver is not functioning properly, or if you have had an allergic reaction to it.

Special warnings about this medication

Remember that liver failure is possible when taking Depakene (see *Most important fact about this drug*). Your doctor should test your liver function at regular intervals.

Also keep in mind the threat of damage to the pancreas (see *Most important fact about this drug*). This problem can develop rapidly, so contact your doctor immediately if you experience any symptoms.

In people with a rare set of genetic abnormalities called urea cycle disorders, Depakene may adversely affect the brain. Signs of a developing problem include lack of energy, repeated attacks of vomiting, and mental changes. If you suspect a problem, see your doctor immediately. Depakene may have to be discontinued.

Depakene has also been known to cause a very rare but potentially fatal skin condition. Contact your doctor if you notice any changes in your skin.

Some side effects are more likely if you have manic episodes or suffer from migraines. Your doctor will monitor your care closely if you have one of these conditions.

Because of the potential for side effects involving blood disorders, your doctor will probably test your blood before prescribing Depakene and at regular intervals while you are taking it. Bruising, hemorrhaging, or clotting disorders usually mean the dosage should be reduced or the drug should be stopped altogether.

Depakene may cause drowsiness, especially in older adults. You should not drive a car, operate heavy machinery, or engage in hazardous activity until you know how you react to the drug.

Do not abruptly stop taking this medicine without first consulting your doctor. A gradual reduction in dosage is usually required to prevent major seizures.

This drug can also increase the effect of painkillers and anesthetics. Before any surgery or dental procedure, make sure the doctor knows you are taking Depakene.

Possible food and drug interactions when taking this medication

If Depakene is taken with certain other drugs, the effects of either could be increased, decreased, or altered. It is especially important to check with your doctor before combining Depakene with the following:

Amitriptyline (Elavil)
Aspirin
Barbiturates such as phenobarbital and Seconal
Blood-thinning drugs such as Coumadin and Dicumarol
Carbamazepine (Tegretol)
Clonazepam (Klonopin)
Diazepam (Valium)
Ethosuximide
Felbamate (Felbatol)
Lamotrigine (Lamictal)
Merrem IV (meropenem for injection)
Nortriptyline (Pamelor)
Phenytoin (Dilantin)
Primidone (Mysoline)
Rifampin (Rifater)
Tolbutamide (Orinase)
Zidovudine (Retrovir)

Extreme drowsiness and other serious effects may occur if Depakene is taken with alcohol or other central nervous system depressants such as Halcion, Restoril, or Xanax.

Special information if you are pregnant or breastfeeding

If taken during pregnancy, Depakene may harm the baby. The drug is not recommended for pregnant women unless the benefits of therapy clearly outweigh the risks. In fact, women in their childbearing years should take Depakene only if it has been shown to be essential in the control of seizures. Since Depakene appears in breast milk, nursing mothers should use it only with caution.

Recommended dosage

ADULTS AND CHILDREN 10 YEARS AND OLDER

The usual starting dose is 10 to 15 milligrams per 2.2 pounds of body weight per day. Your doctor may increase the dose at weekly intervals by 5 to 10 milligrams per 2.2 pounds per day until seizures are controlled or side effects become too severe. If stomach upset develops, the dose may be increased more slowly. The daily dose should not exceed 60 milligrams per 2.2 pounds per day.

OLDER ADULTS

Older adults generally are prescribed reduced starting doses, and receive dosage increases more gradually than younger people.

Overdosage

Any medication taken in excess can have serious consequences. An overdose of Depakene can be fatal. If you suspect an overdose, seek medical help immediately.

■ *Symptoms of Depakene overdose may include:*
Coma, extreme drowsiness, heart problems

DEPAKOTE

Pronounced: DEP-uh-coat
Generic name: Divalproex sodium (Valproic acid)

Why is this drug prescribed?

Depakote, in both delayed-release tablet and capsule form, is used to treat certain types of seizures and convulsions. It may be prescribed alone or with other epilepsy medications.

The delayed-release tablets are also used to control the manic episodes—periods of abnormally high spirits and energy—that occur in bipolar disorder (manic depression).

An extended-release form of this drug, Depakote ER, is prescribed to prevent migraine headaches. The delayed-release tablets are also used for this purpose.

Most important fact about this drug

Depakote can cause serious or even fatal liver damage, especially during the first 6 months of treatment. Children under 2 years of age are the most vulnerable, especially if they are also taking other anticonvulsant medicines and have certain other disorders such as mental retardation.

The risk of liver damage decreases with age; but you should always be alert for the following symptoms: loss of seizure control, weakness, dizziness, drowsiness, a general feeling of ill health, facial swelling, loss of appetite, vomiting, and yellowing of the skin and eyes. If you suspect a liver problem, call your doctor immediately.

Depakote has also been known to cause life-threatening damage to the pancreas. This problem can surface at any time, even after years of treatment. Call your doctor immediately if you develop any of the following warning signs: abdominal pain, loss of appetite, nausea, or vomiting.

How should you take this medication?

Take the tablet with water and swallow it whole (don't chew it or crush it). It has a special coating to avoid upsetting your stomach.

If you are taking the sprinkle capsule, you can swallow it whole or open it and sprinkle the contents on a teaspoon of soft food such as applesauce or pudding. Swallow it immediately, without chewing. The sprinkle capsules are large enough to be opened easily.

Depakote can be taken with meals or snacks to avoid stomach upset. Take it exactly as prescribed.

■ *If you miss a dose...*
If you take Depakote once a day, take your dose as soon as you remember. If you don't remember until the next day, skip the missed dose and return to your regular schedule. Never take 2 doses at the same time.

If you take more than one dose a day, take your dose right away if it's within 6 hours of the scheduled time, and take the rest of the day's doses at equal intervals during the day. Never take 2 doses at the same time.

■ *Storage instructions...*
Store at room temperature.

What side effects may occur?

Side effects cannot be anticipated. If any develop or change in intensity, inform your doctor as soon as possible. Because Depakote is often used with other antiseizure drugs, it may not be possible to determine whether a side effect is due to Depakote alone. Only your doctor can determine if it is safe for you to continue taking Depakote.

■ *Side effects may include:*
Abdominal pain, abnormal thinking, breathing difficulty, bronchitis, bruising, constipation, depression, diarrhea, dizziness, emotional changeability, fever, flu symptoms, hair loss, headache, incoordination, indigestion, infection, insomnia, loss of appetite, memory loss, nasal inflammation, nausea, nervousness, ringing in the ears, sleepiness, sore throat, tremor, vision problems, vomiting, weakness, weight loss or gain

Why should this drug not be prescribed?

You should not take this medication if you have liver disease or your liver is not functioning well, or if you have a genetic abnormality known as urea cycle disorder (UCD).

If you are sensitive to or have ever had an allergic reaction to Depakote, you should not take this medication.

Special warnings about this medication

This medication can severely damage the liver (see *Most important fact about this drug*). Your doctor will test your liver function before you begin taking this medication and at regular intervals thereafter.

Also remember that the drug can damage the pancreas (see *Most important fact about this drug*). This problem can worsen very rapidly, so be sure to contact your doctor immediately if you develop any symptoms.

In people with a rare set of genetic abnormalities called urea cycle disorders, Depakote may adversely effect the brain. Signs of a developing problem include lack of energy, repeated attacks of vomiting, and mental changes. If you suspect a problem, see your doctor immediately. Depakote may have to be discontinued.

Depakote causes some people to become drowsy or less alert. You should not drive or operate dangerous machinery or participate in any hazardous activity that requires full mental alertness until you are certain the drug does not have this effect on you.

Do not abruptly stop taking this medicine without first consulting your doctor. A gradual reduction in dosage is usually required.

Depakote prolongs the time it takes blood to clot, which increases your chances of serious bleeding.

This drug can also increase the effect of painkillers and anesthetics. Before any surgery or dental procedure, make sure the doctor knows you are taking Depakote.

If you are taking Depakote to prevent migraine, remember that it will not cure a headache once it has started.

Some coated particles from the capsules may appear in your stool. This is to be expected, and need not worry you.

Possible food and drug interactions when taking this medication

Depakote depresses activity of the central nervous system, and may increase the effects of alcohol. Do not drink alcohol while taking this medication.

If Depakote is taken with certain other drugs, the effects of either could be increased, decreased, or altered. It is especially important to check with your doctor before combining Depakote with the following:

Amitriptyline (Elavil)
Aspirin
Barbiturates such as phenobarbital and Seconal

Blood thinners such as Coumadin
Cyclosporine (Sandimmune, Neoral)
Merrem IV (meropenem for injection)
Nortriptyline (Pamelor)
Other seizure medications, including carbamazepine (Tegretol),
   clonazepam (Klonopin), ethosuximide (Zarontin), felbamate
   (Felbatol), lamotrigine (Lamictal), phenytoin (Dilantin), and
   Primidone (Mysoline)
Rifampin (Rifater, Rimactane)
Sleep aids such as Halcion
Tolbutamide (Orinase)
Tranquilizers such as Valium and Xanax
Zidovudine (Retrovir)

Special information if you are pregnant or breastfeeding

Depakote may produce birth defects if it is taken during pregnancy. If you
are pregnant or plan to become pregnant, inform your doctor immediately.
Depakote appears in breast milk and could affect a nursing infant. If Depakote is essential to your health, your doctor may advise you to discontinue breastfeeding until your treatment with this medication is finished.

Recommended dosage

EPILEPSY

Dosage for adults and children 10 years of age or older is determined by
body weight. The usual recommended starting dose is 10 to 15 milligrams per 2.2 pounds per day, depending on the type of seizure. Your
doctor may increase the dose at 1-week intervals by 5 to 10 milligrams
per 2.2 pounds per day until your seizures are controlled or the side effects become too severe. The most you should take is 60 milligrams per
2.2 pounds per day. If your total dosage is more than 250 milligrams a
day, your doctor will divide it into smaller individual doses.

Older adults usually begin taking this medication at lower dosages,
and the dosage is increased more slowly.

MANIC EPISODES

The usual starting dose for those aged 18 and over is 750 milligrams a
day, divided into smaller doses. Your doctor will adjust the dose for best
results.

MIGRAINE PREVENTION

Delayed-Release Tablets
The usual starting dose for those aged 16 and over is 250 milligrams
twice a day. Your doctor will adjust the dose, up to a maximum of 1,000
milligrams a day.

Extended-Release Tablets
The usual starting dose is 500 milligrams once a day for 1 week. The dose may then be increased to 1,000 milligrams once a day.

Depakote delayed-release and extended-release tablets work differently, so you cannot substitute one type for the other.

Researchers have not established the safety and effectiveness of Depakote for prevention of migraines in children or in adults over 65.

Overdosage

Any medication taken in excess can have serious consequences. An overdose of Depakote can be fatal. If you suspect an overdose, seek medical attention immediately.

■ *Symptoms of Depakote overdose may include:*
Coma, extreme sleepiness, heart problems

DEPO-PROVERA

Pronounced: DE-po pro-VEH-ra
Generic name: Medroxyprogesterone acetate

Why is this drug prescribed?

Depo-Provera Contraceptive Injection is given in the buttock or upper arm to prevent pregnancy. It is more than 99 percent effective; your chances of becoming pregnant during the first year of use are less than 1 in 100. The injection is given every 3 months (13 weeks) by your doctor. Depo-Provera works by preventing the release of hormones called gonadotropins from the pituitary gland in the brain. Without these hormones, the monthly release of an egg from the ovary cannot occur. If no egg is released, pregnancy is impossible. Depo-Provera also causes changes in the lining of the uterus that make pregnancy less likely even if an egg is released.

In higher doses, Depo-Provera is also used in the treatment of certain cancers, including cancer of the endometrium (lining of the uterus) and kidney cancer.

Most important fact about this drug

Because Depo-Provera is a long-acting form of birth control, it will take a while for the effects of your last injection to wear off. In medical studies, only 68 percent of women became pregnant within 12 months after stopping Depo-Provera. However, within 18 months, 93 percent had become pregnant. If you think you will want to get pregnant shortly after you stop using birth control, Depo-Provera may not be the ideal method for you. The amount of time you use Depo-Provera does not affect the delay in becoming pregnant when you stop.

How should you take this medication?

Depo-Provera is given by a doctor. To make sure you are not pregnant when you receive your first injection, it is given only during the first 5 days after your menstrual period, when it is very unlikely that you could be pregnant. If you are breastfeeding, Depo-Provera is given 6 weeks after childbirth to reduce the infant's exposure to the drug through breast milk. If you are not breastfeeding, it is given within 5 days of childbirth.

Depo-Provera must be taken every 3 months (13 weeks), on schedule. Although the birth-control effects of the drug generally take time to wear off, there is still a possibility of becoming pregnant right away if you miss your scheduled injection.

■ *If you miss a dose...*
If you allow more than 13 weeks to elapse before your next injection, your doctor will do a test to make sure you are not pregnant before giving you another injection.

■ *Storage instructions...*
Depo-Provera is always given at a doctor's office or clinic, never at home.

What side effects may occur?

Side effects cannot be anticipated. If any develop or change in intensity, inform your doctor as soon as possible. Only your doctor can determine if it is safe for you to continue taking Depo-Provera.

By far, the most common side effect of Depo-Provera is unpredictable menstrual bleeding. In fact, most women have some change in their menstrual pattern. For example, when first taking Depo-Provera, it is common to have spotting between menstrual periods, or an increase or decrease in the amount of bleeding when menstrual periods occur. With continued use, many women stop having their menstrual periods altogether.

By 12 months (or four injections), 55 percent of women report not having periods, and by 24 months, 68 percent no longer have periods. Going without a menstrual period is not an indication that something is wrong, however.

■ *Side effects may include:*
Abdominal pain or discomfort, dizziness, headache, nervousness, unpredictable menstrual bleeding, weakness or fatigue, weight gain or loss

Why should this drug not be prescribed?

You should not use Depo-Provera if you know or suspect you are pregnant, or if you have unusual vaginal bleeding that has not been diagnosed by a doctor.

Also avoid Depo-Provera if you know or suspect you have breast cancer, or if you have liver disease.

Do not use this method of birth control if you have thrombophlebitis (inflammation of a vein with development of a blood clot), or have ever had any blood clotting disorders, such as a stroke, or disease of the blood vessels in the brain.

You should not take Depo-Provera if you have ever had an allergic reaction to it or to any of its ingredients.

Special warnings about this medication

Call your doctor immediately if any of these problems occurs after an injection of Depo-Provera: sharp chest pain, coughing up blood, sudden shortness of breath, sudden severe headache or vomiting, dizziness or fainting, problems with your eyesight or speech, weakness or numbness in an arm or leg, severe pain or swelling in the calf, unusually heavy vaginal bleeding, severe pain or tenderness in the lower abdominal area, migraine headache, or persistent pain, pus, or bleeding at the injection site.

Studies indicate that using Depo-Provera may make you more prone to osteoporosis, or brittle-bone disease. The rate at which bone loss occurs is greatest during the early years of Depo-Provera use, and the risk decreases to normal over time.

Studies of women who have used Depo-Provera for a long time have found virtually no increased risk of cancers of the breast, ovaries, liver, or cervix (mouth of the uterus). Some studies do show a slight increased risk of breast cancer in women younger than 35 years old who have taken Depo-Provera for a short time, but the increase is about three additional cases of breast cancer per 10,000 women. At the same time, Depo-Provera helps *reduce* the chance of cancer of the endometrium, or lining of the uterus.

Depo-Provera may cause fluid retention, so if you have conditions that may be worsened by fluid retention, such as epilepsy, migraine headaches, asthma, heart disease, or kidney disease, make sure your doctor is aware of it.

Depo-Provera tends to alter levels of blood sugar, so diabetic women need to be carefully observed by their doctors when taking Depo-Provera.

If you develop jaundice (a yellowing of the skin and whites of the eyes caused by liver disease), you probably should not receive Depo-Provera again.

Most women gain weight while they are using Depo-Provera.

While it is an excellent birth control method, Depo-Provera does not protect you against AIDS or other sexually transmitted diseases. If you are concerned about AIDS or other STDs, be sure your partner uses a condom during intercourse (or, for absolute safety, abstain from sex).

Before you start using Depo-Provera, be sure to tell your doctor if you or anyone in your family has ever had breast cancer; if you have ever had any problems with your breasts; if your menstrual periods have ever been irregular or spotty; if you have kidney disease, high blood pressure, migraine headaches, asthma, epilepsy, or a history of depression; if you or anyone in your family has or has had diabetes; or if you are taking any prescription or over-the-counter drugs.

Possible food and drug interactions when taking this medication

If Depo-Provera is taken with aminoglutethimide (Cytadren), a drug used to treat a disorder of the adrenal glands called Cushing's syndrome, it could make the Depo-Provera less potent, which could lead to unexpected pregnancy. Check with your doctor before taking Cytadren if you are on Depo-Provera.

Special information if you are pregnant or breastfeeding

Depo-Provera is not given to pregnant women. If an unexpected pregnancy occurs 1 to 2 months after a Depo-Provera injection, the baby is more likely to have a low birth weight or other health problems; birth defects are possible if you use the drug during the first 3 months of pregnancy. Children born to women who were taking Depo-Provera show no signs of poor health or development. Because Depo-Provera does not prevent the breasts from producing milk, it can be used by women who are breastfeeding. However, to minimize the amount of Depo-Provera that is passed to the infant during the first weeks of life, the drug is not given until 6 weeks after childbirth. Studies show that Depo-Provera is not harmful to the infant then or later in life.

Recommended dosage

Depo-Provera is given as a single 150-milligram injection every 3 months (13 weeks).

Overdosage

An overdose of Depo-Provera is highly unlikely, since it is given as a single injection by your doctor. However, if you suspect you have received an overdose, seek medical attention immediately.

Desipramine See Norpramin, page 973.

Desloratadine See Clarinex, page 297.

Desmopressin See DDAVP, page 390.

Desogen See Oral Contraceptives, page 1000.

Desonide See Tridesilon, page 1484.

DesOwen See Tridesilon, page 1484.

Desoximetasone See Topicort, page 1465.

DESOXYN

Pronounced: des-OK-sin
Generic name: Methamphetamine hydrochloride

Why is this drug prescribed?

Desoxyn is used to treat Attention Deficit Hyperactivity Disorder (ADHD). This drug is given as part of a total treatment program that includes psychological, educational, and social measures. Symptoms of ADHD include continual problems with moderate to severe distractibility, short attention span, hyperactivity, emotional instability, and impulsiveness.

Desoxyn also may be used for a short time as part of an overall diet plan for weight reduction. Desoxyn is given only when other weight-loss drugs and weight-loss programs have been unsuccessful.

Most important fact about this drug

Excessive doses of this medication can produce addiction. Individuals who stop taking this medication after taking high doses for a long time may suffer withdrawal symptoms, including extreme tiredness, depression, and sleep disorders. Signs of excessive use of Desoxyn include severe skin inflammation, difficulty sleeping, irritability, hyperactivity, personality changes, and psychiatric problems.

Desoxyn can lose its effectiveness in decreasing the appetite after a few weeks. If this happens, you should stop taking the medication. Do not take more than the recommended dose in an attempt to increase its effect.

How should you take this medication?

Follow your doctor's directions carefully. Your doctor will prescribe the lowest effective dose of Desoxyn; never increase it without approval. Do not take this medication late in the evening; it can cause difficulty sleeping.

■ *If you miss a dose...*
Take it as soon as you remember. If it is almost time for the next dose, skip the one that you missed and go back to your regular schedule. Never take 2 doses at the same time.

■ *Storage instructions...*
Store at room temperature.

What side effects may occur?

Side effects cannot be anticipated. If any develop or change in intensity, inform your doctor as soon as possible. Only your doctor can determine if it is safe to continue taking Desoxyn.

■ *Side effects may include:*
Changes in sex drive, constipation, diarrhea, dizziness, dry mouth, exaggerated feeling of well-being, headache, hives, impaired growth, im-

potence, increased blood pressure, overstimulation, rapid or irregular heartbeat, restlessness, sleeplessness, stomach or intestinal problems, tremor, unpleasant taste, worsening of tics, and Tourette's syndrome (severe twitching)

Why should this drug not be prescribed?

You should not take Desoxyn if you are also taking a monoamine oxidase (MAO) inhibitor drug such as Nardil or Parnate. Allow 14 days between stopping an MAO inhibitor and beginning therapy with Desoxyn.

You should not take Desoxyn if you have glaucoma, advanced hardening of the arteries, heart disease, moderate to severe high blood pressure, thyroid problems, or sensitivity to this type of drug. This medication should not be taken by anyone who suffers from tics (repeated, involuntary twitches) or Tourette's syndrome or who has a family history of these conditions.

People who are in an agitated state or who have a history of drug abuse should not take this medication.

Desoxyn should not be used to treat children whose symptoms may be caused by stress or a psychiatric disorder.

Special warnings about this medication

Desoxyn is not appropriate for all children with symptoms of ADHD. Your doctor will do a complete history and evaluation before prescribing this medication. The doctor will take into account the duration and severity of the symptoms as well as your child's age.

This type of medication can affect the growth of children, so your doctor will watch your child carefully while he or she is taking this drug. The long-term effects of this type of medication in children have not been established.

Desoxyn should be used with caution if you have mild high blood pressure.

Desoxyn may affect your ability to perform potentially hazardous activities, such as operating machinery or driving a car.

Desoxyn should not be used to combat fatigue or to replace rest.

Possible food and drug interactions when taking this medication

If Desoxyn is taken with certain other drugs, the effects of either could be increased, decreased, or changed. It is especially important to check with your doctor before combining Desoxyn with the following:

Antidepressants classified as tricyclics, such as Elavil, Pamelor, and Tofranil

Drugs classified as monoamine oxidase (MAO) inhibitors, such as the antidepressants Nardil and Parnate

Drugs classified as phenothiazines, such as the antipsychotic medications chlorpromazine and prochlorperazine

Guanethidine
Insulin

Special information if you are pregnant or breastfeeding

Infants born to women taking this type of drug have a risk of prematurity and low birth weight. Drug dependence may occur in newborns when the mother has taken this drug prior to delivery. If you are pregnant or plan to become pregnant, tell your doctor immediately.

Desoxyn makes its way into breast milk. Do not breastfeed while taking this medication.

Recommended dosage

ATTENTION DEFICIT HYPERACTIVITY DISORDER

For children 6 years and older, the usual starting dose is 5 milligrams of Desoxyn taken once or twice a day. Your doctor may increase the dose by 5 milligrams a week until the child responds to the medication. The typical effective dose is 20 to 25 milligrams a day, usually divided into 2 doses.

Your doctor may periodically discontinue this drug in order to re-assess the child's condition and see whether therapy is still needed.

Desoxyn should not be given to children under 6 years of age to treat attention deficit disorder; the safety and effectiveness in this age group have not been established.

WEIGHT LOSS

For adults and children 12 years and older, the usual starting dose is 5 milligrams taken one-half hour before each meal. Treatment should not continue for longer than a few weeks. The safety and effectiveness of Desoxyn for weight loss have not been established in children under age 12.

Overdosage

Any drug taken in excess can have dangerous consequences. If you suspect an overdose, seek medical attention immediately.

■ *Symptoms of Desoxyn overdose may include:*
Abdominal cramps, agitation, blood pressure changes, confusion, convulsions (may be followed by coma), depression, diarrhea, exaggerated reflexes, fatigue, hallucinations, high fever, irregular heartbeat, kidney failure, muscle aches and weakness, nausea, panic attacks, rapid breathing, restlessness, shock, tremor, vomiting

DESQUAM-E

Pronounced: DES-kwam ee
Generic name: Benzoyl peroxide
Other brand names: Benzac W, Benzagel, BenzaShave,
Clinac BPO, Triaz

Why is this drug prescribed?

Desquam-E gel is used to treat acne. It can be used alone or with other treatments, including antibiotics and products that contain retinoic acid, sulfur, or salicylic acid.

Most important fact about this drug

Significant clearing of the skin should occur after 2 to 3 weeks of treatment with Desquam-E.

How should you use this medication?

Cleanse the affected area thoroughly before applying the medication. Desquam-E should then be gently rubbed in.

■ *If you miss a dose...*
  Apply it as soon as you remember. Then go back to your regular schedule.
■ *Storage instructions...*
  Store at room temperature.

What side effects may occur?

Side effects cannot be anticipated. If any develop or change in intensity, notify your doctor as soon as possible. Only your doctor can determine whether it is safe for you to continue using Desquam-E.

■ *Side effects may include:*
  Allergic reaction (itching, rash in area where the medication was applied), excessive drying (red and peeling skin and possible swelling)

Why should this drug not be prescribed?

Do not use Desquam-E if you are sensitive to or allergic to benzoyl peroxide or any other components of the drug.

Special warnings about this medication

Desquam-E is for external use only. Avoid contact with your eyes, nose, lips, and throat. If the drug does touch these areas accidentally, rinse with water.

If you are sensitive to medications derived from benzoic acid (including certain topical anesthetics) or to cinnamon, you may also be sensitive to Desquam-E.

If your skin becomes severely irritated, stop using the drug and call your doctor.

Desquam-E can bleach or discolor hair or colored fabric.

Stay out of the sun as much as possible, and use a sunscreen.

Possible food and drug interactions when using this medication

When used with sunscreens containing PABA (para-aminobenzoic acid), Desquam-E may cause temporary skin discoloration.

Special information if you are pregnant or breastfeeding

The effects of Desquam-E during pregnancy have not been adequately studied. It should be used only if clearly needed. If you are pregnant or plan to become pregnant, inform your doctor immediately. This medication may appear in breast milk and could affect a nursing infant. If this medication is essential to your health, your doctor may advise you to stop breastfeeding until your treatment with Desquam-E is finished.

Recommended dosage

ADULTS AND CHILDREN 12 YEARS AND OVER

Gently rub Desquam-E gel into all affected areas once or twice a day. If you are fair-skinned or live in an excessively dry climate, you should probably start with one application a day. You can continue to use Desquam-E for as long as your doctor thinks it is necessary.

Overdosage

Overdosage of Desquam-E can result in excessive scaling of the skin, reddening skin, or swelling due to fluid retention. Any medication taken in excess can have serious consequences. If you suspect an overdose, seek medical attention.

DESYREL

Pronounced: DES-ee-rel
Generic name: Trazodone hydrochloride

Why is this drug prescribed?

Desyrel is prescribed for the treatment of depression.

Most important fact about this drug

Desyrel does not provide immediate relief. It may take up to 4 weeks before you begin to feel better, although most patients notice improvement within 2 weeks.

How should you take this medication?

Take Desyrel shortly after a meal or light snack. You may be more apt to feel dizzy or light-headed if you take the drug before you have eaten.

Desyrel may cause dry mouth. Sucking on a hard candy, chewing gum, or melting bits of ice in your mouth can relieve the problem.

■ *If you miss a dose...*
Take it as soon as you remember. If it is within 4 hours of your next dose, skip the one you missed and go back to your regular schedule. Never take 2 doses at once.

■ *Storage instructions...*
Store at room temperature in a tightly closed container, away from light and excessive heat.

What side effects may occur?

Side effects cannot be anticipated. If any develop or change in intensity, inform your doctor as soon as possible. Only your doctor can determine if it is safe for you to continue taking Desyrel.

■ *Side effects may include:*
Abdominal or stomach disorder, aches or pains in muscles and bones, anger or hostility, blurred vision, brief loss of consciousness, confusion, constipation, decreased appetite, diarrhea, dizziness or lightheadedness, drowsiness, dry mouth, excitement, fainting, fast or fluttery heartbeat, fatigue, fluid retention and swelling, headache, inability to fall or stay asleep, low blood pressure, nasal or sinus congestion, nausea, nervousness, nightmares or vivid dreams, tremors, uncoordinated movements, vomiting, weight gain or loss

Why should this drug not be prescribed?

If you are sensitive to or have ever had an allergic reaction to Desyrel or similar drugs, you should not take this medication. Make sure your doctor is aware of any drug reactions you have experienced.

Special warnings about this medication

In clinical studies, antidepressants increased the risk of suicidal thinking and behavior in children and adolescents with depression and other psychiatric disorders. Anyone considering the use of Desyrel or any other antidepressant in a child or adolescent must balance this risk with the clinical need. Desyrel has not been studied in children or adolescents and is not approved for treating anyone less than 18 years old.

Additionally, the progression of major depression is associated with a worsening of symptoms and/or the emergence of suicidal thinking or behavior in both adults and children, whether or not they are taking antidepressants. Individuals being treated with Desyrel and their caregivers should watch for any change in symptoms or any new symptoms that appear suddenly—especially agitation, anxiety, hostility, panic, restlessness, extreme hyperactivity, and suicidal thinking or behavior—and report them to the doctor immediately. Be especially observant at the beginning of treatment or whenever there is a change in dose.

Desyrel may cause you to become drowsy or less alert and may affect your judgment. Therefore, you should not drive or operate dangerous machinery or participate in any hazardous activity that requires full mental alertness until you know how this drug affects you.

Desyrel has been associated with priapism, a persistent, painful erection of the penis. Men who experience prolonged or inappropriate erections should stop taking this drug and consult their doctor.

Notify your doctor or dentist that you are taking this drug if you have a medical emergency, and before you have surgery or dental treatment. Your doctor will ask you to stop using the drug if you are going to have elective surgery.

Be careful taking this drug if you have heart disease. Desyrel can cause irregular heartbeats.

Possible food and drug interactions when taking this medication
Desyrel may intensify the effects of alcohol. Do not drink alcohol while taking this medication.

If Desyrel is taken with certain other drugs, the effects of either could be increased, decreased, or altered. It is especially important to check with your doctor before combining Desyrel with the following:

Antidepressant drugs known as MAO inhibitors, including Nardil and Parnate
Barbiturates such as Seconal
Central nervous system depressants such as Demerol and Halcion
Chlorpromazine
Digoxin (Lanoxin)
Drugs for high blood pressure such as Catapres and Wytensin
Other antidepressants such as Prozac and Norpramin
Phenytoin (Dilantin)
Warfarin (Coumadin)

Special information if you are pregnant or breastfeeding
The effects of Desyrel during pregnancy have not been adequately studied. If you are pregnant or planning to become pregnant, inform your doctor immediately. This medication may appear in breast milk. If treatment with this drug is essential to your health, your doctor may advise you to discontinue breastfeeding your baby until your treatment is finished.

Recommended dosage

ADULTS

The usual starting dosage is a total of 150 milligrams per day, divided into 2 or more smaller doses. Your doctor may increase your dose by 50 milligrams per day every 3 or 4 days. Total dosage should not exceed 400 milligrams per day, divided into smaller doses. Once you have responded well to the drug, your doctor may gradually reduce your dose. Because this medication makes you drowsy, your doctor may tell you to take the largest dose at bedtime.

Overdosage

Any medication taken in excess can have serious consequences. An overdose of Desyrel in combination with other drugs can be fatal. If you suspect an overdose, seek medical attention immediately.

■ *Symptoms of a Desyrel overdose may include:*
Breathing failure, drowsiness, irregular heartbeat, prolonged, painful erection, seizures, vomiting

DETROL

Pronounced: DEE-troll
Generic name: Tolterodine tartrate
Other brand name: Detrol LA

Why is this drug prescribed?

Detrol combats symptoms of overactive bladder, including frequent urination, urgency (increased need to urinate), and urge incontinence (inability to control urination). The drug works by blocking the nerve impulses that prompt the bladder to contract.

Most important fact about this drug

In a limited number of people, Detrol causes blurred vision. Take care when driving or operating machinery until you know how the drug affects you.

How should you take this medication?

Detrol can be taken with or without food. Swallow Detrol LA capsules whole.

■ *If you miss a dose...*
Take the forgotten dose as soon as you remember. If it is almost time for your next dose, skip the one you missed and go back to your regular schedule. Do not take 2 doses at once.
■ *Storage instructions...*
Store at room temperature.

What side effects may occur?

Side effects cannot be anticipated. If any develop or change in intensity, inform your doctor as soon as possible. Only your doctor can determine if it is safe for you to continue taking Detrol.

■ *Side effects may include:*
Abdominal pain, blurred vision, constipation, diarrhea, dizziness, drowsiness, dry eyes, dry mouth, fatigue, flu-like symptoms, headache, indigestion, vertigo

Why should this drug not be prescribed?

If you suffer from urinary retention (inability to urinate normally), gastric retention (a blockage in the digestive system), or uncontrolled narrow-angle glaucoma (high pressure in the eyes), you should not take Detrol. You should also avoid this drug if it gives you an allergic reaction.

Special warnings about this medication

Use Detrol with caution if you have a bladder obstruction or digestive disorder that could lead to a complete blockage. Use caution, too, if you are being successfully treated for glaucoma, or have a liver or kidney problem.

Possible food and drug interactions when taking this medication

If you take Detrol with certain other drugs, the effects of either could be increased, decreased, or altered. It is especially important to check with your doctor before combining Detrol with any of the following:

Clarithromycin (Biaxin)
Cyclosporine (Neoral, Sandimmune)
Erythromycin antibiotics such as Ery-Tab, Eryc, and PCE
Itraconazole (Sporanox)
Ketoconazole (Nizoral)
Miconazole
Vinblastine

Special information if you are pregnant or breastfeeding

The use of Detrol during pregnancy has not been adequately studied. If you are pregnant or plan to become pregnant while taking Detrol, tell your doctor immediately.

Researchers are not sure whether Detrol appears in breast milk. Use of the drug is not recommended while breastfeeding.

Recommended dosage

ADULTS

Detrol
The usual starting dosage is 2 milligrams twice a day. Your doctor may decrease the dose to 1 milligram twice a day if the higher dose causes problems. The 1-milligram dose is also recommended if you have liver problems or must take any of the drugs listed in *Possible food and drug interactions when taking this medication.*

Detrol LA
The usual starting dosage is 4 milligrams taken once a day. Your doctor may cut the dose in half if it causes problems. A dose of 2 milligrams once daily is recommended for people with liver problems and those taking drugs that might interact.

Overdosage
Any medication taken in excess can have serious consequences. If you suspect symptoms of an overdose with Detrol, seek medical attention immediately.

■ *Symptoms of Detrol overdose may include:*
Blurred vision, constipation, drowsiness, dry eyes, dry mouth

Dexamethasone *See Decadron Tablets, page 394.*

Dexamethasone with Neomycin *See Neodecadron Ophthalmic Ointment and Solution, page 927.*

DEXEDRINE
Pronounced: DEX-eh-dreen
Generic name: Dextroamphetamine sulfate

Why is this drug prescribed?
Dexedrine, a stimulant drug available in tablet or sustained-release capsule form, is prescribed to help treat the following conditions:

Narcolepsy (recurrent *sleep attacks*)
Attention Deficit Hyperactivity Disorder (the total treatment program should include social, psychological, and educational guidance along with Dexedrine)

Most important fact about this drug
Because it is a stimulant, this drug has high abuse potential. The stimulant effect may give way to a letdown period of depression and fatigue. Although the letdown can be relieved by taking another dose, this soon becomes a vicious circle.

If you habitually take Dexedrine in doses higher than recommended, or if you take it over a long period of time, you may eventually become dependent on the drug and suffer from withdrawal symptoms when it is unavailable.

How should you take this medication?
Take Dexedrine exactly as prescribed. If it is prescribed in tablet form, you may need up to 3 doses a day. Take the first dose when you wake up; take the next 1 or 2 doses at intervals of 4 to 6 hours. You can take the sustained-release capsules only once a day.

Do not take Dexedrine late in the day, since this could cause insomnia. If you experience insomnia or loss of appetite while taking this drug, notify your doctor; you may need a lower dosage.

It is likely that your doctor will periodically take you off Dexedrine to determine whether you still need it.

Do not chew or crush the sustained-release form, Dexedrine Spansules.

Do not increase the dosage, except on your doctor's advice.

Do not use Dexedrine to improve mental alertness or stay awake. Do not share it with others.

■ *If you miss a dose...*
If you take 1 dose a day, take it as soon as you remember, but not within 6 hours of going to bed. If you do not remember until the next day, skip the dose you missed and go back to your regular schedule.

If you take 2 or 3 doses a day, take the dose you missed if it is within an hour or so of the scheduled time. Otherwise, skip the dose and go back to your regular schedule. Never take 2 doses at once.

■ *Storage instructions...*
Store at room temperature in a tightly closed container, away from light.

What side effects may occur?
Side effects cannot be anticipated. If any develop or change in intensity, inform your doctor as soon as possible. Only your doctor can determine if it is safe for you to continue taking Dexedrine.

■ *Side effects may include:*
Excessive restlessness, overstimulation

■ *Effects of chronic heavy abuse of Dexedrine may include:*
Hyperactivity, irritability, personality changes, schizophrenia-like thoughts and behavior, severe insomnia, severe skin disease

Why should this drug not be prescribed?
Do not take Dexedrine if you are sensitive to or have ever had an allergic reaction to it.

Do not take Dexedrine for at least 14 days after taking a monoamine oxidase inhibitor (MAO inhibitor) such as the antidepressants Nardil and Parnate. Dexedrine and MAO inhibitors may interact to cause a sharp, potentially life-threatening rise in blood pressure.

Your doctor will not prescribe Dexedrine for you if you suffer from any of the following conditions:

Agitation
Cardiovascular disease
Glaucoma
Hardening of the arteries

High blood pressure
Overactive thyroid gland
Substance abuse

Special warnings about this medication

Be aware that one of the inactive ingredients in Dexedrine is a yellow food coloring called tartrazine (Yellow No. 5). In a few people, particularly those who are allergic to aspirin, tartrazine can cause a severe allergic reaction.

Dexedrine may impair judgment or coordination. Do not drive or operate dangerous machinery until you know how you react to the medication.

There is some concern that Dexedrine may stunt a child's growth. For the sake of safety, any child who takes Dexedrine should have his or her growth monitored.

Possible food and drug interactions when taking this medication

If Dexedrine is taken with certain foods or drugs, the effects of either could be increased, decreased, or altered. It is especially important to check with your doctor before combining Dexedrine with the following:

■ *Substances that dampen the effects of Dexedrine:*
  Ammonium chloride
  Chlorpromazine (Thorazine)
  Fruit juices
  Glutamic acid hydrochloride
  Guanethidine
  Haloperidol (Haldol)
  Lithium carbonate (Eskalith)
  Methenamine (Urised)
  Reserpine
  Sodium acid phosphate
  Vitamin C (as ascorbic acid)

■ *Substances that boost the effects of Dexedrine:*
  Acetazolamide (Diamox)
  MAO inhibitors such as Nardil and Parnate
  Propoxyphene (Darvon)
  Sodium bicarbonate (baking soda)
  Thiazide diuretics such as Diuril

■ *Substances that have decreased effect when taken
  with Dexedrine:*
  Antihistamines such as Benadryl
  Blood pressure medications such as Catapres, Hytrin, and Minipress
  Ethosuximide (Zarontin)
  Veratrum alkaloids (found in certain blood pressure drugs)

■ *Substances that have increased effect when taken with Dexedrine:*

Antidepressants such as Norpramin
Meperidine (Demerol)
Norepinephrine (Levophed)
Phenobarbital
Phenytoin (Dilantin)

Special information if you are pregnant or breastfeeding

If you are pregnant or plan to become pregnant, inform your doctor immediately. Babies born to women taking Dexedrine may be premature or have low birth weight. They may also be depressed, agitated, or apathetic due to withdrawal symptoms. Since Dexedrine appears in breast milk, it should not be taken by a nursing mother.

Recommended dosage

Take no more Dexedrine than your doctor prescribes. Intake should be kept to the lowest level that proves effective.

NARCOLEPSY

Adults
The usual dose is 5 to 60 milligrams per day, divided into smaller, equal doses.

Children
Narcolepsy seldom occurs in children under 12 years of age; however, when it does, Dexedrine may be used.

The suggested initial dose for children between 6 and 12 years of age is 5 milligrams per day. Your doctor may increase the daily dose in increments of 5 milligrams at weekly intervals until it becomes effective.

Children 12 years of age and older will be started with 10 milligrams daily. The daily dosage may be raised in increments of 10 milligrams at weekly intervals until effective. If side effects such as insomnia or loss of appetite appear, the dosage will probably be reduced.

ATTENTION DEFICIT HYPERACTIVITY DISORDER

This drug is not recommended for children under 3 years of age.

Children 3 to 5 Years Old
The usual starting dose is 2.5 milligrams daily, in tablet form. Your doctor may raise the daily dosage by 2.5 milligrams at weekly intervals until the drug becomes effective.

Children 6 Years and Older
The usual starting dose is 5 milligrams once or twice a day. Your doctor may raise the dose by 5 milligrams at weekly intervals until he or she is

satisfied with the response. Only in rare cases will the child take more than 40 milligrams per day.

Your child should take the first dose when he or she wakes up; the remaining 1 or 2 doses are taken at intervals of 4 to 6 hours. Alternatively, the doctor may prescribe *Spansule* capsules that are taken once a day. Your doctor may interrupt the schedule occasionally to see if behavioral symptoms come back enough to require continued therapy.

Overdosage

An overdose of Dexedrine can be fatal. If you suspect an overdose, seek medical attention immediately.

■ *Symptoms of an acute Dexedrine overdose may include:*
Abdominal cramps, assaultiveness, coma, confusion, convulsions, depression, diarrhea, fatigue, hallucinations, heightened reflexes, high fever, high or low blood pressure, irregular heartbeat, nausea, panic, rapid breathing, restlessness, tremor, vomiting

Dexmethylphenidate *See Focalin, page 596.*

Dextroamphetamine *See Dexedrine, page 427.*

DiaBeta *See Micronase, page 854.*

DIABINESE
Pronounced: dye-AB-in-eez
Generic name: Chlorpropamide

Why is this drug prescribed?

Diabinese is an oral antidiabetic medication used to treat type 2 (non-insulin-dependent) diabetes. Diabetes occurs when the body fails to produce enough insulin or is unable to use it properly. Insulin is believed to work by helping sugar penetrate the cell wall so it can be used by the cell.

There are two forms of diabetes: type 1, insulin-dependent, and type 2, non-insulin-dependent. Type 1 usually requires insulin injections for life, while type 2 diabetes can usually be treated by dietary changes and oral antidiabetic medications such as Diabinese. Apparently, Diabinese controls diabetes by stimulating the pancreas to secrete more insulin. Occasionally, type 2 diabetics must take insulin injections on a temporary basis, especially during stressful periods or times of illness.

Most important fact about this drug

Always remember that Diabinese is an aid to, not a substitute for, good diet and exercise. Failure to follow a sound diet and exercise plan can lead to serious complications, such as dangerously high or low blood sugar levels. Remember, too, that Diabinese is *not* an oral form of insulin, and cannot be used in place of insulin.

How should you take this medication?

Ordinarily, your doctor will ask you to take a single daily dose of Diabinese each morning with breakfast. However, if this upsets your stomach, he or she may ask you to take Diabinese in smaller doses throughout the day.

To prevent low blood sugar levels (hypoglycemia):

- You should understand the symptoms of hypoglycemia
- Know how exercise affects your blood sugar levels
- Maintain an adequate diet
- Keep a source of quick-acting sugar with you all the time

- *If you miss a dose...*
  Take it as soon as you remember. If it is almost time for the next dose, skip the one you missed and go back to your regular schedule. Do not take 2 doses at the same time.
- *Storage instructions...*
  Store at room temperature.

What side effects may occur?

Side effects cannot be anticipated. If any develop or change in intensity, inform your doctor as soon as possible. Only your doctor can determine if it is safe for you to continue taking Diabinese.

Side effects from Diabinese are rare and seldom require discontinuation of the medication.

- *More common side effects include:*
  Diarrhea, hunger, itching, loss of appetite, nausea, stomach upset, vomiting

Diabinese, like all oral antidiabetics, can cause hypoglycemia (low blood sugar). The risk of hypoglycemia is increased by missed meals, alcohol, other medications, and excessive exercise. To avoid hypoglycemia, closely follow the dietary and exercise regimen suggested by your physician.

- *Symptoms of mild hypoglycemia may include:*
  Cold sweat, drowsiness, fast heartbeat, headache, nausea, nervousness

- *Symptoms of more severe hypoglycemia may include:*
  Coma, pale skin, seizures, shallow breathing

Contact your doctor immediately if these symptoms of severe low blood sugar occur.

Why should this drug not be prescribed?

You should not take Diabinese if you have ever had an allergic reaction to it.

Do not take Diabinese if you are suffering from diabetic ketoacidosis (a life-threatening medical emergency caused by insufficient insulin and marked by excessive thirst, nausea, fatigue, pain below the breastbone, and a fruity breath).

Special warnings about this medication

It's possible that drugs such as Diabinese may lead to more heart problems than diet treatment alone, or diet plus insulin. If you have a heart condition, you may want to discuss this with your doctor.

If you are taking Diabinese, you should check your blood and urine periodically for the presence of abnormal sugar levels.

Remember that it is important that you closely follow the diet and exercise regimen established by your doctor.

Even people with well-controlled diabetes may find that stress, illness, surgery, or fever results in a loss of control. If this happens, your doctor may recommend that Diabinese be discontinued temporarily and insulin used instead.

In addition, the effectiveness of any oral antidiabetic, including Diabinese, may decrease with time. This may occur because of either a diminished responsiveness to the medication or a worsening of the diabetes.

Possible food and drug interactions when taking this medication

When you take Diabinese with certain other drugs, the effects of either could be increased, decreased, or altered. It is important that you consult with your doctor before taking Diabinese with the following:

Anabolic steroids
Aspirin in large doses
Barbiturates such as Seconal
Beta-blocking blood pressure medications such as Inderal and
    Tenormin
Calcium-blocking blood pressure medications such as Cardizem and
    Procardia
Chloramphenicol (Chloromycetin)
Coumarin (Coumadin)
Diuretics such as Diuril and HydroDIURIL
Epinephrine (EpiPen)
Estrogen medications such as Premarin
Isoniazid (Nydrazid)
Major tranquilizers such as Mellaril and Thorazine
MAO inhibitor–type antidepressants such as Nardil and Parnate
Nicotinic acid (Niacor, Niaspan)
Nonsteroidal anti-inflammatory agents such as Advil, Motrin,
    Naprosyn, and Nuprin
Oral contraceptives
Phenothiazines
Phenylbutazone
Phenytoin (Dilantin)

Probenecid (Benemid)
Steroids such as prednisone
Sulfa drugs such as Bactrim and Septra
Thyroid medications such as Synthroid

Avoid alcohol since excessive alcohol consumption can cause low blood sugar, breathlessness, and facial flushing.

Special information if you are pregnant or breastfeeding

The effects of Diabinese during pregnancy have not been adequately established. If you are pregnant or plan to become pregnant, you should inform your doctor immediately. Since studies suggest the importance of maintaining normal blood sugar (glucose) levels during pregnancy, your physician may prescribe injected insulin.

To minimize the risk of low blood sugar (hypoglycemia) in newborn babies, Diabinese, if prescribed during pregnancy, should be discontinued at least 1 month before the expected delivery date.

Since Diabinese appears in breast milk, it is not recommended for nursing mothers. If diet alone does not control glucose levels, then insulin should be considered.

Recommended dosage

Dosage levels are determined by each individual's needs.

ADULTS

Usually, an initial daily dose of 250 milligrams is recommended for stable, middle-aged, non-insulin-dependent diabetics. After 5 to 7 days, your doctor may adjust this dosage in increments of 50 to 125 milligrams every 3 to 5 days to achieve the best benefit. People with mild diabetes may respond well to daily doses of 100 milligrams or less of Diabinese, while those with severe diabetes may require 500 milligrams daily. Maintenance doses above 750 milligrams are not recommended.

OLDER ADULTS

People who are old, malnourished, or debilitated and those with impaired kidney and liver function usually take an initial dose of 100 to 125 milligrams.

CHILDREN

Safety and effectiveness have not been established.

Overdosage

An overdose of Diabinese can cause low blood sugar (see *What side effects may occur?* for symptoms).

Eating sugar or a sugar-based product will often correct the condition. If you suspect an overdose, seek medical attention immediately.

DIAMOX

Pronounced: DYE-uh-mocks
Generic name: Acetazolamide

Why is this drug prescribed?

Diamox controls fluid secretion. It is used in the treatment of glaucoma (excessive pressure in the eyes), epilepsy (for both brief and unlocalized seizures), and fluid retention due to congestive heart failure or drugs. It is also used to prevent or relieve the symptoms of acute mountain sickness in climbers attempting a rapid climb and those who feel sick even though they are making a gradual climb.

Most important fact about this drug

This drug is considered to be a sulfa drug because of its chemical properties. Although rare, severe reactions have been reported with sulfa drugs. If you develop a rash, bruises, sore throat, or fever, contact your doctor immediately.

How should you take this medication?

Take this medication exactly as prescribed by your doctor.

■ *If you miss a dose...*
Take it as soon as you remember. If it is almost time for your next dose, skip the one you missed and go back to your regular schedule. Never take 2 doses at the same time.

■ *Storage instructions...*
Store at room temperature.

What side effects may occur?

Side effects cannot be anticipated. If any develop or change in intensity, inform your doctor as soon as possible. Only your doctor can determine if it is safe for you to continue taking Diamox.

■ *Side effects may include:*
Change in taste, diarrhea, increase in amount or frequency of urination, loss of appetite, nausea, ringing in the ears, tingling or pins and needles in hands or feet, vomiting

Why should this drug not be prescribed?

Your doctor will not prescribe this medication for you if your sodium or potassium levels are low, or if you have kidney or liver disease, including cirrhosis.

Diamox should not be used as a long-term treatment for the type of glaucoma called chronic noncongestive angle-closure glaucoma.

Special warnings about this medication

Be very careful about taking high doses of aspirin if you are also taking Diamox. Effects of this combination can range from loss of appetite, sluggishness, and rapid breathing to unresponsiveness; the combination can be fatal.

If you have emphysema or other breathing disorders, use this drug with caution.

If you are taking Diamox to help in rapid ascent of a mountain, you must still come down promptly if you show signs of severe mountain sickness.

Possible food and drug interactions when taking this medication

If Diamox is taken with certain other drugs, the effects of either could be increased, decreased, or altered. It is especially important to check with your doctor before combining Diamox with the following:

Amitriptyline (Elavil)
Amphetamines such as Dexedrine
Aspirin
Cyclosporine (Sandimmune)
Lithium (Lithonate)
Methenamine (Urex)
Oral diabetes drugs such as Micronase
Quinidine (Quinidex)

Special information if you are pregnant or breastfeeding

The effects of Diamox during pregnancy have not been adequately studied. If you are pregnant or plan to become pregnant, inform your doctor immediately. Diamox may appear in breast milk and could affect a nursing infant. If this medication is essential to your health, your doctor may advise you to discontinue breastfeeding until your treatment with Diamox is finished.

Recommended dosage

ADULTS

This medication is available in both oral and injectable form. Dosages are for the oral form only.

Glaucoma

This medication is used as an addition to regular glaucoma treatment. Dosages for open-angle glaucoma range from 250 milligrams to 1 gram per 24 hours in 2 or more smaller doses. Your doctor will supervise your dosage and watch the effect of this medication carefully if you are using it for glaucoma. In secondary glaucoma and before surgery in acute congestive (closed-angle) glaucoma, the usual dosage is 250 milligrams every 4 hours or, in some cases, 250 milligrams twice a day. Some people may take 500 milligrams to start, and then 125 or 250 milligrams every 4 hours. The injectable form of this drug is occasionally used in acute cases.

The usual dosage of Diamox Sequels (sustained-release capsules) is 1 capsule (500 milligrams) twice a day, usually in the morning and evening.

Your doctor may adjust the dosage, as needed.

Epilepsy
The daily dosage is 8 to 30 milligrams per 2.2 pounds of body weight in 2 or more doses. Typical dosage may range from 375 to 1,000 milligrams per day. Your doctor will adjust the dosage to suit your needs; Diamox can be used with other anticonvulsant medication.

Congestive Heart Failure
The usual starting dosage to reduce fluid retention in people with congestive heart failure is 250 to 375 milligrams per day or 5 milligrams per 2.2 pounds of body weight, taken in the morning. Diamox works best when it is taken every other day—or 2 days on, 1 day off—for this condition.

Edema Due to Medication
The usual dose is 250 to 375 milligrams daily for 1 or 2 days, alternating with a day of rest.

Acute Mountain Sickness
The usual dose is 500 to 1,000 milligrams a day in 2 or more doses, using either tablets or sustained-release capsules. Doses of this medication are often begun 1 or 2 days before attempting to reach high altitudes.

CHILDREN

The safety and effectiveness of Diamox in children have not been established. However, doses of 8 to 30 milligrams per 2.2 pounds of body weight have been used in children with various forms of epilepsy.

Overdosage
There is no specific information available on Diamox overdose, but any medication taken in excess can have serious consequences. If you suspect an overdose, seek medical attention immediately.

Diazepam See Valium, page 1543.

Diclofenac See Voltaren, page 1579.

Diclofenac with Misoprostol See Arthrotec, page 129.

Dicyclomine See Bentyl, page 201.

Didanosine See Videx, page 1563.

Diethylpropion See Tenuate, page 1408.

DIFFERIN

Pronounced: DIFF-er-in
Generic name: Adapalene

Why is this drug prescribed?

Differin is prescribed for the treatment of acne.

Most important fact about this drug

Differin makes your skin more sensitive to sunlight. While using this product, keep your exposure to the sun at a minimum, and protect yourself with sunscreen and clothing. Never apply Differin to sunburned skin.

How should you use this medication?

Differin should be applied once a day at bedtime. Wash the affected areas, then apply a thin layer of the gel. Avoid eyes, lips, mouth, and nostrils. If you are using a single-use pledget, remove it from the foil just before using, and discard it after applying the medication. Do not use if the seal is broken.

Use Differin exactly as prescribed. Applying excessive amounts or using the gel more than once a day will not produce better results and may cause severe redness, peeling, and discomfort.

■ *If you miss a dose...*
Don't try to make it up. Simply return to your regular schedule on the following day.
■ *Storage instructions...*
Store at room temperature.

What side effects may occur?

Side effects cannot be anticipated. If any develop or change in intensity, inform your doctor as soon as possible. Only your doctor can determine if it is safe for you to continue using Differin.

Side effects are most likely to occur during the first 2 to 4 weeks and usually diminish with continued treatment. If side effects are severe, your doctor may advise you to reduce the frequency of use or discontinue the drug entirely. Side effects disappear when the drug is stopped.

■ *Side effects may include...*
Acne flare-ups, burning, dryness, irritation, itching, redness, scaling, stinging, sunburn

Why should this drug not be prescribed?

Do not use Differin if you are sensitive to adapalene or any other components of the gel.

Special warnings about this medication

If you have an allergic reaction or severe irritation, stop using the medication and call your doctor.

Remember that Differin increases sensitivity to sunlight. Take measures to protect yourself from overexposure. Wind and cold weather may also be irritating.

Do not apply Differin to cuts, abrasions, eczema, or sunburned skin.

In the first few weeks of treatment, your acne may actually seem to get worse. This just means the medication is working on hidden acne sores. Continue using the product. It can take as much as 8 to 12 weeks before you start to see improvement in your condition.

Differin has not been tested for children under 12 years old.

Possible food and drug interactions when using this medication

Avoid using Differin with any other product that can irritate the skin, such as medicated soaps and cleansers, soaps and cosmetics that have a strong drying effect, and products with high concentrations of alcohol, astringents, spices, and lime.

Special caution is necessary if you have used, or are currently using, any skin product containing sulfur, resorcinol, or salicylic acid. Do not use such a product with Differin. If you have used one of these products recently, do not begin Differin treatment until the effects of the other product have subsided.

Special information if you are pregnant or breastfeeding

The effects of Differin during pregnancy and breastfeeding have not been adequately studied. If you are pregnant or plan to become pregnant, notify your doctor immediately. It is not known whether Differin appears in breast milk. If you are nursing and need to use Differin, your doctor may advise you to discontinue breastfeeding while using the medication.

Recommended dosage

The usual dose is a thin film applied over the acne-affected area just before bedtime.

Overdosage

Any medication taken in excess can have serious consequences. Overuse of Differin can cause redness, peeling, and discomfort. If you suspect an overdose, check with your doctor immediately.

Diflorasone *See Psorcon, page 1200.*

DIFLUCAN

Pronounced: Dye-FLEW-can
Generic name: Fluconazole

Why is this drug prescribed?

Diflucan is used to treat fungal infections called candidiasis (also known as thrush or yeast infections). These include vaginal infections, throat infections, and fungal infections elsewhere in the body, such as infections of the urinary tract, peritonitis (inflammation of the lining of the abdomen), and pneumonia. Diflucan is also prescribed to guard against candidiasis in some people receiving bone marrow transplants, and is used to treat meningitis (brain or spinal cord inflammation) caused by another type of fungus.

In addition, Diflucan is now being prescribed for fungal infections in kidney and liver transplant patients, and fungal infections in patients with AIDS.

Most important fact about this drug

Strong allergic reactions to Diflucan, although rare, have been reported. Symptoms may include hives, itching, swelling, sudden drop in blood pressure, difficulty breathing or swallowing, diarrhea, or abdominal pain. If you experience any of these symptoms, notify your doctor immediately.

How should you take this medication?

You can take Diflucan with or without meals.

Take this medication exactly as prescribed, and continue taking it for as long as your doctor instructs. You may begin to feel better after the first few days; but it takes weeks or even months of treatment to completely cure certain fungal infections.

■ *If you miss a dose...*
Take the forgotten dose as soon as you remember. However, if it is almost time for your next dose, skip the one you missed and return to your regular schedule. Do not take double doses.
■ *Storage instructions...*
Diflucan tablets should be stored at normal room temperature. Avoid exposing them to temperatures above 86 degrees Fahrenheit.

What side effects may occur?

Side effects cannot be anticipated. If any develop or change in intensity, inform your doctor as soon as possible. Only your doctor can determine if it is safe for you to continue taking Diflucan.

The most common side effect for people taking more than one dose is nausea.

For women taking a single dose to treat vaginal infection, the most common side effects are abdominal pain, diarrhea, headache, and nausea; changes in taste, dizziness, and indigestion may occur less often.

■ *Other side effects may include:*
Abdominal pain, diarrhea, headache, irregular heartbeat, skin rash, vomiting

Why should this drug not be prescribed?

Do not take Diflucan if you are sensitive to any of its ingredients or have ever had an allergic reaction to similar drugs, such as Nizoral. Make sure your doctor is aware of any drug reactions you have experienced.

Avoid combining Diflucan with the heartburn medication Propulsid. The combination has been known to trigger heartbeat irregularities and other cardiac problems.

Special warnings about this medication

Your doctor will watch your liver function carefully while you are taking Diflucan.

If your immunity is low and you develop a rash, your doctor should monitor your condition closely. You may have to stop taking Diflucan if the rash gets worse.

In a small group of patients, drugs similar to Diflucan have caused irregular heartbeats. If you develop such symptoms while taking Diflucan, contact your doctor.

Possible food and drug interactions when taking this medication

If Diflucan is taken with certain other drugs, the effects of either could be increased, decreased, or altered. It is especially important to check with your doctor before combining Diflucan with the following:

Antidiabetic drugs such as Orinase, DiaBeta, and Glucotrol
Astemizole (Hismanal)
Blood-thinning drugs such as Coumadin
Cisapride (Propulsid)
Cyclosporine (Sandimmune, Neoral)
Hydrochlorothiazide (HydroDIURIL)
Phenytoin (Dilantin)
Rifabutin (Mycobutin)
Rifampin (Rifadin)
Tacrolimus (Prograf)
Terfenadine (Seldane)
Theophylline (Theo-Dur)
Ulcer medications such as Tagamet

Special information if you are pregnant or breastfeeding

The effects of Diflucan during pregnancy have not been adequately studied. If you are pregnant or plan to become pregnant, inform your doctor immediately. Diflucan appears in breast milk and could affect a nursing infant. If this medication is essential to your health, your doctor may advise you to stop breastfeeding until your treatment with Diflucan is finished.

Recommended dosage

ADULTS

Vaginal Infections
The usual treatment is a single 150-milligram dose.

Throat Infections
The usual dose for candidiasis of the mouth and throat is 200 milligrams on the first day, followed by 100 milligrams once a day. You should see results in a few days, but treatment should continue for at least 2 weeks to avoid a relapse. For candidiasis of the esophagus (gullet), the usual dose is 200 milligrams on the first day, followed by 100 milligrams once a day. A dose of 400 milligrams a day can also be taken if your infection is more severe. Treatment should continue for a minimum of 3 weeks and for at least 2 weeks after symptoms have stopped.

Systemic (Bodywide) Infections
Doses of up to 400 milligrams per day are sometimes prescribed.

Urinary Infections and Peritonitis
Doses range from 50 to 200 milligrams per day.

Cryptococcal Meningitis
The usual dose is 400 milligrams on the first day, followed by 200 milligrams once a day. Treatment should continue for 10 to 12 weeks once tests of spinal fluid come back negative. For AIDS patients, a 200-milligram dose taken once a day is recommended to prevent relapse.

Prevention of Candidiasis During Bone Marrow Transplantation
The usual dose is 400 milligrams once a day.

If you have kidney disease, your doctor may have to reduce your dosage.

CHILDREN

Throat Infections
The usual dose for candidiasis of the mouth and throat is 6 milligrams for each 2.2 pounds of the child's weight on the first day, and 3 milligrams per 2.2 pounds once a day after that.
   The duration of treatment is the same as that for adults.

Yeast Infections of the Esophagus
Candidiasis in the upper digestive canal is usually treated with a dose of 6 milligrams per 2.2 pounds of body weight on the first day, and half that

amount once daily thereafter. Daily doses of up to 12 milligrams per 2.2 pounds of body weight are sometimes prescribed.

Systemic (Bodywide) Infections
The drug has been given at 6 to 12 milligrams per 2.2 pounds of weight per day.

Cryptococcal Meningitis
The usual dose is 12 milligrams per 2.2 pounds of body weight per day on the first day, and 6 milligrams per 2.2 pounds per day after that. Treatment will last 10 to 12 weeks after the fungus disappears.

Overdosage
Any medication taken in excess can have serious consequences. If you suspect an overdose, seek medical treatment immediately.

■ *Symptoms of Diflucan overdose may include:*
Hallucinations, paranoia

Diflunisal *See Dolobid, page 466.*

Digitek *See Lanoxin, page 725.*

Digoxin *See Lanoxin, page 725.*

Dihydrocodeine, Aspirin, and Caffeine *See Synalgos-DC, page 1369.*

Dihydroergotamine *See Migranal, page 859.*

Dilacor XR *See Cardizem, page 249.*

DILANTIN
Pronounced: dye-LAN-tin
Generic name: Phenytoin sodium

Why is this drug prescribed?
Dilantin is an antiepileptic drug, prescribed to control grand mal seizures (a type of seizure in which the individual experiences a sudden loss of consciousness immediately followed by generalized convulsions) and temporal lobe seizures (a type of seizure caused by disease in the cortex of the temporal [side] lobe of the brain affecting smell, taste, sight, hearing, memory, and movement).

Dilantin may also be used to prevent and treat seizures occurring during and after neurosurgery (surgery of the brain and spinal cord).

Most important fact about this drug
If you have been taking Dilantin regularly, do not stop abruptly. This may precipitate prolonged or repeated epileptic seizures without any recovery

of consciousness between attacks—a condition called status epilepticus that can be fatal if not treated promptly.

How should you take this medication?

It is important that you strictly follow the prescribed dosage regimen and tell your doctor about any condition that makes it impossible for you to take Dilantin as prescribed.

If you are given Dilantin Oral Suspension, shake it well before using. Use the specially marked measuring spoon, a plastic syringe, or a small measuring cup to measure each dose accurately.

Swallow Dilantin Kapseals whole. Dilantin Infatabs can be either chewed thoroughly and then swallowed, or swallowed whole. The Infatabs are not to be used for once-a-day dosing.

Do not change from one form of Dilantin to another without consulting your doctor. Different products may not work the same way.

Depending on the type of seizure disorder, your doctor may give you another drug with Dilantin.

■ *If you miss a dose...*
If you take 1 dose a day, take the dose you missed as soon as you remember. If you do not remember until the next day, skip the missed dose and go back to your regular schedule. Do not take 2 doses at once.

If you take more than 1 dose a day, take the missed dose as soon as possible. If it is within 4 hours of your next dose, skip the one you missed and go back to your regular schedule. Do not take 2 doses at once.

If you forget to take your medication 2 or more days in a row, check with your doctor.

■ *Storage instructions...*
Store at room temperature away from light and moisture.

What side effects may occur?

Side effects cannot be anticipated. If any develop or change in intensity, inform your doctor as soon as possible. Only your doctor can determine whether it is safe for you to continue taking Dilantin.

■ *Side effects may include:*
Decreased coordination, involuntary eye movement, mental confusion, slurred speech

Why should this drug not be prescribed?

If you have ever had an allergic reaction to or are sensitive to phenytoin or similar epilepsy medications such as Peganone or Mesantoin, do not take Dilantin. Make sure your doctor is aware of any drug reactions you have experienced.

Special warnings about this medication

Tell your doctor if you develop a skin rash. If the rash is scale-like, characterized by reddish or purplish spots, or consists of (fluid-filled) blisters, your doctor may stop Dilantin and prescribe an alternative treatment. If the rash is more like measles, your doctor may have you stop taking Dilantin until the rash is completely gone.

Because Dilantin is processed by the liver, people with impaired liver function, older adults, and those who are seriously ill may show early signs of drug poisoning.

Practicing good dental hygiene minimizes the development of gingival hyperplasia (excessive formation of the gums over the teeth) and its complications.

Avoid drinking alcoholic beverages while taking Dilantin.

Possible food and drug interactions when taking this medication

If Dilantin is taken with certain other drugs, the effects of either could be increased, decreased, or altered. It is especially important to check with your doctor before combining Dilantin with the following:

Alcohol
Amiodarone (Cordarone)
Antacids containing calcium
Blood-thinning drugs such as Coumadin
Chloramphenicol (Chloromycetin)
Chlordiazepoxide (Librium)
Cimetidine (Tagamet)
Diazepam (Valium)
Dicumarol
Digitoxin (Crystodigin)
Disulfiram (Antabuse)
Doxycycline (Vibramycin)
Estrogens such as Premarin
Ethosuximide (Zarontin)
Felbamate (Felbatol)
Fluoxetine (Prozac)
Furosemide (Lasix)
Isoniazid (Nydrazid)
Major tranquilizers such as Mellaril and Thorazine
Methylphenidate (Ritalin)
Molindone hydrochloride (Moban)
Oral contraceptives
Paroxetine (Paxil)
Phenobarbital
Quinidine (Quinidex)
Reserpine (Diupres)
Rifampin (Rifadin)

Salicylates such as aspirin

Seizure medications such as Depakene, Depakote, Tegretol, and Zarontin

Steroid drugs such as prednisone (Deltasone)

Sucralfate (Carafate)

Sulfa drugs such as Gantrisin

Theophylline (Theo-Dur, others)

Ticlopidine (Ticlid)

Tolbutamide (Orinase)

Trazodone (Desyrel)

Ulcer medications such as Tagamet and Zantac

Tricyclic antidepressants (such as Elavil, Norpramin, and others) may cause seizures in susceptible people, making a dosage adjustment of Dilantin necessary.

Hyperglycemia (high blood sugar) may occur in people taking Dilantin, which blocks the release of insulin. People with diabetes may experience increased blood sugar levels due to Dilantin.

Abnormal softening of the bones may occur in people taking Dilantin because of Dilantin's interference with vitamin D metabolism.

Special information if you are pregnant or breastfeeding

If you are pregnant or plan to become pregnant, inform your doctor immediately. Because of the possibility of birth defects with antiepileptic drugs such as Dilantin, you may need to discontinue the drug. Do not, however, stop taking it without first consulting your doctor. Dilantin appears in breast milk; breastfeeding is not recommended during treatment with this drug.

Recommended dosage

Dosage is tailored to each individual's needs. Your doctor will monitor blood levels of the drug closely, particularly when switching you from one drug to another.

ADULTS

Standard Daily Dosage

If you have not had any previous treatment, your doctor will have you take one 100-milligram Dilantin capsule 3 times daily to start.

On a continuing basis, most adults need 1 capsule 3 to 4 times a day. Your doctor may increase that dosage to 2 capsules 3 times a day, if necessary.

Once-a-Day Dosage

If your seizures are controlled on 100-milligram Dilantin capsules 3 times daily, your doctor may allow you to take the entire 300 milligrams as a single dose once daily.

CHILDREN

The starting dose is 5 milligrams per 2.2 pounds of body weight per day, divided into 2 or 3 equal doses; the most a child should take is 300 milligrams a day. The regular daily dosage is usually 4 to 8 milligrams per 2.2 pounds. Children over 6 years of age and adolescents may need the minimum adult dose (300 milligrams per day).

Overdosage

An overdose of Dilantin can be fatal. If you suspect an overdose, seek medical attention immediately.

■ *Symptoms of Dilantin overdose may include:*
Coma, difficulty in pronouncing words correctly, involuntary eye movement, lack of muscle coordination, low blood pressure, nausea, sluggishness, slurred speech, tremors, vomiting

DILAUDID

Pronounced: Dye-LAW-did
Generic name: Hydromorphone hydrochloride

Why is this drug prescribed?

Dilaudid, a narcotic analgesic, is prescribed for the relief of moderate to severe pain such as that due to:

Biliary colic (pain caused by an obstruction in the gallbladder or
    bile duct)
Burns
Cancer
Heart attack
Injury (soft tissue and bone)
Renal colic (sharp lower back and groin pain usually caused by the
    passage of a stone through the ureter)
Surgery

Most important fact about this drug

High dose tolerance leading to mental and physical dependence can occur with the use of Dilaudid when it is taken repeatedly. Physical dependence (need for continual doses to prevent withdrawal symptoms) can occur after only a few days of narcotic use, although it usually takes several weeks.

How should you take this medication?

Take Dilaudid exactly as prescribed by your doctor. Never increase the amount you take without your doctor's approval.

■ *If you miss a dose...*
Take the forgotten dose as soon as you remember. If it is almost time for the next dose, skip the one you missed and go back to your regular schedule. Never try to catch up by doubling the dose.

■ *Storage instructions...*
Tablets and liquid should be stored at room temperature. Protect from light and extreme cold or heat. Suppositories should be stored in the refrigerator.

What side effects may occur?

Side effects cannot be anticipated. If any develop or change in intensity, inform your doctor as soon as possible. Only your doctor can determine if it is safe for you to continue taking Dilaudid.

■ *Side effects may include:*
Anxiety, constipation, dizziness, drowsiness, fear, impairment of mental and physical performance, inability to urinate, mental clouding, mood changes, nausea, restlessness, sedation, sluggishness, troubled and slowed breathing, vomiting

Why should this drug not be prescribed?

If you are sensitive to or have ever had an allergic reaction to Dilaudid or narcotic painkillers, you should not take this medication. Make sure that your doctor is aware of any drug reactions that you have experienced.

Additionally, you should not take Dilaudid if you suffer from severe, uncontrolled breathing difficulties or uncontrolled asthma.

Dilaudid cannot be used by pregnant women during labor or delivery.

Special warnings about this medication

Do not stop taking this medication without your doctor's approval. Abruptly stopping Dilaudid could cause withdrawal symptoms within the first 24 hours, including restlessness, tearing or watery eyes, dilated pupils, runny nose, yawning, sweating, goosebumps, and restless sleep. These symptoms could increase during the next 72 hours, and new withdrawal symptoms may appear, including irritability, anxiety, weakness, muscle spasms, severe backache, stomach or leg pain, insomnia, vomiting, and diarrhea.

Dilaudid may impair the mental and/or physical abilities required for the performance of potentially hazardous tasks such as driving a car or operating machinery.

Dilaudid should be used with caution if you are in a weakened condition or if you have a severe liver or kidney disorder, hypothyroidism (underactive thyroid gland), Addison's disease (adrenal gland failure), severe lung problems, an enlarged prostate, a urethral stricture (narrowing of the urethra), low blood pressure, or a head injury.

It's important to tell the doctor if you've ever suffered from alcoholism or other drug dependencies. Abusing Dilaudid, or combining it with other nervous system depressants, can cause serious—and possibly life-threatening—side effects.

Dilaudid suppresses the cough reflex; therefore, the doctor will be cautious about prescribing Dilaudid after an operation or for patients with a lung disease.

High doses of Dilaudid may produce labored or slowed breathing. This drug also affects centers that control breathing rhythm and may produce irregular breathing. People who already have breathing difficulties should be very careful about taking Dilaudid. Be especially cautious if you have chronic obstructive pulmonary disease or a condition that reduces oxygen to the tissues (hypoxia) or causes an excess of carbon dioxide in the blood (hypercapnia).

Let the doctor know if you're scheduled to have any surgical procedures involving the biliary tract, since Dilaudid could increase the chance of muscle spasms in this area.

Narcotics such as Dilaudid may mask or hide the symptoms of sudden or severe abdominal conditions, making diagnosis and treatment difficult.

Dilaudid can cause seizures when taken in high doses and, if you have a seizure disorder, can make the seizures worse.

Be sure to tell the doctor if you're sensitive to sulfites (preservatives commonly found in red wine), since Dilaudid contains these substances.

Possible food and drug interactions when taking this medication
Dilaudid is a central nervous system depressant and intensifies the effects of alcohol. Do not drink alcohol while taking this medication.

If Dilaudid is taken with certain other drugs, the effects of either could be increased, decreased, or altered. It is especially important to check with your doctor before combining Dilaudid with the following:

Antiemetics (drugs that prevent or lessen nausea and vomiting such as Compazine and Phenergan)
Antihistamines such as Benadryl
General anesthetics
Opioid antagonists such as naloxone (Narcan) and nelmefene (Revex)
Other central nervous system depressants such as Nembutal, Restoril
Other narcotic analgesics such as Demerol and Percocet
Phenothiazines such as Thorazine
Sedative/hypnotics such as Valium, Halcion
Tranquilizers such as Xanax
Tricyclic antidepressants such as Elavil and Tofranil

Special information if you are pregnant or breastfeeding

Do not take Dilaudid if you are pregnant or plan to become pregnant unless you are directed to do so by your doctor. Drug dependence occurs in newborns when the mother has taken narcotic drugs regularly during pregnancy. Withdrawal signs include irritability and excessive crying, tremors, overactive reflexes, increased breathing rate, increased stools, sneezing, yawning, vomiting, and fever. Dilaudid may appear in breast milk and could affect a nursing infant. If this medication is essential to your health, your doctor may advise you to discontinue breastfeeding your baby until your treatment is finished.

Recommended dosage

ADULTS

Tablets

The usual starting dose of Dilaudid tablets is 2 to 4 milligrams every 4 to 6 hours as determined by your doctor. Severity of pain, your individual response, and your size are used to determine your exact dosage.

Liquid

The usual dose of Dilaudid liquid is one-half to 2 teaspoonfuls every 3 to 6 hours. In some cases, the dosage may be higher.

Suppositories

Dilaudid suppositories (3 milligrams) may provide relief for a longer period of time. The usual adult dose is 1 suppository inserted rectally every 6 to 8 hours or as directed by your doctor.

CHILDREN

The safety and effectiveness of Dilaudid have not been established in children.

OLDER ADULTS

Be very careful when using Dilaudid. Your doctor will prescribe a dose individualized to suit your needs.

Overdosage

■ *Symptoms of Dilaudid overdose include:*
  Bluish tinge to the skin, cold and clammy skin, constricted pupils, coma, extreme sleepiness progressing to a state of unresponsiveness, labored or slowed breathing, limp, weak muscles, low blood pressure, slow heart rate

In severe overdosage, the patient may stop breathing. Shock, heart attack, and death can occur.

If you suspect an overdose, seek emergency medical treatment immediately.

Diltiazem *See Cardizem, page 249.*

DIOVAN
Pronounced: DYE-oh-van
Generic name: Valsartan
Other brand name: Diovan HCT

Why is this drug prescribed?
Diovan is one of a new class of blood pressure medications called angiotensin II receptor antagonists. Diovan works by preventing the hormone angiotensin II from narrowing the blood vessels, which tends to raise blood pressure. Diovan may be prescribed alone or with other blood pressure medications, such as diuretics that help the body get rid of excess water. Diovan HCT provides just such a combination. It contains Diovan plus the common diuretic hydrochlorothiazide.

Diovan also has a stimulative effect on the heart and is prescribed for heart failure in patients who can't tolerate another type of medication called ACE inhibitors.

Most important fact about this drug
You must take Diovan regularly for it to be effective. Since blood pressure declines gradually, it may be several weeks before you get the full benefit of Diovan, and you must continue taking it even if you are feeling well. Diovan does not cure high blood pressure; it merely keeps it under control.

How should you take this medication?
Diovan and Diovan HCT can be taken with or without food. Try to get into the habit of taking the medicine at the same time each day—for example, before or after breakfast. You'll be less likely to forget your dose.

■ *If you miss a dose...*
Take it as soon as possible. If it is almost time for your next dose, skip the one you missed and go back to your regular schedule. Never take 2 doses at the same time.
■ *Storage instructions...*
Store at room temperature. Keep in a tightly closed container, away from moisture.

What side effects may occur?
Side effects cannot be anticipated. If any develop or change in intensity, tell your doctor as soon as possible. Only your doctor can determine if it is safe for you to continue taking Diovan or Diovan HCT.

■ *Side effects may include:*
Abdominal pain, allergic reactions, back pain, blurred vision, cough, diarrhea, dizziness, fainting, fatigue, headache, joint pain, low blood pressure, nausea, runny nose, sinus inflammation, sore throat, swelling, swollen mouth and throat, upper respiratory infections, vertigo, viral infections

Why should this drug not be prescribed?
Do not take Diovan or Diovan HCT while pregnant. Avoid both drugs if they cause an allergic reaction, and do not take Diovan HCT if you have ever had an allergic reaction to a sulfa drug such as Bactrim or Septra. Also avoid Diovan HCT if you have trouble urinating.

Special warnings about this medication
In rare cases, Diovan and Diovan HCT can cause a severe drop in blood pressure. The problem is more likely if your body's supply of water has been depleted by high doses of diuretics. Symptoms include lightheadedness or faintness, and are more likely when you first start taking the drug. Diovan HCT can also cause dry mouth, weakness, drowsiness, muscle cramps, nausea, and vomiting. Call your doctor if any of these symptoms occurs. You may need to have your dosage adjusted.

Use Diovan HCT with caution if you have a history of allergy or bronchial asthma, or suffer from the condition called lupus erythematosus. Report a rapid or irregular pulse to your doctor.

If you have liver or kidney disease, Diovan and Diovan HCT must be used with caution. Be sure the doctor is aware of either problem. Also let the doctor know if you suffer from gout or diabetes.

The safety and effectiveness of Diovan and Diovan HCT have not been studied in children.

Possible food and drug interactions when taking this medication
Check with your doctor before combining Diovan with salt substitutes that contain potassium, or with diuretics that leave potassium in the body, including the following:

Amiloride (Midamor)
Spironolactone (Aldactone)
Triamterene (Dyrenium)

The hydrochlorothiazide in Diovan HCT may interact with a variety of drugs. Be sure to check with your doctor before combining Diovan HCT with the following:

Alcohol
Cholestyramine (Questran)
Colestipol (Colestid)
Corticosteroids such as hydrocortisone and prednisone

Glipizide (Glucotrol)
Glyburide (Diabeta, Micronase)
Insulin
Lithium (Lithobid, Lithonate)
Nonsteroidal anti-inflammatory drugs such as Advil, Aleve, Motrin, and Naprosyn
Other blood pressure medications such as Cardizem, Lopressor, and Procardia
Phenobarbital
Narcotic drugs such as morphine or codeine products

Special information if you are pregnant or breastfeeding

Drugs such as Diovan and Diovan HCT can cause injury or even death to the unborn child when used during the last 6 months of pregnancy. As soon as you find out that you're pregnant, stop taking the drug and call your doctor. Both of these drugs may also appear in breast milk and could affect the nursing infant. If the medication is essential to your health, your doctor may advise you to avoid breastfeeding while you are taking Diovan or Diovan HCT.

Recommended dosage

DIOVAN

High Blood Pressure

The usual starting dose is 80 or 160 milligrams or more once a day. If your blood pressure does not go down, your doctor may increase the dose or add a diuretic to your regimen. The maximum recommended dose is 320 milligrams a day.

Heart Failure

The usual starting dose is 40 milligrams taken twice a day. The doctor may increase the dose to 80 or 160 milligrams twice daily depending on your tolerance for the drug. The maximum dose is 320 milligrams daily.

DIOVAN HCT

The usual starting dose when switching from Diovan to Diovan HCT is one 80-milligram/12.5-milligram or one 160-milligram/12.5-milligram tablet daily. Daily dosage may be increased to a maximum of 160 milligrams of valsartan and 25 milligrams of hydrochlorothiazide.

Overdosage

There has been little experience with overdosage. However, the most likely results would be extremely low blood pressure and an abnormally slow or rapid heartbeat. If you suspect an overdose, seek medical attention immediately.

Diovan HCT *See Diovan, page 451.*

DIPENTUM
Pronounced: dye-PENT-um
Generic name: Olsalazine sodium

Why is this drug prescribed?
Dipentum is an anti-inflammatory drug used to maintain long-term freedom from symptoms of ulcerative colitis (chronic inflammation and ulceration of the large intestine and rectum). It is prescribed for people who cannot take sulfasalazine (Azulfidine).

Most important fact about this drug
If you have kidney disease, Dipentum could cause further damage. You'll need regular checks on your kidney function, so be sure to keep all regular appointments with your doctor.

How should you take this medication?
Take Dipentum for as long as your doctor has directed, even if you feel better.

Take Dipentum with food.

◼ *If you miss a dose...*
Take it as soon as you remember. If it is almost time for your next dose, skip the one you missed and go back to your regular schedule. Do not take 2 doses at once.

◼ *Storage instructions...*
Store at room temperature.

What side effects may occur?
Side effects cannot be anticipated. If any develop or change in intensity, inform your doctor as soon as possible. Only your doctor can determine if it is safe for you to continue taking Dipentum.

◼ *Side effects may include:*
Diarrhea or loose stools

Rare cases of hepatitis have been reported in people taking Dipentum. Symptoms may include aching muscles, chills, fever, headache, joint pain, loss of appetite, vomiting, and yellowish skin.

Why should this drug not be prescribed?
You should not use Dipentum if you are allergic to salicylates such as aspirin.

Special warnings about this medication
If diarrhea occurs, contact your doctor.

Possible food and drug interactions when taking this medication
If Dipentum is taken with certain other drugs, the effects of either could be increased, decreased, or altered. It is especially important to check with your doctor before combining Dipentum with warfarin (Coumadin).

Special information if you are pregnant or breastfeeding
The effects of Dipentum in pregnancy have not been adequately studied. Pregnant women should use Dipentum only if the possible gains warrant the possible risks to the unborn child. Women who breastfeed an infant should use Dipentum cautiously, because it is not known whether this drug appears in breast milk and what effect it might have on a nursing infant.

Recommended dosage

ADULTS

The usual dose is a total of 1 gram per day, divided into 2 equal doses.

CHILDREN

The safety and effectiveness of Dipentum have not been established in children.

Overdosage
There have been no reports of Dipentum overdose. However, should you suspect one, seek medical help immediately.

Diphenoxylate with Atropine *See Lomotil, page 769.*

Dipivefrin *See Propine, page 1176.*

DIPROLENE

Pronounced: dye-PROH-leen
Generic name: Betamethasone dipropionate
Other brand names: Diprosone

Why is this drug prescribed?
Diprolene, a synthetic cortisone-like steroid available in cream, gel, lotion, or ointment form, is used to treat certain itchy rashes and other inflammatory skin conditions. Its sister product Diprosone is available only as a cream.

Most important fact about this drug
When you use Diprolene, you inevitably absorb some of the medication through your skin and into the bloodstream. Too much absorption can lead to unwanted side effects elsewhere in the body. To keep this problem

to a minimum, avoid using large amounts of Diprolene over large areas, and do not cover it with airtight dressings such as plastic wrap or adhesive bandages.

How should you use this medication?

Apply Diprolene in a thin film, exactly as prescribed by your doctor. A typical regimen is 1 or 2 applications per day. Do not use the medication for longer than prescribed.

Diprolene is for use only on the skin. Be careful to keep it out of your eyes.

Once you have applied Diprolene, never cover the skin with an airtight bandage or other tight dressing.

For a fungal or bacterial skin infection, you will need antifungal or antibacterial medication in addition to Diprolene. If improvement is not prompt, you should stop using Diprolene until the infection is visibly clearing.

■ *If you miss a dose...*
Apply it as soon as you remember. If it is almost time for the next dose, skip the one you missed and go back to your regular schedule.

■ *Storage instructions...*
Store at room temperature.

What side effects may occur?

Side effects cannot be anticipated. A possible side effect of Diprolene is stinging or burning of the skin where the medication is applied.

■ *Other side effects on the skin may include:*
Acne-like eruptions, atrophy, broken capillaries (fine reddish lines), cracking or tightening, dryness, excess hair growth, infected hair follicles, inflammation, irritation, itching, prickly heat, rash, redness, sensitivity to touch

Diprolene can be absorbed and produce side effects elsewhere in the body; see the *Overdosage* section below.

Why should this drug not be prescribed?

Do not use Diprolene if you are sensitive to it or any other steroid medication.

Special warnings about this medication

Do not use Diprolene to treat any condition other than the one for which it was prescribed.

Possible food and drug interactions when using this medication

Do not use Diprolene with any other steroid-containing product. Such combinations increase the chance of absorption and side effects.

Special information if you are pregnant or breastfeeding

It is not known whether Diprolene, when applied to skin, causes any problem during pregnancy or while breastfeeding. It's considered best for pregnant women to avoid the product unless its possible benefits outweigh the potential risk. If it must be used, it should not be applied extensively, in large amounts, or for a long period of time.

Recommended dosage

ADULTS

Diprolene products are not to be used with airtight dressings.

Cream or Ointment
Apply a thin film to the affected skin areas once or twice daily. Treatment should be limited to 45 grams per week.

Lotion
Apply a few drops of Diprolene Lotion to the affected area once or twice daily and massage lightly until the lotion disappears.

Treatment must be limited to 14 days; do not use more than 50 milliliters per week.

Gel
Apply a thin layer of Diprolene Gel to the affected area once or twice daily and rub in gently and completely.

Treatment must be limited to 14 days; do not use more than 50 grams per week.

CHILDREN

Use of Diprolene is not recommended for children 12 and under. For those 13 and over, use no more than necessary to obtain results.

Overdosage

With copious or prolonged use of Diprolene, hormone absorbed into the bloodstream may cause high blood sugar, sugar in the urine, and a group of symptoms called Cushing's syndrome.

■ *Symptoms of Cushing's syndrome may include:*
Acne, depression, excessive hair growth, fractures, high blood pressure, humped upper back, infections, insomnia, moon-faced appearance, muscle weakness, obese trunk, paranoia, retardation of growth, stretch marks, susceptibility to bruising, wasted limbs

Cushing's syndrome may also trigger the development of diabetes mellitus. Left uncorrected, the syndrome may become serious. If you suspect your use of Diprolene has led to this problem, seek medical attention immediately.

Diprosone *See Diprolene, page 455.*

Dipyridamole *See Persantine, page 1082.*

Dirithromycin *See Dynabac, page 488.*

DISALCID
Pronounced: dye-SAL-sid
Generic name: Salsalate

Why is this drug prescribed?
Disalcid, a nonsteroidal anti-inflammatory drug, is used to relieve the symptoms of rheumatoid arthritis, osteoarthritis (the most common form of arthritis), and other rheumatic disorders (conditions that involve pain and inflammation in joints and the tissues around them).

Most important fact about this drug
Disalcid contains salicylate, an ingredient that may be associated with the development of Reye's syndrome (a disorder that causes abnormal brain and liver function). It occurs mostly in children who have taken aspirin or other medications containing salicylate to relieve symptoms of the flu or chickenpox. Do not take Disalcid if you have flu symptoms or chickenpox.

How should you take this medication?
Take Disalcid exactly as prescribed. Food may slow its absorption. However, your doctor may ask you to take Disalcid with food in order to avoid stomach upset.

■ *If you miss a dose...*
   Take it as soon as you remember. If it is almost time for your next dose, skip the one you missed and go back to your regular schedule. Never take 2 doses at once.
■ *Storage instructions...*
   Store at room temperature. Keep out of the reach of children.

What side effects may occur?
Side effects cannot be anticipated. If any develop or change in intensity, inform your doctor as soon as possible. Only your doctor can determine if it is safe for you to continue taking Disalcid.

■ *Side effects may include:*
   Hearing impairment, nausea, rash, ringing in the ears, vertigo

Why should this drug not be prescribed?
Disalcid should not be taken if you are sensitive to or have ever had an allergic reaction to salsalate.

Special warnings about this medication

Use Disalcid with extreme caution if you have chronic kidney disease or a peptic ulcer.

Salicylates occasionally cause asthma in people who are sensitive to aspirin. Although Disalcid contains a salicylate, it is less likely than aspirin to cause this reaction.

Possible food and drug interactions when taking this medication

If Disalcid is taken with certain other drugs, the effects of either could be increased, decreased, or altered. It is especially important to check with your doctor before combining Disalcid with the following:

ACE-inhibitor-type blood pressure drugs such as Capoten and Vasotec
Acetazolamide (Diamox)
Aspirin and other drugs containing salicylates such as Bufferin and Empirin
Blood-thinning medications such as Coumadin
Medications for gout such as Zyloprim and Benemid
Methotrexate (Rheumatrex)
Naproxen (Anaprox, Naprosyn)
Oral diabetes drugs such as Glucotrol and Tolinase
Penicillin (Pen-Vee K)
Phenytoin (Dilantin)
Steroids such as Deltasone and Decadron
Sulfinpyrazone (Anturane)
Thyroid medications such as Synthroid

Special information if you are pregnant or breastfeeding

The effects of Disalcid during pregnancy have not been adequately studied. If you are pregnant or plan to become pregnant, inform your doctor immediately. Disalcid may appear in breast milk and could affect a nursing infant. If this medication is essential to your health, your doctor may advise you to stop breastfeeding until your treatment with Disalcid is finished.

Recommended dosage

You may not feel the full benefit of this medication for 3 to 4 days.

ADULTS

The usual dosage is 3,000 milligrams daily, divided into smaller doses as follows:

2 doses of two 750-milligram tablets, or
2 doses of three 500-milligram tablets or capsules, or
3 doses of two 500-milligram tablets or capsules

CHILDREN

The safety and effectiveness of Disalcid use in children have not been established.

OLDER ADULTS

A lower dosage may be sufficient to achieve desired blood levels without the more common side effects.

Overdosage

Any medication taken in excess can have serious consequences. Deaths have occurred from salicylate overdose. If you suspect an overdose, seek medical treatment immediately.

■ *Symptoms of Disalcid overdose may include:*
Confusion
dehydration
diarrhea
drowsiness
headache
high body temperature
hyperventilation
ringing in the ears
sweating
vertigo
vomiting

Disopyramide See Norpace, page 970.

DITROPAN

Pronounced: *DYE-tro-pan*
Generic name: *Oxybutynin chloride*
Other brand name: *Ditropan XL*

Why is this drug prescribed?

Ditropan and Ditropan XL, the extended-release form of the drug, treat symptoms of overactive bladder, including frequent urination, urgency (increased need to urinate), and urge incontinence (inability to control urination). The drug works by blocking the nerve impulses that prompt the bladder to contract. Ditropan is also used to treat the urgency, frequency, leakage, incontinence, and painful or difficult urination caused by a neurogenic bladder (altered bladder function due to a nervous system abnormality).

Ditropan XL can also be prescribed for children 6 years of age and

older who are suffering from urinary urge incontinence due to a neurological condition such as spina bifida.

Most important fact about this drug

Ditropan can cause heat prostration (fever and heat stroke due to decreased sweating) in high temperatures. If you live in a hot climate or will
be exposed to high temperatures, take appropriate precautions.

How should you take this medication?

Ditropan may be taken with or without food. Take it exactly as prescribed.

Ditropan can make your mouth dry. Sucking hard candies or melting
bits of ice in your mouth can remedy the problem.

Ditropan tablets and syrup must be taken 2 or 3 times a day. Ditropan
XL, a long-acting form of the drug, is available for once-a-day dosing.
Ditropan XL tablets should be swallowed whole with plenty of fluid. Do
not chew, crush, or break them.

■ *If you miss a dose...*
Take the forgotten dose as soon as you remember. If it is almost time
for your next dose, skip the one you missed and go back to your regular schedule. Never take 2 doses at once.

■ *Storage instructions...*
Keep this medication in a tightly closed container and store it at room
temperature. Protect the syrup from direct light. Protect the extended-
release tablets from moisture and humidity.

What side effects may occur?

Side effects cannot be anticipated. If any develop or change in intensity,
inform your doctor as soon as possible. Only your doctor can determine
if it is safe for you to continue taking Ditropan.

■ *Side effects may include:*
Constipation, decreased production of tears, decreased sweating, difficulty falling or staying asleep, dilation of the pupil of the eye, dim
vision, dizziness, drowsiness, dry mouth, eye paralysis, hallucinations, impotence, inability to urinate, nausea, palpitations, rapid heartbeat, rash, restlessness, suppression of milk production, weakness

Why should this drug not be prescribed?

You should not take Ditropan if you have certain types of untreated glaucoma (excessive pressure in the eye), partial or complete blockage of the
gastrointestinal tract, or paralytic ileus (obstructed bowel). Ditropan
should also be avoided if you have severe colitis (inflamed colon), myasthenia gravis (abnormal muscle weakness), or urinary tract obstruction
(inability to urinate). This drug is usually not prescribed for the elderly or
debilitated.

Do not take this medication if you are sensitive or have ever had an allergic reaction to it. Make sure your doctor is aware of any allergic reactions you have experienced.

Special warnings about this medication

If you have an ileostomy or colostomy (an artificial opening to the bowel) and develop diarrhea while taking Ditropan, inform your doctor immediately.

Ditropan may cause drowsiness or blurred vision. Driving or operating dangerous machinery or participating in any hazardous activity that requires full mental alertness is not recommended until you know how this medication affects you.

Your doctor will prescribe Ditropan with caution if you have liver disease, kidney disease, digestive problems such as reflux disease, or a nervous system disorder.

Ditropan may aggravate the symptoms of overactive thyroid, heart disease or congestive heart failure, irregular or rapid heartbeat, high blood pressure, or enlarged prostate.

After taking Ditropan XL, you may notice something like a tablet in your stool. This is not a cause for concern. The outer coating of the extended release tablet sometimes fails to dissolve along with the contents.

Possible food and drug interactions when taking this medication

If Ditropan is taken with certain other drugs, the effects of either may be increased, decreased or altered. It is especially important to check with your doctor before combining Ditropan with alcohol or sedatives such as Halcion or Restoril because increased drowsiness may occur. You should also check with your doctor if you are taking any of the following:

Alendronate (Fosamax)
Antibiotics such as erythromycin (E-Mycin, Ery-Tab) and
   clarithromycin (Biaxin)
Antifungal medication such as itraconazole (Sporanox), ketoconazole
   (Nizoral), and miconazole (Monistat)
Drugs that ease spasms, including Bentyl, Levsin, Pro-Banthine, and
   Robinul
Risedronate (Actonel)

Special information if you are pregnant or breastfeeding

The effects of Ditropan during pregnancy have not been adequately studied. If you are pregnant or plan to become pregnant, inform your doctor immediately. Ditropan may appear in breast milk and could affect a nursing infant. If this medication is essential to your health, your doctor may advise you to stop breastfeeding until your treatment is finished.

Recommended dosage

DITROPAN

Adults
The usual dose is one 5-milligram tablet or 1 teaspoonful of syrup taken 2 to 3 times a day, but not more than 4 times a day.

Children over 5 Years Old
The usual dose is one 5-milligram tablet or 1 teaspoonful of syrup taken 2 times a day, but not more than 3 times a day. Ditropan is not recommended for children under 5.

DITROPAN XL

Adults
The recommended starting dose is 5 or 10 milligrams once a day. If this proves insufficient, the doctor may increase the dose by 5 milligrams at weekly intervals, up to a maximum of 30 milligrams a day.

CHILDREN 6 YEARS AND OLDER

The recommended starting dose is 5 milligrams once a day. If this proves insufficient, the doctor may increase the dose by 5-milligram increments, up to a maximum of 20 milligrams a day.

Overdosage

Any medication taken in excess can have serious consequences. If you suspect an overdose, seek medical attention immediately.

■ *Symptoms of Ditropan overdose may include:*
Coma, convulsions, delirium, dehydration, difficulty breathing, fever, flushing, hallucinations, irritability, low or high blood pressure, nausea, paralysis, rapid heartbeat, restlessness, tremor, urinary tract obstruction, vomiting

DIURIL
Pronounced: DYE-your-il
Generic name: Chlorothiazide

Why is this drug prescribed?

Diuril is used in the treatment of high blood pressure and other conditions that require the elimination of excess fluid (water) from the body. These conditions include congestive heart failure, cirrhosis of the liver, corticosteroid and estrogen therapy, and kidney disease. When used for high blood pressure, Diuril can be used alone or with other high blood pressure medications. Diuril contains a form of thiazide, a diuretic that prompts your body to eliminate more fluid, which helps lower blood pressure.

Most important fact about this drug

If you have high blood pressure, you must take Diuril regularly for it to be effective. Since blood pressure declines gradually, it may be several weeks before you get the full benefit of Diuril; and you must continue taking it even if you are feeling well. Diuril does not cure high blood pressure; it merely keeps it under control.

How should you take this medication?

Take Diuril exactly as prescribed. Stopping Diuril suddenly could cause your condition to worsen.

■ *If you miss a dose...*
Take it as soon as you remember. If it is almost time for your next dose, skip the one you missed and go back to your regular schedule. Never take 2 doses at the same time.

■ *Storage instructions...*
Store at room temperature in a tightly closed container. Protect from moisture and freezing.

What side effects may occur?

Side effects cannot be anticipated. If any develop or change in intensity, inform your doctor as soon as possible. Only your doctor can determine if it is safe for you to continue taking Diuril.

■ *Side effects may include:*
Abdominal cramps, anemia, changes in blood sugar, constipation, diarrhea, difficulty breathing, dizziness, dizziness on standing up, fever, fluid in lungs, hair loss, headache, high levels of sugar in urine, hives, hypersensitivity reactions, impotence, inflammation of the pancreas, inflammation of the salivary glands, light-headedness, loss of appetite, low blood pressure, low potassium (leading to symptoms such as dry mouth, excessive thirst, weak or irregular heartbeat, muscle pain or cramps), lung inflammation, muscle spasms, nausea, rash, reddish or purplish spots on skin, restlessness, sensitivity to light, Stevens-Johnson syndrome, stomach irritation, stomach upset, tingling or pins and needles, vertigo, vision changes, vomiting, weakness, yellow eyes and skin

Why should this drug not be prescribed?

If you are unable to urinate, you should not take this medication. If you are sensitive to or have ever had an allergic reaction to Diuril or other thiazide-type diuretics, or if you are sensitive to sulfa drugs, you should not take this medication.

Special warnings about this medication

Diuretics can cause your body to lose too much potassium. Signs of an excessively low potassium level include muscle weakness and rapid or irregular heartbeat. To boost your potassium level, your doctor may recommend eating potassium-rich foods or taking a potassium supplement.

If you are taking Diuril, your doctor will do a complete assessment of your kidney function and continue to monitor it. Use with caution if you have severe kidney disease.

If you have liver disease, diabetes, gout, or the connective tissue disease lupus erythematosus, your doctor will prescribe Diuril cautiously.

If you have bronchial asthma or a history of allergies, you may be at greater risk for an allergic reaction to this medication.

Dehydration, excessive sweating, severe diarrhea, or vomiting could deplete your body's fluids and lower your blood pressure too much. Be careful when exercising and in hot weather.

Notify your doctor or dentist that you are taking Diuril if you have a medical emergency, and before you have surgery or dental treatment.

Possible food and drug interactions when taking this medication

Diuril may increase the effects of alcohol. Do not drink alcohol while taking this medication.

If Diuril is taken with certain other drugs, the effects of either may be increased, decreased, or altered. It is especially important to check with your doctor before combining Diuril with the following:

Barbiturates such as phenobarbital and Seconal
Cholesterol-lowering drugs such as Questran and Colestid
Drugs to treat diabetes such as insulin and Micronase
Lithium (Eskalith)
Narcotic painkillers such as Percocet
Nonsteroidal anti-inflammatory drugs such as Naprosyn and Motrin
Norepinephrine (Levophed)
Other drugs for high blood pressure such as Capoten and
    Procardia XL
Steroids such as prednisone

Special information if you are pregnant or breastfeeding

The effects of Diuril during pregnancy have not been adequately studied. If you are pregnant or plan to become pregnant, inform your doctor immediately. Diuril appears in breast milk and could affect a nursing infant. If this medication is essential to your health, your doctor may advise you to discontinue breastfeeding until your treatment is finished.

Recommended dosage

ADULTS

Diuril comes in tablets, an oral suspension, and an intravenous preparation, reserved for emergencies. Dosages below are for the oral preparations.

Swelling Due to Excess Water
The usual dose is 0.5 gram to 1 gram 1 or 2 times per day. Your doctor may have you take this medication on alternate days or on some other on-off schedule.

High Blood Pressure
The starting dose is 0.5 gram to 1 gram per day, taken as 1 dose or 2 or more smaller doses. Your doctor will adjust the dosage to suit your needs.

CHILDREN

Dosages for children are adjusted according to weight, generally 10 milligrams per pound of body weight daily in 2 doses.

Under 6 Months
Dosage may be up to 15 milligrams per pound of body weight per day in 2 doses.

Under 2 Years
The usual dosage is 125 to 375 milligrams per day in 2 doses. The liquid form of this drug may be used in children under 2 years of age at a dosage of ½ to 1½ teaspoons (2.5 to 7.5 milliliters) per day.

2 to 12 Years
The usual dosage is 375 milligrams to 1 gram daily in 2 doses. The liquid form of this medication may be used in children 2 to 12 years at a dosage of 1½ to 4 teaspoons (7.5 to 20 milliliters) per day.

Overdosage

Any medication taken in excess can have serious consequences. If you suspect an overdose, seek medical attention immediately.

■ *Signs of Diuril overdose may include:*
Dehydration and symptoms of low potassium (dry mouth, excessive thirst, weak or irregular heartbeat, muscle pain or cramps)

Divalproex See Depakote, page 410.

Docusate See Colace, page 317.

DOLOBID
Pronounced: DOLL-oh-bid
Generic name: Diflunisal

Why is this drug prescribed?

Dolobid, a nonsteroidal anti-inflammatory drug, is used to treat mild to moderate pain and relieve the inflammation, swelling, stiffness, and joint pain associated with rheumatoid arthritis and osteoarthritis (the most common form of arthritis).

Most important fact about this drug

You should have frequent checkups with your doctor if you take Dolobid regularly. Ulcers or internal bleeding can occur without warning.

How should you take this medication?

Dolobid should be taken with food or food together with an antacid, and with a full glass of water or milk. Never take it on an empty stomach.

Tablets should be swallowed whole, not chewed or crushed.

Take this medication exactly as prescribed by your doctor. If you are using Dolobid for arthritis, it should be taken regularly.

■ *If you miss a dose...*
Take it as soon as you remember. If it is almost time for your next dose, skip the one you missed and go back to your regular schedule. Never take 2 doses at the same time.

■ *Storage instructions...*
Do not store in damp places like the bathroom.

What side effects may occur?

Side effects cannot be anticipated. If any develop or change in intensity, inform your doctor as soon as possible. Only your doctor can determine if it is safe for you to continue taking Dolobid.

■ *Side effects may include:*
Abdominal pain, constipation, diarrhea, dizziness, fatigue, gas, headache, inability to sleep, indigestion, nausea, rash, ringing in ears, sleepiness, vomiting

Why should this drug not be prescribed?

If you are sensitive to or have had an allergic reaction to Dolobid, aspirin, or similar drugs, or if you have had asthma attacks caused by aspirin or other drugs of this type, you should not take this medication. Make sure that your doctor is aware of any drug reactions that you have experienced.

Special warnings about this medication

Stomach ulcers and bleeding can occur without warning, especially if you are 65 or older. These and other side effects are also more likely if you have poor kidney function.

This drug should be used with caution if you have kidney or liver disease; and it can cause liver inflammation in some people.

Do not take aspirin or any other anti-inflammatory medications while taking Dolobid, unless your doctor tells you to do so.

Nonsteroidal anti-inflammatory drugs such as Dolobid can hide the signs and symptoms of infection. Be sure your doctor knows about any infection you may have.

Dolobid can cause vision problems. If you experience any changes in your vision, inform your doctor.

Dolobid may prolong bleeding time. If you are taking blood-thinning medication, take Dolobid with caution.

If you have heart disease or high blood pressure, use Dolobid with caution. It can increase water retention.

Dolobid may cause you to become drowsy or less alert; therefore, driving or operating dangerous machinery or participating in any hazardous activity that requires full mental alertness is not recommended.

Possible food and drug interactions when taking this medication

If Dolobid is taken with certain other drugs, the effects of either could be increased, decreased, or altered. It is especially important to check with your doctor before combining Dolobid with the following:

Acetaminophen (Tylenol)
Antacids taken regularly
Aspirin
Cyclosporine (Sandimmune)
Methotrexate (Rheumatrex)
Oral anticoagulants (blood thinners)
Other nonsteroidal anti-inflammatory drugs (Advil, Motrin,
    Naprosyn, others)
The arthritis medication sulindac (Clinoril)
The diuretic hydrochlorothiazide

Special information if you are pregnant or breastfeeding

The effects of Dolobid during pregnancy have not been adequately studied. If you are pregnant or plan to become pregnant, inform your doctor immediately. Dolobid appears in breast milk and could affect a nursing infant. If this medication is essential to your health, your doctor may advise you to discontinue breastfeeding until your treatment with Dolobid is finished.

Recommended dosage

ADULTS

Mild to Moderate Pain
Starting dose is 1,000 milligrams, followed by 500 milligrams every 8 to 12 hours, depending on the individual. Your physician may adjust your dosage according to your age and weight, and the severity of your symptoms.

Osteoarthritis and Rheumatoid Arthritis
The usual dose is 500 to 1,000 milligrams per day in 2 doses of 250 milligrams or 500 milligrams. Use no more than necessary to relieve the pain.
The maximum recommended dosage is 1,500 milligrams per day.

CHILDREN

The safety and effectiveness of Dolobid have not been established in children under 12 years of age. The drug is not recommended for this age group.

Overdosage
Any medication taken in excess can cause symptoms of overdose. If you suspect an overdose, seek medical attention immediately.

■ *Symptoms of Dolobid overdose may include:*
Abnormally rapid heartbeat, coma, diarrhea, disorientation, drowsiness, hyperventilation, nausea, ringing in the ears, stupor, sweating, vomiting

Donepezil See Aricept, page 123.

DONNATAL
Pronounced: DON-nuh-tal
Generic ingredients: Phenobarbital, Hyoscyamine sulfate,
*   Atropine sulfate, Scopolamine hydrobromide*
Other brand name: Bellatal

Why is this drug prescribed?
Donnatal is a mild antispasmodic medication; it has been used with other drugs for relief of cramps and pain associated with various stomach, intestinal, and bowel disorders, including irritable bowel syndrome, acute colitis, and duodenal ulcer.
One of its ingredients, phenobarbital, is a mild sedative.

Most important fact about this drug
Phenobarbital, one of the ingredients of Donnatal, can be habit-forming. If you have ever been dependent on drugs, do not take Donnatal.

How should you take this medication?
Take Donnatal one-half hour to 1 hour before meals. Use it exactly as prescribed.

■ *If you miss a dose...*
Take it as soon as you remember. If it is almost time for your next dose, skip the one you missed and go back to your regular schedule. Never take 2 doses at the same time.

■ *Storage instructions...*
Store at room temperature in a tightly closed container. Protect from light.

What side effects may occur?

Side effects cannot be anticipated. If any develop or change in intensity, inform your doctor as soon as possible. Only your doctor can determine if it is safe for you to continue taking Donnatal.

■ *Side effects may include:*
Agitation, allergic reaction, bloated feeling, blurred vision, constipation, decreased sweating, difficulty sleeping, difficulty urinating, dilation of the pupil of the eye, dizziness, drowsiness, dry mouth, excitement, fast or fluttery heartbeat, headache, hives, impotence, muscular and bone pain, nausea, nervousness, rash, reduced sense of taste, suppression of lactation, vomiting, weakness

Why should this drug not be prescribed?

Do not take Donnatal if you suffer from the eye condition called glaucoma, diseases that block the urinary or gastrointestinal tracts, or myasthenia gravis, a condition in which the muscles become progressively paralyzed. Also, you should not use Donnatal if you have intestinal atony (loss of strength in the intestinal muscles), unstable cardiovascular status, severe ulcerative colitis (chronic inflammation and ulceration of the bowel), or hiatal hernia (a rupture in the diaphragm above the stomach). You should also avoid Donnatal if you have acute intermittent porphyria—a disorder of the metabolism in which there is severe abdominal pain and sensitivity to light.

If you are sensitive to or have ever had an allergic reaction to Donnatal, its ingredients, or similar drugs, you should not take this medication. Also avoid Donnatal if phenobarbital makes you excited or restless, instead of calming you down. Make sure your doctor is aware of any drug reactions you have experienced.

Special warnings about this medication

Be cautious in using Donnatal if you suffer from high blood pressure, overactive thyroid (hyperthyroidism), irregular or rapid heartbeat, or heart, kidney, or liver disease.

Donnatal can decrease sweating. If you are exercising or are subjected to high temperatures, be alert for heat prostration.

If you develop diarrhea, especially if you have an ileostomy or colostomy (artificial openings to the bowel), check with your doctor.

If you have a gastric ulcer, use this medication with caution.

Donnatal may cause you to become drowsy or less alert. You should not drive or operate dangerous machinery or participate in any hazardous activity that requires full mental alertness until you know how this drug affects you.

Possible food and drug interactions when taking this medication

Donnatal may intensify the effects of alcohol. Check with your doctor before using alcohol with this medication.

Avoid taking antacids within 1 hour of a dose of Donnatal; they may reduce its effectiveness.

If Donnatal is taken with certain other drugs, the effects of either could be increased, decreased, or altered. It is especially important to check with your doctor before combining Donnatal with the following:

Antidepressants known as MAO inhibitors, including Nardil and Parnate
Antidepressants such as Elavil and Tofranil
Antihistamines such as Benadryl
Antispasmodic drugs such as Bentyl and Cogentin
Barbiturates such as Seconal
Blood-thinning drugs such as Coumadin
Diarrhea medications containing Kaolin or attapulgite
Digitalis (Lanoxin)
Narcotics such as Percocet
Potassium (Slow-K, K-Dur, others)
Steroids such as Medrol and Deltasone
Tranquilizers such as Valium

Special information if you are pregnant or breastfeeding

The effects of Donnatal during pregnancy have not been adequately studied. If you are pregnant or plan to become pregnant, this drug should be used only when prescribed by your doctor. It is not known whether Donnatal appears in breast milk. If this medication is essential to your health, your doctor may advise you to discontinue breastfeeding until your treatment is finished.

Recommended dosage

ADULTS

Your doctor will adjust the dosage to your needs.

Tablets or Capsules
The usual dosage is 1 or 2 tablets or capsules, 3 or 4 times a day.

Liquid
The usual dosage is 1 or 2 teaspoonfuls, 3 or 4 times a day.

Donnatal Extentabs
The usual dosage is 1 tablet every 12 hours. Your doctor may tell you to take 1 tablet every 8 hours, if necessary.

CHILDREN

Dosage of the elixir is determined by body weight; it can be given every 4 to 6 hours. Follow your doctor's instructions carefully when giving this medication to a child.

Overdosage

Any medication taken in excess can cause symptoms of overdose. If you suspect an overdose, seek medical attention immediately.

■ *The symptoms of Donnatal overdose may include:*
Blurred vision
central nervous system stimulation
difficulty swallowing
dilated pupils
dizziness
dry mouth
headache
hot and dry skin
nausea
vomiting

DORAL

Pronounced: DOHR-al
Generic name: Quazepam

Why is this drug prescribed?

Doral, a sleeping medication available in tablet form, is taken as short-term treatment for insomnia. Symptoms of insomnia may include difficulty falling asleep, frequent awakening throughout the night, or very early morning awakening.

Most important fact about this drug

Doral is a chemical cousin of Valium and is potentially addictive. Over time, your body will get used to the prescribed dosage of Doral, and you will no longer derive any benefit from it. If you were to increase the dosage against medical advice, the drug would again work as a sleeping pill—but only until your body adjusted to the higher dosage. This is a vicious circle that can lead to addiction. To avoid this danger, use Doral only as prescribed.

How should you take this medication?

Take Doral exactly as prescribed by your doctor—1 dose per day, at bedtime. Keep in touch with your doctor; if you respond very well, it may be possible to cut your dosage in half after the first few nights. The older or more run-down you are, the more desirable it is to try for this early dosage reduction.

If you have been taking Doral regularly for 6 weeks or so, you may experience withdrawal symptoms if you stop suddenly, or even if you reduce the dosage without specific instructions on how to do it. Always follow your doctor's advice for tapering off gradually from Doral.

■ *If you miss a dose...*
Take this medication only if needed.
■ *Storage instructions...*
Store at room temperature, away from moisture.

What side effects may occur?
Side effects cannot be anticipated. If any develop or change in intensity, inform your doctor as soon as possible. Only your doctor can determine if it is safe for you to continue taking Doral.

■ *Side effects may include:*
Drowsiness during the day, headache

In rare instances, Doral produces agitation, sleep disturbances, hallucinations, or stimulation—exactly the opposite of the desired effect. If this should happen to you, tell your doctor; he or she will take you off the medication.

Why should this drug not be prescribed?
Do not take Doral if you are sensitive to it, or if you have ever had an allergic reaction to it or to another Valium-type medication.

You should not take Doral if you know or suspect that you have sleep apnea (short periods of interrupted breathing that occur during sleep).

You should not take Doral if you are pregnant.

Special warnings about this medication
Because Doral may decrease your daytime alertness, do not drive, climb, or operate dangerous machinery until you find out how the drug affects you. In some cases, Doral's sedative effect may last for several days after the last dose.

If you are suffering from depression, Doral may make your depression worse.

If you have ever abused alcohol or drugs, you are at special risk for addiction to Doral.

Never increase the dosage of Doral on your own. Tell your doctor right away if the medication no longer seems to be working.

Possible food and drug interactions when taking this medication
If Doral is taken with certain other drugs, the effects of either could be increased, decreased, or altered. It is especially important to check with your doctor before combining Doral with the following:

Antihistamines such as Benadryl
Antipsychotic drugs such as chlorpromazine and Clozaril
Antiseizure medications such as Dilantin and Tegretol
Tranquilizers such as Xanax and Valium

Do not drink alcohol while taking Doral; it can increase the drug's effects.

Special information if you are pregnant or breastfeeding

Because Doral may cause harm to the unborn child, it should not be taken during pregnancy. If you want to have a baby, tell your doctor, and plan to discontinue taking Doral before getting pregnant.

Babies whose mothers are taking Doral at the time of birth may experience withdrawal symptoms from the drug. Such babies may be "floppy" (flaccid) instead of having normal muscle tone.

Since Doral does appear in breast milk, you should not take this medication if you are nursing a baby.

Recommended dosage

ADULTS

The recommended initial dose is 15 milligrams daily. Your doctor may later reduce this dosage to 7.5 milligrams.

CHILDREN

The safety and efficacy of Doral in children under 18 years old have not been established.

OLDER ADULTS

You may be more sensitive to this drug, and the doctor may reduce the dosage after only 1 or 2 nights.

Overdosage

Any medication taken in excess can have serious consequences. If you suspect an overdose of Doral, seek medical attention immediately.

■ *Symptoms of an overdose of Doral may include:*
Coma, confusion, extreme sleepiness

DORYX

Pronounced: DORE-icks
Generic name: Doxycycline hyclate
Other brand names: Vibramycin, Vibra-Tabs

Why is this drug prescribed?

Doxycycline is a broad-spectrum tetracycline antibiotic used against a wide variety of bacterial infections, including Rocky Mountain spotted fever and other fevers caused by ticks, fleas, and lice; urinary tract infections; trachoma (chronic infections of the eye); and some gonococcal infections in adults. It is an approved treatment for inhalational anthrax. It is also used with other medications to treat severe acne and amoebic dysentery (diarrhea caused by severe parasitic infection of the intestines).

Doxycycline may also be taken for the prevention of malaria on foreign trips of less than 4 months' duration.

Occasionally doctors prescribe doxycycline to treat early Lyme disease and to prevent traveler's diarrhea. These are not yet officially approved uses for this drug.

Most important fact about this drug

Generally, children under 8 years old and women in the last half of pregnancy should not take this medication. It may cause developing teeth to become permanently discolored. (However, children under 8 may be given this drug for inhalational anthrax.)

How should you take this medication?

Take doxycycline with a full glass of water or other liquid to avoid irritating your throat or stomach. Doxycycline can be taken with or without food. However, if the medicine does upset your stomach, you may wish to take it with a glass of milk or after you have eaten.

Doxycycline tablets should be swallowed whole. If you have difficulty swallowing pills, you can take this medication by opening the capsule and sprinkling the entire contents onto a spoonful of cool, soft applesauce. Be careful not to spill any of the contents. If you do, you will not be able to use this dose and will have to start over with a new mixture. Swallow the mixture immediately, without chewing, followed by a cool 8-ounce glass of water. Discard the mixture if you are not able to use it immediately; do not store it to use later.

Your doctor will only prescribe doxycycline to treat a bacterial infection; it will not cure a viral infection, such as the common cold. It's important to take the full dosage schedule of doxycycline, even if you're feeling better in a few days. Not completing the full dosage schedule may decrease the drug's effectiveness and increase the chances that the bacteria may become resistant to doxycycline and similar antibiotics.

If you are taking an oral suspension form of doxycycline, shake the bottle well before using. Do not use outdated doxycycline.

■ If you miss a dose...
Take the forgotten dose as soon as you remember. If it is almost time for the next dose, put it off for several hours after taking the missed dose. Specifically, if you are taking 1 dose a day, take the next one 10 to 12 hours after the missed dose. If you are taking 2 doses a day, take the next one 5 to 6 hours after the missed dose. If you are taking 3

doses a day, take the next one 2 to 4 hours after the missed dose. Then return to your regular schedule.

■ *Storage instructions...*
Doxycycline can be stored at room temperature. Protect from light and excessive heat.

What side effects may occur?

Side effects cannot be anticipated. If any develop or change in intensity, inform your doctor as soon as possible. Only your doctor can determine if it is safe for you to continue taking doxycycline.

■ *Side effects may include:*
Angioedema (chest pain; swelling of face, around lips, tongue and throat, arms and legs; difficulty swallowing), bulging foreheads in infants, diarrhea, difficulty swallowing, discolored teeth in infants and children (more common during long-term use of tetracycline), inflammation of the tongue, loss of appetite, nausea, rash, rectal or genital itching, severe allergic reaction (hives, itching, and swelling), skin sensitivity to light, vomiting

Why should this drug not be prescribed?

If you are sensitive to or have ever had an allergic reaction to doxycycline or drugs of this type, you should not take this medication. Make sure your doctor is aware of any drug reactions that you have experienced.

Special warnings about this medication

As with other antibiotics, treatment with doxycycline may result in a growth of bacteria that do not respond to this medication and can cause a secondary infection. An overgrowth of certain bacteria in the colon could cause mild to severe—and rarely, life-threatening—diarrhea. If you develop this symptom, call your doctor immediately.

Bulging foreheads in infants and headaches in adults have occurred. These symptoms disappeared when doxycycline was discontinued.

You may become more sensitive to sunlight while taking doxycycline. Be careful if you are going out in the sun or using a sunlamp. If you develop a skin rash, notify your doctor immediately.

Birth control pills that contain estrogen may not be as effective while you are taking tetracycline drugs. Ask your doctor or pharmacist if you should use another form of birth control while taking doxycycline.

Doxycycline syrup (Vibramycin) contains a sulfite that may cause allergic reactions in certain people. This reaction happens more frequently to people with asthma.

Possible food and drug interactions when taking this medication

If doxycycline is taken with certain other drugs, the effects of either could be increased, decreased, or altered. It is especially important to check with your doctor before combining doxycycline with the following:

Antacids containing aluminum, calcium, or magnesium, and iron-
   containing preparations such as Maalox, Mylanta, and others
Barbiturates such as phenobarbital
Bismuth subsalicylate (Pepto-Bismol)
Blood-thinning medications such as Coumadin
Carbamazepine (Tegretol)
Oral contraceptives
Penicillin (V-Cillin K, Pen-vee K, others)
Phenytoin (Dilantin)
Sodium bicarbonate

Special information if you are pregnant or breastfeeding

Doxycycline should not be used during pregnancy. Tetracycline can damage developing teeth during the last half of pregnancy. If you are pregnant
or plan to become pregnant, inform your doctor immediately. Tetracyclines such as doxycycline appear in breast milk and can affect a nursing
infant. If this medication is essential to your health, your doctor may advise you to discontinue breastfeeding until your treatment is finished.

Recommended dosage

ADULTS

The usual dose of oral doxycycline is 200 milligrams on the first day of
treatment (100 milligrams every 12 hours) followed by a maintenance
dose of 100 milligrams per day. The maintenance dose may be taken as a
single dose or as 50 milligrams every 12 hours.

Your doctor may prescribe 100 milligrams every 12 hours for severe
infections such as chronic urinary tract infection.

Uncomplicated Gonorrhea
(Except Anorectal Infections in Men)

The usual dose is 100 milligrams by mouth, twice a day for 7 days. An
alternate, single-day treatment is 300 milligrams, followed in 1 hour by a
second 300-milligram dose.

Primary and Secondary Syphilis

The usual dose is 200 milligrams a day, divided into smaller, equal doses
for 14 days.

Inhalational Anthrax

To prevent or combat infection after exposure, the usual dose is 100 milligrams taken by mouth twice a day for 60 days. Treatment can be started
intravenously, but should be switched to oral doses as soon as possible.

Prevention of Malaria

The usual dose is 100 milligrams a day. Treatment should begin 1 to 2
days before travel to the area where malaria is found, then continue daily
during travel in the area and 4 weeks after leaving.

CHILDREN

For children above 8 years of age, the recommended dosage schedule for those weighing 100 pounds or less is 2 milligrams per pound of body weight, divided into 2 doses, on the first day of treatment, followed by 1 milligram per pound of body weight given as a single daily dose or divided into 2 doses on subsequent days.

For more severe infections, up to 2 milligrams per pound of body weight may be used.

For inhalational anthrax in children weighing less than 100 pounds, the usual dose is 1 milligram per pound of body weight twice daily for 60 days.

For prevention of malaria, the recommended dose is 2 milligrams per 2.2 pounds of body weight up to 100 milligrams.

For children over 100 pounds, the usual adult dose should be used.

Overdosage

Any medication taken in excess can have serious consequences. If you suspect an overdose, seek medical treatment immediately.

Dorzolamide with Timolol See Cosopt, page 348.

DOVONEX

Pronounced: DOH-va-necks
Generic name: Calcipotriene

Why is this drug prescribed?

Dovonex is prescribed to help clear up the scaly skin condition known as psoriasis. A synthetic form of vitamin D, it is available in cream and ointment form, and in a liquid for the scalp.

Most important fact about this drug

You're likely to begin seeing improvement after 2 weeks of therapy. After 8 weeks of twice-daily application to the skin, 70 percent of patients enjoy marked improvement, and over 10 percent clear up completely.

How should you take this medication?

Dovonex is for external use only. Avoid contact with the face or eyes.

For psoriasis on the skin, gently and completely rub a thin layer of the cream or ointment into the affected areas.

For psoriasis on the scalp, first comb the hair to remove scaly debris, then gently and completely rub the scalp solution into the affected areas. Avoid getting the solution on your forehead or unaffected parts of the scalp.

Wash your hands after each application.

■ *If you miss a dose…*
Apply the forgotten dose as soon as you remember. However, if it is almost time for your next dose, skip the one you missed and return to your regular schedule.

■ *Storage instructions…*
All forms of Dovonex may be stored at room temperature. Do not freeze. Keep the scalp lotion away from sunlight.

What side effects may occur?

Side effects cannot be anticipated. If any develop or change in intensity, tell your doctor as soon as possible. Only your doctor can determine if it is safe to continue using Dovonex.

■ *Side effects may include:*
Burning, itching, skin irritation, tingling

Why should this drug not be prescribed?

Do not use Dovonex on the face. Avoid this drug if it causes an allergic reaction, if you are suffering from vitamin D toxicity, or if you have high levels of calcium in the blood.

Special warnings about this medication

Dovonex should be used only for psoriasis. If skin irritation develops, stop using the drug and check with your doctor immediately.
Dovonex is not approved for use in children.

Possible food and drug interactions when using this medication

No interactions with Dovonex have been reported.

Special information if you are pregnant or breastfeeding

The effects of Dovonex during pregnancy have not been adequately studied. If you are pregnant or plan to become pregnant, inform your doctor immediately.
It's not known whether Dovonex appears in breast milk. Because it may, you should use Dovonex with caution while breastfeeding.

Recommended dosage

ADULTS

Ointment
Apply a thin layer to affected areas once or twice daily.

Cream and Scalp Solution
Apply to affected areas twice a day.

Overdosage
Excessive use of Dovonex can lead to elevated levels of calcium in the blood. Warning signs of this condition include loss of appetite, nausea, vomiting, and frequent urination. If you suspect an overdose, check with your doctor immediately.

Doxazosin *See Cardura, page 252.*

Doxepin *See Sinequan, page 1312.*

Doxycycline *See Doryx, page 474.*

Duloxetine *See Cymbalta, page 372.*

DURAGESIC
Pronounced: door-uh-JEEZ-ic
Generic name: Fentanyl

Why is this drug prescribed?
Duragesic patches deliver a continuous dose of the potent narcotic painkiller fentanyl for a period of three days. The patches are prescribed for chronic pain when short-acting narcotics and other types of painkillers fail to provide relief.

Most important fact about this drug
When wearing a Duragesic patch, check with your doctor before drinking alcohol or taking any other drugs that slow the nervous system. The combined effect can impair breathing, reduce blood pressure, and lead to coma. Drugs in this category include the following:

    Antipsychotic drugs such as Compazine, Mellaril, Stelazine, and
       Thorazine
    Muscle relaxants such as Flexeril, Robaxin, and Skelaxin
    Narcotic painkillers such as Demerol, Percodan, OxyContin, and
       Vicodin
    Sleep aids such as Ambien, Halcion, and Sonata
    Sleep-inducing antihistamines such as Benadryl and Phenergan
    Tranquilizers such as Ativan, Librium, Valium, and Xanax

How should you take this medication?
Apply the patch to a flat surface such as the chest, back, side, or upper arm. Children should have the patch applied to their upper back to discourage them from removing it. Hair at the site should be clipped (but not shaved). If the skin needs to be washed, use clear water. Do not use soaps, oils, lotions, alcohol, or any other cleanser that could irritate the skin. Allow the skin to dry completely.

Apply the patch as soon as you open the sealed package. Do not cut or tear the patch. Press it firmly in place with the palm of your hand for 30 seconds. Make sure that contact with the skin is complete, especially around the edges.

After 3 days (72 hours), remove the patch, fold the adhesive side together, and flush the patch down the toilet.

■ *If you miss a dose...*
If needed, after a used patch is removed a fresh patch can be applied at a different site on the skin.

■ *Storage instructions...*
Store below 77 degrees Fahrenheit. Keep out of reach of children. Unused patches should be removed from their package and flushed down the toilet.

What side effects may occur?

Side effects cannot be anticipated. If any develop or change in intensity, tell your doctor as soon as possible. Only your doctor can determine if it is safe to continue using Duragesic.

■ *Side effects may include:*
Abdominal pain, anxiety, confusion, constipation, depression, diarrhea, dizziness, dry mouth, exaggerated high spirits, hallucinations, headache, impaired or interrupted breathing, indigestion, itching, loss of appetite, nausea, nervousness, shortness of breath, sleepiness, sweating, urinary retention, vomiting, weakness

Why should this drug not be prescribed?

Duragesic should never be used in situations where the right dosage hasn't been established in advance—for instance, after an operation or an accident. It should not be used for mild or intermittent pain that responds to other painkillers.

Duragesic should not be given to children under 2 years old or children who are not tolerant to narcotic painkillers.

The drug should also be avoided if it causes an allergic reaction.

Special warnings about this medication

Heat can increase the release of fentanyl from the Duragesic patch, thereby increasing the risk of impaired breathing and other side effects. Do not expose the patch to heating pads, electric blankets, heated water beds, heat lamps, saunas, hot tubs, or other external sources of heat. Alert your doctor if you develop a high fever (104 degrees Fahrenheit or more).

Like other narcotic painkillers, Duragesic can impair your reactions. Do not drive or operate dangerous machinery until you are certain you can tolerate the drug.

Extended use of Duragesic can lead to physical and psychological dependence, but may be necessary to control chronic pain. Your doctor will take this into account when prescribing this drug.

If your breathing is already impaired by chronic pulmonary disease, Duragesic's tendency to reduce respiration can be especially dangerous. The doctor will determine your dosage with extra caution.

Duragesic is not recommended for people with head injuries and other conditions that increase pressure on the brain, or for those who are semi-conscious or in a coma. It should be used with caution by people with brain tumors.

Use Duragesic with caution if you have an irregular heartbeat; Duragesic can make the problem worse. Caution is also advised if you have kidney or liver disease.

Possible food and drug interactions when using this medication
Remember to check with your doctor before taking any other drugs that slow the nervous system (see *Most important fact about this drug*). The dose of such drugs should be reduced by at least half.

Certain other drugs can increase the effects of Duragesic, triggering the need for a dosage reduction. They include:

Antifungal medications such as Diflucan, Nizoral, and Sporanox
HIV drugs classified as protease inhibitors, including Agenerase,
Crixivan, Fortovase, Invirase, Kaletra, Norvir, and Viracept
Macrolide antibiotics such as erythromycin, Biaxin, and Zithromax

Some drugs may have the opposite impact, decreasing the effects of Duragesic. They include:

Carbamazepine (Tegretol)
Phenytoin (Dilantin)
Rifampin (Rifadin)

Special information if you are pregnant or breastfeeding
The effects of Duragesic during pregnancy have not been adequately studied. Make sure the doctor knows if you are pregnant or planning to become pregnant.

The active ingredient fentanyl does make its way into breast milk, and Duragesic is not recommended for nursing women.

Recommended dosage
The Duragesic patch comes in four sizes: Duragesic-25, -50, -75, and -100. If you have not been taking a narcotic painkiller prior to Duragesic, the doctor will start with the smallest size. If this proves inadequate, the size will be increased after the first 3 days. If necessary, further increases can be made every 6 days thereafter.

For people who are already taking a narcotic painkiller, the dosage of Duragesic is determined by the type of painkiller they've been using, its potency, and the size of the dose. Older adults and the debilitated generally receive a smaller dose of Duragesic.

When Duragesic is to be discontinued, the doctor will reduce the dose gradually to avoid withdrawal symptoms.

Overdosage

An overdose of Duragesic can severely impair breathing. If you suspect an overdose, seek emergency medical attention immediately.

DURICEF

Pronounced: DUHR-i-sef
Generic name: Cefadroxil monohydrate

Why is this drug prescribed?

Duricef, a cephalosporin antibiotic, is used in the treatment of nose, throat, urinary tract, and skin infections that are caused by specific bacteria, including staph, strep, and *E. coli.*

Most important fact about this drug

If you are allergic to either penicillin or cephalosporin antibiotics in any form, consult your doctor *before* taking Duricef. An allergy to either type of medication may signal an allergy to Duricef; and if a reaction occurs, it could be extremely severe. If you take the drug and feel signs of a reaction, seek medical attention immediately.

How should you take this medication?

Take this medication exactly as prescribed. It is important that you finish all of it to obtain the maximum benefit.

Duricef may be taken with or without food. If the drug upsets your stomach, you may find that taking it with meals helps to relieve the problem.

If you are taking the liquid suspension, shake it thoroughly before each use.

■ *If you miss a dose...*
Take it as soon as you remember. If it is almost time for the next dose and you take it once a day, take the one you missed and the next dose 10 to 12 hours later. If you take 2 doses a day, take the one you missed and the next dose 5 to 6 hours later. If you take it 3 or more times a day, take the one you missed and the next dose 2 to 4 hours later. Then go back to your regular schedule.

■ *Storage instructions...*
Store capsules and tablets at room temperature. The liquid form should be kept in the refrigerator in a tightly closed bottle. Discard any unused medication after 14 days.

What side effects may occur?

Side effects cannot be anticipated. If any develop or change in intensity, inform your doctor as soon as possible. Only your doctor can determine if it is safe for you to continue taking Duricef.

■ *Side effects may include:*
Diarrhea, inflammation of the bowel (colitis), nausea, redness and swelling of skin, skin rash and itching, vaginal inflammation, vomiting

Why should this drug not be prescribed?

If you are sensitive to or have ever had an allergic reaction to a cephalosporin antibiotic, you should not take Duricef.

Special warnings about this medication

If you have allergies, particularly to drugs, or often develop diarrhea when taking other antibiotics, you should tell your doctor before taking Duricef.

Also be sure to let the doctor know if you have a kidney disorder. Duricef should be used with caution under these circumstances, and the doctor may want to prescribe a lower dose.

Use Duricef with caution if you have a history of gastrointestinal disease, particularly inflammation of the bowel (colitis).

Continued or prolonged use of Duricef may result in the growth of bacteria that do not respond to this medication and can cause a second infection.

Possible food and drug interactions when taking this medication

No significant interactions have been reported.

Special information if you are pregnant or breastfeeding

The effects of Duricef during pregnancy have not been adequately studied. If you are pregnant or plan to become pregnant, inform your doctor immediately. Duricef may appear in breast milk and could affect a nursing infant. If this medication is essential to your health, your doctor may advise you to stop nursing your baby until your treatment time with Duricef is finished.

Recommended dosage

ADULTS

Urinary Tract Infections
The usual dosage for uncomplicated infections is a total of 1 to 2 grams per day in a single dose or 2 smaller doses. For all other urinary tract infections, the usual dosage is a total of 2 grams per day taken in 2 doses.

Skin and Skin Structure Infections
The usual dose is a total of 1 gram per day in a single dose or 2 smaller doses.

Throat Infections—Strep Throat and Tonsillitis
The usual dosage is a total of 1 gram per day in a single dose or 2 smaller doses for 10 days.

CHILDREN

For urinary tract and skin infections, the usual dose is 30 milligrams per 2.2 pounds of body weight per day, divided into 2 doses and taken every 12 hours. For throat infections, the recommended dose per day is 30 milligrams per 2.2 pounds of body weight in a single dose or 2 smaller doses. In the treatment of strep throat, the dose should be taken for at least 10 days.

OLDER ADULTS

Your dose may be reduced by your doctor.

Overdosage

Duricef is generally safe. However, large amounts may cause seizures or the side effects listed above. If you suspect an overdose of Duricef, seek medical attention immediately.

Dutasteride *See Avodart, page 169.*

DYAZIDE

Pronounced: DYE-uh-zide
Generic ingredients: Hydrochlorothiazide, Triamterene
Other brand names: Maxzide, Maxzide-25 MG

Why is this drug prescribed?

Dyazide is a combination of diuretic drugs used in the treatment of high blood pressure and other conditions that require the elimination of excess fluid from the body. When used for high blood pressure, Dyazide can be taken alone or with other high blood pressure medications. Diuretics help your body produce and eliminate more urine, which helps lower blood pressure. Triamterene, one of the ingredients of Dyazide, helps to minimize the potassium loss that can be caused by the other component, hydrochlorothiazide. Maxzide and Maxzide-25 MG contain the same combination of ingredients.

Most important fact about this drug

If you have high blood pressure, you must take Dyazide regularly for it to be effective. Since blood pressure declines gradually, it may be several weeks before you get the full benefit of Dyazide; and you must continue taking it even if you are feeling well. Dyazide does not cure high blood pressure; it merely keeps it under control.

How should you take this medication?

Dyazide should be taken early in the day. To avoid stomach upset, take it with food.

■ *If you miss a dose...*
Take it as soon as you remember. If it is almost time for the next dose, skip the one you missed and go back to your regular schedule. Do not take 2 doses at the same time.

■ *Storage instructions...*
Store at room temperature, away from light.

What side effects may occur?

Side effects cannot be anticipated. If any occur or change in intensity, inform your doctor as soon as possible. Only your doctor can determine if it is safe for you to continue taking Dyazide.

■ *Side effects may include:*
Abdominal pain, anemia, breathing difficulty, change in potassium level (causing symptoms such as numbness, tingling, muscle weakness, slow heart rate, shock), constipation, diabetes, diarrhea, dizziness, dizziness when standing up, dry mouth, fatigue, headache, hives, impotence, irregular heartbeat, kidney stones, muscle cramps, nausea, rash, sensitivity to light, strong allergic reaction (localized hives, itching, and swelling or, in severe cases, shock), vomiting, weakness, yellow eyes and skin

Why should this drug not be prescribed?

If you are unable to urinate or have any serious kidney disease, if you have high potassium levels in your blood, or if you are taking other drugs that prevent loss of potassium, you should not take Dyazide.

If you are sensitive to or have ever had an allergic reaction to triamterene (Dyrenium), hydrochlorothiazide (Oretic), or sulfa drugs such as Gantrisin, you should not take this medication.

Special warnings about this medication

When taking Dyazide, do not use potassium-containing salt substitutes. Take potassium supplements only if specifically directed to by your doctor. Your potassium level should be checked frequently.

If you are taking Dyazide and have kidney disease, your doctor should monitor your kidney function closely.

If you have liver disease, cirrhosis of the liver, heart failure, or kidney stones, this medication should be used with care. Diabetics may find that the drug increases their blood sugar levels, altering their insulin requirements.

Possible food and drug interactions when taking this medication

Dyazide should be used with caution if you are taking a type of blood pressure medication called an ACE inhibitor, such as Vasotec or Capoten.

If Dyazide is taken with certain other drugs, the effects of either could be increased, decreased, or altered. It is especially important to check with your doctor before combining Dyazide with the following:

Blood-thinning medications such as Coumadin
Corticosteroids such as Deltasone
Drugs for diabetes such as Micronase
Gout medications such as Zyloprim
Laxatives
Lithium (Lithonate)
Methenamine (Urised)
Nonsteroidal anti-inflammatory drugs such as Indocin and Dolobid
Other drugs that minimize potassium loss or contain potassium
Other high blood pressure medications such as Minipress
Salt substitutes containing potassium
Sodium polystyrene sulfonate (Kayexalate)

Special information if you are pregnant or breastfeeding

The effects of Dyazide during pregnancy have not been adequately studied. If you are pregnant or plan to become pregnant, inform your doctor immediately. Dyazide appears in breast milk and could affect a nursing infant. If this medication is essential to your health, your doctor may advise you to discontinue breastfeeding until your treatment is finished.

Recommended dosage

ADULTS

The usual dose of Dyazide is 1 or 2 capsules once daily, with appropriate monitoring of blood potassium levels by your doctor. The usual dose of Maxzide is 1 tablet daily. The recommendation for Maxzide-25 MG is 1 or 2 tablets daily taken in a single dose.

CHILDREN

Safety and effectiveness in children have not been established.

Overdosage

Any medication taken in excess can have serious consequences. If you suspect an overdose, seek medical treatment immediately.

■ *Symptoms of Dyazide overdose may include:*
Fever, flushed face, nausea, production of large amounts of pale urine, vomiting, weakness, weariness

DYNABAC

Pronounced: DYE-na-bak
Generic name: Dirithromycin

Why is this drug prescribed?

Dynabac cures certain mild to moderate skin infections and respiratory infections such as strep throat, tonsillitis, pneumonia, and flare-ups of chronic bronchitis. Dynabac is part of the same family of drugs as the commonly prescribed antibiotic erythromycin.

Most important fact about this drug

Like all antibiotics, Dynabac should be taken until the entire prescription is finished, even if you begin to feel better after the first few days. If you stop taking this medicine too soon, the strongest germs may survive and cause a relapse.

How should you take this medication?

Take Dynabac with food or within 1 hour after a meal. Swallow the tablet whole; do not crush, chew, or break it.

■ *If you miss a dose...*
Take it as soon as you remember. If you don't remember until the next day, skip the forgotten dose and go back to your regular schedule. Never try to catch up by doubling the dose.

■ *Storage instructions...*
Store Dynabac at room temperature.

What side effects may occur?

Side effects cannot be anticipated. If any develop or change in intensity, tell your doctor as soon as possible. Only your doctor can determine if it is safe for you to continue taking Dynabac.

■ *Side effects may include:*
Abdominal pain, diarrhea, headache, nausea, vomiting

Why should this drug not be prescribed?

If you have ever had an allergic reaction to Dynabac or to similar antibiotics such as erythromycin (E.E.S., PCE, and others), do not take this medication.

Special warnings about this medication

Dynabac, like certain other antibiotics, may cause a potentially life-threatening form of diarrhea called pseudomembranous colitis. A mild case may clear up on its own when the drug is stopped. For a more severe case, your doctor may need to prescribe fluids, electrolytes, and another antibiotic.

If you have liver disease, use Dynabac with caution and only if absolutely necessary.

Possible food and drug interactions when taking this medication
If Dynabac is taken with certain other drugs, the effects of either could be increased, decreased, or altered. It is especially important to check with your doctor before combining Dynabac with the following:

Antacids (Maalox, Mylanta)
Cimetidine (Tagamet)
Famotidine (Pepcid)
Nizatidine (Axid)
Ranitidine (Zantac)
Theophylline drugs such as Bronkodyl, Slo-Phyllin, Theo-Dur, and
    others

The following medications can interact with the related drug erythromycin:

Astemizole (Hismanal)
Blood-thinning drugs such as Coumadin
Bromocriptine (Parlodel)
Carbamazepine (Tegretol)
Cyclosporine (Sandimmune and Neoral)
Digoxin (Lanoxin)
Disopyramide (Norpace)
Ergot-containing drugs such as Cafergot and D.H.E.
Lovastatin (Mevacor)
Phenytoin (Dilantin)
Triazolam (Halcion)
Valproate (Depakene, Depakote)

Special information if you are pregnant or breastfeeding
If you are pregnant or plan to become pregnant, tell your doctor immediately. You should take Dynabac during pregnancy only if it is clearly needed. It is not known whether Dynabac appears in breast milk. If this medication is essential to your health, your doctor may advise you to stop breastfeeding until your treatment is finished.

Recommended dosage

ADULTS AND CHILDREN 12 YEARS AND OLDER

Bronchitis and Skin Infections
The usual dose is 500 milligrams (2 tablets) once a day for 5 to 7 days.

Pneumonia
The usual dose is 500 milligrams (2 tablets) once a day for 14 days.

Strep Throat and Tonsillitis
The usual dose is 500 milligrams (2 tablets) once a day for 10 days.

CHILDREN UNDER 12 YEARS OLD

The safety and effectiveness of Dynabac in children under the age of 12 have not been established.

Overdosage
Any medication taken in excess can have serious consequences. If you suspect an overdose, seek medical attention immediately.

■ *Symptoms of Dynabac overdose may include:*
Diarrhea, nausea, stomach problems, vomiting

Dynacin *See Minocin, page 867.*

DYNACIRC
Pronounced: DYE-na-serk
Generic name: Isradipine
Other brand name: DynaCirc CR

Why is this drug prescribed?
DynaCirc, a type of medication called a calcium channel blocker, is pre-scribed for the treatment of high blood pressure. It is effective when used alone or with a thiazide-type diuretic to flush excess water from the body. Calcium channel blockers ease the workload of the heart by slowing down the passage of nerve impulses through the heart muscle, thereby slowing the beat. This improves blood flow through the heart and throughout the body and reduces blood pressure. A controlled-release version of this drug (DynaCirc CR) maintains lower blood pressure for 24 hours.

Most important fact about this drug
You must take DynaCirc regularly for it to be effective. Since blood pres-sure declines gradually, it may be several weeks before you get the full benefit of DynaCirc; and you must continue taking it even if you are feel-ing well. DynaCirc does not cure high blood pressure; it merely keeps it under control.

How should you take this medication?
Take this medication exactly as prescribed, even if your symptoms have disappeared. Try not to miss any doses. If DynaCirc is not taken regularly, your condition may worsen.
    Swallow the capsule or tablet whole, without crushing or chewing it.

■ *If you miss a dose...*
Take it as soon as you remember. If it is almost time for your next dose, skip the one you missed and go back to your regular schedule. Never take 2 doses at the same time.

■ *Storage instructions...*
Store at room temperature, away from light, in a tightly closed container.

What side effects may occur?

Side effects cannot be anticipated. If any develop or change in intensity, inform your doctor as soon as possible. Only your doctor can determine if it is safe for you to continue taking DynaCirc.

■ *Side effects may include:*
Dizziness, fluid retention, flushing, headache, pounding heartbeat

Why should this drug not be prescribed?

If you are sensitive to or have ever had an allergic reaction to DynaCirc or other calcium channel blockers such as Vascor and Procardia, you should not take this medication. Tell your doctor about any drug reactions you have experienced.

Special warnings about this medication

DynaCirc can cause your blood pressure to become too low. If you feel light-headed or faint, contact your doctor.

This medication should be carefully monitored if you have congestive heart failure, especially if you are also taking a beta-blocking medication such as Tenormin or Inderal.

Before having surgery, including dental surgery, tell the doctor that you are taking DynaCirc.

Possible food and drug interactions when taking this medication

If DynaCirc is taken with certain other drugs, the effects of either could be increased, decreased, or altered. It is especially important to check with your doctor before combining DynaCirc with the following:

Beta-blocking blood pressure drugs such as Tenormin, Inderal, and Lopressor
Cimetidine (Tagamet)
Rifampin (Rifadin)

Special information if you are pregnant or breastfeeding

The effects of DynaCirc during pregnancy have not been adequately studied. If you are pregnant or plan to become pregnant, consult your doctor immediately. DynaCirc may appear in breast milk and could affect a nursing infant. If this medication is essential to your health, your doctor may advise you to discontinue breastfeeding until your treatment with DynaCirc is finished.

Recommended dosage

DYNACIRC

Your dosage will be adjusted to meet your individual needs.

The usual starting dose is 2.5 milligrams, 2 times a day, either alone or in combination with a thiazide diuretic drug. DynaCirc may lower blood pressure 2 to 3 hours after taking the first dose, but the full effect of the drug may not take place for 2 to 4 weeks.

After a 2- to 4-week trial, your doctor may increase the dosage by 5 milligrams per day every 2 to 4 weeks until a maximum dose of 20 milligrams per day is reached. Side effects may increase or become more common after a 10-milligram dose.

If you are an older adult or have kidney or liver disease, you should still begin treatment with a 2.5-milligram dose 2 times per day; however, your doctor will monitor you closely, since your condition may alter the effects of this drug.

DYNACIRC CR

The usual starting dose is 5 milligrams once a day, either alone or in combination with a thiazide diuretic. A starting dose of 5 milligrams once a day is also recommended for older adults and those with mild liver and kidney problems.

As with regular DynaCirc, the dosage may be increased to a maximum of 20 milligrams per day.

Overdosage

Although there is little information on DynaCirc, overdose has resulted in sluggishness, low blood pressure, and rapid heartbeat. The symptoms of overdose with other calcium channel blockers include drowsiness, severe low blood pressure, and rapid heartbeat.

If you suspect a DynaCirc overdose, seek medical attention immediately.

Echothiophate See *Phospholine Iodide, page 1095*.

EC-Naprosyn See *Naprosyn, page 914*.

Econazole See *Spectazole Cream, page 1330*.

Ecotrin See *Aspirin, page 132*.

Edex See *Caverject, page 257*.

E.E.S. See *Erythromycin, Oral, page 520*.

Efalizumab See Raptiva, page 1217.

Efavirenz See Sustiva, page 1362.

EFFEXOR

Pronounced: ef-ECKS-or
Generic name: Venlafaxine hydrochloride
Other brand name: Effexor XR

Why is this drug prescribed?

Effexor is prescribed for the treatment of depression—that is, a continuing depression that interferes with daily functioning. The symptoms usually include changes in appetite, sleep habits, and mind/body coordination, decreased sex drive, increased fatigue, feelings of guilt or worthlessness, difficulty concentrating, slowed thinking, and suicidal thoughts.

Effexor XR is also prescribed to relieve abnormal anxiety (generalized anxiety disorder and social anxiety disorder). Generalized anxiety disorder is marked by persistent anxiety for a period of at least 6 months, accompanied by at least 3 of these 6 symptoms: restlessness, fatigue, poor concentration, irritability, muscle tension, and sleep disturbances.

Social anxiety disorder is marked by a persistent fear (avoidance, anxiousness, or distress) of social situations, exposure to unfamiliar people, or possible scrutiny by others. Social anxiety is considered abnormal if it causes someone to alter an otherwise normal routine or interferes with daily functioning. The disorder can also cause panic attacks.

Effexor must be taken 2 or 3 times daily. The extended-release form, Effexor XR, permits once-a-day dosing.

Most important fact about this drug

Serious, sometimes fatal reactions have occurred when Effexor is used in combination with other drugs known as MAO inhibitors, including the antidepressants Nardil and Parnate. Never take Effexor with one of these drugs; and do not begin therapy with Effexor within 14 days of discontinuing treatment with one of them. Also, allow at least 7 days between the last dose of Effexor and the first dose of an MAO inhibitor.

How should you take this medication?

Take Effexor with food, exactly as prescribed. It may take several weeks before you begin to feel better. Your doctor should check your progress periodically.

Take Effexor XR once a day at the same time each day. Swallow the capsule whole with water. Do not divide, crush, or chew it. However, if you have trouble swallowing pills, you may take Effexor XR by carefully opening the capsule and sprinkling the entire contents on a spoonful of applesauce, followed by a glass of water.

■ *If you miss a dose...*
It is not necessary to make it up. Skip the missed dose and continue with your next scheduled dose. Do not take 2 doses at once.

■ *Storage instructions...*
Store in a tightly closed container at room temperature. Protect from excessive heat and moisture.

What side effects may occur?

Side effects cannot be anticipated. If any develop or change in intensity, tell your doctor as soon as possible. Only your doctor can determine if it is safe for you to continue taking Effexor.

■ *Side effects of Effexor may include:*
Abnormal ejaculation/orgasm, anxiety, blurred vision, constipation, dizziness, dry mouth, impotence, insomnia, nausea, nervousness, sleepiness, sweating, tremor, vomiting, weakness, weight loss

■ *Side effects of Effexor XR may include:*
Abnormal dreams, abnormal ejaculation, constipation, dizziness, dry mouth, headache, insomnia, nausea, nervousness, sleepiness, sweating, weakness, weight loss

Why should this drug not be prescribed?

Never take Effexor while taking other drugs known as MAO inhibitors (see *Most important fact about this drug*). Also avoid this drug if it has ever given you an allergic reaction.

Special warnings about this medication

In clinical studies, antidepressants increased the risk of suicidal thinking and behavior in children and adolescents with depression and other psychiatric disorders. Anyone considering the use of Effexor or any other antidepressant in a child or adolescent must balance this risk with the clinical need. Effexor has not been studied in children or adolescents and is not approved for treating anyone less than 18 years old.

Additionally, the progression of major depression is associated with a worsening of symptoms and/or the emergence of suicidal thinking or behavior in both adults and children, whether or not they are taking antidepressants. Individuals being treated with Effexor and their caregivers should watch for any change in symptoms or any new symptoms that appear suddenly—especially agitation, anxiety, hostility, panic, restlessness, extreme hyperactivity, and suicidal thinking or behavior—and report them to the doctor immediately. Be especially observant at the beginning of treatment or whenever there is a change in dose.

Your doctor will prescribe Effexor with caution if you have high blood pressure, heart, liver, or kidney disease or a history of seizures or mania (extreme agitation or excitability). You should discuss all of your medical problems with your doctor before taking Effexor.

Effexor sometimes causes an increase in blood pressure. If this happens, your doctor may need to reduce your dose or discontinue the drug.

Effexor also tends to increase the heart rate, especially at higher doses. Use Effexor with caution if you've recently had a heart attack, suffer from heart failure, or have an overactive thyroid gland.

Effexor may also cause cholesterol levels to rise in some patients who take it for 3 months or longer. This effect is more common among patients taking higher doses of Effexor.

Antidepressants such as Effexor may cause fluid retention, especially if you are an older adult.

Effexor may cause you to feel drowsy or less alert and may affect your judgment. Therefore, avoid driving or operating dangerous machinery or participating in any hazardous activity that requires full mental alertness until you know how this drug affects you.

Your doctor will check you regularly if you have glaucoma (high pressure in the eye), or you are at risk of developing it.

If you have ever been addicted to drugs, tell your doctor before you start taking Effexor.

If you develop a skin rash or hives while taking Effexor, notify your doctor. Effexor may also cause bleeding or bruising of the skin.

Do not stop taking the drug without consulting your doctor. If you stop suddenly, you may have withdrawal symptoms, even though this drug does not seem to be habit-forming. Your doctor will have you taper off gradually.

Possible food and drug interactions when taking this medication
Combining Effexor with MAO inhibitors could cause a fatal reaction (see *Most important fact about this drug*).

Although Effexor does not interact with alcohol, the manufacturer recommends avoiding alcohol while taking this medication.

If you have high blood pressure or liver disease, or are elderly, check with your doctor before combining Effexor with cimetidine (Tagamet).

You should consult your doctor before combining Effexor with other drugs that affect the central nervous system, including lithium, migraine medications such as Imitrex, narcotic painkillers, sleep aids, weight loss products such as phentermine, tranquilizers, antipsychotic medicines such as Haldol, and other antidepressants such as Celexa, Prozac, Tofranil, and Zoloft.

Effexor has been found to reduce blood levels of the HIV drug Crixivan. It's best to check with your doctor before combining Effexor with any other drug or herbal product.

Special Information if you are pregnant or breastfeeding
The effects of Effexor during pregnancy have not been adequately studied. If you are pregnant or are planning to become pregnant, tell your doc-

tor immediately. Effexor should be used during pregnancy only if clearly needed.

If Effexor is taken shortly before delivery, the baby may suffer withdrawal symptoms. It's also known that Effexor appears in breast milk and can cause serious side effects in a nursing infant. You'll need to choose between nursing your baby or continuing your treatment with Effexor.

Recommended dosage

EFFEXOR

The usual starting dose is 75 milligrams a day, divided into 2 or 3 smaller doses, and taken with food. If needed, your doctor may gradually increase your daily dose, in steps of no more than 75 milligrams at a time, up to a maximum of 375 milligrams per day.

If you have kidney or liver disease or are taking other medications, your doctor will adjust your dosage accordingly.

EFFEXOR XR

For both depression and anxiety, the usual starting dose is 75 milligrams once daily taken with food, although some people begin with a dose of 37.5 milligrams for the first 4 to 7 days. Your doctor may gradually increase the dose, in steps of no more than 75 milligrams at a time, up to a maximum of 225 milligrams daily. As with regular Effexor, the doctor will make adjustments in your dosage if you have kidney or liver disease.

Overdosage

An overdose of Effexor, combined with other drugs or alcohol, can be fatal. If you suspect an overdose, seek medical attention immediately.

■ *Symptoms of Effexor overdose include:*
  Coma, low blood pressure, rapid or slow heartbeat, seizures, sleepiness, vertigo

EFUDEX
Pronounced: EFF-you-decks
Generic name: Fluorouracil
Other brand name: Carac

Why is this drug prescribed?

Efudex and Carac are prescribed for the treatment of actinic or solar keratoses (small red horny growths or flesh-colored wartlike growths caused by overexposure to ultraviolet radiation or the sun). Such growths may develop into skin cancer. When conventional methods are impractical—as when the affected sites are hard to get at—the 5 percent strength of Efudex is useful in the treatment of superficial basal cell carcinomas or slow-growing malignant tumors of the face, usually found at the edge of the nostrils, eyelids, or lips. Efudex is available in cream and solution forms. Carac comes in cream form only.

Most important fact about this drug

If you use an airtight dressing to cover the skin being treated, there may be inflammatory reactions in the normal skin around the treated area. If it is necessary to cover the treated area, use a porous gauze dressing to avoid skin reactions.

How should you take this medication?

Use care when applying these products around the eyes, nose, and mouth. Wash your hands immediately after applying this medication.

■ *If you miss a dose...*
Apply it as soon as you remember. If more than a few hours have passed, skip the dose you missed and go back to your regular schedule. If you miss more than 1 dose, contact your doctor.

■ *Storage instructions...*
Store away from heat, light, and moisture.

What side effects may occur?

Side effects cannot be anticipated. If any develop or change in intensity, inform your doctor as soon as possible. Only your doctor can determine if it is safe for you to continue using Efudex.

■ *Side effects may include:*
Burning, discoloration of the skin, itching, pain

If you develop symptoms of a severe allergic reaction—including abdominal pain, bloody diarrhea, vomiting, fever, and chills—stop taking Efudex and contact your doctor immediately. You may have a condition known as DPD enzyme deficiency.

Why should this drug not be prescribed?

If you are sensitive to or have ever had an allergic reaction to Efudex, Carac or similar drugs, you should not take this medication. Make sure your doctor is aware of any drug reactions you have experienced.

People with a condition called DPD enzyme deficiency should also avoid these products. The active ingredient can give them a life-threatening reaction marked by abdominal pain, bloody diarrhea, vomiting, fever, and chills.

Special warnings about this medication

Avoid prolonged exposure to ultraviolet rays while you are under treatment with these products.

Skin may be unsightly during treatment with this drug and, in some cases, for several weeks after treatment has ended.

If your solar keratoses do not clear up with use of this drug, your doctor will probably order a biopsy (removal of a small amount of tissue to be examined under a microscope) to confirm the skin disease.

Your doctor will perform follow-up biopsies if you are being treated for superficial basal cell carcinoma.

Possible food and drug interactions when taking this medication
There are no reported food or drug interactions.

Special information if you are pregnant or breastfeeding
Efudex can harm a developing baby, and should not be used by women who are—or even may become—pregnant. If you do become pregnant while using Efudex, check with your doctor immediately.

Because it's not known whether Efudex could find its way into breast milk and harm a nursing infant, you'll need to choose between breastfeeding your baby and undergoing treatment with Efudex.

Recommended dosage
When Efudex is applied to affected skin, the skin becomes abnormally red, blisters form, and the surface skin wears away. A lesion or sore forms at the affected site, and the diseased or cancerous skin cells die before a new layer of skin forms.

ADULTS

Actinic or Solar Keratosis
Apply Efudex cream or solution 2 times a day, or Carac cream once a day, in an amount sufficient to cover the affected area. Continue using the medication until the inflammatory response reaches the stage where the skin wears away, a sore or lesion forms, and the skin cells die; your doctor will then have you stop using the medication. The usual length of treatment is from 2 to 4 weeks. You may not see complete healing of the affected area for 1 to 2 months after ending the treatment.

Superficial Basal Cell Carcinomas
For this condition, use only the 5% strength of Efudex. Twice a day, apply enough cream or solution to cover the affected area. Continue the treatment for at least 3 to 6 weeks; it may take 10 to 12 weeks of application before the lesions are gone.

Your doctor will want to monitor your condition to make sure it has been cured.

Overdosage
Although no specific information is available on Efudex overdosage, any medication used in excess can have serious consequences. If you suspect an overdosage, seek medical attention immediately.

ELAVIL

Pronounced: ELL-uh-vil
Generic name: Amitriptyline hydrochloride

Why is this drug prescribed?

Elavil is prescribed for the relief of symptoms of mental depression. It is a member of the group of drugs called tricyclic antidepressants. Some doctors also prescribe Elavil to treat bulimia (an eating disorder), to control chronic pain, to prevent migraine headaches, and to treat a pathological weeping and laughing syndrome associated with multiple sclerosis.

Most important fact about this drug

You may need to take Elavil regularly for several weeks before it becomes fully effective. Do not skip doses, even if they seem to make no difference or you feel you don't need them.

How should you take this medication?

Take Elavil exactly as prescribed. You may experience side effects, such as mild drowsiness, early in therapy. However, they usually disappear after a few days. Beneficial effects may take as long as 30 days to appear.

Elavil may cause dry mouth. Sucking a hard candy, chewing gum, or melting bits of ice in your mouth can provide relief.

■ *If you miss a dose...*
Take it as soon as you remember. If it is almost time for your next dose, skip the one you missed and go back to your regular schedule. Never take 2 doses at the same time.

If you take a single daily dose at bedtime, do not make up for it in the morning. It may cause side effects during the day.

■ *Storage instructions...*
Keep Elavil in a tightly closed container. Store at room temperature. Protect from light and excessive heat.

What side effects may occur?

Side effects cannot be anticipated. If any develop or change in intensity, inform your doctor as soon as possible. Only your doctor can determine if it is safe for you to continue taking Elavil.

Older adults are especially liable to certain side effects of Elavil, including rapid heartbeat, constipation, dry mouth, blurred vision, sedation, and confusion, and are in greater danger of sustaining a fall.

■ *Side effects may include:*
Blurred vision, bone marrow depression, bowel problems, breast enlargement (in males and females), constipation, dry mouth, hair loss, heart attack, high body temperature, problems urinating, rash, seizure, stroke, swelling of the testicles, water retention

- *Side effects due to a rapid decrease in dose or abrupt withdrawal from Elavil include:*
  Headache, nausea, vague feeling of bodily discomfort
- *Side effects due to gradual dosage reduction may include:*
  Dream and sleep disturbances, irritability, restlessness

These side effects do not signify an addiction to the drug.

Why should this drug not be prescribed?

If you are sensitive to or have ever had an allergic reaction to Elavil or similar drugs such as Norpramin and Tofranil, you should not take this medication. Make sure your doctor is aware of any drug reactions you have experienced.

Do not take Elavil while taking other drugs known as MAO inhibitors. Drugs in this category include the antidepressants Nardil and Parnate.

Unless you are directed to do so by your doctor, do not take this medication if you are recovering from a heart attack.

Special warnings about this medication

In clinical studies, antidepressants increased the risk of suicidal thinking and behavior in children and adolescents with depression and other psychiatric disorders. Anyone considering the use of Elavil or any other antidepressant in a child or adolescent must balance this risk with the clinical need. Elavil is not approved for treating children less than 12 years old.

Additionally, the progression of major depression is associated with a worsening of symptoms and/or the emergence of suicidal thinking or behavior in both adults and children, whether or not they are taking antidepressants. Individuals being treated with Elavil and their caregivers should watch for any change in symptoms or any new symptoms that appear suddenly—especially agitation, anxiety, hostility, panic, restlessness, extreme hyperactivity, and suicidal thinking or behavior—and report them to the doctor immediately. Be especially observant at the beginning of treatment or whenever there is a change in dose.

Do not stop taking Elavil abruptly, especially if you have been taking large doses for a long time. Your doctor probably will want to decrease your dosage gradually. This will help prevent a possible relapse and will reduce the possibility of withdrawal symptoms.

Elavil may make your skin more sensitive to sunlight. Try to stay out of the sun, wear protective clothing, and apply a sun block.

Elavil may cause you to become drowsy or less alert; therefore, you should not drive or operate dangerous machinery or participate in any hazardous activity that requires full mental alertness until you know how this drug affects you.

While taking this medication, you may feel dizzy or light-headed or actually faint when getting up from a lying or sitting position. If getting up slowly doesn't help or if this problem continues, notify your doctor.

Use Elavil with caution if you have ever had seizures, urinary retention, glaucoma or other chronic eye conditions, a heart or circulatory system disorder, or liver problems. Be cautious, too, if you are receiving thyroid medication. You should discuss all of your medical problems with your doctor before starting Elavil therapy.

Before having surgery, dental treatment, or any diagnostic procedure, tell the doctor that you are taking Elavil. Certain drugs used during surgery, such as anesthetics and muscle relaxants, and drugs used in certain diagnostic procedures may react badly with Elavil.

Possible food and drug interactions when taking this medication
Elavil may intensify the effects of alcohol. Do not drink alcohol while taking this medication.

If Elavil is taken with certain other drugs, the effects of either could be increased, decreased, or altered. It is especially important that you consult with your doctor before taking Elavil in combination with the following:

Airway-opening drugs such as Proventil and Sudafed
Antidepressants that raise serotonin levels, such as Paxil, Prozac, and Zoloft
Antihistamines such as Benadryl and Tavist
Barbiturates such as phenobarbital
Certain blood pressure medicines such as Catapres
Cimetidine (Tagamet)
Disulfiram (Antabuse)
Drugs that control spasms, such as Bentyl and Donnatal
Estrogen drugs such as Premarin and oral contraceptives
Ethchlorvynol (Placidyl)
Major tranquilizers such as Mellaril and Thorazine
MAO inhibitors, such as Nardil and Parnate
Medications for irregular heartbeat such as Rythmol and Tambocor
Other antidepressants, such as amoxapine
Painkillers such as Demerol and Percocet
Parkinsonism drugs such as Cogentin and Larodopa
Quinidine (Quinidex)
Seizure medications such as Dilantin and Tegretol
Sleep medicines such as Dalmane and Halcion
Thyroid hormones (Synthroid)
Tranquilizers such as Librium and Xanax
Warfarin (Coumadin)

Special information if you are pregnant or breastfeeding
The effects of Elavil during pregnancy have not been adequately studied. If you are pregnant or planning to become pregnant, inform your doctor immediately. This medication appears in breast milk. If Elavil is essential

to your health, your doctor may advise you to discontinue breastfeeding until your treatment is finished.

Recommended dosage

ADULTS

The usual starting dosage is 75 milligrams per day divided into 2 or more smaller doses. Your doctor may gradually increase this dose to 150 milligrams per day. The total daily dose is generally never higher than 200 milligrams.

Alternatively, your doctor may want you to start with 50 to 100 milligrams at bedtime. He or she may increase this bedtime dose by 25 or 50 milligrams, up to a total of 150 milligrams a day.

For long-term use, the usual dose ranges from 40 to 100 milligrams taken once daily, usually at bedtime.

CHILDREN

The use of Elavil is not recommended for children under 12 years of age.

The usual dose for adolescents 12 years of age and over is 10 milligrams, 3 times a day, with 20 milligrams taken at bedtime.

OLDER ADULTS

The usual dose is 10 milligrams taken 3 times a day, with 20 milligrams taken at bedtime.

Overdosage

An overdose of Elavil can prove fatal. If you suspect an overdose, seek medical attention immediately.

■ *Symptoms of Elavil overdose may include:*
   Abnormally low blood pressure, confusion, convulsions, dilated pupils and other eye problems, disturbed concentration, drowsiness, hallucinations, impaired heart function, rapid or irregular heartbeat, reduced body temperature, stupor, unresponsiveness or coma

■ *Symptoms contrary to the effect of this medication are:*
   Agitation, extremely high body temperature, overactive reflexes, rigid muscles, vomiting

ELDEPRYL
Pronounced: ELL-dep-rill
Generic name: Selegiline hydrochloride

Why is this drug prescribed?

Eldepryl is prescribed along with Sinemet (levodopa/carbidopa) for people with Parkinson's disease. It is used when Sinemet no longer seems to be working well. Eldepryl has no effect when taken by itself; it works only in combination with Larodopa (levodopa) or Sinemet.

Parkinson's disease, which causes muscle rigidity and difficulty with walking and talking, involves the progressive degeneration of a particular type of nerve cell. Early on, Larodopa or Sinemet alone may alleviate the symptoms of the disease. In time, however, these medications work less well; their effectiveness seems to switch on and off at random, and the individual may begin to experience side effects such as involuntary movements and "freezing" in mid-motion.

Eldepryl may be prescribed at this stage of the disease to help restore the effectiveness of Larodopa or Sinemet. When you begin to take Eldepryl, you may need a reduced dosage of the other medication.

Most important fact about this drug

Eldepryl belongs to a class of drugs known as MAO inhibitors. These drugs can interact with certain foods—including aged cheeses and meats, pickled herring, beer, and wine—to cause a life-threatening surge in blood pressure. At the dose recommended for Eldepryl, this interaction is not a problem. But for safety's sake, you may want to watch your diet; and you should never take more Eldepryl than the doctor prescribes.

How should you take this medication?

Take Eldepryl and your other Parkinson's medication exactly as prescribed.

■ *If you miss a dose...*
Take it as soon as you remember. If you do not remember until late afternoon or evening, skip the dose you missed and go back to your regular schedule. Never take 2 doses at once.
■ *Storage instructions...*
Store at room temperature.

What side effects may occur?

Side effects cannot be anticipated. If any develop or change in intensity, inform your doctor as soon as possible. Only your doctor can determine if it is safe for you to continue taking Eldepryl.

■ *Side effects may include:*
Abdominal pain, confusion, dizziness, dry mouth, fainting, hallucinations, nausea, light-headedness

Why should this drug not be prescribed?

Do not take Eldepryl if you are sensitive to or have ever had an allergic reaction to it. Do not take narcotic painkillers such as Demerol while you are taking Eldepryl.

Special warnings about this medication

Never take Eldepryl at a higher dosage than prescribed; doing so could put you at risk for a dangerous rise in blood pressure. If you develop a severe headache or any other unusual symptoms, contact your doctor immediately.

You may suffer a severe reaction if you combine Eldepryl with tricyclic antidepressants such as Elavil and Tofranil, or with antidepressants that affect serotonin levels, such as Prozac and Paxil. Wait at least 14 days after taking Eldepryl before beginning therapy with any of these drugs. If you have been taking antidepressants such as Prozac and Paxil, you should wait at least *5 weeks* before taking Eldepryl. This much time is needed to clear the antidepressant completely from your system.

Possible food and drug interactions when taking this medication

If Eldepryl is taken with certain other drugs, the effects of either could be increased, decreased, or altered. It is especially important to check with your doctor before combining Eldepryl with the following:

Antidepressant medications classified as tricyclics, such as Elavil and Tofranil
Antidepressant medications that raise serotonin levels, such as Paxil, Prozac, and Zoloft
Narcotic painkillers such as Demerol, Percocet, and Tylenol with Codeine

Eldepryl may worsen side effects caused by your usual dosage of levodopa.

Special information if you are pregnant or breastfeeding

The effects of Eldepryl during pregnancy have not been adequately studied. If you are pregnant or plan to become pregnant, inform your doctor immediately. Although Eldepryl is not known to cause specific birth defects, it should not be taken during pregnancy unless it is clearly needed. It is not known whether Eldepryl appears in breast milk. As a general rule, a nursing mother should not take any drug unless it is clearly necessary.

Recommended dosage

ADULTS

The recommended dose of Eldepryl is 10 milligrams per day divided into 2 smaller doses of 5 milligrams each, taken at breakfast and lunch. There is no evidence of additional benefit from higher doses, and they increase the risk of side effects.

CHILDREN

The use of Eldepryl in children has not been evaluated.

Overdosage

Although no specific information is available about Eldepryl overdosage, it is assumed, because of chemical similarities, that the symptoms would resemble those of overdose with an MAO inhibitor antidepressant.

■ *Symptoms of MAO inhibitor overdose may include:*
Agitation, chest pain, clammy skin, coma, convulsions, dizziness, drowsiness, extremely high fever, faintness, fast and irregular pulse, hallucinations, headache (severe), high blood pressure, hyperactivity, inability to breathe, irritability, lockjaw, low blood pressure (severe), shallow breathing, spasm of the entire body, sweating

It is important to note that after a large overdose, symptoms may not appear for up to 12 hours and may not reach their full force for 24 hours or more. An overdose can be fatal. If you suspect an Eldepryl overdose, seek medical attention immediately. Hospitalization is recommended, with continuous observation and monitoring for at least 2 days.

ELESTAT

Pronounced: ELL-eh-stat
Generic name: Epinastine hydrochloride

Why is this drug prescribed?

Elestat is an antihistamine prescribed to relieve the itchy eyes caused by an allergic trigger such as pollen or animal dander. It starts to work within 3 to 5 minutes of placing the drops in the eye, and its effects usually last for 8 hours.

Most important fact about this drug

Do not use Elestat to treat eye irritation that isn't caused by allergies.

How should you take this medication?

Use Elestat solution only in the eyes; never swallow it. Elestat is packaged in a bottle with a dropper tip. To prevent contamination of the solution, do not touch the dropper tip to any surface, to your eyelids, or to the surrounding area of the eye.

If you wear soft contact lenses and your eyes are not red, wait at least 10 minutes after using Elestat before inserting your lenses. This will prevent them from absorbing the preservative in Elestat. You should not wear contact lenses if your eyes are red.

■ *If you miss a dose...*
Take it as soon as you remember. If it is almost time for your next dose, skip the one you missed and go back to your regular schedule. Never take 2 doses at the same time.

■ *Storage instructions*...
Store upright at room temperature. Keep the bottle tightly closed.

What side effects may occur?
Side effects cannot be anticipated. If any develop or change in intensity, tell your doctor as soon as possible. Only your doctor can determine if it is safe to continue using Elestat.

■ *Side effects may include:*
Bloodshot eyes, burning sensation in the eye, cold-like symptoms, inflammation of eyelid follicles (folliculosis), itching of the eye, upper respiratory infection

Some of these side effects are similar to the symptoms of seasonal allergies.

Why should this drug not be prescribed?
Do not use Elestat if you are allergic to any of its ingredients. If you take Elestat and an allergic reaction occurs, you will have to stop using it.

Special warnings about this medication
If you wear contact lenses, remember that Elestat should not be used to treat eye irritation caused by your lenses.

The safety and effectiveness of Elestat have not been studied in children younger than 3 years old.

Possible food and drug interactions when taking this medication
No interactions with Elestat have been reported.

Special information if you are pregnant or breastfeeding
The effects of Elestat during pregnancy have not been adequately studied. If you are pregnant or plan to become pregnant, inform your doctor immediately.

It is not known whether Elestat appears in breast milk. If this drug is essential to your health, your doctor may advise you to stop nursing until your treatment is finished.

Recommended dosage
The recommended dosage is one drop in each affected eye twice a day. You should continue using Elestat until you are no longer exposed to the allergic trigger (for example, until the pollen season is over), even if you do not have itchy eyes.

Overdosage
There is no information on Elestat overdose. However, any medication taken in excess can have serious consequences. If you suspect an overdose, seek medical attention immediately.

Eletriptan *See Relpax, page 1229.*

ELIDEL
Pronounced: ELL-ih-dell
Generic name: Pimecrolimus

Why is this drug prescribed?
Elidel is a nonsteroidal cream that relieves mild to moderate symptoms of eczema, a skin condition marked by itchy red patches that often crust, scale, and ooze. Elidel is approved for use in adults and children over 2 years old; it can be used for short-term treatment or on-and-off treatment over longer periods of time. Elidel is considered an effective alternative for people who cannot tolerate or do not respond to conventional eczema therapies.

Most important fact about this drug
Because Elidel may make your skin more sensitive to ultraviolet light, you should minimize your exposure to sunlight and tanning beds while using this product.

How should you take this medication?
Apply a thin layer of Elidel to the affected skin twice daily and rub in gently and completely. Do not wrap the treated area with bandages or other coverings unless your doctor tells you to do so.

Elidel is for use on the skin only. Be careful to keep it out of your eyes.

- *If you miss a dose...*
  Apply the cream as soon as you remember. If it is almost time for your next application, skip the one you missed and go back to your regular schedule.
- *Storage instructions...*
  Store at room temperature. Do not freeze.

What side effects may occur?
Side effects cannot be anticipated. If any develop or change in intensity, inform your doctor as soon as possible. Only your doctor can determine if it is safe for you to continue using Elidel.

- *Side effects may include:*
  Allergic reaction, bronchitis, burning or warmth at the application site, constipation, cough, diarrhea, fever, flu, headache, herpes infection, inflammation of the throat and nasal passages, inflammation of the tonsils, nausea, painful menstruation, scabby skin eruptions, sore throat, stomach pain, stomach and intestinal inflammation, viral infection, vomiting

Why should this drug not be prescribed?

If you find that Elidel causes an allergic reaction, you'll be unable to use it.

Elidel is not recommended for people with Netherton's syndrome (a congenital disorder marked by scaly, reddened skin) or those with weak immune systems.

Special warnings about this medication

Elidel may cause skin reactions including mild to moderate feelings of warmth or burning. These reactions are more common during the first few days of treatment and usually last no more than 5 days. If the reaction is severe, however, or lasts more than 1 week, call your doctor immediately.

Avoid wrapping treated areas with bandages and other coverings unless your doctor says to do so. Remember to avoid or minimize your exposure to sunlight and tanning beds while using this medication. Elidel may foster development of sunlight-induced skin tumors.

Check with your doctor if your eczema gets worse or your symptoms go away; treatment usually should be stopped. Your doctor may also stop the treatment if your skin hasn't improved after 6 weeks.

Use Elidel only on non-infected skin. It's important to note that eczema—and possibly Elidel treatment—can make you more prone to skin infections such as herpes, chickenpox, and shingles. Be sure to tell your doctor if you develop any new symptoms such as blisters or red spots. He or she may decide to stop your treatment with Elidel.

Very rare cases of enlarged lymph nodes have occurred during Elidel treatment; skin warts have also been reported. Call your doctor immediately if you develop either of these symptoms, since they may mean you have an infection.

Possible food and drug interactions when taking this medication

If Elidel is used with certain other drugs, the effects of either could be increased, decreased, or altered. It is especially important to check with your doctor before combining Elidel with the following:

Calcium-blocking blood pressure drugs such as Calan, Cardizem, and Procardia
Cimetidine (Tagamet)
Erythromycin (E-Mycin, Erythrocin)
Fluconazole (Diflucan)
Itraconazole (Sporanox)
Ketoconazole (Nizoral)

Special information if you are pregnant or breastfeeding

If you are pregnant or plan to become pregnant, tell your doctor immediately. Elidel should be used during pregnancy only if clearly needed.

It is not known whether Elidel appears in breast milk. Because the drug could harm an infant, you'll need to choose between Elidel therapy or nursing your baby.

Recommended dosage

ADULTS AND CHILDREN OVER 2 YEARS

Apply a thin layer of Elidel to the affected area 2 times a day. Rub in gently and completely. Elidel can be applied to all skin areas, including the head, neck, and skin folds (such as between the toes).

Overdosage

There are no studies about the effects of an Elidel overdose. However, any medication taken in excess can have serious consequences. If you suspect an overdose, or accidentally swallow some Elidel, seek medical attention immediately.

ELOCON
Pronounced: ELL-oh-con
Generic name: Mometasone furoate

Why is this drug prescribed?
Elocon is a cortisone-like steroid available in cream, ointment, and lotion form. It is used to treat certain itchy rashes and other inflammatory skin conditions.

Most important fact about this drug
When you use Elocon, you inevitably absorb some of the medication through your skin and into the bloodstream. Too much absorption can lead to unwanted side effects elsewhere in the body. To keep this problem to a minimum, avoid using large amounts of Elocon over large areas, and do not cover it with airtight dressings such as plastic wrap or adhesive bandages unless specifically told to by your doctor.

How should you use this medication?
Apply a thin film of the cream or ointment or a few drops of the lotion to the affected skin once a day. Massage it in until it disappears.

Elocon is for use only on the skin. Be careful to keep it out of your eyes.

For the most effective and economical use of Elocon lotion, hold the tip of the bottle very close to (but not touching) the affected skin and squeeze the bottle gently.

Once you have applied Elocon, never cover the skin with an airtight bandage, a tight diaper, plastic pants, or any other airtight dressing. This could encourage excessive absorption of the medication into your bloodstream.

Be careful not to use Elocon for a longer time than prescribed. If you do, you may disrupt your ability to make your own natural adrenal corticoid hormones (hormones secreted by the outer layer of the adrenal gland).

■ *If you miss a dose...*
Apply it as soon as you remember. If it is almost time for your next dose, skip the one you missed and go back to your regular schedule.
■ *Storage instructions...*
Store at room temperature.

What side effects may occur?
Side effects cannot be anticipated. If any develop or change in intensity, notify your doctor as soon as possible. Only your doctor can determine if it is safe for you to continue using Elocon.

■ *Side effects may include:*
Acne-like pimples, allergic skin rash, boils, burning, damaged skin, dryness, excessive hairiness, infected hair follicles, infection of the skin, irritation, itching, light-colored patches on skin, prickly heat, rash around the mouth, skin atrophy and wasting, softening of the skin, stretch marks, tingling or stinging

Why should this drug not be prescribed?
Do not use Elocon if you have ever had an allergic reaction to it or any other steroid medication.

Special warnings about this medication
Remember, Elocon is for external use only. Avoid getting it into your eyes. Do not use it to treat anything other than the condition for which it was prescribed.

If your skin becomes irritated, call your doctor.

If you have any kind of skin infection, tell your doctor before you start using Elocon.

Do not use Elocon cream or ointment on your face, underarms, or groin area unless your doctor tells you to.

If your condition doesn't improve in 2 weeks, call your doctor.

Possible food and drug interactions when using this medication
No interactions have been noted.

Special information if you are pregnant or breastfeeding
If you are pregnant or plan to become pregnant, inform your doctor immediately. Elocon should not be used during pregnancy unless the benefit outweighs the potential risk to the unborn child.

You should not use Elocon while breastfeeding, since absorbed hormone could make its way into the breast milk and perhaps harm the nursing baby. If you are a new mother, you should contact your doctor, who will help you decide between breastfeeding and using Elocon.

Recommended dosage

ADULTS

Apply once daily.

CHILDREN

Use should be limited to the smallest amount necessary. Use of steroids over a long period of time may interfere with growth and development.

Elocon cream and ointment may be used for children aged 2 and older, but not for more than 3 weeks.

Overdosage

With extensive or long-term use of Elocon, hormone absorbed into the bloodstream may cause a group of symptoms called Cushing's syndrome.

■ *Symptoms of Cushing's syndrome may include:*
Acne, depression, excessive hair growth, high blood pressure, humped upper back, insomnia, moon-faced appearance, muscle weakness, obese trunk, paranoia, stretch marks, stunted growth (in children), susceptibility to bruising, fractures, and infections, wasted limbs

Cushing's syndrome may also trigger diabetes mellitus.

If it is left uncorrected, Cushing's syndrome may become serious. If you suspect your long-term use of Elocon has led to this problem, seek medical attention immediately.

Empirin *See Aspirin, page 132.*

E-Mycin *See Erythromycin, Oral, page 520.*

Enalapril *See Vasotec, page 1551.*

Enalapril with Felodipine *See Lexxel, page 753.*

Enalapril with Hydrochlorothiazide *See Vaseretic, page 1548.*

ENBREL

Pronounced: EN-brell
Generic name: Etanercept

Why is this drug prescribed?

Enbrel is used to relieve the symptoms and slow the progress of moderate to severe rheumatoid arthritis. It's also prescribed to relieve the symptoms of psoriatic arthritis. It can be added to methotrexate (Rheumatrex) therapy when methotrexate fails to provide adequate relief. Prescribed alone, it is also used for juvenile rheumatoid arthritis when other drugs have failed.

Enbrel is the first in a class of drugs designed to block the action of tumor necrosis factor (TNF), a naturally occurring protein responsible for much of the joint inflammation that plagues the victims of rheumatoid arthritis. In clinical trials, Enbrel provided the majority of patients with significant relief.

Enbrel is also used to reduce the symptoms of active ankylosing spondylitis, an inflammatory condition that results in stiffness and immobility and can sometimes cause joints and bones to fuse together.

In addition, Enbrel is used to treat chronic, moderate to severe plaque psoriasis, a condition where the skin is red and covered with silvery scales and inflammation (patches of round or oval red plaques that itch or burn).

Most important fact about this drug

TNF plays a significant role in the immune system, so blocking its action can lower your resistance to infection. Serious—and even fatal—infections have been known to occur, especially in people whose immune systems have already been weakened by advancing age, conditions such as heart failure or diabetes, or drugs such as Imuran, Prograf, Cellcept, Neoral, and Sandimmune. Due to the possibility of lowered resistance, children with juvenile rheumatoid arthritis should be brought up to date with all immunizations before starting Enbrel therapy.

How should you take this medication?

Enbrel is given by injection under the skin of the thigh, abdomen, or upper arm. Your doctor will instruct you in the proper drug preparation and injection technique and supervise your first injection in the office. You should rotate injection sites and make each new injection at least 1 inch from an older one. Never inject into areas where the skin is tender, bruised, red, or hard.

Do not shake Enbrel solution. Avoid handling the needle cover if you have a latex allergy. Never reuse a syringe. Throw it away in a puncture-proof container immediately after using it.

■ *If you miss a dose...*
Take it as soon as you remember. If it is almost time for your next dose, skip the one you missed and return to your regular schedule. Do not take 2 doses at once.

■ *Storage instructions...*
Store Enbrel powder in the refrigerator. Do not freeze. Discard after the expiration date stamped on the dose tray. After the powder has been mixed with sterile water, it can be stored under refrigeration for up to 14 days.

What side effects may occur?
Side effects cannot be anticipated. If any develop or change in intensity inform your doctor as soon as possible. Only your doctor can determine if it is safe for you to continue taking Enbrel.

■ *Side effects may include:*
Abdominal pain, cough, dizziness, headache, indigestion, infections, injection site reaction, nausea, rash, respiratory problems, respiratory tract infection, serious infections such as cellulitis and pneumonia, sinus and nasal inflammation, sore throat, vomiting, weakness

Why should this drug not be prescribed?
If Enbrel gives you an allergic reaction, you will not be able to continue using it. Do not start taking it during any kind of infection.

Think carefully about using this drug if you are prone to repeated infections or have a condition that encourages infections, such as diabetes. Be cautious, too, if you have a disease of the nervous system such as multiple sclerosis or a seizure disorder; such problems have been known to develop or get worse during Enbrel therapy. Enbrel should also be used with caution if you are prone to blood disorders, since they have occasionally appeared during treatment with Enbrel.

Special warnings about this medication
If you develop an infection, stop taking Enbrel and call your doctor immediately. Children exposed to chickenpox during Enbrel therapy may have to temporarily discontinue the drug and get preventive treatments.

Enbrel may worsen congestive heart failure. If you have this condition, make sure the doctor knows about it; Enbrel should be used with caution.

Enbrel has been known to trigger a condition similar to lupus. If you develop warning signs such as raised patches of red skin, see the doctor immediately. Enbrel therapy may have to be stopped.

Also check with your doctor immediately if you develop warning signs of a blood disorder, including such symptoms as persistent fever, bruising, bleeding, or paleness. You may have to stop taking Enbrel.

Possible food and drug interactions when taking this medication
The immune system–blocking action of Enbrel can lower your resistance to infection. Combining Enbrel with other rheumatoid arthritis drugs, such as Kineret, can lower your resistance even more, possibly leading to a severe infection. Make sure your doctor is aware of any drugs you are taking.

You should also avoid getting vaccinations that contain active, live viruses while taking Enbrel. However, other types of vaccines (such as those with inactive viruses) may be given during treatment with Enbrel.

Special information if you are pregnant or breastfeeding
The effects of Enbrel during pregnancy have not been studied. If you are pregnant or plan to become pregnant, inform your doctor immediately.

It is not known whether Enbrel appears in breast milk, but because there is a possible risk to the infant, you should either give up nursing while taking Enbrel or discontinue the drug. Discuss the problem with your doctor.

Recommended dosage

ADULTS 18 YEARS AND OLDER

Rheumatoid Arthritis, Psoriatic Arthritis,
Ankylosing Spondylitis
The total dose is 50 milligrams per week, given as two 25-milligram injections at separate sites. The injections are given under the skin either on the same day or 3 to 4 days apart.

Plaque Psoriasis
The recommended dose is one 50-milligram injection given under the skin twice weekly (3 or 4 days apart) for 3 months. The medication will be reduced to one 50-milligram dose once a week.

CHILDREN 4 TO 17 YEARS OLD

Rheumatoid Arthritis
The recommended dose is 0.4 milligrams per 2.2 pounds of body weight, up to a maximum of 25 milligrams, injected under the skin twice a week. The safety of Enbrel has not been studied in children less than 4 years old.

Overdosage
High doses of Enbrel do not appear to have any toxic effects. Nevertheless, if you suspect an overdose, you should notify your doctor.

Endocet *See Percocet, page 1073.*

Entacapone *See Comtan, page 333.*

ENTOCORT EC

Pronounced: EN-toe-cort
Generic name: Budesonide

Why is this drug prescribed?

Entocort EC is used to treat Crohn's disease, a chronic intestinal inflammation that causes sustained diarrhea and abdominal pain. The drug contains the anti-inflammatory steroid budesonide in a special formulation that concentrates in the intestines, thereby reducing its impact on the rest of the body.

Most important fact about this drug

Although Entocort EC isn't released until it reaches the intestines, it can still produce some of the side effects typical of other steroid medications, including reduced resistance to infection. Common diseases such as chickenpox and measles can be much more severe in people taking steroids. Be careful to avoid anyone who has such an infection. If, despite caution, you are exposed to one of these diseases, see your doctor immediately. You can be given a protective shot of immune globulin.

How should you take this medication?

Entocort EC capsules should be swallowed whole; do not chew or break the capsules.

■ *If you miss a dose...*
Take it as soon as you remember. If it is almost time for your next dose, skip the one you missed and resume your regular schedule.
■ *Storage instructions...*
Store at room temperature. Keep the container tightly closed.

What side effects may occur?

Side effects cannot be anticipated. If any develop or change in intensity, inform your doctor as soon as possible. Only your doctor can determine if it is safe for you to continue taking Entocort EC.

■ *Side effects may include:*
Abdominal pain, back pain, dizziness, fatigue, gas, headache, indigestion, nausea, pain, respiratory infection, vomiting

Why should this drug not be prescribed?

You cannot take Entocort EC if you have ever had an allergic reaction to it.

Special warnings about this medication

A high level of steroids in the system can lead to symptoms such as acne, easy bruising, swollen ankles, an increase in the size of the face and neck, excessive facial hair growth, irregular menstrual periods, and skin discoloration. If you develop any of these symptoms, alert your doctor.

Also check with your doctor immediately if you develop itching, rash, fever, swelling in the face or throat, or trouble breathing. These could be signs of an allergic reaction.

Because Entocort EC's effects are largely restricted to the intestines, switching to this medication from a steroid that affects the entire body can allow previously suppressed allergies to reappear. If you develop symptoms such as a runny nose or eczema, tell your doctor about it.

Make sure your doctor knows if you have tuberculosis, high blood pressure, osteoporosis, ulcers, cataracts, or high pressure in the eyes (glaucoma), or if anyone in your family has had diabetes or glaucoma. Steroids should be used with caution under these circumstances.

Also make sure the doctor knows if you have a liver condition; you may need a lower dose of Entocort EC.

Because steroids can reduce the body's natural ability to cope with stress, you may need a higher dose when you undergo any type of surgery.

Possible food and drug interactions when taking this medication
Grapefruit juice can increase the amount of Entocort EC in your blood stream. Do not drink grapefruit juice during your course of therapy with Entocort EC.

If Entocort EC is taken with certain other drugs, the effects of either could be increased, decreased, or altered. It is especially important to check with your doctor before combining Entocort EC with the following:

Antifungal medications such as Nizoral and Sporanox
Erythromycin (E.E.S., Ery-Tab, PCE)
Indinavir (Crixivan)
Ritonavir (Norvir)
Saquinavir (Invirase, Fortovase)

Special information if you are pregnant or breastfeeding
This drug should be used during pregnancy only if its benefits outweigh the possibility of harm to the developing baby. If you are pregnant or plan to become pregnant, notify your doctor immediately.

Steroid medications do appear in breast milk. This drug is not recommended for nursing mothers.

Recommended dosage

ADULTS

The recommended dosage is 9 milligrams (three 3-milligram capsules) every morning for up to 8 weeks. Your doctor may reduce the dose to 6 milligrams per day for the last 2 weeks of treatment. If symptoms return, the doctor can prescribe another 8-week course of therapy.

Overdosage

High doses of steroids taken for long periods can produce the symptoms summarized under *Special warnings about this medication*. Single massive overdoses are rare, but can have serious consequences. If you suspect an overdose, seek medical attention immediately.

Epinastine See *Elestat, page 505*.

Epitol See *Tegretol, page 1395*.

EPIVIR

Pronounced: EPP-ih-veer
Generic name: Lamivudine

Why is this drug prescribed?

Epivir is one of the drugs used to fight infection with the human immunodeficiency virus (HIV), the deadly cause of AIDS. Doctors turn to Epivir as the infection gets worse. The drug is taken along with Retrovir, another HIV medication.

HIV does its damage by slowly destroying the immune system, eventually leaving the body defenseless against infections. Like other drugs for HIV, Epivir interferes with the virus's ability to reproduce. This staves off the collapse of the immune system.

Most important fact about this drug

The Epivir/Retrovir combination does not completely eliminate HIV or totally restore the immune system. There is still a danger of serious infections, so you should be sure to see your doctor regularly for monitoring and tests.

How should you take this medication?

It's important to keep adequate levels of Epivir in your bloodstream at all times, so you need to keep taking this medication regularly, just as prescribed, even when you're feeling better. Epivir may be taken with or without food.

■ *If you miss a dose...*
  Take it as soon as you remember. If it is almost time for the next dose, skip the one you missed and go back to your regular schedule. Do not take 2 doses at once.
■ *Storage instructions...*
  Store at room temperature. Keep the bottle tightly closed.

What side effects may occur?

Side effects cannot be anticipated. If any develop or change in intensity, inform your doctor as soon as possible. Only your doctor can determine if it is safe for you to continue taking Epivir.

■ *Side effects may include:*
Abdominal cramps and pains, allergic reaction, anemia, chills, cough, depression, diarrhea, dizziness, enlarged lymph nodes, enlarged spleen, fatigue, fever, general feeling of illness, hair loss, headache, hives, insomnia and other sleep problems, itching, joint pain, liver damage, lost appetite, mouth sores, muscle and bone pain, muscle weakness or wasting, nasal problems, nausea, pancreatitis, prickling or tingling sensation, skin rashes, stomach upset, vomiting, weakness, wheezing

Why should this drug not be prescribed?

If Epivir gives you an allergic reaction, you cannot take this drug.

Special warnings about this medication

The Epivir tablets and liquid used to treat HIV are not interchangeable with Epivir-HBV, a low-dose form of the drug used to treat the chronic liver disease hepatitis B. If you have both HIV and hepatitis B, you should be treated with the high-strength form of the drug along with other HIV medications. Treatment with Epivir-HBV could promote drug-resistant strains of HIV. Note that when you stop taking Epivir, the hepatitis B may come back.

Remember that Epivir does not eliminate HIV from the body. The infection can still be passed to others through sexual contact or blood contamination.

Epivir can cause an enlarged liver and the chemical imbalance known as lactic acidosis. This serious and sometimes fatal side effect is more likely in women, people who are overweight, and those who have been taking drugs such as Epivir for an extended period. Signs of lactic acidosis include fatigue, nausea, abdominal pain, and a feeling of unwellness. Contact your doctor if you experience any of these symptoms. Treatment with Epivir may have to be discontinued.

The Epivir/Retrovir combination should be given to a child with a history of pancreatitis (inflammation of the pancreas) only when there is no alternative. If any signs of a pancreas problem develop while the child is taking this combination, treatment should be stopped immediately. The chief signs of pancreatitis are bouts of severe abdominal pain—usually lasting for days—accompanied by nausea and vomiting.

Some people receiving drugs for HIV experience a redistribution of body fat, leading to extra fat around the middle, a "buffalo hump" on the back, and wasting in the arms, legs, and face. Researchers don't know whether this represents a long-term health problem or not.

Possible food and drug interactions when taking this medication
Combining Epivir with the HIV drug Hivid is not recommended. Check with your doctor before combining Epivir with Bactrim or Septra.

While no other interactions with Epivir have been reported, its companion drug, Retrovir, can interact with a number of medications.

Special information if you are pregnant or breastfeeding
The effects of Epivir during pregnancy have not been adequately studied, but there is reason to suspect some risk. If you are pregnant or plan to become pregnant, notify your doctor immediately.

Since HIV can be passed to your baby through breast milk, you should not plan on breastfeeding.

Recommended dosage

ADULTS

The usual dose (either tablets or liquid) is 150 milligrams twice daily or 300 milligrams once a day. Your doctor may adjust the dosage if you have kidney problems or weigh less than 110 pounds.

CHILDREN AGED 3 MONTHS TO 16 YEARS

The usual dose is 4 milligrams per 2.2 pounds of body weight twice a day, up to a maximum of 150 milligrams twice daily. The safety of Epivir in combination with antiretroviral drugs other than Retrovir has not been established in children.

Overdosage
The symptoms of Epivir overdose are unknown at this time. However, any medication taken in excess can have serious consequences. If you suspect an overdose, seek medical attention immediately.

Eplerenone See Inspra, page 686.

Eprosartan See Teveten, page 1425.

Eprosartan and Hydrochlorothiazide See Teveten HCT, page 1427.

Ergoloid mesylates See Hydergine, page 655.

Ergotamine with Caffeine See Cafergot, page 227.

Erycette See Erythromycin, Topical, page 524.

ERYC See Erythromycin, Oral, page 520.

Ery-Tab See Erythromycin, Oral, page 520.

Erythrocin See Erythromycin, Oral, page 520.

Erythromycin ethylsuccinate with Sulfisoxazole
See Pediazole, page 1052.

ERYTHROMYCIN, ORAL

Pronounced: er-ITH-row-MY-sin
Brand names: E.E.S., E-Mycin, ERYC, Ery-Tab,
Erythrocin, PCE

Why is this drug prescribed?

Erythromycin is an antibiotic used to treat many kinds of infections, including:

Acute pelvic inflammatory disease
Gonorrhea
Intestinal parasitic infections
Legionnaires' disease
Listeriosis
Pinkeye
Rectal infections
Reproductive tract infections
Skin infections
Syphilis
Upper and lower respiratory tract infections
Urinary tract infections
Whooping cough

Erythromycin is also prescribed to prevent rheumatic fever in people who are allergic to penicillin and sulfa drugs. It is prescribed before colorectal surgery to prevent infection.

Most important fact about this drug

Erythromycin, like any other antibiotic, works best when there is a constant amount of drug in the blood. To help keep the drug amount constant, it is important not to miss any doses. Also, it is advisable to take the doses at evenly spaced times around the clock.

How should you take this medication?

Some forms of erythromycin are most effective when taken on an empty stomach. Your doctor may advise you to take each dose at least ½ hour and preferably 2 hours before meals. Delayed-release formulations may be taken with or without food. If the drug upsets your stomach, taking it with meals may help. Ask your doctor whether this is advisable for you.

Chewable forms of erythromycin should be crushed or chewed before being swallowed.

Delayed-release brands and tablets and capsules that are coated to slow their breakdown should be swallowed whole. Do not crush or break.

If you are not sure about the form of erythromycin you are taking, ask your pharmacist.

The liquid should be shaken well before each use.

■ *If you miss a dose...*
Take it as soon as you remember. If it is almost time for your next dose, and you take 2 doses a day, space the missed dose and the next dose 5 to 6 hours apart; if you take 3 or more doses a day, space the missed dose and the next one 2 to 4 hours apart. Never take 2 doses at the same time.

■ *Storage instructions...*
The liquid form of erythromycin should be kept in the refrigerator; use E.E.S. within 10 days. Do not freeze. Store tablets and capsules at room temperature in a tightly closed container.

What side effects may occur?

Side effects cannot be anticipated. If any develop or change in intensity, inform your doctor as soon as possible. Only your doctor can determine whether it is safe to continue taking this medication.

■ *Side effects may include:*
Abdominal pain, diarrhea, loss of appetite, nausea, vomiting

Why should this drug not be prescribed?

You should not use erythromycin if you have ever had an allergic reaction to it or are sensitive to it.

Special warnings about this medication

As with other antibiotics, treatment with erythromycin may result in a growth of bacteria that do not respond to this medication and can cause a secondary infection.

If you have ever had liver disease, consult your doctor before taking erythromycin.

If a new infection (called superinfection) develops, talk to your doctor. You may need to be treated with a different antibiotic.

This drug may cause a severe form of intestinal inflammation. If you develop diarrhea, contact your doctor immediately. If you have myasthenia gravis (muscle weakness), it can be aggravated by erythromycin.

When erythromycin is used to treat syphilis in pregnant women, it does not prevent the disease from infecting their babies. The infants should be treated after birth with penicillin.

Prolonged or repeated use of erythromycin may result in the growth of bacteria or fungi that do not respond to this medication and can cause a second infection.

Possible food and drug interactions when taking this medication

Combining erythromycin with lovastatin (Mevacor) can cause severe muscle wasting and damage to the kidneys. If you are taking both of these drugs, your doctor will monitor you closely for warning signs of this interaction.

If erythromycin is taken with certain other drugs, the effects of either could be increased, decreased, or altered. It is especially important to check with your doctor before combining erythromycin with the following:

Benzodiazepines such as Halcion and Versed
Blood-thinning drugs such as Coumadin
Bromocriptine (Parlodel)
Carbamazepine (Tegretol)
Cyclosporine (Sandimmune, Neoral)
Digoxin (Lanoxin)
Dihydroergotamine (D.H.E. 45)
Disopyramide (Norpace)
Ergotamine (Cafergot)
Hexobarbital
Seizure medications such as Depakene, Depakote, and Dilantin
Tacrolimus (Prograf)
Theophylline (Theo-Dur)

Special information if you are pregnant or breastfeeding

There is no evidence that erythromycin will harm a developing baby, but the possibility has not been completely ruled out. If you are pregnant or plan to become pregnant, inform your doctor immediately.

Erythromycin appears in breast milk and could affect a nursing infant. If this medication is essential to your health, your doctor may advise you to discontinue breastfeeding until your treatment is finished.

Recommended dosage

Dosage instructions are determined by the type (and severity) of infection being treated and may vary slightly for different brands of erythromycin. The following are recommended dosages for PCE, one of the most commonly prescribed brands.

ADULTS

Streptococcal Infections

The usual dose is 333 milligrams every 8 hours, or 500 milligrams every 12 hours. Depending on the severity of the infection, the dose may be increased to a total of 4 grams a day. However, when the daily dosage is larger than 1 gram, twice-a-day doses are not recommended, and the drug should be taken more often in smaller doses.

To treat streptococcal infections of the upper respiratory tract (tonsillitis or strep throat), erythromycin should be taken for at least 10 days.

To prevent repeated infections in people who have had rheumatic fever, the usual dosage is 250 milligrams twice a day.

Urinary Tract Infections Due to Chlamydia Trachomatis During Pregnancy
The usual dosage is 500 milligrams of erythromycin orally 4 times a day or 666 milligrams every 8 hours on an empty stomach for at least 7 days. For women who cannot tolerate this regimen, a decreased dose of 500 milligrams every 12 hours or 333 milligrams every 8 hours a day should be used for at least 14 days.

Uncomplicated Urinary, Reproductive Tract, or Rectal Infections Caused by Chlamydia Trachomatis When Tetracycline Cannot Be Taken
The usual oral dosage is 500 milligrams of erythromycin 4 times a day or 666 milligrams every 8 hours for at least 7 days.

Nongonococcal Urethral Infections When Tetracycline Cannot Be Taken
The usual dosage is 500 milligrams of erythromycin by mouth 4 times a day or 666 milligrams orally every 8 hours for at least 7 days.

Acute Pelvic Inflammatory Disease Caused by Neisseria gonorrhoeae
The usual treatment is three days of intravenous erythromycin followed by 500 milligrams orally every 12 hours or 333 milligrams orally every 8 hours for 7 days.

Syphilis
The usual dosage is 30 to 40 grams divided into smaller doses over a period of 10 to 15 days.

Intestinal Infections
The usual dosage is 500 milligrams every 12 hours, or 333 milligrams every 8 hours, for 10 to 14 days.

Legionnaires' Disease
The usual dosage ranges from 1 to 4 grams daily, divided into smaller doses.

CHILDREN

Age, weight, and severity of the infection determine the correct dosage.

The usual dosage is from 30 to 50 milligrams daily for each 2.2 pounds of body weight, divided into equal doses for 10 to 14 days. For pneumonia in infants due to chlamydia, treatment lasts at least 3 weeks.

For more severe infections, this dosage may be doubled, but it should not exceed 4 grams per day.

Children weighing over 44 pounds should follow the recommended adult dose schedule.

For prevention of bacterial endocarditis, the children's dosage is 10 milligrams per 2.2 pounds of body weight 2 hours before dental work or surgery, followed by 5 milligrams per 2.2 pounds 6 hours later.

Overdosage

Any medication taken in excess can have serious consequences. If you suspect an overdose, seek medical help immediately.

■ *Symptoms of erythromycin overdose may include:*
Diarrhea, nausea, stomach cramps, vomiting

ERYTHROMYCIN, TOPICAL

Pronounced: er-ITH-row-MY-sin
Brand names: A/T/S, Erycette, T-Stat

Why is this drug prescribed?

Topical erythromycin (applied directly to the skin) is used for the treatment of acne.

Most important fact about this drug

For best results, you should continue the treatment for as long as prescribed, even if your acne begins to clear up. This medicine is not an instant cure.

How should you use this medication?

Use exactly as prescribed by your doctor.

Thoroughly wash the affected area with soap and water and pat dry before applying medication.

Moisten the applicator or pad with the medication and lightly spread it over the affected area. A/T/S Topical Gel should not be rubbed in.

■ *If you miss a dose...*
Apply the forgotten dose as soon as you remember. If it is almost time for the next application, skip the one you missed and go back to your regular schedule.
■ *Storage instructions...*
This medicine can be stored at room temperature.

What side effects may occur?

Side effects cannot be anticipated. If any develop or change in intensity, inform your doctor as soon as possible. Only your doctor can determine if it is safe for you to continue using topical erythromycin.

■ *Side effects may include:*
Burning sensation, dryness, hives, irritation of the eyes, itching, oiliness, peeling, scaling, tenderness, unusual redness of the skin

Why should this drug not be prescribed?

Erythromycin should not be used if you are sensitive to or have ever had an allergic reaction to any of the ingredients.

Special warnings about this medication

This type of erythromycin is for external use only. Do not use it in the eyes, nose, or mouth.

If the acne does not improve after 6 to 8 weeks of treatment, or if it gets worse, stop using the topical erythromycin preparation and call your doctor.

The use of antibiotics can stimulate the growth of other bacteria that are resistant to the antibiotic you are taking. If new infections (called superinfections) occur, talk to your doctor. You may need to be treated with a different antibiotic drug.

If you develop diarrhea, let your doctor know right away. Drugs such as erythromycin can cause a potentially serious intestinal inflammation.

The use of other topical acne medications in combination with topical erythromycin may cause irritation, especially with the use of peeling, scaling, or abrasive medications.

The safety and effectiveness of A/T/S and Erycette have not been established in children.

Possible food and drug interactions when using this medication

If topical erythromycin is used with certain other drugs, the effects of either could be increased, decreased, or altered. It is especially important to check with your doctor before combining topical erythromycin with other topical acne medications.

Special information if you are pregnant or breastfeeding

The effects of topical erythromycin during pregnancy have not been adequately studied. If you are pregnant or plan to become pregnant, inform your doctor immediately. Erythromycin may appear in breast milk and could affect a nursing infant. If this medication is essential to your health, your doctor may advise you to stop breastfeeding until your treatment with erythromycin is finished.

Recommended dosage

Apply solution to the affected area 2 times a day. Moisten the applicator or a pad, then spread over the affected area. Use additional pads as needed. Apply gel products as a thin film over the affected area once or twice a day.

Make sure the area is thoroughly washed with soap and water and patted dry before applying medication. Thoroughly wash your hands after application of the medication.

Reducing the frequency of applications may reduce peeling and drying.

Overdosage

Although overdosage is unlikely, any medication used in excess can have serious consequences. If you suspect an overdose, seek medical treatment immediately.

Erythromycin with Benzoyl peroxide *See Benzamycin, page 206.*

Eryzole *See Pediazole, page 1052.*

Escitalopram *See Lexapro, page 746.*

Esclim *See Estrogen Patches, page 538.*

Esgic *See Fioricet, page 565.*

Esidrix *See HydroDIURIL, page 658.*

ESKALITH

*Pronounced: ESS-kuh-li*s*h*
Generic name: Lithium carbonate
Other brand names: Eskalith CR, Lithobid

Why is this drug prescribed?

Eskalith is used to treat the manic episodes of manic-depressive illness, a condition in which a person's mood swings from depression to excessive excitement. A manic episode may involve some or all of the following symptoms:

> Aggressiveness
> Elation
> Fast, urgent talking
> Frenetic physical activity
> Grandiose, unrealistic ideas
> Hostility
> Little need for sleep
> Poor judgment

Once the mania subsides, Eskalith treatment may be continued over the long term, at a somewhat lower dosage, to prevent or reduce the intensity of future manic episodes.

Some doctors also prescribe lithium for premenstrual tension, eating disorders such as bulimia, certain movement disorders, and sexual addictions.

Most important fact about this drug

If the Eskalith dosage is too low, you will derive no benefit; if it is too high, you could suffer lithium poisoning. You and your doctor will need to work together to find the correct dosage. Initially, this means frequent blood tests to find out how much of the drug is actually circulating in your bloodstream. As long as you take Eskalith, you will need to watch for side effects. Signs of lithium poisoning include vomiting, unsteady walking, diarrhea, drowsiness, tremor, and weakness. Stop taking the drug and call your doctor if you have any of these symptoms.

How should you take this medication?

To avoid stomach upset, take Eskalith immediately after meals or with food or milk.

Do not change from one brand of lithium to another without consulting your doctor or pharmacist. Take the drug exactly as prescribed.

While taking Eskalith, you should drink 10 to 12 glasses of water or fluid a day. To minimize the risk of harmful side effects, eat a balanced diet that includes some salt and lots of liquids. If you have been sweating a great deal or have had diarrhea, make sure you get extra liquids and salt.

If you develop an infection with a fever, you may need to cut back on your Eskalith dosage or even quit taking it temporarily. While you are ill, keep in close touch with your doctor.

Long-acting forms of lithium, such as Eskalith CR or Lithobid, should be swallowed whole. Do not chew, crush, or break.

■ *If you miss a dose...*
  Ask your doctor what to do; requirements vary for each individual. Do not take 2 doses at once.
■ *Storage instructions...*
  Store at room temperature.

What side effects may occur?

The possibility of side effects varies with the level of lithium in your bloodstream. If you experience unfamiliar symptoms of any kind, inform your doctor as soon as possible.

■ *Side effects that may occur when you start taking lithium include:*
  Discomfort, frequent urination, hand tremor, mild thirst, nausea
■ *Other side effects may include:*
  Diarrhea, drowsiness, lack of coordination, muscle weakness, vomiting

Why should this drug not be prescribed?

Although your doctor will be cautious under certain conditions, lithium may be prescribed for anyone.

Special warnings about this medication

Eskalith may affect your judgment or coordination. Do not drive, climb, or perform hazardous tasks until you find out how this drug affects you.

Your doctor will prescribe Eskalith with extra caution if you have a heart or kidney problem, a brain or spinal cord disease, or a weak, run-down, or dehydrated condition.

Also make sure your doctor is aware of any medical problems you may have, including diabetes, epilepsy, thyroid problems, Parkinson's disease, and difficulty urinating.

You should be careful in hot weather to avoid activities that cause you to sweat heavily. Also avoid drinking large amounts of coffee, tea, or cola, which can cause dehydration through increased urination. Do not make a major change in your eating habits or go on a weight loss diet without consulting your doctor. The loss of water and salt from your body could lead to lithium poisoning.

Possible food and drug interactions when taking this medication

If Eskalith is taken with certain other drugs, the effects of either could be increased, decreased, or altered. It is especially important to check with your doctor before combining Eskalith with the following:

ACE-inhibitor blood pressure drugs such as Capoten or Vasotec
Acetazolamide (Diamox)
Amphetamines such as Dexedrine
Antidepressant drugs that boost serotonin levels, including Paxil, Prozac, and Zoloft
Antipsychotic drugs such as Haldol and chlorpromazine
Bicarbonate of soda
Caffeine (No-Doz)
Calcium-blocking blood pressure drugs such as Calan and Cardizem
Carbamazepine (Tegretol)
Diuretics such as Lasix or HydroDIURIL
Fluoxetine (Prozac)
Iodine-containing preparations such as potassium iodide (Quadrinal)
Methyldopa (Aldomet)
Metronidazole (Flagyl)
Nonsteroidal anti-inflammatory drugs such as Advil, Celebrex, Feldene, and Indocin
Phenytoin (Dilantin)
Sodium bicarbonate
Tetracyclines such as Achromycin V and Sumycin
Theophylline (Theo-Dur, Quibron, others)

Special information if you are pregnant or breastfeeding

The use of Eskalith during pregnancy can harm the developing baby. If you are pregnant or plan to become pregnant, inform your doctor immediately.

Eskalith appears in breast milk and is considered potentially harmful to a nursing infant. If this medication is essential to your health, your doctor may advise you to discontinue breastfeeding while you are taking it.

Recommended dosage

ADULTS

Acute Episodes
The usual dosage is a total of 1,800 milligrams per day. Immediate-release forms are taken in 3 or 4 doses per day; long-acting forms are taken twice a day.

Your doctor will individualize your dosage according to the levels of the drug in your blood. Your blood levels will be checked at least twice a week when the drug is first prescribed and on a regular basis thereafter.

Long-term Control
Dosage will vary from one individual to another, but a total of 900 to 1,200 milligrams per day is typical. Immediate-release forms are taken in 3 or 4 doses per day; long-acting forms are taken twice a day.

Blood levels in most cases should be checked every 2 months.

CHILDREN

The safety and effectiveness of Eskalith in children under 12 years of age have not been established.

OLDER ADULTS

Older people often need less Eskalith and may show signs of overdose at a dosage younger people can handle well.

Overdosage

Any medication taken in excess can have serious consequences. If you suspect symptoms of an overdose of Eskalith, seek medical attention immediately.

The harmful levels are close to those that will treat your condition. Watch for early signs of overdose, such as diarrhea, drowsiness, lack of coordination, vomiting, and weakness. If you develop any of these signs, stop taking the drug and call your doctor.

Esomeprazole *See Nexium, page 934.*

Estazolam *See ProSom, page 1180.*

Esterified estrogens and Methyltestosterone
See Estratest, page 533.

Estraderm *See Estrogen Patches, page 538.*

Estradiol *See Estrogen Patches, page 538.*

Estradiol acetate *See Femring, page 560.*

Estradiol and Norethindrone acetate *See CombiPatch, page 323.*

Estradiol topical lotion See Estrasorb, below.

Estradiol vaginal ring See Estring, page 536.

Estradiol vaginal tablets See Vagifem, page 1538.

ESTRASORB
Pronounced: ES-trah-sorb
Generic name: Estradiol topical lotion

Why is this drug prescribed?
Estrasorb is a topical lotion that contains the hormone estrogen. It's used to reduce the symptoms of moderate to severe hot flashes associated with menopause. The most common symptoms during a hot flash include sudden sweating, intense feelings of body heat, and sudden feelings of warmth spreading to the face, neck, and chest.

Most important fact about this drug
Because estrogens have been linked with an increased risk of endometrial cancer (cancer in the lining of the uterus), it is essential to have regular checkups and to report any unusual vaginal bleeding to your doctor immediately.

How should you take this medication?
Estrasorb lotion is packaged in foil pouches. Do not open the pouches until just before you're ready to use the medication.

Apply Estrasorb in the morning. Be sure your skin is dry before applying the lotion, and do not rub it on skin that is red or irritated. Cut or tear open one pouch and apply the contents to your left thigh. Rub the lotion into your entire left thigh and calf for 3 minutes until the medication is absorbed. You can rub any excess lotion remaining on your hands onto your buttocks. When you're done with the left leg, cut or tear open a second pouch and follow the same procedure on your right thigh and calf. Be sure to use all of the lotion in each pouch.

Wash your hands with soap and water when you're finished. Allow the application sites to dry completely before putting on clothes.

The legs are the only application sites recommended by the drug's manufacturer. It is not known if the medication will be absorbed as well if it's applied to other parts of the body.

Do not apply Estrasorb and sunscreen at the same time, since sunscreen may affect how much of the medication you absorb.

■ *If you miss a dose…*
  If you forget to apply Estrasorb in the morning, do it as soon as you remember. Do not apply Estrasorb more than once a day.

■ *Storage instructions…*
Store the pouches at room temperature.

What side effects may occur?

Side effects cannot be anticipated. If any develop or change in intensity, tell your doctor as soon as possible. Only your doctor can determine if it is safe to continue using Estrasorb.

■ *Side effects may include:*
Abdominal cramps, bloating, breast pain, hair loss, headache, infection, irregular vaginal bleeding or spotting, itchy spots, nausea and vomiting, problems with the lining of the uterus (endometrium), sinus inflammation, skin irritation at the application site

Why should this drug not be prescribed?

You should not use estrogen products, including Estrasorb, if you have any of the following:

■ Unexplained genital bleeding
■ A history of breast cancer or any other cancer stimulated by estrogen (or a possibility that you have this type of cancer)
■ A history of blood clots, especially in the legs or lungs
■ Active or recent (within the past year) blood-vessel disease such as stroke or heart attack
■ Liver disease or poor liver function
■ Known or suspected pregnancy
■ Allergic reaction to Estrasorb or any of its ingredients

Special warnings about this medication

Estrogen therapy may increase the risk of heart disease, stroke, and blood clots. It could also increase the risk of certain cancers, including breast, uterine, and ovarian cancer. (Combination products that also contain progestin pose less risk of uterine cancer, but increase the risk of breast cancer.) If you are in danger of developing any of these, your doctor should take a complete medical and family history—and do a complete physical exam—before prescribing Estrasorb. As a general rule, you should have an examination at least once a year while using this product.

Estrogen therapy may also increase the risk of gallbladder disease and high calcium levels (hypercalcemia).

Serious eye problems, including blood clots in the retina, have been reported during estrogen therapy. Contact your doctor immediately if you suddenly lose all or part of your vision or you develop any eye problems. Also tell your doctor if you suddenly develop migraines, which could be related to eye problems.

Use Estrasorb with caution if you have a history of high blood pressure, endometriosis, liver problems, jaundice, or low calcium levels (hypocalcemia). Also be cautious if you have cholesterol problems, since using estrogen could trigger a spike in your triglyceride levels and possibly damage the pancreas.

While taking estrogen, get in touch with your doctor right away if you notice any of the following:

Abdominal pain, tenderness, or swelling
Abnormal bleeding from the vagina
Breast lumps
Coughing up blood
Difficulty with speech
Dizziness or fainting
Pain in your chest or calves
Severe headache or vomiting
Sudden shortness of breath
Vision changes
Weakness or numbness of an arm or leg
Yellowing of the skin or eyes

Because estrogen can affect the ability to handle blood sugar, diabetic women should use this product with caution. Be alert, too, for signs of fluid retention, which can be especially harmful for people with a heart condition or kidney problems. Estrogen can also worsen the symptoms of asthma, epilepsy, migraine, lupus, and the genetic disorder porphyria.

Estrogen could interfere with thyroid hormone metabolism. Tell your doctor if you have thyroid problems or are taking thyroid hormone, since you may need your dosage increased.

If you're having surgery or need long periods of bed rest, you should stop taking Estrasorb at least 4 to 6 weeks beforehand to avoid the risk of blood clots.

Possible food and drug interactions when using this medication

If you take certain other drugs while using estrogen, the effects of either could be increased, decreased, or altered. It is especially important to check with your doctor before taking the following:

Carbamazepine (Tegretol)
Clarithromycin (Biaxin)
Erythromycin (E-Mycin, Ery-Tab, Erythrocin)
Grapefruit juice
Itraconazole (Sporanox)
Ketoconazole (Nizoral)
Phenobarbital
Rifampin (Rifadin)
Ritonavir (Norvir)
St. John's wort

Special information if you are pregnant or breastfeeding

Estrasorb must not be used during pregnancy.

Estrasorb does appear in breast milk. If this drug is essential to your health, you may have to quit breastfeeding until your treatment is finished.

Recommended dosage

The recommended daily dose is 2 lotion-filled pouches, one applied to each leg every morning. Two pouches deliver 3.48 grams of estrogen.

Overdosage

No serious side effects have been reported after oral overdoses of estrogen-containing products. An oral overdose of estrogen could be expected to cause nausea, vomiting, or vaginal bleeding.

ESTRATEST

Pronounced: ESS-truh-test
Generic name: Esterified estrogens and Methyltestosterone

Why is this drug prescribed?

Estratest tablets quell the flushing, sweating, hot flashes, and vaginal irritation that trouble three-quarters of all women when they reach menopause. Estratest works by replacing some of the estrogen that is lost when the reproductive system shuts down. Although it relieves the physical symptoms of menopause, it won't help emotional symptoms such as depression if the physical symptoms are absent. It combines supplemental estrogen with a synthetic form of the male hormone testosterone, and is prescribed when estrogen alone fails to relieve menopausal symptoms.

Most important fact about this drug

Estrogen replacement therapy increases the risk of endometrial cancer (cancer in the lining of the uterus). It is also important to note that estrogen replacement therapy will not prevent heart disease; in fact, it is possible that it could increase your risk for heart attack and stroke.

The higher the dose and the longer the treatment, the greater the risks. It's wise, therefore, to limit yourself to the smallest dose that provides relief, and to stop the treatment as soon as you can. It's also essential to have regular checkups and to report any unusual vaginal bleeding to your doctor immediately.

How should you take this medication?

Take Estratest cyclically—a dose a day for 3 weeks, then no tablets for 1 week.

■ *If you miss a dose...*
Take it as soon as you remember. However, if it almost time for your next dose, skip the one you missed and return to your regular schedule. Do not take 2 doses at once.

■ *Storage instructions...*
Store at room temperature.

What side effects may occur?

Side effects cannot be anticipated. If any develop or change in intensity, tell your doctor as soon as possible. Only your doctor can determine if it is safe to continue using Estratest.

■ *Side effects may include:*
Abdominal cramps, acne, allergic reactions, anxiety, bladder problems, bloating, breast discharge, breast swelling and tenderness, brown patches on the face, cervical changes, clotting disorders, deepening of the voice, depression, dizziness, enlarged clitoris, enlarged fibroids, gallbladder disease, hair loss on scalp, hair growth on face, headache, high blood sugar, high cholesterol, intolerance to contact lenses, liver disorders, menstrual problems, migraine, nausea, sex drive changes, skin eruptions, swelling, tingling, twitching, vaginal yeast infection, vision changes, vomiting, weight changes, yellowing of skin and eyes

Why should this drug not be prescribed?

You should avoid Estratest if you have any of the following conditions:

■ Breast cancer or any other type of cancer that's stimulated by estrogen (except in certain special circumstances)
■ Known or suspected pregnancy
■ Unexplained vaginal bleeding
■ A clotting disorder such as phlebitis, or clotting problems during previous estrogen therapy
■ Severe liver damage
■ Breastfeeding

Special warnings about this medication

Long-term estrogen replacement therapy definitely increases the risk of endometrial cancer and may increase the risk of breast cancer as well. If you have a family history of breast cancer, or if you have breast nodules or abnormal mammograms, be sure to have frequent breast exams.

Estrogen replacement drugs have been associated with an increased risk of heart disease, such as heart attack and stroke, as well as blood clots in the brain, heart, or lungs. You are at a higher risk for heart disease if you have high blood pressure or diabetes, or if you smoke cigarettes, have high cholesterol, or are overweight. If you are having surgery, you will need to discontinue estrogen therapy at least 4 to 6 weeks prior to the procedure because the risk for blood clots becomes higher due to the time you may be immobilized. Because estrogen replacement poses a slight theoretical danger of clotting disorders, and testosterone has been known to cause fluid retention and heart failure in people with heart, liver, or kidney disease, take Estratest with caution if you have any of these conditions or have ever suffered a stroke. Also let the doctor know if you have asthma, epilepsy, migraines, or bone disease.

Estrogen replacement also increases the risk of gallbladder disease. Women who take birth-control pills, which have the same effect, suffer an increase in gallbladder problems after 2 years of use.

Both estrogen and testosterone can cause liver problems, including benign tumors, cancers, and hepatitis. Be sure to report any pain, tenderness, or swelling in the abdomen to your doctor immediately. If you develop signs of liver disease, such as yellowing of the skin and eyes, stop taking Estratest and see your doctor at once.

Estrogen can cause an increase in blood pressure, so the doctor will monitor it closely. Estrogen also can raise blood sugar levels. If you have diabetes, use Estratest cautiously.

Estrogen therapy occasionally causes symptoms of hormonal overload, such as breast tenderness and excessive uterine bleeding. Estrogen can also foster an increase in the size of uterine fibroids (benign tumors) and may increase the risk of mental depression.

High doses of the testosterone in Estratest can cause a woman's voice to deepen and can promote the growth of facial hair. To prevent a permanent change, the hormone must be discontinued. Inform your doctor immediately if you develop hoarseness, acne, or hair on the face. Also report any nausea, vomiting, changes in skin color, or swelling in the ankles.

Possible food and drug interactions when taking this medication

If Estratest is taken with certain other drugs, their effects may be altered. It is especially important to check with your doctor before combining Estratest with the following:

Blood thinners such as Coumadin
Insulin

Special information if you are pregnant or breastfeeding

Estrogen and testosterone both can cause birth defects, and estrogen taken during pregnancy increases the child's risk of certain vaginal and cervical cancers later in life. Do not take Estratest if there's any chance that you're pregnant, and avoid it when nursing a baby.

Recommended dosage

WOMEN IN MENOPAUSE

Estratest is available in full- and half-strength tablets (Estratest H.S.). The tablets are taken cyclically (3 weeks on and 1 week off). The usual daily dosage is 1 tablet of Estratest or 1 to 2 tablets of Estratest H.S.

Overdosage

Any medication taken in excess can have serious consequences. If you suspect an overdose of Estratest, seek medical attention immediately.

■ *Symptoms of overdose may include:*
  Nausea, vaginal bleeding

ESTRING

Pronounced: ESST-ring
Generic name: Estradiol vaginal ring

Why is this drug prescribed?

Estring is an estrogen replacement system for relief of the vaginal problems that often occur after menopause, including vaginal dryness, burning, and itching, and difficult or painful intercourse. Estring is also prescribed for postmenopausal urinary problems such as difficulty urinating or urinary urgency.

Most important fact about this drug

Estrogens increase the risk of cancer in the lining of the uterus, called the endometrium. Because estrogen replacement therapy is not advisable if you are in any danger of developing cancer, your doctor should take a complete medical and family history, and perform a complete physical exam, before prescribing Estring. It is important to have regular checkups (at least once a year) and to report any unusual vaginal bleeding to your doctor immediately.

Estring and other estrogen drugs, with or without progesterone, should not be used to prevent heart disease. Recent studies have confirmed an increased rate of heart attack, stroke, and dangerous blood clots among women taking estrogen or estrogen combinations for 5 years. Blood clots can lead to phlebitis, stroke, heart attack, a loss of blood supply to the lungs, a blockage in the blood vessels leading to the eye, and other serious disorders.

How should you use this medication?

Each Estring is left in place for 3 months. Press the Estring into an oval and insert it as deeply as possible into the upper third of the vagina. The exact position is unimportant as long as you don't feel the ring. If the ring causes discomfort, it is probably not far enough inside.

If the ring slips down into the lower part of the vagina, push it back up with your finger. If it falls out, rinse it in warm water and reinsert it. When replacing the ring, simply hook a finger through it and pull it out.

■ *If you miss a dose...*
If the ring is not replaced after 90 days, the dose of estrogen will gradually decline and your symptoms will return.
■ *Storage instructions...*
Store at room temperature.

What side effects may occur?
Side effects cannot be anticipated. If any develop or change in intensity, tell your doctor as soon as possible. Only your doctor can determine if it is safe for you to continue using Estring.

■ *Side effects may include:*
Abdominal pain, arthritis, back pain, flu-like symptoms, headaches, insomnia, joint pain, nausea, sinus inflammation, upper respiratory tract infections, vaginal discharge, vaginal discomfort or pain, vaginal inflammation or bleeding, yeast infection

Why should this drug not be prescribed?
Do not use Estring if you have unexplained vaginal bleeding. Also avoid Estring if there is a possibility that you are pregnant.

Do not use Estring if there is any chance that you have breast cancer or any other cancer stimulated by estrogen. You will also have to avoid Estring if it causes an allergic reaction.

Special warnings about this medication
Estrogen replacement therapy increases the risk of developing cancer of the lining of the uterus. The risk increases with longer use and higher doses. Therefore, you should use Estring for as short a time and at as low a dose as is necessary to relieve your symptoms. Report any unusual vaginal bleeding to you doctor immediately.

Using estrogen may also increase the risk of breast cancer, ovarian cancer, heart attack, stroke, blood clots, and gallbladder disease.

Use estrogen with caution if you have severely low blood levels of calcium (hypocalcemia).

Tell your doctor if you've ever had liver problems, high cholesterol, high blood pressure, thyroid problems, or visions problems. Using estrogen could make these conditions worse.

Estrogens can cause water retention. If you have a condition that could be affected by this—such as heart or kidney problems—your doctor will monitor you closely.

While using Estring, contact your doctor right away if you develop any of the following:

Abdominal pain, tenderness, or swelling
Abnormal bleeding from the vagina
Breast lumps
Coughing up blood
Difficulty with speech
Dizziness or faintness
Pains in your chest or calves
Severe headache or vomiting
Sudden shortness of breath
Vision changes
Weakness or numbness of an arm or leg
Yellowing of skin or whites of the eyes (could signal a liver problem)

Any vaginal infection should be cleared up before you begin Estring therapy. If an infection develops after you begin, you'll need to remove the ring during treatment.

Possible food and drug interactions when using this medication
No interactions have been reported, but Estring should be removed during treatment with other vaginally administered drugs.

Special information if you are pregnant or breastfeeding
Estring must not be used during pregnancy and is not intended for nursing mothers.

Recommended dosage
Insert a new ring every 3 months.

Overdosage
An overdose from Estring is unlikely. An oral overdose of estrogen could be expected to cause the symptoms listed below.

■ *Symptoms of estrogen overdose may include:*
Nausea, vomiting, vaginal bleeding

ESTROGEN PATCHES
Generic name: Estradiol
Brand names: Alora, Climara, Esclim, Estraderm, Vivelle,
    Vivelle-Dot

Why is this drug prescribed?
All of these products are used to reduce symptoms of menopause, including feelings of warmth in the face, neck, and chest; the sudden intense episodes of heat and sweating known as hot flashes; dry, itchy

external genitals; and vaginal irritation. They are also prescribed for other conditions that cause low levels of estrogen, and some doctors prescribe them for teenagers who fail to mature at the usual rate.

Along with diet, calcium supplements, and exercise, Alora, Estraderm, Climara, Vivelle, and Vivelle-Dot are prescribed to prevent osteoporosis, a condition in which the bones become brittle and easily broken.

Most important fact about this drug

Because estrogens have been linked with an increased risk of breast, uterine, and endometrial cancer (cancer in the lining of the uterus), it is essential to have regular mammograms and checkups. Report any unusual vaginal bleeding to your doctor immediately.

Hormone replacement therapy using estrogens, with or without progestin, should not be used to prevent heart disease. Recent studies have confirmed an increased rate of heart attack, stroke, and dangerous blood clots among women taking estrogen or estrogen combinations for 5 years. Blood clots can lead to phlebitis, stroke, heart attack, a loss of blood supply to the lungs, a blockage in the blood vessels serving the eye, and other serious disorders. Because of these risks, hormone replacement therapy should be given at the lowest effective dose for the shortest possible time. Your doctor will determine the dosage that is best for you.

How should you take this medication?

Each patch is individually sealed in a protective pouch and is applied directly to the skin.

A stiff protective liner covers the adhesive side of the patch. Remove the liner by sliding it sideways between your thumb and index finger. Holding the patch at one edge, remove the protective liner and discard it. Try to avoid touching the adhesive. Use immediately after removing the liner. If you are using Alora, Vivelle, or Vivelle-Dot, peel off one side of the protective liner and discard it. Use the other half of the liner as a handle until you have applied the sticky area, then fold back the remaining side of the patch, pull off the rest of the liner, and smooth the second half of the patch onto your skin.

Apply the adhesive side to a clean, dry area of your skin on the trunk of your body (including the buttocks and abdomen). Do not apply to your breasts or waist. Firmly press the patch in place with the palm of your hand for about 10 seconds, to make sure the edges are flat against your skin. When first using Alora, start on the lower abdomen. Climara is applied only to the abdomen or upper buttock, and is pressed in place with the fingers.

Remove the patch slowly and carefully to avoid irritating your skin. If any adhesive remains, let it dry for 15 minutes, then gently rub the area with an oil-based cream or lotion to remove the adhesive residue. The used patch still contains active hormone. To dispose of it properly, fold it in half so it sticks to itself before throwing it away.

Contact with water during bathing, swimming, or showering will not affect the patch.

The application site must be rotated. Allow an interval of at least 1 week between applications to a particular site.

Alora, Esclim, Estraderm, Vivelle, and Vivelle-Dot patches should be replaced twice a week; Climara once weekly.

■ *If you miss a dose...*
If you forget to apply a new patch when you are supposed to, do it as soon as you remember. If it is almost time to change patches anyway, skip the one you missed and go back to your regular schedule. Do not apply more than the prescribed number of patches at a time.

■ *Storage instructions...*
Store the patches at room temperature, in their sealed pouches.

What side effects may occur?

Side effects cannot be anticipated. If any develop or change in intensity, notify your doctor as soon as possible. Only your doctor can determine if it is safe for you to continue using the estrogen patch.

■ *Side effects may include:*
Anxiety, back pain, breakthrough bleeding, breast tenderness, constipation, depression, flu-like symptoms, headache, high blood pressure, hot flushes, insomnia, indigestion, nausea, neck pain, sinus problems; skin redness and irritation at the site of the patch, upper respiratory tract infection, weight increase

Why should this drug not be prescribed?

Estrogen patches should not be used during pregnancy. You should also avoid this product if you have:

■ Unexplained vaginal bleeding
■ Known or suspected breast cancer
■ Any type of tumor stimulated by estrogen
■ Phlebitis, blood clots in the lung, or any other clotting disorder
■ Active or recent (within the last year) heart disease, heart attack, or stroke
■ Liver disease or liver problems
■ An allergy to any component of the patch

Special warnings about this medication

Estrogen has the potential of causing clot-related disorders, including heart attack and stroke, pulmonary embolism (a clot in the lungs), and thrombophlebitis (a clot in the veins). A complete medical and family history should be taken by your doctor before starting any estrogen therapy, especially if you have a history of deep vein thrombosis (a clot in the legs) or a history of thrombosis in your family. The chance of developing a clot-related problem can be reduced by using the lowest dose of estrogen that still proves effective. If a problem surfaces anyway, you'll have to stop using the patch. Likewise, you should discontinue the patch and call your doctor immediately if you suffer a loss of vision, any other eye problems, or a migraine headache.

Some experts suspect that high doses of estrogen, with or without a progestin, may increase the risk of ovarian, breast, and endometrial cancer. The risk may increase with prolonged use.

Hormone therapy occasionally causes a rise in blood pressure. If you have a blood pressure problem, use the patch with caution and have your pressure checked regularly.

If you suffer from liver problems or liver disease, you may not be able to use hormone therapy.

If you are on hormone therapy, you may need to have your thyroid medication adjusted and your thyroid tested more frequently.

Hormones also tend to cause fluid retention. If you have a condition that could be aggravated by excess fluid, such as asthma, epilepsy, migraine headaches, heart disease, or kidney problems, use the patch with caution.

If you suffer from endometriosis, a condition where the endometrium (the lining of the uterus) doesn't shed properly and attaches to the outside of the uterus or other areas such as the ovaries or bowels, hormone therapy may cause a worsening of this condition.

Because estrogen can increase triglyceride levels, you'll need to be closely monitored if your triglycerides tend to be high. If you have diabetes, estrogen may also affect your blood sugar levels.

Estrogen therapy occasionally causes abnormal uterine bleeding or breast pain. In view of concerns about cancer, you should have these symptoms checked by your doctor. In general, you should not take estrogen for more than 1 year without a follow-up physical exam. Ideally, you should have a checkup every 3 to 6 months.

Women who take oral estrogen after menopause face a two- to fourfold increase in the odds of gallbladder disease.

For teenagers who fail to mature at the usual rate, large doses of estrogen taken for an extended period may affect growth. In girls, it may cause the early start of menstruation or early breast development.

While taking estrogen, get in touch with your doctor right away if you notice any of the following:

Abdominal pain, tenderness, or swelling
Abnormal bleeding of the vagina
Breast lumps
Coughing up blood
Difficulty with speech
Pain in your chest or calves
Severe headache, dizziness, or faintness

Skin irritation, redness, or rash
Sudden shortness of breath
Vision changes
Weakness or numbness of an arm or leg
Yellowing of the skin or eyes

Possible food and drug interactions when taking this medication

If you take certain other drugs while using estrogen, the effects of either could be increased, decreased, or altered. It is especially important to check with your doctor before taking the following:

Alcohol
Barbiturates such as phenobarbital and Seconal
Blood thinners such as Coumadin
Cimetidine (Tagamet)
Clarithromycin (Biaxin)
Dantrolene (Dantrium)
Epilepsy drugs such as Tegretol and Dilantin
Erythromycin (E-Mycin, Ery-Tab)
Grapefruit juice
Itraconazole (Sporanox)
Ketoconazole (Nizoral)
Rifampin (Rifadin)
Ritonavir (Norvir)
St. John's wort
Steroids such as Deltasone
Tricyclic antidepressants such as Elavil and Tofranil

Special information if you are pregnant or breastfeeding

Estrogens should not be used during pregnancy or immediately after childbirth. Use of estrogens during pregnancy has been linked to reproductive tract problems in the children. If you are pregnant or plan to become pregnant, notify your doctor immediately. Estrogens decrease the quantity and quality of breast milk. If this medication is essential to your health, your doctor may advise you to discontinue breastfeeding until your treatment is finished.

Recommended dosage

If you are a postmenopausal woman with a uterus, progestin may be prescribed as well in order to reduce the risk of endometrial cancer. Your doctor will determine the dosage that is right for you. Typically, hormone replacement therapy should be started at the lowest possible dose and for the shortest duration needed to relieve your symptoms. You should be evaluated every 3 to 6 months.

ALORA AND ESTRADERM

The usual starting dose is one 0.05-milligram patch applied to the skin 2 times a week. (For osteoporosis, the doctor may prescribe a 0.025-milligram patch.)

CLIMARA

The usual starting dose is one 0.025-milligram patch applied to the skin once a week. (For osteoporosis, the doctor may prescribe a 0.025-milligram patch.)

ESCLIM

The usual starting dose is one 0.025-milligram patch applied to the skin 2 times a week.

VIVELLE AND VIVELLE-DOT

The usual starting dose to relieve symptoms of menopause is one 0.0375-milligram patch applied to the skin 2 times a week. (For osteoporosis, the doctor may prescribe a 0.025-milligram patch.) The patch may be used continuously, or left off every fourth week.

Overdosage

Any medication taken in excess can have serious consequences. If you suspect an overdose, seek medical attention immediately.

■ *Symptoms of estrogen overdose may include:*
Nausea, vomiting, withdrawal bleeding

Estrogen with Progestin *See Activella and femhrt, page 26.*

Estropipate *See Ogen, page 991.*

Estrostep *See Oral Contraceptives, page 1000.*

Etanercept *See Enbrel, page 512.*

Ethinyl estradiol and Norelgestromin *See Ortho Evra, page 1010.*

Ethotoin *See Peganone, page 1055.*

Etodolac *See Lodine, page 767.*

Etonogestrel and Ethinyl estradiol *See NuvaRing, page 985.*

EULEXIN

Pronounced: you-LEKS-in
Generic name: Flutamide

Why is this drug prescribed?

Eulexin is used along with drugs such as Lupron to treat prostate cancer. Eulexin belongs to a class of drugs known as antiandrogens. It blocks the effect of the male hormone testosterone. Giving Eulexin with Lupron, which reduces the body's testosterone levels, is one way of treating prostate cancer. For some forms of prostate cancer, radiation therapy is given along with the drugs.

Most important fact about this drug

Taking Eulexin and Lupron together is essential in this form of treatment. You should not interrupt their doses or stop taking either of these medications without consulting your doctor.

How should you take this medication?

Take Eulexin exactly as prescribed. Do not use more or less, and do not take it more often than instructed.

If you develop diarrhea—a relatively common side effect of therapy—you may find the following measures helpful: drink plenty of fluids; avoid dairy products; increase your intake of whole grains, fruits, and vegetables; avoid laxatives; and take nonprescription antidiarrhea medicine. If the diarrhea continues or becomes severe, contact your doctor.

■ *If you miss a dose...*
Take it as soon as you remember. If it is almost time for your next dose, skip the one you missed and go back to your regular schedule. Never take 2 doses at once.

■ *Storage instructions...*
Store at room temperature.

What side effects may occur?

Side effects cannot be anticipated. If any develop or change in intensity, inform your doctor immediately. Since Eulexin is always given with another antiandrogen drug, when a side effect develops, it is difficult to know which drug is responsible. Only your doctor can determine if it is safe for you to continue taking Eulexin.

■ *Side effects may include:*
Breast tissue swelling and tenderness, diarrhea, hot flashes, impotence, loss of sex drive, nausea, vomiting

When the drugs are used along with radiation therapy, additional side effects may include bladder inflammation, bleeding from the rectum, blood in the urine, and intestinal problems.

Why should this drug not be prescribed?

This drug is not intended for women, and should not be used by anyone with serious liver disease. You'll also be unable to take it if it gives you an allergic reaction.

Special warnings about this medication

Eulexin has been known to cause liver failure in some patients, in rare cases leading to death. Your doctor will do blood tests to check your liver function before you start treatment with Eulexin, and at regular intervals thereafter. If a liver problem does develop, you may need to take less Eulexin or stop taking the drug altogether. Report any signs or symptoms that might suggest liver damage to your doctor right away. Warning signs include dark urine, itching, flu-like symptoms, jaundice (a yellowing of the skin and eyes), persistent appetite loss, and persistent tenderness on the right side of the upper abdomen.

Possible food and drug interactions when taking this medication

If you are already taking the anticoagulant drug warfarin (Coumadin), you will need to be monitored especially closely after treatment with Eulexin begins. Your doctor may need to lower your dosage of warfarin.

Special information if you are pregnant or breastfeeding

Eulexin can harm a developing baby. Women should never take this drug, either during pregnancy or at any other time.

Recommended dosage

The recommended adult Eulexin dosage is 2 capsules 3 times a day at 8-hour intervals for a total daily dosage of 750 milligrams.

Overdosage

You may notice breast development or tenderness with an overdose of Eulexin. Any medication taken in excess can have serious consequences. If you suspect an overdose, seek medical attention immediately.

EVISTA

Pronounced: Eve-IST-ah
Generic name: Raloxifene hydrochloride

Why is this drug prescribed?

Evista is prescribed to treat and prevent osteoporosis, the brittle bone disease that strikes some women after menopause. A variety of factors promote osteoporosis. The more factors that apply to you, the greater your chances of developing the disease. These factors include:

- Caucasian or Asian descent
  Slender build

Early menopause
Smoking
Drinking
A diet low in calcium
An inactive lifestyle
Osteoporosis in the family

Most important fact about this drug

Like estrogen, Evista reduces bone loss and increases bone density. However, Evista does not have estrogen-like effects on the uterus and breasts, and therefore is unlikely to increase the risk of cancer, as estrogen therapy sometimes can do.

Although Evista has been shown to increase bone density over the course of a two-year study, its longer-term ability to prevent bone fractures has not yet been proven.

How should you use this medication?

Take Evista once daily, at any time, with or without food. Take calcium and vitamin D supplements as well, if you do not get enough in your diet. Avoid alcohol and tobacco. Do weight-bearing exercises to strengthen your bones.

■ *If you miss a dose...*
Take it as soon as you remember. If it is almost time for your next dose, skip the one you missed and go back to your regular schedule. Never take a double dose.

■ *Storage instructions...*
Store at room temperature.

What side effects may occur?

Evista has one very positive side effect: It lowers total cholesterol and LDL ("bad") cholesterol. It does not affect HDL ("good") cholesterol or triglyceride levels.

The unwanted side effects of Evista cannot be predicted. If any develop or change in intensity, inform your doctor as soon as possible. Only your doctor can determine if it is safe for you to continue taking Evista.

■ *Side effects may include:*
Abdominal pain, arthritis, breast pain, bronchitis, chest pain, depression, diarrhea, dizziness, fever, flu symptoms, gas, gynecological problems, headache, hot flashes, increased cough, indigestion, infection, insomnia, joint pain, leg cramps, muscle ache, nasal inflammation, nausea, rash, sinusitis, sore throat, stomach and intestinal problems, sweating, swelling, tendon soreness, uterine discharge, urinary tract infection, vomiting, weight gain

Why should this drug not be prescribed?

Evista is not for use by women who are—or could become—pregnant. You should also avoid this drug if you have a history of blood clot formation, including deep vein thrombosis (blood clot in the legs), pulmonary embolism (blood clot in the lungs), and retinal vein thrombosis (blood clot in the retina of the eye), since Evista increases the risk of clots. Avoid the drug, too, if it gives you an allergic reaction.

Special warnings about this medication

Because of Evista's tendency to promote clots, you should not take it during long periods of immobilization such as recovery from surgery or prolonged bed rest, or for 72 hours beforehand. If you are scheduled for surgery, make sure the doctor is aware that you are taking Evista.

For the same reason, if you are going on a trip where your movement will be restricted, make a point of periodically getting up and walking around.

Evista is not needed prior to menopause and shouldn't be taken until menopause has passed. It has not been studied in premenopausal women and its use is not recommended.

Use Evista with caution if you have congestive heart failure, a liver condition, or cancer. Be cautious, too, if you've had breast cancer in the past; the drug's effect in this situation is unknown.

If you develop unusual uterine bleeding or breast problems while taking Evista, tell your doctor immediately.

Evista will not cure hot flashes. (In fact, it may cause them.) Nevertheless, never combine Evista with estrogen hormones.

If you've had a problem with high blood triglyceride levels when taking estrogen, Evista may cause the same problem. However, it tends to lower cholesterol levels by 6 to 11 percent.

Possible food and drug interactions when taking this medication

If Evista is taken with certain other drugs, the effects of either could be increased, decreased, or altered. It is especially important to check with your doctor before combining Evista with the following:

Cholestyramine (Questran)
Clofibrate (Atromid-S)
Diazepam (Valium)
Diazoxide (Proglycem)
Ibuprofen (Advil, Motrin, Nuprin)
Indomethacin (Indocin)
Naproxen (Aleve, Anaprox, Naprosyn)
Warfarin (Coumadin)

Special information if you are pregnant or breastfeeding

Evista can harm a developing baby. Do not use if you are or may become pregnant. Also avoid breastfeeding while taking Evista.

Recommended dosage

POSTMENOPAUSAL WOMEN

The recommended dosage is one 60-milligram tablet once a day.

Overdosage

There have not been any reports of overdose with Evista. However, any medication taken in excess can have serious consequences. If you suspect an overdose, seek medical attention immediately.

EXELON

Pronounced: ECKS-ell-on
Generic name: Rivastigmine tartrate

Why is this drug prescribed?

Exelon is used in the treatment of mild to moderate Alzheimer's disease. Alzheimer's disease causes physical changes in the brain that disrupt the flow of information and interfere with memory, thinking, and behavior. By boosting levels of the chemical messenger acetylcholine, Exelon can temporarily improve brain function in some Alzheimer's sufferers, though it does not halt the progress of the underlying disease. Exelon may become less effective as the disease progresses.

Most important fact about this drug

Patience is in order when starting this drug. It can take up to 12 weeks before Exelon's full benefits appear.

How should you take this medication?

Exelon should be taken with food in the morning and in the evening.

■ *If you miss a dose...*
 Give the forgotten dose as soon as you remember. If it is almost time for the next dose, skip the one you missed and go back to the regular schedule. Never double the dose.
■ *Storage instructions...*
 Store at room temperature in a tightly closed container.

What side effects may occur?

Side effects from Exelon cannot be anticipated. If any side effects develop or change in intensity, inform your doctor as soon as possible. Only your doctor can determine if it is safe to continue taking Exelon.

■ *Side effects may include:*
 Abdominal pain, accidental injury, anxiety, aggression, confusion, constipation, depression, diarrhea, dizziness, drowsiness, fainting, fatigue, flu-like symptoms, gas, hallucinations, headache, high blood

pressure, increased sweating, indigestion, inflamed nasal passages, insomnia, loss of appetite, nausea, tremor, unwell feeling, urinary infection, vomiting, weakness, weight loss

Why should this drug not be prescribed?
Exelon cannot be used if it causes an allergic reaction.

Special warnings about this medication
Exelon often causes nausea and vomiting, especially at the beginning of treatment. The problem is more likely in women, but it can lead to significant weight loss in both women and men. Tell your doctor immediately if these side effects occur.

The chance of severe vomiting increases when Exelon is given after an interruption of several days. Do not start giving the drug again without first checking with the doctor. Dosage may need to be reduced to the lowest starting level.

Exelon may aggravate asthma and other breathing problems and can increase the risk of seizures. Other drugs of its type are also known to increase the chance of ulcers, stomach bleeding, and urinary obstruction, although these problems have not been noted with Exelon. Drugs in this category can also slow the heartbeat, possibly causing fainting in people who have a heart condition. Contact your doctor if any of these problems occur.

Exelon has not been tested in children.

Possible food and drug interactions when taking this medication
If Exelon is taken with certain other drugs, the effects of either could be increased, decreased, or altered. It is especially important to check with your doctor before combining Exelon with the following:

Bethanechol (Urecholine)
Drugs that control spasms, such as Bentyl, Donnatal, and Levsin

Special information if you are pregnant or breastfeeding
Exelon is not intended for women of childbearing age, and its effects during pregnancy and breastfeeding have not been studied.

Recommended dosage

ADULTS

The usual starting dose is 1.5 milligrams 2 times a day for at least 2 weeks. At 2-week intervals, your doctor may then increase the dose to 3 milligrams, 4.5 milligrams, and finally 6.0 milligrams 2 times a day. Higher doses tend to be more effective. The maximum dosage is 12 milligrams daily.

If side effects such as nausea and vomiting begin to develop, your doctor may recommend skipping a few doses, then starting again at the same or the next lowest dosage.

Overdosage

Any medication taken in excess can have serious consequences. If you suspect an overdose, seek emergency medical attention immediately.

■ *Symptoms of Exelon overdose may include:*
Collapse, convulsions, breathing difficulty, extreme muscle weakness (possibly ending in death if breathing muscles are affected), low blood pressure, salivation, severe nausea, slow heartbeat, sweating, vomiting

Ex-Lax Stool Softener *See Colace, page 317.*

Ezetimibe *See Zetia, page 1627.*

Ezetimibe and Simvastatin *See Vytorin, page 1582.*

FACTIVE
Pronounced: FAK-tiv
Generic Name: Gemifloxacin

Why is this drug prescribed?

Factive is an antibiotic that is used to treat infections of the respiratory tract, such as bronchitis and pneumonia.

Most important fact about this drug

Medications similar to Factive have been known to cause dangerous allergic reactions as soon as you take the first dose. Stop taking the drug and call your doctor immediately if you develop any of the following warning signs while taking Factive:

Abnormal or rapid heartbeat
Difficulty swallowing or breathing
Fainting spells
Heart palpitations
Skin rash, hives, or any skin reaction
Swelling of the face, lips, tongue, or throat

How should you take this medication?

Factive should be taken once daily at the same time each day. It can be taken with or without food. Do not take more than 1 dose per day.

Swallow the tablet whole with plenty of fluids. Do not chew the tablet.

Take your complete prescription exactly as prescribed, even if you begin to feel better. If you stop taking Factive too soon, the infection may come back.

■ *If you miss a dose...*
If you miss a dose, take it as soon as you remember. If it is almost time for your next dose, skip the one you missed and go back to your regular schedule. Do not take 2 doses at once.

■ *Storage instructions...*
Store at room temperature and protect from light.

What side effects may occur?

Side effects cannot be anticipated. If any develop or change in intensity, inform your doctor as soon as possible. Only your doctor can determine if it is safe for you to continue taking Factive.

■ *Side effects may include:*
Diarrhea, headache, nausea, rash

Why should this drug not be prescribed?

You cannot take Factive if you have ever had an allergic reaction to it or to other fluoroquinolone antibiotics, including: ciprofloxacin (Cipro), enoxacin (Penetrex), gatifloxacin (Tequin), levofloxacin (Levaquin), lomefloxacin (Maxaquin), moxifloxacin (Avelox), norfloxacin (Noroxin), ofloxacin (Floxin), soarfloxacin (Zagam), trovafloxacin (Trovan tablets), and alatrofloxacin (Trovan intravenous).

Special warnings about this medication

Do not use Factive if you have had a recent heart attack or if you have a history of irregular heartbeat, obstructed blood vessels or arteries, a very slow heartbeat, or a family history of heart rhythm problems.

Use Factive with caution if you have epilepsy or a history of convulsions. Antibiotics such as Factive have infrequently caused serious nervous system problems, including convulsions. These antibiotics have also caused tremors, restlessness, anxiety, lightheadedness, confusion, hallucinations, paranoia, depression, insomnia, and suicidal thoughts. Call your doctor immediately if you develop any of these symptoms.

Do not take Factive if you have low potassium or magnesium levels, since this increases the possibility of having convulsions.

Tell your doctor immediately if you have heart palpitations or fainting spells while taking Factive. These symptoms could signal a rare—but serious—heart problem associated with the drug.

Like all antibiotics, Factive could cause severe inflammation of the bowels. Tell your doctor right away if you develop diarrhea while taking this drug.

Factive may cause dizziness. Do not drive or operate dangerous machinery until you know how the medication affects you.

Antibiotics such as Factive may cause tendon problems in certain people, especially athletes, those taking steroids, and the elderly. Call your doctor immediately if you feel pain or tenderness in a tendon or rupture any tendons, and be sure to rest and avoid exercise until the injury has been evaluated.

Because Factive increases sensitivity to sunlight, use sunblock when outdoors and avoid sunlamps.

Antibiotics such as Factive have been known to thin the blood. If you take blood thinners such as warfarin (Coumadin), your doctor will monitor you closely.

The safety and effectiveness of Factive have not been studied in pregnant or breastfeeding women, or in children less than 18 years old.

Possible food and drug interactions when taking this medication
If Factive is taken with certain other drugs, the effects of either could be increased, decreased, or altered. It is especially important to check with your doctor before combining Factive with the following:

> Antiarrhythmics (heartbeat-regulating drugs) such as amiodarone (Cordarone), procainamide (Procan), quinidine (Quinidex), and sotalol (Betapace)
> Antidepressants such as Elavil
> Antipsychotics such as Risperdal
> Diuretics (water pills) such as hydrochlorothiazide or Lasix
> Erythromycin
> Probenecid
> Steroids such as Prednisone

Be sure to tell your doctor if you are taking any over-the-counter drugs or dietary supplements.

Factive should be taken at least 2 hours before sucralfate (Carafate).

The following medications should not be taken within 3 hours before or 2 hours after taking Factive:

> Antacids that contain aluminum and magnesium, such as Maalox
> Didanosine (Videx)
> Iron pills (ferrous sulfate)
> Multivitamins that contain zinc

Special information if you are pregnant or breastfeeding
The safety and effectiveness of Factive in pregnant and breastfeeding women have not been established. The drug should not be used unless the potential benefit to the mother outweighs the risk to the baby.

Recommended dosage

ADULTS

The recommended dosage is one 320-milligram tablet once a day for 5 days if you have bronchitis and for 7 days if you have pneumonia.

Patients with kidney problems may need a lower dosage.

The safety and effectiveness of Factive have not been evaluated in children less than 18 years old.

Overdosage

Any medication taken in excess can have serious consequences. If you suspect an overdose, seek medical attention immediately.

Famciclovir See Famvir, below.

Famotidine See Pepcid, page 1070.

FAMVIR

Pronounced: FAM-veer
Generic name: Famciclovir

Why is this drug prescribed?

Famvir tablets are used to treat herpes zoster, commonly referred to as shingles, in adults. Shingles is a painful rash with raised, red pimples on the trunk of the body, usually the back. Because it is caused by the same virus that causes chickenpox, only people who have had chickenpox can get shingles. When prescribed for shingles, Famvir works best in people age 50 or over.

Famvir is also prescribed to treat attacks of genital herpes and to prevent future flare-ups. For people with HIV infections, it is used as a treatment for both genital and oral herpes.

Most important fact about this drug

Famvir is most effective if started within the first 48 hours after shingles first appears; treatment should be started at the first sign or symptom of genital herpes. Famvir treatment may not be effective if it is delayed more than 72 hours after the herpes zoster rash first appears or more than 6 hours after genital herpes becomes evident. Thus, it is important to see your doctor as soon as possible after symptoms appear.

How should you take this medication?

For maximum benefit, take Famvir for the full time of treatment, even if your symptoms begin to clear up. Do not, however, take Famvir more often or for a longer time than your doctor directs.

You may take Famvir with meals or in between.

■ *If you miss a dose...*
Take the forgotten dose as soon as you remember. If it is almost time for your next dose, skip the one you missed and go back to your regular schedule. Never take 2 doses at the same time.

■ *Storage instructions...*
Store at room temperature.

What side effects may occur?

Side effects cannot be anticipated. If any develop or change in intensity, inform your doctor as soon as possible. Only your doctor can determine if it is safe for you to continue taking Famvir.

■ *Side effects may include:*
Constipation, diarrhea, dizziness, fatigue, fever, headache, nausea, vomiting

Why should this drug not be prescribed?

Do not take Famvir if you are sensitive to it or have ever had an allergic reaction to it. Also avoid Famvir if you are sensitive to Denavir (penciclovir cream).

Special warnings about this medication

Famvir speeds healing of shingles and genital herpes, but it is not a cure. It may not prevent transmission of genital herpes to others, so you should avoid sexual intercourse whenever you have symptoms of the disease.

If you have any kidney problems, be sure your doctor knows about them before prescribing Famvir for you.

Possible food and drug interactions when taking this medication

If Famvir is taken with certain other drugs, the effects of either could be increased, decreased, or altered. It is especially important to check with your doctor before combining Famvir with probenecid (Benemid), a drug used to treat gout (a type of arthritis).

Special information if you are pregnant or breastfeeding

The effects of Famvir during pregnancy have not been adequately studied. If you are pregnant or plan to become pregnant, inform your doctor immediately. Famvir should be used during pregnancy only when the benefit to the mother clearly outweighs the potential risk to the baby. Famvir may appear in breast milk, and could affect a nursing infant. If this drug is essential to your health, your doctor may advise you to discontinue breastfeeding until your treatment with Famvir is finished.

Recommended dosage

ADULTS

Herpes Zoster
The usual adult dose is 500 milligrams every 8 hours for 7 days.

Recurrent Genital Herpes Treatment
The usual dose is 125 milligrams twice a day for 5 days.

DRUG IDENTIFICATION GUIDE

Use this section to quickly verify the identity of a capsule, tablet, or other solid oral medication. More than 200 leading tablets and capsules are shown in actual size and color, organized alphabetically by brand name. Each is labeled with its generic name, as well as its strength and the name of its supplier.

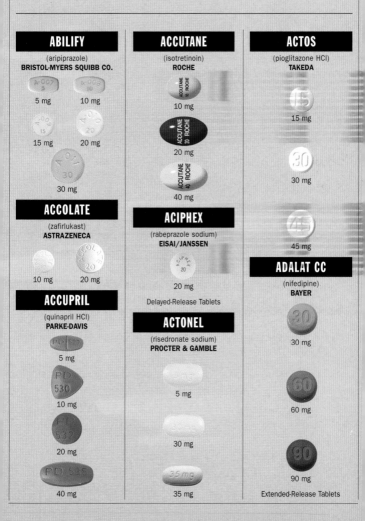

ABILIFY
(aripiprazole)
BRISTOL-MYERS SQUIBB CO.

5 mg   10 mg

15 mg   20 mg

30 mg

ACCOLATE
(zafirlukast)
ASTRAZENECA

10 mg   20 mg

ACCUPRIL
(quinapril HCl)
PARKE-DAVIS

5 mg

10 mg

20 mg

40 mg

ACCUTANE
(isotretinoin)
ROCHE

10 mg

20 mg

40 mg

ACIPHEX
(rabeprazole sodium)
EISAI/JANSSEN

20 mg

Delayed-Release Tablets

ACTONEL
(risedronate sodium)
PROCTER & GAMBLE

5 mg

30 mg

35 mg

ACTOS
(pioglitazone HCl)
TAKEDA

15 mg

30 mg

45 mg

ADALAT CC
(nifedipine)
BAYER

30 mg

60 mg

90 mg

Extended-Release Tablets

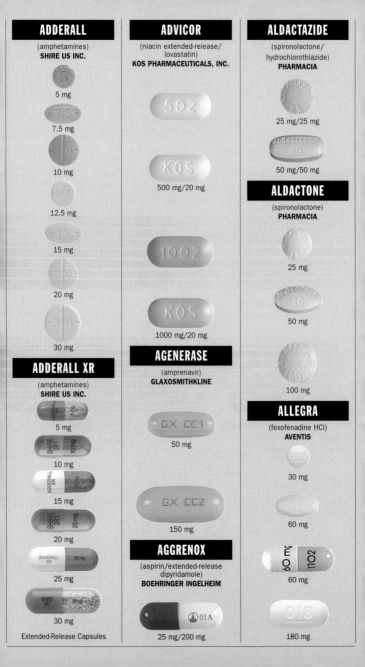

ADDERALL

(amphetamines)
SHIRE US INC.

5 mg

7.5 mg

10 mg

12.5 mg

15 mg

20 mg

30 mg

ADDERALL XR

(amphetamines)
SHIRE US INC.

5 mg

10 mg

15 mg

20 mg

25 mg

30 mg

Extended-Release Capsules

ADVICOR

(niacin extended-release/
lovastatin)
KOS PHARMACEUTICALS, INC.

502

KOS

500 mg/20 mg

1002

KOS

1000 mg/20 mg

AGENERASE

(amprenavir)
GLAXOSMITHKLINE

GX CC1

50 mg

GX CC2

150 mg

AGGRENOX

(aspirin/extended-release
dipyridamole)
BOEHRINGER INGELHEIM

01A

25 mg/200 mg

ALDACTAZIDE

(spironolactone/
hydrochlorothiazide)
PHARMACIA

25 mg/25 mg

50 mg/50 mg

ALDACTONE

(spironolactone)
PHARMACIA

25 mg

50 mg

100 mg

ALLEGRA

(fexofenadine HCl)
AVENTIS

30 mg

60 mg

60 mg

180 mg

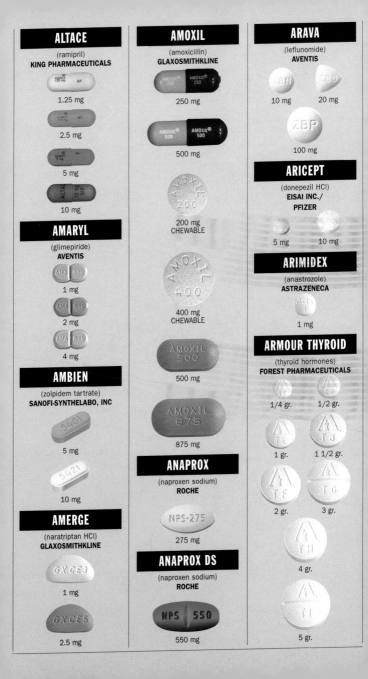

ALTACE
(ramipril)
KING PHARMACEUTICALS

1.25 mg

2.5 mg

5 mg

10 mg

AMARYL
(glimepiride)
AVENTIS

1 mg

2 mg

4 mg

AMBIEN
(zolpidem tartrate)
SANOFI-SYNTHELABO, INC

5 mg

10 mg

AMERGE
(naratriptan HCl)
GLAXOSMITHKLINE

1 mg

2.5 mg

AMOXIL
(amoxicillin)
GLAXOSMITHKLINE

250 mg

500 mg

200 mg
CHEWABLE

400 mg
CHEWABLE

500 mg

875 mg

ANAPROX
(naproxen sodium)
ROCHE

275 mg

ANAPROX DS
(naproxen sodium)
ROCHE

550 mg

ARAVA
(leflunomide)
AVENTIS

10 mg   20 mg

100 mg

ARICEPT
(donepezil HCl)
**EISAI INC./
PFIZER**

5 mg   10 mg

ARIMIDEX
(anastrozole)
ASTRAZENECA

1 mg

ARMOUR THYROID
(thyroid hormones)
FOREST PHARMACEUTICALS

1/4 gr.   1/2 gr.

1 gr.   1 1/2 gr.

2 gr.   3 gr.

4 gr.

5 gr.

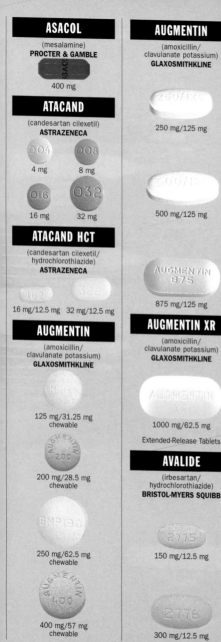

ASACOL

(mesalamine)
PROCTER & GAMBLE

400 mg

ATACAND

(candesartan cilexetil)
ASTRAZENECA

004
4 mg

008
8 mg

016
16 mg

032
32 mg

ATACAND HCT

(candesartan cilexetil/
hydrochlorothiazide)
ASTRAZENECA

162
16 mg/12.5 mg

322
32 mg/12.5 mg

AUGMENTIN

(amoxicillin/
clavulanate potassium)
GLAXOSMITHKLINE

125 mg/31.25 mg
chewable

AUGMENTIN
200
200 mg/28.5 mg
chewable

BMP190
250 mg/62.5 mg
chewable

AUGMENTIN
400
400 mg/57 mg
chewable

AUGMENTIN

(amoxicillin/
clavulanate potassium)
GLAXOSMITHKLINE

250/125
250 mg/125 mg

500/125
500 mg/125 mg

AUGMENTIN
875
875 mg/125 mg

AUGMENTIN XR

(amoxicillin/
clavulanate potassium)
GLAXOSMITHKLINE

AUGMENTIN
XR
1000 mg/62.5 mg

Extended-Release Tablets

AVALIDE

(irbesartan/
hydrochlorothiazide)
BRISTOL-MYERS SQUIBB

2775
150 mg/12.5 mg

2776
300 mg/12.5 mg

AVANDAMET

(rosiglitazone maleate/
metformin HCl)
GLAXOSMITHKLINE

1/500
1 mg/500 mg

2/500
2 mg/500 mg

2/1000
2 mg/1000 mg

4/500
4 mg/500 mg

4/1000
4 mg/1000 mg

AVANDIA

(rosiglitazone maleate)
GLAXOSMITHKLINE

2 mg

4
4 mg

8 mg

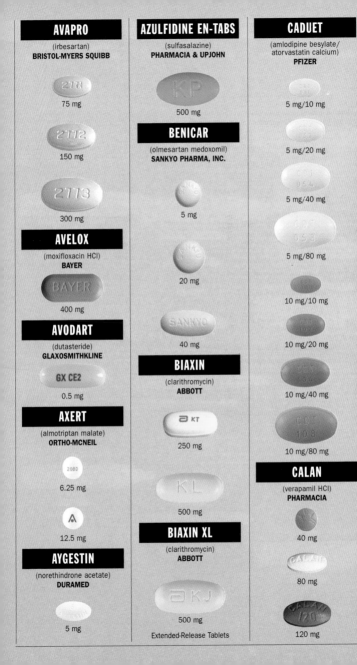

AVAPRO
(irbesartan)
BRISTOL-MYERS SQUIBB

2771
75 mg

2772
150 mg

2773
300 mg

AVELOX
(moxifloxacin HCl)
BAYER

BAYER
400 mg

AVODART
(dutasteride)
GLAXOSMITHKLINE

GX CE2
0.5 mg

AXERT
(almotriptan malate)
ORTHO-MCNEIL

2080
6.25 mg

A
12.5 mg

AYGESTIN
(norethindrone acetate)
DURAMED

5
5 mg

AZULFIDINE EN-TABS
(sulfasalazine)
PHARMACIA & UPJOHN

KP
500 mg

BENICAR
(olmesartan medoxomil)
SANKYO PHARMA, INC.

SANKYO
5 mg

SANKYO
20 mg

SANKYO
40 mg

BIAXIN
(clarithromycin)
ABBOTT

a KT
250 mg

KL
500 mg

BIAXIN XL
(clarithromycin)
ABBOTT

a KJ
500 mg
Extended-Release Tablets

CADUET
(amlodipine besylate/
atorvastatin calcium)
PFIZER

5 mg/10 mg

5 mg/20 mg

CDT
054
5 mg/40 mg

CDT
058
5 mg/80 mg

10 mg/10 mg

10 mg/20 mg

CDT
10 mg/40 mg

CDT
108
10 mg/80 mg

CALAN
(verapamil HCl)
PHARMACIA

40 mg

CALAN
80 mg

CALAN
120
120 mg

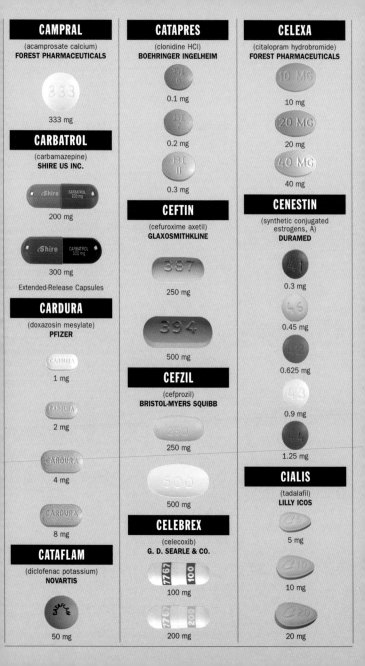

CAMPRAL
(acamprosate calcium)
FOREST PHARMACEUTICALS

333 mg

CARBATROL
(carbamazepine)
SHIRE US INC.

200 mg

300 mg

Extended-Release Capsules

CARDURA
(doxazosin mesylate)
PFIZER

1 mg

2 mg

4 mg

8 mg

CATAFLAM
(diclofenac potassium)
NOVARTIS

50 mg

CATAPRES
(clonidine HCl)
BOEHRINGER INGELHEIM

0.1 mg

0.2 mg

0.3 mg

CEFTIN
(cefuroxime axetil)
GLAXOSMITHKLINE

250 mg

500 mg

CEFZIL
(cefprozil)
BRISTOL-MYERS SQUIBB

250 mg

500 mg

CELEBREX
(celecoxib)
G. D. SEARLE & CO.

100 mg

200 mg

CELEXA
(citalopram hydrobromide)
FOREST PHARMACEUTICALS

10 mg

20 mg

40 mg

CENESTIN
(synthetic conjugated estrogens, A)
DURAMED

0.3 mg

0.45 mg

0.625 mg

0.9 mg

1.25 mg

CIALIS
(tadalafil)
LILLY ICOS

5 mg

10 mg

20 mg

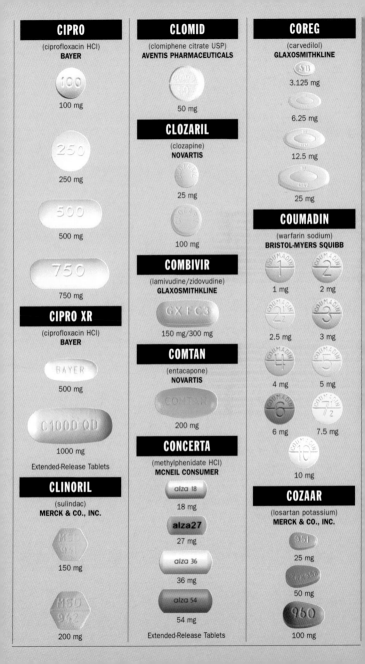

CIPRO
(ciprofloxacin HCl)
BAYER

100 mg

250 mg

500 mg

750 mg

CIPRO XR
(ciprofloxacin HCl)
BAYER

500 mg

1000 mg

Extended-Release Tablets

CLINORIL
(sulindac)
MERCK & CO., INC.

150 mg

200 mg

CLOMID
(clomiphene citrate USP)
AVENTIS PHARMACEUTICALS

50 mg

CLOZARIL
(clozapine)
NOVARTIS

25 mg

100 mg

COMBIVIR
(lamivudine/zidovudine)
GLAXOSMITHKLINE

150 mg/300 mg

COMTAN
(entacapone)
NOVARTIS

200 mg

CONCERTA
(methylphenidate HCl)
MCNEIL CONSUMER

18 mg

27 mg

36 mg

54 mg

Extended-Release Tablets

COREG
(carvedilol)
GLAXOSMITHKLINE

3.125 mg

6.25 mg

12.5 mg

25 mg

COUMADIN
(warfarin sodium)
BRISTOL-MYERS SQUIBB

1 mg

2 mg

2.5 mg

3 mg

4 mg

5 mg

6 mg

7.5 mg

10 mg

COZAAR
(losartan potassium)
MERCK & CO., INC.

25 mg

50 mg

100 mg

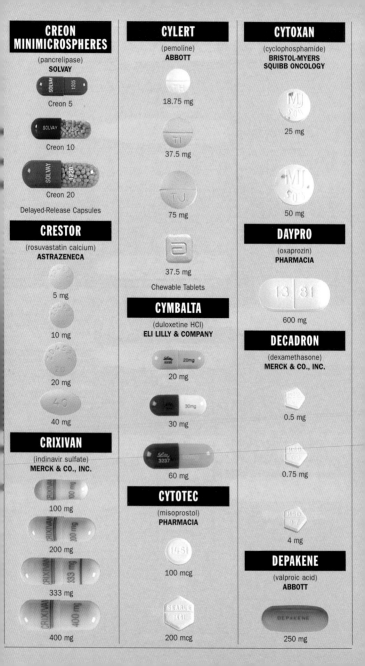

CREON MINIMICROSPHERES

(pancrelipase)
SOLVAY

Creon 5

Creon 10

Creon 20

Delayed-Release Capsules

CRESTOR

(rosuvastatin calcium)
ASTRAZENECA

5 mg

10 mg

20 mg

40 mg

CRIXIVAN

(indinavir sulfate)
MERCK & CO., INC.

100 mg

200 mg

333 mg

400 mg

CYLERT

(pemoline)
ABBOTT

18.75 mg

37.5 mg

75 mg

37.5 mg

Chewable Tablets

CYMBALTA

(duloxetine HCl)
ELI LILLY & COMPANY

20 mg

30 mg

60 mg

CYTOTEC

(misoprostol)
PHARMACIA

100 mcg

200 mcg

CYTOXAN

(cyclophosphamide)
BRISTOL-MYERS SQUIBB ONCOLOGY

25 mg

50 mg

DAYPRO

(oxaprozin)
PHARMACIA

600 mg

DECADRON

(dexamethasone)
MERCK & CO., INC.

0.5 mg

0.75 mg

4 mg

DEPAKENE

(valproic acid)
ABBOTT

250 mg

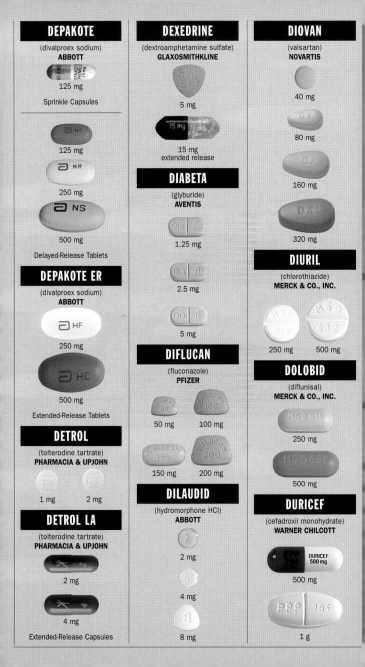

DEPAKOTE
(divalproex sodium)
ABBOTT

125 mg
Sprinkle Capsules

125 mg

250 mg

500 mg
Delayed-Release Tablets

DEPAKOTE ER
(divalproex sodium)
ABBOTT

250 mg

500 mg
Extended-Release Tablets

DETROL
(tolterodine tartrate)
PHARMACIA & UPJOHN

1 mg   2 mg

DETROL LA
(tolterodine tartrate)
PHARMACIA & UPJOHN

2 mg

4 mg
Extended-Release Capsules

DEXEDRINE
(dextroamphetamine sulfate)
GLAXOSMITHKLINE

5 mg

15 mg
extended release

DIABETA
(glyburide)
AVENTIS

1.25 mg

2.5 mg

5 mg

DIFLUCAN
(fluconazole)
PFIZER

50 mg   100 mg

150 mg   200 mg

DILAUDID
(hydromorphone HCl)
ABBOTT

2 mg

4 mg

8 mg

DIOVAN
(valsartan)
NOVARTIS

40 mg

80 mg

160 mg

320 mg

DIURIL
(chlorothiazide)
MERCK & CO., INC.

250 mg   500 mg

DOLOBID
(diflunisal)
MERCK & CO., INC.

250 mg

500 mg

DURICEF
(cefadroxil monohydrate)
WARNER CHILCOTT

500 mg

1 g

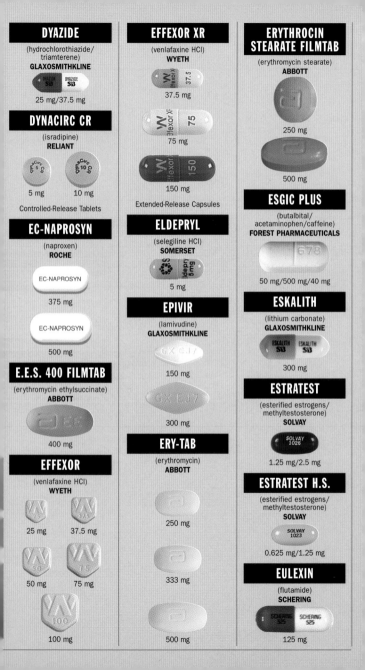

DYAZIDE

(hydrochlorothiazide/
triamterene)
GLAXOSMITHKLINE

25 mg/37.5 mg

DYNACIRC CR

(isradipine)
RELIANT

5 mg   10 mg

Controlled-Release Tablets

EC-NAPROSYN

(naproxen)
ROCHE

EC-NAPROSYN

375 mg

EC-NAPROSYN

500 mg

E.E.S. 400 FILMTAB

(erythromycin ethylsuccinate)
ABBOTT

400 mg

EFFEXOR

(venlafaxine HCl)
WYETH

25 mg   37.5 mg

50 mg   75 mg

100 mg

EFFEXOR XR

(venlafaxine HCl)
WYETH

37.5 mg

75 mg

150 mg

Extended-Release Capsules

ELDEPRYL

(selegiline HCl)
SOMERSET

5 mg

EPIVIR

(lamivudine)
GLAXOSMITHKLINE

150 mg

300 mg

ERY-TAB

(erythromycin)
ABBOTT

250 mg

333 mg

500 mg

ERYTHROCIN STEARATE FILMTAB

(erythromycin stearate)
ABBOTT

250 mg

500 mg

ESGIC PLUS

(butalbital/
acetaminophen/caffeine)
FOREST PHARMACEUTICALS

50 mg/500 mg/40 mg

ESKALITH

(lithium carbonate)
GLAXOSMITHKLINE

300 mg

ESTRATEST

(esterified estrogens/
methyltestosterone)
SOLVAY

1.25 mg/2.5 mg

ESTRATEST H.S.

(esterified estrogens/
methyltestosterone)
SOLVAY

0.625 mg/1.25 mg

EULEXIN

(flutamide)
SCHERING

125 mg

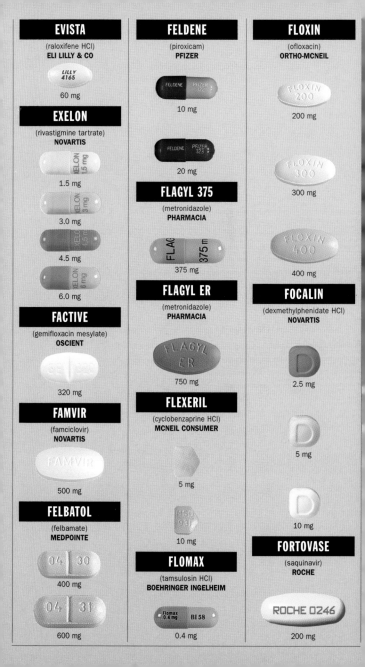

EVISTA
(raloxifene HCl)
ELI LILLY & CO

LILLY 4165

60 mg

EXELON
(rivastigmine tartrate)
NOVARTIS

EXELON 1.5 mg
1.5 mg

EXELON 3 mg
3.0 mg

EXELON 4.5 mg
4.5 mg

EXELON 6 mg
6.0 mg

FACTIVE
(gemifloxacin mesylate)
OSCIENT

GE 320
320 mg

FAMVIR
(famciclovir)
NOVARTIS

FAMVIR
500 mg

FELBATOL
(felbamate)
MEDPOINTE

04 30
400 mg

04 31
600 mg

FELDENE
(piroxicam)
PFIZER

FELDENE PFIZER 323
10 mg

FELDENE PFIZER 323
20 mg

FLAGYL 375
(metronidazole)
PHARMACIA

FLAG 375 m
375 mg

FLAGYL ER
(metronidazole)
PHARMACIA

FLAGYL ER
750 mg

FLEXERIL
(cyclobenzaprine HCl)
MCNEIL CONSUMER

5 mg

MSD 931
10 mg

FLOMAX
(tamsulosin HCl)
BOEHRINGER INGELHEIM

Flomax 0.4 mg   BI 58
0.4 mg

FLOXIN
(ofloxacin)
ORTHO-MCNEIL

FLOXIN 200
200 mg

FLOXIN 300
300 mg

FLOXIN 400
400 mg

FOCALIN
(dexmethylphenidate HCl)
NOVARTIS

D
2.5 mg

D
5 mg

D
10 mg

FORTOVASE
(saquinavir)
ROCHE

ROCHE 0246
200 mg

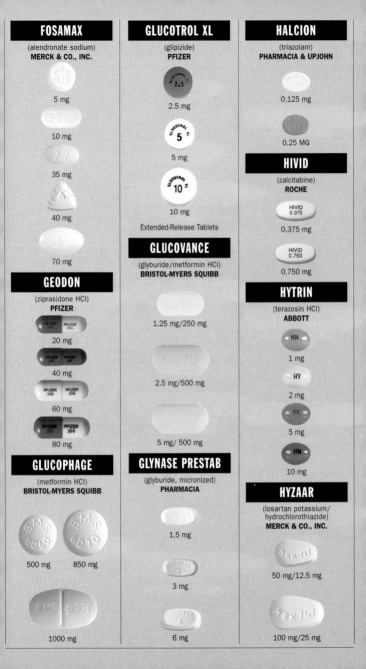

FOSAMAX
(alendronate sodium)
MERCK & CO., INC.

5 mg

10 mg

35 mg

40 mg

70 mg

GEODON
(ziprasidone HCl)
PFIZER

20 mg

40 mg

60 mg

80 mg

GLUCOPHAGE
(metformin HCl)
BRISTOL-MYERS SQUIBB

500 mg   850 mg

1000 mg

GLUCOTROL XL
(glipizide)
PFIZER

2.5 mg

5 mg

10 mg

Extended-Release Tablets

GLUCOVANCE
(glyburide/metformin HCl)
BRISTOL-MYERS SQUIBB

1.25 mg/250 mg

2.5 mg/500 mg

5 mg/ 500 mg

GLYNASE PRESTAB
(glyburide, micronized)
PHARMACIA

1.5 mg

3 mg

6 mg

HALCION
(triazolam)
PHARMACIA & UPJOHN

0.125 mg

0.25 MG

HIVID
(zalcitabine)
ROCHE

0.375 mg

0.750 mg

HYTRIN
(terazosin HCl)
ABBOTT

1 mg

2 mg

5 mg

10 mg

HYZAAR
(losartan potassium/
hydrochlorothiazide)
MERCK & CO., INC.

50 mg/12.5 mg

100 mg/25 mg

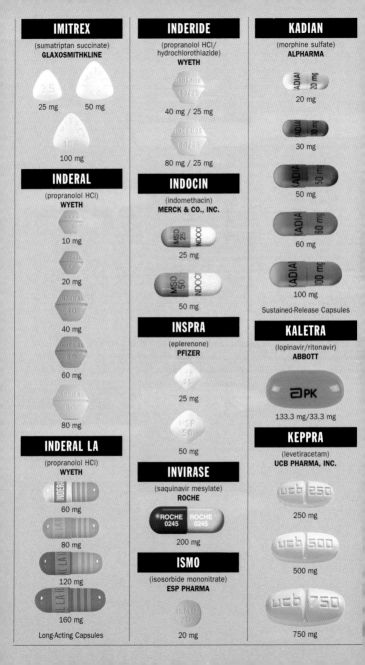

IMITREX

(sumatriptan succinate)
GLAXOSMITHKLINE

25 mg   50 mg

100 mg

INDERAL

(propranolol HCl)
WYETH

10 mg

20 mg

40 mg

60 mg

80 mg

INDERAL LA

(propranolol HCl)
WYETH

60 mg

80 mg

120 mg

160 mg

Long-Acting Capsules

INDERIDE

(propranolol HCl/
hydrochlorothiazide)
WYETH

40 mg / 25 mg

80 mg / 25 mg

INDOCIN

(indomethacin)
MERCK & CO., INC.

25 mg

50 mg

INSPRA

(eplerenone)
PFIZER

25 mg

50 mg

INVIRASE

(saquinavir mesylate)
ROCHE

200 mg

ISMO

(isosorbide mononitrate)
ESP PHARMA

20 mg

KADIAN

(morphine sulfate)
ALPHARMA

20 mg

30 mg

50 mg

60 mg

100 mg

Sustained-Release Capsules

KALETRA

(lopinavir/ritonavir)
ABBOTT

133.3 mg/33.3 mg

KEPPRA

(levetiracetam)
UCB PHARMA, INC.

250 mg

500 mg

750 mg

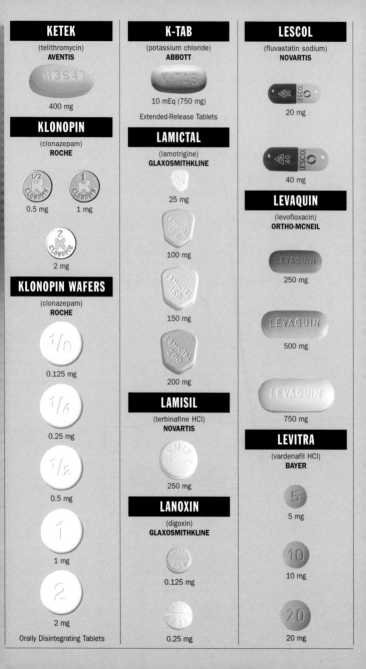

KETEK
(telithromycin)
AVENTIS

400 mg

KLONOPIN
(clonazepam)
ROCHE

0.5 mg   1 mg

2 mg

KLONOPIN WAFERS
(clonazepam)
ROCHE

0.125 mg

0.25 mg

0.5 mg

1 mg

2 mg

Orally Disintegrating Tablets

K-TAB
(potassium chloride)
ABBOTT

10 mEq (750 mg)

Extended-Release Tablets

LAMICTAL
(lamotrigine)
GLAXOSMITHKLINE

25 mg

100 mg

150 mg

200 mg

LAMISIL
(terbinafine HCl)
NOVARTIS

250 mg

LANOXIN
(digoxin)
GLAXOSMITHKLINE

0.125 mg

0.25 mg

LESCOL
(fluvastatin sodium)
NOVARTIS

20 mg

40 mg

LEVAQUIN
(levofloxacin)
ORTHO-MCNEIL

250 mg

500 mg

750 mg

LEVITRA
(vardenafil HCl)
BAYER

5 mg

10 mg

20 mg

LEVOTHROID

(levothyroxine sodium)
FOREST PHARMACEUTICALS

25 mcg	50 mcg
75 mcg	88 mcg
100 mcg	112 mcg
125 mcg	137 mcg
150 mcg	175 mcg
200 mcg	300 mcg

LEVOXYL

(levothyroxine sodium)
KING PHARMACEUTICALS

25 mcg	50 mcg
75 mcg	88 mcg
100 mcg	112 mcg
125 mcg	137 mcg
150 mcg	175 mcg
200 mcg	300 mcg

LEVSIN SL

(hyoscyamine sulfate)
SCHWARZ PHARMA

0.125 mg

LEXAPRO

(escitalopram oxalate)
FOREST PHARMACEUTICALS

5 mg	10 mg
20 mg	

LEXIVA

(fosamprenavir calcium)
GLAXOSMITHKLINE

700 mg

LEXXEL

(enalapril maleate/
felodipine ER)
ASTRAZENECA LP

5 mg/2.5 mg	5 mg/5 mg

LIPITOR

(atorvastatin calcium)
PARKE-DAVIS

10 mg	20 mg
40 mg	
80 mg	

LODINE

(etodolac)
WYETH

200 mg

300 mg

400 mg

500 mg

LOPRESSOR

(metoprolol tartrate)
NOVARTIS

50 mg

100 mg

LOPRESSOR HCT

(metoprolol tartrate/
hydrochorothazide)
NOVARTIS

50 mg/25 mg

100 mg/25 mg

100 mg/50 mg

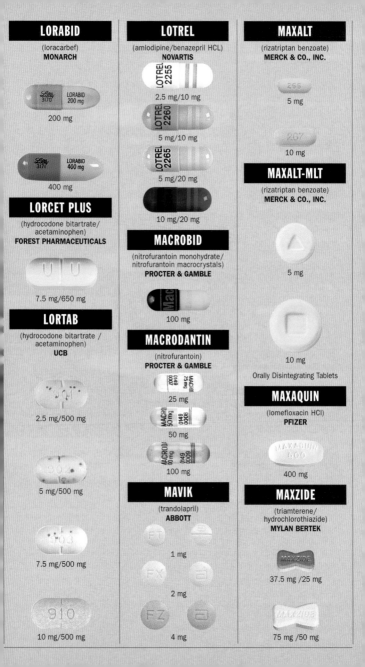

LORABID

(loracarbef)
MONARCH

200 mg

400 mg

LORCET PLUS

(hydrocodone bitartrate/
acetaminophen)
FOREST PHARMACEUTICALS

7.5/650 mg

LORTAB

(hydrocodone bitartrate /
acetaminophen)
UCB

2.5/500 mg

5 mg/500 mg

7.5/500 mg

10 mg/500 mg

LOTREL

(amlodipine/benazepril HCL)
NOVARTIS

2.5 mg/10 mg

5 mg/10 mg

5 mg/20 mg

10 mg/20 mg

MACROBID

(nitrofurantoin monohydrate/
nitrofurantoin macrocrystals)
PROCTER & GAMBLE

100 mg

MACRODANTIN

(nitrofurantoin)
PROCTER & GAMBLE

25 mg

50 mg

100 mg

MAVIK

(trandolapril)
ABBOTT

1 mg

2 mg

4 mg

MAXALT

(rizatriptan benzoate)
MERCK & CO., INC.

5 mg

10 mg

MAXALT-MLT

(rizatriptan benzoate)
MERCK & CO., INC.

5 mg

10 mg

Orally Disintegrating Tablets

MAXAQUIN

(lomefloxacin HCl)
PFIZER

400 mg

MAXZIDE

(triamterene/
hydrochlorothiazide)
MYLAN BERTEK

37.5 mg /25 mg

75 mg /50 mg

Recurrent Genital Herpes Prevention
The usual dose is 250 milligrams twice a day for up to 1 year. Famvir therapy to prevent genital herpes has not been tested for periods exceeding 1 year.

Recurrent Oral or Genital Herpes in HIV-infected Individuals
The usual dose is 500 milligrams twice a day for 7 days. Smaller doses are prescribed for people with damaged kidneys.

CHILDREN

Safety and effectiveness in children under the age of 18 have not been established.

Overdosage
Any medication taken in excess can have serious consequences. If you suspect an overdose, seek medical attention immediately.

Felbamate *See Felbatol, below.*

FELBATOL
Pronounced: FELL-ba-tohl
Generic name: Felbamate

Why is this drug prescribed?
Felbatol, a relatively new epilepsy medication, is used alone or with other drugs to treat partial seizures with or without generalization (seizures in which consciousness may be retained or lost). It is also used with other medications to treat seizures associated with Lennox-Gastaut syndrome (a childhood condition characterized by brief loss of awareness and muscle tone).

Felbatol is prescribed only when other medications have failed to control severe cases of epilepsy.

Most important fact about this drug
When taking Felbatol, be alert for signs of a very rare but dangerous side effect called aplastic anemia, in which the red blood cell count declines drastically. Warning signs include weakness, fatigue, and a tendency to easily bruise or bleed.

Felbatol has also been known to cause fatal cases of liver failure. Warning signs of a liver problem include dark urine, loss of appetite, stomach upset, and yellow skin or eyes. Alert the doctor immediately if you develop these symptoms. The sooner Felbatol is discontinued, the better your chances of recovery.

How should you take this medication?

Take this medication exactly as prescribed by your doctor. Felbatol should not be stopped suddenly. This could increase the frequency of your seizures.

If you are taking Felbatol liquid, shake well before using.

■ *If you miss a dose...*
Take the forgotten dose as soon as you remember. If it is almost time for your next dose, skip the one you missed and go back to your regular schedule. Never take a double dose.

■ *Storage instructions...*
Felbatol should be stored in a tightly closed container, at room temperature, away from excessive heat and moisture.

What side effects may occur?

Side effects cannot be anticipated. If any develop or change in intensity, notify your doctor as soon as possible. Only your doctor can determine if it is safe for you to continue taking Felbatol.

■ *Side effects in adults taking Felbatol alone may include:*
Acne, anxiety, constipation, diarrhea, double vision, ear infection, facial swelling, fatigue, headache, inability to fall or stay asleep, indigestion, loss of appetite, menstrual irregularities, nausea, nasal inflammation, rash, upper respiratory infection, urinary tract infection, vomiting, weight decrease

■ *Side effects in adults taking Felbatol with other medication may include:*
Abdominal pain, abnormal stride, abnormal taste, abnormal vision, anxiety, chest pain, constipation, depression, diarrhea, dizziness, double vision, dry mouth, fatigue, fever, headache, inability to fall or stay asleep, indigestion, lack of muscle coordination, loss of appetite, muscle pain, nausea, nervousness, pins and needles, rash, sinus inflammation, sleepiness, sore throat, stupor, tremor, upper respiratory infection, vomiting

■ *Side effects in children taking Felbatol with other medication may include:*
Abnormal stride, abnormal thinking, abnormally small pupils (pinpoint pupils), constipation, coughing, diarrhea, ear infection, fatigue, fever, headache, hiccups, inability to control urination, inability to fall or stay asleep, indigestion, lack of muscle coordination, loss of appetite, mood changes, nausea, nervousness, pain, rash, red or purple spots on skin, sleepiness, sore throat, taste changes, unstable emotions, upper respiratory infection, vomiting, weight decrease

Why should this drug not be prescribed?

If you are sensitive to or have ever had an allergic reaction to Felbatol or similar drugs, or if you have ever had any blood abnormalities or liver problems, do not take this medication. Make sure your doctor is aware of any drug reactions you have experienced.

Special warnings about this medication

Remember to watch for signs of aplastic anemia (see *Most important fact about this drug*). If you have ever had liver problems, be sure to tell your doctor. '

Expect your doctor to monitor your response carefully when you start taking Felbatol and to check your liver function every 1 or 2 weeks.

Possible food and drug interactions when taking this medication

If you are taking Felbatol with certain other drugs, the effects of either could be increased, decreased, or altered. It is especially important to check with your doctor before combining Felbatol with other epilepsy drugs, such as Dilantin, Depakene, Depakote, Tegretol, and phenobarbital.

Special information if you are pregnant or breastfeeding

The effects of Felbatol during pregnancy have not been adequately studied. If you are pregnant or plan to become pregnant, inform your doctor immediately. Felbatol appears in breast milk and could affect a nursing infant. If this medication is essential to your health, your doctor may advise you to discontinue breastfeeding until your treatment is finished.

Recommended dosage

ADULTS 14 YEARS AND OLDER

Whether Felbatol is taken alone or with other antiepileptic drugs, the usual starting dose is 1,200 milligrams per day divided into smaller doses and taken 3 or 4 times daily. Your doctor may gradually increase your daily dose to as much as 3,600 milligrams.

If you are already taking a drug to control your epilepsy, your doctor will reduce its dosage when you add Felbatol.

CHILDREN WITH LENNOX-GASTAUT SYNDROME (2 TO 14 YEARS)

The usual dose is 15 milligrams per 2.2 pounds of body weight per day divided into smaller doses taken 3 or 4 times daily. Your doctor may gradually increase your child's dose to 45 milligrams per 2.2 pounds of body weight per day. The doctor will reduce the amount of any other epilepsy drug your child is taking when starting Felbatol.

Overdosage

Any medication taken in excess can have serious consequences. If you suspect an overdose, seek medical treatment immediately.

■ *Symptoms of Felbatol overdose may include:*
Mild stomach upset, unusually fast heartbeat

FELDENE
Pronounced: FELL-deen
Generic name: Piroxicam

Why is this drug prescribed?
Feldene, a nonsteroidal anti-inflammatory drug, is used to relieve the inflammation, swelling, stiffness, and joint pain associated with rheumatoid arthritis and osteoarthritis (the most common form of arthritis). It is prescribed both for sudden flare-ups and for long-term treatment.

Most important fact about this drug
In a few patients on long-term therapy, Feldene can cause stomach ulcers and bleeding. Warning signs include severe abdominal or stomach cramps, pain or burning in the stomach, and black, tarry stools. Inform your doctor immediately if you develop any of these symptoms.

How should you take this medication?
To avoid digestive side effects, take Feldene with food or an antacid, and with a full glass of water. Never take it on an empty stomach.

Take this medication exactly as prescribed by your doctor. Avoid alcohol and aspirin while taking this drug.

■ *If you miss a dose...*
If you forget to take a dose, take it as soon as you remember. If it is almost time for your next dose, skip the one you missed and go back to your regular schedule. Never take 2 doses at the same time.

■ *Storage instructions...*
Store at room temperature. Protect from light and heat.

What side effects may occur?
Side effects cannot be anticipated. If any develop or change in intensity, inform your doctor as soon as possible. Only your doctor can determine if it is safe for you to continue taking Feldene.

■ *Side effects may include:*
Abdominal pain or discomfort, anemia, constipation, diarrhea, dizziness, fluid retention, gas, general feeling of ill health, headache, heartburn, itching, kidney problems, loss of appetite, nausea, rash, ringing in ears, sleepiness, stomach ulcers or bleeding, stomach upset, vertigo, vomiting

This side effects list is not complete. If you have any questions about side effects, you should consult your doctor. Report any new or continuing symptoms to your doctor right away.

Why should this drug not be prescribed?

If you are sensitive to or have ever had an allergic reaction to Feldene, aspirin, or similar drugs, or if you have had asthma attacks caused by aspirin or other drugs of this type, you should not take this medication. If you develop breathing difficulties or allergic symptoms after taking Feldene, seek emergency treatment immediately.

Special warnings about this medication

The chances that Feldene will cause a stomach ulcer or bleeding are dramatically higher if you've had such problems previously. Severe stomach reactions are also more likely among older adults, those in poor health, smokers, heavy drinkers, and people taking steroids or blood thinners.

If you have heart disease, high blood pressure, or other conditions that cause fluid retention, use this drug with caution. Feldene can increase water retention.

Feldene has been known to damage the kidneys, and is not recommended for people with advanced kidney disease. Feldene can also cause liver damage. If you develop warning signs of liver dysfunction such as fatigue, itchiness, yellow skin or eyes, a flu-like feeling, and pain in the upper right abdomen, stop taking Feldene and see your doctor immediately.

Drugs such as Feldene may cause eye disturbances in some people. If you develop visual problems, notify your eye doctor.

Possible food and drug interactions when taking this medication

If Feldene is taken with certain other drugs, the effects of either could be increased, decreased, or altered. It is especially important to check with your doctor before combining Feldene with the following:

Anticoagulants (blood thinners such as Coumadin)
Aspirin
Blood pressure medications known as ACE inhibitors, including
    Accupril, Altace, Mavik, Prinivil, and Zestril
Furosemide (Lasix)
Lithium (Lithobid, Lithonate)
Methotrexate (Rheumatrex)
Thiazide-type water pills such as HydroDIURIL

Special information if you are pregnant or breastfeeding

Feldene is not recommended for use in nursing mothers or pregnant women. If you are pregnant or plan to become pregnant, inform your doctor immediately.

Recommended dosage

ADULTS

Rheumatoid Arthritis and Osteoarthritis
The usual dose is 20 milligrams a day in one dose. Your doctor may want you to divide this dose into smaller ones. You will not feel Feldene's full effects for 7 to 12 days, although some relief of symptoms will start to occur soon after you take the medication.

CHILDREN

The safety and effectiveness of Feldene have not been established in children.

Overdosage

Any medication taken in excess can have serious consequences. If you suspect an overdose, seek medical attention immediately.

■ *Symptoms of Feldene overdose may include:*
Drowsiness, nausea, stomach pain, vomiting

Felodipine See Plendil, page 1110.

femhrt See Activella and femhrt, page 26.

FEMRING
Pronounced: FEM-ring
Generic name: Estradiol acetate

Why is this drug prescribed?

Femring is an estrogen replacement system used to relieve moderate to severe hot flashes that occur during menopause. Hot flashes are marked by feelings of warmth in the face, neck, and chest or sudden intense episodes of heat and sweating.

Femring also provides relief for the vaginal dryness and irritation that can accompany menopause. However, when vaginal symptoms occur without hot flashes, your doctor will most likely prescribe a treatment other than Femring.

Most important fact about this drug

Estrogens increase the risk of cancer in the lining of the uterus, called the endometrium. Because estrogen replacement therapy is not advisable if you are in any danger of developing cancer, your doctor should take a complete medical and family history, and perform a complete physical exam, before prescribing Femring. It is important to have regular checkups (at least once a year) and to report any unusual vaginal bleeding to your doctor immediately.

Femring and other estrogen drugs, with or without progesterone, should not be used to prevent heart disease. Recent studies have confirmed an increased rate of heart attack, stroke, and dangerous blood clots among women taking estrogen or estrogen combinations for 5 years. Blood clots can lead to phlebitis, stroke, heart attack, a loss of blood supply to the lungs, a blockage in the blood vessels leading to the eye, and other serious disorders.

How should you take this medication?
Each Femring is left in place for 3 months. Press the Femring into an oval or a figure 8 and insert it as deeply as possible into the upper third of the vagina. The exact position is unimportant as long as you don't feel the ring. If Femring causes discomfort, it is probably not far enough inside. There is no danger of pushing the ring too far up in the vagina, or of it getting lost.

If the ring slips down into the lower part of the vagina, push it back up with your finger. If it falls out, rinse it in warm water and reinsert it. When replacing the ring, simply hook a finger through it and pull it out.

Femring should not interfere with sexual intercourse. It can also be left in place if you need to use medication for a vaginal infection.

■ *If you miss a dose...*
   If the ring is not replaced after 90 days, the dose of estrogen will gradually decline and your symptoms are likely to return.
■ *Storage instructions...*
   Store at room temperature.

What side effects may occur?
Side effects cannot be anticipated. If any develop or change in intensity, tell your doctor as soon as possible. Only your doctor can determine if it is safe to continue using Femring.

■ *Side effects may include:*
   Abdominal cramps, back pain, bloating, breast tenderness, hair loss, headache, high blood pressure, high blood sugar, irregular vaginal bleeding or spotting, liver problems, nausea and vomiting, uterine pain (due to enlargement of benign tumors known as fibroids), vaginal yeast infections, water retention

Why should this drug not be prescribed?
You should not use Femring if you have ever had breast cancer or another cancer stimulated by estrogen. Also, do not use Femring if you have ever had blot clots, or if you've had a stroke or heart attack in the past year.

Do not use Femring if you have unexplained vaginal bleeding. You must also avoid it if you are pregnant.

You will not be able to use Femring if it causes an allergic reaction.

Special warnings about this medication

If Femring does not stay in place and comes out often, tell your doctor. Femring may not be right for you.

Estrogen replacement therapy increases the risk of developing cancer of the lining of the uterus. The risk increases with longer use and higher doses. Therefore, you should use Femring for as short a time and at as low a dose as is necessary to relieve your symptoms. Report any unusual bleeding to your doctor immediately.

Using estrogen may also increase your chances of breast cancer, ovarian cancer, heart attack, stroke, blood clots, and gallbladder disease.

Use estrogen with caution if you have severely low blood levels of calcium (hypocalcemia).

Your doctor may also prescribe a drug containing the hormone progesterone while you are using Femring. Combining estrogen and progesterone reduces the risk of endometrial cancer caused by estrogen alone. This combination is not recommended for women who have had a hysterectomy (removal of the uterus), since they are not at risk for endometrial cancer. Combining estrogen and progesterone could increase their risk of breast cancer, raise cholesterol levels, and cause blood sugar problems.

Tell your doctor if you've ever had liver problems, high cholesterol, high blood pressure, thyroid problems, or vision problems. Using estrogen could make these conditions worse.

Estrogens can cause water retention. If you have a condition that could be affected by this—such as heart or kidney problems—your doctor will monitor you closely.

Using estrogen could worsen certain conditions, including endometriosis, asthma, diabetes, epilepsy, migraine, or the genetic disorder porphyria. Be sure your doctor is aware of any medical problems you have.

While using Femring, contact your doctor right away if you develop any of the following:

Abdominal cramps or swelling
Abnormal vaginal bleeding
Breast lumps
Dizziness and fainting
Pains in your chest or legs
Problems with speech
Severe headache or vomiting
Shortness of breath
Vision changes
Yellowing of the skin or whites of the eyes

Let your doctor know if you're going to have surgery or will be on bed rest; you may need to stop taking estrogens.

Possible food and drug interactions when taking this medication
If you use Femring while taking certain other drugs, the effects of either could be increased, decreased, or altered. It is especially important to check with your doctor before using Femring with any of the following:

Carbamazepine (Tegretol)
Clarithromycin (Biaxin)
Erythromycin (E-Mycin, Erytab, Erythrocin, and others)
Itraconazole (Sporanox)
Ketoconazole (Nizoral)
Phenobarbital
Rifampin (Rifadin, Rifamate, Rimactane)
Ritonavir (Norvir)
St. John's wort

Also, drinking large amounts of grapefruit juice could alter the effects of Femring.

Special information if you are pregnant or breastfeeding
Femring should not be used during pregnancy. Notify your doctor immediately if you are pregnant or plan to become pregnant.

The estrogens in Femring can show up in breast milk. Because estrogens may decrease the quantity and quality of breast milk, your doctor may advise you not to breastfeed while using Femring.

Recommended dosage
There are two doses of Femring available: 0.05 milligram a day and 0.10 milligram a day. Each ring should remain in the vagina for 3 months.

Femring should only be used as long as medically necessary. Your doctor will examine you periodically and recommend when to end treatment.

Overdosage
It is difficult to overdose on Femring because of how it is administered. If you suspect an overdose, seek emergency treatment immediately.

■ *Symptoms of estrogen overdose may include:*
Nausea, vomiting, withdrawal bleeding

Fenofibrate See Tricor, page 1482.

Fentanyl See Duragesic, page 480.

Fexofenadine See Allegra, page 72.

FINACEA

Pronounced: Fin-AY-shuh
Generic name: Azelaic acid

Why is this drug prescribed?

Finacea is an ointment used to treat mild to moderate rosacea (a skin condition marked by red eruptions, usually on the cheeks and nose). In advanced cases—and usually only in men—the nose becomes red and bulbous. Doctors aren't sure what causes rosacea, but the condition may be aggravated by stress, infection, vitamin deficiencies, and hormonal problems.

Most important fact about this drug

You should keep using Finacea regularly, even if you see no immediate improvement. It may take a few weeks before you see results.

How should you take this medication?

Use Finacea once in the morning and again in the evening. Wash the areas to be treated with very mild soap or a soapless cleansing lotion and pat dry with a soft towel. Apply a thin film of the medication and gently but thoroughly massage it into the skin. Wash your hands afterwards. You can apply makeup after the medication has dried.

Do not put bandages or dressings over the treated areas. Avoid getting the medication into the eyes, mouth, or nose. If any of it does get into your eyes, wash it out with large amounts of water. Call your doctor if your eyes remain irritated.

Be sure to avoid things that make your face turn red or flushed. Typical offenders include hot or spicy foods, hot drinks such as tea or coffee, and alcohol. You should also avoid using cleansers and other facial products that contain alcohol, astringents, abrasive ingredients, or peeling agents.

■ *If you miss a dose...*
  Apply it as soon as you remember. If it is almost time for the next application, skip the one you missed and go back to your regular schedule.
■ *Storage instructions...*
  Store at room temperature.

What side effects may occur?

Side effects cannot be anticipated. Skin irritations—burning, stinging, and itchy spots—are most likely to occur during the first few weeks of treatment. If any side effects develop or change in intensity, inform your doctor as soon as possible. Only your doctor can determine if it is safe for you to continue using this medication.

■ *Side effects may include:*
  Burning, itching, itchy spots, scaling or dry skin, stinging, tingling

Why should this drug not be prescribed?

Do not use Finacea if it causes an allergic reaction or if you're allergic to propylene glycol (an additive in many facial products).

Special warnings about this medication

This medicine may cause some itching, burning, or stinging when you first begin treatment. You can expect this to stop as treatment continues. If it doesn't, you should check with your doctor. You may have to cut back to a single application daily, or even temporarily stop using this medication.

This medicine has been known to occasionally have a bleaching effect on the skin. Report any abnormal changes in skin color to your doctor.

Possible food and drug interactions when taking this medication

No interactions have been reported.

Special information if you are pregnant or breastfeeding

The effects of this medication during pregnancy and breastfeeding have not been adequately studied. If you are pregnant or plan to become pregnant, notify your doctor immediately. Small amounts of the drug could appear in breast milk. If you are nursing, use this medication with caution.

Recommended dosage

The usual dose of Finacea is a thin film applied twice a day, once in the morning and again in the evening.

Overdosage

An overdose is unlikely. However, if your skin becomes severely irritated, you should stop applying the medication and call your doctor.

Finasteride for baldness See Propecia, page 1174.

Finasteride for prostate problems See Proscar, page 1178.

Finevin See Azelex, page 179.

FIORICET

Pronounced: fee-OAR-i-set
Generic ingredients: Butalbital, Acetaminophen, Caffeine
Other brand names: Anolor 300, Esgic, Esgic-Plus

Why is this drug prescribed?

Fioricet, a strong, non-narcotic pain reliever and relaxant, is prescribed for the relief of tension headache symptoms caused by muscle contractions in the head, neck, and shoulder area. It combines a sedative barbiturate (butalbital), a non-aspirin pain reliever (acetaminophen), and caffeine.

Most important fact about this drug

Mental and physical dependence can occur with the use of barbiturates such as butalbital when these drugs are taken in higher than recommended doses over long periods of time.

How should you take this medication?

Take Fioricet exactly as prescribed. Do not increase the amount you take without your doctor's approval.

- *If you miss a dose...*
  Take it as soon as you remember. If it is almost time for your next dose, skip the one you missed and go back to your regular schedule. Never take 2 doses at the same time.
- *Storage instructions...*
  Store at room temperature in a tight, light-resistant container.

What side effects may occur?

Side effects cannot be anticipated. If any develop or change in intensity, inform your doctor as soon as possible. Only your doctor can determine if it is safe for you to continue taking Fioricet.

- *Side effects may include:*
  Abdominal pain, dizziness, drowsiness, intoxicated feeling, lightheadedness, nausea, sedation, shortness of breath, vomiting

Why should this drug not be prescribed?

If you are sensitive to or have ever had an allergic reaction to barbiturates, acetaminophen, or caffeine, you should not take this medication. Make sure that your doctor is aware of any drug reactions that you have experienced.

Unless you are directed to do so by your doctor, do not take this medication if you have porphyria (an inherited metabolic disorder affecting the liver or bone marrow).

Special warnings about this medication

Fioricet may cause you to become drowsy or less alert; therefore, driving or operating dangerous machinery or participating in any hazardous activity that requires full mental alertness is not recommended until you know your response to this drug.

If you are being treated for severe depression or have a history of severe depression or drug abuse, consult with your doctor before taking Fioricet.

Use this drug with caution if you are elderly or in a weakened condition, if you have liver or kidney problems, or if you have severe abdominal trouble.

Possible food and drug interactions when taking this medication

Butalbital slows the central nervous system (CNS) and intensifies the effects of alcohol and other CNS depressants. Use of alcohol with this drug may also cause overdose symptoms. Avoid alcoholic beverages while taking Fioricet.

If Fioricet is taken with certain other drugs, the effects of either could be increased, decreased, or altered. It is especially important to check with your doctor before combining Fioricet with the following:

Antihistamines such as Benadryl
Drugs known as monoamine oxidase inhibitors, including the
   antidepressants Nardil and Parnate
Drugs to treat depression such as Elavil
Major tranquilizers such as Haldol and Thorazine
Muscle relaxants such as Flexeril
Narcotic pain relievers such as Darvon
Sleep aids such as Halcion
Tranquilizers such as Xanax and Valium

Special information if you are pregnant or breastfeeding

If you are pregnant or plan to become pregnant, inform your doctor immediately. Fioricet can affect a developing baby. It also appears in breast milk. If this medication is essential to your health, your doctor may advise you to discontinue breastfeeding your baby until your treatment is finished.

Recommended dosage

ADULTS

The usual dose of Fioricet is 1 or 2 tablets taken every 4 hours as needed. Do not exceed a total dose of 6 tablets per day.

The usual dose of Esgic-Plus is 1 tablet every 4 hours as needed. Do not take more than 6 tablets a day.

CHILDREN

The safety and effectiveness of Fioricet have not been established in children under 12 years of age.

OLDER ADULTS

Fioricet may cause excitement, depression, and confusion in older people. Therefore, your doctor will prescribe a dose individualized to suit your needs.

Overdosage

Symptoms of Fioricet overdose can be due to its barbiturate or its acetaminophen component.

■ *Symptoms of barbiturate poisoning may include:*
Coma, confusion, drowsiness, low blood pressure, shock, slow or troubled breathing
Overdose due to the acetaminophen component of Fioricet may cause kidney and liver damage, blood disorders, or coma due to low blood sugar. Massive doses may cause liver failure.
■ *Symptoms of liver damage include:*
Excess perspiration, feeling of bodily discomfort, nausea, vomiting
If you suspect an overdose, seek emergency medical treatment immediately.

FIORINAL

Pronounced: fee-OR-i-nahl
Generic ingredients: Butalbital, Aspirin, Caffeine

Why is this drug prescribed?

Fiorinal, a strong, non-narcotic pain reliever and muscle relaxant, is prescribed for the relief of tension headache symptoms caused by stress or muscle contraction in the head, neck, and shoulder area. It combines a non-narcotic, sedative barbiturate (butalbital) with a pain reliever (aspirin) and a stimulant (caffeine).

Most important fact about this drug

Barbiturates such as butalbital can be habit-forming if you take them over long periods of time.

How should you take this medication?

For best relief, take Fiorinal as soon as a headache begins.
Take the medication with a full glass of water or food to reduce stomach irritation. Do not take this medication if it has a strong odor of vinegar.
Take Fiorinal exactly as prescribed. Do not increase the amount you take without your doctor's approval, or take the drug for longer than prescribed.

■ *If you miss a dose...*
If you take Fiorinal on a regular schedule, take the forgotten dose as soon as you remember. If it is almost time for your next dose, skip the one you missed and go back to your regular schedule. Do not take 2 doses at once.
■ *Storage instructions...*
Store at room temperature. Keep the container tightly closed.

What side effects may occur?

Side effects cannot be anticipated. If any develop or change in intensity, inform your doctor as soon as possible. Only your doctor can determine if it is safe for you to continue taking Fiorinal.

■ *Side effects may include:*
Dizziness, drowsiness

Why should this drug not be prescribed?

If you are sensitive to or have ever had an allergic reaction to barbiturates, aspirin, caffeine, or other sedatives and pain relievers, you should not take this medication. The aspirin in Fiorinal, in particular, can cause a severe reaction in someone allergic to it. Make sure your doctor is aware of any drug reactions you have experienced.

Unless you are directed to do so by your doctor, do not take this medication if you have porphyria (an inherited metabolic disorder affecting the liver or bone marrow).

Because aspirin, when given to children and teenagers suffering from flu or chickenpox, can cause a dangerous neurological disease called Reye's syndrome, do not use Fiorinal under these circumstances.

Fiorinal contains aspirin. If you have a stomach (peptic) ulcer or a disorder affecting the blood clotting process, you should not take Fiorinal. Aspirin may irritate the stomach lining and may cause bleeding.

Special warnings about this medication

Fiorinal may make you drowsy or less alert; therefore, you should not drive or operate dangerous machinery or participate in any hazardous activity that requires full mental alertness until you know your response to this drug.

Taking more of this drug than your doctor has prescribed may cause dependence and symptoms of overdose.

Be especially careful with Fiorinal if you are an older person or in a weakened condition, if you have any kidney, liver, or intestinal problems or an enlarged prostate gland, or if you have had a head injury. Also be cautious if you have a thyroid problem, blood clotting difficulties, or a urinary disorder.

Possible food and drug interactions when taking this medication

Butalbital decreases the activity of the central nervous system and intensifies the effects of alcohol. Avoid drinking alcohol while you are taking Fiorinal.

If Fiorinal is taken with certain other drugs, the effects of either could be increased, decreased, or altered. It is especially important to check with your doctor before combining Fiorinal with the following:

Acetazolamide (Diamox)
Beta-blocking blood pressure drugs such as Inderal and Tenormin

Blood-thinning drugs such as Coumadin
Drugs known as MAO inhibitors, such as the antidepressants Nardil and Parnate
Insulin
Mercaptopurine (Purinethol)
Methotrexate (Rheumatrex)
Narcotic pain relievers such as Darvon and Percocet
Nonsteroidal anti-inflammatory drugs such as Naprosyn, Motrin
Oral contraceptives
Oral diabetes drugs such as Micronase
Probenecid (Benemid)
Sleep aids such as Halcion and Nembutal
Steroid medications such as prednisone
Sulfinpyrazone (Anturane)
Theophylline (Theo-Dur, others)
Tranquilizers such as Librium, Valium, and Xanax
Valproic acid (Depakene, Depakote)

Special information if you are pregnant or breastfeeding

The effects of Fiorinal during pregnancy have not been adequately studied. If you are pregnant or plan to become pregnant, inform your doctor immediately. If you take aspirin late in your pregnancy, it could cause bleeding in you or your baby, or could delay the baby's birth. Aspirin, butalbital, and caffeine appear in breast milk. If this medication is essential to your health, your doctor may advise you to discontinue breastfeeding until your treatment with this medication is finished.

Recommended dosage

ADULTS

The usual dose of Fiorinal is 1 or 2 tablets or capsules taken every 4 hours. You should not take more than 6 tablets or capsules in a day.

CHILDREN

The safety and effectiveness of Fiorinal have not been established in children.

Overdosage

Any medication taken in excess can have serious consequences. If you suspect an overdose, seek medical attention immediately.

■ *Symptoms of an overdose of Fiorinal are attributed mainly to its barbiturate component. These symptoms may include:* Coma, confusion, drowsiness, low blood pressure, shock, slow or troubled breathing

■ *Symptoms attributed to the aspirin and caffeine components of Fiorinal may include:*
Abdominal pain, deep, rapid breathing, delirium, high fever, inability to fall or stay asleep, rapid or irregular heartbeat, restlessness, ringing in the ears, seizures, tremor, vomiting

FIORINAL WITH CODEINE

Pronounced: fee-OR-i-nahl with KO-deen
Generic ingredients: Butalbital, Codeine phosphate, Aspirin, Caffeine

Why is this drug prescribed?

Fiorinal with Codeine, a strong narcotic pain reliever and muscle relaxant, is prescribed for the relief of tension headache caused by stress and muscle contraction in the head, neck, and shoulder area. It combines a sedative barbiturate (butalbital), a narcotic pain reliever and cough suppressant (codeine), a non-narcotic pain and fever reliever (aspirin), and a stimulant (caffeine).

Most important fact about this drug

Barbiturates such as butalbital and narcotics such as codeine can be habit-forming when taken in higher than recommended doses over long periods of time.

How should you take this medication?

Take Fiorinal with Codeine with a full glass of water or food to reduce stomach irritation. Do not take this medication if it has a strong odor of vinegar.

Take Fiorinal with Codeine exactly as prescribed. Do not increase the amount you take without your doctor's approval.

Do not take it more frequently than your doctor has prescribed.

■ *If you miss a dose...*
If you take the drug on a regular schedule, take the forgotten dose as soon as you remember. If it is almost time for your next dose, skip the one you missed and go back to your regular schedule. Do not take 2 doses at once.

■ *Storage instructions...*
Store at room temperature. Keep the container tightly closed.

What side effects may occur?

Side effects cannot be anticipated. If any develop or change in intensity, inform your doctor as soon as possible. Only your doctor can determine if it is safe for you to continue taking Fiorinal with Codeine.

- *Side effects may include:*
Abdominal pain, dizziness, drowsiness, nausea
- *Additional side effects, which can be caused by this drug's components, may include:*
Anemia, blocked air passages, hepatitis, high blood sugar, internal bleeding, intoxicated feeling, irritability, kidney damage, lack of clotting, light-headedness, peptic ulcer, stomach upset, tremors

Why should this drug not be prescribed?

If you are sensitive to or have ever had an allergic reaction to butalbital, codeine, aspirin, caffeine, or other pain relievers, you should not take this medication. Make sure your doctor is aware of any drug reactions you have experienced.

Unless you are directed to do so by your doctor, do not take this medication if you have: a tendency to bleed too much, severe vitamin K deficiency, severe liver damage, nasal polyps (growths or nodules), asthma due to aspirin or other nonsteroidal anti-inflammatory drugs such as Motrin, swelling due to fluid retention, peptic ulcer, or porphyria (an inherited metabolic disorder affecting the liver and bone marrow).

Because aspirin, when given to children and teenagers with chickenpox or flu, can cause a dangerous neurological disease called Reye's syndrome, do not use Fiorinal with Codeine under these circumstances.

Special warnings about this medication

Fiorinal with Codeine may make you drowsy or less alert; therefore, you should not drive or operate dangerous machinery or participate in any hazardous activity that requires full mental alertness until you know how this drug affects you.

Codeine may cause unusually slow or troubled breathing and may increase the pressure caused by fluid surrounding the brain and spinal cord in people with head injury. Codeine also affects brain and spinal cord function and makes it hard for a doctor to see how people with head injuries are doing.

If you have chronic (long-lasting or frequently recurring) tension headaches and your prescribed dose of Fiorinal with Codeine does not relieve the pain, consult with your doctor. Taking more of this drug than your doctor has prescribed may cause dependence and symptoms of overdose.

Aspirin can cause internal bleeding in people with ulcers or bleeding disorders.

Codeine can hide signs of severe abdominal problems.

If you have ever developed dependence on a drug, consult with your doctor before taking Fiorinal with Codeine.

If you are being treated for a kidney, liver, or blood clotting disorder, consult with your doctor before taking Fiorinal with Codeine.

If you are older or in a weakened condition, be very careful taking Fiorinal with Codeine. You should also be careful if you have Addison's disease (an adrenal gland disorder), if you have difficulty urinating, if your prostate gland is enlarged, or if your thyroid gland is not working well.

Possible food and drug interactions when taking this medication

Fiorinal with Codeine reduces the activity of the central nervous system and intensifies the effects of alcohol. Use of alcohol with this drug may also cause overdose symptoms. Therefore, use of alcohol should be avoided.

If Fiorinal with Codeine is taken with certain other drugs, the effects of either could be increased, decreased, or altered. It is especially important to check with your doctor before combining Fiorinal with Codeine with the following:

Acetazolamide (Diamox)
Antidepressant drugs such as Elavil, Nardil, and Parnate
Antigout medications such as Benemid and Anturane
Antihistamines such as Benadryl
Beta-blocking blood pressure drugs such as Inderal and Tenormin
Blood-thinning drugs such as Coumadin
Divalproex (Depakote)
Insulin
6-Mercaptopurine (Purinethol)
Methotrexate (Rheumatrex)
Narcotic pain relievers such as Darvon and Vicodin
Nonsteroidal anti-inflammatory drugs such as Motrin and Indocin
Oral contraceptives
Oral diabetes drugs such as Micronase
Sleep aids such as Nembutal and Halcion
Steroid drugs such as prednisone
Theophylline (Theo-Dur, others)
Tranquilizers such as Librium, Xanax, and Valium
Valproic acid (Depakene)

Special information if you are pregnant or breastfeeding

The effects of Fiorinal with Codeine during pregnancy have not been adequately studied. If you are pregnant or plan to become pregnant, inform your doctor immediately. Butalbital, aspirin, caffeine, and codeine appear in breast milk. If this medication is essential to your health, your doctor may advise you to discontinue breastfeeding until your treatment with this medication is finished.

Recommended dosage

ADULTS

The usual dose of Fiorinal with Codeine is 1 or 2 capsules taken every 4 hours. Do not take more than 6 capsules per day.

CHILDREN

The safety and effectiveness of butalbital have not been established in children under 12 years of age.

Overdosage

Symptoms of an overdose of Fiorinal with Codeine are mainly attributed to its barbiturate and codeine ingredients.

- *Symptoms attributed to the barbiturate ingredient of Fiorinal with Codeine may include:*
  Coma, confusion, dizziness, drowsiness, low blood pressure, shock, slow or troubled breathing
- *Symptoms attributed to the codeine ingredient of Fiorinal with Codeine may include:*
  Convulsions, loss of consciousness, pinpoint pupils, troubled and slowed breathing
- *Symptoms attributed to the aspirin ingredient of Fiorinal with Codeine may include:*
  Abdominal pain, deep, rapid breathing, delirium, high fever, restlessness, ringing in the ears, seizures, vomiting

Though caffeine poisoning occurs only at very high doses, it can cause delirium, insomnia, irregular heartbeat, rapid heartbeat, restlessness, and tremor.

If you suspect an overdose of Fiorinal with Codeine, seek emergency medical treatment immediately.

FLAGYL

Pronounced: FLAJ-ill
Generic name: Metronidazole

Why is this drug prescribed?

Flagyl is an antibacterial drug prescribed for certain vaginal and urinary tract infections in men and women; amebic dysentery and liver abscess; and infections of the abdomen, skin, bones and joints, brain, lungs, and heart caused by certain bacteria.

Most important fact about this drug

Do not drink alcoholic beverages while taking Flagyl. The combination can cause abdominal cramps, nausea, vomiting, headaches, and flushing. It can also change the taste of the alcoholic beverage. When you have stopped taking Flagyl, wait at least 72 hours (3 days) before consuming any alcohol. Also avoid over-the-counter medications containing alcohol, such as certain cough and cold products.

How should you take this medication?

Flagyl works best when there is a constant amount in the blood. Take your doses at evenly spaced intervals, day and night, and try to avoid missing any.

If you are being treated for the sexually transmitted genital infection called trichomoniasis, your doctor may want to treat your partner at the same time, even if there are no symptoms. Try to avoid sexual intercourse until the infection is cured. If you do have sex, use a condom.

Flagyl can be taken with or without food. It may cause dry mouth. Hard candy, chewing gum, or bits of ice can help to relieve the problem.

■ *If you miss a dose...*
Take it as soon as you remember. If it is almost time for your next dose skip the one you missed and go back to your regular schedule. Do not take 2 doses at once.

■ *Storage instructions...*
Store at room temperature. Protect from light.

What side effects may occur?

Side effects cannot be anticipated. If any develop or change in intensity, tell your doctor immediately. Only your doctor can determine whether it is safe for you to continue taking Flagyl.

Two serious side effects that have occurred with Flagyl are seizures and numbness or tingling in the arms, legs, hands, and feet. If you experience either of these symptoms, stop taking the medication and call your doctor immediately.

■ *Side effects may include:*
Abdominal cramps, constipation, diarrhea, headache, loss of appetite, nausea, upset stomach, vomiting

Why should this drug not be prescribed?

Flagyl should not be used during the first 3 months of pregnancy to treat vaginal infections. Do not take Flagyl if you have ever had an allergic reaction to or are sensitive to metronidazole or similar drugs. Tell your doctor about any drug reactions you have experienced.

Special warnings about this medication

If you experience seizures or numbness or tingling in your arms, legs, hands, or feet, remember that you should stop taking Flagyl and call your doctor immediately.

If you have liver disease, make sure the doctor is aware of it. Flagyl should be used with caution.

Active or undiagnosed yeast infections may appear or worsen when you take Flagyl.

Possible food and drug interactions when taking this medication
Do not drink alcohol while taking Flagyl and for at least 72 hours after your last dose.

If Flagyl is taken with certain other drugs, the effects of either could be increased, decreased, or altered. It is especially important to check with your doctor before combining Flagyl with any of the following:

Blood thinners such as Coumadin
Cholestyramine (Questran)
Cimetidine (Tagamet)
Disulfiram (Antabuse)
Lithium (Eskalith)
Phenobarbital
Phenytoin (Dilantin)

Special information if you are pregnant or breastfeeding
The effects of Flagyl in pregnancy have not been adequately studied. If you are pregnant or plan to become pregnant, notify your doctor. This medication should be used during pregnancy only if it is clearly needed. Flagyl appears in breast milk and could affect a nursing infant. If Flagyl is essential to your health, your doctor may advise you to stop breastfeeding until your treatment is finished.

Recommended dosage

ADULT

Trichomoniasis
One-day treatment: 2 grams of Flagyl, taken as a single dose or divided into 2 doses (1 gram each) taken in the same day.

Seven-day course of treatment: 250 milligrams 3 times daily for 7 consecutive days.

Acute Intestinal Amebiasis (Acute Amebic Dysentery)
The usual dose is 750 milligrams taken by mouth 3 times daily for 5 to 10 days.

Amebic Liver Abscess
The usual dose is 500 milligrams or 750 milligrams taken by mouth 3 times daily for 5 to 10 days.

Anaerobic Bacterial Infections
The usual adult oral dosage is 7.5 milligrams per 2.2 pounds of body weight every 6 hours.

CHILDREN

Amebiasis
The usual dose is 35 to 50 milligrams for each 2.2 pounds of body weight per day, divided into 3 doses taken for 10 days.

The safety and efficacy of Flagyl for any other condition in children have not been established.

OLDER ADULTS

Your doctor will test to see how much medication is in your blood and will adjust your dosage if necessary.

Overdosage

Any medication taken in excess can have serious consequences. If you suspect an overdose, seek medical treatment immediately.

■ *Symptoms of Flagyl overdose may include:*
Lack of muscle coordination, nausea, vomiting

Flavoxate *See Urispas, page 1534.*

Flecainide *See Tambocor, page 1382.*

FLEXERIL

Pronounced: FLEX-eh-rill
Generic name: Cyclobenzaprine hydrochloride

Why is this drug prescribed?

Flexeril is a muscle relaxant prescribed to relieve muscle spasms resulting from injuries such as sprains, strains, or pulls. Combined with rest and physical therapy, Flexeril provides relief of muscular stiffness and pain.

Most important fact about this drug

Flexeril is not a substitute for the physical therapy, rest, or exercise that your doctor orders for proper healing. Although Flexeril relieves the pain of strains and sprains, it is not useful for other types of pain.

How should you take this medication?

Flexeril may be taken with or without food.

Flexeril should be used only for short periods (no more than 3 weeks). Since the type of injury that Flexeril treats should improve in a few weeks, there is no reason to use it for a longer period.

Flexeril may cause dry mouth. Sucking a hard candy, chewing gum, or melting ice chips in your mouth can provide temporary relief.

■ *If you miss a dose...*
Take it as soon as you remember, if it is within an hour or so of your scheduled time. If you do not remember until later, skip the missed dose and go back to your regular schedule. Do not take 2 doses at once.

■ *Storage instructions...*
Store away from heat, light, and moisture.

What side effects may occur?

Side effects cannot be anticipated. If any develop or change in intensity, inform your doctor as soon as possible. Only your doctor can determine if it is safe for you to continue taking Flexeril.

■ *Side effects may include:*
Dizziness, drowsiness, dry mouth

Why should this drug not be prescribed?

You should not take this drug if you are taking an antidepressant drug known as an MAO inhibitor (such as Nardil or Parnate) or have taken an MAO inhibitor within the last 2 weeks. Also avoid Flexeril if you have ever had an allergic reaction to it, or if your thyroid gland is overactive.

In addition, you should not take Flexeril if you have recently had a heart attack or if you have congestive heart failure, or suffer from irregular heartbeat.

Special warnings about this medication

Flexeril may cause you to become drowsy or less alert; therefore, you should not drive or operate dangerous machinery or participate in any hazardous activity that requires full mental alertness until you know how this drug affects you.

You should use Flexeril with caution if you have ever been unable to urinate or if you have ever had the eye condition called glaucoma.

Possible food and drug interactions when taking this medication

Serious, potentially fatal reactions may occur if you take Flexeril with an antidepressant drug known as an MAO inhibitor (such as Nardil or Parnate) or if it has been less than 2 weeks since you last took an MAO inhibitor. You should closely follow your doctor's advice regarding discontinuation of MAO inhibitors before taking Flexeril.

Avoid alcoholic beverages while taking Flexeril.

If Flexeril is taken with certain other drugs, the effects of either could be increased, decreased, or altered. It is especially important to check with your doctor before combining Flexeril with the following:

Barbiturates such as phenobarbital
Guanethidine and other high blood pressure drugs

Other drugs that slow the central nervous system, such as Halcion and Xanax

Tramadol (Ultram)

Special information if you are pregnant or breastfeeding

The effects of Flexeril during pregnancy have not been adequately studied. If you are pregnant or plan to become pregnant, inform your doctor immediately. It is not known if Flexeril appears in breast milk. However, cyclobenzaprine is related to tricyclic antidepressants, and some of those drugs do appear in breast milk. If this medication is essential to your health, your doctor may advise you to discontinue breastfeeding your baby until your treatment is finished.

Recommended dosage

ADULTS

The usual dose is 10 milligrams 3 times a day. You should not take more than 60 milligrams a day.

CHILDREN

Safety and effectiveness of Flexeril have not been established for children under the age of 15.

Overdosage

Any medication taken in excess can have serious consequences. If you suspect a Flexeril overdose, seek medical attention immediately.

■ *Symptoms of Flexeril overdose may include:*
Agitation, coma, confusion, congestive heart failure, convulsions, dilated pupils, disturbed concentration, drowsiness, hallucinations, high or low temperature, increased heartbeats, irregular heart rhythms, muscle stiffness, overactive reflexes, severe low blood pressure, stupor, vomiting

High doses also may cause any of the conditions listed in *What side effects may occur?*

FLOMAX

Pronounced: FLOW-maks
Generic name: Tamsulosin hydrochloride

Why is this drug prescribed?

Flomax is used to treat the symptoms of an enlarged prostate—a condition technically known as benign prostatic hyperplasia or BPH. The walnut-sized prostate gland surrounds the urethra (the duct that drains the bladder). If the gland becomes enlarged, it can squeeze the urethra, interfering with the flow of urine. This can cause difficulty in starting urination, a weak flow of urine, and the need to urinate urgently or more frequently. Flomax doesn't shrink the prostate. Instead, it relaxes the muscle around it, freeing the flow of urine and decreasing urinary symptoms.

Most important fact about this drug

Flomax can cause dizziness, especially when you first stand up. Be careful about driving, operating machinery, and performing any other hazardous task until you know how you react to the drug.

How should you take this medication?

Take Flomax once daily, half an hour after the same meal each day. Do not crush, chew, or open the capsule.

■ *If you miss a dose...*
Take it as soon as you remember. If it is almost time for your next dose, skip the one you missed and go back to your regular schedule. Do not take 2 doses at once.

   If you miss several doses in a row, resume treatment with a dose of 1 capsule daily and check with your doctor on how to proceed.

■ *Storage instructions...*
Store at room temperature.

What side effects may occur?

Side effects cannot be anticipated. If any develop or change in intensity, inform your doctor as soon as possible. Only your doctor can determine if it is safe for you to continue taking Flomax.

■ *Side effects may include:*
Abnormal ejaculation, back pain, chest pain, cough, diarrhea, dizziness, headache, infection, nausea, runny nose, sinus problems, sleepiness, sore throat, weakness

Why should this drug not be prescribed?

If Flomax gives you an allergic reaction, you cannot take the drug.

Special warnings about this medication

Remember that, in a few men, Flomax can cause a drop in blood pressure upon first standing up, which in turn can lead to dizziness or fainting. Avoid driving and other hazardous tasks for 12 hours after your first dose or a dosage increase, and be careful to stand up slowly until you're sure the drug won't make you dizzy. If you do become dizzy, sit down until it passes.

   Although the problem is extremely rare (affecting perhaps 1 in

50,000), Flomax has been known to cause priapism—a painful, persistent erection unrelated to sexual activity. If you develop this side effect, call your doctor without delay. The condition can lead to permanent impotence if not treated immediately.

Possible food and drug interactions when taking this medication

If Flomax is taken with certain other drugs, the effects of either could be increased, decreased, or altered. It is especially important to check with your doctor before combining Flomax with any of the following:

Blood pressure drugs classified as alpha-blockers, such as Catapres
Cimetidine (Tagamet)
Warfarin (Coumadin)

Special information if you are pregnant or breastfeeding

Flomax is for use only by men.

Recommended dosage

ADULT MEN

The recommended starting dose of Flomax is 1 capsule (0.4 milligram) daily, half an hour following the same meal each day. Your doctor may increase the dose to 2 capsules (0.8 milligram) once a day if needed.

Overdosage

Any medication taken in excess can have serious consequences. If you suspect an overdose, seek medical treatment immediately.

■ *Symptoms of Flomax overdose may include:*
Dizziness, fainting, headache

Flonase See Fluticasone, page 586.

Flovent See Fluticasone, page 586.

FLOXIN

Pronounced: FLOCKS-in
Generic name: Ofloxacin

Why is this drug prescribed?

Floxin is an antibiotic. Floxin tablets have been used effectively to treat lower respiratory tract infections, including chronic bronchitis and pneumonia, sexually transmitted diseases (except syphilis), pelvic inflammatory disease, and infections of the urinary tract, prostate gland, and skin. Floxin Otic solution is used to treat ear infections.

Most important fact about this drug

Floxin kills a variety of bacteria and is frequently used to treat infections in many parts of the body. However, you should stop taking the drug and notify your doctor immediately at the first sign of a skin rash or any other allergic reaction. Although rare, serious and occasionally fatal allergic reactions have been reported, some after only one dose. Signs of an impending reaction include swelling of the face and throat, shortness of breath, difficulty swallowing, rapid heartbeat, tingling, itching, and hives.

How should you take this medication?

You may take Floxin tablets with or without food. Be sure to drink plenty of fluids while taking the tablets.

Do not take mineral supplements, vitamins with iron or minerals, Videx chewable tablets and pediatric powder, or antacids containing calcium, aluminum, or magnesium within 2 hours of taking Floxin tablets.

To administer Floxin Otic:
1. Wash hands.
2. Clean the outer ear of any discharge. Do not insert any object into the ear canal.
3. Warm the drops by holding the bottle in your hand for one or two minutes.
4. Have the individual receiving the drops lie on his or her side with the affected ear up.
5. Place the prescribed number of drops in the ear.
6. Do not touch the applicator to the ear or your fingers.
7. If a middle ear infection is involved, gently press the flap in front of the ear canal 4 times to help push the drops inward. For an outer ear canal infection, gently pull the ear upward and backward while giving the drops.
8. Keep the ear facing upward for 5 minutes to allow the drops to be absorbed into the ear.

Take Floxin exactly as prescribed. You need to complete the full course of therapy to obtain best results and decrease the risk of a recurrence of the infection.

■ *If you miss a dose...*
Take it as soon as you remember. If it is almost time for your next dose, skip the one you missed and go back to your regular schedule. Never take 2 doses at the same time.

■ *Storage instructions...*
Store at room temperature in a tightly closed container, away from light.

What side effects may occur?

Side effects cannot be anticipated. If any develop or change in intensity, inform your doctor as soon as possible. Only your doctor can determine if it is safe for you to continue taking Floxin.

FLOXIN TABLETS

■ *Side effects may include:*
Diarrhea, difficulty sleeping, dizziness, headache, itching of genital area in women, nausea, vaginal inflammation, vomiting

FLOXIN OTIC SOLUTION

■ *Side effects may include:*
Abnormal or bitter taste, itching

Why should this drug not be prescribed?
Do not take Floxin if you are sensitive to or have ever had an allergic reaction to it or other quinolone antibiotics such as Cipro and Noroxin.

Special warnings about this medication
Floxin tablets, used in high doses for short periods of time, may hide or delay the symptoms of syphilis but are not effective in treating syphilis. If you are taking Floxin for gonorrhea, your doctor will test you for syphilis and then perform a follow-up test after 3 months of treatment.

Convulsions, increased pressure in the head, psychosis, tremors, restlessness, light-headedness, nervousness, confusion, depression, nightmares, insomnia, and hallucinations have occasionally been reported with this type of antibiotic. If you experience any of these symptoms, stop taking the drug and contact your doctor immediately.

Like all antibiotics, Floxin has been known to cause serious inflammation of the bowels. Notify your doctor if you develop diarrhea during or after a course of therapy with this drug.

Floxin can cause a rupture in the muscle tendons in your hand, shoulder, or heel. If you notice any pain and inflammation in a tendon, rest and avoid exercise until you have seen your doctor.

If you are prone to seizures due to kidney disease, a brain disorder, or epilepsy, make sure your doctor knows about it. Floxin tablets should be used with caution under these conditions.

If you have liver or kidney disease, your doctor will watch you closely while you are taking Floxin tablets.

Avoid being in the sun too much; you can develop sun poisoning while you are taking Floxin tablets.

Floxin tablets may make you feel dizzy or light-headed. Be careful driving, operating machinery, or doing any activity that requires full mental alertness until you know how you react to this medication.

Never put Floxin eardrops in the eyes or mouth. When placed in the ear, the drops may cause dizziness if they have not been sufficiently warmed.

Floxin tablets have not been tested in children under 18 years old. Floxin eardrops have not been tested in children under 1 years old.

Possible food and drug interactions when taking this medication
If Floxin is taken with certain other drugs, the effects of either could be increased, decreased, or altered. It is especially important to check with your doctor before combining Floxin with the following:

Antacids containing calcium, magnesium, or aluminum
Blood thinners such as Coumadin
Calcium supplements such as Caltrate
Cimetidine (Tagamet)
Cyclosporine (Sandimmune, Neoral)
Didanosine (Videx)
Insulin
Iron supplements such as Feosol
Multivitamins containing zinc
Nonsteroidal anti-inflammatory drugs such as Motrin and Naprosyn
Oral diabetes drugs such as Diabinese and Micronase
Probenecid (Benemid)
Sucralfate (Carafate)
Theophylline-containing drugs, such as Theo-Dur

Special information if you are pregnant or breastfeeding
The effects of Floxin during pregnancy have not been adequately studied. If you are pregnant or plan to become pregnant, inform your doctor immediately. This medication should not be used during pregnancy unless your doctor has determined that the benefit to you outweighs the risk to the unborn baby. Floxin appears in breast milk and could affect a nursing infant. If this medication is essential to your health, your doctor may advise you to stop breastfeeding until your treatment with Floxin is finished.

Recommended dosage

FLOXIN TABLETS

Worsening of Chronic Bronchitis
The usual dose is 400 milligrams every 12 hours for 10 days, for a total daily dose of 800 milligrams.

Pneumonia
The usual dose is 400 milligrams every 12 hours for 10 days, for a total daily dose of 800 milligrams.

Gonorrhea
The usual dose is 400 milligrams taken once.

Sexually Transmitted Infections of the Cervix or Urethra
The usual dose is 300 milligrams every 12 hours for 7 days, for a total daily dose of 600 milligrams.

Pelvic Inflammatory Disease
The usual dose is 400 milligrams every 12 hours for 10 to 14 days, for a total daily dose of 800 milligrams.

Mild to Moderate Skin Infections
The usual dose is 400 milligrams every 12 hours for 10 days, for a total daily dose of 800 milligrams.

Bladder Infections
The usual dose is 200 milligrams every 12 hours for a total daily dose of 400 milligrams. This dose is taken for 3 days for infections due to E. coli or K. pneumoniae. For infections due to other microbes, it is taken for 7 days.

Complicated Urinary Tract Infections
The usual dose is 200 milligrams every 12 hours for 10 days, for a total daily dose of 400 milligrams.

Prostatitis
The usual dose is 300 milligrams every 12 hours for 6 weeks, for a total daily dose of 600 milligrams.

FLOXIN OTIC SOLUTION

Otitis Externa (Swimmer's Ear)
For adults and children over 13, the usual dose is 10 drops in the affected ear once a day for 7 days. For children from 1 to 12 years of age, the usual dose is 5 warmed drops in the affected ear once a day for 7 days.

Acute Otitis Media (Severe Middle Ear Infection) in Children with Ear Tubes
For children from 1 to 12 years of age, the usual dose is 5 warmed drops in the affected ear 2 times a day for 10 days.

Chronic Otitis Media with Perforated Eardrum and Pus
For adults and children over 12, the usual dose is 10 warmed drops in the affected ear 2 times a day for 14 days.

Overdosage
Any medication used in excess can have serious consequences. If you suspect an overdose, seek medical treatment immediately.

■ Symptoms of Floxin overdose may include:
Disorientation, dizziness, drowsiness, hot and cold flashes, nausea, slurring of speech, swelling and numbness in the face.

Fluconazole See Diflucan, page 440.

Flunisolide See AeroBid, page 49.

Fluocinonide See Lidex, page 761.

Fluorometholone See FML, page 594.

Fluorouracil See Efudex, page 496.

Fluoxetine See Prozac, page 1195.

Flurazepam See Dalmane, page 382.

Flurbiprofen See Ansaid, page 111.

Flutamide See Eulexin, page 544.

FLUTICASONE

Pronounced: flue-TICK-uh-zone
Brand names: Flonase, Flovent, Flovent Diskus,
   Flovent Rotadisk

Why is this drug prescribed?

Flonase nasal spray is a remedy for the stuffy, runny, itchy nose that plagues many allergy sufferers. It can be used either for seasonal attacks of hay fever or for year-round allergic conditions. Flonase is a steroid medication. It works by relieving inflammation within the nasal passages.

The Flovent, Flovent Rotadisk, and Flovent Diskus oral inhalers are used to prevent flare-ups of asthma. (They will not, however, relieve an acute attack.) They sometimes serve as a replacement for the steroid tablets that many people take to control asthma.

Most important fact about this drug

Fluticasone is not an instant cure. It may take a few days for the medication to start working; and you need to keep taking it regularly in order to maintain its benefits. While you are waiting for fluticasone to take effect, neither increase the dose nor stop taking the medication.

How should you take this medication?

Flonase is taken in the nostrils. For best effect, take the prescribed doses at regular intervals. First, blow your nose. Then shake the spray bottle gently, prime the pump 6 times if it hasn't been used during the past week, tilt your head back, press one nostril closed, and insert the tip of the bottle a short way into the other nostril. Spray once, pull the tip of the bottle away from your nose, and inhale deeply through the treated nostril. Repeat with the other nostril. Avoid spraying into your eyes.

Flovent inhalation aerosol is taken orally. Shake the canister before each use. Take a deep breath and exhale. Then, as you begin to inhale, put your lips around the mouthpiece and depress the canister. Rinse your mouth with water after each use of the inhaler. Avoid spraying the contents into your eyes.

Flovent Rotadisk inhalation powder is also taken orally. Assemble the Rotadisk Diskhaler according to package instructions. To use, exhale, then place the Diskhaler mouthpiece between your teeth (without biting down) and close your lips firmly around it. (Be careful to avoid covering the small air holes on either side of the mouthpiece.) Breathe in through your mouth as deeply as you can, then hold your breath while you remove the Diskhaler. Continue to hold your breath as long as you comfortably can, up to a maximum of 10 seconds.

Flovent Diskus is a disposable oral inhaler that contains 60 inhalations. It must be kept dry. Do not wash it or attempt to take it apart. Always activate the inhaler in a level, horizontal position. Do not exhale into it. Do not use a spacer.

■ *If you miss a dose…*
Take it as soon as you remember. If it is almost time for your next dose, skip the one you missed and go back to your regular schedule. Do not take 2 doses at once.

■ *Storage instructions…*
Flonase may be stored at room temperature or in the refrigerator.

Flovent inhalation aerosol may be stored at room temperature away from sunlight, or in the refrigerator.

Flovent Rotadisk inhalation powder should be stored at room temperature in a dry place. Use the Rotadisk blisters within 2 months after opening the foil overwrap or before the expiration date, whichever comes first. Do not puncture the blisters until you are ready to use them in the Diskhaler.

The Flovent Diskus disposable inhaler should be stored at room temperature in a dry place, away from direct heat or sunlight. Once removed from its foil pouch, the device should be discarded after 2 months if not used up (after 6 weeks for the 50-microgram inhaler).

What side effects may occur?
Side effects cannot be anticipated. If any develop or change in intensity, inform your doctor as soon as possible. Only your doctor can determine if it is safe for you to continue taking fluticasone.

■ *Side effects may include:*
Abdominal pain, aches and pains, agitation, aggression, anaphylactic reaction, back problems, bad taste in mouth, brittle bones, bronchitis, bruising, cataracts, congestion, cough, depression, diarrhea, dizziness, dry mouth, dry nose, eye problems, facial changes, fever, flu, headache, hives, hoarseness, indigestion, itching, loss of speech, mouth infection or swelling, nasal congestion, nasal irritation or burning, nasal sores, nausea, nosebleeds, rash, respiratory tract infection, runny nose, shortness of breath, sinus problems, sneezing, sore or irritated throat, stunted growth, swelling of the face and tongue, vomiting, weight gain, wheezing, worsening of asthma

Why should this drug not be prescribed?

If you have ever had an allergic reaction to Flonase or similar steroid inhalants such as Flovent, you should not take this medication.

Flovent is not to be used to treat status asthmaticus or acute asthma attacks.

Under very rare circumstances Flovent Rotadisk may cause an anaphylactic reaction in people with a severe milk protein allergy.

Special warnings about this medication

If your symptoms do not improve after the first few days of fluticasone therapy, check with your doctor. Never take more than the recommended dose. High doses of steroid medications such as fluticasone can cause a condition known as Cushing's syndrome. Warning signs of this problem include weight gain and changes in the appearance of the face.

If you are being switched from an oral steroid tablet to fluticasone, you may experience joint pain, muscle pain, weakness, depression, or fatigue while your body adjusts to the absence of steroid tablets and increases its own production of steroids. You may also experience eye inflammation, eczema, arthritis, and nasal inflammation.

People taking steroid medications run an increased risk of infections such as chickenpox and measles, and when an infection develops, it's more likely to be serious. If you've never had these diseases and have not been vaccinated against them, avoid anyone who may have them. If by chance you're exposed, contact your doctor immediately.

In rare cases, fluticasone can also cause a fungal infection in the nose and throat. Steroid treatment can also make an existing infection worse. Be sure the doctor is aware of any infections you may have, including TB and viral infections of the eye.

Steroid medications can stunt growth. If your child is on fluticasone therapy, the doctor should periodically check height and weight. In rare cases, people using Flovent have developed a serious lung condition marked by worsening asthma, heart problems, and numbness. If you start to notice any of these symptoms, report them to your doctor immediately.

If you develop wheezing and an asthma attack after inhaling any form of Flovent, use an emergency medicine such as an inhaled bronchodilator and call your doctor immediately. Also alert your doctor immediately if emergency medications fail to work as well once you've started Flovent therapy.

In rare cases, inhaled steroids such as Flovent have caused cataracts or increased pressure in the eye (glaucoma). Alert your doctor if you suffer from either problem.

If you have recently had a nasal injury or ulcer, or had surgery on your nose, you should wait until you are fully healed before using Flonase.

Possible food and drug interactions when taking this medication
The risk of developing Cushing's syndrome and other side effects increases when you take other steroid medications while using fluticasone. Prednisone and dexamethasone are examples of oral steroid medications. Certain other asthma inhalers, skin creams, eyedrops, and eardrops also may contain steroids.

Also be sure to check with your doctor before combining fluticasone with ketoconazole (Nizoral) or HIV drugs known as protease inhibitors, including Agenerase, Crixivan, Fortovase, Norvir, and Viracept.

Special information if you are pregnant or breastfeeding
The effects of this drug during pregnancy have not been adequately studied. If you are pregnant or plan to become pregnant, inform your doctor immediately. It is not known whether fluticasone appears in breast milk. If the drug is essential to your health, your doctor may advise you to stop nursing until your treatment is finished.

Recommended dosage

FLONASE

Adults
The usual starting dose is 2 sprays in each nostril once daily. (Some doctors may prescribe 1 spray in each nostril every 12 hours.) Once your symptoms are under control, your doctor may reduce the dose to 1 spray in each nostril once daily.

Some people (12 and over) with seasonal allergies find that it's sufficient to use Flonase only on days when their symptoms flare up. If you use Flonase this way, take no more than 2 sprays per nostril on any given day.

Children
Flonase is not recommended for children under the age of 4. The recommended starting dose is 1 spray in each nostril once a day. If symptoms do not improve in a few days, the dose can be increased to 2 sprays in each nostril once a day, or 1 spray in each nostril twice a day. The dose should be reduced again once symptoms have subsided.

FLOVENT INHALATION AEROSOL

Adults and Children 12 and Older
If you are currently using an inhaled bronchodilator, the recommended starting dose is 88 micrograms twice a day. The maximum dose is 440 micrograms twice a day.

If you are currently using another steroid inhaler, the starting dose ranges from 88 to 220 micrograms twice daily. The maximum dose is 440 micrograms twice a day.

If you are taking oral steroid tablets, the doctor will start you at 880 micrograms of Flovent twice a day. He will slowly decrease your dose of steroid tablets, then lower your dose of Flovent.

Children Under 12

Flovent inhalation aerosol is not recommended.

FLOVENT ROTADISK AND FLOVENT DISKUS

Adults and Children 12 and Older

If you are currently using an inhaled bronchodilator, the recommended starting dose is 100 micrograms twice a day. The maximum dose is 500 micrograms twice a day.

If you are currently using another steroid inhaler, the starting dose ranges from 100 to 250 micrograms twice daily. The maximum dose is 500 micrograms twice a day.

If you are taking oral steroid tablets, the doctor will start you at 1000 micrograms of Flovent twice a day. He will slowly decrease your dose of steroid tablets, then lower your dose of Flovent.

Children 4 to 11 Years Old

For children already taking an inhaled bronchodilator or steroid, the recommended starting dose is 50 micrograms twice daily. The maximum dose is 100 micrograms twice a day.

Children Under 4

Not recommended.

Overdosage

Any medication taken in excess can have serious consequences. If you habitually use too much fluticasone, you run the risk of developing Cushing's syndrome (see *Special warnings about this medication*).

Fluticasone, topical See *Cutivate*, page 367.

Fluticasone and Salmeterol See *Advair Diskus*, page 43.

Fluvastatin See *Lescol*, page 731.

FLUVOXAMINE MALEATE

Pronounced: FLUE-vox-uh-mean

Why is this drug prescribed?

Fluvoxamine is prescribed for obsessive-compulsive disorder. An obsession is marked by continual, unwanted thoughts that prevent proper functioning in everyday living. Compulsive behavior is typified by ritualistic actions such as repetitious washing, repeating certain phrases, completing steps in a process over and over, counting and recounting, checking and rechecking to make sure that something has not been forgotten, excessive neatness, and hoarding of useless items.

Fluvoxamine is thought to work by increasing levels of serotonin, a brain chemical associated with mood and thinking. It belongs to a class of drugs known as selective serotonin re-uptake inhibitors (SSRIs), which also includes antidepressants such as Paxil and Prozac.

Most important fact about this drug

Before starting therapy with fluvoxamine, be sure your doctor knows what medications you are taking—both prescription and over-the-counter—since combining fluvoxamine with certain drugs may cause serious or even life-threatening effects. You should never take fluvoxamine with thioridazine (Mellaril) or pimozide (Orap). You should also avoid taking fluvoxamine within 14 days of taking any antidepressant drug classified as an MAO inhibitor, including Nardil and Parnate.

How should you take this medication?

Take this medication only as directed by your doctor.

Fluvoxamine may be taken with or without food.

■ *If you miss a dose...*
If you are taking 1 dose a day, skip the missed dose and go back to your regular schedule. If you are taking 2 doses a day, take the missed dose as soon as possible, then go back to your regular schedule. Never take 2 doses at the same time.

■ *Storage instructions...*
Store at room temperature and protect from humidity.

What side effects may occur?

Side effects cannot be anticipated. If any develop or change in intensity, tell your doctor immediately. Only your doctor can determine if it is safe for you to continue taking fluvoxamine.

■ *Side effects may include:*
Abnormal ejaculation, agitation, anxiety, diarrhea, dizziness, dry mouth, headache, indigestion, insomnia, nausea, nervousness, sleepiness, sweating, tremor, vomiting, weakness, weight loss

Why should this drug not be prescribed?

If you are sensitive to or have ever had an allergic reaction to fluvoxamine or similar drugs, such as Prozac and Zoloft, do not take this medication. Make sure your doctor is aware of any drug reactions you have experienced.

Never combine fluvoxamine with Mellaril or Orap, or take it within 14 days of taking an MAO inhibitor such as Nardil or Parnate (see *Most important fact about this drug*).

Special warnings about this medication

In clinical studies, SSRI antidepressants increased the risk of suicidal thinking and behavior in children and adolescents with depression and other psychiatric disorders. Anyone considering the use of fluvoxamine or any other antidepressant in a child or adolescent must balance this risk with the clinical need. Fluvoxamine must be used with caution in children with depression. Fluvoxamine is approved for treating obsessive-compulsive disorder only in children 8 years and older.

Additionally, the progression of major depression is associated with a worsening of symptoms and/or the emergence of suicidal thinking or behavior in both adults and children, whether or not they are taking antidepressants. Individuals being treated with fluvoxamine and their caregivers should watch for any change in symptoms or any new symptoms that appear suddenly—especially agitation, anxiety, hostility, panic, restlessness, extreme hyperactivity, and suicidal thinking or behavior—and report them to the doctor immediately. Be especially observant at the beginning of treatment or whenever there is a change in dose.

You should discuss all your medical problems with your doctor before starting therapy with fluvoxamine, as certain physical conditions or diseases may affect your reaction to it.

If you suffer from seizures, use this medication cautiously. If you experience a seizure while taking fluvoxamine, stop taking the drug and call your doctor immediately.

If you have a history of mania (excessively energetic, out-of-control behavior), use this medication cautiously.

If you have liver disease, your doctor will adjust the dosage.

Fluvoxamine may cause you to become drowsy or less alert and may affect your judgment. Therefore, avoid driving, operating dangerous machinery, or participating in any hazardous activity that requires full mental alertness until you know your reaction to this medication.

Fluvoxamine can also deplete the body's supply of salt, especially in older adults and people who take diuretics or suffer from dehydration. Under these conditions, your doctor will check your salt levels regularly.

If you develop a rash or hives, or any other allergic-type reaction, notify your physician immediately.

Possible food and drug interactions when taking this medication

Do not drink alcohol while taking this medication. If you smoke, be sure to tell your doctor before starting fluvoxamine therapy, as your dosage may need adjustment.

If fluvoxamine is taken with certain other drugs, the effects of either could be increased, decreased, or altered. It is especially important to check with your doctor before combining fluvoxamine with the following:

Anticoagulant drugs such as Coumadin

Antidepressant medications such as Anafranil, Elavil, and Tofranil,
    as well as the MAO inhibitors Nardil and Parnate

Blood pressure medications known as beta-blockers, including
    Inderal and Lopressor

Carbamazepine (Tegretol)

Clozapine (Clozaril)

Diltiazem (Cardizem)

Lithium (Eskalith, Lithobid)

Methadone (Dolophine)

Mexiletine (Mexitil)

Phenytoin (Dilantin)

Pimozide (Orap)

Quinidine (Quinidex)

Sumatriptan (Imitrex)

Tacrine (Cognex)

Theophylline (Theo-Dur)

Thioridazine (Mellaril)

Tranquilizers and sedatives such as Halcion, Valium, Versed,
    and Xanax

Tryptophan

Special information if you are pregnant or breastfeeding

The effects of fluvoxamine in pregnancy have not been adequately studied. If you are pregnant or plan to become pregnant, consult your doctor
immediately. Fluvoxamine passes into breast milk and may cause serious
reactions in a nursing baby. If this medication is essential to your health,
your doctor may advise you to discontinue breastfeeding until your treatment with fluvoxamine is finished.

Recommended dosage

OBSESSIVE-COMPULSIVE DISORDER

Adults

The usual starting dose is one 50-milligram tablet taken at bedtime. Your
doctor may increase your dose, depending upon your response. The
maximum daily dose is 300 milligrams. If you take more than 100 milligrams a day, your doctor will divide the total amount into 2 doses; if the
doses are not equal, you should take the larger dose at bedtime. Older
adults and people with liver problems may need a reduced dosage.

Children

For children ages 8 to 17, the recommended starting dose is 25 milligrams taken at bedtime. The dose may be increased to a maximum of
200 milligrams daily for children under 11, and 300 milligrams for chil-

dren aged 11 to 17. Young girls sometimes respond to lower doses than boys do. Larger daily dosages are divided in two, as for adults.

Overdosage
Any medication taken in excess can have serious consequences. An overdose of fluvoxamine can be fatal. If you suspect an overdose, seek medical help immediately.

■ *Common symptoms of fluvoxamine overdose include:*
Breathing difficulties, coma, nausea, rapid heartbeat, sleepiness, vomiting

Other possible symptoms include convulsions, tremor, diarrhea, exaggerated reflexes, and slow or irregular heartbeat. After recovery, some overdose victims have been left with kidney complications, bowel damage, an unsteady gait, or dilated pupils.

FML
Generic name: Fluorometholone

Why is this drug prescribed?
FML is a steroid (cortisone-like) eye ointment that is used to treat inflammation of the eyelid and the eye itself.

Most important fact about this drug
Do not use FML more often or for a longer period of time than your doctor orders. Overuse can increase the risk of side effects and lead to eye damage. Also, if your eye problems return, do not use any leftover FML without first consulting your doctor.

How should you use this medication?
FML may increase the chance of infection from contact lenses. Your doctor may advise you to stop wearing your contacts while using this medication.

Use FML exactly as prescribed. Do not stop until your doctor advises you to do so. To avoid spreading infection, do not let anyone else use your prescription.

To administer FML eyedrops:
1. Wash your hands thoroughly.
2. Shake well before using.
3. Gently pull your lower eyelid down to form a pocket between your eye and eyelid.
4. Hold the eyedrop bottle on the bridge of your nose or on your forehead.
5. Do not touch the applicator tip to any surface, including your eye.

6. Tilt your head back and squeeze the medication into your eye.
7. Close your eyes gently. Keep them closed for 1 to 2 minutes.
8. Do not rinse the dropper.
9. Wait for 5 to 10 minutes before using a second eye medication.

■ *If you miss a dose…*
Apply it as soon as you remember. If it is almost time for your next dose, skip the one you missed and return to your regular schedule. Do not apply a double dose.

■ *Storage instructions…*
Store at room temperature. Protect from extreme heat.

What side effects may occur?
Side effects cannot be anticipated. If any develop or change in intensity, inform your doctor as soon as possible. Only your doctor can determine if it is safe for you to continue using FML.

■ *Side effects may include:*
Allergic reactions, blurred vision, burning/stinging, cataract formation, corneal ulcers, dilation of the pupil, drooping eyelids, eye inflammation and infection including pinkeye, eye irritation, glaucoma, increased eye pressure, slow wound healing, taste alterations

Why should this drug not be prescribed?
Do not use FML if you have ever had an allergic reaction to or are sensitive to fluorometholone or similar drugs (anti-inflammatories and steroids) such as Decadron. Tell your doctor about any drug reactions you have experienced.

FML is not prescribed for patients with certain viral, fungal, and bacterial infections of the eye.

Special warnings about this medication
Prolonged use of FML may result in glaucoma (elevated pressure in the eye causing optic nerve damage and loss of vision), cataract formation (an eye disorder causing the lens of the eye to cloud up), or the development or worsening of eye infections.

Steroids such as FML have been known to cause punctures when used in the presence of diseases that cause thinning of the cornea or the sclera (the tough, opaque covering at the back of the eyeball).

The use of a corticosteroid medication could hide the presence of a severe eye infection or cause the infection to become worse.

Internal pressure of the eye should be checked frequently by your doctor.

This medication should be used with caution after cataract surgery.

If pain or inflammation lasts longer than 48 hours, or becomes worse, discontinue use of FML and notify your doctor.

Possible food and drug interactions when taking this medication
No interactions with food or other drugs have been reported.

Special information if you are pregnant or breastfeeding
The effects of FML in pregnancy have not been adequately studied. If you are pregnant or plan to become pregnant, tell your doctor immediately. FML may appear in breast milk and could affect a nursing infant. If using FML is essential to your health, your doctor may advise you to stop breastfeeding until your treatment is finished.

Recommended dosage

ADULTS

FML Ointment
Apply a small amount of ointment (a half-inch ribbon) between the lower eyelid and eyeball 1 to 3 times a day. During the first 24 to 48 hours, your doctor may increase the dosage to 1 application every 4 hours.

FML Liquifilm
Place 1 drop of suspension between the lower eyelid and eyeball 2 to 4 times a day. During the first 24 to 48 hours, the dosage may be increased to 1 application every 4 hours.

CHILDREN

The safety and effectiveness of FML have not been established in children under 2 years of age.

Overdosage
Overdosage with FML will not ordinarily cause severe problems. If FML is accidentally swallowed, drink fluids to dilute the medication.

FOCALIN
Pronounced: FOKE-ah-lin
Generic name: Dexmethylphenidate hydrochloride

Why is this drug prescribed?
Focalin is a mild central nervous system stimulant used to treat Attention Deficit Hyperactivity Disorder (ADHD) in children. The drug is a modified version of Ritalin (a common medication for attention disorders) and contains only the most active component of Ritalin. Because of this special formulation, the usual dose of Focalin is half the amount of the Ritalin dose.

Focalin should be given as part of a total treatment program that includes psychological, educational, and social measures. Symptoms of attention deficit disorders include continual problems with moderate to severe distractibility, short attention span, hyperactivity, emotional changeability, and impulsiveness.

Most important fact about this drug

Excessive doses of Focalin over a long period of time can produce addiction. It is also possible to develop tolerance to the drug, so that larger doses are needed to produce the original effect. Because of these dangers, be sure to check with your doctor before making any change in dosage; and withdraw the drug only under your doctor's supervision.

How should you take this medication?

Focalin can be taken with or without food. The drug is usually taken twice a day, at least 4 hours apart, but your doctor may adjust the schedule depending on your child's response.

■ *If you miss a dose...*
Give it to the child as soon as you remember. If it is almost time for the next dose, skip the one you missed and return to your regular schedule. Never give 2 doses at the same time.

■ *Storage instructions...*
Keep out of reach of children. Store below 86 degrees Fahrenheit in a tightly closed, light-resistant container. Do not store in hot, damp, or humid places.

What side effects may occur?

Side effects cannot be anticipated. If any develop or change in intensity, inform your doctor as soon as possible. Only your doctor can determine if it is safe for your child to continue taking Focalin.

■ *Side effects may include:*
Fever, insomnia, loss of appetite, nausea, nervousness, stomach pain

The most common side effects reported for drugs that are similar to Focalin (including Ritalin) are nervousness and the inability to fall asleep or stay asleep. In children, loss of appetite, stomach pain, weight loss during long-term treatment, inability to fall asleep or stay asleep, and abnormally fast heartbeat are the more common side effects.

Why should this drug not be prescribed?

Focalin should not be used by people who suffer from anxiety, tension, and agitation, since the drug may aggravate these symptoms.

If Focalin, or similar drugs such as Ritalin, cause an allergic reaction, the drug should be avoided. It should not be taken by anyone with the eye condition known as glaucoma. It should also be avoided by anyone who suffers from motion tics (repeated, uncontrollable twitches) or verbal tics (uncontrollable repetition of words or sounds), or someone who suffers from, or has a family history of, Tourette's syndrome (severe and multiple tics).

Focalin should not be taken with drugs classified as monoamine oxidase (MAO) inhibitors, such as the antidepressants Nardil and Parnate, or within 14 days of stopping this type of medication.

Special warnings about this medication

Your doctor will do a complete history and evaluation before prescribing Focalin. It is important to remember that the drug is only part of the overall management of ADHD, and your doctor may also recommend counseling or other therapy.

There is no information about the safety and effectiveness of long-term Focalin treatment in children. However, suppression of growth has been seen with the long-term use of stimulants, so your doctor will watch your child carefully while he or she is taking this drug. If your child is not growing or gaining weight as expected, the doctor may stop Focalin treatment. This drug should not be given to children under 6 years of age; its safety and effectiveness in this age group have not been established.

Blood pressure should be monitored in anyone taking Focalin, especially those with high blood pressure or abnormal heart rate or rhythm. Caution is also advised in those with heart or thyroid problems.

Be sure to tell the doctor if your child has blurred vision while taking Focalin; some people have reported visual disturbances while taking stimulants similar to this drug.

The use of Focalin by anyone with a seizure disorder or psychosis (abnormal thinking and hallucinations) is not recommended. Caution is also advisable for anyone with a history of emotional instability or substance abuse, due to the danger of addiction. Focalin should not be used for the prevention or treatment of normal fatigue, nor should it be used for the treatment of severe depression.

Do not share Focalin with anyone else, and give your child only the number of tablets prescribed by your doctor. Keep track of the number of tablets in a bottle so you will notice if any are missing. Not using Focalin correctly can lead to dependence; call the doctor *immediately* if you seem to be using more than the prescribed amount.

Possible food and drug interactions when taking this medication

If Focalin is taken with certain other drugs, the effects of either can be increased, decreased, or altered. It is especially important to check with your doctor before combining Focalin with the following:

Antidepressant drugs, including MAO inhibitors (Nardil, Parnate), tricyclics (Elavil, Tofranil), and serotonin reuptake inhibitors (Prozac, Paxil)
Antiseizure drugs such as phenobarbital, Dilantin, and Mysoline
Blood pressure drugs such as Catapres

Blood thinners such as Coumadin
Herbal remedies such as ephedra and St. John's wort

Special information if you are pregnant or breastfeeding

The effects of Focalin during pregnancy have not been adequately studied. If you are pregnant or plan to become pregnant, tell your doctor immediately. Focalin should be used during pregnancy only if clearly needed.

It is not known whether Focalin appears in breast milk. Caution is advised if you are nursing a baby.

Recommended dosage

For people who are not currently taking Ritalin, the usual starting dose is 5 milligrams a day. For those who are switching from Ritalin, the starting Focalin dose is half the amount of the Ritalin dose. In either case, the total daily dose of Focalin should be divided into 2 doses taken at least 4 hours apart.

Depending on the response, your doctor may increase the dose by 2.5 to 5 milligrams a day, up to a maximum daily dose of 20 milligrams (10 milligrams twice a day). Increases are usually made at weekly intervals.

Overdosage

If you suspect an overdose, seek medical attention immediately.

■ *Symptoms of Focalin overdose may include:*
Abnormal reflexes, agitation, confusion, convulsions (may be followed by coma), delirium, dryness of mucous membranes, enlarged pupils in the eyes, exaggerated feeling of elation, extremely elevated body temperature, flushing, hallucinations, headache, high blood pressure, irregular or rapid heartbeat, muscle twitching, palpitations, sweating, tremors, vomiting

FORADIL

Pronounced: FOUR-a-dil
Generic name: Formoterol

Why is this drug prescribed?

Foradil relaxes the muscles in the walls of the airways, allowing them to expand. Taken on a twice-daily basis, it helps to control asthma in people who need regular treatment with short-acting inhalers, including people with nighttime asthma. Regular twice-daily use can also relieve tightening of the airways in people with Chronic Obstructive Pulmonary Disease, including chronic bronchitis and emphysema.

Taken on an as-needed basis, Foradil can also be used to prevent exercise-induced tightening of the airways (also called exercise-induced asthma) in adults and children 12 years of age and older.

Most important fact about this drug

Foradil is used to *prevent* asthma attacks, and should not be used for the relief of acute asthma symptoms. Your doctor will prescribe a short-acting inhaler such as Proventil or Ventolin to use for acute asthma attacks.

How should you take this medication?

Foradil capsules are intended for use only with the Aerolizer inhaler; they should not be swallowed.

To use the system, place a capsule in the well of the Aerolizer, then press and release the buttons on the side of the device. This will pierce the capsule. The medication is dispersed into the air stream when you inhale rapidly and deeply through the mouthpiece. Do not exhale into the device and do not use a spacer with this medication. Detailed instructions are supplied with your prescription. If you have any questions, ask your doctor or pharmacist.

One rare occasions, the capsule may break into small pieces, which could reach the throat or mouth during inhalation. You can reduce the chance of breakage by storing the capsules in a dry place, keeping them in their blister pack until just before use, and piercing them only once.

Be sure your hands are dry before handling the capsules, and be careful to keep the Aerolizer dry, too—do not wash any part of the device. Discard the aerolizer when your prescription is finished. Replace it with the new one that comes with each refill.

■ *If you miss a dose...*
Take it as soon as you remember. If it is almost time for your next dose, skip the one you missed and go back to your regular schedule.

■ *Storage instructions...*
Store at room temperature, away from heat and moisture. Leave the capsules in the blister pack until needed for use.

What side effects may occur?

Side effects cannot be anticipated. If any develop or change in intensity, inform your doctor as soon as possible. Only your doctor can determine if it is safe for you to continue taking Foradil.

■ *Side effects may include:*
Abdominal pain, allergic reaction, anxiety, back pain, bronchitis, chest infection, chest pain, difficulty breathing, difficulty speaking, dizziness, dry mouth, fatigue, fever, headache, high blood sugar, high or low blood pressure, inability to sleep, increased sputum, indigestion, irregular heartbeat, itching, muscle cramps, nausea, nervousness, rash, runny nose, sinusitis, sore throat, stomach upset, tonsillitis, tremor, unwell feeling, upper respiratory and viral infections, worsening of asthma

Why should this drug not be prescribed?

Foradil cannot be used for acute episodes of asthma that require intensive therapy. You'll also be unable to use Foradil if it gives you an allergic
reaction.

Special warnings about this medication

Your doctor will probably prescribe additional medications for use along
with Foradil. Steroid inhalers such as Beclovent and Flovent fight inflammation in the airways. Short-acting airway openers such as Proventil and
Ventolin relieve acute attacks. Be sure to use these medications exactly as
prescribed. Do not change the dosage or stop using them without consulting your doctor.

Be sure to keep track of how often you use your short-acting inhaler for
relief of acute asthma symptoms. Your doctor will use this information to
help determine how well Foradil is working. Notify your doctor if your
symptoms worsen, if you need more inhalations of the short-acting inhaler than usual, or if Foradil seems to be getting less effective. Keep
track of your peak flow readings, too. Call your doctor if you notice a drop
in this measurement of lung capacity.

Do not use Foradil more often than prescribed. Excessive use can
cause heart irregularities. Use Foradil with caution if you have any kind of
heart disorder or high blood pressure. Notify your doctor immediately if
you experience palpitations, chest pain, rapid heart rate, or tremor.

Do not use Foradil in combination with Serevent, Advair Diskus, or
other long-acting inhalers. They contain the same type of active ingredient and will provide no extra benefit. If you've been using a short-acting
inhaler on a routine basis, you should stop using it regularly and reserve
it for occasional relief of acute attacks.

Call your doctor immediately if you develop hives, rash, or swelling, or
if you have an asthma attack that does not respond to your usual medication. Foradil has been known to cause allergic reactions and acute
asthma attacks.

Possible food and drug interactions when taking this medication

If Foradil is taken with certain other drugs, the effect of either may be increased, decreased, or altered. It is especially important to check with
your doctor before combining Foradil with the following:

Antidepressants categorized as tricyclics, such as Elavil and Tofranil
Antidepressants classified as monoamine oxidase inhibitors, such as
  Nardil and Parnate
Beta-blockers (drugs such as Inderal and Tenormin that are used to
  control blood pressure and treat various heart conditions)
Steroids such as prednisone and hydrocortisone
Theophylline (Theo-Dur, Slo-Phyllin)
Water pills (diuretics) such as HydroDIURIL or Lasix

Special information if you are pregnant or breastfeeding

The possibility of harm during pregnancy has not been ruled out. Foradil is recommended for pregnant women only if the potential benefit outweighs the potential risk. Inform your doctor immediately if you are pregnant or plan to become pregnant.

It's not known whether Foradil appears in breast milk. Use this medication with caution if you are nursing.

Recommended dosage

ASTHMA

For the long-term control of asthma in adults and children 5 years of age and older, the recommended dosage is 1 capsule every 12 hours. Do not use more than 2 capsules per day.

PREVENTION OF EXERCISE-INDUCED ASTHMA

For adults and children 12 years of age and older, the recommended dosage is 1 capsule at least 15 minutes before exercise. If a second dose is needed the same day, it must be taken at least 12 hours after the first dose. Do not exceed 2 capsules per day. If you are already taking Foradil on a regular twice-daily basis, do not take additional doses before exercise.

CHRONIC OBSTRUCTIVE PULMONARY DISEASE

The usual dosage is 1 capsule every 12 hours. Do not use more than 2 capsules a day. If your customary dosage fails to provide the usual relief, check with your doctor immediately. Other treatments may have to be added to your regimen.

Overdosage

Any medication taken in excess can have serious consequences. If you suspect an overdose, seek medical attention immediately.

■ *Symptoms of Foradil overdose may include:*
  Chest pain, dizziness, dry mouth, fast or irregular heartbeat, fatigue, general feeling of illness, headache, heart palpitations, inability to sleep, muscle cramps, nausea, nervousness, seizures, tremor

Formoterol *See Foradil, page 599.*

FORTOVASE

Pronounced: FORT-o-vace
Generic name: Saquinavir
Other brand name: Invirase

Why is this drug prescribed?

Fortovase is used in the treatment of advanced human immunodeficiency virus (HIV) infection. HIV causes the immune system to break down so that it can no longer fight off other infections. This leads to the fatal disease known as acquired immune deficiency syndrome (AIDS).

Fortovase belongs to a class of HIV drugs called protease inhibitors, which work by interfering with an important step in the virus's reproductive cycle. Fortovase is used in combination with other HIV drugs called nucleoside analogues (Retrovir or Hivid, for example). The combination produces an increase in the immune system's vital CD4 cells (white blood cells) and reduces the amount of virus in the bloodstream. Fortovase should not be used by itself.

The active ingredient in Invirase is saquinavir mesylate, and although it's similar to the active ingredient in Fortovase, the two drugs are *not* interchangeable (see *Most important fact about this drug*). However, the drug information provided here about Fortovase also applies to Invirase.

Most important fact about this drug

Fortovase will not cure an HIV infection. You will continue to face the possibility of complications, including opportunistic infections (rare infections that develop only when the immune system falters, such as certain types of pneumonia, tuberculosis, and fungal infections). Therefore, it is important that you remain under the care of a doctor and keep all your follow-up appointments.

Although they contain a similar ingredient, Fortovase and Invirase are *not* interchangeable.

When using saquinavir as the sole protease inhibitor in a combination drug regimen, Fortovase is the recommended brand. Invirase may be used only if it is combined with ritonavir (Norvir). Any switch from Invirase to Fortovase or vice versa should be made only under the supervision of your doctor.

How should you take this medication?

Take this medication exactly as prescribed by your doctor. Do not share this medication with anyone, and do not exceed your recommended dosage. Take Fortovase with a meal or within 2 hours afterwards. This allows the drug to be properly absorbed by your body. Your doctor will perform laboratory tests before you start therapy with Fortovase and at regular intervals during your therapy to see how you are reacting to the medication.

■ *If you miss a dose...*
Take it as soon as possible. If it is almost time for your next dose, skip the one you missed and go back to your regular schedule. Never take a double dose.

■ *Storage instructions...*
Store Fortovase in the refrigerator in a tightly closed bottle. The capsules should be used within 3 months if they've been allowed to reach room temperature.

What side effects may occur?

Side effects cannot be anticipated. If any develop or change in intensity, tell your doctor as soon as possible. Only your doctor can determine if it is safe for you to continue taking Fortovase.

■ *Side effects may include:*
Abdominal discomfort and pain, appetite disturbance, depression, diarrhea, dizziness, fatigue, gas, headache, indigestion, mouth sores, muscle and bone pain, nausea, numbness in the arms and legs, tingling or pins and needles sensation, vomiting, weakness

Why should this drug not be prescribed?

You should not use Fortovase if you have severe liver impairment. Also, you should not take certain medications while using Fortovase (see *Possible food and drug interactions when taking this medication*).

If you suffer an allergic reaction to Fortovase or any of its components, you will not be able to use this drug.

Invirase may be used only when it's combined with ritonavir (Norvir); it cannot be added to regimens that don't contain Norvir.

Special warnings about this medication

Fortovase may increase blood sugar levels. If you have diabetes, be sure to let the doctor know. Your dosage of diabetes medication may need adjustment.

Fortovase may aggravate mild to moderate liver problems and should be used with caution if you have such liver disorders as hepatitis or cirrhosis. Also use the drug with caution if you have severe kidney problems.

Fortovase may cause bleeding in people with hemophilia type A or B.

Patients taking protease inhibitors such as Fortovase sometimes undergo a redistribution of body fat, gaining weight around the waist, developing a pad of fat on the upper back, and losing weight in the arms and legs. The long-term health effects of these changes are still unknown.

High cholesterol and triglyceride levels have been observed in people taking Fortovase or Invirase combined with ritonavir (Norvir). If you're taking this drug combination, your doctor will do periodic blood tests to check for problems.

This medication does not reduce the risk of transmission of HIV to others through sexual contact or blood contamination. Therefore, you should continue to avoid practices that could give HIV to others.

Possible food and drug interactions when taking this medication

Combining certain medications with Fortovase could cause serious or life-threatening reactions. The following drugs should never be used while you're taking Fortovase:

Amiodarone (Cordarone)
Astemizole
Bepridil
Certain migraine drugs, including D.H.E. 45 injection, Cafergot, Ergostat, and Migranal Nasal Spray
Cisapride
Flecainide (Tambocor)
Midazolam (Versed)
Pimozide
Propafenone (Rythmol)
Quinidine (Quinidex)
Terfenadine
Triazolam (Halcion)

The manufacturer also warns against combining Fortovase with the following:

Cholesterol-lowering drugs known as statins, such as Lipitor, Mevacor, and Zocor
Garlic
Rifampin (Rifadin)
St. John's wort

If Fortovase is taken with certain other drugs, the effects of either could be increased, decreased, or altered. It is especially important to check with your doctor before combining Fortovase with the following:

Antidepressants known as tricyclics, such as Elavil and Tofranil
Carbamazepine (Tegretol)
Calcium channel blockers, including Cardene, Cardizem, and Verelan
Delavirdine (Rescriptor)
Dexamethasone (Decadron)
Efavirenz (Sustiva)
Erectile dysfunction medications such as Cialis, Levitra, and Viagra
Immunosuppressants such as Rapamune, Prograf, and Sandimmune
Lidocaine
Methadone
Nevirapine (Viramune)

Oral contraceptives
Other protease inhibitors such as Crixivan, Norvir, and Viracept
Phenobarbital (Donnatal)
Phenytoin (Dilantin)
Rifabutin (Mycobutin)
Sedatives such as Tranxene, Valium, and Xanax
Warfarin (Coumadin)

Be sure to tell your doctor and pharmacist about all the medications (both prescription and over-the-counter) that you are presently taking. Alert them, too, whenever you stop taking a medication.

Special information if you are pregnant or breastfeeding
The effects of Fortovase during pregnancy have not been adequately studied. If you are pregnant or plan to become pregnant, tell your doctor immediately. Do not breastfeed. HIV appears in breast milk and can be passed to a nursing infant.

Recommended dosage

ADULTS AND CHILDREN 16 YEARS AND OLDER

Fortovase Combined with Other Anti-HIV Drugs
The recommended dosage is 1,200 milligrams (six 200-milligram capsules), taken 3 times a day with a meal or within 2 hours afterwards. Daily doses lower than 1,200 milligrams 3 times a day are not recommended, since they will not have the same antiviral activity. You should also be taking Retrovir, Hivid, or another antiviral drug as directed.

Invirase Combined with Ritonavir
The recommended dosage is 1,000 milligrams (five 200-milligram capsules) taken 2 times a day with a meal or within 2 hours afterwards. Ritonavir (Norvir) should be taken at the same time as Invirase. Daily doses lower than 1,000 milligrams (along with 100 milligrams of Norvir) 2 times a day are not recommended, since they will not have the same antiviral activity.

CHILDREN LESS THAN 16 YEARS OLD

Fortovase and Invirase have not been studied in children younger than 16 years old.

Overdosage
There have been no reports of Fortovase poisoning. However, any medication taken in excess can have serious consequences. If you suspect an overdose, seek emergency medical treatment immediately.

FOSAMAX

Pronounced: FAH-suh-max
Generic name: Alendronate sodium

Why is this drug prescribed?

Fosamax is prescribed for the prevention and treatment of osteoporosis, the brittle bone disease, in postmenopausal women. It is also used to increase bone mass in men with osteoporosis, and is prescribed for both men and women who have developed a form of osteoporosis sometimes caused by steroid medications such as prednisone. This drug can also be used to relieve Paget's disease of bone, a painful condition that weakens and deforms the bones.

Most important fact about this drug

For Fosamax to be effective, you must take the tablets without food or other medications, exactly as directed.

How should you use this medication?

Fosamax is effective only when each tablet or bottle of oral solution is taken with a full glass of plain water first thing in the morning, at least 30 minutes before the first food, beverage, or other medication. If you can wait longer before eating or drinking, the medication will be absorbed better. Do not lie down after taking Fosamax until at least 30 minutes have passed and you've had something to eat.

Avoid chewing or sucking on the tablet; it can cause mouth sores.

You should take calcium and vitamin D supplements if you don't get enough in your diet. Avoid smoking and alcohol. Weight-bearing exercise can also strengthen bones.

■ *If you miss a dose...*
  If you are taking Fosamax on a daily basis, do not take a missed dose later in the day. Instead, skip it and go back to your regular schedule the next morning.

  If you are taking Fosamax once a week, take 1 tablet or 1 bottle of oral solution the morning after you remember, then return to your original once-weekly schedule on the chosen day. Do not take 2 doses on the same day.

■ *Storage instructions...*
  Keep the container tightly closed and store at room temperature. Do not freeze the oral solution.

What side effects may occur?

Side effects cannot be anticipated. If any develop or change in intensity, inform your doctor as soon as possible. Only your doctor can determine if it is safe for you to continue using Fosamax.

■ *Side effects may include:*
Abdominal pain, acid regurgitation, bone and joint pain, constipation, diarrhea, gas, indigestion, muscle pain, nausea

Why should this drug not be prescribed?

You should not take Fosamax if the calcium level in your blood is low. Avoid Fosamax if it causes an allergic reaction.

You will not be able to take Fosamax if you are unable to stand or sit upright for at least 30 minutes. You must also avoid the drug if your esophagus is not working properly due to strictures or achalasia (a swallowing disorder).

If you're prone to swallowing air or choking when you drink something, you should not use the oral solution.

Special warnings about this medication

Fosamax is not recommended for women on hormone replacement therapy, or for women with kidney problems.

Be sure to tell your doctor if you have trouble swallowing or have any digestive problems, including heartburn or ulcers. Fosamax may cause problems in your esophagus such as inflammation, ulcers, bleeding, and in rare cases, blockage or perforation.

Possible food and drug interactions when taking this medication

Combining aspirin with a Fosamax dose of more than 10 milligrams per day will increase the likelihood of stomach upset.

Calcium supplements such as Caltrate, antacids such as Riopan, and some other oral medications will interfere with the absorption of Fosamax, so wait at least 30 minutes after taking Fosamax before you take anything else.

Special information if you are pregnant or breastfeeding

The effects of Fosamax during pregnancy and breastfeeding have not been adequately studied. If you are pregnant or plan to become pregnant, notify your doctor immediately. It is not known whether Fosamax appears in breast milk. The drug is not recommended for nursing mothers.

Recommended dosage

TREATMENT OF POSTMENOPAUSAL OSTEOPOROSIS

The usual dose is one 10-milligram tablet once a day, or one 70-milligram tablet or bottle of oral solution once a week. Treatment continues for years.

PREVENTION OF POSTMENOPAUSAL OSTEOPOROSIS

The usual dose is one 5-milligram tablet once a day or one 35-milligram tablet once a week.

OSTEOPOROSIS IN MEN

The usual dose is one 10-milligram tablet once a day, or one 70-milligram tablet or bottle of oral solution once a week.

STEROID-INDUCED OSTEOPOROSIS

The usual dose is one 5-milligram tablet once a day, except for postmenopausal women not taking estrogen, who should take one 10-milligram tablet once daily.

PAGET'S DISEASE

The usual dose is 40 milligrams once a day for 6 months.

Overdosage

Any medication taken in excess can have serious consequences. If you suspect an overdose, seek medical attention immediately.

■ *Symptoms of Fosamax overdose may include:*
Heartburn, inflammation of the esophagus or stomach, ulcer, upset stomach

Fosamprenavir See Lexiva, page 749.

Fosfomycin See Monurol, page 893.

Fosinopril See Monopril, page 887.

Fosinopril with Hydrochlorothiazide See Monopril-HCT, page 891.

FROVA
Pronounced: FROE-va
Generic name: Frovatriptan succinate

Why is this drug prescribed?

Frova is used to relieve attacks of migraine headache. It's helpful whether or not the headache is preceded by an aura (visual disturbances such as seeing halos or flickering lights).

Experts think that migraines are caused by the expansion of blood vessels serving the brain, and that this expansion is triggered by a decline in the level of serotonin, one of the brain's chief chemical messengers. Frova works by restoring serotonin levels to normal. It belongs to a class of drugs called serotonin agonists.

Most important fact about this drug

Frova can quell migraine attacks once they've begun, but it won't prevent them before they start. It should not be used for certain rare types of migraine called hemiplegic migraine or basilar migraine, and it is not recommended for the cluster headaches that tend to affect older men.

How should you take this medication?

One Frova tablet can be taken any time after the onset of a headache. If the headache goes away and comes back you can take a second tablet after 2 hours. A third tablet can be taken 2 hours or more after the last dose. Do not take more than 3 tablets in one day.

■ *If you miss a dose...*
Frova is not for regular use. Take it only during an attack.
■ *Storage instructions...*
Store Frova tablets at room temperature away from moisture and light.

What side effects may occur?

Side effects cannot be anticipated. If any develop or change in intensity, inform your doctor as soon as possible. Only your doctor can determine if it is safe for you to continue taking Frova.

■ *Side effects may include:*
Bone pain, dizziness, dry mouth, fatigue, flushing, headache, hot or cold sensation, joint pain, tingling feeling

Why should this drug not be prescribed?

If you have heart disease, you must avoid Frova. You also cannot take this drug if you have had a stroke, suffer mini-strokes, or have any other kind of circulation problem. Avoid it, too, if you have high blood pressure that is not under control.

Remember that Frova should not be used for hemiplegic migraine or basilar migraine. Do not use it again if it causes an allergic reaction, and do not take it for 24 hours after using another serotonin agonist or an ergot-based migraine medication. Serotonin agonists include Amerge, Axert, Imitrex, Maxalt, and Zomig. Ergot medications include such drugs as Cafergot, DHE, Sansert, and Wigraine.

Special warnings about this medication

In people with heart disease, medications similar to Frova have been known to cause serious problems, including heart attacks and strokes. If you have heart disease, or know of any factors that make undetected heart disease a possibility, be sure to tell the doctor. Risk factors include high blood pressure, high cholesterol, diabetes, excess weight, smoking, a history of heart disease in your family, and menopause in women or age over 40 in men.

If there's any chance of a heart problem, your doctor may administer the first dose of Frova in the office and monitor your response. After later doses, call your doctor immediately if you develop pain, tightness, heaviness, and pressure in your throat, chest, neck, or jaw.

Frova is not recommended for children under age 18.

Possible food and drug interactions when taking this medication

Remember that Frova must never be combined with other serotonin-agonist or ergot-based migraine drugs (see *Why should this drug not be prescribed?*).

If Frova is taken with certain other drugs, the effects of either could be increased, decreased, or altered. It is especially important to check with your doctor before combining Frova with the following:

Antidepressants and anti-anxiety drugs that boost serotonin levels, including Luvox, Paxil, Prozac, and Zoloft
Propranolol (Inderal)

Special information if you are pregnant or breastfeeding

Frova has not been studied in pregnant women. If you are pregnant or if you plan to become pregnant, inform your doctor right away so you can discuss your treatment options.

It is not known if Frova appears in breast milk. Caution is advised if you plan on nursing.

Recommended dosage

ADULTS

Take one 2.5-milligram tablet with a liquid at the onset of headache. If one dose does not work, do not take a second dose, as it is not likely to work either.

If the headache comes back later, a second tablet can be taken 2 hours or more after the first tablet. Do not take more than three 2.5-milligram tablets in one day.

Overdosage

Although little is known about the effects of an overdose of Frova, any medication taken in excess can have serious consequences. If you suspect an overdose, seek medical attention immediately.

Frovatriptan See *Frova, page 609.*

Fulvicin P/G See *Gris-PEG, page 633.*

Furosemide See *Lasix, page 729.*

Gabapentin See *Neurontin, page 931.*

Galantamine See *Razadyne, page 1220.*

GANTRISIN

Pronounced: GAN-tris-in
Generic name: Sulfisoxazole acetyl

Why is this drug prescribed?

Gantrisin is a children's medication prescribed for the treatment of severe, repeated, or long-lasting urinary tract infections. These include pyelonephritis (bacterial kidney inflammation), pyelitis (inflammation of the part of the kidney that drains urine into the ureter), and cystitis (inflammation of the bladder).

This drug is also used to treat bacterial meningitis, and is prescribed as a preventive measure for children who have been exposed to meningitis.

Some middle ear infections are treated with Gantrisin in combination with penicillin or erythromycin.

Toxoplasmosis (parasitic disease transmitted by infected cats, their feces or litter boxes, and by undercooked meat) can be treated with Gantrisin in combination with pyrimethamine (Daraprim).

Malaria that does not respond to the drug chloroquine (Aralen) can be treated with Gantrisin in combination with other drug treatment.

Gantrisin is also used in the treatment of bacterial infections such as trachoma and inclusion conjunctivitis (eye infections), nocardiosis (bacterial disease affecting the lungs, skin, and brain), and chancroid (venereal disease causing enlargement and ulceration of lymph nodes in the groin).

Most important fact about this drug

Notify your doctor at the first sign of a reaction such as skin rash, sore throat, fever, joint pain, cough, shortness of breath, or other breathing difficulties, abnormal skin paleness, reddish or purplish skin spots or yellowing of the skin or whites of the eyes.

Rare but severe reactions, sometimes fatal, have occurred with the use of sulfa drugs such as Gantrisin. These reactions include sudden and severe liver damage, agranulocytosis (a severe blood disorder), and Stevens-Johnson syndrome (severe blistering).

Children taking sulfa drugs such as Gantrisin should have frequent blood counts.

How should you take this medication?

Be sure your child takes Gantrisin exactly as prescribed. It is important that the child drink plenty of fluids while taking this medication in order to prevent crystals in the urine and the formation of stones.

Gantrisin is available as a suspension and should be shaken well before each dose. To ensure an accurate dose, ask your pharmacist for a specially marked measuring spoon.

Gantrisin, like other antibacterials, works best when there is a constant amount in the blood and urine. To help keep a constant level, try to make sure that your child does not miss any doses and takes them at evenly spaced intervals, around the clock.

■ *If you miss a dose...*
Give it as soon as you remember. If it is almost time for the next dose, skip the one you missed and go back to the regular schedule. Never give 2 doses at the same time.

■ *Storage instructions...*
Keep this medication in the container it came in, tightly closed. Store it at room temperature, away from moist places and direct light.

What side effects may occur?

Side effects cannot be anticipated. If any develop or change in intensity, inform your doctor as soon as possible. Only your doctor can determine if it is safe for your child to continue taking Gantrisin.

■ *Side effects may include:*
Abdominal bleeding, abdominal pain, allergic reactions, anemia and other blood disorders, angioedema (swelling of face, lips, tongue and throat), anxiety, bluish discoloration of the skin, chills, colitis, convulsions, cough, dark, tarry stools, depression, diarrhea, disorientation, dizziness, drowsiness, enlarged salivary glands, enlarged thyroid, exhaustion, fainting, fatigue, fever, flushing, gas, hallucinations, headache, hearing loss, hepatitis, hives, inability to fall or stay asleep, inability to urinate, increased urination, inflammation of the mouth or tongue, itching, joint pain, kidney failure, lack of feeling or concern, lack of muscle coordination, lack or loss of appetite, low blood sugar, muscle pain, nausea, palpitations, presence of blood or crystals in urine, rapid heartbeat, reddish or purplish skin spots, retention of urine, ringing in the ears, sensitivity to light, serum sickness (fever, painful joints, enlarged lymph nodes, skin rash), severe skin welts or swelling, shortness of breath, skin eruptions, skin rash, swelling due to fluid retention, tingling or pins and needles, vertigo, vomiting, weakness, yellow eyes and skin

Why should this drug not be prescribed?

If your child is sensitive to or has ever had an allergic reaction to Gantrisin or other sulfa drugs, do not use this medication. Make sure your doctor is aware of any drug reactions the child has experienced.

Except in rare cases, doctors do not prescribe Gantrisin for infants less than 2 months of age. In addition, Gantrisin should never be taken by women at the end of pregnancy or those nursing a baby under 2 months.

Special warnings about this medication

If your child has impaired kidney or liver function, or severe allergies or bronchial asthma, make sure your doctor knows about it. Caution should be exercised when taking Gantrisin.

An analysis of urine and kidney function should be performed by your doctor during treatment with Gantrisin, especially if your child has a kidney problem.

If your child develops a skin rash, stop Gantrisin therapy and call your doctor. Also notify the doctor if your child develops diarrhea.

Possible food and drug interactions when taking this medication
If Gantrisin is taken with certain other drugs, the effects of either could be increased, decreased, or altered. It is especially important to check with your doctor before combining this drug with the following:

Blood-thinning drugs such as Coumadin
Methotrexate, an anticancer drug
Oral diabetes drugs such as Micronase

Special information if you are pregnant or breastfeeding
There are no adequate and well-controlled studies in pregnant women. This medication should never be used during pregnancy unless the doctor has determined that the benefits outweigh the potential risks. Gantrisin appears in breast milk. If this medication is essential, the doctor may recommend against breastfeeding until treatment with this drug is finished.

Recommended dosage

CHILDREN

This medication should not be prescribed for infants under 2 months of age except in the treatment of congenital toxoplasmosis (a parasitic infection contracted by pregnant women and passed along to the fetus).

The usual dose for children 2 months of age or older is 150 milligrams per 2.2 pounds of body weight divided into 4 to 6 doses taken over 24 hours.

The usual starting dose is one-half of the regular dose, or 75 milligrams per 2.2 pounds of body weight divided into 4 to 6 doses taken over 24 hours. Doses should not exceed 6 grams over 24 hours.

Gantrisin pediatric suspension supplies a half-gram (500 milligrams) in each teaspoonful.

Overdosage
Any medication taken in excess can have serious consequences. If you suspect an overdose, seek emergency medical treatment immediately.

■ *Symptoms of an overdose of Gantrisin include:*
Blood or sediment in the urine, blue tinge to the skin, colic, dizziness, drowsiness, fever, headache, lack or loss of appetite, nausea, unconsciousness, vomiting, yellowing of skin and whites of the eyes

GARAMYCIN OPHTHALMIC
Pronounced: gar-uh-MY-sin
Generic name: Gentamicin sulfate

Why is this drug prescribed?
Garamycin Ophthalmic, an antibiotic, is applied to the eye for treatment of infections such as conjunctivitis (pinkeye) and other eye infections.

Most important fact about this drug
To help clear up your infection completely, keep using Garamycin eye-drops or ointment for the full time of treatment, even if your symptoms have disappeared. Do not allow anyone else to use this medication, and do not save it for use on another infection.

How should you use this medication?
Use this medication exactly as prescribed.

To administer Garamycin eyedrops:
1. Wash your hands thoroughly.
2. Gently pull your lower eyelid down to form a pocket between your eye and the lid.
3. Brace the eyedrop bottle on your forehead or on the bridge of your nose.
4. Do not touch the applicator tip to your eye or any other surface.
5. Close your eyes gently and keep them closed for a minute or two.
6. Do not rinse the dropper.
7. If you are using a second type of eyedrop, wait 5 to 10 minutes before applying it.

To administer Garamycin eye ointment:
1. Wash your hands thoroughly.
2. Pull your lower eyelid down away from the eye to form a pocket.
3. Squeeze a thin strip of ointment into the pouch.
4. Avoid touching the tip of the tube to your eye or any other surface.
5. Close your eyes for a couple of minutes.
6. Wipe the tip of the tube with tissue and immediately replace the cap tightly.

Your vision may be blurred for a few minutes following application of the ointment.

■ *If you miss a dose...*
Apply it as soon as you remember. If it is almost time for your next dose, skip the one you missed and go back to your regular schedule.
■ *Storage instructions...*
Store away from heat and light. Do not freeze.

What side effects may occur?

Occasional eye irritation—with itching, redness and swelling—may occur with use of the eyedrops. Occasional burning or stinging in the eye may occur with use of the ointment.

Why should this drug not be prescribed?

If you are sensitive to or have ever had an allergic reaction to Garamycin or certain other antibiotics, such as Tobrex, you should not take this medication. Make sure your doctor is aware of any drug reactions you have experienced.

Special warnings about this medication

Continued or prolonged use of this drug may result in a growth of bacteria or fungi that do not respond to this medication and can cause a second infection. Should this occur, notify your doctor.

Ophthalmic ointments may slow corneal healing.

Possible food and drug interactions with this medication

No interactions have been reported.

Special information if you are pregnant or breastfeeding

There are no special recommendations for this medication. If you are pregnant or plan to become pregnant, ask your doctor for the best advice in your personal situation.

Recommended dosage

ADULTS AND CHILDREN

Garamycin Ophthalmic Solution

Put 1 or 2 drops into the affected eye every 4 hours. For severe infections, your doctor may increase your dosage up to a maximum of 2 drops once every hour.

Garamycin Ophthalmic Ointment

Apply a thin strip—about one-third inch—of ointment to the affected eye 2 or 3 times a day.

Overdosage

Although there is no information on overdose with Garamycin ophthalmic products, any medication taken in excess can have serious consequences. If you suspect an overdose, seek medical attention immediately.

Gatifloxacin *See Tequin, page 1410.*

Gatifloxacin eyedrops *See Zymar, page 1668.*

Gaviscon *See Antacids, page 114.*

Gemfibrozil *See Lopid, page 772.*

Gemifloxacin *See Factive, page 550.*

Gentamicin *See Garamycin Ophthalmic, page 615.*

Genuine Bayer *See Aspirin, page 132.*

GEODON
Pronounced: GEE-oh-dahn
Generic name: Ziprasidone hydrochloride

Why is this drug prescribed?
Geodon is prescribed to treat schizophrenia. It is also used for the short-term treatment of mania associated with bipolar disorder. Researchers believe that it works by opposing the action of serotonin and dopamine, two of the brain's major chemical messengers. Because of its potentially serious side effects, Geodon is typically prescribed only after other medications have proved inadequate.

Geodon is usually taken in capsule form. An injectable version is available for quick relief of agitated patients. Injectable Geodon is generally used for no more than a few days.

Most important fact about this drug
In some people with heart problems or a slow heartbeat, Geodon can cause serious and potentially fatal heartbeat irregularities. The chance of a problem is greater if you are taking a water pill (diuretic) or a medication that prolongs a part of the heartbeat known as the QT interval. Many of the drugs prescribed for heartbeat irregularities prolong the QT interval and should never be combined with Geodon. Other drugs to avoid when taking Geodon include Anzemet, Avelox, Halfan, Inapsine, Lariam, Mellaril, Nebupent, Orap, Orlaam, Pentam, Probucol, Prograf, Serentil, Tequin, Thorazine, Trisenox, and Zagam. If you're uncertain about the risks of any drug you're taking, be sure to check with your doctor before combining it with Geodon.

Drugs such as Geodon may increase the risk of death in elderly people with dementia-related psychosis. Geodon is not approved for use in such patients.

How should you take this medication?
Geodon capsules should be taken twice a day with food.

■ *If you miss a dose...*
   Take it as soon as you remember. If it is almost time for your next dose, skip the one you missed and go back to your regular schedule. Do not take 2 doses at once.

■ *Storage instructions…*
Store at room temperature.

What side effects may occur?

Side effects cannot be anticipated. If any develop or change in intensity, inform your doctor as soon as possible. Only your doctor can determine if it is safe for you to continue taking Geodon.

■ *Side effects may include:*
Accidental injury, cold symptoms, constipation, cough, diarrhea, dizziness, drowsiness, dry mouth, headache, indigestion, involuntary muscle contractions, muscle tightness, nausea, rash, stuffy and runny nose, upper respiratory infection, vision problems, vomiting, weakness

Why should this drug not be prescribed?

Do not take Geodon if you have the heartbeat irregularity known as QT prolongation, have had a recent heart attack, or suffer from heart failure. You'll also need to avoid this drug if it gives you an allergic reaction.

Special warnings about this medication

Remember that Geodon can cause dangerous—even fatal—heartbeat irregularities. Warning signs include dizziness, palpitations, and fainting. Tell your doctor immediately if you experience any of these symptoms. Be careful to avoid drugs that prolong the QT interval of the heartbeat. Check with your doctor before combining any other medication with Geodon.

Particularly during the first few days of therapy, Geodon can cause low blood pressure, with accompanying dizziness, fainting, and rapid heartbeat. Tell your doctor if you experience any of these side effects. To minimize such problems, your doctor will increase your dose gradually. If you are prone to low blood pressure, take blood pressure medicine, become dehydrated, or have heart disease or poor circulation in the brain, use Geodon with caution.

Geodon may cause drowsiness and can impair your judgment, thinking, and motor skills. Use caution while driving and don't operate potentially dangerous machinery until you know how this drug affects you.

Geodon poses a very slight risk of seizures, especially if you are over age 65, have a history of seizures, or have Alzheimer's disease.

Drugs such as Geodon sometimes cause a condition called Neuroleptic Malignant Syndrome (NMS). Symptoms include high fever, muscle rigidity, irregular pulse or blood pressure, rapid heartbeat, excessive perspiration, and changes in heart rhythm. If these symptoms appear, tell your doctor immediately. You'll need to stop taking Geodon while the condition is under treatment.

There also is the risk of developing tardive dyskinesia, a condition marked by slow, rhythmical, involuntary movements. This problem is more likely to occur in mature adults, especially older women. When it does, use of Geodon is usually stopped.

Geodon can suppress the cough reflex; you may have trouble clearing your airway. Some people taking Geodon also develop a rash. Tell your doctor when this happens. If the rash doesn't clear up with treatment, you may have to discontinue the drug.

Other antipsychotic medications have been known to interfere with the body's temperature-regulating mechanism, causing the body to overheat. Although this problem has not occurred with Geodon, caution is still advisable. Avoid exposure to extreme heat, strenuous exercise, and dehydration. There also is a remote chance that this medication may cause abnormal, prolonged, and painful erections.

Certain antipsychotic drugs are associated with an increased risk of developing high blood sugar, which on rare occasions has led to coma or death. There have been only a few reports of diabetes or blood sugar problems occurring in people using Geodon. Still, it's important to see your doctor if you develop signs of high blood sugar, including dry mouth, unusual thirst, increased urination, and tiredness. If you have diabetes or have a high risk of developing it, see your doctor regularly for blood sugar testing.

Geodon is prescribed for the short-term treatment of rapid-onset bipolar mania; it is not approved for preventing future episodes. The effectiveness of the drug for treating mania for more than 3 weeks has not been studied.

Animal studies suggest that Geodon may increase the risk of breast cancer, although human studies have not confirmed such a risk. If you have a history of breast cancer, see your doctor regularly for checkups.

The safety and effectiveness of Geodon have not been studied in children.

Possible food and drug interactions when taking this medication

Remember that you must never combine Geodon with any drug that prolongs the part of the heartbeat known as the QT interval (see *Most important fact about this drug*). Check with your doctor or pharmacist if you have any doubts about a drug you're taking.

If Geodon is taken with certain other drugs, the effects of either could be increased, decreased, or altered. It is especially important to check with your doctor before combining Geodon with the following:

Carbamazepine (Tegretol)
Certain blood pressure medications
Drugs that affect the brain and nervous system, such as sedatives, tranquilizers, and antidepressants
Drugs that boost the effects of dopamine, such as Mirapex, Parlodel, Permax, and Requip
Ketoconazole (Nizoral)
Levodopa (Larodopa, Sinemet)

Special information if you are pregnant or breastfeeding
Geodon has caused fetal harm when tested in animals. It should be taken during pregnancy only if the benefits outweigh the potential risk. Notify your doctor as soon as you become pregnant or plan to become pregnant.

It is not known whether Geodon appears in breast milk, and breastfeeding is not recommended.

Recommended dosage

SCHIZOPHRENIA

Adults
The usual starting dose is 20 milligrams twice a day. If needed, the dosage may be increased at several-week intervals up to a maximum of 80 milligrams twice a day.

BIPOLAR MANIA (SHORT-TERM TREATMENT
OF ACUTE EPISODES)

Adults
For the first day of treatment, the usual dose is 40 milligrams twice a day. The doctor will then increase the dose on the second day to 60 or 80 milligrams twice a day. Based on your body's response, the dose can be adjusted as needed within the range of 40 to 80 milligrams twice a day.

Overdosage
Any medication taken in excess can have serious consequences. If you suspect an overdose, seek medical help immediately.

■ *Symptoms of Geodon overdose may include:*
   Drowsiness, high blood pressure, slurred speech

Glimepiride See Amaryl, page 86.

Glipizide See Glucotrol, page 625.

Glipizide with Metformin See Metaglip, page 827.

GLUCOPHAGE
Pronounced: GLEW-co-fahj
Generic name: Metformin hydrochloride

Why is this drug prescribed?
Glucophage is an oral antidiabetic medication used to treat type 2 (non-insulin-dependent) diabetes. Diabetes develops when the body proves

unable to burn sugar and the unused sugar builds up in the bloodstream. Glucophage lowers the amount of sugar in your blood by decreasing sugar production and absorption and helping your body respond better to its own insulin, which promotes the burning of sugar. It does not, however, increase the body's production of insulin.

Glucophage is sometimes prescribed along with insulin or certain other oral antidiabetic drugs such as Micronase or Glucotrol. It is also used alone.

Standard Glucophage tablets are taken two or three times daily. An extended-release form (Glucophage XR) is available for once-daily dosing.

Always remember that Glucophage is an aid to, not a substitute for, good diet and exercise. Failure to follow a sound diet and exercise plan can lead to serious complications such as dangerously high or low blood sugar levels. Remember, too, that Glucophage is not an oral form of insulin and cannot be used in place of insulin.

Most important fact about this drug

Glucophage could cause a very rare—but potentially fatal—side effect known as lactic acidosis. It is caused by a buildup of lactic acid in the blood. The problem is most likely to occur in people whose liver or kidneys are not working well, and in those who have multiple medical problems, take several medications, or have congestive heart failure. The risk also is higher if you are an older adult or drink alcohol. Lactic acidosis is a medical emergency that must be treated in a hospital. Notify your doctor immediately if you experience any of the following:

■ *Symptoms of lactic acidosis may include:*
Dizziness, extreme weakness or tiredness, light-headedness, low body temperature, rapid breathing or trouble breathing, sleepiness, slow or irregular heartbeat, unexpected or unusual stomach discomfort, unusual muscle pain

How should you take this medication?

Do not take more or less of this medication than directed by your doctor. The drug should be taken with food to reduce the possibility of nausea or diarrhea, especially during the first few weeks of therapy.

If taking Glucophage XR, be sure to swallow the tablet whole; do not crush it or chew it. The inactive ingredients in the tablet may occasionally appear in the stool. This is not a cause for concern.

■ *If you miss a dose...*
Take it as soon as you remember. If it is almost time for your next dose, skip the one you missed and go back to your regular schedule. Never take 2 doses at the same time.
■ *Storage instructions...*
Store it at room temperature.

What side effects may occur?

Side effects cannot be anticipated. If any develop or change in intensity, tell your doctor as soon as possible. Only your doctor can determine if it is safe for you to continue taking Glucophage.

If side effects from Glucophage occur, they usually happen during the first few weeks of therapy. Most side effects are minor and will go away after you've taken Glucophage for a while.

■ *Side effects may include:*
Abdominal discomfort, diarrhea, gas, headache, indigestion, nausea, vomiting, weakness

Why should this drug not be prescribed?

Glucophage is processed primarily by the kidneys, and can build up to excessive levels in the body if the kidneys aren't working properly. It should be avoided if you have kidney disease or your kidney function has been impaired by a condition such as shock, blood poisoning, or a heart attack.

You should not use Glucophage if you need to take medicine for congestive heart failure.

Do not take Glucophage if you have ever had an allergic reaction to metformin.

Do not take Glucophage if you have metabolic or diabetic ketoacidosis (a life-threatening medical emergency caused by insufficient insulin and marked by excessive thirst, nausea, fatigue, pain below the breastbone, and fruity breath). Diabetic ketoacidosis should be treated with insulin.

Special warnings about this medication

Before you start therapy with Glucophage, and at least once a year thereafter, your doctor will do a complete assessment of your kidney function. If you develop kidney problems while on Glucophage, your doctor will discontinue this medication. If you are an older person, you will need to have your kidney function monitored more frequently, and your doctor may want to start you at a lower dosage.

You should not take Glucophage for 2 days before and after having an X-ray procedure (such as an angiogram) that uses an injectable dye. Also, if you are going to have surgery, except minor surgery, you should stop taking Glucophage. Once you have resumed normal food and fluid intake, your doctor will tell you when you can start drug therapy again.

Avoid drinking too much alcohol while taking Glucophage. Heavy drinking increases the danger of lactic acidosis and can also trigger an attack of low blood sugar.

Because poor liver function could increase the risk of lactic acidosis, your doctor may decide to check your liver function before prescribing Glucophage and periodically thereafter. If you develop liver problems, your doctor may stop treatment with Glucophage.

If you are taking Glucophage, you should check your blood or urine periodically for abnormal sugar (glucose) levels. Your doctor will do annual blood checks to see if Glucophage is causing a vitamin B_{12} deficiency or any other blood problem.

Glucophage does not usually cause hypoglycemia (low blood sugar). However, it remains a possibility, especially in older, weak, and undernourished people and those with kidney, liver, adrenal, or pituitary gland problems. The risk of low blood sugar increases when Glucophage is combined with other diabetes medications. The risk is also boosted by missed meals, alcohol, and excessive exercise. To avoid low blood sugar, you should closely follow the diet and exercise plan suggested by your doctor.

If your blood sugar becomes unstable due to the stress of a fever, injury, infection, or surgery, your doctor may temporarily take you off Glucophage and ask you to take insulin instead.

You should stop taking Glucophage if you become seriously dehydrated, since this increases the likelihood of developing lactic acidosis. Tell your doctor if you lose a significant amount of fluid due to vomiting, diarrhea, fever, or some other condition.

The effectiveness of any oral antidiabetic, including Glucophage, may decrease with time. This may occur because of either a diminished responsiveness to the medication or a worsening of the diabetes.

Possible food and drug interactions when taking this medication

If Glucophage is taken with certain other drugs, the effects of either could be increased, decreased, or altered. It is especially important to check with your doctor before combining Glucophage with the following:

Amiloride (Moduretic)
Calcium channel blockers (heart medications) such as Calan, Isoptin, and Procardia
Cimetidine (Tagamet)
Decongestant, airway-opening drugs such as Sudafed and Ventolin
Digoxin (Lanoxin)
Estrogens such as Premarin
Furosemide (Lasix)
Glyburide (Micronase)
Isoniazid (Rifamate), a drug used for tuberculosis
Major tranquilizers such as Thorazine
Morphine
Niacin (Niaspan)
Nifedipine (Adalat, Procardia)
Oral contraceptives
Phenytoin (Dilantin)
Procainamide (Procanbid, Pronestyl)
Quinidine (Quinidex)
Quinine

Ranitidine (Zantac)
Steroids such as prednisone (Deltasone)
Thyroid hormones such as Synthroid
Triamterene (Dyazide, Dyrenium)
Trimethoprim (Bactrim, Septra)
Vancomycin (Vancocin)
Water pills (diuretics) such as HydroDIURIL, Dyazide, and Moduretic

Do not drink too much alcohol, since excessive alcohol consumption can cause low blood sugar and alcohol enhances some effects of this drug.

Special information if you are pregnant or breastfeeding

If you are pregnant or plan to become pregnant, tell your doctor immediately. Glucophage should not be taken during pregnancy. Since studies suggest the importance of maintaining normal blood sugar (glucose) levels during pregnancy, your doctor may prescribe insulin injections instead.

It is not known whether Glucophage appears in human breast milk. Therefore, women should discuss with their doctors whether to discontinue the medication or to stop breastfeeding. If the medication is discontinued and if diet alone does not control glucose levels, then your doctor may consider insulin injections.

Recommended dosage

Your doctor will tailor your dosage to your individual needs.

ADULTS

Glucophage

The usual starting dose is one 500-milligram tablet twice a day, taken with morning and evening meals. Your doctor may increase your daily dose by 500 milligrams at weekly intervals, based on your response, up to a total of 2,000 milligrams.

An alternative starting dose is one 850-milligram tablet a day, taken with the morning meal. Your doctor may increase this by 850 milligrams at 14-day intervals, to a maximum of 2,550 milligrams a day.

The usual maintenance dose ranges from 1,500 to 2,550 milligrams daily. If you take more than 2,000 milligrams a day, your doctor may recommend that the medication be divided into three doses, taken with each meal.

Glucophage XR

The usual starting dose is one 500-milligram tablet once daily with the evening meal. Your doctor may increase your dose by 500 milligrams at weekly intervals, up to a maximum dosage of 2,000 milligrams a day. If a single 2,000-milligram dose fails to control your blood sugar, you may be asked to take 1,000-milligram doses twice a day. If you need more than 2,000 milligrams a day, the doctor will switch you to regular Glucophage.

CHILDREN

Glucophage
For children 10 to 16 years old, the usual starting dose is one 500-milligram tablet twice a day with meals. The dosage may be increased by 500 milligrams at weekly intervals up to a maximum of 2,000 milligrams daily. Glucophage has not been tested in children younger than 10.

Glucophage XR
This form of the drug has not been tested in children younger than 17.

OLDER ADULTS

Older people and those who are malnourished or in a weakened state are generally given lower doses of Glucophage because their kidneys may be weaker, making side effects more likely.

Overdosage

An overdose of Glucophage can cause lactic acidosis (see *Most important fact about this drug*). If you suspect a Glucophage overdose, seek emergency treatment immediately.

GLUCOTROL

Pronounced: GLUE-kuh-troll
Generic name: Glipizide
Other brand name: Glucotrol XL

Why is this drug prescribed?

Glucotrol is an oral antidiabetic medication used to treat type 2 (non-insulin-dependent) diabetes. In diabetics either the body does not make enough insulin or the insulin that is produced no longer works properly.

There are actually two forms of diabetes: type 1 (insulin-dependent) and type 2 (non-insulin-dependent). Type 1 usually requires insulin injections for life, while type 2 diabetes can usually be treated by dietary changes and/or oral antidiabetic medications such as Glucotrol. Apparently, Glucotrol controls diabetes by stimulating the pancreas to secrete more insulin. If you suffer from type 1 diabetes, you will need to use insulin and will not be able to use Glucotrol. Occasionally, type 2 diabetics must take insulin injections on a temporary basis, especially during stressful periods or times of illness.

Most important fact about this drug

Always remember that Glucotrol is an aid to, not a substitute for, good diet and exercise. Failure to follow a sound diet and exercise plan can lead to serious complications, such as dangerously high or low blood sugar levels. Remember, too, that Glucotrol is *not* an oral form of insulin, and cannot be used in place of insulin.

How should you take this medication?

In general, to achieve the best control over blood sugar levels, Glucotrol should be taken 30 minutes before a meal. However, the exact dosing schedule as well as the dosage amount must be determined by your physician.

Glucotrol XL should be taken with breakfast. Swallow the tablets whole; do not chew, crush, or divide them. Do not be alarmed if you notice something that looks like a tablet in your stool—it will be the empty shell that has been eliminated.

■ *If you miss a dose...*
Take it as soon as you remember. If it is almost time for your next dose, skip the one you missed and go back to your regular schedule. Never take 2 doses at the same time.

■ *Storage instructions...*
Glucotrol should be stored at room temperature and protected from moisture and humidity.

What side effects may occur?

Side effects from Glucotrol are rare and seldom require discontinuation of the medication.

■ *Side effects may include:*
Constipation, diarrhea, dizziness, drowsiness, gas, headache, hives, itching, low blood sugar, nervousness, sensitivity to light, skin rash and eruptions, stomach pain, tremor

Glucotrol and Glucotrol XL, like all oral antidiabetic drugs, can cause low blood sugar. This risk is increased by missed meals, alcohol, other diabetes medications, and excessive exercise. Low blood sugar is also more likely in older people, those with kidney or liver problems, and those with poorly functioning adrenal or pituitary glands. To avoid low blood sugar, you should closely follow the dietary and exercise regimen suggested by your physician.

■ *Symptoms of mild low blood sugar may include:*
Blurred vision, cold sweats, dizziness, fast heartbeat, fatigue, headache, hunger, light-headedness, nausea, nervousness
■ *Symptoms of more severe low blood sugar may include:*
Coma, disorientation, pale skin, seizures, shallow breathing

Ask your doctor what steps you should take if you experience mild hypoglycemia. If symptoms of severe low blood sugar occur, contact your doctor immediately. Severe hypoglycemia should be considered a medical emergency, and prompt medical attention is essential.

Why should this drug not be prescribed?

You should not take Glucotrol if you have had an allergic reaction to it previously.

Glucotrol will be stopped if you are suffering from diabetic ketoacidosis (a life-threatening medical emergency caused by insufficient insulin and marked by excessive thirst, nausea, fatigue, pain below the breastbone, and a fruity breath).

Special warnings about this medication

It's possible that drugs such as Glucotrol may lead to more heart problems than diet treatment alone, or diet plus insulin. If you have a heart condition, you may want to discuss this with your doctor.

If you are taking Glucotrol, you should check your blood and urine periodically for the presence of abnormal sugar (glucose) levels.

Even people with well-controlled diabetes may find that injury, infection, surgery, or fever results in a lack of control over their diabetes. In these cases, the physician may recommend that you stop taking Glucotrol temporarily and use insulin instead.

Glucotrol may not work well in patients with poor kidney or liver function.

In addition, the effectiveness of any oral antidiabetic, including Glucotrol, may decrease with time. This may occur because of either a diminished responsiveness to the medication or a worsening of the diabetes.

Be careful taking the extended-release form of the drug, Glucotrol XL, if you have any narrowing in your stomach or intestines. Also, if you have any stomach or intestinal disease, Glucotrol XL may not work as well.

Possible food and drug interactions when taking this medication

It is essential that you closely follow your physician's dietary guidelines and that you inform your physician of any medication, either prescription or nonprescription, that you are taking. Specific medications that affect Glucotrol include:

Airway-opening drugs such as Sudafed
Antacids such as Mylanta
Aspirin
Chloramphenicol (Chloromycetin)
Cimetidine (Tagamet)
Clofibrate (Atromid-S)
Corticosteroids such as prednisone (Deltasone)
Diuretics such as HydroDIURIL
Estrogens such as Premarin
Fluconazole (Diflucan)
Gemfibrozil (Lopid)
Heart and blood pressure medications called beta-blockers, such as
    Tenormin and Lopressor

Heart medications called calcium channel blockers, such as
  Cardizem and Procardia XL
Isoniazid (Rifamate, Rimactane)
Itraconazole (Sporanox)
Major tranquilizers such as Thorazine and Mellaril
MAO inhibitors (antidepressant drugs such as Nardil and Parnate)
Miconazole (Monistat)
Nicotinic acid (Nicobid)
Nonsteroidal anti-inflammatory drugs such as Motrin and Naprosyn
Oral contraceptives
Phenytoin (Dilantin)
Probenecid (Benemid)
Rifampin (Rifadin)
Sulfa drugs such as Bactrim and Septra
Thyroid medications such as Synthroid
Warfarin (Coumadin)

Alcohol must be used carefully, since excessive alcohol consumption can
cause low blood sugar.

Special information if you are pregnant or breastfeeding

The effects of Glucotrol during pregnancy have not been adequately studied. Therefore, if you are pregnant, or planning to become pregnant, you
should take Glucotrol only on the advice of your physician. Since studies
suggest the importance of maintaining normal blood sugar (glucose)
levels during pregnancy, your physician may prescribe insulin during
pregnancy. To minimize the risk of low blood sugar in newborn babies,
Glucotrol, if taken during pregnancy, should be discontinued at least one
month before the expected delivery date.

Although it is not known if Glucotrol appears in breast milk, other oral
antidiabetics do. Because of the potential for hypoglycemia in nursing
infants, your doctor may advise you either to discontinue Glucotrol or to
stop nursing. If Glucotrol is discontinued and if diet alone does not control glucose levels, your doctor may prescribe insulin.

Recommended dosage

Dosage levels must be determined by each patient's needs.

ADULTS

Glucotrol
The usual recommended starting dose is 5 milligrams taken before
breakfast. Depending upon blood glucose response, your doctor may increase the initial dose in increments of 2.5 to 5 milligrams. The maximum
recommended daily dose is 40 milligrams; total daily dosages above 15
milligrams are usually divided into 2 equal doses that are taken before
meals.

Glucotrol XL

The usual starting dose is 5 milligrams each day at breakfast. After 3 months, your doctor may increase the dose to 10 milligrams daily. The maximum recommended daily dose is 20 milligrams.

CHILDREN

The safety and effectiveness of this drug in children have not been established.

OLDER ADULTS

Older people or those with liver disease usually start Glucotrol therapy with 2.5 milligrams. They can start Glucotrol XL treatment with 5 milligrams.

Overdosage

An overdose of Glucotrol can cause low blood sugar (see *What side effects may occur?*). Eating sugar or a sugar-based product will often correct the condition. Otherwise, seek medical attention immediately.

GLUCOVANCE

Pronounced: GLUE-coe-vance
Generic ingredients: Glyburide, Metformin

Why is this drug prescribed?

Glucovance is used in the treatment of type 2 (non-insulin-dependent) diabetes. Diabetes develops when the body's ability to burn sugar declines and the unused sugar builds up in the bloodstream. Ordinarily, sugar is moved out of the blood and into the body's cells by the hormone insulin. A buildup occurs when the body either fails to make enough insulin or doesn't respond to it properly.

Glucovance is a combination of 2 drugs—glyburide (DiaBeta, Micronase) and metformin (Glucophage)—that attack high blood sugar levels in several ways. The glyburide component stimulates the pancreas to produce more insulin and helps the body use it properly. The metformin component also encourages proper insulin utilization, and in addition works to decrease sugar production and absorption.

Glucovance is prescribed when diet and exercise prove insufficient to keep blood sugar levels under control. Glucovance can also be combined with other diabetes drugs such as Avandia.

Most important fact about this drug

Very rarely, Glucovance has been known to cause a dangerous condition called lactic acidosis, a buildup of lactic acid in the blood. Lactic acidosis is a medical emergency that requires immediate treatment in the hospital.

Notify your doctor without delay if you experience any of the following symptoms: a slow or irregular heartbeat; a cold, dizzy, or light-headed feeling; a weak, tired, or uncomfortable feeling; stomach discomfort; trouble breathing; unusual muscle pain.

How should you take this medication?

Glucovance is taken once or twice a day with meals.

■ *If you miss a dose...*
Take it as soon as you remember. If it is almost time for your next dose, skip the one you missed and go back to your regular schedule. Never take 2 doses at the same time.

■ *Storage instructions...*
Store at room temperature and protect from light.

What side effects may occur?

Side effects cannot be anticipated. If any develop or change in intensity, inform your doctor as soon as possible. Only your doctor can determine if it is safe for you to continue taking Glucovance.

■ *Side effects may include:*
Cold sweats, diarrhea, dizziness, headache, hunger, nausea, shakiness, stomach pain, upper respiratory infections, vomiting

Why should this drug not be prescribed?

Glucovance is processed primarily by the kidneys, and can build up to excessive levels in the body if the kidneys aren't working properly. It should be avoided if you have kidney disease or your kidney function has been impaired by a condition such as shock, blood poisoning, or a heart attack. It should also be avoided if you need to take medicine for congestive heart failure, and you'll probably be unable to use it if you have liver disease.

If you need to have an X-ray procedure done, find out if it requires injection of a contrast agent. If so, Glucovance will have to be temporarily discontinued. (Check with your doctor for instructions; do not discontinue the drug on your own.)

If you have ever had an allergic reaction to metformin, glyburide, or diabetes medications similar to glyburide, you should not take Glucovance. It also should not be prescribed if you have acute or chronic metabolic acidosis.

Special warnings about this medication

Avoid excessive alcohol intake while taking Glucovance. Heavy drinking increases the danger of lactic acidosis and can also trigger an attack of low blood sugar (hypoglycemia).

Missed meals, malnutrition, general debility, liver or kidney problems, other medications, and overexertion also increase the risk of hypoglycemia. Symptoms of a mild case include cold sweats, dizziness, shakiness, and hunger. Severe hypoglycemia can lead to seizures and coma. If you notice any of the warning signs, check with your doctor immediately.

Lactic acidosis also becomes more likely when you become dehydrated. If you experience severe vomiting, diarrhea, or fever, or if your fluid intake is significantly reduced, tell your doctor.

Taking Glucovance with certain diabetes drugs, such as Avandia, can increase the risk of hypoglycemia, weight gain, and liver problems. Your doctor will periodically test your liver function to guard against any problems.

Glucovance occasionally causes a mild deficiency of vitamin B_{12}. Your doctor will check annually and may prescribe a supplement if necessary.

Some experts suspect that the glyburide component of Glucovance may lead to more heart problems than treatment with diet alone. In a long-term trial of a similar drug, researchers noted an increase in heart-related deaths (though the overall mortality rate remained unchanged). If you have a heart condition, you may want to discuss this potential risk with your doctor.

Possible food and drug interactions when taking this medication

If Glucovance is taken with certain other drugs, the effects of either drug could be increased, decreased, or altered. It is especially important to check with your doctor before combining Glucovance with the following:

Airway-opening drugs such as Proventil and Ventolin
Beta-blockers (heart and blood-pressure drugs such as Inderal and Tenormin)
Birth control pills
Calcium channel blockers (heart medications) such as Calan, Isoptin, and Procardia
Chloramphenicol (Chloromycetin)
Ciprofloxacin (Cipro)
Estrogens such as Premarin
HydroDiuril, Lasix, and other diuretics
Isoniazid (Rifamate)
Major tranquilizers such as Compazine, Stelazine, and Thorazine
MAO inhibitors such as the antidepressants Nardil and Parnate
Niacin (Niacor, Niaspan)
Nonsteroidal anti-inflammatory drugs such as Advil, Motrin, Naprosyn, and Voltaren
Phenytoin (Dilantin)
Probenecid
Steroids such as prednisone (Deltasone)
Sulfa drugs such as Bactrim
Thyroid medications such as Synthroid
Warfarin (Coumadin)

Special information if you are pregnant or breastfeeding

Glucovance is not recommended during pregnancy. To control blood sugar during this crucial period, most doctors prefer insulin instead of Glucovance. If you are pregnant or plan to become pregnant, inform your doctor immediately.

You'll also need to avoid Glucovance while breastfeeding. If blood sugar becomes a problem, your doctor can prescribe insulin.

Recommended dosage

ADULTS

Your doctor will start therapy at a low dose and increase it until your blood sugar levels are under control.

Patients Not Previously Treated with Diabetes Medications
The recommended starting dose is 1.25 milligrams of glyburide with 250 milligrams of metformin once or twice daily with meals. The dosage can be increased every two weeks until blood sugar levels are controlled. The maximum recommended daily dosage of Glucovance for previously un-treated patients is 10 milligrams of glyburide with 2,000 milligrams of metformin.

Patients Previously Treated with Glyburide
(or a Similar Drug) or Metformin
The recommended starting dose of Glucovance is either 2.5 or 5 milli-grams of glyburide with 500 milligrams of metformin twice daily with meals. The maximum recommended daily dosage of Glucovance for pre-viously treated patients is 20 milligrams of glyburide with 2,000 milli-grams of metformin.

CHILDREN

Glucovance is not for use in children.

OLDER ADULTS

Since kidney function declines with age, it should be closely monitored in people taking Glucovance after age 65. Older patients are usually not pre-scribed the maximum recommended dose of Glucovance.

Overdosage

An overdose of Glucovance can cause an attack of hypoglycemia requir-ing immediate treatment. If you experience any of the symptoms listed in *Special warnings about this medication,* see a doctor immediately.

An excessive dose of Glucovance can also trigger lactic acidosis. If you begin to notice the warning signs listed in *Most important fact about this drug,* seek emergency treatment.

Glyburide See Micronase, page 854.

Glyburide with Metformin *See Glucovance, page 629.*

Glynase *See Micronase, page 854.*

Goserelin *See Zoladex, page 1644.*

Griseofulvin *See Gris-PEG, below.*

GRIS-PEG

Pronounced: GRISS-peg
Generic name: Griseofulvin
Other brand name: Fulvicin P/G

Why is this drug prescribed?

Gris-PEG is prescribed for the treatment of the following ringworm infections:

> Athlete's foot
> Barber's itch (inflammation of the facial hair follicles)
> Ringworm of the body
> Ringworm of the groin and thigh
> Ringworm of the nails
> Ringworm of the scalp

Because Gris-PEG is effective for only certain types of fungal infections, before treatment your doctor may perform tests to identify the source of infection.

Most important fact about this drug

To clear up your infection completely, continue taking Gris-PEG as prescribed until your doctor tells you to stop. Although some improvement may appear within a few days, you need to take Gris-PEG for an extended period.

How should you take this medication?

To minimize stomach irritation and help your body absorb the drug, take Gris-PEG at mealtimes or with food or whole milk. If you are on a low-fat diet, check with your doctor.

Observe good hygiene during treatment to help control infection and prevent reinfection.

■ *If you miss a dose...*
Take it as soon as you remember. If it is almost time for your next dose, skip the one you missed and go back to your regular schedule. Do not take 2 doses at once.

■ *Storage instructions...*
Store at room temperature in a tightly closed container. Protect from light. Keep the liquid from freezing.

What side effects may occur?

Side effects cannot be anticipated. If any develop or change in intensity, inform your doctor as soon as possible. Only your doctor can determine if it is safe for you to continue taking Gris-PEG.

■ *Side effects may include:*
Hives, skin rashes

Why should this drug not be prescribed?

If you are sensitive to or have ever had an allergic reaction to Gris-PEG or other drugs of this type, you should not take this medication. Make sure your doctor is aware of any drug reactions you have experienced.

Unless you are directed to do so by your doctor, do not take this medication if you have liver damage or porphyria (an inherited disorder of the liver or bone marrow).

Do not take Gris-PEG while pregnant.

Special warnings about this medication

Gris-PEG is similar to penicillin. Although penicillin-sensitive people have used Gris-PEG without difficulty, notify your doctor if you are sensitive to or allergic to penicillin.

Because Gris-PEG can make you sensitive to light, avoid exposure to intense natural or artificial sunlight.

Notify your doctor if you develop lupus erythematosus (a form of rheumatism) or a lupus-like condition. Signs and symptoms of lupus include arthritis, red "butterfly" rash over the nose and cheeks, tiredness, weakness, sensitivity to sunlight, and skin eruptions.

If you are being treated with Gris-PEG for an extended period of time, your doctor should perform regular tests, including periodic monitoring of kidney function, liver function, and blood cell production.

Gris-PEG has not been proved safe and effective for the prevention of fungal infections.

Gris-PEG may decrease the effectiveness of birth control pills. Use additional protection while you are taking Gris-PEG.

Men should wait at least 6 months after finishing therapy with griseofulvin before they father a child.

Women should avoid becoming pregnant while they are taking the drug.

Possible food and drug interactions when taking this medication

Gris-PEG may intensify the effects of alcohol. If you drink alcohol while taking this medication, your heart may start beating faster and your skin may be flushed.

If Gris-PEG is taken with certain other drugs, the effects of either could be increased, decreased, or altered. It is especially important to check with your doctor before combining Gris-PEG with the following:

Barbiturates such as phenobarbital
Blood-thinning drugs such as Coumadin
Oral contraceptives

Special information if you are pregnant or breastfeeding

Do not take Gris-PEG if you are pregnant. If you become pregnant while taking this drug, notify your doctor immediately. There is a potential hazard to the developing baby.

If you are breastfeeding, consult with your doctor before taking Gris-PEG.

Recommended dosage

The usual treatment periods for various ringworm infections are:

Ringworm of the scalp: 4 to 6 weeks
Ringworm of the body: 2 to 4 weeks
Athlete's foot: 4 to 8 weeks

The usual treatment period, depending on the rate of growth, for ringworm of the fingernails is at least 4 months and for ringworm of the toenails at least 6 months.

ADULTS

Ringworm of the Body, Groin and Thigh, Scalp
The usual dosage is 375 milligrams a day taken as a single dose or divided into smaller doses, as determined by your doctor.

Athlete's Foot, Ringworm of the Nails
The usual dosage is 750 milligrams a day divided into smaller doses, as determined by your doctor.

CHILDREN

A single daily dose is effective in children with ringworm of the scalp.

The usual dosage is 3.3 milligrams per pound of body weight per day. This means that children weighing 35 to 60 pounds will take 125 to 187.5 milligrams a day, and children weighing more than 60 pounds will take 187.5 to 375 milligrams a day.

No dosage has been established for children 2 years of age and under.

Overdosage

Any medication taken in excess can have dangerous consequences. If you suspect an overdose of Gris-PEG, seek emergency medical treatment immediately.

Guaifenesin with Codeine *See Tussi-Organidin NR,*
page 1510.

GUANABENZ ACETATE
Pronounced: GWAHN-ah-benz

Why is this drug prescribed?
This drug is used in the treatment of high blood pressure. It is effective used alone or in combination with a thiazide type of diuretic. Guanabenz begins to lower blood pressure within 60 minutes after taking a single dose and may slow your pulse rate slightly.

Most important fact about this drug
You must take guanabenz regularly for it to be effective. Since blood pressure declines gradually, it may be several weeks before you get the full benefit of guanabenz; and you must continue taking it even if you are feeling well. Guanabenz does not cure high blood pressure; it merely keeps it under control.

How should you take this medication?
Guanabenz may be taken with or without food. Take it exactly as prescribed.

■ *If you miss a dose...*
Take it as soon as you remember. If it is almost time for the next dose, skip the one you missed and go back to your regular schedule. Do not take 2 doses at the same time. If you forget the medication 2 or more times in a row, contact your doctor.

■ *Storage instructions...*
Store at room temperature, in a tightly closed container, away from light.

What side effects may occur?
Side effects cannot be anticipated. If any develop or change in intensity, inform your doctor as soon as possible. Only your doctor can determine if it is safe for you to continue taking guanabenz.

■ *Side effects may include:*
Dizziness, drowsiness, dry mouth, headache, weakness

Why should this drug not be prescribed?
Do not take guanabenz if you are sensitive to it or have ever had an allergic reaction to it.

Special warnings about this medication
Guanabenz can make you drowsy or less alert. Driving or operating dangerous machinery or participating in any hazardous activity that requires full mental alertness is not recommended until you know how this drug affects you.

If you have severe heart disease, stroke or related disorders, or severe liver or kidney failure, or if you have recently had a heart attack, this drug should be used with caution.

Your doctor will monitor your blood pressure if you have disorders of the kidney or liver.

Possible food and drug interactions when taking this medication

Guanabenz may intensify the effects of alcohol. Use of alcohol should be avoided.

If guanabenz is taken with certain other drugs, the effects of either could be increased, decreased, or altered. It is especially important to check with your doctor before combining guanabenz with the following:

Antihistamines such as Benadryl, Chlor-Trimeton, and Tavist
Drugs that depress the central nervous system, such as Halcion, Valium, and phenobarbital

Special information if you are pregnant or breastfeeding

The effects of guanabenz during pregnancy have not been adequately studied, but it may affect the fetus. If you are pregnant or plan to become pregnant, inform your doctor immediately. Guanabenz may appear in breast milk and could affect a nursing infant. If this medication is essential to your health, your doctor may advise you to discontinue breastfeeding until your treatment is finished.

Recommended dosage

ADULTS

Your doctor will adjust the dosage of this medication to meet your individual needs.

The usual starting dose is 4 milligrams 2 times per day, whether guanabenz is used alone or with a thiazide type of diuretic.

Your doctor may increase the dosage in increments of 4 to 8 milligrams per day every 1 to 2 weeks, depending on your response.

The maximum reported dose has been 32 milligrams twice daily, but doses as high as this are rarely needed.

CHILDREN

The safety and effectiveness of this drug have not been established in children under 12 years of age.

OLDER ADULTS

Older adults should use this drug with caution.

Overdosage

Any medication taken in excess can have serious consequences. If you suspect an overdose, seek medical attention immediately.

■ *Symptoms of guanabenz overdose may include:*
Excessive contraction of the pupils, irritability, low blood pressure, sleepiness, slow heartbeat, sluggishness

GUANFACINE HYDROCHLORIDE
Pronounced: GWAHN-fah-seen

Why is this drug prescribed?
Guanfacine is given to help control high blood pressure. This medication reduces nerve impulses to the heart and arteries; this slows the heartbeat, relaxes the blood vessels, and thus reduces blood pressure. Guanfacine may be given alone or in combination with other high blood pressure medications, especially thiazide diuretics, such as Diuril, Esidrix, or Naturetin.

Most important fact about this drug
You must take guanfacine regularly for it to be effective. Since blood pressure declines gradually, it may be several weeks before you get the full benefit of guanfacine; and you must continue taking it even if you are feeling well. Guanfacine does not cure high blood pressure; it merely keeps it under control.

How should you take this medication?
Take guanfacine exactly as prescribed by your doctor—usually 1 dose per day. Guanfacine should be taken at bedtime, since it will probably cause drowsiness.

After 3 or 4 weeks, if your blood pressure is still too high, your doctor may raise the dosage of guanfacine. In some cases, you may take 2 evenly spaced doses per day rather than a single dose at bedtime.

■ *If you miss a dose...*
Take the forgotten dose as soon as you remember. This will help to keep the proper amount of medicine in your body. However, if it is almost time for the next dose, skip the one you missed and go back to your regular schedule. Never try to catch up by doubling the dose. If you miss taking guanfacine for 2 or more days in a row, check with your doctor.

■ *Storage instructions...*
Store guanfacine at room temperature. Use the container it came in.

What side effects may occur?
Side effects cannot be anticipated. If any develop or change in intensity, inform your doctor as soon as possible. Only your doctor can determine whether it is safe for you to continue taking guanfacine. This medication will probably make you drowsy, especially when you first begin to take it.

■ *Side effects may include:*
Constipation, dizziness, dry mouth, fatigue, headache, impotence, sleepiness, weakness

Some of these side effects may lessen or disappear as your body gets used to guanfacine.

Why should this drug not be prescribed?
Do not take guanfacine if you are sensitive to it or have ever had an allergic reaction to it.

Guanfacine is not recommended for controlling the severe high blood pressure that accompanies toxemia of pregnancy (a disorder of pregnant women characterized by a rise in blood pressure, swelling, and leakage of protein into urine).

Special warnings about this medication
While taking guanfacine, you should be monitored very closely by your doctor if you have any of the following medical conditions:

Chronic kidney or liver failure
Heart disease
History of stroke
Recent heart attack

Since guanfacine causes drowsiness and may also make you dizzy, do not drive, climb, or perform hazardous tasks until you find out exactly how the medication affects you.

While taking guanfacine, use alcoholic beverages with care; you may feel intoxicated after drinking only a small amount of alcohol.

If you have kidney damage and also take the antiseizure drug phenytoin (Dilantin), your body may process and eliminate guanfacine rather quickly; in that case, you may need fairly frequent doses of guanfacine to lower your blood pressure adequately.

If you have been taking guanfacine for a while, do not stop taking it without consulting your doctor. Discontinuing abruptly may result in nervousness, rapid pulse, anxiety, heartbeat irregularities, and so-called rebound high blood pressure (higher than before you started taking guanfacine). If you do have rebound high blood pressure, it will probably develop 2 to 4 days after your last dose of guanfacine. Rebound high blood pressure, if it occurs, will usually diminish and then disappear over a period of 2 to 4 days.

Possible food and drug interactions when taking this medication
If guanfacine is taken with certain other drugs, the effects of either could be increased, decreased, or altered. It is especially important to check with your doctor before combining guanfacine with the following:

Barbiturates such as Amytal, Seconal, Tuinal, and others
Benzodiazepines such as Tranxene, Valium, Xanax, and others
Phenothiazines such as Mellaril, Stelazine, Thorazine, and others
Phenytoin (Dilantin)

Special information if you are pregnant or breastfeeding

If you are pregnant or plan to become pregnant, notify your doctor immediately. Guanfacine should be taken during pregnancy only if clearly needed. It is not known whether guanfacine appears in breast milk. Check with your doctor if you plan to breastfeed.

Recommended dosage

ADULTS

The usual recommended dose of guanfacine is 1 milligram daily, taken at bedtime. If necessary, after 3 to 4 weeks your doctor may increase the daily dosage to 2 milligrams.

CHILDREN

The safety and effectiveness of guanfacine have not been established in children under 12 years of age.

Overdosage

Any medication taken in excess can have serious consequences. If you suspect an overdose of guanfacine, seek medical attention immediately.

■ *Symptoms of guanfacine overdose may include:*
   Drowsiness, lethargy, slowed heartbeat, very low blood pressure

GYNE-LOTRIMIN

Pronounced: GUY-nuh-LOW-trim-in
Generic name: Clotrimazole
Other brand names: Lotrimin, Mycelex, Mycelex-7

Why is this drug prescribed?

Clotrimazole, the active ingredient in these medications, is used to treat fungal infections. In preparations for the skin, it is effective against ringworm, athlete's foot, and jock itch. In vaginal creams and tablets, it is used against vaginal yeast infections. In lozenge form, it is prescribed to treat oral yeast infections and to prevent them in people with weak immune systems.

Most important fact about this drug

Keep using this medicine for the full time of treatment, even if the infection seems to have disappeared. If you stop too soon, the infection could return. You should continue using the vaginal forms of this medicine even during your menstrual period.

How should you take this medication?

Keep all forms of this medicine away from your eyes.

Before applying the skin preparations, be sure to wash your hands. Massage the medication gently into the affected area and the surrounding skin.

If you are taking Mycelex troches, place the lozenge in your mouth and let it dissolve slowly for 15 to 30 minutes. Do not chew the lozenge or swallow it whole.

To administer a vaginal cream or tablet:
1. Load the applicator to the fill line with cream, or unwrap a tablet, wet it with warm water, and place it in the applicator as shown in the instructions you receive with the product.
2. Lie on your back with your knees drawn up.
3. Gently insert the applicator high into the vagina and push the plunger.
4. Withdraw the applicator and discard it if disposable, or wash with soap and water.

To keep the vaginal medication from getting on your clothing, wear a sanitary napkin. Do not use a tampon because it will absorb the medicine. Wear underwear or pantyhose with a cotton crotch—avoid synthetic fabrics such as nylon or rayon. Do not douche unless your doctor tells you to do so.

■ *If you miss a dose...*
Make up for it as soon as you remember. If it is almost time for the next dose, skip the one you missed and go back to your regular schedule.
■ *Storage instructions...*
Store at room temperature, away from heat, light, and moisture.

What side effects may occur?

Side effects cannot be anticipated. If any develop or change in intensity, inform your doctor as soon as possible. Only your doctor can determine if it is safe for you to continue using this medication.

■ *Side effects may include:*
Blistering, burning, hives, irritated skin, itching, peeling, reddened skin, stinging, swelling due to fluid retention

■ *Side effects of clotrimazole vaginal preparations may include:*
Abdominal/stomach cramps/pain, burning/irritation of penis of sexual partner, headache, hives, pain during sexual intercourse, skin rash, vaginal burning, vaginal irritation, vaginal itching, vaginal soreness during sexual intercourse

An unpleasant mouth sensation has been reported by some people taking Mycelex.

Why should this drug not be prescribed?

You should not be using this medication if you have had an allergic reaction to any of its ingredients.

Special warnings about this medication

Contact your doctor if you experience increased skin irritations (such as redness, itching, burning, blistering, swelling, or oozing).

Check with your doctor before using this medication on a child.

In general, if your symptoms have not improved within 2 to 4 weeks of treatment, notify your doctor.

Clotrimazole vaginal preparations should not be used if you have abdominal pain, fever, or a foul-smelling vaginal discharge. Contact your doctor immediately.

While using the vaginal preparations, either avoid sexual intercourse or make sure your partner uses a condom. This will prevent reinfection. Oils used in some vaginal preparations can weaken latex condoms or diaphragms. To find out whether you can use your medication with latex products, check with your pharmacist.

Possible food and drug interactions when taking this medication

None has been reported.

Special information if you are pregnant or breastfeeding

The use of clotrimazole during the first trimester of pregnancy has not been adequately studied. It should be used during the first trimester only if clearly needed. Do not use clotrimazole at any time during pregnancy without the advice and supervision of your doctor.

It is not known whether clotrimazole appears in breast milk. Nursing mothers should use this medication cautiously and only when clearly needed.

Recommended dosage

LOTRIMIN

Adults and Children

Wash your hands before and after you use Lotrimin. Apply in the morning and evening. Use enough Lotrimin to massage into the affected area.

Symptoms usually improve during the first week of treatment with Lotrimin.

GYNE-LOTRIMIN CREAM

ADULTS
Fill the applicator with the cream and insert 1 applicatorful into the vagina every day, preferably at bedtime. Repeat this procedure for 7 consecutive days.

MYCELEX TROCHE

ADULTS
The recommended dosage is 1 troche slowly dissolved in the mouth 5 times daily for 14 consecutive days. For prevention, the recommended dose is 1 troche 3 times daily.

Overdosage
Although any medication used in excess can have serious consequences, an overdose of clotrimazole is unlikely. If you suspect an overdose, however, seek medical help immediately.

Habitrol *See Nicotine Patches, page 939*.

HALCION
Pronounced: HAL-see-on
Generic name: Triazolam

Why is this drug prescribed?
Halcion is used for short-term treatment of insomnia. It is a member of the benzodiazepine class of drugs, many of which are used as tranquilizers.

Most important fact about this drug
Sleep problems are usually temporary, requiring treatment for only a short time, usually 1 or 2 days and no more than 1 to 2 weeks. Insomnia that lasts longer than this may be a sign of another medical problem. If you find you need this medicine for more than 7 to 10 days, be sure to check with your doctor.

How should you take this medication?
Take this medication exactly as directed; never take more than your doctor has prescribed.

■ *If you miss a dose...*
Take Halcion only as needed.

■ *Storage instructions...*
Keep this medication in the container it came in, tightly closed, and out of reach of children. Store it at room temperature.

What side effects may occur?
Side effects cannot be anticipated. If any develop or change in intensity, inform your doctor as soon as possible. Only your doctor can determine if it is safe for you to continue taking Halcion.

■ *Side effects may include:*
Coordination problems, dizziness, drowsiness, headache, light-headedness, nausea/vomiting, nervousness

Why should this drug not be prescribed?
You should not take this drug if you are pregnant or if you have had an allergic reaction to it or to other benzodiazepine drugs such as Valium.

Also avoid Halcion if you are taking the antifungal medications Nizoral or Sporanox, or the antidepressant Serzone.

Special warnings about this medication
When Halcion is used every night for more than a few weeks, it loses its effectiveness to help you sleep. This is known as tolerance. Also, it can cause dependence, especially when it is used regularly for longer than a few weeks or at high doses.

Abrupt discontinuation of Halcion should be avoided, since it has been associated with withdrawal symptoms (convulsions, cramps, tremor, vomiting, sweating, feeling ill, perceptual problems, and insomnia). A gradual dosage-tapering schedule is usually recommended for patients taking more than the lowest dose of Halcion for longer than a few weeks. The usual treatment period is 7 to 10 days.

If you develop unusual and disturbing thoughts or behavior—including increased anxiety or depression—during treatment with Halcion, you should discuss them with your doctor immediately.

Traveler's amnesia has been reported by patients who took Halcion to induce sleep while traveling. To avoid this condition, do not take Halcion on an overnight airplane flight of less than 7 to 8 hours.

You may suffer increased anxiety during the daytime while taking Halcion.

When you first start taking Halcion, until you know whether the medication will have any carryover effect the next day, use extreme care while doing anything that requires complete alertness such as driving a car or operating machinery.

After discontinuing the drug, you may experience rebound insomnia for the first 2 nights—that is, insomnia may be worse than before you took the sleeping pill.

You should be aware that anterograde amnesia (forgetting events after an injury) has been associated with benzodiazepine drugs such as Halcion.

You should be cautious about using this drug if you have liver or kidney problems, lung problems, or a tendency to temporarily stop breathing while you are asleep.

Possible food and drug interactions when taking this medication

Avoid alcoholic beverages and grapefruit juice.

If Halcion is taken with certain other drugs, the effects of either could be increased, decreased, or altered. It is especially important to check with your doctor before combining Halcion with the following:

Amiodarone (Cordarone)
Antidepressant medications, including tricyclic drugs such as Elavil
   and MAO inhibitors such as Nardil and Parnate
Antihistamines such as Benadryl and Tavist
Barbiturates such as phenobarbital and Seconal
Cimetidine (Tagamet)
Clarithromycin (Biaxin)
Cyclosporine (Sandimmune Neoral)
Diltiazem (Cardizem)
Ergotamine (Cafergot)
Erythromycin (E.E.S., PCE, E-Mycin, others)
Fluvoxamine
Isoniazid (Nydrazid)
Itraconazole (Nizoral)
Ketoconazole (Sporanox)
Narcotic painkillers such as Demerol
Major tranquilizers such as Mellaril and chlorpromazine
Nefazodone
Nicardipine (Cardene)
Nifedipine (Adalat)
Other tranquilizers such as BuSpar, Valium, and Xanax
Oral contraceptives
Paroxetine (Paxil)
Ranitidine (Zantac)
Seizure medications such as Dilantin and Tegretol
Sertraline (Zoloft)
Verapamil (Calan)

Special information if you are pregnant or breastfeeding

Since benzodiazepines have been associated with damage to the developing baby, you should not take Halcion if you are pregnant, think you may be pregnant, or are planning to become pregnant; or if you are breastfeeding.

Recommended dosage

ADULTS

The usual dose is 0.25 milligram before bedtime. The dose should never be more than 0.5 milligram.

CHILDREN

The safety and effectiveness of Halcion for children under the age of 18 have not been established.

OLDER ADULTS

To decrease the possibility of oversedation, dizziness, or impaired coordination, the usual starting dose is 0.125 milligram. This may be increased to 0.25 milligram if necessary.

Overdosage

Any medication taken in excess can have serious consequences. Severe overdosage of Halcion can be fatal. If you suspect an overdose, seek medical help immediately.

■ *Symptoms of Halcion overdose may include:*
Apnea (temporary cessation of breathing), coma, confusion, excessive sleepiness, problems in coordination, seizures, shallow or difficult breathing, slurred speech

HALDOL
Pronounced: HAL-dawl
Generic name: Haloperidol

Why is this drug prescribed?
Haldol is used to reduce the symptoms of mental disorders such as schizophrenia. It is also prescribed to control tics (uncontrolled muscle contractions of face, arms, or shoulders) and the unintended utterances that mark Tourette's syndrome. In addition, it is used in short-term treatment of children with severe behavior problems, including hyperactivity and combativeness.

Some doctors also prescribe Haldol to relieve severe nausea and vomiting caused by cancer drugs, to treat drug problems such as LSD flashback and PCP intoxication, and to control symptoms of hemiballismus, a condition that causes involuntary writhing of one side of the body.

Most important fact about this drug
Haldol may cause tardive dyskinesia—a condition characterized by involuntary muscle spasms and twitches in the face and body. This condition can be permanent, and appears to be most common among the elderly,

especially women. Ask your doctor for information about this possible risk.

How should you take this medication?

Haldol may be taken with food or after eating. If taking Haldol in a liquid concentrate form, you will need to dilute it with milk or water.

You should not take Haldol with coffee, tea, or other caffeinated beverages, or with alcohol.

Haldol causes dry mouth. Sucking on a hard candy or ice chips may help alleviate the problem.

■ *If you miss a dose...*
Take it as soon as you remember. Take the rest of the doses for that day at equally spaced intervals. Do not take 2 doses at once.

■ *Storage instructions...*
Store away from heat, light, and moisture in a tightly closed container. Do not freeze the liquid.

What side effects may occur?

Side effects cannot be anticipated. If any side effects develop or change in intensity, inform your doctor as soon as possible. Only your doctor can determine if it is safe for you to continue taking Haldol.

■ *Side effects may include:*
Breast development in men, breathing problems, cataracts, constipation, drowsiness, dry mouth, insomnia, involuntary muscle contractions, skin reactions, tardive dyskinesia (see *Most important fact about this drug*), tightening of the throat muscles, weight loss

Why should this drug not be prescribed?

You should not take Haldol if you have Parkinson's disease or are sensitive to or allergic to the drug.

Special warnings about this medication

You should use Haldol cautiously if you have ever had breast cancer, a severe heart or circulatory disorder, chest pain, the eye condition known as glaucoma, seizures, or any drug allergies.

Temporary muscle spasms and twitches may occur if you suddenly stop taking Haldol. Follow your doctor's instructions closely when discontinuing the drug.

This drug may impair your ability to drive a car or operate potentially dangerous machinery. Do not participate in any activities that require full alertness if you are unsure of your reaction to Haldol.

Haldol may make your skin more sensitive to sunlight. When spending time in the sun, use a sunscreen or wear protective clothing.

Avoid exposure to extreme heat or cold. Haldol interferes with the body's temperature-regulating mechanism, so you could become over-heated or suffer severe chills.

Possible food and drug interactions when taking this medication
Extreme drowsiness and other potentially serious effects can result if Haldol is combined with alcohol, narcotics, painkillers, sleeping medications, or other drugs that slow down the central nervous system.

If Haldol is taken with certain other drugs, the effects of either could be increased, decreased, or altered. It is especially important to check with your doctor before combining Haldol with the following:

Antiseizure drugs such as Dilantin and Tegretol
Antispasmodic drugs such as Bentyl and Cogentin
Blood-thinning medications such as Coumadin
Certain antidepressants, including Elavil, Tofranil, and Prozac
Epinephrine (EpiPen)
Lithium (Eskalith, Lithobid)
Methyldopa (Aldomet)
Propranolol (Inderal)
Rifampin (Rifadin)

Special information if you are pregnant or breastfeeding
The effects of Haldol during pregnancy have not been adequately studied. Pregnant women should use Haldol only if clearly needed. If you are pregnant or plan to become pregnant, inform your doctor immediately. Haldol should not be used by women who are breastfeeding an infant.

Recommended dosage

ADULTS

Moderate Symptoms
The usual dosage is 1 to 6 milligrams daily. This amount should be divided into 2 or 3 smaller doses.

Severe Symptoms
The usual dosage is 6 to 15 milligrams daily, divided into 2 or 3 smaller doses.

CHILDREN

Children younger than 3 years old should not take Haldol.

For children between the ages of 3 and 12, weighing approximately 33 to 88 pounds, doses should start at 0.5 milligram per day. Your doctor will increase the dose if needed.

Psychotic Disorders
The daily dose may range from 0.05 milligram to 0.15 milligram for every 2.2 pounds of body weight.

Non-Psychotic Behavior Disorders and Tourette's Syndrome
The daily dose may range from 0.05 milligram to 0.075 milligram for every 2.2 pounds of body weight.

OLDER ADULTS

In general, older people take dosages of Haldol in the lower ranges. Older adults (especially older women) may be more susceptible to tardive dyskinesia, a possibly irreversible condition marked by involuntary muscle spasms and twitches in the face and body. Consult your doctor for information about these potential risks.

Doses may range from 1 to 6 milligrams daily.

Overdosage

Any medication taken in excess can have serious consequences. If you suspect an overdose, seek medical help immediately.

■ *Symptoms of Haldol overdose may include:*
Catatonic (unresponsive) state, coma, decreased breathing, low blood pressure, rigid muscles, sedation, tremor, weakness

Halfprin *See Aspirin, page 132.*

Halobetasol *See Ultravate, page 1524.*

Haloperidol *See Haldol, page 646.*

HELIDAC THERAPY

Pronounced: HEL-i-dak
Generic ingredients: Bismuth subsalicylate, Metronidazole,
*   Tetracycline hydrochloride*

Why is this drug prescribed?

Helidac is a drug combination that cures the infection responsible for most stomach ulcers. Although ulcers used to be blamed on stress and spicy food, doctors now know that a germ called *Helicobacter pylori* is the actual culprit in a majority of cases.

Most important fact about this drug

You need to take all of the Helidac pills 4 times each day for 14 days. (You should also be taking an acid blocker such as Zantac, Pepcid, or Tagamet.) If you fail to stick to this regimen, the infection may not be cured.

How should you take this medication?

There are four pills in each dose of Helidac. The two pink tablets (bismuth subsalicylate) should be chewed and swallowed. The white tablet (metronidazole) and the orange and white capsule (tetracycline) should be swallowed whole. Be sure to drink at least 8 ounces of fluid with each dose—especially at bedtime—to prevent irritation.

■ *If you miss a dose...*
Take the next dose at the appointed time and continue with your regular schedule until the medication is used up. Do not try to catch up by doubling a dose. If you miss more than 4 doses, contact your physician.

■ *Storage instructions...*
Store at room temperature.

What side effects may occur?
Side effects cannot be anticipated. If any develop or change in intensity, inform your doctor as soon as possible. Only your doctor can determine if it is safe for you to continue taking Helidac.

■ *Side effects may include:*
Abdominal pain, diarrhea, nausea

Why should this drug not be prescribed?
Do not take Helidac if you have ever had an allergic reaction to any of the following medications:

Aspirin
Flagyl (metronidazole)
Pepto-Bismol (bismuth subsalicylate)
Tetracycline
Vibramycin (doxycycline)

Helidac is not for use by children and pregnant or nursing women. The tetracycline part of the therapy can harm a developing baby, stunt a child's growth, and interfere with tooth development.

You should also avoid Helidac if you have kidney or liver disease.

Special warnings about this medication
Don't be alarmed if your tongue and/or bowel movements turn black while you are taking Helidac. This is a harmless side effect of the bismuth subsalicylate part of the therapy.

The tetracycline part of Helidac therapy increases the risk of getting a bad sunburn. Limit your exposure to the sun. If you notice a reddening of your skin, stop taking Helidac and call your doctor.

If you develop a headache and blurred vision, numbness and tingling in the arms and legs, or seizures, stop taking Helidac and call your doctor immediately. Also report any infection that develops and be sure your doctor is aware of any infection or blood disorder you already have.

Possible food and drug interactions when taking this medication
Combining aspirin with Helidac sometimes causes ringing in the ears. If this happens, check with your doctor. You may need to temporarily stop taking aspirin.

During Helidac therapy, alcoholic beverages can cause abdominal cramps, nausea, vomiting, headache, and flushing. Avoid alcohol until at least 1 day after finishing Helidac.

For 1 hour before and 2 hours after each dose of Helidac, avoid eating dairy products. They can interfere with the medication's absorption.

Since Helidac can interfere with oral contraceptives, you should use an additional form of birth control during Helidac therapy.

Do not start Helidac therapy if you have taken the anti-alcohol drug Antabuse within the past 2 weeks.

Certain other drugs may also interact. Check with your doctor before combining Helidac with any of the following:

Antacids containing aluminum, calcium, or magnesium
Blood-thinning drugs such as warfarin (Coumadin)
Cimetidine (Tagamet)
Diabetes medications such as insulin and glyburide (Micronase)
Iron (including vitamins that contain iron)
Lithium (Eskalith, Lithobid)
Penicillin
Phenobarbital
Phenytoin (Dilantin)
Probenecid (Benemid)
Sodium bicarbonate (baking soda)
Sulfinpyrazone (Anturane)
Zinc (including vitamins that contain zinc)

Special information if you are pregnant or breastfeeding
Do not undertake Helidac therapy during this period.

Recommended dosage

ADULTS

Take all 4 Helidac pills 4 times daily, with each meal and at bedtime.

Overdosage
An overdose of the bismuth subsalicylate part of Helidac can be fatal. The other components can have serious consequences as well.

■ *Symptoms of Helidac overdose may include:*
Confusion, coma, convulsions, coordination problems, diarrhea, fast heartbeat, high fever, lethargy, nausea, numbness or pain in the arms and legs, rapid breathing, ringing in the ears, severe heart and lung problems, vomiting

If you suspect an overdose, seek medical attention immediately.

HIVID

Pronounced: HIV-id
Generic name: Zalcitabine

Why is this drug prescribed?

Hivid is one of the drugs used against the human immunodeficiency virus (HIV)—the deadly cause of AIDS. HIV does its damage by slowly undermining the immune system, finally leaving the body without any defense against infection. Hivid staves off collapse of the immune system by interfering with the virus's ability to reproduce.

Hivid is often combined with a protease inhibitor (Crixivan, Invirase, and Norvir) as part of the regimen of drugs that has proven so effective in halting or even reversing the progress of HIV. Hivid can also be combined with the HIV drug Retrovir, provided you have not already been taking Retrovir for more than 3 months. For people with advanced cases of HIV, Hivid is sometimes prescribed by itself when other drugs don't work or can't be tolerated.

Most important fact about this drug

Although Hivid can slow the progress of HIV, it is not a cure. You may continue to develop complications, including frequent infections. Even if you feel better, regular physical exams and blood counts by your doctor are highly advisable. Also be sure to notify your doctor immediately if you experience any changes in your general health.

How should you take this medication?

Hivid should be taken every 8 hours, exactly as prescribed. It is important to keep levels of the drug in your body as constant as possible, so be sure to take every scheduled dose. Never take more than the prescribed dose; nerve disorders could result.

■ *If you miss a dose...*
Take it as soon as you remember. If it is almost time for the next dose, skip the one you missed and go back to your regular schedule. Never take 2 doses at once.

■ *Storage instructions...*
Store at room temperature in a tightly closed bottle.

What side effects may occur?

Although side effects can never be predicted, they are more likely—and more apt to be severe—in people with an advanced case of HIV. If any side effects develop or change in intensity, inform your doctor as soon as possible. Only your doctor can determine if it is safe for you to continue using Hivid.

■ *Side effects may include:*
Abdominal pain, fatigue, hives, itching, mouth sores and inflammation, nausea and vomiting, rash, tingling, burning, numbness, or pain in the hands and feet

There have been isolated reports of an extremely wide variety of additional problems occurring during Hivid therapy. Whether these problems were caused by the drug remains unclear. Nevertheless, it's wise to check with your doctor whenever any unexplained symptom develops.

Why should this drug not be prescribed?
If Hivid gives you an allergic reaction, you cannot use this medication.

Special warnings about this medication
If you have an advanced case of HIV, there is a one-in-three chance that Hivid will cause a serious nerve disorder called peripheral neuropathy. The first signs of this problem are numbness, tingling, and burning pain in the hands and feet. Check with your doctor as soon as any of these symptoms develops. If you continue to take Hivid, they will be followed by episodes of intense, sharp, shooting pain or severe, continuous, burning pain—and the condition could become irreversible. If Hivid is stopped promptly, the symptoms will gradually disappear.

Much more rarely, Hivid has been known to cause a dangerous inflammation of the pancreas (pancreatitis), especially in people who have previously had the problem. The chief signs are bouts of severe abdominal pain—usually lasting for days—accompanied by nausea and vomiting. If these symptoms develop, call your doctor without delay. Hivid therapy must be discontinued permanently.

Other rare but dangerous side effects to watch for include liver failure, weakening of the heart, and ulcers in the mouth and the canal to the stomach (esophagus). Kidney disease increases the risk of these side effects. If you've ever had kidney, liver, or heart problems, have hepatitis, or tend to abuse alcohol, be sure your doctor is aware of the situation. If you develop a liver problem, treatment with Hivid may have to be stopped.

Like other HIV drugs, Hivid sometimes causes a redistribution of body fat, resulting in added weight around the waist, a "buffalo hump" of fat on the upper back, breast enlargement, and wasting of the face, arms, and legs. It's not known why this occurs, or what long-term effects it might have.

Remember that Hivid does not eliminate HIV from the body. The infection can still be passed to others through sexual contact or blood contamination.

Possible food and drug interactions when taking this medication
A number of drugs can cause peripheral neuropathy and should not be taken with Hivid. The list includes:

Chloramphenicol (Chloromycetin)
Cisplatin (Platinol)
Dapsone
Disulfiram (Antabuse)
Ethionamide (Trecator-SC)
Glutethimide
Gold
Hydralazine
Iodoquinol (Yodoxin)
Isoniazid (Nydrazid)
Metronidazole (Flagyl)
Nitrofurantoin (Macrodantin)
Phenytoin (Dilantin)
Ribavirin (Virazole)
Vincristine (Oncovin)

Several other drugs should be either avoided or taken with caution while on Hivid therapy. Check with your doctor before taking the following:

Aminoglycoside antibiotics such as Garamycin
Amphotericin B (Fungizone)
Antacids containing magnesium and aluminum, including Maalox
    and Mylanta
Cimetidine (Tagamet)
Didanosine (Videx)
Foscarnet (Foscavir)
Lamivudine (Epivir)
Metoclopramide
Pentamidine (Pentam)
Probenecid

Special information if you are pregnant or breastfeeding

The safety of Hivid during pregnancy has not been adequately studied. Take contraceptive measures while using Hivid. If you are pregnant or plan to become pregnant, notify your doctor immediately.

Do not breastfeed your baby. HIV can be passed to an infant through breast milk.

Recommended dosage

ADULTS

The usual dose is one 0.750-milligram tablet every 8 hours. Your doctor may adjust the dosage if you have kidney problems. Hivid is recommended for use in combination with other HIV medications.

CHILDREN

The safety and effectiveness of Hivid have not been established for children under 13.

Overdosage

Any medication taken in excess can have serious consequences. If you suspect an overdose, seek medical attention immediately.

■ *Symptoms of Hivid overdose may include:*
Drowsiness, vomiting, numbness, tingling, burning, and pain in the arms and legs

Humalog *See Insulin, page 689.*

Humulin *See Insulin, page 689.*

HYDERGINE
Pronounced: HY-der-jeen
Generic name: Ergoloid mesylates

Why is this drug prescribed?

Hydergine helps relieve symptoms of declining mental capacity, thought to be related to aging or dementia, seen in some people over age 60. The symptoms include reduced understanding and motivation, and a decline in self-care and interpersonal skills.

Most important fact about this drug

It may take several weeks or more for Hydergine to produce noticeable results. In fact, your doctor may need up to 6 months to determine whether the drug is right for you. Keep taking your regular doses even if you feel no effect.

How should you take this medication?

Take Hydergine exactly as prescribed.

■ *If you miss a dose...*
Skip the dose you missed and go back to your regular schedule Do not take 2 doses at once. If you miss 2 or more doses in a row, consult your doctor.
■ *Storage instructions...*
Store at room temperature. Protect from heat and light. Do not freeze capsules or oral solution.

What side effects may occur?

Side effects cannot be anticipated. If any develop or change in intensity, notify your doctor as soon as possible. Only your doctor can determine whether it is safe to continue taking Hydergine.

■ *Side effects may include:*
Stomach upset, temporary nausea

Why should this drug not be prescribed?
Do not use Hydergine if you have ever had an allergic reaction to or are sensitive to the drug, or if you have a mental disorder.

Special warnings about this medication
Since the symptoms treated with Hydergine are of unknown origin and may change or evolve into a specific disease, your doctor will make a careful diagnosis before prescribing Hydergine and then watch closely for any changes in your condition.

Possible food and drug interactions when taking this medication
No interactions have been reported.

Special information if you are pregnant or breastfeeding
Hydergine is not intended for use by women of childbearing age.

Recommended dosage

ADULTS

The usual dose of Hydergine is 1 milligram, 3 times a day.

Overdosage
Any medication taken in excess can have serious consequences. If you suspect an overdose of Hydergine, seek medical attention immediately.

Hydrocet See Vicodin, page 1557.

Hydrochlorothiazide See HydroDIURIL, page 658.

Hydrochlorothiazide with Triamterene See Dyazide, page 485.

Hydrocodone with Acetaminophen See Vicodin, page 1557.

Hydrocodone with Chlorpheniramine polistirex
    See Tussionex, page 1508.

Hydrocodone with Ibuprofen See Vicoprofen, page 1560.

HYDROCORTISONE SKIN PREPARATIONS
Pronounced: hi-droh-COURT-i-zone
Brand names: Cetacort, Hytone, Nutracort

Why is this drug prescribed?
Hydrocortisone creams and lotions contain a steroid medication that relieves a variety of itchy rashes and inflammatory skin conditions.

Most important fact about this drug

When you apply a hydrocortisone cream or lotion, you inevitably absorb some of the medication through your skin and into the bloodstream. Too much absorption can lead to unwanted side effects elsewhere in the body. To keep this problem to a minimum, avoid using large amounts of hydrocortisone over extensive areas, and do not cover it with airtight dressings such as plastic wrap or adhesive bandages unless specifically told to by your doctor.

How should you use this medication?

Use hydrocortisone exactly as directed, and only to treat the condition for which your doctor prescribed it.

Apply the medication directly to the affected area. Hydrocortisone cream and lotion are for use only on the skin. Be careful to keep them out of your eyes.

If you are using hydrocortisone for psoriasis or a condition that has been difficult to cure, your doctor may advise you to use a bandage or covering over the affected area. If an infection develops, remove the bandage and contact your doctor.

■ *If you miss a dose...*
Apply it as soon as you remember. If it is almost time for the next dose, skip the one you missed and go back to your regular schedule.
■ *Storage instructions...*
Keep the container tightly closed, and store it at room temperature, away from heat. Protect from freezing.

What side effects may occur?

Side effects cannot be anticipated. If any develop or change in intensity, inform your doctor as soon as possible. Only your doctor can determine if it is safe for you to continue using hydrocortisone.

■ *Side effects may include:*
Acne-like skin eruptions, burning, dryness, growth of excessive hair, inflammation of the hair follicles, inflammation around the mouth, irritation, itching, peeling skin, prickly heat, secondary infection, skin inflammation, skin softening, stretch marks, unusual lack of skin color

Why should this drug not be prescribed?

Do not use hydrocortisone if it has ever given you an allergic reaction.

Special warnings about this medication

Avoid covering a treated area with waterproof diapers or plastic pants. They can increase unwanted absorption of hydrocortisone.

If you use this medication over large areas of skin for prolonged periods of time—or cover the treated area—the amount of the hormone absorbed into your bloodstream may eventually lead to Cushing's syndrome: a moon-faced appearance, fattened neck and trunk, and purplish streaks on the skin. You can also develop glandular problems or high blood sugar, or show sugar in your urine. Children, because of their relatively larger ratio of skin surface area to body weight, are particularly susceptible to overabsorption of hydrocortisone.

Long-term treatment of children with steroids such as hydrocortisone may interfere with growth and development.

If an irritation develops, stop using the medication and contact your doctor.

Possible food and drug interactions when using this medication
No interactions have been reported.

Special information if you are pregnant or breastfeeding
The effects of hydrocortisone during pregnancy have not been adequately studied. If you are pregnant or plan to become pregnant, inform your doctor immediately. It is not known whether this medication appears in breast milk in sufficient amounts to affect a nursing baby. To avoid any possible harm to your baby, use hydrocortisone sparingly, and only with your doctor's permission, when breastfeeding.

Recommended dosage

ADULTS

Apply hydrocortisone cream or lotion to the affected area 2 to 4 times a day, depending on the severity of the condition.

CHILDREN

Limit use to the least amount necessary, as directed by your doctor.

Overdosage
Extensive or long-term use can cause Cushing's syndrome (see *Special warnings about this medication*), glandular problems, higher than normal amounts of sugar in the blood, and high amounts of sugar in the urine. If you suspect an overdose of hydrocortisone, seek medical treatment immediately.

HYDRODIURIL

Pronounced: High-dro-DYE-your-il
Generic name: Hydrochlorothiazide
Other brand name: Esidrix

Why is this drug prescribed?
HydroDIURIL is used in the treatment of high blood pressure and other conditions that require the elimination of excess fluid (water) from the

body. These conditions include congestive heart failure, cirrhosis of the liver, corticosteroid and estrogen therapy, and kidney disorders. When used for high blood pressure, HydroDIURIL can be used alone or with other high blood pressure medications. HydroDIURIL contains a form of thiazide, a diuretic that prompts your body to produce and eliminate more urine, which helps lower blood pressure.

Most important fact about this drug

If you have high blood pressure, you must take HydroDIURIL regularly for it to be effective. Since blood pressure declines gradually, it may be several weeks before you get the full benefit of HydroDIURIL; and you must continue taking it even if you are feeling well. HydroDIURIL does not cure high blood pressure; it merely keeps it under control.

How should you take this medication?

Take HydroDIURIL exactly as prescribed by your doctor.

■ *If you miss a dose...*
If you forget a dose, take it as soon as you remember. If it is almost time for your next dose, skip the one you missed and go back to your regular schedule. Never take 2 doses at the same time.

■ *Storage instructions...*
Keep container tightly closed. Protect from light, moisture, and freezing cold. Store at room temperature.

What side effects may occur?

Side effects cannot be anticipated. If any develop or change in intensity, inform your doctor as soon as possible. Only your doctor can determine if it is safe for you to continue taking HydroDIURIL.

■ *Side effects may include:*
Abdominal cramping, diarrhea, dizziness upon standing up, headache, loss of appetite, low blood pressure, low potassium (leading to symptoms such as dry mouth, excessive thirst, muscle pain or cramps, weak or irregular heartbeat), stomach irritation, stomach upset, weakness

■ *Less common or rare side effects may include:*
Anemia, blood disorders, changes in blood sugar, constipation, difficulty breathing, dizziness, fever, fluid in the lung, hair loss, high levels of sugar in the urine, hives, hypersensitivity reactions, impotence, inflammation of the lung, inflammation of the pancreas, inflammation of the salivary glands, kidney failure, muscle spasms, nausea, rash, reddish or purplish spots on the skin, restlessness, sensitivity to light, skin disorders including Stevens-Johnson syndrome (blisters in the mouth and eyes), skin peeling, tingling or pins and needles, vertigo, vision changes, vomiting, yellow eyes and skin

Why should this drug not be prescribed?

If you are unable to urinate, you should not take this medication.

If you are sensitive to or have ever had an allergic reaction to HydroDIURIL or similar drugs, or if you are sensitive to sulfa or other sulfonamide-derived drugs, you should not take this medication.

Special warnings about this medication

Diuretics can cause your body to lose too much potassium. Signs of an excessively low potassium level include muscle weakness and rapid or irregular heartbeat. To boost your potassium level, your doctor may recommend eating potassium-rich foods or taking a potassium supplement.

If you are taking HydroDIURIL, your kidney function should be given a complete assessment, and should continue to be monitored.

If you have liver disease, diabetes, gout, or lupus erythematosus (a form of rheumatism), HydroDIURIL should be used with caution.

If you have bronchial asthma or a history of allergies, you may be at greater risk for an allergic reaction to this medication.

Dehydration, excessive sweating, severe diarrhea or vomiting could deplete your body's fluids and cause your blood pressure to become too low. Be careful when exercising and in hot weather.

Possible food and drug interactions when taking this medication

HydroDIURIL may increase the effects of alcohol. Do not drink alcohol while taking this medication.

If HydroDIURIL is taken with certain other drugs, the effects of either could be increased, decreased, or altered. It is especially important to check with your doctor before combining HydroDIURIL with the following:

Barbiturates such as phenobarbital
Cholestyramine (Questran)
Colestipol (Colestid)
Corticosteroids such as prednisone and ACTH
Digoxin (Lanoxin)
Drugs to treat diabetes such as insulin or Micronase
Lithium (Lithonate)
Narcotics such as Percocet
Nonsteroidal anti-inflammatory drugs such as Naprosyn
Norepinephrine (Levophed)
Other high blood pressure medications such as Aldomet
Skeletal muscle relaxants, such as tubocurarine

Special information if you are pregnant or breastfeeding

The effects of HydroDIURIL during pregnancy have not been adequately studied. If you are pregnant or plan to become pregnant, inform your doctor immediately. HydroDIURIL appears in breast milk and could affect a nursing infant. If this medication is essential to your health, your doctor may advise you to discontinue breastfeeding until your treatment is finished.

Recommended dosage

Dosage should be adjusted to each individual's needs. The smallest dose that is effective should be used.

ADULTS

Water Retention
The usual dose is 25 to 100 milligrams per day. Your doctor may tell you to take the drug in a single dose or to divide the total amount into more than one dose. Your doctor may put you on a day on, day off schedule or some other alternate day schedule to suit your needs.

High Blood Pressure
The usual dose is 25 milligrams as a single dose. Your doctor may increase the dose to 50 milligrams, as a single dose or divided into 2 doses. Dosages should be adjusted when used with other high blood pressure medications.

CHILDREN

Dosages for children should be adjusted according to weight, generally 0.5 to 1 milligram per pound of body weight in 1 or 2 doses per day. Infants under 2 years should not receive more than 37.5 milligrams per day, and children aged 2 to 12 should not get more than 100 milligrams a day. Infants under 6 months may need 1.5 milligrams per pound per day in 2 doses.

Under 2 years
Based on age and body weight, the daily dosage is 12.5 to 37.5 milligrams per day.

2 to 12 years
The daily dosage, based on body weight, is 37.5 to 100 milligrams.
    HydroDIURIL tablets come in strengths of 25, 50 and 100 milligrams.

Overdosage

Any medication taken in excess can cause symptoms of overdose. If you suspect an overdose, seek medical attention immediately.

■ *Symptoms of HydroDIURIL overdose may include:*
    Dry mouth, excessive thirst, muscle pain or cramps, nausea and vomiting, weak or irregular heartbeat, weakness and dizziness

Hydromorphone *See Dilaudid, page 447.*

Hydroxychloroquine *See Plaquenil, page 1104.*

Hydroxyzine *See Atarax, page 142.*

Hyoscyamine *See Levsin, page 742.*

Hytone *See Hydrocortisone Skin Preparations, page 656.*

HYTRIN

Pronounced: HIGH-trin
Generic name: Terazosin hydrochloride

Why is this drug prescribed?

Hytrin is prescribed to reduce high blood pressure. It may be used alone or in combination with other blood pressure–lowering drugs, such as HydroDIURIL (a diuretic) or Inderal, a beta-blocker.

Hytrin is also prescribed to relieve the symptoms of benign prostatic hyperplasia or BPH. BPH is an enlargement of the prostate gland that surrounds the urinary canal. It leads to the following symptoms:

- Weak or interrupted stream when urinating
- Feeling that you cannot empty your bladder completely
- Feeling of delay when you start to urinate
- Need to urinate often, especially at night
- Feeling that you must urinate right away

Hytrin relaxes the tightness of a certain type of muscle in the prostate and at the opening of the bladder. This can reduce the severity of the symptoms.

Most important fact about this drug

If you have high blood pressure, you must take Hytrin regularly for it to be effective. Since blood pressure declines gradually, it may be several weeks before you get the full benefit of Hytrin; and you must continue taking it even if you are feeling well. Hytrin does not cure high blood pressure; it merely keeps it under control.

How should you take this medication?

You may take Hytrin with or without food. Take your first dose at bedtime. Do not take more than the 1 milligram your doctor has prescribed.

- *If you miss a dose...*
  Take it as soon as you remember. If it is almost time for the next dose, skip the one you missed and go back to your regular schedule. Do not take 2 doses at the same time.
- *Storage instructions...*
  Store at room temperature in a cool, dry place. Protect from light.

What side effects may occur?

Side effects cannot be anticipated. If any develop or change in intensity, inform your doctor as soon as possible. Only your doctor can determine if it is safe for you to continue taking Hytrin.

■ *Side effects may include:*
Difficult or labored breathing, dizziness, headache, heart palpitations, light-headedness upon standing, nausea, pain in the arms and legs, sleepiness, stuffy nose, swollen wrists and ankles, weakness

If these symptoms persist, tell your doctor. Your dosage of Hytrin may be higher than needed.

Why should this drug not be prescribed?

Do not take Hytrin if you are sensitive to it or have ever had an allergic reaction to it.

Special warnings about this medication

When your blood pressure falls in response to Hytrin, you may faint. Other less severe reactions include dizziness, heart palpitations, light-headedness, and drowsiness. You are also likely to feel dizzy or faint whenever you rise from a sitting or lying position; this should disappear as your body becomes accustomed to Hytrin. If your occupation is such that these symptoms might cause serious problems, make sure your doctor knows this from the start; he or she will increase your Hytrin dosage very cautiously.

Regardless of your occupation, avoid driving, climbing, and other hazardous tasks at the following times:

■ For 12 hours after your first dose of Hytrin
■ With each new dosage increase
■ When you restart Hytrin after any treatment interruption

If you are taking Hytrin for benign prostatic hyperplasia, remember that although Hytrin helps relieve the symptoms of BPH, it does NOT change the size of the prostate, which may continue to grow. You may still need surgery in the future. In addition, it *is* possible to have BPH and prostate cancer at the same time.

If you develop the side effect called priapism—a painful erection that last for hours—call your doctor without delay. The condition can lead to impotence if not treated immediately.

Possible food and drug interactions when taking this medication

If Hytrin is taken with certain other drugs, the effects of either could be increased, decreased, or altered. It is especially important to check with your doctor before combining Hytrin with the following:

Nonsteroidal anti-inflammatory painkillers such as Motrin and Naprosyn

Other blood pressure medications, such as Dyazide, Vasotec, Calan, and Verelan

Special information if you are pregnant or breastfeeding

The effects of Hytrin during pregnancy have not been adequately studied. If you are pregnant or plan to become pregnant, notify your doctor immediately. Hytrin is not recommended during pregnancy unless the benefit outweighs the potential risk to the unborn baby. It is not known whether Hytrin appears in breast milk. Because many drugs do appear in breast milk, your doctor may advise you to stop breastfeeding until your treatment with this drug is finished.

Recommended dosage

ADULTS

High Blood Pressure
The usual initial dose is 1 milligram at bedtime. Your doctor may slowly increase the dose until your blood pressure has been lowered sufficiently. The usual recommended dosage range is 1 to 5 milligrams taken once a day; however, some people may benefit from doses as high as 20 milligrams per day.

Benign Prostatic Hyperplasia
The starting dose is 1 milligram at bedtime. Your doctor will gradually increase the dose to 10 milligrams, taken once a day, usually for at least 4 to 6 weeks. A few men have needed a dose of 20 milligrams a day.

If you stop taking Hytrin for several days or longer, your doctor will restart your treatment with 1 milligram at bedtime.

CHILDREN

The safety and effectiveness of Hytrin in children have not been established.

Overdosage

If you take too much Hytrin, dizziness, light-headedness, and fainting may occur within 90 minutes. A large overdose may lead to shock. If you suspect an overdose of Hytrin, seek medical attention immediately.

HYZAAR

Pronounced: HIGH-zahr
*Generic ingredients: Losartan potassium and
    Hydrochlorothiazide*

Why is this drug prescribed?

Hyzaar is a combination medication used in the treatment of high blood pressure. One component, losartan, belongs to a new class of blood pressure medications that work by preventing the hormone angiotensin II from constricting the blood vessels, thus allowing blood to flow more freely and keeping the blood pressure down. The other component, hydrochlorothiazide, is a diuretic that increases the output of urine, removing excess fluid from the body and thus lowering blood pressure.

Most important fact about this drug

You must take Hyzaar regularly for it to be effective. Since blood pressure declines gradually, it may be several weeks before you get the full benefit of Hyzaar, and you must continue taking it even if you are feeling well. Hyzaar does not cure high blood pressure; it merely keeps it under control.

How should you take this medication?

Hyzaar may be taken with or without food. Take Hyzaar exactly as directed. Try to take it at the same time each day so that it is easier to remember.

■ *If you miss a dose...*
Take the forgotten dose as soon as you remember. If it is almost time for your next dose, skip the one you missed and go back to your regular schedule.

■ *Storage instructions...*
Keep in a tightly closed container at room temperature. Protect from light.

What side effects may occur?

Side effects cannot be anticipated. If any develop or change in intensity, inform your doctor as soon as possible. Only your doctor can determine if it is safe for you to continue taking Hyzaar.

■ *Side effects include:*
Dizziness, upper respiratory infection

Why should this drug not be prescribed?

If you have ever had an allergic reaction to losartan, hydrochlorothiazide, or sulfa drugs, you should not take this medication. If you are unable to urinate, do not take Hyzaar.

Special warnings about this medication

If you are taking Hyzaar and have kidney disease, your doctor will watch your kidney function carefully.

Hyzaar can cause low blood pressure, especially if you are also taking another diuretic. You may feel light-headed or faint, especially during the first few days of therapy. If these symptoms occur, contact your doctor. Your dosage may need to be adjusted or discontinued. If you actually faint, stop taking the medication until you have talked to your doctor.

If you have liver or kidney disease, diabetes, gout, or lupus erythematosus, Hyzaar should be used with caution. This drug may bring out hidden diabetes. If you are already taking insulin or oral diabetes drugs, your medication may have to be adjusted. If you have bronchial asthma or a history of allergies, you may be at greater risk for an allergic reaction to this medication.

Excessive sweating, severe diarrhea, or vomiting could deplete your body fluids and cause your blood pressure to drop too low. Be careful when exercising and in hot weather. Call your doctor if your mouth becomes dry, you feel weak or tired or sluggish, you are unusually thirsty, you feel restless or confused, you ache all over, your heart starts beating faster, or you are nauseated. Rare but serious allergic reactions to Hyzaar have been reported. If you develop swelling of the face, lips, or throat, call your doctor immediately. Serious swelling could obstruct your breathing.

Possible food and drug interactions when taking this medication
Hyzaar may increase the effects of alcohol. Avoid alcohol while taking this medication.

If Hyzaar is taken with certain other drugs, the effects of either could be increased, decreased, or altered. It is especially important to check with your doctor before taking Hyzaar with the following:

Barbiturates such as phenobarbital and Seconal
Cholestyramine (Questran)
Colestipol (Colestid)
Corticosteroids (Prednisone)
Diuretics that leave potassium in the body, such as Aldactone,
    triamterene, and amiloride
Indomethacin (Indocin)
Insulin
Ketoconazole (Nizoral)
Lithium (Eskalith, Lithobid)
Narcotic painkillers such as Demerol, Tylenol with Codeine, and
    Percocet
Nonsteroidal anti-inflammatory drugs such as Aleve, Anaprox, and
    Motrin
Other blood pressure–lowering drugs such as Procardia XL and
    Tenormin
Oral diabetes drugs such as Diabinese, DiaBeta, and Glucotrol
Potassium supplements such as Slow-K
Salt substitutes containing potassium
Sulfaphenazole
Troleandomycin (Tao)

Special information if you are pregnant or breastfeeding
When used in the second or third trimester of pregnancy, Hyzaar can cause injury or even death to the unborn child. Stop taking Hyzaar as

soon as you know you are pregnant. If you are pregnant or plan to become pregnant, tell your doctor immediately. Hyzaar appears in breast milk and can affect the nursing infant. If this medication is essential to your health, your doctor may advise you to stop breastfeeding while you are taking Hyzaar.

Recommended dosage

ADULTS

Hyzaar comes in two strengths, 50-12.5 (50 milligrams of losartan and 12.5 milligrams of hydrochlorothiazide) and 100-25 (a double dose of each component). The usual starting dose is one 50-12.5 tablet per day.

If your blood pressure does not respond to this dose, after about 3 weeks the doctor may increase the dose to two 50-12.5 tablets once daily, or one 100-25 tablet a day.

CHILDREN

The safety and effectiveness of Hyzaar in children have not been studied.

Overdosage

Any medication taken in excess can have serious consequences. Information concerning Hyzaar overdosage is limited. However, extremely low blood pressure and abnormally rapid or slow heartbeat may be signs of an overdose. Other signs may include dryness and thirst, overall weakness and tiredness, restlessness and confusion, muscle pains, nausea, and vomiting.

If you suspect an overdose, seek medical attention immediately.

Ibuprofen See *Motrin, page 895.*

Iletin See *Insulin, page 689.*

IMDUR
Pronounced: IM-duhr
Generic name: Isosorbide mononitrate
Other brand names: Ismo, Monoket

Why is this drug prescribed?
Imdur is prescribed to prevent angina pectoris (crushing chest pain that results when partially clogged arteries restrict the flow of needed oxygen-rich blood to the heart muscle). This medication does not relieve angina attacks already under way.

Most important fact about this drug
Imdur may cause severe low blood pressure (possibly marked by dizziness or fainting), especially when you are standing or if you sit up quickly.

People taking blood pressure medication and those who have low blood pressure should use Imdur with caution.

How should you take this medication?

To maintain this drug's protective effect, it is important that you take it exactly as prescribed.

Take Imdur once a day, when you get up in the morning. It may be taken with or without food. Imdur tablets should not be crushed or chewed. Swallow them with half a glass of liquid.

Do not switch to another brand of isosorbide mononitrate without consulting your doctor or pharmacist.

■ *If you miss a dose...*
Take it as soon as you remember. If it is almost time for your next dose, skip the one you missed and go back to your regular schedule. Do not take 2 doses at the same time.

■ *Storage instructions...*
Store at room temperature.

What side effects may occur?

Side effects cannot be anticipated. If any develop or change in intensity, tell your doctor as soon as possible. Only your doctor can determine if it is safe for you to continue taking Imdur.

Headache is the most common side effect; usually, aspirin or acetaminophen will relieve the pain. The headaches associated with Imdur usually subside within a short time after treatment with the drug begins. Check with your doctor if your headaches persist or become more intense. Another common side effect is dizziness.

Why should this drug not be prescribed?

You should not take Imdur if you have had a previous allergic reaction to it or to other heart medications containing nitrates or nitrites. Your doctor will probably not prescribe Imdur if you have recently had a heart attack or congestive heart failure. If the doctor decides that this medication is essential, your heart function and blood pressure will need to be closely monitored to avoid potential side effects.

Special warnings about this medication

Do not abruptly stop taking this medication. Follow your doctor's plan for a gradual withdrawal.

Since Imdur can cause dizziness, you should be careful while driving, operating machinery, or performing other tasks that demand concentration.

Nitrate-type medications such as Imdur may aggravate angina caused by certain heart conditions.

Do not try to avoid a headache by changing your dose. If your headache stops, it may mean the drug has lost its effectiveness.

Be sure to tell your doctor about any medical conditions you have before starting Imdur therapy.

Possible food and drug interactions when taking this medication

If Imdur is taken with certain other drugs, the effects of either could be increased, decreased, or altered. Extremely low blood pressure with dizziness and fainting upon standing up may occur if Imdur is taken with the impotence drug Viagra or calcium-blocking blood pressure medications such as Calan, Cardizem, and Procardia.

Alcohol may interact with Imdur and cause a swift decrease in blood pressure, possibly resulting in light-headedness.

Special information if you are pregnant or breastfeeding

The effects of Imdur during pregnancy have not been adequately studied. If you are pregnant or plan to become pregnant, tell your doctor immediately. Imdur should be used during pregnancy only if it is clearly needed.

It is not known whether Imdur appears in breast milk. If the drug is essential to your health, your doctor may advise you to stop nursing until your treatment is finished.

Recommended dosage

ADULTS

The usual starting dose is 30 milligrams (taken as a single 30-milligram tablet or as one-half of a 60-milligram tablet) or 60 milligrams once a day.

After several days, your doctor may increase the dose to 120 milligrams (a single 120-milligram tablet or two 60-milligram tablets) once daily.

Your doctor may further adjust the dosage according to your response to the medication.

CHILDREN

The safety and effectiveness of Imdur in children have not been established.

Overdosage

Any medication taken in excess can have serious consequences. Severe overdosage of Imdur can be fatal. If you suspect an overdose, seek medical help immediately.

■ *Symptoms of Imdur overdose may include:*
Air hunger, bloody diarrhea, coma, confusion, difficulty breathing, fainting, fever, nausea, palpitations, paralysis, pressure in the head, profuse sweating, seizures, skin either cold and clammy or flushed, slow heartbeat, throbbing headache, vertigo, visual disturbances, vomiting

Imipramine *See Tofranil, page 1448.*

IMITREX

Pronounced: IM-i-trex
Generic name: Sumatriptan succinate

Why is this drug prescribed?

Imitrex is prescribed for the treatment of a migraine attack with or without the presence of an aura (visual disturbances, usually sensations of halos or flickering lights, which precede an attack). The injectable form is also used to relieve cluster headache attacks. (Cluster headaches come on in waves, then disappear for long periods of time. They are limited to one side of the head, and occur mainly in men.)

Imitrex cuts headaches short. It will not reduce the number of attacks you experience.

Most important fact about this drug

Imitrex should be used only to treat an acute, classic migraine attack or a cluster headache. It should not be used for certain unusual types of migraine.

How should you take this medication?

Imitrex should be taken as soon as your symptoms appear, but may be used at any time during an attack. It is available in three forms: injection, tablets, and nasal spray.

Imitrex injection is administered just below the skin with an autoinjector (self-injection device). Choose a site where the skin is thick enough to take the full length of the needle (¼ inch). Avoid injecting Imitrex into a muscle or a vein. Your doctor should instruct you on how to use the autoinjector and how to dispose of the empty syringes. You should also read the instruction pamphlet that comes with the medication.

You can take a second injection if your headache returns; however, never take more than 2 injections within 24 hours, and be sure to wait 1 hour between doses.

Imitrex tablets should be swallowed whole, with liquid. If you have had no relief 2 hours after taking Imitrex tablets, you may take a second dose of up to 100 milligrams, if your doctor advises it. If the headache returns, you may take additional doses at intervals of at least 2 hours. You should not take more than 300 milligrams in one day. If your headache returns after you have had an Imitrex injection, you may take single Imitrex tablets, at intervals of at least 2 hours, up to a maximum of 200 milligrams in a day.

Imitrex nasal spray is packaged in single-dose bottles containing either 5 or 20 milligrams of the drug. The usual dosage is a single spray in one nostril. If the headache returns, you may repeat the dose once after 2 hours. Do not take more than 40 milligrams a day.

■ *If you miss a dose...*
Imitrex is *not* for regular use. Take it only during an attack.
■ *Storage instructions...*
Store Imitrex away from heat and light, at room temperature, in the case provided. If your medication has expired (the expiration date is printed on the treatment pack), throw it away as instructed, but keep the autoinjector. If your doctor decides to stop your treatment, do not keep any leftover medicine unless your doctor tells you to. Throw away your medicine as instructed.

What side effects may occur?
Side effects cannot be anticipated. If any develop or change in intensity, inform your doctor as soon as possible. Only your doctor can determine if it is safe for you to continue taking Imitrex.

■ *Side effects may include:*
Burning sensation, dizziness or vertigo, feeling of heaviness, feeling of tightness, flushing, mouth and tongue discomfort, muscle weakness, nausea (nasal spray), neck pain and stiffness, numbness, pressure sensation, redness at the site of injection, sinus or nasal discomfort (nasal spray), sore throat, tingling, unusual taste (nasal spray), vomiting (nasal spray), warm/cold sensation

In addition to the above side effects, people taking Imitrex for cluster headache may experience nausea, a pins and needles sensation, vomiting, or wheezing.

Why should this drug not be prescribed?
Imitrex should not be used for the hemiplegic or basilar forms of migraine. You must also avoid Imitrex if it gives you an allergic reaction.

In addition, the drug should not be prescribed if you have certain types of heart or blood vessel disease, including angina (crushing chest pain) or a history of heart attack, stroke, mini-strokes, or other circulatory problems. It should not be used if you have severe liver disease or uncontrolled high blood pressure. It must not be used within 24 hours of taking an ergotamine-based migraine remedy (such as D.H.E. 45 Injection or Sansert) or any drug in the same class as Imitrex (such as Amerge, Maxalt, or Zomig). And it must not be used for 2 weeks after taking an MAO inhibitor drug such as the antidepressants Nardil and Parnate.

Special warnings about this medication
Although the danger is minimal, Imitrex has triggered serious heart problems in people with heart disease. For that reason, the doctor may want

you to take your first dose of Imitrex in the office, where you can be closely watched for ill effects.

Be sure to tell the doctor if you have any conditions that increase your risk of heart disease, such as high blood pressure, high cholesterol, or diabetes. Also let him know if you smoke, have heart disease in the family, or have gone through menopause. Patients at risk of heart disease should have periodic cardiac evaluations as long as they continue using Imitrex. If you develop pain or tightness in the chest, throat, or jaw after taking a dose, consult your doctor before taking any more.

If you develop severe chest pain, call the doctor immediately. Also seek immediate attention if you suffer sudden, severe abdominal pain after a dose of Imitrex. It could signal a blood vessel problem.

Be careful not to inject Imitrex into a vein. This can cause a serious heart irregularity.

If your fingers turn pale, then blue, after a dose of Imitrex, you may have a circulatory problem such as hardening of the arteries. Be sure to let your doctor know.

This medication should not be used for other types of migraine headache. If the first dose does not relieve your symptoms, your doctor will re-evaluate you; you may not have migraine or cluster headache.

If your headache does not feel like any you have been experiencing, do not take Imitrex.

Use Imitrex cautiously if you have liver or kidney disease. Also, if you have any trouble with your eyes, tell your doctor.

Imitrex is not recommended for adults over 65. It has not been tested in children.

Although very rare, severe and even fatal allergic reactions have occurred in people taking Imitrex. Such reactions are more likely in people who have several allergies.

In rare cases, people have suffered seizures after taking Imitrex. Use the drug with caution if you have epilepsy or any condition that increases your risk of having a seizure.

Possible food and drug interactions when taking this medication

If Imitrex is taken with certain other drugs, the effects of either may be increased, decreased, or altered. It is important to check with your doctor before combining Imitrex with the following:

Drugs classified as MAO inhibitors, including the antidepressants Nardil and Parnate
Ergot-containing drugs such as Cafergot and Ergostat
Fluoxetine (Prozac)
Fluvoxamine (Luvox)
Paroxetine (Paxil)
Sertraline (Zoloft)

Special information if you are pregnant or breastfeeding
The effects of Imitrex during pregnancy have not been adequately studied. If you are pregnant or plan to become pregnant, inform your doctor
immediately. Imitrex does appear in breast milk and could affect a nursing infant. If this medication is essential to your health, your doctor may
advise you to discontinue breastfeeding until your treatment with Imitrex
is finished.

Recommended dosage

IMITREX INJECTION

The maximum single recommended adult dose is 6 milligrams injected
under the skin.
    The maximum recommended dose that may be given within 24 hours
is two 6 milligram injections taken at least 1 hour apart.

IMITREX TABLETS

The usual adult dose is one 25-, 50-, or 100-milligram tablet taken with
water or other liquid. The most you should take at one time is 100 milligrams, and the most you should take in 1 day is 200 milligrams. Doses
should be spaced at least 2 hours apart.
    If you have liver disease, you should not take more than 50 milligrams
of Imitrex tablets at one time.

IMITREX NASAL SPRAY

The recommended adult dose ranges from 5 to 20 milligrams taken when
the attack begins and repeated once, if necessary, 2 hours later. Doses are
usually taken as a single spray in one nostril, but if a 10-milligram dose
works best for you, you can take it as a 5-milligram spray in each nostril.
Do not use more than 20 milligrams at a time, or take more than 40 milligrams a day.

Overdosage
Any medication taken in excess can have serious consequences. If you
suspect an overdose, seek medical attention immediately.

- ■ *Symptoms of Imitrex overdose may include:*
    Bluish tinge to the skin, convulsions, dilated pupils, inactivity, lack of
    coordination, paralysis, redness in the arms and legs, skin changes at
    the site of injection, slow breathing, sluggishness, tremor

IMODIUM

Pronounced: i-MOH-dee-um
Generic name: Loperamide hydrochloride

Why is this drug prescribed?

Imodium controls symptoms of diarrhea, including traveler's diarrhea. It works by slowing the activity of the intestines and affecting the movement of water and chemicals through the bowel. It can be purchased over the counter in liquid and capsule form under the brand name Imodium A-D.

Most important fact about this drug

If your diarrhea does not stop after a couple of days, or your symptoms get worse, notify your doctor immediately.

How should you take this medication?

Do not take more than the prescribed dose of this medication.

Imodium may cause dryness of the mouth. Sucking on a hard candy or chewing gum can help relieve the problem.

■ *If you miss a dose...*
Take only after each loose stool as directed.
■ *Storage instructions...*
Store at room temperature.

What side effects may occur?

Side effects reported from the use of Imodium are difficult to distinguish from symptoms associated with diarrhea. Those reported, however, were more commonly observed during the treatment of long-lasting diarrhea.

■ *Side effects may include:*
Abdominal distention, abdominal pain or discomfort, allergic reactions, including skin rash, constipation, dizziness, drowsiness, dry mouth, nausea and vomiting, tiredness

Why should this drug not be prescribed?

If you are sensitive to or have ever had an allergic reaction to Imodium, you should not take this medication. Avoid it, too, if you have black or bloody stools.

Special warnings about this medication

If you suffer from a liver condition, have a fever, or have mucus in the stool, check with your doctor before using this drug.

Too much Imodium may cause drowsiness and/or dizziness. You should exercise extra caution while driving or performing tasks requiring mental alertness.

Dehydration can be a problem when you have diarrhea. It is important that you drink plenty of fluids while taking Imodium.

Use special caution when giving Imodium to a young child. Response to the drug can be unpredictable.

Possible food and drug interactions when taking this medication
There are no reported food or drug interactions.

Special information if you are pregnant or breastfeeding
The effects of Imodium during pregnancy have not been adequately studied. If you are pregnant, plan to become pregnant, or want to breastfeed, check with your doctor.

Recommended dosage

ADULTS

For adults and children 12 and over, the usual dosage is 2 caplets or 4 teaspoonfuls after the first loose stool, then 1 caplet or 2 teaspoonfuls after each loose stool that follows. Take no more than 4 caplets or 8 teaspoonfuls in 24 hours.

CHILDREN

Ages 9 to 11 (60 to 95 Pounds)
The usual dosage is 1 caplet or 2 teaspoonfuls after the first loose stool, then ½ caplet or 1 teaspoonful after each loose stool that follows. Give no more than 3 caplets or 6 teaspoonfuls in 24 hours.

Ages 6 to 8 (48 to 59 Pounds)
The usual dosage is 1 caplet or 2 teaspoonfuls after the first loose stool, then ½ caplet or 1 teaspoonful after each loose stool that follows. Give no more than 2 caplets or 4 teaspoonfuls in 24 hours.

Ages 2 to 5 (24 to 47 Pounds)
The usual dosage is 1 teaspoonful after the first loose stool, then 1 teaspoonful after each loose stool that follows. Give no more than 3 teaspoonfuls in 24 hours.

Imodium is not recommended in children under 2 years of age.

Overdosage
Any medication taken in excess can have serious consequences. If you suspect an Imodium overdose, seek medical attention immediately.

■ *Symptoms of an Imodium overdose may include:*
Constipation, drowsiness, lethargy, nausea

Indapamide *See Lozol, page 796.*

INDERAL

Pronounced: IN-der-al
Generic name: Propranolol hydrochloride
Other brand name: Inderal LA

Why is this drug prescribed?

Inderal, a type of medication known as a beta-blocker, is used in the treatment of high blood pressure, angina pectoris (chest pain, usually caused by lack of oxygen to the heart due to clogged arteries), changes in heart rhythm, prevention of migraine headache, hereditary tremors, hypertrophic subaortic stenosis (a condition related to exertional angina), and tumors of the adrenal gland. It is also used to reduce the risk of death from recurring heart attack.

When used for the treatment of high blood pressure, it is effective alone or combined with other high blood pressure medications, particularly thiazide-type diuretics. Beta-blockers decrease the force and rate of heart contractions, reducing the heart's demand for oxygen and lowering blood pressure.

Most important fact about this drug

If you have high blood pressure, you must take Inderal regularly for it to be effective. Since blood pressure declines gradually, it may be several weeks before you get the full benefit of Inderal; and you must continue taking it even if you are feeling well. Inderal does not cure high blood pressure; it merely keeps it under control.

How should you take this medication?

Inderal works best when taken before meals. Take it exactly as prescribed, even if your symptoms have disappeared.

Try not to miss any doses. If this medication is not taken regularly, your condition may worsen.

■ *If you miss a dose...*
Take it as soon as you remember. If it is within 8 hours of your next scheduled dose, skip the one you missed and go back to your regular schedule. Never take 2 doses at the same time.

■ *Storage instructions...*
Store at room temperature in a tightly closed, light-resistant container. Protect from freezing or excessive heat.

What side effects may occur?

Side effects cannot be anticipated. If any develop or change in intensity, inform your doctor as soon as possible. Only your doctor can determine if it is safe for you to continue taking Inderal.

■ *Side effects may include:*

Abdominal cramps, colitis, congestive heart failure, constipation, decreased sexual ability, depression, diarrhea, difficulty breathing, disorientation, dry eyes, fever with sore throat, hair loss, hallucinations, headache, light-headedness, low blood pressure, lupus erythematosus (a disease of the connective tissue), nausea, rash, reddish or purplish spots on the skin, short-term memory loss, slow heartbeat, tingling, prickling in hands, tiredness, trouble sleeping, upset stomach, visual changes, vivid dreams, vomiting, weakness, worsening of certain heartbeat irregularities

Why should this drug not be prescribed?

If you have inadequate blood supply to the circulatory system (cardiogenic shock), certain types of irregular heartbeat, a slow heartbeat, bronchial asthma, or severe congestive heart failure, you should not take this medication.

Special warnings about this medication

If you have a history of congestive heart failure, your doctor will prescribe Inderal cautiously.

Inderal should not be stopped suddenly. This can cause increased chest pain and heart attack. Dosage should be gradually reduced.

If you suffer from asthma or other bronchial conditions, coronary artery disease, or kidney or liver disease, this medication should be used with caution.

Ask your doctor if you should check your pulse while taking Inderal. This medication can cause your heartbeat to become too slow.

This medication may mask the symptoms of low blood sugar or alter blood sugar levels. In addition, diabetics who experience a severe drop in blood sugar after taking insulin may suffer a spike in blood pressure if they are also taking Inderal.

Notify your doctor or dentist that you are taking Inderal if you have a medical emergency, and before you have surgery or dental treatment.

Possible food and drug interactions when taking this medication

If Inderal is taken with certain other drugs, the effects of either could be increased, decreased, or altered. It is especially important to check with your doctor before combining Inderal with the following:

Alcohol
Aluminum hydroxide gel (Amphojel)
Antipyrine (Auralgan)
Calcium-blocking blood pressure drugs such as Cardizem, Procardia, and Calan
Certain high blood pressure medications such as Diupres and Ser-Ap-Es

Chlorpromazine (Thorazine)
Cimetidine (Tagamet)
Epinephrine (EpiPen)
Haloperidol (Haldol)
Insulin
Lidocaine (Xylocaine)
Nonsteroidal anti-inflammatory drugs such as Motrin and Naprosyn
Oral diabetes drugs such as Micronase
Phenobarbitone
Phenytoin (Dilantin)
Rifampin (Rifadin)
Theophylline (Theo-Dur and others)
Thyroid medications such as Synthroid

Special information if you are pregnant or breastfeeding

The effects of Inderal during pregnancy have not been adequately studied. If you are pregnant or plan to become pregnant, inform your doctor immediately. Inderal appears in breast milk and could affect a nursing infant. If this medication is essential to your health, your doctor may advise you to discontinue breastfeeding until your treatment with this medication is finished.

Recommended dosage

ADULTS

All dosages of Inderal, for any problem, must be tailored to the individual. Your doctor will determine when and how often you should take this drug. If you are over 65, the doctor will probably start with a relatively low dosage. Remember to take it exactly as directed.

Hypertension

The usual starting dose is 40 milligrams 2 times a day. This dose may be in combination with a diuretic. Dosages are gradually increased to between 120 and 240 milligrams per day for maintenance. In some cases, a dose of 640 milligrams per day may be needed. Depending on the individual, the maximum effect of this drug may not be reached for a few days or even several weeks. Some people may do better taking this medication 3 times a day.

Angina Pectoris

The usual daily dosage is 80 to 320 milligrams, divided into 2, 3, or 4 smaller doses. When your treatment is being discontinued, your doctor will reduce the dosage gradually over a period of several weeks.

Irregular Heartbeat

The usual dose is 10 to 30 milligrams 3 or 4 times a day, before meals and at bedtime.

Heart Attack
The usual daily dosage is 180 to 240 milligrams divided into smaller doses. The usual maximum dose is 240 milligrams, although your doctor may increase the dose when treating heart attack with angina or high blood pressure.

Migraine
The usual starting dosage is 80 milligrams per day divided into smaller doses. Dosages can be increased gradually to between 160 and 240 milligrams per day. If this dose does not relieve your symptoms in 4 to 6 weeks, your doctor will slowly take you off the drug.

Tremors
The usual starting dose is 40 milligrams, 2 times per day. Symptoms will usually be relieved with a dose of 120 milligrams per day; however, on occasion, dosages of 240 to 320 milligrams per day may be necessary.

Hypertrophic Subaortic Stenosis
The usual dose is 20 to 40 milligrams, 3 to 4 times a day, before meals and at bedtime.

Before Adrenal Gland Surgery
The usual dose is 60 milligrams a day divided into smaller doses for 3 days before surgery in combination with an alpha-blocker drug.

Inderal may also be taken by people with inoperable tumors in doses of 30 milligrams a day, divided into smaller doses.

CHILDREN
Inderal will be carefully individualized for use in children and is used only for high blood pressure. Doses in children are calculated by body weight, and range from 2 to 4 milligrams per 2.2 pounds daily, divided into 2 equal doses. The maximum dose is 16 milligrams per 2.2 pounds per day.

If treatment is stopped, this drug must be gradually reduced over a 7- to 14-day period.

Inderal is also available in a sustained-release formulation, called Inderal LA, for once-a-day dosing.

Overdosage
No specific information on Inderal overdosage is available; however, overdose symptoms with other beta-blockers include:

Extremely slow heartbeat, irregular heartbeat, low blood pressure, severe congestive heart failure, seizures, wheezing

Any medication taken in excess can have serious consequences. If you suspect an overdose, seek medical attention immediately.

INDERIDE

Pronounced: IN-deh-ride
Generic ingredients: Inderal (Propranolol hydrochloride),
   Hydrochlorothiazide
Other brand name: Inderide LA

Why is this drug prescribed?

Inderide is used in the treatment of high blood pressure. It combines a
beta-blocker (Inderal) with a thiazide diuretic (hydrochlorothiazide).
Beta-blockers decrease the force and rate of heart contractions, thus lowering blood pressure. Diuretics help your body produce and eliminate
more urine, which also helps lower blood pressure.

Most important fact about this drug

You must take Inderide regularly for it to be effective. Since blood pressure declines gradually, it may be several weeks before you get the full
benefit of Inderide; and you must continue taking it even if you are feeling
well. Inderide does not cure high blood pressure; it merely keeps it under
control.

How should you take this medication?

Take Inderide exactly as prescribed, even if your symptoms have disappeared.

Try not to miss any doses. If this medication is not taken regularly,
your condition may worsen.

■ *If you miss a dose...*
   Take it as soon as you remember. If the next dose is within 8 hours,
   skip the one you missed and go back to your regular schedule. Do not
   take 2 doses at the same time.
■ *Storage instructions...*
   Store at room temperature in a tightly closed container, protected from
   moisture, freezing, and excessive heat.

What side effects may occur?

Side effects cannot be anticipated. If any develop or change in intensity,
inform your doctor as soon as possible. Only your doctor can determine
if it is safe for you to continue taking Inderide.

■ *Side effects may include:*
   Allergic reactions, blood disorders, congestive heart failure, depression, inflammation of the pancreas, light-headedness, low blood pressure, nausea, slow heartbeat, vomiting

Why should this drug not be prescribed?

If you have inadequate blood supply to the circulatory system (cardiogenic shock), certain types of irregular heartbeat, slow heartbeat, bronchial asthma, or congestive heart failure, you should not take this medication.

Do not take Inderide if you are unable to urinate or if you are sensitive to or have ever had an allergic reaction to any of its ingredients or to sulfa drugs.

Special warnings about this medication

Inderide should not be stopped suddenly. This can cause chest pain and even heart attack. Dosage should be gradually reduced.

Diuretics can cause your body to lose too much potassium. Signs of an excessively low potassium level include muscle weakness and rapid or irregular heartbeat. To boost your potassium level, your doctor may recommend eating potassium-rich foods or taking a potassium supplement.

If you suffer from asthma, seasonal allergies or other bronchial conditions, or kidney or liver disease, your doctor will prescribe this medication with caution.

This medication may mask the symptoms of low blood sugar or alter blood sugar levels. If you are diabetic, discuss this with your doctor.

If you have a history of allergies or bronchial asthma, you are more likely to have an allergic reaction to Inderide.

Inderide may interfere with the screening test for glaucoma (excessive pressure in the eyes) and pressure within the eyes may increase when the medication is stopped.

Notify your doctor or dentist that you are taking Inderide if you have a medical emergency, and before you have surgery or dental treatment.

Possible food and drug interactions when taking this medication

If Inderide is taken with certain other drugs, the effects of either could be increased, decreased, or altered. It is especially important to check with your doctor before combining Inderide with the following:

ACTH (adrenocorticotropic hormone)
Alcohol
Aluminum hydroxide gel (Amphojel)
Antipyrine (Auralgan)
Calcium-blocking blood pressure drugs such as Calan, Cardizem, and Procardia XL
Certain blood pressure medications such as Diupres and Ser-Ap-Es
Chlorpromazine (Thorazine)
Cimetidine (Tagamet)
Corticosteroids such as prednisone
Digitalis (Lanoxin)
Epinephrine (EpiPen)
Haloperidol (Haldol)

Insulin
Lidocaine (Xylocaine)
Nonsteroidal anti-inflammatory drugs such as Motrin
Norepinephrine (Levophed)
Oral diabetes drugs such as Micronase
Phenobarbitone
Phenytoin (Dilantin)
Rifampin (Rifadin)
Theophylline (Theo-Dur)
Thyroid medications such as Synthroid

Special information if you are pregnant or breastfeeding

The effects of Inderide during pregnancy have not been adequately studied. If you are pregnant or plan to become pregnant, inform your doctor immediately. Inderide appears in breast milk and could affect a nursing infant. If Inderide is essential to your health, your doctor may advise you to discontinue breastfeeding until your treatment is finished.

Recommended dosage

ADULTS

Your doctor will tailor your dosage according to your response to Inderide's main ingredients.

The usual dose is 1 Inderide tablet 2 times per day.

Your doctor may use this medication in combination with other high blood pressure drugs to achieve the desired effect.

This drug is also available in a sustained-release formulation, called Inderide LA, for once-a-day dosing.

CHILDREN

The safety and effectiveness of Inderide in children have not been established.

OLDER ADULTS

Your doctor will adjust your dosage with extra caution.

Overdosage

Any medication taken in excess can have severe consequences. If you suspect an overdose, seek medical attention immediately.

■ *Symptoms of Inderide overdose may include:*
Coma, extremely slow heartbeat, heart failure, increased urination, irritation and overactivity of the stomach and intestines, low blood pressure, sluggishness, stupor, wheezing

Indinavir *See Crixivan, page 361.*

INDOCIN

Pronounced: IN-doh-sin
Generic name: Indomethacin

Why is this drug prescribed?

Indocin, a nonsteroidal anti-inflammatory drug, is used to relieve the inflammation, swelling, stiffness and joint pain associated with moderate or severe rheumatoid arthritis and osteoarthritis (the most common form of arthritis), and ankylosing spondylitis (arthritis of the spine). It is also used to treat bursitis, tendinitis (acute painful shoulder), acute gouty arthritis, and other kinds of pain.

Most important fact about this drug

You should have frequent checkups by your doctor if you take Indocin regularly. Ulcers or internal bleeding can occur without warning.

How should you take this medication?

Indocin should be taken with food or an antacid, and with a full glass of water. Never take on an empty stomach.

Take this medication exactly as prescribed by your doctor.

If you are using Indocin for arthritis, it should be taken regularly.

If you are taking the liquid form of this medicine, shake the bottle well before each use.

Indocin SR capsules should be swallowed whole, not crushed or broken.

Do not lie down for about 20 to 30 minutes after taking Indocin. This helps prevent irritation that could lead to trouble in swallowing.

If you are using the suppository form of this medicine:

1. If the suppository is too soft to insert, hold it under cool water or chill it before removing the wrapper.
2. Remove the foil wrapper and moisten your rectal area with cool tap water.
3. Lie down your side and use your finger to push the suppository well up into the rectum. Hold your buttocks together for a few seconds.
4. Indocin suppositories should be kept inside the rectum for at least 1 hour so that all of the medicine can be absorbed by your body.

■ *If you miss a dose...*
Take the forgotten dose as soon as you remember. If it is time for your next dose, skip the one you missed and return to your regular schedule. Never take a double dose.

■ *Storage instructions...*
The liquid and suppository forms of Indocin may be stored at room temperature. Keep both forms from extreme heat, and protect the liquid from freezing.

What side effects may occur?

Side effects cannot be anticipated. If any develop or change in intensity inform your doctor as soon as possible. Only your doctor can determine if it is safe for you to continue taking Indocin.

■ *Side effects may include:*
Abdominal pain, constipation, depression, diarrhea, dizziness, fatigue, headache, heartburn, indigestion, nausea, ringing in the ears, sleepiness or excessive drowsiness, stomach pain, stomach upset, vertigo, vomiting

Why should this drug not be prescribed?

If you are sensitive to or have ever had an allergic reaction to Indocin, aspirin, or similar drugs, or if you have had asthma attacks caused by aspirin or other drugs of this type, you should not take this medication. Make sure that your doctor is aware of any drug reactions that you have experienced.

Do not use Indocin suppositories if you have a history of rectal inflammation or recent rectal bleeding.

Special warnings about this medication

Indocin prolongs bleeding time. If you are taking blood-thinning medication, this drug should be taken with caution.

Your doctor should prescribe the lowest possible effective dose. The incidence of side effects increases as dosage increases.

Peptic ulcers and bleeding can occur without warning, especially in people over 65.

This drug should be used with caution if you have kidney or liver disease, and it can cause liver inflammation in some people.

Do not take aspirin or any other anti-inflammatory medications while taking Indocin, unless your doctor tells you to do so.

If you have heart disease or high blood pressure, this drug can increase water retention.

This drug can mask the symptoms of an existing infection.

Indocin may cause you to become drowsy or less alert; therefore, driving or operating dangerous machinery or participating in any hazardous activity that requires full mental alertness is not recommended. Indocin may also cause confusion and, rarely, psychosis, especially in older adults.

Possible food and drug interactions when taking this medication

If Indocin is taken with certain other drugs, the effects of either could be increased, decreased, or altered. It is especially important to check with your doctor before combining Indocin with the following:

Aspirin
Beta-blockers such as the blood pressure medications Tenormin and Inderal

Blood-thinning medicines such as Coumadin
Captopril (Capoten)
Cyclosporine (Sandimmune)
Diflunisal (Dolobid)
Digoxin (Lanoxin)
Lithium (Eskalith)
Loop diuretics (Lasix)
Other nonsteroidal anti-inflammatory drugs such as Advil, Aleve,
    and Motrin
Potassium-sparing water pills such as Aldactone
Probenecid (Benemid, ColBenemid)
The anticancer drug methotrexate
Thiazide-type water pills such as Diuril
Triamterene (Dyazide)

Special information if you are pregnant or breastfeeding

The effects of Indocin during pregnancy have not been adequately studied. If you are pregnant or plan to become pregnant inform your doctor immediately. Indocin appears in breast milk and could affect a nursing infant. If this medication is essential to your health, your doctor may advise you to discontinue breastfeeding until your treatment with this medication is finished.

Recommended dosage

ADULTS

This medication is available in liquid, capsule, and suppository form. The following dosages are for the capsule form. If you prefer the liquid form, ask your doctor to make the proper substitution. Do not try to convert the medication or dosage yourself.

Moderate to Severe Rheumatoid Arthritis, Osteoarthritis, Ankylosing Spondylitis

The usual dose is 25 milligrams 2 or 3 times a day, increasing to a total daily dose of 150 to 200 milligrams. Your doctor should monitor you carefully for side effects when you are taking this drug.

Your doctor may prescribe a single daily 75-milligram capsule of Indocin SR in place of regular Indocin.

Bursitis or Tendinitis

The usual dose is 75 to 150 milligrams daily divided into 3 to 4 small doses for 1 to 2 weeks, until symptoms disappear.

Acute Gouty Arthritis

The usual dose is 50 milligrams 3 times a day until pain is reduced to a tolerable level (usually 3 to 5 days). Your doctor will advise you when to stop taking this drug for this condition. Keep him informed of its effects on your symptoms.

CHILDREN

The safety and effectiveness of Indocin have not been established in children under 14 years of age. However, your doctor may decide that the benefits of this medication outweigh any potential risks.

OLDER ADULTS

Your doctor will adjust the dosage as needed.

Overdosage

Any medication taken in excess can cause symptoms of overdose. If you suspect an overdose seek medical attention immediately.

■ *The symptoms of Indocin overdose may include:*
Convulsions, disorientation, dizziness, intense headache, lethargy, mental confusion, nausea, numbness, tingling or pins and needles, vomiting

Indomethacin See Indocin, page 683.

INSPRA
Pronounced: IN-sprah
Generic name: Eplerenone

Why is this drug prescribed?

Inspra is prescribed to improve survival in patients who have congestive heart failure and left ventricular systolic dysfunction following a heart attack. It is also used to treat high blood pressure. Inspra may be used alone or with other antihypertensive agents. Inspra lowers blood pressure by blocking the actions of the hormone aldosterone.

Most important fact about this drug

Inspra can increase the levels of potassium in your blood, resulting in a potentially serious condition called hyperkalemia. Your doctor will order periodic blood tests to check the amount of potassium in your blood. Be sure to avoid potassium supplements and salt substitutes that contain potassium. Make sure your doctor knows about every medication you are taking. Call your doctor immediately if you experience nausea, diarrhea, or weakness, as these may be signs of hyperkalemia.

How should you take this medication?

Take Inspra exactly as prescribed; higher than recommended doses provide no additional benefit. Inspra may be taken with or without food.

■ *If you miss a dose…*
Take the forgotten dose as soon as you remember. However, if it is almost time for your next dose, skip the one you missed and return to your regular schedule. Do not take 2 doses at once.

■ *Storage instructions…*
Store at room temperature.

What side effects may occur?

Side effects cannot be anticipated. If any develop or change in intensity, tell your doctor as soon as possible. Only your doctor can determine if it is safe to continue using Inspra.

■ *Side effects may include:*
Chest pain, dizziness, headache, high cholesterol and triglyceride levels, increased blood potassium level, increased risk for heart attack, kidney problems

This side effects list is not complete. If you have any questions about side effects you should consult your doctor. Report any new or continuing symptoms to your doctor right away.

Why should this drug not be prescribed?

If your doctor determines that you have high blood potassium levels or severe kidney impairment, you cannot take Inspra. You must also avoid this drug if you are taking certain medications that affect the liver (see *Possible food and drug interactions when taking this medication*).

You cannot take Inspra for high blood pressure if you also take potassium-sparing diuretics such as amiloride (Moduretic), spironolactone (Aldactone), and triamterene (Dyazide, Dyrenium, Maxzide). Likewise, this drug cannot be used to treat high blood pressure if you have type 2 diabetes along with high protein levels in the urine (known as microalbuminuria), a condition that could signal kidney problems.

Special warnings about this medication

Inspra could cause potentially dangerous increases of blood potassium levels. Your doctor will monitor you closely to guard against this problem, especially if you also have diabetes or mild kidney or liver problems.

Use Inspra with caution if you have severe liver impairment. The drug's safety has not been studied in such people.

In clinical studies, Inspra did not appear to benefit people 75 years and older who were being treated for congestive heart failure following a heart attack. However, when treated for high blood pressure, those 65 and older experienced the same benefits as younger people.

Possible food and drug interactions when taking this medication

Be sure to check with your doctor about the medications that should never be taken with Inspra, including:

Clarithromycin (Biaxin)
Itraconazole (Sporanox)
Ketoconazole (Nizoral)
Nefazodone (Serzone)
Nelfinavir (Viracept)
Ritonavir (Norvir)
Troleandomycin (Tao)

You should never take Inspra for high blood pressure if you're also taking potassium-sparing diuretics, including:

Amiloride (Moduretic)
Spironolactone (Aldactone)
Triamterene (Dyazide, Dyrenium, Maxzide)

If Inspra is taken with certain other drugs, the effects of either drug could be increased, decreased, or altered. It is especially important to check with your doctor before combining Inspra with the following:

Blood pressure drugs known as ACE inhibitors, such as Prinivil and Zestril
Blood pressure drugs known as angiotensin II receptor antagonists, such as Avapro, Cozaar, and Diovan
Erythromycin (Ery-Tab)
Fluconazole (Diflucan)
Lithium (Eskalith, Lithobid, Lithonate)
Nonsteroidal anti-inflammatory drugs such as Motrin and Advil
Potassium supplements including K-Tabs, K-Dur, and Slow-K
Saquinavir (Invirase)
Verapamil (Calan, Isoptin)

You should also consult your doctor before using salt substitutes that contain potassium.

Special information if you are pregnant or breastfeeding

The effects of Inspra during pregnancy have not been adequately studied. If you are pregnant or planning to become pregnant, inform your doctor immediately.

It is not known whether Inspra appears in human breast milk. If this drug is essential to your health, your doctor may advise you to stop nursing until your treatment is finished.

Recommended dosage

ADULTS

Congestive Heart Failure After a Heart Attack
The recommended daily dose is 50 milligrams. Your doctor will start you at 25 milligrams once a day and gradually increase the dose to 50 milligrams once a day over a period of 4 weeks.

Your doctor will test your blood potassium levels during the first week of treatment and again after 1 month. Depending on the results, the doctor may change your dosage and continue monitoring your potassium levels.

High Blood Pressure

The recommended starting dose is 50 milligrams once a day. Based on your response, the doctor may increase the dose to a maximum of 50 milligrams twice a day. If you're taking certain drugs that affect the liver, the doctor may start you at a dose of 25 milligrams once a day.

Overdosage

No cases of overdose have been reported. However, any medication taken in excess can have serious consequences. If you suspect an overdose, seek emergency treatment immediately.

■ *Symptoms of an Inspra overdose may include:*
Diarrhea, dizziness, feeling faint or light-headed, nausea, weakness

INSULIN

Pronounced: IN-suh-lin
Brand names: Apidra, Humalog, Humulin, Iletin, Novolin

Why is this drug prescribed?

Insulin is prescribed for diabetes mellitus when diet modifications and oral medications fail to correct the condition. Insulin is a hormone produced by the pancreas, a large gland that lies near the stomach. This hormone is necessary for the body's correct use of food, especially sugar. Insulin apparently works by helping sugar penetrate the cell wall, where it is then utilized by the cell. In people with diabetes, the body either does not make enough insulin, or the insulin that is produced cannot be used properly.

There are actually two forms of diabetes: type 1 (insulin-dependent) and type 2 (non-insulin-dependent). Type 1 usually requires insulin injection for life, while type 2 diabetes can usually be treated by dietary changes and/or oral antidiabetic medications such as Diabinese, Glucotrol, and Glucophage. Occasionally, type 2 diabetics must take insulin injections on a temporary basis, especially during stressful periods or times of illness.

The various available types of insulin differ in several ways: in the source (animal, human, or genetically engineered), in the time requirements for the insulin to take effect, and in the length of time the insulin remains working.

Regular insulin is manufactured from beef and pork pancreas, begins working within 30 to 60 minutes, and lasts for 6 to 8 hours. Variations of insulin have been developed to satisfy the needs of individual patients.

For example, zinc suspension insulin is an intermediate-acting insulin that starts working within 1 to 1½ hours and lasts approximately 24 hours. Insulin combined with zinc and protamine is a longer-acting insulin that takes effect within 4 to 6 hours and lasts up to 36 hours. The time and course of action may vary considerably in different individuals or at different times in the same individual. Genetically engineered insulin works faster and for a shorter length of time than regular human insulin and should be used along with a longer-acting insulin. It is available only by prescription.

Animal-based insulin is a very safe product. However, some components may cause an allergic reaction (see *What side effects may occur?*). Therefore, genetically engineered human insulin has been developed to lessen the chance of an allergic reaction. It is structurally identical to the insulin produced by your pancreas. However, some human insulin may be produced in a semi-synthetic process that begins with animal-based ingredients, and may cause an allergic reaction.

Most important fact about this drug

Regardless of the type of insulin your doctor has prescribed, you should follow carefully the dietary and exercise guidelines he or she has recommended. Failure to follow these guidelines or to take your insulin as prescribed may result in serious and potentially life-threatening complications such as hypoglycemia (lowered blood sugar levels).

How should you take this medication?

Take your insulin exactly as prescribed, being careful to follow your doctor's dietary and exercise recommendations. Before taking your injection, carefully read and follow the manufacturer's instructions on how to prepare your prefilled pen or syringe.

■ *If you miss a dose...*
Your doctor should tell you what to do if you miss an insulin injection or meal.

■ *Storage instructions...*
Store insulin in a refrigerator (but not in the freezer) or in another cool, dark place. Do not expose insulin to heat or direct sunlight.

Some brands of prefilled syringes can be kept at room temperature for a week or a month. The vial or cartridge of the genetically engineered insulin lispro can be kept unrefrigerated for up to 28 days. Check your product's label. Never use insulin after the expiration date printed on the label and carton.

What side effects may occur?

While side effects from insulin use are rare, allergic reactions or low blood sugar (sometimes called an insulin reaction) may pose significant health risks. Your doctor should be notified if any of the following occurs:

■ *Mild allergic reactions:*
 Swelling, itching or redness at the injection site (usually disappears within a few days or weeks)
■ *More serious allergic reactions:*
 Fast pulse, low blood pressure, perspiration, rash over the entire body, shortness of breath, shallow breathing, or wheezing

Other side effects are virtually eliminated when the correct dose of insulin is matched with the proper diet and level of physical activity. Low blood sugar may develop in poorly controlled or unstable diabetes. Consuming sugar or a sugar-containing product will usually correct the condition, which can be brought about by taking too much insulin, missing or delaying meals, exercising or working more than usual, an infection or illness, a change in the body's need for insulin, drug interactions, or consuming alcohol.

■ *Symptoms of low blood sugar include:*
 Abnormal behavior, anxiety, blurred vision, cold sweat, confusion, depressed mood, dizziness, drowsiness, fatigue, headache, hunger, inability to concentrate, light-headedness, nausea, nervousness, personality changes, rapid heartbeat, restlessness, sleep disturbances, slurred speech, sweating, tingling in the hands, feet, lips, or tongue, tremor, unsteady movement

Contact your physician if these symptoms persist.

■ *Symptoms of more severe low blood sugar include:*
 Coma, disorientation

 Remember, too, the symptoms associated with an under-supply of insulin, which can be brought on by taking too little of it, overeating, or fever and infection.

■ *Symptoms of insufficient insulin include:*
 Drowsiness, flushing, fruity breath, heavy breathing, loss of appetite, rapid pulse, thirst

If you are ill, you should check your urine for ketones (acetone), and notify your doctor if the test is positive. This condition can be life-threatening.

Why should this drug not be prescribed?
Insulin should be used only to correct diabetic conditions.

Special warnings about this medication
Wear personal identification that states clearly that you are diabetic. Carry a sugar-containing product such as hard candy to offset any symptoms of low blood sugar.
 Do not change the type of insulin or even the model and brand of

syringe or needle you use without your physician's instruction. Failure to use the proper syringe may lead to improper dosage levels of insulin.

If you become ill from any cause, especially with nausea and vomiting or fever, your insulin requirements may change. It is important to eat as normally as possible. If you have trouble eating, drink fruit juices, soda, or clear soups, or eat small amounts of bland foods. Test your urine and/or blood sugar and tell your doctor at once. If you have severe and prolonged vomiting, seek emergency medical care.

If you are taking insulin, you should check your glucose levels with home blood and urine testing devices. If your blood tests consistently show above-normal sugar levels or your urine tests consistently show the presence of sugar, your diabetes is not properly controlled, and you should tell your doctor.

To avoid infection or contamination, use disposable needles and syringes or sterilize your reusable syringe and needle carefully.

Always keep handy an extra supply of insulin as well as a spare syringe and needle.

Possible food and drug interactions when taking this medication

Follow your physician's dietary guidelines as closely as you can and inform your physician of any medication, either prescription or nonprescription, that you are taking. Specific medications, depending on the amount present, that affect insulin levels or its effectiveness include:

ACE inhibitors such as the blood pressure medications Accupril and Lotensin
Anabolic steroids such as Anadrol-50
Appetite suppressants such as Tenuate
Aspirin
Beta-blocking blood pressure medicines such as Tenormin and Lopressor
Diuretics such as Lasix and Dyazide
Epinephrine (EpiPen)
Estrogens such as Premarin
Isoniazid (Nydrazid)
Major tranquilizers such as Mellaril and Thorazine
MAO inhibitors (drugs such as the antidepressants Nardil and Parnate)
Niacin (Nicobid)
Octreotide (Sandostatin)
Oral contraceptives
Oral drugs for diabetes such as Diabinese and Orinase
Phenytoin (Dilantin)
Steroid medications such as prednisone
Sulfa antibiotics such as Bactrim and Septra
Thyroid medications such as Synthroid

Use alcohol carefully, since excessive alcohol consumption can cause low blood sugar. Don't drink unless your doctor has approved it.

Special information if you are pregnant or breastfeeding

Insulin is considered safe for pregnant women, but pregnancy may make managing your diabetes more difficult.

Properly controlled diabetes is essential for the health of the mother and the developing baby; therefore, it is extremely important that pregnant women follow closely their physician's dietary and exercise guidelines and prescribing instructions.

Since insulin does not pass into breast milk, it is safe for nursing mothers. It is not known whether the genetically engineered insulin lispro appears in breast milk.

Recommended dosage

Your doctor will specify which insulin to use, how much, when, and how often to inject it. Your dosage may be affected by changes in food, activity, illness, medication, pregnancy, exercise, travel, or your work schedule. Proper control of your diabetes requires close and constant cooperation with your doctor. Failure to use your insulin as prescribed may result in serious and potentially fatal complications.

Some insulins should be clear, and some have a cloudy precipitate. Find out what your insulin should look like and check it carefully before using.

Genetically engineered insulin lispro injection should not be used by children under age 12.

Overdosage

- *An overdose of insulin can cause low blood sugar (hypoglycemia). Symptoms include:*
  Depressed mood, dizziness, drowsiness, fatigue, headache, hunger, inability to concentrate, irritability, nausea, nervousness, personality changes, rapid heartbeat, restlessness, sleep disturbances, slurred speech, sweating, tingling, tremor, unsteady movements
- *Symptoms of more severe low blood sugar include:*
  Coma, disorientation, pale skin, seizures

Your doctor should be contacted immediately if these symptoms of severe low blood sugar occur.

Eating sugar or a sugar-based product will often correct the condition. If you suspect an overdose, seek medical attention immediately.

INTAL

Pronounced: IN-tahl
Generic name: Cromolyn sodium
Other brand name: Nasalcrom

Why is this drug prescribed?

Intal contains the antiasthmatic/antiallergic medication cromolyn sodium.

Different forms of the drug are used to manage bronchial asthma, to prevent asthma attacks, and to prevent and treat seasonal and chronic allergies.

The drug works by preventing certain cells in the body from releasing substances that can cause allergic reactions or prompt too much bronchial activity. It also helps prevent bronchial constriction caused by exercise, aspirin, cold air, and certain environmental pollutants such as sulfur dioxide.

Most important fact about this drug

Intal does not help an acute asthma attack. When taken to prevent severe bronchial asthma, it can be 4 weeks before you feel its maximum benefit, though some people get relief sooner. Do not discontinue the inhalation capsules or nasal solution abruptly without the advice of your doctor.

How should you take this medication?

Intal capsules should not be swallowed. They are for inhalation using the Spinhaler turbo-inhaler. The contents of 1 capsule are usually inhaled 4 times daily at regular intervals. Wash the Spinhaler in warm water at least once a week; dry thoroughly. Replace the Spinhaler every 6 months.

Intal nebulizer solution should be inhaled using a power-operated nebulizer equipped with an appropriate face mask or mouthpiece. Hand-operated nebulizers are not suitable. It is important that the solution be inhaled at regular intervals, usually 4 times per day.

Intal aerosol spray can be used either for chronic asthma or to prevent an asthma attack. For chronic asthma, it must be inhaled at regular intervals, as directed by your doctor, usually 2 sprays inhaled 4 times daily. To prevent an asthma attack caused by exercise, cold air, or other irritants, the usual dose of 2 inhalation sprays should be taken between 10 and 60 minutes before exercising or exposure to cold or pollutants.

Nasalcrom nasal solution should be used with a metered nasal spray device, which should be replaced every 6 months. Blow your nose to clear your nasal passages before administering the spray. The nasal solution is used for nasal congestion due to seasonal or chronic allergies. For seasonal allergies, treatment is more effective if begun before the start of the allergy season. Treatment should then continue throughout the season. For year-round allergies, treatment may be required for up to 4 weeks before results are seen. Your doctor may find it necessary to add other allergy medications, such as antihistamines or decongestants, during initial treatment.

■ *If you miss a dose...*
Take it as soon as you remember. Then take the rest of that day's doses at equally spaced intervals. Do not take 2 doses at once.

■ *Storage instructions...*
Store at room temperature, away from light and heat. Keep the ampules in their foil pouch until you are ready to use them.

What side effects may occur?
Side effects cannot be anticipated. If any develop or change in intensity, inform your doctor as soon as possible. Only your doctor can determine if it is safe for you to continue taking Intal.

■ *Side effects may include:*
Cough, nasal congestion or irritation, nausea, sneezing, throat irritation, wheezing

Why should this drug not be prescribed?
If you are sensitive to or have ever had an allergic reaction to cromolyn sodium or lactose, you should not take this medication. Make sure your doctor is aware of any drug reactions you have experienced.

Special warnings about this medication
Asthma symptoms may recur if the recommended dosage of Intal is reduced or discontinued. Intal has no role in the treatment of an acute asthmatic attack once it has begun. Obtain medical help immediately if you experience a severe attack.

If you have liver or kidney problems, your doctor may have to reduce the dosage or even take you off the drug altogether.

When using the capsules, you may accidentally inhale some powder, which can irritate your throat or make you cough. Try rinsing your mouth or taking a drink of water immediately before and/or after using the Spinhaler.

If your heartbeat is ever irregular or if you have any other kind of heart trouble, be sure your doctor knows about it before you use Intal aerosol spray.

Intal aerosol spray may not help you if your attack has been brought on by exercise.

Possible food and drug interactions when taking this medication
If you are taking other prescription or nonprescription drugs, discuss this with your doctor to determine if these drugs would interact with Intal.

Special information if you are pregnant or breastfeeding

The effects of Intal during pregnancy have not been adequately studied. If you are pregnant or plan to become pregnant, inform your doctor immediately. It is not known whether Intal appears in breast milk. As with all medication, a nursing woman should use this drug only after careful consultation with her doctor.

Recommended dosage

INTAL CAPSULES FOR INHALATION AND INTAL NEBULIZER SOLUTION

Adults and Children 2 Years Old and Over
For management of bronchial asthma, the usual dosage is 20 milligrams (1 capsule or ampule) inhaled 4 times daily at regular intervals, using the Spinhaler turbo-inhaler or power-operated nebulizer. If you have chronic asthma, this drug's effectiveness depends on your taking it regularly, as directed, and only after an attack has been controlled and you can inhale adequately.

For the prevention of an acute attack following exercise or exposure to cold, dry air or environmental irritants, the usual dose is 1 capsule or ampule inhaled shortly before exposure to the irritant. You may repeat the inhalation as needed for continued protection during prolonged exposure.

INTAL INHALER AEROSOL SPRAY

Adults and Children 5 Years Old and Over
For the management of bronchial asthma, the usual starting dose is 2 metered sprays taken at regular intervals, 4 times daily. This is the maximum dose that should be taken, and lower dosages may be effective in children. This drug should be used only after an asthma attack has been controlled and you can inhale adequately.

For the prevention of an acute asthma attack following exercise, exposure to cold air or environmental agents, the usual dose is inhalation of 2 metered sprays shortly (10 to 15 minutes but not more than 60 minutes) before exposure to the irritant.

NASALCROM NASAL SOLUTION

Adults and Children 6 Years Old and Over
For the prevention and treatment of allergies caused by exposure to certain irritants, the usual dosage is 1 spray in each nostril 3 to 4 times per day at regular intervals, using the metered spray device. Your doctor may have you use the spray 6 times a day if you need it.

Overdosage
Any medication taken in excess can have serious consequences. If you suspect an overdose, seek medical attention immediately.

■ *Symptoms of Intal overdose may include:*
Difficulty breathing, heart failure, low blood pressure, slow heartbeat

Invirase *See Fortovase, page 603.*

Ionamin *See Adipex-P, page 40.*

Ipratropium *See Atrovent, page 147.*

Ipratropium with Albuterol *See Combivent, page 327.*

Irbesartan *See Avapro, page 163.*

Irbesartan with Hydrochlorothiazide *See Avalide, page 153.*

Ismo *See Imdur, page 667.*

Isometheptene, Dichloralphenazone, and Acetaminophen *See Midrin, page 858.*

Isoptin *See Calan, page 229.*

Isopto Carpine *See Pilocar, page 1098.*

ISORDIL
Pronounced: ICE-or-dill
Generic name: Isosorbide dinitrate
Other brand name: Sorbitrate

Why is this drug prescribed?
Isordil is prescribed to relieve or prevent angina pectoris (suffocating chest pain). Angina pectoris occurs when the arteries and veins become constricted and sufficient oxygen does not reach the heart. Isordil dilates the blood vessels by relaxing the muscles in their walls. Oxygen flow improves as the vessels relax, and chest pain subsides.

In swallowed capsules or tablets, Isordil helps to increase the amount of exercise you can do before chest pain begins.

In chewable or sublingual (held under the tongue) tablets, Isordil can help relieve chest pain that has already started or prevent pain expected from a strenuous activity such as walking up a hill or climbing stairs.

Most important fact about this drug
Isordil may cause severe low blood pressure (possibly marked by dizziness or fainting), especially when you stand or sit up quickly. People tak-

ing diuretic medication or those who have low blood pressure should use Isordil with caution.

How should you take this medication?

Swallowed capsules or tablets should be taken on an empty stomach. While regular tablets may be crushed for easier use, sustained- or prolonged-release products should not be chewed, crushed or altered.

Chewable tablets should be chewed thoroughly and held in the mouth for a couple of minutes. Do not eat, drink, smoke, or use chewing tobacco while a sublingual tablet is dissolving.

This drug's effectiveness is closely linked to the dose, so follow your doctor's instructions carefully.

■ *If you miss a dose...*
If you are taking this drug regularly, take the forgotten dose as soon as you remember. If your next dose is within 2 hours—or 6 hours for controlled-release tablets and capsules—skip the one you missed and go back to your regular schedule. Do not take 2 doses at once.

■ *Storage information...*
Store at room temperature in a tightly closed container, away from light.

What side effects may occur?

Side effects cannot be anticipated. If any develop or change in intensity, inform your doctor as soon as possible. Only your doctor can determine if it is safe for you to continue taking Isordil.

Headache is the most common side effect; usually, standard headache treatments with over-the-counter pain products will relieve the pain. The headaches associated with Isordil usually subside within 2 weeks after treatment with the drug begins. Do not change your dose to avoid the headache. At a dose that eliminates headaches, the drug may not be as effective against angina.

Why should this drug not be prescribed?

You should not take Isordil if you have had a previous allergic reaction to it or to other nitrates or nitrites.

Special warnings about this medication

You should use Isordil with caution if you have anemia, the eye condition called glaucoma, a previous head injury or heart attack, heart disease, low blood pressure, or thyroid disease.

If you stop using Isordil, you should follow your doctor's plan for a gradual withdrawal schedule. Abruptly stopping this medication could result in additional chest pain.

Some people may develop a tolerance to Isordil, which causes its effects to be reduced over time. Tell your doctor if you think Isordil is starting to lose its effectiveness.

Possible food and drug interactions when taking this medication
If Isordil is taken with certain other drugs, the effects of either could be increased, decreased, or altered.

Extremely low blood pressure (marked by dizziness, fainting, and numbness) may occur if you take Isordil with certain other high blood pressure drugs such as Cardizem and Procardia, as well as the impotence remedy Viagra.

Alcohol may interact with Isordil and produce a swift decrease in blood pressure, possibly causing dizziness and fainting.

Special information if you are pregnant or breastfeeding
The effects of Isordil in pregnancy have not been adequately studied. Isordil should be used only when the benefits of therapy clearly outweigh the potential risks to the developing baby. If you are pregnant or plan to become pregnant, inform your doctor immediately. It is not known if Isordil appears in breast milk; therefore, nursing mothers should use Isordil with caution.

Recommended dosage
Because you can develop a tolerance to this drug, your doctor may schedule a daily period of time when you do not take any drug.

ADULTS

The usual sublingual starting dose for the treatment of angina pectoris is 2.5 to 5 milligrams. Your doctor will increase this initial dose gradually until the pain subsides or side effects prove bothersome.

The usual sublingual starting dose for the prevention of an impending attack of angina pectoris is usually 5 or 10 milligrams every 2 to 3 hours.

To prevent chronic stable angina pectoris, the usual starting dose for swallowed, immediately released Isordil is 5 to 20 milligrams. Your doctor may increase this initial dose to 10 to 40 milligrams every 6 hours.

To prevent chronic stable angina pectoris with controlled-release Isordil, the usual initial dose is 40 milligrams. Your doctor may increase this dose from 40 to 80 milligrams given every 8 to 12 hours.

CHILDREN

The safety and effectiveness of Isordil have not been established for children.

Overdosage
Any medication taken in excess can have serious consequences. Severe overdosage of Isordil can be fatal. If you suspect an overdose, seek medical help immediately.

■ *Symptoms of Isordil overdose may include:*
Bloody diarrhea, coma, confusion, convulsions, fainting, fever, flushed and perspiring skin (later cold and blue), nausea, palpitations, paralysis, rapid decrease in blood pressure, rapid, then difficult and slow breathing, slow pulse, throbbing headache, vertigo, visual disturbances, vomiting

Isosorbide dinitrate *See Isordil, page 697.*

Isosorbide mononitrate *See Imdur, page 667.*

Isotretinoin *See Accutane, page 12.*

Isradipine *See DynaCirc, page 490.*

Itraconazole *See Sporanox, page 1337.*

Kadian *See MS Contin, page 898.*

KALETRA
Pronounced: cuh-LEE-tra
Generic ingredients: Lopinavir, Ritonavir

Why is this drug prescribed?
Kaletra combats the human immunodeficiency virus (HIV). HIV is the deadly virus that undermines the infection-fighting capacity of the body's immune system, eventually leading to AIDS.

Kaletra is a combination of two drugs, lopinavir and ritonavir (Norvir), both of which fall into the drug category known as protease inhibitors. When taken along with other HIV drugs, Kaletra lowers the amount of the virus circulating in the bloodstream. However, it does not completely eradicate the virus, and you may continue to develop the rare infections that attack when the immune system weakens. It's also important to remember that Kaletra does not eliminate the danger of transmitting the virus to others.

Most important fact about this drug
Combining Kaletra with certain other medications can cause serious, even life-threatening, reactions. Never take Kaletra with the following:

Flecainide (Tambocor)
Midazolam (Versed)
Migraine remedies based on ergot, including Cafergot, D.H.E. 45, Methergine, Migranal, and Wigraine
Pimozide (Orap)
Propafenone (Rythmol)
Triazolam (Halcion)

How should you take this medication?

Kaletra is used in combination with other HIV drugs. It should be taken twice a day, in the morning and evening, with food. Do not change the dose or discontinue therapy without consulting your doctor first.

If your doctor has also prescribed Videx (didanosine), you must take Kaletra one hour before or two hours after Videx.

■ *If you miss a dose...*
Take it as soon as you remember. If it is almost time for your next dose, skip the one you missed and return to your normal schedule. Never double a dose.

■ *Storage instructions...*
If Kaletra capsules and Kaletra oral solution are kept in the refrigerator, they can be used until the expiration date imprinted on the bottle. If they are stored at room temperature, they should be used within 2 months of opening. Avoid exposing the medication to excessive heat.

What side effects may occur?

Side effects cannot be anticipated. If any develop or change in intensity, inform your doctor as soon as possible. Only your doctor can determine if it is safe for you to continue taking Kaletra.

■ *Side effects may include:*
Abdominal pain, diarrhea, headache, nausea, rash, vomiting, weakness

Why should this drug not be prescribed?

You will not be able to use Kaletra if you prove to be allergic to either lopinavir or ritonavir. Remember, too, that Kaletra must never be combined with drugs listed under *Most important fact about this drug*.

Special warnings about this medication

In some patients Kaletra causes a substantial increase in cholesterol and triglyceride levels, so the doctor will check yours periodically. High triglycerides can lead to a serious condition called pancreatitis. Call your doctor if you develop symptoms of this problem, such as nausea, vomiting, and abdominal pain.

Kaletra has been known to raise blood sugar levels, and can even cause diabetes. If you already have diabetes, be sure to monitor your blood sugar carefully and to notify your doctor if your blood sugar becomes difficult to control.

Liver failure, including some fatalities, has been reported among patients on Kaletra. Be sure your doctor knows if you have a history of liver disease, including hepatitis. You will need to be monitored carefully.

Some patients taking HIV medications find that their body fat gets redistributed. They may develop a fatty "buffalo hump" on their upper back, suffer breast enlargement, and gain weight in the abdomen. At the same time, they often lose weight in the face, arms, and legs.

During treatment with drugs similar to Kaletra, some patients with hemophilia have experienced increased bleeding.

Possible food and drug interactions when taking this medication

Kaletra interacts with a wide variety of other medications. Be careful to avoid combining it with any of the drugs listed under *Most important fact about this drug.* Also be especially careful when taking Viagra. Kaletra can increase this drug's side effects, and has been known to cause potentially damaging erections that last for more than 4 hours. If this happens to you, call your doctor immediately.

Kaletra also decreases the effectiveness of birth control pills. Check with your doctor about additional contraceptive measures you may want to take while using Kaletra.

Listed below are some of the other drugs that may interact with Kaletra. However, because interactions are so likely, it's best to check with your doctor before combining Kaletra with any medication, including over-the-counter products and herbal remedies.

Anticonvulsants such as Dilantin, Phenobarbital, Tegretol
Antifungals such as Nizoral and Sporanox
Atovaquone (Mepron)
Certain cholesterol-lowering agents, including Lipitor, Mevacor, and Zocor
Certain HIV drugs such as Sustiva, Videx, Viramune
Clarithromycin (Biaxin)
Dexamethasone (Decadron)
Disulfuram (Antabuse)
Drugs used to treat heart arrhythmias, such as Cordarone, Lidocaine, Quinidex, Rhythmol
Drugs used to treat tuberculosis, such as Mycobutin, Rifadin, Rifater
Heart medications such as Adalat, Cardene, Plendil, Procardia
Immunosuppressants such as Neoral and Prograf
Methadone
Metronidazole (Flagyl)
St. John's wort (also called *Hypericum perforatum*)
Warfarin (Coumadin)

Special information if you are pregnant or breastfeeding

Kaletra has not been studied in pregnant women and should be used only if the potential benefit to the mother outweighs the possible risk to the developing baby.

HIV can be passed to your baby in breast milk, so breastfeeding is not advised.

Recommended dosage

ADULTS

Kaletra Capsules
The usual dose is 3 capsules twice daily with food. The dose may be increased to 4 capsules twice daily if Kaletra is used in conjunction with Sustiva or Viramune.

Kaletra Oral Solution
Take 5 milliliters (1 teaspoonful) twice daily with food. The dose may be increased to 6.5 milliliters twice daily if Kaletra is used in conjunction with Sustiva or Viramune.

CHILDREN

Aged 6 Months to 12 Years
The dose of Kaletra for children is based on body weight. It should be taken twice a day with food and should be administered using a calibrated dosing syringe. The dose may be increased if the child is also taking Sustiva or Viramune.

Overdosage

Little is known about Kaletra overdose. Any medication taken in excess can have serious consequences. If you suspect an overdose, seek medical attention immediately.

Kaletra oral solution contains a high percentage of alcohol, which could be dangerous to a young child. If a child swallows more than the recommended dose, contact your local poison control center immediately.

Kaon-CL *See Micro-K, page 851.*

K-Dur *See Micro-K, page 851.*

KEFLEX

Pronounced: KEF-lecks
Generic name: Cephalexin hydrochloride
Other brand name: Keftab

Why is this drug prescribed?

Keflex and Keftab are cephalosporin antibiotics. They are prescribed for bacterial infections of the respiratory tract, the middle ear, the bones, the skin, and the reproductive and urinary systems. Because they are effective for only certain types of bacterial infections, before beginning treatment your doctor may perform tests to identify the organisms causing the infection.

Keflex is available in capsules and an oral suspension form for use in children. Keftab, available only in tablet form, is prescribed exclusively for adults.

Most important fact about this drug

If you are allergic to either penicillin or cephalosporin antibiotics in any form, consult your doctor *before taking Keflex*. There is a possibility that you are allergic to both types of medication, and if a reaction occurs, it could be extremely severe. If you take the drug and feel signs of a reaction, seek medical attention immediately.

How should you take this medication?

Keflex may be taken with or without meals. However, if the drug upsets your stomach, you may want to take it after you have eaten.

Take Keflex at even intervals around the clock as prescribed by your doctor.

If you are taking the liquid form of Keflex, use the specially marked spoon to measure each dose accurately.

Your doctor will prescribe Keflex only to treat a bacterial infection; it will not cure a viral infection, such as the common cold. It's important to take the full dosage schedule of Keflex, even if you're feeling better in a few days. Not completing the full dosage schedule may decrease the drugs' effectiveness and increase the chances that the bacteria may become resistant to Keflex and similar antibiotics.

■ *If you miss a dose...*
Take it as soon as you remember. If it is almost time for the next dose, and you take 2 doses a day, take the one you missed and the next dose 5 to 6 hours later. If you take 3 or more doses a day, take the one you missed and the next dose 2 to 4 hours later, or double the next dose. Then go back to your regular schedule.

■ *Storage instructions...*
Store capsules and tablets at room temperature. Store the liquid suspension in a refrigerator; discard any unused medication after 14 days.

What side effects may occur?

Side effects cannot be anticipated. If any develop or change in intensity, inform your doctor as soon as possible. Only your doctor can determine if it is safe for you to continue taking Keflex.

■ *Side effects may include:*
Diarrhea

Why should this drug not be prescribed?

If you are sensitive to or have ever had an allergic reaction to the cephalosporin group of antibiotics, you should not use this medication. Make sure your doctor is aware of any drug reactions you have experienced.

Special warnings about this medication

If you have a history of stomach or intestinal disease, especially colitis, check with your doctor before taking Keflex.

If you have ever had an allergic reaction, particularly to drugs, be sure to tell your doctor.

If diarrhea occurs while taking cephalexin, check with your doctor before taking a remedy. Certain diarrhea medications (for instance, Lomotil) may increase your diarrhea or make it last longer.

Prolonged use of Keflex may result in an overgrowth of bacteria that do not respond to the medication, causing a secondary infection. Your doctor will monitor your use of this drug on a regular basis.

If you have a kidney disorder, check with your doctor before taking Keflex. You may need a reduced dose.

If you are diabetic, it is important to note that Keflex may cause false results in tests for urine sugar. Notify your doctor that you are taking this medication before being tested. Do not change your diet or dosage of diabetes medication without first consulting with your doctor.

If your symptoms do not improve within a few days, or if they get worse, notify your doctor immediately.

Do not give this medication to other people or use it for other infections before checking with your doctor.

Possible food and drug interactions when taking this medication

If Keflex is taken with certain other drugs, the effects of either could be increased, decreased, or altered. It is especially important to check with your doctor before combining Keflex with the following:

Certain diarrhea medications such as Lomotil
Oral contraceptives

Special information if you are pregnant or breastfeeding

The effects of Keflex during pregnancy have not been adequately studied. If you are pregnant or plan to become pregnant, notify your doctor immediately. Keflex appears in breast milk and could affect a nursing infant. If this medication is essential to your health, your doctor may advise you to discontinue breastfeeding until your treatment is finished.

Recommended dosage

ADULTS

Throat, Skin, and Urinary Tract Infections
The usual adult dosage is 500 milligrams taken every 12 hours. Cystitis (bladder infection) therapy should be continued for 7 to 14 days.

Other Infections
The usual recommended dosage is 250 milligrams taken every 6 hours. For more severe infections, larger doses may be needed, as determined by your doctor.

CHILDREN UNDER 15 YEARS OLD

Keflex
The usual dose is 25 to 50 milligrams for each 2.2 pounds of body weight per day, divided into smaller doses.

For strep throat in children over 1 year of age and for skin infections, the dose may be divided into 2 doses taken every 12 hours. For strep infections, the medication should be taken for at least 10 days. Your doctor may double the dose if your child has a severe infection.

For middle ear infection, the dose is 75 to 100 milligrams per 2.2 pounds per day, divided into 4 doses.

Keftab
Safety and effectiveness have not been established in children.

Overdosage
Any medication taken in excess can have serious consequences.

If you suspect an overdose, seek emergency medical treatment immediately.

■ *Symptoms of Keflex overdose may include:*
Blood in the urine, diarrhea, nausea, upper abdominal pain, vomiting

Keftab *See Keflex, page 703.*

KEPPRA
Pronounced: KEP-rah
Generic name: Levetiracetam

Why is this drug prescribed?
Keppra helps reduce the frequency of partial epileptic seizures, a form of epilepsy in which neural disturbances are limited to a specific region of the brain and the victim remains conscious throughout the attack. The drug is used along with other epilepsy medications, never by itself.

Most important fact about this drug
Keppra can cause dizziness and drowsiness. Do not drive, operate machinery, or engage in other hazardous activities until you're sure the drug won't interfere.

How should you take this medication?

Keppra may be taken with or without food.

Do not stop taking this drug on your own. If the doctor decides to discontinue Keppra, he will tell you how to taper off slowly. Abrupt discontinuation of Keppra can increase the frequency of seizures.

■ *If you miss a dose...*
Take it as soon as you remember. If it is almost time for your next dose, skip the one you missed and go back to your regular schedule. Never take 2 doses at the same time.
■ *Storage instructions...*
Store this prescription at room temperature.

What side effects may occur?

Side effects cannot be anticipated. If any develop or change in intensity, inform your doctor as soon as possible. Only your doctor can determine if it is safe for you to continue taking Keppra.

■ *Side effects may include:*
Depression, dizziness, drowsiness, headache, infection, loss of muscle coordination, nervousness, pain, runny nose, sore throat, weakness

Why should this drug not be prescribed?

You will not be able to use Keppra if it gives you an allergic reaction.

Special warnings about this medication

Especially during the first few weeks of treatment, Keppra sometimes triggers psychological problems, including psychosis, hallucinations, aggression, agitation, anger, hostility, irritability, anxiety, apathy, emotional instability, depression, and attempted suicide. These problems usually pass, but be sure to alert your doctor if you feel one developing; your doctor may have to discontinue the drug or change your dosage.

At the start of treatment, Keppra also can cause extreme drowsiness, unusual weakness, and coordination difficulties. Bring such symptoms to your doctor's attention. In a few patients, therapy must be stopped or reduced.

This drug has not been tested in children under age 16.

Possible food and drug interactions when taking this medication

No unwanted interactions have been identified to date.

Special information if you are pregnant or breastfeeding

In animal tests, Keppra has produced fetal abnormalities. Accordingly, Keppra is recommended for pregnant women only if its potential benefits outweigh the potential risk to the baby. Notify your physician immediately if you are pregnant or plan to become pregnant.

Keppra makes its way into breast milk and could cause serious reactions in a nursing infant. Do not take this drug while breastfeeding.

Recommended dosage

ADULTS

For adults and children over 16, the usual starting dosage of Keppra is 500 milligrams twice a day. The dose may be increased every 2 weeks up to a maximum dose of 1,500 milligrams twice a day. If you have kidney disease, your dosage will be lower.

Overdosage

Any medication taken in excess can have serious consequences. If you suspect an overdose, seek medical attention immediately.

■ *Symptoms of Keppra overdose may include:*
Aggression, agitation, coma, drowsiness, reduced consciousness, slowed breathing

KETEK

Pronounced: KEE-tek
Generic name: Telithromycin

Why is this drug prescribed?

Ketek is a new type of antibiotic known as a ketolide. It is used to treat bacterial infections in the lungs and sinuses, specifically:

Acute (severe or sudden) flare-ups of chronic bronchitis
Acute sinusitis
Aneumonia

Most important fact about this drug

Like all antibiotics, Ketek can cause a severe inflammation of the colon (known as pseudomembranous colitis). It results from bacterial overgrowth in the colon and ranges in severity from mild to life-threatening. Contact your doctor right away if you develop any of the following:

Abdominal cramps
Bloody stools
Frequent bowel movements
Low-grade fever
Watery diarrhea

How should you take this medication?

Try to take Ketek at the same time every day. It may be taken with or without food.

Your doctor will prescribe Ketek only to treat a bacterial infection; it will not cure a viral infection, such as the common cold. It's important to take the full dosage schedule of Ketek, even if you're feeling better in a few days. Not completing the full dosage schedule may decrease the drug's effectiveness and increase the chances that the bacteria may become resistant to Ketek and other antibiotics.

■ *If you miss a dose...*
Take the forgotten dose as soon as you remember. However, if it is almost time for your next dose, skip the one you missed and return to your regular schedule. Do not take two doses at once.

■ *Storage instructions...*
Store at room temperature.

What side effects may occur?

Side effects cannot be anticipated. If any develop or change in intensity, tell your doctor as soon as possible. Only your doctor can determine if it is safe to continue using Ketek.

■ *Side effects may include:*
Diarrhea, dizziness, headache, nausea

Why should this drug not be prescribed?

You should not use Ketek if you have ever had an allergic reaction to it or to macrolide antibiotics such as erythromycin (E-Mycin, Erytab, Erythrocin, and others), Zithromax, and Biaxin.

You should not use Ketek if you are currently taking the medications pimozide (Orap) or cisapride.

Special warnings about this medication

Use Ketek with caution if you have myasthenia gravis. The drug can worsen your symptoms and cause severe—and even life-threatening—reactions. Be sure to tell your doctor if you have this illness.

Ketek may cause visual problems, including blurred vision or difficulty focusing. These episodes can last for several hours. Problems with vision are most likely to occur after the first or second dose, although they can occur anytime during treatment. If visual problems occur, avoid driving a motor vehicle, operating heavy machinery, and engaging in other hazardous activities. Also avoid looking quickly from one object to another. If you have vision problems that interfere with your daily activities, notify your doctor.

Ketek could potentially affect heart rhythm and cause changes on an electrocardiogram (ECG or EKG). Tell the doctor if you develop an irregular heartbeat or if you faint while taking the drug. Use Ketek cautiously, if at all, if you have a condition that makes you susceptible to heartbeat irregularities, such as low potassium or magnesium levels, a severely slow heartbeat, or a congenital heart rhythm disturbance.

There have been reports of liver function problems in people taking Ketek. Use this drug cautiously if you've ever had liver problems, including hepatitis or jaundice (yellowing of the skin or whites of the eyes).

Possible food and drug interactions when taking this medication

Ketek should never be combined with the drugs pimozide (Orap) or cisapride.

Ketek could alter levels of certain cholesterol-lowering drugs, including atorvastatin (Lipitor), lovastatin (Mevacor, Altocor), and simvastatin (Zocor). This could increase the risk of drug-induced muscle damage. Therapy with these cholesterol drugs should generally be stopped until treatment with Ketek is finished.

Ketek should also be avoided if you're taking medication to correct an abnormal heart rhythm. Examples include quinidine, procainamide (Procanbid), and dofetilide (Tikosyn).

When Ketek is taken together with certain other drugs, the effects of either could be increased, decrease, or altered. It is especially important to check with your doctor before combining Ketek with the following:

Carbamazepine (Tegretol)
Cyclosporine (Sandimmune)
Digoxin (Lanoxin)
Diuretics (water pills) such as furosemide (Lasix) or
   hydrochlorothiazide (HydroDIURIL, Esidrix)
Ergot-containing drugs such as Cafergot
Hexobarbital
Itraconazole (Sporanox)
Ketoconazole (Nizoral)
Metoprolol (Lopressor, Toprol-XL)
Midazolam (Versed)
Phenytoin (Dilantin)
Rifampin (Rifadin, Rifamate, Rimactane)
Sirolimus (Rapamune)
Tacrolimus (Prograf)
Theophylline (Theo-Dur)

Special information if you are pregnant or breastfeeding

The effects of Ketek during pregnancy have not been adequately studied. Ketek should be used only if the benefits outweigh the potential risks to the baby. Notify your doctor right away if you become pregnant or plan to become pregnant while taking this drug.

It is not known whether Ketek appears in human breast milk. However, it did appear when given to breastfeeding animals. If this medication is essential to your health, the doctor may advise you to stop breastfeeding until your treatment is finished.

Recommended dosage

ADULTS 18 YEARS AND OLDER

The usual dose is two 400-milligram tablets (for a total of 800 milligrams) taken once a day at the same time. For acute flare-ups of chronic bronchitis or acute sinusitis, treatment lasts 5 days. For pneumonia, treatment lasts 7 to 10 days.

Safety and effectiveness in children have not been studied.

Overdosage

Although no specific information on Ketek overdose is available, any medication taken in excess can have serious consequences. If you suspect an overdose, seek emergency treatment immediately.

Ketoconazole *See Nizoral, page 956.*

Ketoprofen *See Orudis, page 1016.*

Ketorolac *See Toradol, page 1467.*

Ketorolac, ocular *See Acular, page 34.*

Ketotifen *See Zaditor, page 1606.*

KINERET
Pronounced: KIN-eh-ret
Generic name: Anakinra

Why is this drug prescribed?

Kineret is used to relieve the symptoms of rheumatoid arthritis. It is usually prescribed after other antirheumatic drugs have failed to make an improvement. Kineret can be prescribed alone or in combination with other drugs for rheumatoid arthritis.

Kineret works by blocking the effects of interleukin-1, an inflammatory compound released by the immune system. While fighting inflammation, Kineret may also affect the immune system's ability to fight infection.

Most important fact about this drug

Because of Kineret's potential impact on immunity, make sure your doctor knows if you have a condition that weakens your immune system. If you develop an infection while taking Kineret, notify your doctor immediately.

How should you take this medication?

Kineret is taken as an injection beneath the skin. Take it at the same time each day. Follow your doctor's instructions on how to administer this drug. Inspect the medication in the syringe before administering it. If the

Kineret solution is discolored or has particles in it, do not use the medication.

Do not save any unused portion of the medication. Do not use any medication that is beyond the expiration date. Dispose of the used needles in a puncture-resistant container. Never reuse a needle or syringe.

■ *If you miss a dose...*
Take it as soon as you remember. If it is almost time for your next dose, skip the one you missed and go back to your regular schedule. Do not take 2 doses at once.

■ *Storage instructions...*
Do not use Kineret beyond the expiration date shown on the carton. Store Kineret in a refrigerator (but not in the freezer) and protect from light. Do not shake.

What side effects may occur?
Side effects cannot be anticipated. If any develop or change in intensity, inform your doctor as soon as possible. Only your doctor can determine if it is safe for you to continue taking Kineret.

The most common side effect of Kineret is a reaction at the injection site, including redness, swelling, inflammation, and pain. These reactions usually disappear after the first month.

■ *Other side effects may include:*
Abdominal pain, bone and joint infections, diarrhea, flu-like symptoms, headache, nausea, serious infections such as cellulitis and pneumonia, sinus inflammation, upper respiratory infections

Why should this drug not be prescribed?
You should not take Kineret if you are sensitive to or have ever had an allergic reaction to this medication.

Special warnings about this medication
Because of Kineret's effect on the immune system, it has not been tested in people with immune disorders or chronic infections. Do not start taking this drug while you have an infection. Stop taking it and contact your doctor if you develop an infection. People with asthma have a higher risk of infection while using Kineret. Older adults are more prone to infections, and should use Kineret with caution.

Do not take a live vaccine while using Kineret; it's possible that you could contract the disease, although there's no evidence of this happening to date. It's also possible that Kineret could render any vaccination—live or killed—ineffective.

Use Kineret with caution if you have kidney disease. This condition makes a reaction to the drug more likely.

Kineret has not been tested in children under 18.

Possible food and drug interactions when taking this medication

Arthritis drugs classified as tumor necrosis factor (TNF)-blocking agents increase the risk of infection just as Kineret does, and taking the two types of drug together further increases the risk. Therefore, combining Kineret and a TNF-blocking agent is not recommended. TNF-blocking agents include:

Etanercept (Enbrel)
Infliximab (Remicade)

Special information if you are pregnant or breastfeeding

The effects of Kineret during pregnancy have not been adequately studied. If you are pregnant or plan to become pregnant, tell your doctor. Kineret should be used during pregnancy only if clearly needed.

It is not known whether Kineret appears in breast milk. Use the drug with caution while breastfeeding.

Recommended dosage

ADULTS

The dosage is one prefilled, 100-milligram syringe each day. Higher doses have no greater effect.

If you suffer from kidney problems, your doctor will lower the dose to 100 milligrams every other day.

Overdosage

Kineret overdose has produced no serious reactions. However any medication taken in excess can have serious consequences. If you suspect an overdose, seek medical help immediately.

KLONOPIN

Pronounced: KLON-uh-pin
Generic name: Clonazepam

Why is this drug prescribed?

Klonopin is used alone or along with other medications to treat convulsive disorders such as epilepsy. It is also prescribed for panic disorder—unexpected attacks of overwhelming panic accompanied by fear of recurrence. Klonopin belongs to a class of drugs known as benzodiazepines.

Most important fact about this drug

Klonopin works best when there is a constant amount in the bloodstream. To keep blood levels as constant as possible, take your doses at regularly spaced intervals and try not to miss any.

How should you take this medication?

Take Klonopin exactly as prescribed. If you are taking it for panic disorder and you find it makes you sleepy, your doctor may recommend a single dose at bedtime.

■ *If you miss a dose...*
If it is within an hour after the missed time, take the dose as soon as you remember. If you do not remember until later, skip the dose and go back to your regular schedule. Never take 2 doses at the same time.

■ *Storage instructions...*
Store at room temperature away from heat, light, and moisture.

What side effects may occur?

Side effects cannot be anticipated. If any develop or change in intensity, inform your doctor as soon as possible. Only your doctor can determine if it is safe for you to continue taking Klonopin.

■ *Side effects in seizure disorders may include:*
Behavior problems, drowsiness, lack of muscular coordination

■ *Side effects in panic disorder may include:*
Allergic reaction, constipation, coordination problems, depression, dizziness, fatigue, inflamed sinuses or nasal passages, flu, memory problems, menstrual problems, nervousness, reduced thinking ability, respiratory infection, sleepiness, speech problems, vaginal inflammation

Klonopin can also cause aggressive behavior, agitation, anxiety, excitability, hostility, irritability, nervousness, nightmares, sleep disturbances, and vivid dreams.

■ *Side effects due to a rapid decrease in dose or abrupt withdrawal from Klonopin may include:*
Abdominal and muscle cramps, behavior disorders, convulsions, depressed feeling, hallucinations, restlessness, sleeping difficulties, tremors

Why should this drug not be prescribed?

If you are sensitive to or have ever had an allergic reaction to Klonopin or similar drugs, such as Librium and Valium, you should not take this medication. Make sure your doctor is aware of any reactions you have experienced.

You should not take this medication if you have severe liver disease or the eye condition known as acute narrow-angle glaucoma.

Special warnings about this medication

Klonopin may cause you to become drowsy or less alert; therefore, you should not drive or operate dangerous machinery or participate in any hazardous activity that requires full mental alertness until you know how this drug affects you.

If you have several types of seizures, this drug may increase the possibility of grand mal seizures (epilepsy). Inform your doctor if this occurs. Your doctor may wish to prescribe an additional anticonvulsant drug or increase your dose.

Klonopin can be habit-forming and can lose its effectiveness as you build up a tolerance to it. You may experience withdrawal symptoms—such as convulsions, hallucinations, tremor, and abdominal and muscle cramps—if you stop using this drug abruptly. Discontinue or change your dose only in consultation with your doctor.

Possible food and drug interactions when taking this medication

Klonopin slows the nervous system, and its effects may be intensified by alcohol. Do not drink while taking this medication.

If Klonopin is taken with certain other drugs, the effects of either could be increased, decreased, or altered. It is especially important to check with your doctor before combining Klonopin with the following:

Antianxiety drugs such as Valium
Antidepressant drugs such as Elavil, Nardil, Parnate, and Tofranil
Barbiturates such as phenobarbital
Carbamazepine (Tegretol)
Major tranquilizers such as Haldol, Navane, and Thorazine
Narcotic pain relievers such as Demerol and Percocet
Oral antifungal drugs such as Fungizone, Mycelex, and Mycostatin
Other anticonvulsants such as Dilantin, Depakene, and Depakote
Sedatives such as Halcion

Special information if you are pregnant or breastfeeding

Avoid Klonopin if at all possible during the first 3 months of pregnancy; there is a risk of birth defects. When taken later in pregnancy, the drug can cause other problems, such as withdrawal symptoms in the newborn. If you are pregnant or plan to become pregnant, inform your doctor immediately. Klonopin appears in breast milk and could affect a nursing infant. Mothers taking this medication should not breastfeed.

Recommended dosage

SEIZURE DISORDERS

Adults

The starting dose should be no more than 1.5 milligrams per day, divided into 3 doses. Your doctor may increase your daily dosage by 0.5 to 1 milligram every 3 days until your seizures are controlled or the side effects become too bothersome. The most you should take in 1 day is 20 milligrams.

Children
The starting dose for infants and children up to 10 years old or up to 66 pounds should be 0.01 to 0.03 milligram—no more than 0.05 milligram—per 2.2 pounds of body weight daily. The daily dosage should be given in 2 or 3 smaller doses. Your doctor may increase the dose by 0.25 to 0.5 milligram every 3 days until seizures are controlled or side effects become too bad. If the dose cannot be divided into 3 equal doses, the largest dose should be given at bedtime. The maximum maintenance dose is 0.1 to 0.2 milligram per 2.2 pounds daily.

PANIC DISORDER

Adults
The starting dose is 0.25 milligram twice a day. After 3 days, your doctor may increase the dose to 1 milligram daily. Some people need as much as 4 milligrams a day.

Children
For panic disorder, safety and effectiveness have not been established in children under age 18.

Older Adults
Klonopin tends to build up in the body if the kidneys are weak—a common problem among older adults. Higher doses of the drug also tend to cause more drowsiness and confusion in older patients. People over age 65 are therefore started on low doses of Klonopin and watched with extra care.

Overdosage
Any medication taken in excess can have serious consequences. If you suspect an overdose, seek medical attention immediately.

■ *The symptoms of Klonopin overdose may include:*
    Coma, confusion, sleepiness, slowed reaction time

Klor-Con *See Micro-K, page 851.*

K-Tab *See Micro-K, page 851.*

Labetalol *See Normodyne, page 964.*

LAC-HYDRIN
Pronounced: lack-HIGH-drin
Generic name: Ammonium lactate

Why is this drug prescribed?
Lac-Hydrin is used in the treatment of dry, scaly skin, including the genetic condition called ichthyosis vulgaris. Available in cream and lotion form, the drug moisturizes the skin and breaks up the scales.

Most important fact about this drug

Keep areas treated with Lac-Hydrin out of the sun as much as possible. If you must go outdoors, protect treated areas with clothing.

How should you take this medication?

Shake the lotion well. Apply cream or lotion to the affected areas and rub in thoroughly.

- *If you miss a dose...*
  Apply it as soon as you remember. However, if it almost time for your next dose, skip the one you missed and return to your regular schedule.
- *Storage instructions...*
  Store at room temperature.

What side effects may occur?

Side effects cannot be anticipated. If any develop or change in intensity, tell your doctor as soon as possible. Only your doctor can determine if it is safe to continue using Lac-Hydrin.

- *Side effects may include:*
  Burning, dryness, eczema, irritation, itching, peeling, rash, skin discoloration, small spots on the skin, stinging

Why should this drug not be prescribed?

If Lac-Hydrin causes an allergic reaction, you will not be able to use it.

Special warnings about this medication

Use Lac-Hydrin only on the skin. Avoid contact with eyes, lips, and mucous membranes.

If the skin condition worsens, stop using Lac-Hydrin immediately and call your doctor.

Lac-Hydrin may cause stinging and burning when applied to raw or broken skin. Due to the possibility of irritation, use caution when you apply it to the face.

Possible food and drug interactions when taking this medication

No interactions are known.

Special information if you are pregnant or breastfeeding

The effects of Lac-Hydrin during pregnancy have not been adequately studied. If you are pregnant or plan to become pregnant, inform your doctor immediately. The drug should be used only if clearly needed.

Use Lac-Hydrin with caution when nursing a baby.

Recommended dosage

Doctors usually recommend rubbing the medication into the affected areas twice a day.

Overdosage

Lac-Hydrin is relatively non-toxic and an overdose is unlikely. Nevertheless, if you suspect a problem, don't hesitate to check with your doctor.

Lactulose See Chronulac Syrup, page 282.

LAMICTAL

Pronounced: LAM-ic-tal
Generic name: Lamotrigine
Other brand name: Lamictal CD

Why is this drug prescribed?

Lamictal is prescribed to control partial seizures in people with epilepsy. It is also used to control a serious form of epilepsy known as Lennox-Gastaut syndrome. Lamictal is used in combination with other antiepileptic medications or as a replacement for a medication such as Tegretol, Dilantin, phenobarbital, or Mysoline.

In addition, Lamictal is used to help prevent the manic and/or depressive phases of bipolar disorder.

Most important fact about this drug

You may develop a rash during the first 2 to 8 weeks of Lamictal therapy, particularly if you are also taking Depakene or Depakote. If this happens, notify your doctor immediately. The rash could become severe and even dangerous, particularly in children. Signs of a more serious reaction include hives, fever, swollen lymph glands, painful sores in the mouth or around the eyes, or swelling of the lips or tongue. A slight possibility of this problem remains for up to 6 months.

How should you take this medication?

Take Lamictal exactly as prescribed by your doctor. Taking more than the prescribed amount can increase your risk of developing a serious rash. Do not stop taking this medication without first discussing it with your doctor. An abrupt halt could increase your seizures. Your doctor can schedule a gradual reduction in dosage.

Lamictal Chewable Dispersible (CD) tablets may be swallowed whole, chewed, or dissolved in liquid. When chewing the tablets, drink a small amount of water or diluted fruit juice to aid in swallowing. When dissolving the tablets, add them to a small amount of water or diluted fruit juice (about 1 teaspoonful), and wait 1 minute, until the tablets are completely dissolved. Swirl the solution and drink immediately. Do not try to cut the dose by drinking only part of the solution.

■ *If you miss a dose...*
Take it as soon as you remember. If it is almost time for your next dose, skip the one you missed and go back to your regular schedule. Do not take 2 doses at once.

■ *Storage instructions...*
Store in a tightly closed container at room temperature. Keep dry and protect from light.

What side effects may occur?

Side effects cannot be anticipated. If any develop or change in intensity, tell your doctor as soon as possible. Only your doctor can determine if it is safe for you to continue taking Lamictal.

■ *Side effects may include:*
Abdominal pain, back pain, blurred vision, constipation, dizziness, double vision, dry mouth, fatigue, headache, increased cough, insomnia, nausea, rash, runny nose, sleepiness, sore throat, uncoordinated movements, vomiting

■ *Additional side effects in children may include:*
Bronchitis, convulsions, ear problems, eczema, facial swelling, hemorrhage, infection, indigestion, light sensitivity, lymph node problems, nervousness, penis disorder, sinus infection, swelling, tooth problems, urinary tract infection, vertigo, vision problems

Why should this drug not be prescribed?

If you are sensitive to or have ever had an allergic reaction to Lamictal, you should not take this medication. Make sure your doctor is aware of any drug reactions you have experienced.

Special warnings about this medication

Lamictal may cause some people to become drowsy, dizzy, or less alert. Do not drive or operate dangerous machinery or participate in any activity that requires full mental alertness until you are certain the drug does not have this kind of effect on you. Remember to be alert for development of any type of rash, especially during the first 2 to 8 weeks of treatment (see *Most important fact about this drug*).

Be sure to tell your doctor about any medical problems you have before starting therapy with Lamictal. If you have kidney or liver disease, or heart problems, Lamictal should be used with caution.

Lamictal may cause vision problems. If any develop, notify your doctor immediately. Also be quick to call your doctor if you develop a fever or have any other signs of an allergic reaction. Notify your doctor, too, if your seizures get worse.

If you're taking Lamictal for bipolar disorder, be aware that the drug should not be used to stop an episode of mania or depression once it has started.

There are no clinical studies to prove the safety and effectiveness of Lamictal for treating bipolar disorder in children less than 18 years old.

Possible food and drug interactions when taking this medication

If Lamictal is taken with certain other drugs, the effects of either could be increased, decreased, or altered. It is especially important to check with your doctor before combining Lamictal with the following:

Carbamazepine (Tegretol)
Drugs that inhibit folate metabolism, such as methotrexate and
   Septra
Oral contraceptives
Phenobarbital
Phenytoin (Dilantin)
Primidone (Mysoline)
Valproic acid (Depakene, Depakote)

Special information if you are pregnant or breastfeeding

The effects of Lamictal during pregnancy have not been adequately studied. If you are pregnant or plan to become pregnant, tell your doctor immediately. Lamictal should be used during pregnancy only if clearly needed. Lamictal appears in breast milk. Because the effects of Lamictal on an infant exposed to this medication are unknown, breastfeeding is not recommended.

Recommended dosage

ADULTS

Seizures

*Lamictal combined with Tegretol, Dilantin, Phenobarbital,
or Mysoline*
One 50-milligram dose per day for 2 weeks, then two 50-milligram doses per day, for 2 weeks. After that, your doctor will have you take a total of 300 milligrams to 500 milligrams a day, divided into 2 doses.

*Lamictal combined with Depakene or Depakote,
whether taken alone or with any of the above medications*
One 25-milligram dose every *other* day for 2 weeks, then 25 milligrams once a day for 2 weeks. After that, the doctor will prescribe a total of 100 milligrams to 400 milligrams a day, taken in 1 or 2 doses.

*Lamictal as a replacement for Tegretol, Dilantin,
Phenobarbital, Mysoline, or Valproate*
While you continue to take Tegretol, Dilantin, phenobarbital, or Mysoline, your doctor will add Lamictal, starting at a dose of 50 milligrams per day,

then gradually increasing the daily dose. Once you've reached a dosage of 500 milligrams per day divided into 2 doses, the doctor will then begin gradually reducing the dosage of the other drug until, after 4 weeks, it has been completely eliminated. If you're switching from valproate, your doctor will have you follow a slightly different regimen.

Bipolar Disorder

Lamictal NOT combined with Depakene, Depakote, Tegretol, Dilantin, Phenobarbital, or Mysoline
One 25-milligram dose of Lamictal per day for weeks 1 and 2, then 50 milligrams per day for weeks 3 and 4, then 100 milligrams a day for week 5. After that, your doctor will have you take a total of 200 milligrams a day.

Lamictal combined with Depakene or Depakote
One 25-milligram dose of Lamictal every *other* day for weeks 1 and 2, then 25 milligrams once a day for weeks 3 and 4, then 50 milligrams a day for week 5. After that, your doctor will have you take a total of 100 milligrams a day.

Lamictal combined with Tegretol, Dilantin, Phenobarbital, or Mysoline
One 50-milligram dose of Lamictal per day for weeks 1 and 2, then 50 milligrams twice a day for weeks 3 and 4, then 100 milligrams twice a day for week 5. After that, your doctor will have you take a total of 300 to 400 milligrams a day, divided into 2 doses.

If you are currently taking Lamictal and the doctor tells you to stop taking any of the medications listed above—or you start or stop taking oral contraceptives or psychiatric drugs—the doctor may need to adjust your Lamictal dose accordingly.

Because there is little data on the use of Lamictal in people with liver or kidney impairment, the drug should be used with caution. The doctor may have you take less than the usual dose and raise it based on your body's response.

CHILDREN 2 YEARS OF AGE AND OLDER

Seizures
Lamictal can be added to other epilepsy drugs prescribed for children under 16 who have partial seizures or a serious form of epilepsy known as Lennox-Gastaut syndrome. Doses for children under 12 are based on the child's weight. Children 12 and older receive the adult dose. Doses are increased gradually from a low starting level to limit the risk of severe rash. Lamictal is not used as a replacement drug for children under 16.

Bipolar Disorder
Due to the lack of clinical studies, Lamictal is not recommended for treating bipolar disorder in children under 18 years old.

Overdosage

A massive overdose of Lamictal can be fatal. If you suspect an overdose, seek medical treatment immediately.

■ *Symptoms of Lamictal overdose may include:*
Coma, decreased level of consciousness, delayed heartbeat, increased seizures, lack of coordination, rolling eyeballs

LAMISIL

Pronounced: LAM-ih-sill
Generic name: Terbinafine hydrochloride

Why is this drug prescribed?

Lamisil fights fungal infections. In tablet form, it's used for fungus of the toenail or fingernail. The cream and the solution are used for other fungal infections such as athlete's foot, jock itch, and ringworm. The solution is also used to treat tinea versicolor, a fungal infection that produces brown, tan, or white spots on the trunk of the body.

Most important fact about this drug

Lamisil does not produce instant results. You won't see the full effect of the tablets for several months, until a healthy new nail has grown out. The cream and solution also work gradually. It usually takes a week for results to appear, and improvement often continues for 2 to 6 weeks after treatment has stopped. However, if you see no change at all after a full week of applying the cream or solution, notify your doctor. The problem may be other than fungal.

How should you take this medication?

Before applying Lamisil solution, clean and dry the infected area thoroughly. Use enough solution to wet the entire area fully. When using either the solution or the cream, do not cover the treated area with dressings unless directed by your doctor.

Continue using Lamisil for the full amount of time your doctor prescribes, even if your symptoms begin to improve.

■ *If you miss a dose...*
Take it as soon as you remember. If it is almost time for your next dose, skip the one you missed and return to your regular schedule. Do not take 2 doses at one time.
■ *Storage instructions...*
Store the tablets at room temperature, away from light in a tight container. The cream and solution should be stored at room temperature, and not refrigerated.

What side effects may occur?

Side effects cannot be anticipated. If any develop or change in intensity, inform your doctor as soon as possible. Only your doctor can determine if it is safe for you to continue taking Lamisil.

Side effects of the cream and solution are uncommon. They include burning or irritation, itching, dryness, peeling, and rash.

The tablets are a bit more likely to cause a reaction.

■ *Side effects of the tablets may include:*
Diarrhea, headache, indigestion, rash

Why should this drug not be prescribed?

Do not use Lamisil if it has ever given you an allergic reaction.

Special warnings about this medication

Changes in the lens and retina of the eye have been reported in people taking Lamisil tablets. If you notice any changes in your vision while taking the tablets, notify your doctor.

Lamisil tablets have been known to cause rare cases of liver damage. If you develop warning signs such as nausea, loss of appetite, or fatigue, alert your doctor. Lamisil tablets are not recommended if you have liver disease or kidney problems.

If you suffer from the autoimmune disorder lupus erythematosus, you will not be able to take Lamisil.

Lamisil tablets have also, in rare instances, caused very severe skin reactions. If you develop a steadily worsening rash, stop taking the tablets and call your doctor immediately.

If you develop another kind of infection while taking Lamisil tablets, tell your doctor. Lamisil may decrease your ability to fight infection.

Do not use Lamisil cream or solution in the eyes, mouth, nose, or vagina. In case of accidental contact with the eyes, rinse them thoroughly with running water and call your doctor if symptoms continue.

If you develop skin irritation, redness, itching, burning, blistering, swelling, or oozing while using the cream or solution, notify your doctor. Do not cover the treated area with dressings unless directed by your doctor.

Lamisil has not been tested for safety in children.

Possible food and drug interactions when taking this medication

If Lamisil is taken with certain other drugs, the effects of either could be increased, decreased, or altered. It is especially important to check with your doctor before combining Lamisil tablets with the following:

Antidepressants such as Elavil, Nardil, Norpramin, Pamelor, Parnate, Paxil, Prozac, Tofranil, and Zoloft
Cimetidine (Tagamet)
Cyclosporine (Neoral, Sandimmune)

Drugs classified as beta-blockers, such as the heart and blood
  pressure medications Inderal, Sectral, and Tenormin
Rifampin (Rifadin, Rimactane)

Special information if you are pregnant or breastfeeding

The safety of Lamisil during pregnancy has not been conclusively proven.
Treatment with the tablets should not be started during pregnancy, and
the cream and solution should be used only if clearly needed.

Lamisil from the tablets does appear in breast milk, so the drug is not
recommended while breastfeeding. Do not apply Lamisil cream or solution to the breast.

Recommended dosage

TABLETS

Fungal Infection of the Fingernails
The recommended dose is one 250-milligram tablet once a day for 6
weeks.

Fungal Infection of the Toenails
The recommended dose is one 250-milligram tablet once a day for 12
weeks.

CREAM

Athlete's Foot, Jock Itch, and Ringworm
Apply to the affected and closely surrounding areas twice a day until
signs and symptoms improve. Use for a minimum of 7 days, but no more
than 4 weeks.

For athlete's foot found only on the soles of the feet and not between
the toes, use the cream twice a day for 2 weeks.

SOLUTION

Athlete's Foot and Tinea Versicolor
Apply to the affected and closely surrounding areas twice a day for 1
week.

Jock Itch and Ringworm
Apply to the affected and closely surrounding areas once a day for 1
week.

Overdosage

Any medication taken in excess can have serious consequences. If you
suspect an overdose with Lamisil tablets, seek medical treatment immediately.

■ *Symptoms of overdose with Lamisil tablets may include:*
Abdominal pain, dizziness, frequent urination, headache, nausea, rash, vomiting

Lamivudine *See Epivir, page 517.*

Lamivudine and Zidovudine *See Combivir, page 330.*

Lamotrigine *See Lamictal, page 718.*

LANOXIN

Pronounced: *la-NOCKS-in*
Generic name: *Digoxin*
Other brand name: *Digitek*

Why is this drug prescribed?

Lanoxin is used in the treatment of congestive heart failure, certain types of irregular heartbeat, and other heart problems. It improves the strength and efficiency of your heart, which leads to better circulation of blood and reduction of the uncomfortable swelling that is common in people with congestive heart failure. Lanoxin is usually prescribed along with a water pill (to help relieve swelling) and a drug called an ACE inhibitor (to further improve circulation). It belongs to a class of drugs known as digitalis glycosides.

Most important fact about this drug

You should not stop taking Lanoxin without first consulting your doctor. A sudden absence of the drug could cause a serious change in your heart function. You will probably have to take Lanoxin for a long time—possibly for the rest of your life.

How should you take this medication?

Lanoxin usually is taken once daily. To help you remember your dose, try to take it at the same time every day, for instance when brushing your teeth in the morning or going to bed at night.

Lanoxin is available in tablet, capsule, liquid, and injectable forms. If you are taking the liquid form, use the specially marked dropper that comes with it.

It's best to take this medicine on an empty stomach. However, if this upsets your stomach, you can take Lanoxin with food.

Avoid taking this medicine with high-bran/high-fiber foods, such as certain breakfast cereals.

Do not change from one brand of this drug to another without first consulting your doctor or pharmacist.

Your doctor may ask you to check your pulse rate while taking Lanoxin.

Slowing or quickening of your pulse could mean you are developing side effects to your prescribed dose. The amount of Lanoxin needed to help most people is very close to the amount that could cause serious problems from overdose, so monitoring your pulse can be very important.

■ *If you miss a dose...*
If you remember within 12 hours, take it immediately. If you remember later, skip the dose you missed and go back to your regular schedule. Never take 2 doses at the same time. If you miss doses 2 or more days in a row, consult your doctor.

■ *Storage instructions...*
Store this medication at room temperature in the container it came in, tightly closed, and away from moist places and direct light. Keep out of reach of children. Digitalis-type drugs such as Lanoxin are a major cause of accidental poisoning in the young.

What side effects may occur?
Side effects cannot be anticipated. If any develop or change in intensity, inform your doctor as soon as possible. Only your doctor can determine if it is safe for you to continue taking Lanoxin.

■ *Side effects may include:*
Apathy, blurred vision, breast development in males, change in heartbeat, confusion, diarrhea, dizziness, headache, loss of appetite, lower stomach pain, nausea, psychosis, rash, vomiting, weakness, yellow vision

Why should this drug not be prescribed?
If you are sensitive to or have ever had an allergic reaction to Lanoxin or other digitalis preparations, you should not take this medication. Make sure your doctor is aware of any drug reactions you have experienced.

Lanoxin should not be taken by people with the heart irregularity known as ventricular fibrillation.

Lanoxin should not be used, alone or with other drugs, for weight reduction. It can cause irregular heartbeat and other dangerous, even fatal, reactions.

Special warnings about this medication
Your doctor will prescribe Lanoxin with caution—if at all—in the presence of certain heart disorders, including sinus node disease, AV block, certain disorders of the left ventricle, and Wolff-Parkinson-White syndrome. Caution is also advised if you have poor kidneys, a thyroid disorder, or an imbalance in your calcium, potassium, or magnesium levels.

Tell the doctor that you are taking Lanoxin if you have a medical emergency and before you have surgery or dental treatment.

Even if you have no symptoms, do not change your dose or discontinue the use of Lanoxin before consulting with your doctor.

Possible food and drug interactions when taking this medication
In general, you should avoid nonprescription medicines, such as antacids; laxatives; cough, cold, and allergy remedies; and diet aids, except on professional advice.

If Lanoxin is taken with certain other drugs, the effects of either can be increased, decreased, or altered. It is especially important to check with your doctor before combining Lanoxin with the following:

Airway-opening drugs such as Proventil and Ventolin
Alprazolam (Xanax)
Amiloride (Midamor)
Amiodarone (Cordarone)
Antacids such as Maalox and Mylanta
Antibiotics such as neomycin, tetracycline, erythromycin, and
    clarithromycin
Beta-blocking blood pressure drugs such as Tenormin and
    Inderal
Calcium (injectable form)
Calcium-blocking blood pressure drugs such as Calan SR,
    Cardizem, and Procardia
Certain anticancer drugs such as Neosar
Cholestyramine (Questran)
Colestipol (Colestid)
Cyclosporine (Sandimmune)
Diphenoxylate (Lomotil)
Disopyramide (Norpace)
Heartbeat-regulating drugs such as Quinidex
Indomethacin (Indocin)
Itraconazole (Sporanox)
Kaolin-pectin
Metoclopramide (Reglan)
Propafenone (Rythmol)
Propantheline (Pro-Banthine)
Rifampin (Rifadin)
Spironolactone (Aldactone)
Steroids such as Decadron and Deltasone
Succinylcholine (Anectine)
Sucralfate (Carafate)
Sulfasalazine (Azulfidine)
Thyroid hormones such as Synthroid
Water pills such as Lasix

Special information if you are pregnant or breastfeeding
The effects of Lanoxin during pregnancy have not been adequately studied. If you are pregnant or plan to become pregnant, inform your doctor immediately. Lanoxin appears in breast milk and could affect a nursing in-

fant. If this medication is essential to your health, your doctor may advise you to discontinue breastfeeding.

Recommended dosage

Your doctor will determine your dosage based on several factors: (1) the disease being treated; (2) your body weight; (3) your kidney function; (4) your age; and (5) other diseases you have or drugs you are taking.

If you are receiving Lanoxin for the first time, you may be rapidly dosed (a larger first dose may be taken, followed by smaller maintenance doses), or gradually dosed (maintenance doses only), depending on your doctor's recommendation.

ADULTS

If your doctor feels you need rapid digitalization, your first few doses may be given intravenously. You'll then be switched to tablets or capsules for long-term maintenance. A typical maintenance dose might be a 0.125-milligram or 0.25-milligram tablet once daily, but individual requirements vary widely. The exact dose will be determined by your doctor, based on your needs.

CHILDREN

Infants and young children usually have their daily dose divided into smaller doses; children over age 10 need adult dosages in proportion to body weight as determined by your doctor.

Overdosage

Suspected overdoses of Lanoxin must be treated immediately; you should contact your doctor or emergency room without delay.

■ *Symptoms of Lanoxin overdose include:*
Abdominal pain, diarrhea, irregular heartbeat, loss of appetite, nausea, very slow pulse, vomiting
In infants and children, irregular heartbeat is the most common sign of overdose.

Lansoprazole See Prevacid, page 1143.

Lansoprazole and Naproxen See Prevacid NapraPAC, page 1147.

LASIX

Pronounced: LAY-six
Generic name: Furosemide

Why is this drug prescribed?

Lasix is used in the treatment of high blood pressure and other conditions that require the elimination of excess fluid (water) from the body. These conditions include congestive heart failure, cirrhosis of the liver, and kidney disease. When used to treat high blood pressure, Lasix is effective alone or in combination with other high blood pressure medications. Diuretics help your body produce and eliminate more urine, which helps lower blood pressure. Lasix is classified as a "loop diuretic" because of its point of action in the kidneys.

Lasix is also used with other drugs in people with fluid accumulation in the lungs.

Most important fact about this drug

Lasix acts quickly, usually within 1 hour. However, since blood pressure declines gradually, it may be several weeks before you get the full benefit of Lasix; and you must continue taking it even if you are feeling well. Lasix does not cure high blood pressure; it merely keeps it under control.

How should you take this medication?

Take this medication exactly as prescribed by your doctor.

■ *If you miss a dose...*
Take the forgotten dose as soon as you remember. If it is almost time for your next dose, skip the one you missed and go back to your regular schedule. Never take 2 doses at the same time.

■ *Storage instructions...*
Keep this medication in the container it came in, tightly closed, and away from direct light. Store at room temperature.

What side effects may occur?

Side effects cannot be anticipated. If any develop or change in intensity, inform your doctor as soon as possible. Only your doctor can determine if it is safe for you to continue taking Lasix.

■ *Side effects may include:*
Anemia, blood disorders, blurred vision, constipation, cramping, diarrhea, dizziness, dizziness upon standing, fever, headache, hearing loss, high blood sugar, hives, itching, loss of appetite, low potassium (leading to symptoms like dry mouth, excessive thirst, weak or irregular heartbeat, muscle pain or cramps), muscle spasms, nausea, rash, reddish or purplish spots on the skin, restlessness, ringing in the ears, sensitivity to light, skin eruptions, skin inflammation and flaking,

stomach or mouth irritation, tingling or pins and needles, vertigo, vision changes, vomiting, weakness, yellow eyes and skin

Why should this drug not be prescribed?

If you are sensitive to or have ever had an allergic reaction to Lasix or diuretics, or if you are unable to urinate, you should not take this medication.

Special warnings about this medication

Lasix can cause your body to lose too much potassium. Signs of an excessively low potassium level include muscle weakness and rapid or irregular heartbeat. To improve your potassium level, your doctor may prescribe a potassium supplement or recommend potassium-rich foods, such as bananas, raisins, and orange juice.

Make sure the doctor knows if you have kidney disease, liver disease, diabetes, gout, or the connective tissue disease, lupus erythematosus. Lasix should be used with caution.

If you are allergic to sulfa drugs, you may also be allergic to Lasix.

If you have high blood pressure, avoid over-the-counter medications that may increase blood pressure, including cold remedies and appetite suppressants.

Your skin may be more sensitive to the effects of sunlight.

Possible food and drug interactions when taking this medication

If Lasix is taken with certain other drugs, the effects of either could be increased, decreased, or altered. It is especially important to consult with your doctor before taking Lasix with any of the following:

Aminoglycoside antibiotics such as Garamycin
Aspirin and other salicylates
Ethacrynic acid (Edecrin)
Indomethacin (Indocin)
Lithium (Lithonate)
Norepinephrine (Levophed)
Other high blood pressure medications such as Hytrin and Cardura
Sucralfate (Carafate)

Special information if you are pregnant or breastfeeding

The effects of Lasix during pregnancy have not been adequately studied. If you are pregnant or plan to become pregnant, inform your doctor immediately. Lasix appears in breast milk and could affect a nursing infant. If this medication is essential to your health, your doctor may advise you to discontinue breastfeeding until your treatment is finished.

Recommended dosage

Your doctor will adjust the dosages of this strong diuretic to meet your specific needs.

ADULTS

Fluid Retention

You will probably be started at a single dose of 20 to 80 milligrams. If needed, the same dose can be repeated 6 to 8 hours later, or the dose may be increased. Your doctor may raise the dosage by 20 milligrams or 40 milligrams with each successive administration—each 6 to 8 hours after the previous dose—until the desired effect is achieved. This dosage is then taken once or twice daily thereafter. Your doctor should monitor you carefully using laboratory tests. The maximum daily dose is 600 milligrams.

High Blood Pressure

The usual starting dose is 80 milligrams per day, divided into 2 doses. Your doctor will adjust the dosages and may add other high blood pressure medications if Lasix is not enough.

CHILDREN

The usual initial dose is 2 milligrams per 2.2 pounds of body weight given in a single oral dose. The doctor may increase subsequent doses by 1 to 2 milligrams per 2.2 pounds. Doses are spaced 6 to 8 hours apart. A child's dosage will be adjusted to the lowest needed to achieve maximum effect, and should not exceed 6 milligrams per 2.2 pounds.

Overdosage

Any medication taken in excess can have serious consequences. An overdose of Lasix can cause symptoms of severe dehydration. If you suspect an overdose, seek medical attention immediately.

■ *Symptoms of Lasix overdose may include:*
   Dry mouth, excessive thirst, low blood pressure, muscle pain or cramps, nausea and vomiting, weak or irregular heartbeat, weakness or drowsiness

Latanoprost *See Xalatan, page 1592.*

Leflunomide *See Arava, page 121.*

LESCOL

Pronounced: LESS-cahl
Generic name: Fluvastatin sodium

Why is this drug prescribed?

Lescol reduces "bad" LDL cholesterol—and increases "good" HDL cholesterol—in the blood, and can lower your chances of developing clogged arteries and heart disease. It is also prescribed to slow the accumulation of plaque in the arteries of people who already have coronary heart disease, and may be prescribed for you when you are released from the hospital after a heart attack.

Also, if you have coronary heart disease you may be prescribed Lescol to reduce the risk of undergoing coronary revascularization procedures (angioplasty, bypass surgery, or stent insertion).

Your doctor will prescribe Lescol only if you have been unable to reduce your blood cholesterol level sufficiently with a low-fat, low-cholesterol diet alone. For people at high risk of heart disease, current guidelines call for considering drug therapy when LDL levels reach 130. For people at lower risk, the cutoff is 160. For those at little or no risk, it's 190.

Most important fact about this drug

Lescol is usually prescribed only if diet, exercise, and weight loss fail to bring your cholesterol levels under control. It's important to remember that Lescol is a supplement—not a substitute—for those other measures. To get the full benefit of the medication, you need to stick to the diet and exercise program prescribed by your doctor. All these efforts to keep your cholesterol levels normal are important because together they may lower your risk of heart disease.

How should you take this medication?

Lescol is available in standard capsules and extended-release tablets (Lescol XL).

If you are taking standard Lescol capsules and you've been prescribed a small, single dose per day, take it at bedtime. A large dosage (80 milligrams) may be divided into 2 smaller doses and taken twice a day.

Lescol XL tablets should be taken once a day at bedtime. The tablets should be swallowed whole, never crushed or chewed. You may take Lescol with or without food.

■ *If you miss a dose...*
If you miss a dose of this medication, take it as soon as you remember. However, if it is almost time for your next dose, skip the one you missed and go back to your regular schedule. Do not take 2 doses at the same time.

■ *Storage instructions...*
Store at room temperature in a tightly closed container. Protect from direct light and excessive heat.

What side effects may occur?

Side effects cannot be anticipated. If any develop or change in intensity, tell your doctor as soon as possible. Only your doctor can determine if it is safe for you to continue taking Lescol.

■ *Side effects may include:*
Abdominal pain, accidental injury, diarrhea, flu-like symptoms, headache, indigestion, joint diseases, muscle pain, nasal inflammation, nausea

This side effects list is not complete. If you have any questions about side effects you should consult your doctor. Report any new or continuing symptoms to your doctor right away.

Why should this drug not be prescribed?

Do not take Lescol while pregnant or nursing. Also avoid Lescol if you are experiencing liver problems, or if you have ever been found to be excessively sensitive to it. A variety of conditions that raise cholesterol levels should be ruled out before you turn to Lescol therapy. These problems include diabetes, kidney disease, poor thyroid function, liver disease, and alcoholism.

Special warnings about this medication

Because Lescol may damage the liver, your doctor may order a blood test to check your liver enzyme levels before you start taking this medication. Blood tests will probably be done 12 weeks after you start Lescol therapy, whenever your dose is increased, and periodically after that. If your liver enzymes rise too high, your doctor may tell you to stop taking Lescol. Your doctor will monitor you especially closely if you have ever had liver disease or if you are, or have ever been, a heavy drinker.

Since Lescol may cause damage to muscle tissue, be sure to tell your doctor of any unexplained muscle pain, tenderness, or weakness right away, especially if you also have a fever or feel sick. Your doctor may want to do a blood test to check for signs of muscle damage. If your blood test shows signs of muscle damage, your doctor may suggest discontinuing this medication.

If your risk of muscle and/or kidney damage suddenly increases because of major surgery or injury, or conditions such as low blood pressure, severe infection, or seizures, your doctor may tell you to stop taking Lescol for a while.

Possible food and drug interactions when taking this medication

If you take Lescol with certain drugs, the effects of either could be increased, decreased, or altered. It is especially important to check with your doctor before combining Lescol with the following:

Cholestyramine (Questran)
Cimetidine (Tagamet)
Clofibrate (Atromid-S)
Cyclosporine (Sandimmune, Neoral)

Diclofenac (Voltaren)
Digoxin (Lanoxin, Lanoxicaps)
Erythromycin (E-Mycin, E.E.S.)
Gemfibrozil (Lopid)
Glyburide (Micronase)
Niacin (Niaspan)
Omeprazole (Prilosec)
Phenytoin (Dilantin)
Ranitidine (Zantac)
Rifampin (Rifadin)

Special information if you are pregnant or breastfeeding

You must not become pregnant while taking Lescol. This medication lowers cholesterol, and cholesterol is needed for a baby to develop properly. Because of the possible risk of birth defects, your doctor will prescribe Lescol only if you are highly unlikely to get pregnant while taking this medication. If you do become pregnant while taking Lescol, stop taking the drug and notify your doctor right away.

Lescol does appear in breast milk. Therefore, Lescol could cause severe side effects in a nursing baby. Do not take Lescol while breastfeeding your baby.

Recommended dosage

Your doctor will put you on a cholesterol-lowering diet before starting treatment with Lescol. You should continue on this diet while you are taking Lescol.

ADULTS

Lescol Capsules

The usual starting dose is 20 to 40 milligrams per day taken as a single dose at bedtime. The usual range after that is 20 to 80 milligrams per day. At the 80-milligram level, the dosage will be split into two 40-milligram doses taken 2 times a day. If you have kidney disease, doses over 40 milligrams should be used with caution. After 4 weeks of therapy with Lescol, your doctor will check your cholesterol level and adjust your dosage if necessary.

Lescol XL Tablets

The usual starting dose is one 80-milligram XL tablet taken as a single dose at bedtime. After 4 months of therapy with Lescol XL, your doctor will check your cholesterol level and adjust your dosage if necessary.

Combined Drug Therapy

If you are taking Lescol capsules with another cholesterol medication such as Questran, make sure you take the other drug at least 2 hours before your dose of Lescol.

CHILDREN

Do not give Lescol to children under 18 years of age.

Overdosage

Excessive doses of Lescol can cause a variety of stomach and intestinal problems. If you suspect an overdose, seek medical treatment immediately.

Leuprolide See Lupron Depot, page 800.

Levalbuterol See Xopenex, page 1602.

LEVAQUIN

Pronounced: LEAV-ah-kwin
Generic name: Levofloxacin

Why is this drug prescribed?

Levaquin cures a variety of bacterial infections, including several types of sinus infection and pneumonia. It is also prescribed for flare-ups of chronic bronchitis, acute kidney infections, certain urinary or chronic prostate infections, and skin infections. Levaquin is a member of the quinolone family of antibiotics.

Most important fact about this drug

Levaquin has been known to cause dangerous allergic reactions as soon as you take the first dose. Stop taking the drug and call your doctor immediately if you develop any of the following warning signs:

Difficulty swallowing or breathing
Rapid heartbeat
Skin rash, hives, or any other skin reaction
Swelling of the face, lips, tongue, or throat

How should you take this medication?

Take your complete prescription exactly as directed, even if you begin to feel better. If you stop taking Levaquin too soon, the infection may come back.

You may take Levaquin at mealtimes or in between, but you should avoid taking it within 2 hours of the following:

Aluminum or magnesium antacids such as Maalox, Mylanta,
   or Gaviscon
Any multivitamin preparation containing zinc
Iron supplements such as Ferro-Sequels or Feosol
The ulcer medication Carafate
Videx chewable tablets or pediatric powder

Be sure to drink plenty of fluid while taking Levaquin.

■ *If you miss a dose...*
Take it as soon as you remember. If it is almost time for your next dose, skip the one you missed and go back to your regular schedule. Do not take 2 doses at once.

■ *Storage instructions...*
Store at room temperature. Keep container tightly closed.

What side effects may occur?

Side effects cannot be anticipated. If any develop or change in intensity, tell your doctor as soon as possible. Only your doctor can determine if it is safe for you to continue taking Levaquin.

■ *More common side effects may include:*
Constipation, diarrhea, difficulty sleeping, headache, nausea

■ *Less common or rare side effects may include:*
Abdominal pain, abnormal dreams, abnormal or double vision, aggressiveness, agitation, anemia, angina, anxiety, asthma, back pain, blood abnormalities, blood clots, changeable emotions, chest pain, circulatory failure, colitis, coma, confusion, depression, difficulty in or obstructed breathing, difficulty concentrating, disorientation, dizziness, emotional or mental problems, exaggerated sense of well-being, fainting, fungal infection, gangrene or other infections, gas, genital infection and itching, hallucination, heart attack, heart failure, heartbeat irregularities, high or low blood pressure, high or low blood sugar, hives, impaired thinking, indigestion, intestinal bleeding, intestinal inflammation or blockage, irregular heartbeat, itching, kidney disorders, lack of muscle coordination, liver disorders, lung problems or inflammation, muscle pain weakness, pancreatitis, paralysis, pneumonia, rapid or slow heartbeat, rash, seizures, swelling of face or extremities, swollen tongue, tendon inflammation, tumor, vaginal inflammation, vertigo, vomiting, yellowing of eyes and skin

Why should this drug not be prescribed?

If any other quinolone antibiotic—such as Cipro, Floxin, Maxaquin, Noroxin, or Penetrex—has ever given you an allergic reaction, avoid Levaquin.

Special warnings about this medication

In rare cases, Levaquin has caused convulsions and other nervous disorders. If you develop any warning signs of a nervous reaction—ranging from restlessness and tremors to depression and hallucinations—stop taking this medication and call your doctor.

Levaquin may cause dizziness or light-headedness. Do not drive or operate machinery until you know how this drug affects you.

Hypersensitivity to quinolone antibiotics can, in rare instances, lead to severe illnesses ranging from blood disorders to liver or kidney failure. The first sign of a developing problem is often a rash, so you should stop taking Levaquin and check with your doctor when any type of skin disorder appears. Remember, too, that an immediate allergic reaction is also a possibility (see *Most important fact about this drug*).

A case of diarrhea during Levaquin therapy could signal development of the potentially dangerous condition known as pseudomembranous colitis, an inflammation of the bowel. Call your doctor for treatment at the first sign of a problem.

Stop taking Levaquin, avoid exercise, and call your doctor if you develop pain, inflammation, or a rupture in a tendon. Quinolone antibiotics have been known to cause tendon rupture during and after therapy. The danger of this is greater when quinolones are combined with steroid medications, especially among older adults.

In rare cases, Levaquin has been known to cause heartbeat irregularities. Avoid this drug if you are taking other medications that can change the heartbeat, or if you have a condition that predisposes you to this problem, such as a weak heart, a slow heartbeat, or low potassium.

If you have a kidney condition, make sure the doctor is aware of it. Your dosage may need to be lowered.

Possible food and drug interactions when taking this medication

Nonsteroidal anti-inflammatory drugs such as Advil, Motrin, and Naprosyn can increase the risk of a nervous reaction to Levaquin. Also, check with your doctor before combining Levaquin with an oral diabetes drug such as Glucotrol, Micronase, or Orinase; changes in blood sugar levels could result.

If you are taking the asthma drug theophylline or the blood-thinning drug, Coumadin, make sure your doctor is aware of it. Other quinolone antibiotics have been known to interact with these medications.

Special information if you are pregnant or breastfeeding

The possibility that Levaquin might harm a developing baby has not been ruled out. It should be used during pregnancy only if the potential benefit outweighs the possible risk. If you are pregnant or plan to become pregnant, inform your doctor immediately. Levaquin is likely to appear in breast milk and could harm a nursing infant. If the drug is essential to your health, your doctor may advise you to stop nursing until your treatment is finished.

Recommended dosage

ADULTS

Respiratory and Uncomplicated Skin Infections, and Chronic Prostate Infections
The usual dose is 500 milligrams once a day. For certain types of pneumonia, the dose is 750 milligrams once a day. Treatment of respiratory in-

fections typically lasts 5 to 14 days; for uncomplicated skin infections, expect 7 to 10 days of treatment; for chronic prostate infections, treatment lasts for 28 days.

Complicated Skin Infections
The usual dose is 750 milligrams once a day. Treatment typically lasts for 7 to 14 days.

Kidney and Urinary Infections
The usual dose is 250 milligrams once a day. Treatment lasts 3 to 10 days.

CHILDREN

Not for children under 18. Levaquin might damage developing bones and joints.

Overdosage
Levaquin is not especially poisonous. However, an overdose could still be dangerous. If you suspect one, seek emergency treatment immediately.

■ *Symptoms of Levaquin overdose may include:*
Breathlessness, collapse, convulsions, lack of movement, poor coordination, tremors

Levbid *See Levsin, page 742.*

Levetiracetam *See Keppra, page 706.*

LEVITRA
Pronounced: Luh-VEE-trah
Generic name: Vardenafil

Why is this drug prescribed?
Levitra is an oral drug for male impotence, also known as erectile dysfunction (ED). It works by dilating blood vessels in the penis, allowing the inflow of blood needed for an erection.

Most important fact about this drug
Levitra causes erections only during sexual excitement. It does not work in the absence of arousal and does not increase sexual desire.

How should you take this medication?
Take one Levitra tablet about one hour before sexual activity, with or without food.

■ *If you miss a dose...*
Take Levitra only before sexual activity, but no more than once a day. Do not take 2 doses at once.

■ *Storage instructions...*
Store at room temperature.

What side effects may occur?

Side effects cannot be anticipated. If any develop or change in intensity, tell your doctor as soon as possible. Only your doctor can determine if it is safe to continue using Levitra.

■ *Side effects may include:*
Flu-like symptoms, flushing, headache, indigestion, runny nose, sinus inflammation

This side effects list is not complete. If you have any questions about side effects you should consult your doctor. Report any new or continuing symptoms to your doctor right away.

Why should this drug not be prescribed?

Do not take Levitra if you are taking any nitrate-based drug, including nitroglycerin patches (Nitro-Dur, Transderm-Nitro), nitroglycerin ointment (Nitro-Bid, Nitrol), nitroglycerin pills (Nitro-Bid, Nitrostat), and isosorbide pills (Dilatrate-SR, Isordil, Sorbitrate). This also includes street drugs known as "poppers," including amyl nitrate and butyl nitrate. Combining Levitra with any of these drugs can cause a dangerous drop in blood pressure.

Likewise, do not take Levitra with certain blood pressure and prostate drugs known as alpha-blockers, including Cardura (doxazosin), Flomax (tamsulosin), Hytrin (terazosin), Minipress (prazosin), and Uroxatral (alfuzosin).

If Levitra gives you an allergic reaction, do not use it again.

Special warnings about this medication

If you have heart problems severe enough to make sexual activity a danger, you should avoid using Levitra. If you take this drug and develop cardiac symptoms (for example, dizziness, nausea, and chest pain) during sexual activity, do not continue. Alert your doctor to the problem as soon as possible.

Because Levitra has not been studied in people with cardiovascular disease, it's best to avoid this drug if you've recently had a stroke or heart failure, or if you've had a heart attack within the past 6 months. Be equally cautious if you have severely high or low blood pressure, heartbeat irregularities, or unstable angina (crushing heart pain that occurs at any time). If you develop angina after taking Levitra, seek medical attention immediately.

If you have severe kidney or liver problems, a bleeding disorder, stomach ulcer, or an inherited retinal disorder such as retinitis pigmentosa, use this medication with caution. Its safety under these circumstances has not yet been studied.

Rare cases of prolonged and sometimes painful erection (known as priapism) have been reported with Levitra. If you develop an erection that lasts more than 4 hours, seek medical treatment immediately. Otherwise, permanent damage and impotence could result.

If you have a condition that might result in long-lasting erections, such as sickle-cell anemia, multiple myeloma (a disease of the bone marrow), or leukemia, use Levitra with caution. Also use caution if you have a genital problem or deformity such as Peyronie's disease.

Remember that Levitra offers no protection from transmission of sexually transmitted diseases, such as HIV, the virus that causes AIDS.

Possible food and drug interactions when taking this medication
Be sure to check with your doctor about the medications that should never be taken with Levitra, including:

Alpha-blocking drugs prescribed for high blood pressure or prostate problems, including doxazosin (Cardura), tamsulosin (Flomax), terazosin (Hytrin), prazosin (Minipress), and alfuzosin (Uroxatral)
Nitrate-based drugs prescribed for chest pain, such as nitroglycerin patches (Nitro-Dur, Transderm-Nitro), nitroglycerin ointment (Nitro-Bid, Nitrol), nitroglycerin pills (Nitro-Bid, Nitrostat), and isosorbide pills (Dilatrate-SR, Isordil, Sorbitrate)
Street drugs known as "poppers," including amyl nitrate and butyl nitrate

If Levitra is taken with certain other drugs, the effects of either could be increased, decreased, or altered. It is especially important to check with your doctor before combining Levitra with the following:

Other impotence drugs including alprostadil (Caverject), sildenafil (Viagra), and tadalafil (Cialis)
Amiodarone (Pacerone)
Erythromycin (E-Mycin, Ery-Tab, PCE)
Indinavir (Crixivan)
Itraconazole (Sporanox)
Ketoconazole (Nizoral)
Nifedipine (Procardia)
Procainamide (Procanbid)
Quinidine (Quinidex)
Ritonavir (Norvir)
Sotalol (Betapace)

Special information about pregnancy and breastfeeding
Levitra should not be used by women. Its effects during pregnancy and breastfeeding have not been studied.

Recommended dosage

ADULT MALES

Doses range from 5 to 20 milligrams, depending on the drug's effect. The recommended starting dose is 10 milligrams for most people. However, if you're 65 or older, the doctor may start you at 5 milligrams.

Take Levitra only before sexual activity. The manufacturer recommends a maximum of 1 dose per day. However, your doctor may need to lower the dose if you're taking certain drugs that affect the liver, including erythromycin, indinavir (Crixivan), itraconazole (Sporanox), ketoconazole (Nizoral), and ritonavir (Norvir).

If you have moderate liver impairment, the recommended starting dose is 5 milligrams, not to exceed a daily dose of 10 milligrams. If your liver problems are mild, no dosage adjustment is required.

Overdosage

A small study found that a single 120-milligram dose of Levitra caused reversible side effects such as vision changes and back and muscle pain. However, any medication taken in excess can have serious consequences. If you suspect an overdose, seek medical attention immediately.

Levlen See *Oral Contraceptives, page 1000.*

Levlite See *Oral Contraceptives, page 1000.*

Levobunolol See *Betagan, page 208.*

Levofloxacin See *Levaquin, page 735.*

Levonorgestrel for emergency contraception See *Plan B, page 1102.*

Levonorgestrel and Ethinyl estradiol See *Preven, page 1150.*

Levora See *Oral Contraceptives, page 1000.*

Levothroid See *Synthroid, page 1375.*

Levothyroxine See *Synthroid, page 1375.*

Levoxyl See *Synthroid, page 1375.*

LEVSIN

Pronounced: LEV-sin
Generic name: Hyoscyamine sulfate
Other brand names: Anaspaz, Levbid, Levsinex, NuLev

Why is this drug prescribed?

Levsin is an antispasmodic medication given to help treat various stomach, intestinal, and urinary tract disorders that involve cramps, colic, or other painful muscle contractions. Because Levsin has a drying effect, it may also be used to dry a runny nose or to dry excess secretions before anesthesia is administered.

Together with morphine or other narcotics, Levsin is prescribed for the pain of gallstones or kidney stones. For inflammation of the pancreas, Levsin may be used to help control excess secretions and reduce pain. Levsin may also be taken in Parkinson's disease to help reduce muscle rigidity and tremors and to help control drooling and excess sweating. The drug is sometimes prescribed during treatment for peptic ulcer.

Doctors also give Levsin as part of the preparation for certain diagnostic X-rays (for example, of the stomach, intestines, or kidneys).

Levsin comes in several forms, including regular tablets, tablets to be dissolved under the tongue, tablets that dissolve on the tongue (NuLev), sustained-release capsules (Levsinex Timecaps) and sustained-release tablets (Levbid), liquid, drops, and an injectable solution.

Most important fact about this drug

Levsin may make you sweat less, causing your body temperature to increase and putting you at the risk of heatstroke. Try to stay inside as much as possible on hot days, and avoid warm places such as very hot baths and saunas.

How should you take this medication?

If you take Levsin for a stomach disorder, you may also need to take antacid medication. However, antacids make it more difficult for the body to absorb Levsin. To minimize this problem, take Levsin before meals and the antacid after meals.

Take Levsin exactly as prescribed. Although the sublingual tablets (Levsin/SL) are designed to be dissolved under the tongue, they may also be chewed or swallowed. The regular tablets should be swallowed. Levbid extended-release tablets should not be crushed or chewed. NuLev tablets should be placed on the tongue, allowed to disintegrate, then swallowed. They can be taken with or without water.

Levsin can cause dry mouth. For temporary relief, suck on a hard candy or chew gum.

■ *If you miss a dose...*
Take it as soon as you remember. If it is almost time for your next dose, skip the one you missed and go back to your regular schedule. Do not take 2 doses at once.

■ *Storage instructions...*
Store at room temperature. Protect NuLev tablets from moisture.

What side effects may occur?

Side effects cannot be anticipated. If any side effects develop or change in intensity, tell your doctor immediately. Only your doctor can determine whether it is safe for you to continue taking Levsin.

■ *Side effects may include:*
Allergic reactions, bloating, blurred vision, confusion, constipation, decreased sweating, dilated pupils, dizziness, drowsiness, dry mouth, excitement, headache, hives, impotence, inability to urinate, insomnia, itching, heart palpitations, lack of coordination, loss of sense of taste, nausea, nervousness, rapid heartbeat, skin reactions, speech problems, vomiting, weakness

Why should this drug not be prescribed?

Do not take Levsin if you have ever had an allergic reaction to it or similar drugs such as scopolamine. Also, you should not be given Levsin if you have any of the following:

Bowel or digestive tract obstruction or paralysis
Glaucoma (excessive pressure in the eyes)
Myasthenia gravis (a disorder in which muscles become weak and tire easily)
Ulcerative colitis (severe bowel inflammation)
Urinary obstruction

Levsin is not appropriate if you have diarrhea, especially if you have a surgical opening to the bowels (an ileostomy or colostomy).

Special warnings about this medication

Be careful using Levsin if you have an overactive thyroid gland, heart disease, congestive heart failure, irregular heartbeats, high blood pressure, or kidney disease.

Because Levsin may make you dizzy or drowsy, or blur your vision, do not drive, operate other machinery, or do any other hazardous work while taking this medication.

While you are taking Levsin, you may experience confusion, disorientation, short-term memory loss, hallucinations, difficulty speaking, lack of coordination, coma, an exaggerated sense of well-being, decreased anxiety, fatigue, sleeplessness and agitation. These symptoms should disappear 12 to 48 hours after you stop taking the drug.

People who must avoid phenylalanine should note that NuLev tablets contain this substance.

Possible food and drug interactions when taking this medication

If Levsin is taken with certain other drugs, the effects of either drug could be increased, decreased, or altered. It is especially important to check with your doctor before combining Levsin with the following:

Amantadine (Symmetrel)
Antacids
Antidepressant drugs such as Elavil, Nardil, Parnate, and Tofranil
Antihistamines such as Benadryl
Major tranquilizers such as Thorazine and Haldol
Other antispasmodic drugs such as Bentyl
Potassium supplements such as Slow-K

Special information if you are pregnant or breastfeeding

If you are pregnant or plan to become pregnant, inform your doctor immediately. Although it is not known whether Levsin can cause birth defects, pregnant women should avoid all drugs except those necessary to health.

Levsin appears in breast milk. Your doctor may ask you to forgo breastfeeding when taking this drug.

Recommended dosage

LEVSIN, LEVSIN/SL, AND NULEV TABLETS

Adults and Children 12 Years and Older
The usual dose is 1 to 2 tablets every 4 hours or as needed. Do not take more than 12 tablets in 24 hours.

Children 2 to 12 Years
The usual dose is ½ to 1 tablet every 4 hours or as needed. Do not give a child more than 6 tablets in 24 hours.

LEVSIN ELIXIR

Adults and Children 12 Years and Older
The recommended dosage is 1 to 2 teaspoonfuls every 4 hours or as needed, but no more than 12 teaspoonfuls in 24 hours.

Children 2 to 12 Years
Dosage is by body weight. Doses may be given every 4 hours or as needed. Do not give a child more than 6 teaspoonfuls in 24 hours.

Weight	Dose
22 pounds	¼ teaspoon
44 pounds	½ teaspoon
88 pounds	¾ teaspoon
110 pounds	1 teaspoon

LEVSIN DROPS

Adults and Children 12 Years and Older
The recommended dosage is 1 to 2 milliliters every 4 hours or as needed, but no more than 12 milliliters in 24 hours.

Children 2 to 12 Years
The usual dosage is ¼ to 1 milliliter every 4 hours or as needed. Do not give a child more than 6 milliliters in 24 hours.

Children Under 2 Years
Your doctor will determine the dosage based on body weight. The doses may be repeated every 4 hours or as needed.

Weight	Usual Dose	Do not Exceed in 24 Hours
7.5 pounds	4 drops	24 drops
11 pounds	5 drops	30 drops
15 pounds	6 drops	36 drops
22 pounds	8 drops	48 drops

LEVSINEX TIMECAPS

Adults and Children 12 Years and Older
The recommended dosage is 1 to 2 capsules every 12 hours. Your doctor may adjust the dosage to 1 capsule every 8 hours if needed. Do not take more than 4 capsules in 24 hours.

LEVBID EXTENDED-RELEASE TABLETS

Adults and Children 12 Years and Older
The dosage is 1 to 2 tablets every 12 hours. The tablets are scored so that you can break them in half if your doctor wants you to. Do not crush or chew them. You should not take more than 4 tablets in 24 hours.

Overdosage
Any medication taken in excess can have serious consequences. If you suspect an overdose, seek medical attention immediately.

■ *Symptoms of Levsin overdose may include:*
Blurred vision, dilated pupils, dizziness, dry mouth, excitement, headache, hot dry skin, nausea, swallowing difficulty, vomiting

Levsinex *See Levsin, page 742.*

LEXAPRO

Pronounced: LEKS-uh-proh
Generic name: Escitalopram oxalate

Why is this drug prescribed?

Lexapro is prescribed for major depression—a persistently low mood that interferes with daily functioning. To be considered major, depression must occur nearly every day for at least 2 weeks, and must include at least 5 of the following symptoms: low mood, loss of interest in usual activities, significant change in weight or appetite, change in sleep patterns, agitation or lethargy, fatigue, feelings of guilt or worthlessness, slowed thinking or lack of concentration, and thoughts of suicide.

Lexapro is also prescribed for generalized anxiety disorder, a condition marked by excessive worry and anxiety that is hard to control and interferes with daily life. To be diagnosed with this disorder, your symptoms must have lasted at least 6 months and you must have at least 3 of the following: restlessness, fatigue, poor concentration, irritability, muscle tension, and sleep disturbances.

Lexapro works by boosting levels of serotonin, one of the chief chemical messengers in the brain. The drug is a close chemical cousin of the antidepressant medication Celexa. Other antidepressants that work by raising serotonin levels include Paxil, Prozac, and Zoloft.

Most important fact about this drug

Do not take Lexapro for 2 weeks before or after taking any drug classified as an MAO inhibitor. Drugs in this category include the antidepressants Marplan, Nardil, and Parnate. Combining these drugs with Lexapro can cause serious and even fatal reactions marked by such symptoms as fever, rigidity, twitching, and agitation leading to delirium and coma.

How should you take this medication?

Take Lexapro exactly as prescribed, even after you begin to feel better. Although improvement usually begins within 1 to 4 weeks, treatment typically continues for several months. Lexapro is available in tablet and liquid forms and can be taken with or without food.

■ *If you miss a dose...*
Take the forgotten dose as soon as you remember. However, if it is almost time for your next dose, skip the one you missed and return to your regular schedule. Do not take 2 doses at once.
■ *Storage instructions...*
Store at room temperature.

What side effects may occur?

Side effects cannot be anticipated. If any develop or change in intensity, tell your doctor as soon as possible. Only your doctor can determine if it is safe to continue using Lexapro.

■ *Side effects may include:*

Constipation, decreased appetite, decreased sex drive, diarrhea, dizziness, dry mouth, ejaculation disorder, fatigue, flu-like symptoms, headache, impotence, indigestion, insomnia, nausea, runny nose, sinusitis, sleepiness, sweating

Why should this drug not be prescribed?

You'll be unable to use Lexapro if it causes an allergic reaction, or if you've ever had an allergic reaction to the related drug Celexa. Remember, too, that you must never take Lexapro while taking an MAO inhibitor such as Marplan, Nardil, or Parnate.

Special warnings about this medication

In clinical studies, antidepressants increased the risk of suicidal thinking and behavior in children and adolescents with depression and other psychiatric disorders. Anyone considering the use of Lexapro or any other antidepressant in a child or adolescent must balance this risk with the clinical need. Lexapro has not been studied in children or adolescents and is not approved for treating anyone less than 18 years old.

Additionally, the progression of major depression is associated with a worsening of symptoms and/or the emergence of suicidal thinking or behavior in both adults and children, whether or not they are taking antidepressants. Individuals being treated with Lexapro and their caregivers should watch for any change in symptoms or any new symptoms that appear suddenly—especially agitation, anxiety, hostility, panic, restlessness, extreme hyperactivity, and suicidal thinking or behavior—and report them to the doctor immediately. Be especially observant at the beginning of treatment or whenever there is a change in dose.

Lexapro makes some people sleepy. Until you know how the drug affects you, use caution when driving a car or operating other hazardous machinery.

In rare cases, Lexapro can trigger mania (unreasonably high spirits and excess energy). If you've ever had this problem, be sure to let the doctor know.

Also make sure that the doctor knows if you have liver problems or severe kidney disease. Your dosage may need adjustment.

Convulsions have been reported during Lexapro treatment. If you have a history of seizures, use this drug with caution.

Serotonin-boosting antidepressants could potentially cause stomach bleeding, especially in older people or those taking nonsteroidal anti-inflammatory drugs (NSAIDs) such as aspirin, ibuprofen (Advil, Motrin), naproxen (Aleve), and ketoprofen (Orudis KT). Consult your doctor before combining Lexapro with NSAIDs or blood-thinning medications.

You should never stop taking Lexapro without consulting your doctor. An abrupt decrease in dose could cause withdrawal symptoms such as mood problems, lethargy, insomnia, and tingling sensations.

Possible food and drug interactions when taking this medication

Do not use Lexapro if you are taking the related drug Celexa. Be sure to avoid MAO inhibitors when taking Lexapro. Although Lexapro does not interact with alcohol, the manufacturer recommends avoiding alcoholic beverages.

If Lexapro is taken with certain other drugs, the effects of either could be increased, decreased, or altered. It is especially important to check with your doctor before combining Lexapro with the following:

Aspirin
Carbamazepine (Tegretol)
Cimetidine (Tagamet)
Desipramine (Norpramin)
Drugs that act on the brain, including antidepressants, painkillers, sedatives, and tranquilizers
Ketoconazole (Nizoral)
Linezolid (Zyvox)
Lithium (Eskalith)
Metoprolol (Lopressor)
Narcotic painkillers
Nonsteroidal anti-inflammatory drugs such as Advil and Motrin
Sumatriptan (Imitrex)
Warfarin (Coumadin)

Special information if you are pregnant or breastfeeding

There have been reports of newborns developing serious complications after exposure to Lexapro late in the last 3 months of pregnancy. If you are pregnant or plan to become pregnant, inform your doctor immediately. Lexapro should be taken during pregnancy only if its benefits outweigh the potential risks.

Lexapro appears in breast milk and can affect a nursing infant. If you decide to breastfeed, Lexapro is not recommended.

Recommended dosage

ADULTS

The recommended dose of Lexapro tablets or oral solution is 10 milligrams once a day. If necessary, the doctor may increase the dose to 20 milligrams after a minimum of 1 week, but the higher dose is not recommended for most older adults and people with liver problems.

Overdosage

A massive overdose of Lexapro can be fatal. If you suspect an overdose, seek emergency treatment immediately.

■ *Typical symptoms of Lexapro overdose include:*
Dizziness, drowsiness, nausea, rapid heartbeat, seizures, sweating, tremors, vomiting

In rare cases, an overdose may also cause memory loss, confusion, coma, breathing problems, muscle wasting, irregular heartbeat, and a bluish tinge to the skin.

LEXIVA

Pronounced: Lex-EE-vah
Generic name: Fosamprenavir calcium

Why is this drug prescribed?

Lexiva is prescribed for adults with human immunodeficiency virus (HIV) infection. HIV undermines the immune system, reducing the body's ability to fight off other infections and eventually leading to the deadly condition known as acquired immune deficiency syndrome (AIDS).

Lexiva slows the progression of HIV by interfering with an important step in the virus's reproductive cycle. The drug is a member of the group of protease inhibitors. Lexiva is prescribed only as part of a drug regimen that attacks the virus on several fronts. It is not to be used alone.

Lexiva is not a cure for HIV infection or AIDS. It does not completely eliminate HIV from the body, nor does it totally restore the immune system. There is still a danger of developing serious opportunistic infections (that is, infections that develop when the immune system falters). It is important, therefore, to continue seeing your doctor for regular blood counts and tests. Notify your healthcare provider immediately of any change in your general health.

Most important fact about this drug

Combining Lexiva with certain drugs can cause serious—and possibly life-threatening—side effects (see *Possible food and drug interactions when taking this medication*). Be sure to tell your doctor and pharmacist what medications you are taking, both prescription and over-the-counter, and let them know when you stop taking any medication.

How should you take this medication?

Lexiva can be taken with or without food. Take Lexiva every day as prescribed. Do not change your dose or stop taking Lexiva without talking to your doctor.

■ *If you miss a dose...*
Take the forgotten dose as soon as you remember, then return to your normal schedule. However, if it is almost time for your next dose, skip the one you missed and return to your regular schedule. Do not take two doses at once.

■ *Storage instructions...*
Store at room temperature. Keep the container tightly closed.

What side effects may occur?

Side effects cannot be anticipated. If any develop or change in intensity, tell your doctor as soon as possible. Only your doctor can determine if it is safe to continue using Lexiva.

■ *Side effects may include:*
Diarrhea, headache, nausea, rash, vomiting

Why should this drug not be prescribed?

If Lexiva causes an allergic reaction, you will not be able to use it. If you have severe liver damage, you should not use Lexiva.

Certain drugs should never be combined with Lexiva due to the risk of serious—and possibly life-threatening—side effects (see *Possible food and drug interactions when taking this medication*).

Special warnings about this medication

There is no reason to believe that taking Lexiva lowers your chances of transmitting HIV to others. Continue to take precautions to prevent transmission of virus.

Lexiva can interfere with oral contraceptives. Use a backup form of birth control to avoid an unwanted pregnancy.

Lexiva must be used with caution if you have liver problems. If you have any liver disorder, make sure your doctor is aware of it.

One serious potential side effect of Lexiva is a rash that occasionally becomes so severe as to be life-threatening. If you notice any signs of rash, inform your doctor immediately. If the rash gets worse or is accompanied by fever, blisters, mouth sores, red eyes, swelling, or flu-like symptoms, stop taking the drug and call your doctor.

Lexiva may trigger diabetes or make it worse. If this occurs, you may have to start taking insulin or oral diabetes drugs, or have your dosage of these medications adjusted. Lexiva plus ritonavir can increase levels of a lipid called triglyceride, possibly resulting in the need for treatment.

Like other HIV drugs, Lexiva sometimes causes a redistribution of body fat, resulting in added weight around the waist, a "buffalo hump" of fat on the upper back, breast enlargement, and wasting of the face, arms, and legs. It's not known why this occurs, or what long-term effects it might have.

Lexiva belongs to the sulfonamide family of drugs. If you have an allergy to sulfa drugs such as Bactrim or Septra, be sure to tell your doctor.

Possible food and drug interactions when taking this medication

Be sure to check with your doctor about the medicines and herbal remedies that should *not* be taken with this drug. Due to the danger of life-threatening side effects, Lexiva should never be combined with any of the following:

Cisapride
Dihydroergotamine (Migranal)
Ergonovine (Ergotrate)
Ergotamine (Cafergot)
Lovastatin (Mevacor)
Methylergonovine (Methergine)
Pimozide (Orap)
Midazolam (Versed)
Simvastatin (Zocor)
Triazolam (Halcion)

Due to the potential for serious or life-threatening side effects, your doctor will monitor you closely if you must take Lexiva with any of the following:

Amiodarone (Cordarone)
Antidepressants known as tricyclics, such as amitriptyline (Elavil) and imipramine (Tofranil)
Bepridil (Vascor)
Certain cholesterol-lowering drugs in the statin family, such as atorvastatin (Lipitor)
Lidocaine (systemic)
Quinidine (Quinidex)

If you are taking both Lexiva and the HIV drug ritonavir (Norvir), you must be careful to avoid the heart medications flecainide (Tambocor) and propafenone (Rythmol).

Rifampin (Rifadin, Rifamate, Rifater) and St. John's wort should never be given with Lexiva because they combat the antiviral effects of Lexiva. Delavirdine should not be given with Lexiva as the combination may lead to resistance to delavirdine.

Be careful about combining Lexiva with Viagra or other erectile dysfunction drugs such as Cialis or Levitra. The combination increases the risk of the side effects of those agents, such as low blood pressure, changes in your vision, and persistent painful erection.

If Lexiva is taken with certain other drugs, the effects of either could be increased, decreased, or altered. It is especially important to check with your doctor before combining Lexiva with the following:

Acid reflux medications classified as *proton pump inhibitors,* such as AcipHex and Nexium

Antifungal medications such as Nizoral and Sporanox

Antiulcer medications classified as H_2-receptor antagonists, such as Zantac and Tagamet

Anxiety medications (tranquilizers) such as Tranxene, Valium, and Xanax

Dexamethasone (Decadron)

Efavirenz (Sustiva)

Flurazepam (Dalmane)

High blood pressure and angina medications (calcium channel blockers), such as Adalat, Calan, Cardene, Cardizem, Dilacor, DynaCirc, Nimotop, Norvasc, Plendil, Procardia, and Sular

HIV medications such as Crixivan and Viracept

Immune-suppressing drugs such as Neoral, Prograf, Rapamune, Sandimmune

Lopinavir/ritonavir (Kaletra)

Methadone

Nevirapine (Viramune)

Oral contraceptives

Rifabutin (Mycobutin)

Ritonavir (Norvir)

Saquinavir (Fortovase)

Seizure medications such as Dilantin, Tegretol, and phenobarbital

Warfarin (Coumadin)

Special information if you are pregnant or breastfeeding

The effects of Lexiva during pregnancy have not been adequately studied. If you are pregnant or plan to become pregnant, tell your doctor immediately.

Since HIV infection can be passed to your baby through breast milk, you should not breastfeed.

Recommended dosage

ADULTS

If you have never taken anti-HIV medication before
Your doctor will prescribe one of the following regimens:

■ Lexiva 1,400 milligrams (two 700-milligram tablets) twice daily (without ritonavir)

■ Lexiva 1,400 milligrams (two 700-milligram tablets) once daily plus ritonavir 200 milligrams once daily

■ Lexiva 700 milligrams (one 700-milligram tablet) twice daily plus ritonavir 100 milligrams twice daily

If you have taken anti-HIV medication anytime before
The recommended dose of Lexiva is 700 milligrams twice daily plus ritonavir 100 milligrams twice daily. HIV-infected persons who have taken protease inhibitors before should *not* take Lexiva plus ritonavir once daily.

If you are taking Lexiva and ritonavir with efavirenz
If you are taking this combination once a day, your doctor will increase the usual dose of ritonavir to 300 milligrams. No dosage adjustment is needed if you are taking this combination twice a day.

CHILDREN

Lexiva is not recommended for use in children.

THOSE WITH REDUCED LIVER FUNCTION

Your doctor may prescribe Lexiva at a reduced dose of 700 milligrams twice daily if you have mild or moderate liver damage and are not also taking ritonavir. Lexiva is not recommended for people with severe liver damage.

Overdosage

Little is known about the symptoms of Lexiva overdose. However, any medication taken in excess can have serious consequences. If you suspect an overdose, seek medical attention immediately.

LEXXEL

Pronounced: LECKS-ell
Generic ingredients: Enalapril maleate, Felodipine

Why is this drug prescribed?

Lexxel is used to treat high blood pressure. It combines two blood pressure drugs: an ACE inhibitor and a calcium channel blocker. The ACE inhibitor (enalapril) lowers blood pressure by preventing a chemical in your blood called angiotensin I from converting to a more potent form that narrows the blood vessels and increases salt and water retention. The calcium channel blocker (felodipine) also works to keep the blood vessels open, and eases the heart's workload by reducing the force and rate of your heartbeat.

Lexxel can be prescribed alone or in combination with other blood pressure medicines, especially water pills (diuretics) such as Hydro-DIURIL or Esidrix.

Most important fact about this drug

Doctors usually prescribe Lexxel for patients who have been taking one of its components—enalapril (Vasotec) or extended-release felodipine (Plendil)—without showing improvement. Like other blood pressure medications, Lexxel must be taken regularly for it to be effective. Since blood pressure declines gradually, it may be 1 or 2 weeks before you get the full benefit of Lexxel; and you must continue taking it even if you are feeling well. Lexxel does not cure high blood pressure; it merely keeps it under control.

How should you take this medication?

Lexxel can be taken with a light meal or without food. Remember, however, that a high-fat meal can reduce its effectiveness, and that grapefruit juice increases its impact.

Swallow Lexxel tablets whole. Do not crush, divide, or chew them.

■ *If you miss a dose...*
Take it as soon as you remember. If it is almost time for your next dose, skip the one you missed and go back to your regular schedule. Never take 2 doses at the same time.

■ *Storage instructions...*
Store at room temperature. Keep the container tightly closed and protect from light and humidity.

What side effects may occur?

Side effects cannot be anticipated. If any develop or change in intensity, inform your doctor as soon as possible. Only your doctor can determine if it is safe for you to continue taking Lexxel.

■ *Side effects may include:*
Dizziness, headache, swelling

Why should this drug not be prescribed?

Avoid Lexxel if you have ever had an allergic reaction to it, or have ever developed a swollen throat and difficulty swallowing (angioedema) while taking similar drugs such as Capoten, Vasotec, or Zestril. Make sure your doctor is aware of the incident.

Special warnings about this medication

Call your doctor immediately if you begin to suffer angioedema while taking Lexxel. Warning signs include swelling of the face, lips, tongue, or throat; swelling of the arms and legs; and difficulty swallowing or breathing.

Bee or wasp venom given to prevent an allergic reaction to stings may cause a severe allergic reaction to Lexxel. Kidney dialysis can also prompt an allergic reaction to the drug.

Lexxel sometimes causes a severe drop in blood pressure. The danger is especially great if you have been taking water pills (diuretics), or if you have heart disease, kidney disease, or a potassium or salt imbalance. Excessive sweating, severe diarrhea, and vomiting are also a threat. They can rob the body of water, causing a dangerous drop in blood pressure. If you feel light-headed or faint, have chest pain, or feel your heart racing, contact your doctor immediately.

Because another of the ACE inhibitors, Capoten, has been known to cause serious blood disorders, your doctor will check your blood regularly while you are taking Lexxel. If you develop signs of infection such as a sore throat or a fever, you should contact your doctor at once—an infection could be a signal of blood abnormalities.

Lexxel may also affect the liver; and your doctor will need to adjust your dosage with extra care if you are over 65 or have liver disease. Report these symptoms of liver problems to your doctor immediately: a generally run-down feeling, pain in the upper right abdomen, or yellowing of the skin or the whites of your eyes.

If you suffer from heart failure or kidney disease, make certain that your doctor knows about it. Lexxel should be used with caution under these circumstances.

Some people taking Lexxel develop a dry, nagging cough. This will go away when you stop taking the drug. Others are troubled by swollen gums. Good dental hygiene makes this less likely.

Possible food and drug interactions when taking this medication

If Lexxel is taken with certain other drugs, the effects of either could be increased, decreased, or altered. It is especially important to check with your doctor before combining Lexxel with the following:

Cimetidine (Tagamet)
Diuretics such as Lasix or HydroDIURIL
Diuretics that leave potassium in the body, such as Aldactone, Midamor, and Dyrenium
Epilepsy medications such as Dilantin, phenobarbital, and Tegretol
Erythromycin (E.E.S., E-Mycin, ERYC, others)
Grapefruit juice
High-fat meals
Itraconazole (Sporanox)
Lithium (Eskalith, Lithobid)
Potassium supplements such as K-Lyte, K-Tabs, and Slow-K

Because Lexxel tends to increase your potassium level, avoid potassium-containing salt substitutes unless your doctor approves.

Special information if you are pregnant or breastfeeding

Do not take Lexxel during pregnancy. When taken during the final 6 months, the ACE inhibitor in Lexxel can cause birth defects, prematurity, and death in the developing or newborn baby. If you are pregnant, inform your doctor immediately.

Lexxel may appear in breast milk and could affect a nursing infant. If this medication is essential to your health, your doctor may advise you to stop breastfeeding.

Recommended dosage

ADULTS

Lexxel is available in two strengths. Lexxel 5-2.5 contains 5 milligrams of enalapril and 2.5 milligrams of felodipine. Lexxel 5-5 contains 5 milligrams of each.

The usual starting dose is 1 tablet of Lexxel 5-5 once a day. If there is no change in your blood pressure after 1 or 2 weeks, the doctor may increase your dose to 2 tablets once a day. If your blood pressure still remains too high, the dose may be increased to 4 tablets of Lexxel once a day. The doctor may also add a water pill (containing a thiazide) to your regimen.

CHILDREN

The safety and effectiveness of Lexxel in children have not been established.

OLDER ADULTS

If you are over 65, your doctor may have to monitor your blood pressure closely at the beginning of treatment, and adjust your dose with care.

Overdosage

Any medication taken in excess can have serious consequences. If you suspect an overdose, seek medical treatment immediately.

■ *Symptoms of Lexxel overdose may include:*
Low blood pressure, rapid heartbeat

LIBRAX

Pronounced: LIB-racks
Generic ingredients: Chlordiazepoxide hydrochloride,
Clidinium bromide

Why is this drug prescribed?

Librax is used, in combination with other therapy, for the treatment of peptic ulcer, irritable bowel syndrome (spastic colon), and acute enterocolitis (inflammation of the colon and small intestine). Librax is a combination of a benzodiazepine (chlordiazepoxide) and an antispasmodic medication (clidinium).

Most important fact about this drug

Because of its sedative effects, you should not operate heavy machinery, drive, or engage in other hazardous tasks that require you to be mentally alert while you are taking Librax.

How should you take this medication?
Take Librax as directed by your doctor. Other therapy may be prescribed to be used at the same time.

Librax can make your mouth dry. For temporary relief, suck a hard candy or chew gum.

Take Librax before meals and at bedtime.

■ *If you miss a dose...*
Take it as soon as you remember. If it is almost time for your next dose, skip the one you missed and go back to your regular schedule. Do not take 2 doses at once.

■ *Storage instructions...*
Store away from heat, light, and moisture.

What side effects may occur?
Side effects cannot be anticipated. If any develop or change in intensity, inform your doctor as soon as possible. Only your doctor can determine if it is safe for you to continue taking Librax.

■ *Side effects may include:*
Blurred vision, changes in sex drive, confusion, constipation, drowsiness, dry mouth, fainting, lack of coordination, liver problems, minor menstrual irregularities, nausea, skin eruptions, swelling due to fluid retention, urinary difficulties, yellowing of skin and eyes

Why should this drug not be prescribed?
You should not take this drug if you have glaucoma (elevated pressure in the eye), prostatic hypertrophy (enlarged prostate), or a bladder obstruction. If you are sensitive to or have ever had an allergic reaction to Librax or any of its ingredients, you should not take this medication. Make sure your doctor is aware of any drug reactions you have experienced.

Special warnings about this medication
Librax can be habit-forming and has been associated with drug dependence and addiction. Be very careful taking this medication if you have ever had problems with alcohol or drug abuse. Never take more than the prescribed amount.

In addition, you should not stop taking Librax suddenly, because of the risk of withdrawal symptoms (convulsions, cramps, tremors, vomiting, sweating, feeling depressed, and insomnia). If you have been taking Librax over a long period of time, your doctor will have you taper off gradually.

The elderly are more likely to develop side effects such as confusion, excessive drowsiness, and uncoordinated movements when taking Librax. The doctor will probably prescribe a low dose.

Long-term treatment with Librax may call for periodic blood and liver function tests.

Possible food and drug interactions when taking this medication
If Librax is taken with certain other drugs, the effects of either can be increased, decreased, or altered. It is especially important to check with your doctor before combining Librax with the following:

Antidepressant drugs known as MAO inhibitors, such as Nardil and Parnate
Blood-thinning drugs such as Coumadin
Certain diarrhea medications such as Donnagel and Kaopectate
Ketoconazole (Nizoral)
Major tranquilizers such as Stelazine and Thorazine
Potassium supplements such as Micro-K

In addition, you may experience excessive drowsiness and other potentially dangerous side effects if you combine Librax with alcohol or other drugs, such as Benadryl and Valium, that make you drowsy.

Special information if you are pregnant or breastfeeding
Several studies have found an increased risk of birth defects if Librax is taken during the first 3 months of pregnancy. Therefore, Librax is rarely recommended for use by pregnant women. If you are pregnant, plan to become pregnant, or are breastfeeding, inform your doctor immediately.

Recommended dosage

ADULTS

The usual dose is 1 or 2 capsules, 3 or 4 times a day before meals and at bedtime.

OLDER ADULTS

Your doctor will have you take the lowest dose that is effective.

Overdosage
Any medication taken in excess can have serious consequences. A severe overdose of Librax can be fatal. If you suspect an overdose, seek medical help immediately.

■ *Symptoms of Librax overdose may include:*
Blurred vision, coma, confusion, constipation, excessive sleepiness, excessively dry mouth, slow reflexes, urinary difficulties

LIBRIUM

Pronounced: LIB-ree-um
Generic name: Chlordiazepoxide

Why is this drug prescribed?

Librium is used in the treatment of anxiety disorders. It is also prescribed for short-term relief of the symptoms of anxiety, symptoms of withdrawal in acute alcoholism, and anxiety and apprehension before surgery. It belongs to a class of drugs known as benzodiazepines.

Most important fact about this drug

Librium is habit-forming, and you can become dependent on it. You could experience withdrawal symptoms if you stop taking it abruptly (see *What side effects may occur?*). You should not discontinue the drug or change your dose without your doctor's approval.

How should you take this medication?

Take this medication exactly as prescribed.

- *If you miss a dose...*
  Take it as soon as you remember if it is within an hour or so of your scheduled time. If you do not remember until later, skip the dose you missed and go back to your regular schedule. Do not take 2 doses at once.
- *Storage instructions...*
  Store away from heat, light, and moisture.

What side effects may occur?

Side effects cannot be anticipated. If any develop or change in intensity, inform your doctor as soon as possible. Only your doctor can determine if it is safe for you to continue taking Librium.

- *Side effects may include:*
  Confusion, constipation, drowsiness, fainting, increased or decreased sex drive, liver problems, lack of muscle coordination, minor menstrual irregularities, nausea, skin rash or eruptions, swelling due to fluid retention, yellow eyes and skin
- *Side effects due to rapid decrease or abrupt withdrawal from Librium may include:*
  Abdominal and muscle cramps, convulsions, exaggerated feeling of depression, sleeplessness, sweating, tremors, vomiting

Why should this drug not be prescribed?

If you are sensitive to or have ever had an allergic reaction to Librium or similar tranquilizers, you should not take this medication.

Anxiety or tension related to everyday stress usually does not require treatment with Librium. Discuss your symptoms thoroughly with your doctor.

Special warnings about this medication

Librium may cause you to become drowsy or less alert; therefore, you should not drive or operate dangerous machinery or participate in any hazardous activity that requires full mental alertness until you know how you react to this drug.

If you are severely depressed or have suffered from severe depression, consult with your doctor before taking this medication.

This drug may cause children to become less alert.

If you have a hyperactive, aggressive child taking Librium, inform your doctor if you notice contrary reactions such as excitement, stimulation, or acute rage.

Consult with your doctor before taking Librium if you are being treated for porphyria (a rare metabolic disorder) or kidney or liver disease.

Possible food and drug interactions when taking this medication

Librium is a central nervous system depressant and may intensify the effects of alcohol or have an additive effect. Do not drink alcohol while taking this medication.

If Librium is taken with certain other drugs, the effects of either can be increased, decreased, or altered. It is especially important to check with your doctor before combining Librium with the following:

Antacids such as Maalox and Mylanta
Antidepressant drugs known as MAO inhibitors, including Nardil and
    Parnate
Antipsychotic medications such as chlorpromazine and
    trifluoperazine
Barbiturates such as phenobarbital
Blood-thinning drugs such as Coumadin
Cimetidine (Tagamet)
Disulfiram (Antabuse)
Levodopa (Larodopa)
Narcotic pain relievers such as Demerol and Percocet
Oral contraceptives

Special information if you are pregnant or breastfeeding

Do not take Librium if you are pregnant or planning to become pregnant. There may be an increased risk of birth defects. This drug may appear in breast milk and could affect a nursing infant. If the medication is essential to your health, your doctor may advise you to discontinue breastfeeding until your treatment with the drug is finished.

Recommended dosage

ADULTS

Mild or Moderate Anxiety
The usual dose is 5 or 10 milligrams, 3 or 4 times a day.

Severe Anxiety
The usual dose is 20 to 25 milligrams, 3 or 4 times a day.

Apprehension and Anxiety Before Surgery
On days preceding surgery, the usual dose is 5 to 10 milligrams, 3 or 4 times a day.

Withdrawal Symptoms of Acute Alcoholism
The usual starting oral dose is 50 to 100 milligrams; the doctor will repeat this dose, up to a maximum of 300 milligrams per day, until agitation is controlled. The dose will then be reduced as much as possible.

CHILDREN

The usual dose for children 6 years of age and older is 5 milligrams, 2 to 4 times per day. Some children may need to take 10 milligrams, 2 or 3 times per day. The drug is not recommended for children under 6.

OLDER ADULTS

Your doctor will limit the dose to the smallest effective amount in order to avoid oversedation or lack of coordination. The usual dose is 5 milligrams, 2 to 4 times per day.

Overdosage

Any medication taken in excess can cause symptoms of overdose. If you suspect an overdose, seek medical attention immediately.

■ *The symptoms of Librium overdose may include:*
  Coma, confusion, sleepiness, slow reflexes

LIDEX

Pronounced: LYE-decks
Generic name: Fluocinonide

Why is this drug prescribed?

Lidex is a steroid medication that relieves the itching and inflammation of a wide variety of skin problems, including redness and swelling.

Most important fact about this drug

When you use Lidex, you inevitably absorb some of the medication through your skin and into the bloodstream. Too much absorption can lead to unwanted side effects elsewhere in the body. To keep this problem to a minimum, avoid using large amounts of Lidex over large areas, and do not cover it with airtight dressings such as plastic wrap or adhesive bandages unless specifically told to by your doctor.

How should you use this medication?

Lidex is for use only on the skin. Be careful to keep it out of your eyes. If the medication gets in your eyes and causes irritation, immediately flush your eyes with a large amount of water.

Apply Lidex as directed by your doctor. Do not use more of the medication than suggested by your doctor.

■ *If you miss a dose...*
Apply it as soon as you remember. If it is almost time for the next dose, skip the one you missed and go back to your regular schedule.
■ *Storage instructions...*
Store at room temperature. Avoid excessive heat.

What side effects may occur?

Side effects cannot be anticipated. If any develop or change in intensity, inform your doctor immediately. Only your doctor can determine if it is safe for you to continue using Lidex.

■ *Side effects may include:*
Acne-like eruptions, burning, dryness, excessive hair growth, infection of the skin, irritation, itching, lack of skin color, prickly heat, skin inflammation, skin loss or softening, stretch marks

Why should this drug not be prescribed?

You should not use Lidex if you are allergic to any of its components.

Special warnings about this medication

Do not use Lidex more often or for a longer time than your doctor ordered. If enough of the drug is absorbed through the skin, it may produce unusual side effects, including increased sugar in your blood and urine and a group of symptoms called Cushing's syndrome, characterized by a moon-shaped face, emotional disturbances, high blood pressure, weight gain, and growth of body hair in women.

Some factors that may increase absorption include:
Using bandages over the area where the medication is applied;
Using the medication over a large area of skin or on broken skin; or
Using the medication for an extended period of time

Children may absorb a proportionally greater amount of steroid drugs and may be more sensitive to the effects of these drugs. Avoid covering a treated area with waterproof diapers or plastic pants. They can increase absorption of Lidex.

Effects experienced by children may include:
  Bulges on the head
  Delayed weight gain
  Headache
  Slow growth

Lidex should be discontinued if irritation develops, and another treatment should be used.

Extended treatment time with any steroid product may cause skin to waste away. This may also occur with short-term use on the face, armpits, and skin creases.

Possible food and drug interactions when taking this medication
No interactions have been reported with Lidex.

Special information if you are pregnant or breastfeeding
Pregnant women should not use steroids on the skin in large amounts or for long periods of time. During pregnancy, these medications should be used only if the possible gains outweigh the possible risks to the baby.

Steroids do appear in breast milk. Women who breastfeed an infant should use them cautiously.

Recommended dosage

ADULTS

Lidex is applied to the affected areas in a thin film 2 to 4 times a day. If hair covers the infected area, part the hair so that the medication can be applied directly.

CHILDREN

Children should be given the smallest effective dose.

Overdosage
Lidex can be absorbed in amounts large enough to have temporary effects on the adrenal, hypothalamic, and pituitary glands.

■ *Some effects of steroid drugs may include:*
  Abnormal sugar levels in urine, excessive blood sugar levels, symptoms of Cushing's syndrome

■ *Symptoms of Cushing's syndrome may include:*
  Easily bruised skin, increased blood pressure, mood swings, water retention, weak muscles, weight gain

If you suspect a Lidex overdose, seek medical help immediately.

Linezolid See Zyvox, page 1678.

LIPITOR

Pronounced: LIP-ih-tor
Generic name: Atorvastatin calcium

Why is this drug prescribed?

Lipitor is a cholesterol-lowering drug. Your doctor may prescribe it along with a special diet if your blood cholesterol or triglyceride level is high and you have been unable to lower your readings by diet alone. The drug works by helping to clear harmful low-density-lipoprotein (LDL) cholesterol out of the blood and by limiting the body's ability to form new LDL cholesterol.

Your doctor may prescribe Lipitor to reduce your chances of having a heart attack or developing heart disease if you have any of the following risk factors:

Are age 55 years or older
Have a family history of early heart disease
Have high blood pressure
Have low levels of HDL (high-density lipoprotein—the good cholesterol)
Smoke

For people at high risk of heart disease, the doctor may suggest a cholesterol-lowering medication if LDL readings are 130 or more. For those at low risk, a medication is considered at readings of 190 or more.

Most important fact about this drug

Lipitor is usually prescribed only if diet, exercise, and weight loss fail to bring your cholesterol levels under control. It's important to remember that Lipitor is a supplement to—not a substitute for—those other measures. To get the full benefit of the medication, you need to stick to the diet and exercise program prescribed by your doctor. All these efforts to keep your cholesterol levels normal are important because they may lower your risk of heart disease.

How should you take this medication?

Lipitor should be taken once a day, with or without food. You can take it in the morning or the evening, but should hold to the same time each day. The drug generally begins working within 2 weeks.

For an even greater cholesterol-lowering effect, your doctor may prescribe Lipitor along with a different kind of lipid-lowering drug such as Questran or Colestid. It's important to avoid taking the two drugs at the same time of day. Take Lipitor at least 1 hour before or 4 hours after the other drug.

■ *If you miss a dose...*
Take the forgotten dose as soon as you remember. If it is almost time for your next dose, skip the one you missed and go back to your regular schedule. Do not take 2 doses at the same time.

■ *Storage instructions...*
Store at room temperature.

What side effects may occur?
Side effects cannot be anticipated. If any develop or change in intensity, inform your doctor as soon as possible. Only your doctor can determine if it is safe for you to continue taking Lipitor.

■ *Side effects may include:*
Abdominal pain, abnormal heartbeat, accidental injury, allergic reaction, arthritis, back pain, bronchitis, chest pain, constipation, diarrhea, dizziness, flu symptoms, fluid retention, gas, headache, indigestion, infection, inflammation of sinus and nasal passages, insomnia, joint pain, muscle aching or weakness, nausea, rash, stomach pain, urinary tract infection, weakness

Why should this drug not be prescribed?
Never take Lipitor during pregnancy or while breastfeeding. You should also avoid Lipitor if you have liver disease, or if the drug gives you an allergic reaction.

Special warnings about this medication
There is a slight chance of liver damage from Lipitor, so your doctor may order a blood test to check your liver function before you start taking the drug, again 12 weeks after you begin therapy or your dosage is increased, and periodically thereafter. If the tests reveal a problem, you may have to stop using the drug.

Drugs like Lipitor have occasionally been known to damage muscle tissue, so be sure to tell your doctor immediately if you notice any unexplained muscle tenderness, weakness, or pain, especially if you also have a fever or feel sick. Your doctor may want to do a blood test to check for signs of muscle damage.

If you are scheduled for major surgery, your doctor will have you stop taking Lipitor a few days before the operation.

Possible food and drug interactions when taking this medication
If you take Lipitor with certain other drugs, the effects of either could be increased, decreased, or altered. It is especially important to check with your doctor before combining Lipitor with any of the following:

Antacids such as Maalox TC Suspension
Clofibrate (Atromid-S)

Colestipol (Colestid)
Cyclosporine (Sandimmune, Neoral)
Digoxin (Lanoxin)
Drugs that suppress the immune system
Erythromycin (E.E.S., Erythrocin, others)
Fenofibrate (Tricor)
Fluconazole (Diflucan)
Gemfibrozil (Lopid)
Itraconazole (Sporanox)
Ketoconazole (Nizoral)
Niacin (Niaspan, Niacor, Slo-Niacin)
Oral contraceptives

Special information if you are pregnant or breastfeeding

Developing babies need plenty of cholesterol, so this cholesterol-lowering drug should never be used during pregnancy. In fact, your doctor is unlikely to prescribe Lipitor if there is even a chance that you may become pregnant. If you do conceive while taking this drug, notify your doctor right away. Lipitor does make its way into breast milk, so you should not take the drug while breastfeeding your baby.

Recommended dosage

You need to follow a standard cholesterol-lowering diet before starting Lipitor, and should continue following it throughout your therapy.

ADULTS

The recommended starting dose is 10 or 20 milligrams once a day. (The doctor may start with 40 milligrams daily if your LDL levels need to be reduced by more than 45 percent.) The doctor will check your cholesterol levels every 2 to 4 weeks and adjust the dose accordingly. The maximum recommended daily dose is 80 milligrams.

CHILDREN 10 TO 17 YEARS OLD

The recommended starting dose is 10 milligrams once a day. The dosage may be increased after 4 weeks, as determined by the doctor, up to a maximum of 20 milligrams a day. Girls must be having regular menstrual cycles before starting therapy with Lipitor.

The safety and effectiveness of Lipitor in children under 10 years old or in doses greater than 20 milligrams a day have not been studied.

Overdosage

Although no specific information about Lipitor overdose is available, any medication taken in excess can have serious consequences. If you suspect an overdose of Lipitor, seek medical attention.

Lisinopril *See Zestril, page 1624.*

Lisinopril with Hydrochlorothiazide *See Zestoretic,*
page 1621.

Lithium carbonate *See Eskalith, page 526.*

Lithobid *See Eskalith, page 526.*

LODINE
Pronounced: LOW-deen
Generic name: Etodolac

Why is this drug prescribed?
Lodine, a nonsteroidal anti-inflammatory drug, is available in regular and
extended-release (Lodine XL) forms. Both forms are used to relieve the
inflammation, swelling, stiffness, and joint pain of osteoarthritis (the
most common form of arthritis) and rheumatoid arthritis. Regular Lodine
is also used to relieve pain in other situations.

Most important fact about this drug
You should have frequent checkups by your doctor if you take Lodine regularly. Ulcers or internal bleeding can occur without warning.

How should you take this medication?
Your doctor may ask you to take Lodine with food or an antacid, and with
a full glass of water. Never take it on an empty stomach.
 Take this medication exactly as prescribed by your doctor.
 You should see results in 1 to 2 weeks.
 If you are using Lodine for arthritis, it should be taken regularly.

■ *If you miss a dose…*
 Take the forgotten dose as soon as you remember. If it is almost time
 for the next dose, skip the one you missed and go back to your regular
 schedule. Never try to catch up by doubling the dose.
■ *Storage instructions…*
 Store at room temperature. Protect capsules from moisture. Protect
 Lodine tablets from light; protect Lodine XL tablets from excessive
 heat and humidity.

What side effects may occur?
Side effects cannot be anticipated. If any develop or change in intensity,
inform your doctor as soon as possible. Only your doctor can determine
if it is safe for you to continue taking Lodine.

■ *Side effects may include:*
 Abdominal pain, black stools, blurred vision, chills, constipation, depression, diarrhea, dizziness, fever, gas, increased frequency of urination, indigestion, itching, nausea, nervousness, painful or difficult
 urination, rash, ringing in ears, vomiting, weakness

Why should this drug not be prescribed?

If you are sensitive to or have ever had an allergic reaction to Lodine, or if you have had asthma attacks, hives, or other allergic reactions caused by aspirin or other nonsteroidal anti-inflammatory drugs such as Motrin, you should not take this medication; it might cause a severe allergic reaction. Make sure your doctor is aware of any drug reactions you have experienced; and be careful about taking this drug if you have asthma—even if you've never had a drug reaction before. If you do suffer an allergic reaction, call for emergency help immediately.

Special warnings about this medication

Peptic ulcers and bleeding can occur without warning. You may have other problems with bleeding as well.

Call your doctor if you have any signs or symptoms of stomach or intestinal ulcers or bleeding, blurred vision or other eye problems, skin rash, weight gain, or fluid retention and swelling.

This drug should be used with caution if you have kidney or liver disease; and it can cause liver inflammation in some people.

Do not take aspirin or any other anti-inflammatory medications while taking Lodine, unless your doctor tells you to do so.

If you are taking Lodine over an extended period of time, your doctor should check your blood for anemia.

This drug can increase water retention. Use with caution if you have heart disease or high blood pressure.

Possible food and drug interactions when taking this medication

If Lodine is taken with certain other drugs, the effects of either could be increased, decreased, or altered. It is especially important to check with your doctor before combining Lodine with the following:

Aspirin
Cyclosporine (Sandimmune, Neoral)
Digoxin (Lanoxin)
Lithium (Lithobid, others)
Methotrexate
Phenylbutazone (Butazolidin)
The blood-thinning drug warfarin (Coumadin)

Special information if you are pregnant or breastfeeding

The effects of Lodine during pregnancy have not been adequately studied. However, you should definitely not take it in late pregnancy. If you are pregnant or plan to become pregnant, inform your doctor immediately. Lodine may appear in breast milk and could affect a nursing infant. If this medication is essential to your health, your doctor may advise you to discontinue breastfeeding until your treatment with this medication is finished.

Recommended dosage

ADULTS

General Pain Relief
Take 200 to 400 milligrams every 6 to 8 hours as needed. Ordinarily, you should not take more than 1,000 milligrams a day, although your doctor may increase the dose to 1,200 milligrams a day if absolutely necessary.

Osteoarthritis and Rheumatoid Arthritis
The starting dose of Lodine is 300 milligrams 2 or 3 times a day, or 400 or 500 milligrams twice a day. The usual daily maximum ranges from 600 to 1,000 milligrams, although your doctor may prescribe as much as 1,200 milligrams a day if necessary.

The usual dose of Lodine XL is 400 to 1,200 milligrams taken once a day.

Your doctor will stick with the lowest dose that proves effective.

CHILDREN

The safety and effectiveness of Lodine have not been established in children.

Overdosage

Any medication taken in excess can cause symptoms of overdose. If you suspect an overdose, seek medical attention immediately.

■ *Symptoms of Lodine overdose may include:*
   Drowsiness, lethargy, nausea, stomach pain, vomiting

Loestrin *See Oral Contraceptives, page 1000.*

Lofibra *See Tricor, page 1482.*

Lomefloxacin *See Maxaquin, page 814.*

LOMOTIL
Pronounced: loe-MOE-till
Generic ingredients: Diphenoxylate hydrochloride,
   Atropine sulfate

Why is this drug prescribed?
Lomotil is used, along with other drugs, in the treatment of diarrhea.

Most important fact about this drug
Lomotil is not a harmless drug, so never exceed your recommended dosage. An overdose could be fatal.

How should you take this medication?

Lomotil can be habit-forming. Take it exactly as prescribed.

Be sure to drink plenty of liquids to replace lost body fluids. Eat bland foods, such as cooked cereals, breads, and crackers.

Lomotil may cause dry mouth. Suck on a hard candy or chew gum to relieve this problem.

■ *If you miss a dose...*
Take it as soon as you remember. If it is almost time for your next dose, skip the one you missed and go back to your regular schedule. Do not take 2 doses at once.

■ *Storage instructions...*
Store away from heat, light, and moisture. Keep the liquid from freezing.

What side effects may occur?

Side effects cannot be anticipated. If any develop or change in intensity, inform your doctor as soon as possible. Only your doctor can determine if it is safe for you to continue taking Lomotil.

■ *Side effects may include:*
Abdominal discomfort, confusion, depression, difficulty urinating, dizziness, dry mouth and skin, exaggerated feeling of elation, fever, flushing, general feeling of not being well, headache, hives, intestinal blockage, itching, lack or loss of appetite, nausea, numbness of arms and legs, rapid heartbeat, restlessness, sedation/drowsiness, severe allergic reaction, sluggishness, swelling due to fluid retention, swollen gums, vomiting

Why should this drug not be prescribed?

If you are sensitive to or have ever had an allergic reaction to the ingredients of Lomotil, diphenoxylate or atropine, you should not take this medication. Make sure your doctor is aware of any drug reactions you have experienced.

Unless you are directed to do so by your doctor, do not take Lomotil if you have obstructive jaundice (a disease in which bile made in the liver does not reach the intestines because of a bile duct obstruction such as gallstones). Do not take Lomotil if you have diarrhea associated with pseudomembranous enterocolitis (inflammation of the intestines) or an infection with enterotoxin-producing bacteria (an enterotoxin is a poisonous substance that affects the stomach and intestines).

Special warnings about this medication

Certain antibiotics such as Ceclor, Cleocin, PCE, and Achromycin V may cause diarrhea. Lomotil can make this type of diarrhea worse and longer-lasting. Check with your doctor before using Lomotil while taking an antibiotic.

Lomotil may cause drowsiness or dizziness. Therefore, you should not drive a car, operate dangerous machinery, or participate in any hazardous activity that requires full mental alertness until you know how this drug affects you.

Lomotil slows activity of the digestive system; this can result in a buildup of fluid in the intestine, which may worsen the dehydration and imbalance in normal body salts that usually occur with diarrhea.

If you have severe ulcerative colitis (an inflammation of the intestines), your doctor will want to monitor your condition while you are taking this drug. If your abdomen becomes distended or enlarged, notify your doctor.

Use Lomotil with extreme caution if you have kidney and liver disease or if your liver is not functioning normally.

Lomotil should be used with caution in children, since side effects may occur even with recommended doses, especially in children with Down syndrome (congenital mental retardation).

Since addiction to diphenoxylate hydrochloride is possible at high doses, you should never exceed the recommended dosage.

Possible food and drug interactions when taking this medication

Lomotil may intensify the effects of alcohol. It's better not to drink alcohol while taking this medication.

If Lomotil is taken with certain other drugs, the effects of either could be increased, decreased, or altered. It is especially important to check with your doctor before combining Lomotil with the following:

Barbiturates (anticonvulsants and sedatives such as phenobarbital)
MAO inhibitors (antidepressants such as Nardil and Parnate)
Tranquilizers (such as Valium and Xanax)

Special information if you are pregnant or breastfeeding

The effects of Lomotil during pregnancy have not been adequately studied. If you are pregnant or plan to become pregnant, notify your doctor immediately. Lomotil appears in breast milk and could affect a nursing infant. If this medication is essential to your health, your doctor may advise you to discontinue breastfeeding until your treatment is finished.

Recommended dosage

ADULTS

The recommended starting dosage is 2 tablets 4 times a day or 2 regular teaspoonfuls (10 milliliters) of liquid 4 times per day.

Once your diarrhea is under control, your doctor may reduce the dosage; you may need as little as 5 milligrams (2 tablets or 10 milliliters of liquid) per day.

You should see improvement within 48 hours. If your diarrhea persists after you have taken 20 milligrams a day for 10 days, the drug is not likely to work for you.

CHILDREN

Lomotil is not recommended in children under 2 years of age.

Your doctor will take into account your child's nutritional status and degree of dehydration before prescribing this drug.

The recommended dose for children 13 to 16 years old is 2 tablets or 2 teaspoonfuls of liquid three times a day.

In children under 13 years of age, use only Lomotil liquid and administer with the plastic dropper. The recommended starting dosage is 0.3 to 0.4 milligram per 2.2 pounds of body weight per day, divided into 4 equal doses. The following table provides approximate starting dosage recommendations for children:

2 years (24–31 pounds):	1.5–3.0 milligrams, 4 times daily
3 years (26–35 pounds):	2.0–3.0 milligrams, 4 times daily
4 years (31–44 pounds):	2.0–4.0 milligrams, 4 times daily
5 years (35–51 pounds):	2.5–4.5 milligrams, 4 times daily
6–8 years (38–71 pounds):	2.5–5.0 milligrams, 4 times daily
9–12 years (51–121 pounds):	3.5–5.0 milligrams, 4 times daily

Your doctor may reduce the dosage as soon as symptoms are controlled. A maintenance dosage may be as low as one-quarter of the starting dose. If your child does not show improvement within 48 hours, Lomotil is unlikely to work.

Overdosage

An overdose of Lomotil can be dangerous and even fatal. If you suspect an overdose, seek medical attention immediately.

■ *Symptoms of Lomotil overdose may include:*
Coma, dry skin and mucous membranes, enlarged pupils of the eyes, extremely high body temperature, flushing, involuntary eyeball movement, lower than normal muscle tone, pinpoint pupils, rapid heartbeat, restlessness, sluggishness, suppressed breathing

Suppressed breathing may be seen as late as 30 hours after an overdose.

Lo/Ovral *See Oral Contraceptives, page 1000.*

Loperamide *See Imodium, page 674.*

LOPID
Pronounced: LOH-pid
Generic name: Gemfibrozil

Why is this drug prescribed?

Lopid is prescribed, along with a special diet, for treatment of people with very high levels of serum triglycerides (a fatty substance in the blood) who are at risk of developing pancreatitis (inflammation of the pancreas) and who do not respond adequately to a strict diet.

This drug can also be used to reduce the risk of coronary heart disease in people who have failed to respond to weight loss, diet, exercise, and other triglyceride- or cholesterol-lowering drugs.

Most important fact about this drug

Lopid is usually prescribed only if diet, exercise, and weight loss fail to bring your cholesterol levels under control. It's important to remember that Lopid is a supplement—not a substitute—for these other measures. To get the full benefit of the medication, you need to stick to the diet and exercise program prescribed by your doctor. All these efforts to keep your cholesterol levels normal are important because together they may lower your risk of heart disease.

How should you take this medication?

Take this medication 30 minutes before the morning and evening meals, exactly as prescribed.

■ *If you miss a dose...*
Take it as soon as you remember. If it is almost time for the next dose, skip the one you missed and go back to your regular schedule. Do not take 2 doses at the same time.
■ *Storage instructions...*
Store at room temperature.

What side effects may occur?

Side effects cannot be anticipated. If any develop or change in intensity, inform your doctor as soon as possible. Only your doctor can determine if it is safe for you to continue taking Lopid.

■ *Side effects may include:*
Abdominal pain, acute appendicitis, constipation, diarrhea, eczema, fatigue, headache, indigestion, nausea/vomiting, rash, vertigo

Why should this drug not be prescribed?

There is a slight possibility that Lopid may cause malignancy, gallbladder disease, abdominal pain leading to appendectomy, or other serious, possibly fatal, abdominal disorders. This drug should not be used by those who have only mildly elevated cholesterol levels, since the benefits do not outweigh the risk of these severe side effects.

If you are sensitive to or have ever had an allergic reaction to Lopid or similar drugs such as Atromid-S, you should not take this medication. Make sure your doctor is aware of any drug reactions you have experienced.

Unless you are directed to do so by your doctor, do not take this medication if you are being treated for severe kidney or liver disorders or gallbladder disease.

Do not combine Lopid with any of the cholesterol-lowering drugs known as statins, including Lescol, Lipitor, Mevacor, Pravachol, and Zocor. This combination increases the danger of serious, muscle-wasting side effects.

Special warnings about this medication

Excess body weight and excess alcohol intake may be important risk factors leading to unusually high levels of fats in the body. Your doctor will probably want you to lose weight and stop drinking before he or she tries to treat you with Lopid.

Your doctor will probably do periodic blood level tests during the first 12 months of therapy with Lopid because of blood diseases associated with the use of this medication.

Liver disorders have occurred with the use of this drug. Therefore, your doctor will probably test your liver function periodically.

If you are being treated for any disease that contributes to increased blood cholesterol, such as an overactive thyroid, diabetes, nephrotic syndrome (kidney and blood vessel disorder), dysproteinemia (excess of protein in the blood), or obstructive liver disease, consult with your doctor before taking Lopid.

Lopid should begin to reduce cholesterol levels during the first 3 months of therapy. If your cholesterol is not lowered sufficiently, this medication should be discontinued. Therefore, it is important that your doctor check your progress regularly.

The use of this medication may cause gallstones leading to possible gallbladder surgery. If you develop gallstones, your doctor will tell you to stop taking the drug.

The use of this drug may be associated with myositis, a muscle disease. If you have muscle pain, tenderness, or weakness, consult with your doctor. If myositis is suspected, your doctor will stop treating you with this drug.

Possible food and drug interactions when taking this medication

To avoid the possibility of severe muscle-wasting side effects, do not use any of the cholesterol-lowering statin drugs while taking Lopid. Drugs in this category include:

Atorvastatin (Lipitor)
Fluvastatin (Lescol)
Lovastatin (Mevacor)
Pravastatin (Pravachol)
Simvastatin (Zocor)

Also be sure to check with your doctor before taking Lopid along with a blood-thinning drug such as Coumadin. The dosage of the blood thinner must be reduced to avoid abnormal bleeding.

You should not start taking Lopid if you are already taking the diabetes medication Prandin. Conversely, you should not start taking Prandin if you are already using Lopid. Combining the two drugs could lead to a dangerous drop in blood sugar. However, if you're already taking both drugs, the doctor will monitor your blood sugar levels closely and adjust the dosages as needed.

Special information if you are pregnant or breastfeeding

The effects of Lopid during pregnancy have not been adequately studied. If you are pregnant or plan to become pregnant, inform your doctor immediately. This medication causes tumors in animals, and it could have an effect on nursing infants. If Lopid is essential to your health, your doctor may advise you to discontinue breastfeeding until your treatment with Lopid is finished.

Recommended dosage

ADULTS

The recommended dose is 1,200 milligrams divided into 2 doses, given 30 minutes before the morning and evening meals.

CHILDREN

Safety and effectiveness of Lopid have not been established for use in children.

OLDER ADULTS

This drug should be used with caution by older adults.

Overdosage

Any medication taken in excess can have serious consequences. If you suspect an overdose, seek medical help immediately.

■ *Symptoms of Lopid overdose may include:*
  Abdominal cramps, diarrhea, joint and muscle pain, nausea, vomiting

Lopinavir and Ritonavir See Kaletra, page 700.

LOPRESSOR

Pronounced: low-PRESS-or
Generic name: Metoprolol tartrate
Other brand name: Toprol-XL

Why is this drug prescribed?

Lopressor, a type of medication known as a beta-blocker, is used in the treatment of high blood pressure, angina pectoris (chest pain, usually caused by lack of oxygen to the heart due to clogged arteries), and heart attack. When prescribed for high blood pressure, it is effective when used alone or in combination with other high blood pressure medications. Beta-blockers decrease the force and rate of heart contractions, thereby reducing the demand for oxygen and lowering blood pressure.

Occasionally doctors prescribe Lopressor for the treatment of aggressive behavior, prevention of migraine headache, and relief of temporary anxiety.

An extended-release form of this drug, called Toprol-XL, is prescribed for high blood pressure, angina, and heart failure.

Most important fact about this drug

If you have high blood pressure, you must take Lopressor regularly for it to be effective. Since blood pressure declines gradually, it may be several weeks before you get the full benefit of Lopressor; and you must continue taking it even if you are feeling well. Lopressor does not cure high blood pressure; it merely keeps it under control.

How should you take this medication?

Lopressor should be taken with food or immediately after you have eaten.

Take Lopressor exactly as prescribed, even if your symptoms have disappeared.

Try not to miss any doses. If this medication is not taken regularly, your condition may worsen.

■ *If you miss a dose...*
If it is within 4 hours of your next dose, skip the one you missed and go back to your regular schedule. Never take 2 doses at the same time.

■ *Storage instructions...*
Store Lopressor at room temperature in a tightly closed container, away from light. Protect from moisture. Store Toprol-XL at room temperature.

What side effects may occur?

Side effects cannot be anticipated. If any develop or change in intensity, inform your doctor as soon as possible. Only your doctor can determine if it is safe for you to continue taking Lopressor.

■ *Side effects may include:*
Depression, diarrhea, dizziness, itching, rash, shortness of breath, slow heartbeat, tiredness

Why should this drug not be prescribed?

If you have a slow heartbeat, certain heart irregularities, low blood pressure, inadequate output from the heart, or heart failure, you should not take this medication.

Special warnings about this medication

If you have a history of congestive heart failure, Lopressor should be used with caution. If you are taking the extended-release form of this drug, Toprol-XL, to relieve heart failure, the condition may temporarily be worsened as your dosage is increased. Be sure to alert your doctor to any signs of worsening heart failure such as weight gain or increasing shortness of breath. If you have peripheral vascular disease, use Toprol-XL with caution.

Do not stop Lopressor abruptly. This can cause increased chest pain and heart attack. Dosage should be gradually reduced.

If you suffer from asthma, seasonal allergies or other bronchial conditions, or liver disease, this medication should be used with caution.

Ask your doctor if you should check your pulse while taking Lopressor. This medication can cause your heartbeat to become too slow.

This medication may mask some symptoms of low blood sugar in diabetics or alter blood sugar levels. If you are diabetic, discuss this with your doctor.

If you have pheochromocytoma and your doctor prescribes Toprol-XL, you will first need to take an alpha-blocking drug (a different type of blood pressure medication).

Lopressor may cause you to become drowsy or less alert; therefore, driving or operating dangerous machinery or participating in any hazardous activity that requires full mental alertness is not recommended until you know how you respond to this medication.

Notify your doctor or dentist that you are taking Lopressor if you have a medical emergency, or before you have surgery or dental treatment.

Notify your doctor if you have any difficulty breathing.

Possible food and drug interactions when taking this medication

If Lopressor is taken with certain other drugs, the effects of either could be increased, decreased, or altered. It is especially important to check with your doctor before combining Lopressor with certain high blood pressure drugs such as reserpine (Ser-Ap-Es).

Other medications that might interact with Lopressor include:

Albuterol (Proventil, Ventolin)
Amiodarone (Cordarone)
Barbiturates such as phenobarbital
Calcium channel blockers such as Calan and Cardizem
Cimetidine (Tagamet)
Ciprofloxacin (Cipro)
Clonidine (Catapres)
Epinephrine (EpiPen)
Fluoxetine (Prozac)
Hydralazine (Apresoline)

Insulin
Nonsteroidal anti-inflammatory drugs such as Motrin and Indocin
Oral diabetes drugs such as Glucotrol and Micronase
Paroxetine (Paxil)
Prazosin (Minipress)
Propafenone (Rythmol)
Quinidine (Quinaglute)
Ranitidine (Zantac)
Rifampin (Rifadin)

Special information if you are pregnant or breastfeeding

The effects of Lopressor during pregnancy have not been adequately studied. If you are pregnant or plan to become pregnant, inform your doctor immediately. Lopressor appears in breast milk and could affect a nursing infant. If this medication is essential to your health, your doctor may advise you to discontinue breastfeeding until your treatment with this medication is finished.

Recommended dosage

ADULTS

Dosages of Lopressor should be individualized by your doctor. It should be taken with or immediately following meals.

High Blood Pressure
The usual starting dosage of Lopressor is a total of 100 milligrams a day taken in 1 or 2 doses, whether taken alone or with a diuretic. The initial dosage of Toprol-XL ranges from 50 to 100 milligrams once a day. Your doctor may gradually increase the dosage up to 400 milligrams a day. Generally, the effectiveness of each dosage increase will be seen within a week.

Angina Pectoris
The usual starting dosage is a total of 100 milligrams a day taken in 2 doses of Lopressor or a single dose of Toprol-XL. Your doctor may gradually increase the dosage up to 400 milligrams a day.

Generally, the effectiveness of each dosage increase will be seen within a week. If treatment is to be discontinued, your doctor will withdraw the drug gradually over a period of 1 to 2 weeks.

Heart Attack
Lopressor can be used for treatment of heart attack both in the hospital during the early phases and after the individual's condition has stabilized. Your doctor will determine the dosage according to your needs.

Heart Failure
The recommended starting dose of Toprol-XL is 25 milligrams once daily for 2 weeks (12.5 milligrams in severe cases). Your doctor will double the

dose every 2 weeks up to the highest level that works without side effects. The maximum recommended dose is 200 milligrams daily.

CHILDREN

The safety and effectiveness of Lopressor have not been established in children.

Overdosage

Any medication taken in excess can cause symptoms of overdose. If you suspect an overdose, seek medical attention immediately.

■ *The symptoms of Lopressor overdose may include:*
Asthma-like symptoms, coma, heart failure, irregular heartbeat, low blood pressure, nausea and vomiting, shock, slow heartbeat, stopped heart

LOPROX

Pronounced: LOW-prox
Generic name: Ciclopirox

Why is this drug prescribed?

Loprox cream, lotion, and topical solution are prescribed for the treatment of the following fungal skin infections:

Athlete's foot
Candidiasis (yeastlike fungal infection of the skin)
Fungal infection of the groin (jock itch)
Fungal infection of non-hairy parts of the skin
Tinea versicolor—infection of the skin that is characterized by
    brown or tan patches on the trunk

Loprox gel is used for athlete's foot, fungal infections of the non-hairy parts of the skin, and certain scalp inflammations (seborrheic dermatitis of the scalp).

Most important fact about this drug

Loprox is for external treatment of skin infections. Do not use Loprox in the eyes.

How should you use this medication?

Use this medication for the full treatment time even if your symptoms have improved. Notify your doctor if there is no improvement after 4 weeks.

Avoid contact with eyes and mucous membranes. Shake Loprox lotion vigorously before each use.

■ *If you miss a dose…*
Apply the forgotten dose as soon as you remember. If it is almost time for your next dose, skip the one you missed and go back to your regular schedule.

■ *Storage instructions…*
Store at room temperature.

What side effects may occur?

Side effects cannot be anticipated. If any develop or change in intensity, inform your doctor as soon as possible. Only your doctor can determine if it is safe for you to continue using Loprox.

When Loprox gel is applied to the scalp, about 15 to 20 percent of patients feel a temporary burning or stinging sensation.

Why should this drug not be prescribed?

If you are sensitive to or have ever had an allergic reaction to ciclopirox or any other ingredient in Loprox, you should not take this medication. Make sure your doctor is aware of any drug reactions you have experienced.

Special warnings about this medication

If the affected area of skin shows signs of increased irritation (redness, itching, burning, blistering, swelling, oozing), notify your doctor.

Avoid the use of airtight dressings or bandages.

Special information if you are pregnant or breastfeeding

The effects of Loprox during pregnancy have not been adequately studied. If you are pregnant or plan to become pregnant, inform your doctor immediately. It is not known whether this drug appears in breast milk. If this medication is essential to your health, your doctor may advise you to discontinue breastfeeding your baby until your treatment is finished.

Recommended dosage

ADULTS

Gently massage Loprox into the affected and surrounding skin areas 2 times a day, in the morning and evening. For most infections, improvement usually begins within the first week of treatment. People with tinea versicolor usually show signs of improvement after 2 weeks of treatment.

CHILDREN

The safety and effectiveness of cream, lotion, and solution have not been established in children under 10 years of age (16 for Loprox gel).

Overdosage

Any medication taken in excess can have serious consequences. If you suspect an overdose, seek medical treatment immediately.

LORABID

Pronounced: LOR-a-bid
Generic name: Loracarbef

Why is this drug prescribed?

Lorabid is used to treat mild to moderate bacterial infections of the lungs, ears, throat, sinuses, skin, urinary tract, and kidneys.

Most important fact about this drug

If you have ever had an allergic reaction to Lorabid, penicillin, cephalo-sporins, or any other drug, be sure your doctor is aware of it before you take Lorabid. You may experience a severe reaction if you are sensitive to penicillin-type medications.

How should you take this medication?

Take Lorabid at least 1 hour before or 2 hours after eating. It is best to take your medication at evenly spaced intervals, day and night.

Do not stop taking your medication even if you begin to feel better after a few days. If you stop taking your medicine too soon, your symptoms may return. If you have a strep infection, you should take your medication for at least 10 days.

■ *If you miss a dose…*
Take it as soon as possible. This will help keep a constant amount of medicine in your system. If it is almost time for your next dose, skip the one you missed and go back to your regular schedule. Do not take 2 doses at once.

■ *Storage instructions…*
Lorabid can be stored at room temperature. The liquid form can be kept in the refrigerator, but not in the freezer. Discard any unused portion.

What side effects may occur?

Side effects cannot be anticipated. If any develop or change in intensity, tell your doctor as soon as possible. Only your doctor can determine if it is safe for you to continue taking Lorabid.

■ *Side effects in children may include:*
Diarrhea, inflamed, runny nose, vomiting
■ *Side effects in adults may include:*
Diarrhea, headache
■ *Side effects of other drugs of this class may include:*
Allergic reactions (sometimes severe), anemia, blood disorders, hemorrhage, kidney problems, seizures, serum sickness (fever, skin rash, joint pain, swollen lymph nodes), skin peeling

Why should this drug not be prescribed?

If you are allergic to penicillin, cephalosporins, or other medications, you should not take Lorabid. Make sure you tell your doctor about any drug reactions you have experienced.

Special warnings about this medication

As with many antibiotics, Lorabid can cause colitis—an inflammation of the bowel. This condition can range from mild to life-threatening. If you develop diarrhea while taking Lorabid, notify your doctor, and do not take any diarrhea medication without your doctor's approval.

Prolonged use of Lorabid may result in development of bacteria that do not respond to the medication, leading to a second infection. Because of this danger, you should not use any leftover Lorabid for later infections, even if they have similar symptoms. Take Lorabid only when your doctor prescribes it for you.

If you have known or suspected kidney problems, your doctor will perform blood tests to check your urine and kidney function before and during Lorabid therapy.

Possible food and drug interactions when taking this medication

If Lorabid is taken with certain other drugs, the effects of either could be increased, decreased, or altered. It is especially important to check with your doctor before combining Lorabid with the following:

Diuretics such as Lasix and Bumex
Probenecid

Special information if you are pregnant or breastfeeding

The effects of Lorabid during pregnancy have not been adequately studied. If you are pregnant or plan to become pregnant, tell your doctor immediately. Lorabid should be used during pregnancy only if clearly needed. It is not known whether Lorabid appears in human breast milk. Your doctor will determine whether it is safe for you to take Lorabid while breastfeeding.

Recommended dosage

ADULTS (13 YEARS AND OLDER)

Bronchitis
The usual dose is 200 to 400 milligrams every 12 hours for 7 days.

Pneumonia
The usual dose is 400 milligrams every 12 hours for 14 days.

Sinusitis
The usual dose is 400 milligrams every 12 hours for 10 days.

Skin and Soft Tissue Infections
The usual dose is 200 milligrams every 12 hours for 7 days.

Streptococcal Pharyngitis (Strep Throat) and Tonsillitis
The usual dose is 200 milligrams every 12 hours for 10 days. For strep throat, take Lorabid for at least 10 days.

Bladder Infections
The usual dose is 200 milligrams every 24 hours for 7 days.

Kidney Infections
The usual dose is 400 milligrams every 12 hours for 14 days.
If you have impaired kidney function, your doctor will adjust the dosage according to your needs.

CHILDREN (6 MONTHS TO 12 YEARS OF AGE)

Otitis Media
This infection of the middle ear should be treated with the suspension. Do not use the pulvules.
The dose is based on body weight. The usual dose is 30 milligrams of liquid per 2.2 pounds of body weight per day in divided doses (half the dose every 12 hours), for 10 days.

Streptococcal Pharyngitis (Strep Throat) and Tonsillitis
The dose is based on body weight. The usual dose is 15 milligrams per 2.2 pounds of body weight per day in divided doses (half the dose every 12 hours), for at least 10 days.

Impetigo (Skin Infection)
The dose is based on body weight. The usual dose is 15 milligrams of liquid per 2.2 pounds of body weight per day in divided doses (half the dose every 12 hours), for 7 days.

Overdosage
Any medication taken in excess can have serious consequences If you suspect an overdose, seek medical attention immediately.

■ *Symptoms of Lorabid overdose may include:*
   Diarrhea, nausea, stomach upset, vomiting

Loracarbef *See Lorabid, page 783.*

Loratadine *See Claritin, page 299.*

Loratadine with Pseudoephedrine *See Claritin-D, page 300.*

Lorazepam *See Ativan, page 144.*

Lorcet *See Vicodin, page 1557.*

Lortab *See Vicodin, page 1557.*

Losartan *See Cozaar, page 355.*

Losartan with Hydrochlorothiazide *See Hyzaar, page 664.*

LOTENSIN

Pronounced: *Lo-TEN-sin*
Generic name: *Benazepril hydrochloride*

Why is this drug prescribed?

Lotensin is used in the treatment of high blood pressure in adults and children 7 to 17 years old. It is effective when used alone or in combination with thiazide diuretics. Lotensin is in a family of drugs called ACE (angiotensin-converting enzyme) inhibitors. It works by preventing a chemical in your blood called angiotensin I from converting into a more potent form that increases salt and water retention in your body. Lotensin also enhances blood flow throughout your blood vessels.

Most important fact about this drug

You must take Lotensin regularly for it to be effective. Since blood pressure declines gradually, it may be several weeks before you get the full benefit of Lotensin; and you must continue taking it even if you are feeling well. Lotensin does not cure high blood pressure; it merely keeps it under control.

How should you take this medication?

Lotensin can be taken with or without food. Do not use salt substitutes containing potassium.

Take Lotensin exactly as prescribed. Suddenly stopping Lotensin could cause your blood pressure to increase.

■ *If you miss a dose...*
Take the forgotten dose as soon as you remember. If it is almost time for the next dose, skip the one you missed and go back to your regular schedule. Never try to catch up by doubling the dose.

■ *Storage instructions...*
Store at room temperature in a tightly closed container. Protect from light.

What side effects may occur?

Side effects cannot be anticipated. If any develop or change in intensity, inform your doctor as soon as possible. Only your doctor can determine if it is safe for you to continue taking Lotensin.

If you develop swelling of your face, around the lips, tongue, or throat;

swelling of arms and legs; or difficulty swallowing, you should contact your doctor immediately. You may need emergency treatment. Be especially wary if you're an African American: your chances of this type of reaction are higher. Severe allergic reactions are also more likely if you are being given bee or wasp venom to guard against future reactions to stings.

■ *Side effects may include:*
Cough, dizziness, headache

Why should this drug not be prescribed?
If you are sensitive to or have ever had an allergic reaction to Lotensin or other angiotensin-converting enzyme (ACE) inhibitors, do not take this medication.

Special warnings about this medication
Your kidney function should be assessed when you start taking Lotensin and then monitored for the first few weeks.

If you have poor kidney function, there is a slight chance that Lotensin may reduce your supply of infection-fighting white blood cells. The risk of this problem rises if you also have a disease such as lupus. If you're on kidney dialysis, your chances of an allergic reaction to the drug are increased.

If you develop abdominal pain with or without nausea and vomiting, contact your doctor. ACE inhibitors such as Lotensin have been known to cause intestinal swelling.

Lotensin can cause low blood pressure, especially if you are also taking a diuretic. You may feel light-headed or faint, especially during the first few days of therapy. If these symptoms occur, contact your doctor. Your dosage may need to be adjusted or discontinued.

If you have congestive heart failure, this drug should be used with caution.

Do not use potassium supplements or salt substitutes containing potassium without talking to your doctor first.

If you develop a sore throat or fever, you should contact your doctor immediately. It could indicate a more serious illness.

Excessive sweating, dehydration, severe diarrhea, or vomiting could make you lose too much water, causing your blood pressure to become too low.

Possible food and drug interactions when taking this medication
If Lotensin is taken with certain other drugs, the effects of either could be increased, decreased, or altered. It is especially important to check with your doctor before combining Lotensin with the following:

Diuretics such as Lasix and HydroDIURIL
Lithium (Lithonate)

Potassium supplements such as Slow-K

Potassium-sparing diuretics such as Moduretic and Dyazide

Special information if you are pregnant or breastfeeding

Lotensin can cause injury or death to developing and newborn babies, especially if taken during the second and third trimesters of pregnancy. If you are pregnant or plan to become pregnant and are taking Lotensin, contact your doctor immediately to discuss the potential hazard to your unborn child. Minimal amounts of Lotensin appear in breast milk. If this medication is essential to your health, your doctor may advise you to discontinue breastfeeding until your treatment with this medication is finished.

Recommended dosage

ADULTS

For people not taking a diuretic drug, the usual starting dose is 10 milligrams, once a day. Regular total dosages range from 20 to 40 milligrams per day either taken in a single dose or divided into 2 equal doses. The maximum dose is 80 milligrams per day. Your doctor will closely monitor the effect of this drug and adjust it according to your individual needs.

For people already taking a diuretic, the diuretic should be stopped, if possible, 2 to 3 days before taking Lotensin. This reduces the possibility of fainting or light-headedness. If blood pressure cannot be controlled by Lotensin alone, then diuretic use should begin again. If the diuretic cannot be discontinued, the starting dosage of Lotensin should be 5 milligrams.

For people with reduced kidney function, the dosages should be individualized according to the amount of reduced function. The usual starting dose in these instances is 5 milligrams per day, adjusted upwards to a maximum of 40 milligrams per day.

CHILDREN 7 TO 16 YEARS OLD

The starting dose of Lotensin alone is 0.2 milligrams per 2.2 pounds of body weight, once daily.

The safety and effectiveness of Lotensin have not been established in children 6 years old and younger or children with kidney disease.

Overdosage

Although there is no specific information available, a sudden drop in blood pressure would most likely be the primary symptom of Lotensin overdose. If you suspect a Lotensin overdose, seek medical attention immediately.

LOTENSIN HCT

Pronounced: lo-TEN-sin
Generic ingredients: Benazepril hydrochloride,
Hydrochlorothiazide

Why is this drug prescribed?

Lotensin HCT combines two types of blood pressure medication. The first, benazepril hydrochloride, is an ACE (angiotensin-converting enzyme) inhibitor. It works by preventing a chemical in your blood called angiotensin I from converting into a more potent form (angiotensin II) that increases salt and water retention in the body and causes the blood vessels to constrict—two actions that tend to increase blood pressure.

To aid in clearing excess water from the body, Lotensin HCT also contains hydrochlorothiazide, a diuretic that promotes production of urine. Diuretics often wash too much potassium out of the body along with the water. However, the ACE inhibitor part of Lotensin HCT tends to keep potassium in the body, thereby canceling this unwanted effect.

Lotensin HCT is not used for the initial treatment of high blood pressure. It is saved for later use, when a single blood pressure medication is not sufficient for the job. In addition, some doctors are using Lotensin HCT along with other drugs to treat congestive heart failure.

Most important fact about this drug

You must take Lotensin HCT regularly for it to be effective. Since blood pressure declines gradually, it may be several weeks before you get the full benefit of Lotensin HCT; and you must continue taking it even if you are feeling well. Lotensin HCT does not cure high blood pressure; it merely keeps it under control.

How should you take this medication?

Take Lotensin HCT exactly as prescribed, and see your doctor regularly to make sure the drug is working properly without unwanted side effects. Do not stop taking this drug without first consulting your doctor.

- ■ *If you miss a dose…*
  Take it as soon as you remember. If it is almost time for your next dose, skip the one you missed and go back to your regular schedule. Never take 2 doses at the same time.
- ■ *Storage instructions…*
  Store at room temperature in a tightly closed container. Protect from moisture and light.

What side effects may occur?

Side effects cannot be anticipated. If any develop or change in intensity, inform your doctor as soon as possible. Only your doctor can determine if it is safe for you to continue taking Lotensin HCT.

■ *Side effects may include:*
Dizziness, fatigue, headache

This side effects list is not complete. If you have any questions about side effects, you should consult your doctor. Report any new or continuing symptoms to your doctor right away.

Why should this drug not be prescribed?

If you are unable to urinate, avoid this medication.

You should not take this medication if you are sensitive to or have ever had an allergic reaction to any of the following: Lotensin, thiazide diuretics such as HydroDIURIL and Esidrix, ACE inhibitors such as captopril and Vasotec, or sulfa or other sulfonamide-derived drugs such as Bactrim and Septra. If you have a history of allergies or asthma, you may be at greater risk for an allergic reaction to this medication. Make sure your doctor is aware of any drug reactions you have experienced.

Special warnings about this medication

If you develop swelling of the face, lips, tongue, or throat, or of your arms and legs, or have difficulty swallowing or breathing, stop taking the medication and contact your doctor immediately. You may be having an allergic reaction and might need emergency treatment.

If you develop abdominal pain with or without nausea and vomiting, contact your doctor. ACE inhibitors such as Lotensin HCT have been known to cause intestinal swelling.

You may feel light-headed, especially during the first few days of Lotensin HCT therapy. If this occurs, notify your doctor. If you actually faint, stop taking the medication until you have consulted with your doctor.

Dehydration, excessive sweating, vomiting, or diarrhea can all deplete your body's fluids and cause your blood pressure to drop. If this leads to light-headedness or fainting, you should check with your doctor.

Inform your doctor or dentist that you are taking Lotensin HCT before undergoing surgery or anesthesia.

Do not use potassium supplements or salt substitutes containing potassium without consulting your doctor.

If you develop a sore throat or fever, contact your doctor immediately. It could indicate a more serious illness.

Your doctor will probably check your kidney function when you start taking Lotensin HCT and do follow-up tests periodically thereafter. For people with severe kidney disease, doctors usually prescribe other blood pressure medications instead of Lotensin HCT.

Caution is warranted, too, if you have liver disease. If you notice a yellow tinge to your skin and the whites of your eyes, stop taking the drug and notify your doctor. This could be a sign of liver damage.

Lotensin HCT may increase your blood sugar levels if you have diabetes. It may cause kidney problems in people with severe congestive heart failure. It can also trigger gout or the connective tissue disease lupus erythematosus. Use Lotensin HCT cautiously if you have any of these problems.

The safety and effectiveness of Lotensin HCT in children have not been established.

Possible food and drug interactions when taking this medication

If Lotensin HCT is taken with certain other drugs, the effects of either could be increased, decreased, or altered. It is especially important to check with your doctor before combining Lotensin HCT with the following:

Barbiturates such as phenobarbital
Cholestyramine (Questran)
Colestipol (Colestid)
Corticosteroids such as prednisone and ACTH
Diabetes medications such as insulin and Micronase
Digoxin (Lanoxin)
Diuretics such as HydroDIURIL and Lasix
Lithium (Eskalith, Lithobid)
Narcotics such as Percocet
Nonsteroidal anti-inflammatory drugs such as Naprosyn
Norepinephrine (Levophed)
Other high blood pressure medications
Potassium-sparing diuretics such as Aldactone, Dyazide, and
    Moduretic
Potassium supplements such as Slow-K and K-Dur
Salt substitutes containing potassium

Alcohol may increase the effect of Lotensin HCT, and could cause dizziness or fainting. Check with your doctor before drinking alcoholic beverages.

Special information if you are pregnant or breastfeeding

ACE inhibitors such as the one in Lotensin HCT have been shown to cause injury and even death to the unborn child when used in pregnancy during the second and third trimesters. If you are pregnant, your doctor should discontinue this medication as soon as possible. If you plan to become pregnant, make sure your doctor knows you are taking this medication. The diuretic component of Lotensin HCT can cause jaundice (yellowing of the skin and whites of the eyes) and abnormal bruising and bleeding in newborns.

Lotensin HCT appears in breast milk and could affect a nursing infant. To avoid potential harm to the baby, you'll need to choose between breastfeeding and continuing your treatment with Lotensin HCT.

Recommended dosage

ADULTS

Lotensin HCT is usually taken once a day. Your doctor will adjust the dosage depending on how your blood pressure responds. The smallest dose that is effective should be used.

Overdosage

Any medication taken in excess can have serious consequences. If you suspect an overdose, seek medical attention immediately.

■ *Symptoms of Lotensin HCT overdose may include:*
A severe drop in blood pressure, dry mouth, excessive thirst, muscle pain or cramps, nausea and vomiting, weak or irregular heartbeat, weakness and dizziness

LOTREL

Pronounced: LOW-trel
Generic names: Amlodipine, Benazepril hydrochloride

Why is this drug prescribed?

Lotrel is used in the treatment of high blood pressure. It is a combination medicine that is used when treatment with a single drug has not been successful or has caused side effects.

One component, amlodipine, is a calcium channel blocker. It eases the workload of the heart by slowing down the passage of nerve impulses and hence the contractions of the heart muscle. This improves blood flow through the heart and throughout the body and reduces blood pressure. The other component, benazepril, is an angiotensin-converting enzyme (ACE) inhibitor. It works by preventing the transformation of a hormone called angiotensin I into a more potent substance that increases salt and water retention in your body.

Most important fact about this drug

You must take Lotrel regularly for it to be effective. Since blood pressure declines gradually, it may take 1 to 2 weeks for the full effect of Lotrel to be seen. Even if you are feeling well, you must continue to take the medication. Lotrel does not cure high blood pressure; it merely keeps it under control.

How should you take this medication?

Take Lotrel exactly as prescribed by your doctor Try to take your medication at the same time each day, such as before or after breakfast, so that it is easier to remember.

■ *If you miss a dose...*
Take it as soon as you remember. However, if it is almost time for your next dose, skip the one you missed and go back to your regular schedule. Do not take 2 doses at once.

■ *Storage instructions...*
Store at room temperature. Store away from moisture and light; avoid excessive heat.

What side effects may occur?

Side effects cannot be anticipated. If any develop or change in intensity, tell your doctor as soon as possible. Only your doctor can determine if it is safe for you to continue taking Lotrel.

If you develop swelling of your face, around the lips, tongue, or throat; swelling of arms and legs; or difficulty swallowing, you should contact your doctor immediately. You may need emergency treatment. Be especially wary if you're an African American: Your chances of this type of reaction are higher. Severe allergic reactions are also more likely if you are being given bee or wasp venom to guard against future reactions to stings.

■ *Side effects may include:*
Cough, dizziness, headache, swelling

Why should this drug not be prescribed?

If you are sensitive to or have ever had an allergic reaction to amlodipine, benazepril, or any angiotensin-converting enzyme (ACE) inhibitor, do not take this medication.

Special warnings about this medication

Your kidney function should be assessed when you start taking Lotrel, then monitored for the first few weeks.

If you have poor kidney function, there is a slight chance that Lotensin may reduce your supply of infection-fighting white blood cells. The risk of this problem rises if you also have a disease such as lupus. If you're on kidney dialysis, your chances of an allergic reaction to the drug are increased.

Contact your doctor if you develop abdominal pain with or without nausea and vomiting. ACE inhibitors such as Lotrel have been known to cause intestinal swelling.

Lotrel can cause low blood pressure, especially if you are taking high doses of diuretics. You may feel light-headed or faint, especially during the first few days of therapy. If these symptoms occur, contact your doctor. Your dosage may need to be adjusted or discontinued.

If you have congestive heart failure, use this drug with caution. If you have kidney disease or severe liver disease, diabetes, lupus erythematosus, or scleroderma (a rare disease affecting the blood vessels or connective tissue), use Lotrel with caution.

Excessive sweating, severe diarrhea, or vomiting could make you lose too much water, causing a severe drop in blood pressure. If you notice a yellow coloring to your skin or the whites of your eyes, stop taking the drug and notify your doctor immediately. You could be developing liver problems.

If you develop a persistent, dry cough, tell your doctor. It may be due to the medication and, if so, will disappear if you stop taking Lotrel. In a medical emergency and before you have surgery, notify your doctor or dentist that you are taking Lotrel.

Possible food and drug interactions when taking this medication

If Lotrel is taken with certain other drugs, the effects of either could be increased, decreased, or altered. It is especially important to check with your doctor before combining Lotrel with the following:

Diuretics such as Diuril, Lasix, and HydroDIURIL
Lithium (Eskalith, Lithobid)
Potassium-sparing diuretics such as Aldactazide, Moduretic, and Maxzide
Potassium supplements (Slow-K)

Special information if you are pregnant or breastfeeding

Lotrel can cause injury or death to developing and newborn babies, especially if taken during the second and third trimesters of pregnancy. If you are pregnant and are taking Lotrel, contact your doctor immediately to discuss the potential hazard to your unborn child. Minimal amounts of benazepril appear in breast milk. If this medication is essential to your health, your doctor may advise you to discontinue breastfeeding while you are taking Lotrel.

Recommended dosage

ADULTS

Your doctor will closely monitor the effects of this drug and adjust the dosage according to your blood pressure response. Lotrel is available in capsules containing 2.5 milligrams of amlodipine and 10 milligrams of benazepril, capsules containing 5 milligrams of amlodipine and 10 or 20 milligrams of benazepril, and capsules containing 10 milligrams of amlodipine and 20 milligrams of benazepril. Small, older, frail, and kidney- or liver-impaired individuals usually start with the lowest dose.

CHILDREN

The safety and effectiveness of Lotrel in children have not been established.

Overdosage

Any medication taken in excess can have serious consequences. Although there is no specific information available, a sudden drop in blood pressure and rapid heartbeat would be the primary symptoms of a Lotrel overdose. If you suspect an overdose, seek medical attention immediately.

Lotrimin *See Gyne-Lotrimin, page 640.*

LOTRISONE

Pronounced: LOE-trih-sone
Generic ingredients: Clotrimazole, Betamethasone
  dipropionate

Why is this drug prescribed?

Lotrisone cream and lotion contain a combination of a steroid (betamethasone) and an antifungal drug (clotrimazole). Lotrisone is used to treat skin infections caused by fungus, such as athlete's foot, jock itch, and ringworm of the body.

Betamethasone treats symptoms (such as itching, redness, swelling, and inflammation) that result from fungus infections, while clotrimazole treats the cause of the infection by inhibiting the growth of certain yeast and fungus organisms. If the infection is not inflamed, your doctor may prescribe a different medication.

Most important fact about this drug

When you use Lotrisone, you inevitably absorb some of the medication through your skin and into the bloodstream. Too much absorption can lead to unwanted side effects elsewhere in the body. To keep this problem to a minimum, avoid using large amounts of Lotrisone cream or lotion over wide areas, and do not cover it with airtight dressings such as plastic wrap or adhesive bandage unless specifically told to by your doctor. If widespread application is unavoidable, your doctor may order periodic tests to make sure your body is not absorbing too much of this medication.

How should you use this medication?

Wash your hands before and after applying Lotrisone. If you are using Lotrisone lotion, shake it well before using. Lotrisone is for use only on the skin. Be careful to keep it out of the eyes, mouth, and vaginal area. Gently massage it into the affected area and surrounding skin twice a day, in the morning and evening.

Use Lotrisone for the full time prescribed, even if your condition has improved.

Lotrisone should be applied sparingly to the groin area, and it should not be used for longer than 2 weeks. Wear loose-fitting clothing.

■ *If you miss a dose...*
Apply it as soon as you remember. If it is almost time for your next dose, skip the one you missed and go back to your regular schedule.

■ *Storage instructions...*
Store at room temperature.

What side effects may occur?
Side effects cannot be anticipated. If any develop or change in intensity, inform your doctor as soon as possible. Only your doctor can determine if it is safe for you to continue using Lotrisone.

■ *Side effects may include:*
Blistering, burning, dry skin, hives, infection, irritated skin, itching, peeling, reddened skin, skin eruptions and rash, stinging, swelling, tingling sensation

Why should this drug not be prescribed?
You should not use Lotrisone if you are sensitive to clotrimazole or betamethasone or any of its other ingredients, or to similar steroid and antifungal medications.

Lotrisone is not recommended for children under 17 years of age. In this age group it is more likely to cause serious side effects such as stunted growth, thinning skin, and the set of symptoms called Cushing's syndrome. (See *Special warnings about this medication* for details.)

Special warnings about this medication
Steroid drugs (such as betamethasone) can affect the functioning of the adrenal, hypothalamic, and pituitary glands and temporarily produce sugar in the urine, excessive blood sugar levels, and a disorder called Cushing's syndrome. Symptoms of Cushing's syndrome include acne, depression, excessive hair growth, humped upper back, insomnia, moon-faced appearance, muscle weakness, obese trunk, paranoia, stretch marks, stunted growth (in children), wasted limbs, and susceptibility to bruising, fractures, and infection.

Do not take Lotrisone cream or lotion internally and be sure to keep it away from your eyes.

If you are using Lotrisone to treat jock itch (tinea cruris) or a fungal infection of the skin called tinea corporis, and there has been no improvement after 1 week, notify your doctor.

If you are using Lotrisone to treat athlete's foot (tinea pedis), notify your doctor if there is no improvement after 2 weeks of treatment.

Do not use Lotrisone for any condition other than the one for which it was prescribed. Do not use Lotrisone in the groin area or on the body for longer than 2 weeks or in the foot area for longer than 4 weeks.

Lotrisone should be used with caution by adults over age 65. In older adults, Lotrisone may cause skin reactions, especially thinning skin.

Possible food and drug interactions when taking this medication
Do not combine Lotrisone with other steroid creams. Use of more than one steroid-containing product increases the chance of side effects.

Special information if you are pregnant or breastfeeding
Pregnant women should not use steroid drugs in large amounts or for prolonged periods of time. The effects of Lotrisone during pregnancy have not been adequately studied. The medication should be used during pregnancy only if the potential benefits justify the potential risk to the developing baby. It is not known whether Lotrisone appears in breast milk. Nursing mothers should use Lotrisone with caution and only when clearly needed.

Recommended dosage

ADULTS AND CHILDREN OVER 17 YEARS OLD

"Jock Itch" (Tinea Cruris) or Fungal Skin Infections (Tinea Corporis)
Gently massage Lotrisone cream or lotion into the affected and surrounding skin areas twice a day, in the morning and the evening, for 2 weeks. Lotrisone should be applied sparingly to the groin area. Notify your doctor if there has been no improvement after 1 week of treatment.

Athlete's Foot (Tinea Pedis)
Gently massage Lotrisone cream or lotion into the affected and surrounding skin areas twice a day, in the morning and the evening, for 4 weeks. Notify your doctor if there has been no improvement after 2 weeks of treatment.

Overdosage
Any medication used in excess can have serious consequences. A life-threatening overdose of Lotrisone, which is applied to the skin, is unlikely. However, misuse or overuse of Lotrisone can cause disorders such as Cushing's syndrome. Be sure to check with your doctor if you suspect such a problem.

Lovastatin *See Mevacor, page 839.*

Lovastatin and Extended-release niacin *See Advicor, page 46.*

Lovastatin, extended release *See Altocor, page 81.*

Low-Ogestrel *See Oral Contraceptives, page 1000.*

LOZOL

Pronounced: LOW-zoll
Generic name: Indapamide

Why is this drug prescribed?

Lozol is used in the treatment of high blood pressure, either alone or in combination with other high blood pressure medications. Lozol is also used to relieve salt and fluid retention. During pregnancy, your doctor may prescribe Lozol to relieve fluid retention caused by a specific condition or when fluid retention causes extreme discomfort that is not relieved by rest.

Most important fact about this drug

If you have high blood pressure, you must take Lozol regularly for it to be effective. Since blood pressure declines gradually, it may be several weeks before you get the full benefit of Lozol; and you must continue taking it even if you are feeling well. Lozol does not cure high blood pressure; it merely keeps it under control.

How should you take this medication?

Take Lozol exactly as prescribed by your doctor. Suddenly stopping Lozol could cause your condition to worsen.

Lozol is best taken in the morning.

■ *If you miss a dose...*
Take the forgotten dose as soon as you remember. If it is almost time for your next dose, skip the one you missed and go back to your regular schedule. Never take 2 doses at the same time.

■ *Storage instructions...*
Store Lozol at room temperature. Protect from excessive heat. Keep the container tightly closed.

What side effects may occur?

Side effects cannot be anticipated. If any side effects develop or change in intensity, tell your doctor immediately. Only your doctor can determine whether it is safe to continue taking Lozol. Most side effects are mild and temporary.

■ *Side effects may include:*
Agitation, anxiety, back pain, dizziness, fatigue, headache, infection, irritability, loss of energy or tiredness, muscle cramps or spasms, nasal inflammation, nervousness, numbness in hands and feet, pain, tension, weakness

Why should this drug not be prescribed?

Avoid using Lozol if you are unable to urinate or if you have ever had an allergic reaction or are sensitive to indapamide or other sulfa-containing drugs.

Special warnings about this medication

Diuretics such as Lozol can cause the body to lose too much salt and potassium, especially among elderly women. Signs of an excessively low potassium level include muscle weakness and rapid or irregular heartbeat. To boost your potassium level, your doctor may recommend eating potassium-rich foods or taking a potassium supplement.

The risk of potassium loss increases when larger doses are used, if you have cirrhosis, or if you are also using corticosteroids or ACTH. Your doctor should check your blood regularly, especially if you have an irregular heartbeat or are taking heart medications.

Lozol should be used with care if you have gout or high uric acid levels, liver disease, diabetes, or lupus erythematosus, a disease of the connective tissue.

This medication should be used with caution if you have severe kidney disease. Your kidney function should be given a complete assessment and should continue to be monitored.

In general, diuretics should not be taken if you are taking lithium, as they increase the risk of lithium poisoning.

Safety and effectiveness in children have not been established.

Possible food and drug interactions when taking this medication

If Lozol is taken with certain other drugs, the effects of either could be increased, decreased, or altered. It is especially important to check with your doctor before combining Lozol with the following:

Lithium (Eskalith)
Norepinephrine (a drug used to treat cardiac arrest and to maintain blood pressure)
Other high blood pressure medications such as Aldomet and Tenormin

Special information if you are pregnant or breastfeeding

If you are pregnant or plan to become pregnant, tell your doctor immediately. No information is available about the safety of Lozol during pregnancy.

Lozol may appear in breast milk and could affect a nursing infant. If Lozol is essential to your health, your doctor may advise you to stop breastfeeding until your treatment is finished.

Recommended dosage

ADULTS

High Blood Pressure
The usual starting dose is 1.25 milligrams as a single daily dose taken in the morning. If Lozol does not seem to be working for you, your doctor may gradually increase your dosage up to 5 milligrams taken once a day.

Fluid Buildup in Congestive Heart Failure
The usual starting dose is 2.5 milligrams as a single daily dose taken in the morning. Your doctor may increase your dosage to 5 milligrams taken once daily.

Overdosage
Any medication taken in excess can have serious consequences. If you suspect an overdose, seek medical treatment immediately.

■ *Symptoms of Lozol overdose may include:*
Electrolyte imbalance (potassium or salt depletion due to too much fluid loss), nausea, stomach disorders, vomiting, weakness

LUMIGAN
Pronounced: LOO-mi-gan
Generic name: Bimatoprost

Why is this drug prescribed?
Lumigan is an eyedrop that combats high pressure inside the eyeball. It is prescribed for a condition called open-angle glaucoma (a gradual increase of pressure in the eye). It is typically used after other remedies have caused problems or fail to work. It lowers pressure by promoting drainage of the fluid (aqueous humor) that fills the eye.

Most important fact about this drug
Lumigan has been known to cause several changes in the appearance of the eyes. The color of the iris occasionally changes to brown, and the eyelids may darken. The eyelashes may also be affected, increasing in length, thickness, and number, and turning a darker shade.

These changes occur slowly, and may take months or years to notice. They may be permanent, and are especially important to patients who will be using Lumigan in only one eye.

How should you take this medication?
This eyedrop is administered once a day. If you wear contact lenses, remove them before using Lumigan. Wait 15 minutes before reinserting

them. If you are using more than one type of eyedrop, space the drugs 5 minutes apart.

To avoid contamination and to reduce the risk of developing an eye infection, do not let the tip of the container touch the eye, face, or fingers.

■ *If you miss a dose...*
Take it as soon as you remember. If it is almost time for your next dose, skip the one you missed and go back to your regular schedule. Never take 2 doses at the same time.

■ *Storage instructions...*
Store at room temperature in the original container.

What side effects may occur?
Side effects cannot be anticipated. If any develop or change in intensity, inform your doctor as soon as possible. Only your doctor can determine if it is safe for you to continue taking Lumigan.

■ *Side effects may include:*
Burning eyes, cataract, darkening of eyelashes, darkening of the skin surrounding the eye, dry eyes, excessive hair growth, eye irritation, eye pain, feeling of a foreign body in the eye, growth of eyelashes, headaches, itchy eyes, red eyelids, respiratory infections, swelling of the eyelids, visual disturbances, weakness

Why should this drug not be prescribed?
You'll be unable to use Lumigan if it causes an allergic reaction.

Special warnings about this medication
Due to the risk of infection if the drops become contaminated, you should check with your doctor about using the dispenser bottle if you suffer any eye injury or are scheduled for eye surgery.

An infection could cause serious damage to the eye. Check with your doctor immediately if you develop any eye reactions, particularly inflamed eyelids.

Your doctor will check for the presence of certain eye conditions such as inflammation in the area of the iris (uveitis) and swelling in the back of the eye (macular edema). Lumigan must be used with caution under these circumstances.

Also be sure the doctor knows if you have kidney disease or liver problems. They are reasons for caution when using Lumigan.

Do not use Lumigan more than once a day. More frequent administration may diminish the effect of the drug.

Possible food and drug interactions when taking this medication
There is no information on interactions with other drugs.

Special information if you are pregnant or breastfeeding

The effects of Lumigan during pregnancy have not been adequately studied. If you are pregnant or plan to become pregnant, inform your doctor immediately.

It is not known whether Lumigan appears in breast milk. Use Lumigan with caution if you are nursing.

Recommended dosage

ADULTS

The recommended dose is 1 drop in the affected eye or eyes once daily in the evening.

Overdosage

Any medication taken in excess can have serious consequences. If you suspect an overdose, seek medical attention immediately.

LUPRON DEPOT
Pronounced: LU-pron DEE-poe
Generic name: Leuprolide acetate

Why is this drug prescribed?

Lupron is a synthetic version of the naturally occurring gonadotropin-releasing hormone (GnRH). Lupron suppresses shedding of the endometrium (lining of the uterus) during menstruation and is used to treat endometriosis, a condition in which cells from the endometrium grow outside the uterus. Endometriosis causes painful growths to form around the outsides of the uterus, fallopian tubes, and ovaries.

Two forms of Lupron—Lupron Depot 3.75 and Lupron Depot 11.25—are prescribed to relieve the pain of endometriosis and shrink the growths. (The hormonal medication norethindrone acetate is often added to the regimen.) Three other forms of Lupron—Lupron Depot 7.5, Lupron Depot 22.5, and Lupron Depot 30—are prescribed to relieve the symptoms of advanced prostate cancer.

The first two forms of Lupron are also used before surgery, along with iron, to treat anemia caused by fibroids (tumors) in the uterus when iron alone is not effective. Some doctors also prescribe Lupron for infertility and for early puberty.

Most important fact about this drug

Lupron lowers estrogen levels, which can lead to a decrease in bone density in both men and women. Decreased bone density could increase your risk of osteoporosis, or brittle bone disease, later in life. Consequently, the drug is not usually given for longer than 6 months at a time.

How should you take this medication?

Lupron must be given under the supervision of a physician. It is given by injection once a month, every 3 months, or every 4 months, depending on the form you've been prescribed.

■ *If you miss a dose...*
Women who miss their monthly injections of Lupron Depot 3.75 may experience resumption of menstrual bleeding.

■ *Storage instructions...*
Lupron does not need to be refrigerated. Protect from freezing.

What side effects may occur?

Side effects cannot be anticipated. If any develop or change in intensity, inform your doctor as soon as possible. Only your doctor can determine if it is safe for you to continue taking Lupron.

WOMEN

Lupron stops menstruation and reduces estrogen levels in your body. Reduced estrogen may cause side effects such as acne, decreased sex drive, headaches, hot flashes, mood swings, muscle pain, a reduction in breast size, and vaginal inflammation and dryness. Your menstrual periods and estrogen levels will return to normal when you stop taking Lupron.

■ *Side effects may include:*
Anxiety, appetite changes, breast tenderness or pain, depression, development of male characteristics, dizziness, fluid retention, general pain, inflammation of the vagina (vaginitis), insomnia or other sleep disorders, joint pain, memory problems, nausea and vomiting, nervousness, skin reactions, stomach or intestinal disorders, unusual burning or prickling sensation of the skin, weakness, weight gain or loss

■ *Additional side effects you may experience if you are taking Lupron for anemia include:*
Body odor, flu symptoms, nail problems, nasal irritation, pinkeye, taste disorders

MEN

Lupron increases male hormone levels.

■ *Side effects may include:*
Breathing problems, dizziness/vertigo, fluid retention, headache, hot flashes, impotence, joint disorders, nausea, pain, skin reaction, sleep disorders, stomach and intestinal disorder, sweats, testicle shrinking, urinary problems, vomiting, weakness

A few other side effects are possible with the Lupron Depot 30 formulation.

Why should this drug not be prescribed?

Lupron should not be used if you are known to be hypersensitive to it, or to any drug containing a form of GnRH.

If you have undiagnosed abnormal vaginal bleeding, you should not take Lupron.

If you are pregnant or might become pregnant, you should not take Lupron. The drug could harm a developing baby. Also avoid Lupron if you are breastfeeding.

Lupron Depot 30 is for use by men only.

Special warnings about this medication

WOMEN

Your doctor will want to make sure you are not pregnant before giving you Lupron. If you become pregnant while taking the drug, stop taking it and notify your doctor immediately.

Even though your menstrual periods stop while you are taking Lupron, there is still a chance you could become pregnant and you should take birth control measures. Use condoms or diaphragms rather than hormonal methods such as birth control pills or Norplant, because hormones will interfere with Lupron treatment.

Notify your doctor if you continue to have menstrual periods. If you miss successive doses of Lupron you may have some bleeding.

Treatment with Lupron can cause an irreversible weakening of the bones (osteoporosis). No more than one course of therapy is recommended for women who develop this problem or who are at risk of bone loss. Adding norethindrone to the treatment regimen reduces bone loss, but increases the risk of other side effects such as clotting problems and fluid retention. If norethindrone is part of your regimen, your doctor will be on the alert for inflamed veins (thrombophlebitis) and other signs of clotting disorders. Norethindrone should be used with caution if you have heart disease risk factors such as high cholesterol or cigarette smoking. The doctor should also monitor you carefully if you have kidney disease, asthma, epilepsy, or other conditions that might be aggravated by fluid retention. Norethindrone may cause depression, and should be discontinued if severe depression occurs. The drug should also be discontinued if you develop vision problems or migraine headaches.

Lupron therapy for endometriosis has not been studied in women under 18 years of age, nor is the product recommended for women over 65.

MEN

Men taking Lupron for prostate cancer may find that their symptoms get worse, or that new symptoms appear, during the first few weeks of treatment. If this happens, let your doctor know immediately. Bone pain may increase temporarily, and in rare cases a blockage in the urinary tract or pressure on the spinal cord may appear. If you already have problems in the spine or urinary tract, the doctor will start Lupron therapy with caution.

Possible food and drug interactions when taking this medication

If Lupron is taken with certain other drugs, the effects of either could be increased, decreased, or altered. It is especially important to check with your doctor before combining Lupron with any type of hormones, such as birth control pills.

No interactions are likely in men.

Special information if you are pregnant or breastfeeding

Do not take Lupron if you are pregnant or breastfeeding.

Recommended dosage

LUPRON DEPOT 3.75

For endometriosis, a single intramuscular injection is given once a month. Norethindrone may be included in the treatment regimen. Treatment lasts 6 months. One additional 6-month course of treatment may be given, provided norethindrone is included in the second regimen.

For anemia due to uterine fibroids, the same dose is given once a month for up to 3 months.

LUPRON DEPOT 7.5

For prostate cancer, a single injection is given once a month.

LUPRON DEPOT 11.25

For endometriosis, a single injection is given every 3 months. Norethindrone may be included in the treatment regimen. Treatment lasts 6 months. One additional 6-month course of treatment may be given, provided norethindrone is included in the second regimen.

For anemia due to fibroids, the usual treatment is a single injection.

LUPRON DEPOT 22.5

For prostate cancer, a single injection is given every 3 months.

LUPRON DEPOT 30

For prostate cancer, a single injection is given every 4 months.

Overdosage

An overdose is extremely unlikely. However, if you suspect overdosage, call your doctor immediately.

LURIDE

Pronounced: LUHR-ide
Generic name: Sodium fluoride

Why is this drug prescribed?

Luride is prescribed to strengthen children's teeth against decay during the period when the teeth are still developing.

Studies have shown that children who live where the drinking water contains a certain level of fluoride have fewer cavities than others. Fluoride helps prevent cavities in three ways: by increasing the teeth's resistance to dissolving on contact with acid, by strengthening teeth, and by slowing down the growth of mouth bacteria.

Luride may be given to children who live where the water fluoride level is 0.6 part per million or less.

Most important fact about this drug

Before Luride is prescribed, it is important for the doctor to know the fluoride content of the water your child drinks every day. Your water company, or a private laboratory, can tell you the level of fluoride in your water.

How should you take this medication?

Give your child Luride exactly as prescribed by your doctor. It is preferable to give the tablet at bedtime after the child's teeth have been brushed. The youngster may chew and swallow the tablet or simply suck on it until it dissolves. The liquid form of this medicine is to be taken by mouth only. It may be dropped directly into the mouth or mixed with water or fruit juice. Always store Luride drops in the original plastic dropper bottle.

■ *If you miss a dose...*
  Give it as soon as you remember. If it is almost time for the next dose, skip the one you missed and go back to your regular schedule. Do not give 2 doses at once.
■ *Storage instructions...*
  Store at room temperature away from heat, light, and moisture. Keep the liquid from freezing.

What side effects may occur?

Side effects cannot be anticipated. If any develop, tell your doctor immediately. Only your doctor can determine whether it is safe for your child to continue taking Luride.

In rare cases, Luride may cause an allergic rash or some other unexpected effect.

Why should this drug not be prescribed?

Your child should not take Luride if he or she is sensitive to it or has had an allergic reaction to sodium fluoride in the past.

Your child should not take the 1-milligram strength of Luride if the drinking water in your area contains 0.3 part per million of fluoride or more. He or she should not take the other forms of Luride if the water contains 0.6 part per million of fluoride or more.

Special warnings about this medication

Do not give full-strength tablets (1 milligram) to children under the age of 6. Do not give the half-strength tablets (0.5 milligram) to children under 3, or to children under 6 when your drinking water fluoride content is 0.3 part per million or more. Do not give the quarter-strength tablets (0.25 milligram) to children under 6 months, or to children under 3 years when fluoride content is 0.3 part per million or more.

Possible food and drug interactions when taking this medication

Avoid giving your child Luride with dairy products. The calcium in dairy products may interact with the fluoride to create calcium fluoride, which the body cannot absorb well.

Recommended dosage

Since this drug is used to supplement water with low fluoride content, consult your physician to determine the proper amount based on the local water content. Also check with your doctor if you move to a new area, change to bottled water, or begin using a water-filtering device. Dosages are determined by both age and the fluoride content of the water.

INFANTS AND CHILDREN

The following daily dosages are recommended for areas where the drinking water contains fluoride at less than 0.3 part per million:

Children 6 Months to 3 Years of Age
1 quarter-strength (0.25-milligram) tablet or half a dropperful of liquid

3 to 6 Years of Age
1 half-strength (0.5-milligram) tablet or 1 dropperful of liquid

6 to 16 Years of Age
1 full-strength (1-milligram) tablet or 2 droppersful of liquid

For areas where the fluoride content of drinking water is between 0.3 and 0.6 part per million, the recommended daily dosage of the tablets is one-half the above dosages. Dosage of the liquid should be reduced to half a dropperful for children ages 3 to 6 and 1 dropperful for children over 6.

Overdosage

Any medication taken in excess can have serious consequences. Taking too much fluoride for a long period of time may cause discoloration of the teeth. Notify your doctor or dentist if you notice white, brown, or black spots on the teeth.

Swallowing large amounts of fluoride can cause burning in the mouth and a sore tongue, followed by diarrhea, nausea, salivation, stomach cramping and pain, and vomiting, sometimes with blood.

Maalox *See Antacids, page 114.*

Macrobid *See Macrodantin, below.*

MACRODANTIN
Pronounced: Mack-row-DAN-tin
Generic name: Nitrofurantoin
Other brand name: Macrobid

Why is this drug prescribed?
Nitrofurantoin, an antibacterial drug, is prescribed for the treatment of urinary tract infections caused by certain strains of bacteria.

Most important fact about this drug
Breathing disorders have occurred in people taking nitrofurantoin. The drug can cause inflammation of the lungs marked by coughing, difficulty breathing, and wheezing. It has also been known to cause pulmonary fibrosis (an abnormal increase in fibrous tissue of the lungs). This condition can develop gradually without symptoms and can be fatal. An allergic reaction to this drug is also possible and may occur without warning. Symptoms include a feeling of ill health and a persistent cough. However, all these reactions occur rarely and generally in those receiving nitrofurantoin therapy for 6 months or longer.

Sudden and severe lung reactions are characterized by fever, chills, cough, chest pain, and difficulty breathing. These acute reactions usually occur within the first week of treatment and subside when therapy with nitrofurantoin is stopped.

Your doctor should monitor your condition closely, especially if you are receiving long-term treatment with this medication.

How should you take this medication?
To improve absorption of the drug, nitrofurantoin should be taken with food.

Your doctor will prescribe Macrodantin only to treat a bacterial infection. Macrodantin will not cure a viral infection such as the common cold. It's important to take all of your medication as instructed by your doctor, even if you're feeling better in a few days. Skipping doses or not finishing the complete dosage of Macrodantin may decrease the drug's effectiveness and increase the chances of bacterial resistance to Macrodantin and similar antibiotics.

This medication works best if your urine is acidic. Ask your doctor whether you should be taking special measures to ensure its acidity.

Nitrofurantoin may turn the urine brown.

■ *If you miss a dose...*
Take the forgotten dose as soon as you remember, then space out the rest of the day's doses at equal intervals.

■ *Storage instructions...*
Store at room temperature. Protect from light and keep the container tightly closed.

What side effects may occur?
Side effects cannot be anticipated. If any develop or change in intensity, inform your doctor as soon as possible. Only your doctor can determine if it is safe for you to continue taking nitrofurantoin.

■ *Side effects may include:*
Lack or loss of appetite, nausea, vomiting

Why should this drug not be prescribed?
If you are sensitive to or have ever had an allergic reaction to nitrofurantoin or other drugs of this type, such as Furoxone, you should not take this medication. Make sure that your doctor is aware of any drug reactions that you have experienced.

Unless you are directed to do so by your doctor, do not take this medication if you have poor kidney function, producing little or no urine.

Nitrofurantoin should not be taken in the last month of pregnancy or during labor and delivery; it should not be given to infants under 1 month of age.

Special warnings about this medication
Tell your doctor if you have any unusual symptoms while you are taking this drug.

Fatalities have been reported from hepatitis (liver disease) during treatment with nitrofurantoin. Long-lasting, active hepatitis can develop without symptoms; therefore, if you are receiving long-term treatment with this drug, your doctor should test your liver function periodically.

Fatalities from peripheral neuropathy—a disease of the nerves—have also been reported in people taking nitrofurantoin. Conditions such as a kidney disorder, anemia, diabetes mellitus, a debilitating disease, or a vitamin B deficiency make peripheral neuropathy more likely. If you develop symptoms such as muscle weakness or lack of sensation, check with your doctor immediately.

If you experience diarrhea, tell your doctor. It may be a sign of serious intestinal inflammation.

Hemolytic anemia (destruction of red blood cells) has occurred in people taking nitrofurantoin.

Continued or prolonged use of this drug may result in growth of bacteria that do not respond to it. This can cause a renewed infection, so it is important that your doctor monitor your condition on a regular basis.

Possible food and drug interactions when taking this medication
If nitrofurantoin is taken with certain other drugs, the effects of either could be increased, decreased, or altered. It is especially important to check with your doctor before combining nitrofurantoin with the following:

Magnesium trisilicate (Gaviscon Antacid Tablets)
The gout drugs probenecid and sulfinpyrazone and other drugs that
    increase the amount of uric acid in the urine

Special information if you are pregnant or breastfeeding
The safety of nitrofurantoin during pregnancy and breastfeeding has not been established. Nitrofurantoin does appear in human breast milk. If you are pregnant or breastfeeding or you plan to become pregnant or breast-feed, inform your doctor immediately.

Recommended dosage
Treatment with nitrofurantoin should be continued for 1 week or for at least 3 days after obtaining a urine specimen free of infection. If your infection has not cleared up, your doctor should re-evaluate your case.

ADULTS

The recommended dosage of Macrodantin is 50 to 100 milligrams taken 4 times a day. For long-term treatment, your doctor may reduce your dosage to 50 to 100 milligrams taken at bedtime.

The recommended dosage of Macrobid is one 100-milligram capsule every 12 hours for 7 days.

CHILDREN

This medication should not be prescribed for children under 1 month of age.

The recommended daily dosage of Macrodantin for infants and children over 1 month of age is 5 to 7 milligrams per 2.2 pounds of body weight, divided into 4 doses over 24 hours.

For the long-term treatment of children, the doctor may prescribe daily doses as low as 1 milligram per 2.2 pounds of body weight taken in 1 or 2 doses per day.

The dosage of Macrobid for children over 12 years of age is one 100 milligram capsule every 12 hours for 7 days. Safety and effectiveness have not been established for children under 12.

OLDER ADULTS

Doctors tend to prescribe lower doses of Macrodantin for older adults. The drug is more likely to cause lung and liver problems in members of this group; and because more older adults have poor kidneys, the risk of toxic reactions to Macrodantin is also greater.

Overdosage

An overdose of nitrofurantoin does not cause any specific symptoms other than vomiting. If vomiting does not occur soon after an excessive dose, it should be induced.

If you suspect an overdose, seek emergency medical treatment immediately.

Magnesium salicylate See Novasal, page 982.

Materna See Prenatal Vitamins, page 1141.

MAVIK

Pronounced: MA-vick
Generic name: Trandolapril

Why is this drug prescribed?

Mavik controls high blood pressure. It is effective when used alone or combined with other high blood pressure medications such as diuretics that help rid the body of excess water. Mavik is also used to treat heart failure or dysfunction following a heart attack.

Mavik is in a family of drugs known as ACE (angiotensin-converting enzyme) inhibitors. It works by preventing a chemical in your blood called angiotensin I from converting into a more potent form that increases salt and water retention in your body. ACE inhibitors also expand your blood vessels, further reducing blood pressure.

Most important fact about this drug

You will get the full benefit of Mavik within a week; but you must continue taking it regularly to maintain the effect. Mavik does not cure high blood pressure; it merely keeps it under control.

How should you take this medication?

Mavik can be taken with or without food. Try to make Mavik part of your regular daily routine. If you take it at the same time each day—for example, right after breakfast—you will be less likely to forget a dose.

- *If you miss a dose…*
  Take it as soon as you remember. However, if it is almost time for your next dose, skip the one you missed and go back to your regular schedule.
- *Storage instructions…*
  Mavik may be stored at room temperature.

What side effects may occur?

Side effects cannot be anticipated. If any develop or change in intensity, tell your doctor as soon as possible. Only your doctor can determine if it is safe for you to continue taking Mavik.

■ *Side effects may include:*

Abdominal pain, anxiety, bloating, chest pain, constipation, cough, cramps, decreased sex drive, diarrhea, difficult or labored breathing, dizziness, drowsiness, fainting, flushing, fluid retention, gout, impotence, indigestion, insomnia, itching, low blood pressure, muscle cramps, nosebleed, pains in arms and legs, palpitations, pins and needles, rash, severe skin disease, slowed heartbeat, swelling of arms or legs, swelling of face and lips, swelling of tongue and throat, throat inflammation, upper respiratory infection, vertigo, vomiting, yellow eyes and skin

Why should this drug not be prescribed?

If you have ever had an allergic reaction to Mavik or similar drugs such as Capoten or Vasotec, you should not take this medication. Make sure your doctor is aware of any drug reactions you have experienced.

Special warnings about this medication

If you develop signs of an allergic reaction, such as swelling of the face, lips, tongue, or throat and difficulty swallowing (or swelling of the arms and legs), you should stop taking Mavik and contact your doctor immediately. You may need emergency treatment. Desensitization treatments with bee or wasp venom make an allergic reaction more likely. Kidney dialysis also increases the danger.

When prescribing Mavik, your doctor will perform a complete assessment of your kidney function and will continue to monitor your kidneys.

If you have congestive heart failure, your blood pressure may drop sharply after the first few doses of Mavik and you may feel light-headed for a time. Your doctor should monitor you closely when you start taking this medication and when your dosage is increased.

High doses of diuretics combined with Mavik may cause excessively low blood pressure. Your doctor may need to reduce your diuretic dose to avoid this problem.

Mavik sometimes affects the liver. If you notice a yellow coloring to your skin or the whites of your eyes, stop taking Mavik and notify your doctor immediately.

Dehydration may cause a drop in blood pressure. If you do not drink enough water, perspire a lot, or suffer from vomiting or diarrhea, notify your doctor immediately.

Also contact your doctor promptly if you develop a sore throat or fever. It could indicate a more serious illness.

If you develop a persistent dry cough, tell your doctor. It may be due to the medication and, if so, will disappear if Mavik is discontinued.

Heart and circulatory problems, diabetes, lupus erythematosus, and kidney disease are all reasons for using Mavik with care. Also be sure to tell your doctor or dentist that you are taking Mavik if you are planning any type of surgery.

Possible food and drug interactions when taking this medication

If Mavik is taken with certain other drugs, the effects of either could be increased, decreased, or altered. It is especially important to check with your doctor before combining Mavik with the following:

Diuretics such as HydroDIURIL
Diuretics that spare the body's potassium, such as Aldactone,
 Dyazide, and Moduretic
Lithium (Eskalith, Lithobid)
Potassium preparations such as Micro-K and Slow-K

Also check with your doctor before using potassium-containing salt substitutes.

Special information if you are pregnant or breastfeeding

ACE inhibitors such as Mavik can cause injury and even death to the developing baby when used during the last 6 months of pregnancy. At the first sign of pregnancy, stop taking Mavik and contact your doctor immediately.

Mavik may appear in breast milk and could affect a nursing infant. Do not take this medication while you are breastfeeding.

Recommended dosage

ADULTS

High Blood Pressure
The usual starting dose if you are not taking a diuretic is 1 milligram once a day; African Americans should start on 2 milligrams once a day.

Depending on your blood pressure response, your doctor may increase your dosage at 1-week intervals, up to 2 to 4 milligrams once a day. If your blood pressure still does not respond, your dosage may be increased to 4 milligrams twice a day and the doctor may add a diuretic to your regimen.

If you are already taking a diuretic, your doctor will have you stop taking it 2 to 3 days before you start treatment with Mavik. If your diuretic should not be stopped, your starting dose of Mavik will be 0.5 milligram. A starting dose of 0.5 milligram daily is also recommended for people with liver or kidney disease.

Treatment After Heart Attack
The usual starting dose is 1 milligram once a day. The doctor will gradually increase the dose up to a maximum of 4 milligrams once a day.

If you have poor kidney function or cirrhosis of the liver, your starting dose, for either high blood pressure or heart attack, will probably be lowered to 0.5 milligram once daily.

CHILDREN

The safety and effectiveness of Mavik in children have not been established.

Overdosage

Any medication taken in excess can have serious consequences. The most likely effects of a Mavik overdose are light-headedness or dizziness due to a sudden drop in blood pressure. If you suspect an overdose, seek medical attention immediately.

MAXALT

Pronounced: MAX-alt
Generic name: Rizatriptan benzoate
Other brand name: Maxalt-MLT

Why is this drug prescribed?

Maxalt is prescribed for the treatment of a migraine attack with or without the presence of an aura (visual disturbances, usually sensations of halos or flickering lights, which precede an attack). It cuts headaches short, but won't prevent attacks.

Most important fact about this drug

Maxalt should be used only for typical migraine headaches. It is not recommended for any other type of headache, or for unusual types of migraine such as hemiplegic or basilar migraine.

How should you take this medication?

Take Maxalt as soon as your first symptoms appear. The drug is available in standard and orally disintegrating tablets (Maxalt-MLT). The standard tablets should be swallowed whole with liquid. No liquid is needed for Maxalt-MLT.

When using Maxalt-MLT, leave each individual blister pack in its foil pouch until needed. When ready, remove the pack from the pouch, peel it open with dry hands, and place the tablet on your tongue. The tablet will dissolve rapidly and can be swallowed with your saliva alone.

If your headache comes back, you may take a second dose as soon as 2 hours have elapsed. If the first dose provides no relief at all, check with your doctor before taking another.

Do not take more than 30 milligrams of Maxalt in a 24-hour period.

Check with your doctor if you need to take the drug more than 4 times a month.

■ *If you miss a dose...*
Maxalt is not for regular use. Take it only during a migraine attack.

■ *Storage instructions...*
Maxalt and Maxalt-MLT may be stored at room temperature. Keep the Maxalt bottle tightly closed. Leave each Maxalt-MLT tablet in its pouch.

What side effects may occur?

Side effects cannot be anticipated. If any develop or change in intensity, inform your doctor as soon as possible. Only your doctor can determine if it is safe for you to continue taking Maxalt.

■ *Side effects may include:*
Chest pain, dizziness, drowsiness, dry mouth, fatigue, nausea, pain, tingling skin, weakness

Why should this drug not be prescribed?

If Maxalt gives you an allergic reaction, you won't be able to use it. You should also avoid this drug if you have certain types of heart or blood vessel disease, including angina (crushing chest pain) or a history of heart attack. Do not use it if you have uncontrolled high blood pressure.

Never take Maxalt within 24 hours of using an ergotamine-type migraine medication such as Cafergot, D.H.E. 45 Injection, Migranal Nasal Spray, or Sansert, or a drug in the same family as Maxalt, such as Amerge, Imitrex, or Zomig. You should also refrain from using Maxalt within 2 weeks of taking an MAO inhibitor such as the antidepressants Marplan, Nardil, and Parnate.

Special warnings about this medication

Because some people with risk factors for heart and blood vessel disease have suffered an irregular heartbeat, a heart attack, or stroke after taking Maxalt, your doctor may ask you to take the first dose in the office, where you can be monitored for cardiac side effects. High blood pressure, high cholesterol, diabetes, smoking, a history of heart disease in your family, and menopause all increase the odds of such side effects.

Maxalt can cause drowsiness and dizziness. Do not participate in any activities that require full alertness until you are certain of the drug's effect. Use Maxalt with caution if you have liver disease or need kidney dialysis. Also alert your doctor if you have an eye condition. There is a theoretical possibility that Maxalt could affect the eyes.

If your first dose of Maxalt has no effect on your symptoms, you may not be suffering from migraine. Ask your doctor for a re-evaluation.

If you have a condition called phenylketonuria, you should be aware that the Maxalt-MLT tablets contain phenylalanine.

Maxalt is not recommended for people under 18.

Possible food and drug interactions when taking this medication

The following drugs may boost or add to the effect of Maxalt and should never be combined with it:

Drugs classified as MAO inhibitors, including the antidepressants Marplan, Nardil, and Parnate

Ergot-containing drugs such as Cafergot, D.H.E. Injection, and Migranal Nasal Spray

Other drugs in the Maxalt family, including Amerge, Imitrex, and Zomig

Certain other drugs may also interact with Maxalt. Check with your doctor before combining it with the following:

Fluoxetine (Prozac)
Fluvoxamine (Luvox)
Paroxetine (Paxil)
Propranolol (Inderal)
Sertraline (Zoloft)

Special information if you are pregnant or breastfeeding

The effects of Maxalt during pregnancy have not been adequately studied. If you are pregnant or plan to become pregnant, inform your doctor immediately. It is not known whether Maxalt appears in breast milk, but because many drugs do, you should use Maxalt with caution while breastfeeding an infant.

Recommended dosage

ADULTS

The usual dose of Maxalt and Maxalt-MLT is one 5- or 10-milligram tablet. Doses should be spaced at least 2 hours apart. Take no more than 30 milligrams a day.

Overdosage

Any medication taken in excess can have serious consequences. If you suspect an overdose, seek medical attention immediately.

■ *Symptoms of Maxalt overdose may include:*
Dizziness, fainting, heart and blood vessel problems, high blood pressure, loss of bowel and bladder control, slow heartbeat, vomiting

MAXAQUIN

Pronounced: MAX-ah-kwin
Generic name: Lomefloxacin hydrochloride

Why is this drug prescribed?

Maxaquin is a quinolone antibiotic used to treat lower respiratory infections, including chronic bronchitis, and urinary tract infections, including cystitis (inflammation of the inner lining of the bladder). Maxaquin is also given before bladder surgery and prostate biopsy to prevent the infections that sometimes follow these operations.

Most important fact about this drug

During and following treatment, Maxaquin causes sensitivity reactions in people exposed to sunlight or sunlamps. The reactions can occur despite the use of sunscreens and sunblocks, and can be prompted by shaded or diffused light or exposure through glass. Avoid even indirect sunlight while taking Maxaquin and for several days following therapy.

How should you take this medication?

It is important to finish your prescription of Maxaquin completely. If you stop taking your medication too soon, your symptoms may return.

Maxaquin may be taken with or without food. Take it with a full 8-ounce glass of water, and be sure to drink plenty of fluids while on this medication.

You can reduce the risk of a reaction to sunlight by taking Maxaquin in the evening (at least 12 hours before you will be exposed to the sun).

■ *If you miss a dose…*
Take it as soon as you remember. If it is almost time for your next dose, skip the one you missed and go back to your regular schedule. Do not take 2 doses at the same time.

■ *Storage instructions…*
Store at room temperature.

What side effects may occur?

Side effects cannot be anticipated. If any develop or change in intensity, tell your doctor as soon as possible. Only your doctor can determine if it is safe for you to continue taking Maxaquin.

■ *Side effects may include:*
Headache, nausea

Why should this drug not be prescribed?

If you are sensitive to or have ever had an allergic reaction to Maxaquin or other quinolone antibiotics such as Cipro and Floxin, you should not take this medication. Make sure your doctor is aware of any drug reactions you have experienced.

Special warnings about this medication

Use Maxaquin cautiously if you have disorders such as epilepsy, severe hardening of the arteries in the brain, and other conditions that can lead to seizures. Maxaquin may cause convulsions.

In rare cases, people taking antibiotics similar to Maxaquin have experienced severe, even fatal reactions, sometimes after only one dose.

These reactions may include confusion, convulsions, difficulty breathing, hallucinations, hives, itching, light-headedness, loss of consciousness, rash, restlessness, swelling in the face or throat, tingling, and tremors. If you develop any of these symptoms, stop taking Maxaquin immediately and seek medical help.

If other antibiotics have given you diarrhea, or it develops while you are taking Maxaquin, be sure to tell your doctor. Maxaquin may cause inflammation of the bowel, ranging from mild to life-threatening.

Maxaquin may cause dizziness or light-headedness and may impair your ability to drive a car or operate potentially dangerous machinery. Do not participate in any activities that require full alertness until you know how Maxaquin affects you.

Maxaquin can cause rupture of muscle tendons. If you notice any pain or inflammation, stop exercising the affected tendon until your doctor has examined you.

Possible food and drug interactions when taking this medication

If Maxaquin is taken with certain other drugs, the effects of either could be increased, decreased, or altered. It is especially important to check with your doctor before combining Maxaquin with the following:

Antacids containing magnesium or aluminum, such as Maalox or Gaviscon
Caffeine (including coffee, tea, and some soft drinks)
Cimetidine (Tagamet)
Cyclosporine (Sandimmune and Neoral)
Didanosine (Videx) chewable tablets or powder for oral solution
Probenecid (Benemid)
Sucralfate (Carafate)
Theophylline (Theo-Dur)
Warfarin (Coumadin)
Vitamins or products containing iron or zinc

Do not take the antacids, Videx preparations, or Carafate within 4 hours before or 2 hours after a dose of Maxaquin.

Special information if you are pregnant or breastfeeding

The effects of Maxaquin in pregnancy have not been adequately studied. If you are pregnant or plan to become pregnant, notify your doctor immediately. It is not known if Maxaquin appears in breast milk. Because many drugs do make their way into breast milk, your doctor may have you stop breastfeeding while you are taking Maxaquin.

Recommended dosage

ADULTS

Chronic Bronchitis
The usual dosage is 400 milligrams once a day for 10 days.

Cystitis
The usual dosage is 400 milligrams once a day for 10 days.

Complicated Urinary Tract Infections
The usual dosage is 400 milligrams once a day for 14 days.

People with Impaired Renal Function or Cirrhosis
Your doctor will adjust the dosage according to your needs.

People on Dialysis
The recommended dosage for people on dialysis is 400 milligrams, followed by daily maintenance doses of 200 milligrams (one half tablet) once a day for the duration of treatment.

CHILDREN

The safety and efficacy of Maxaquin have not been established for children under the age of 18.

Overdosage

There is no information on overdosage with Maxaquin. However, any medication taken in excess can have serious consequences. If you suspect an overdose, seek medical help immediately.

Maxidone *See Vicodin, page 1557.*

Maxzide *See Dyazide, page 485.*

Meclizine *See Antivert, page 119.*

MEDROL
Pronounced: MED-rohl
Generic name: Methylprednisolone

Why is this drug prescribed?

Medrol, a corticosteroid drug, is used to reduce inflammation and improve symptoms in a variety of disorders, including rheumatoid arthritis, acute gouty arthritis, and severe cases of asthma. Medrol may be given to people to treat primary or secondary adrenal cortex insufficiency (inability of the adrenal gland to produce sufficient hormone). It is also given to help treat the following disorders:

Severe allergic conditions (including drug-induced allergic states)
Blood disorders (leukemia and various anemias)
Certain cancers (along with other drugs)
Skin diseases (including severe psoriasis)
Connective tissue diseases such as systemic lupus erythematosus
Digestive tract diseases such as ulcerative colitis
High serum levels of calcium associated with cancer
Fluid retention due to nephrotic syndrome (a condition in which
    damage to the kidney causes loss of protein in urine)
Various eye diseases
Lung diseases such as tuberculosis
Worsening of multiple sclerosis

Most important fact about this drug

Medrol lowers your resistance to infections and can make them harder to treat. Medrol may also mask some of the signs of an infection, making it difficult for your doctor to diagnose the actual problem.

How should you take this medication?

Take Medrol exactly as prescribed. It can be taken every day or every other day, depending on the condition being treated.

Do not abruptly stop taking Medrol without checking with your doctor. If you have been using Medrol for a long time, the dose should be reduced gradually.

Medrol may cause stomach upset. Take Medrol with meals or snacks.

■ *If you miss a dose...*
If you take your dose once a day, take it as soon as you remember. Then go back to your regular schedule. If you don't remember until the next day, skip the one you missed. Do not take 2 doses at once.

If you take it several times a day, take it as soon as you remember. Then go back to your regular schedule. If you don't remember until your next dose, double the dose you take.

If you take your dose every other day, and you remember it the same morning, take it as soon as you remember and go back to your regular schedule. If you don't remember until the afternoon, do not take it until the following morning, then skip a day and go back to your regular schedule.

■ *Storage instructions...*
Store at room temperature.

What side effects may occur?

Side effects cannot be anticipated. If any develop or change in intensity, tell your doctor immediately. Only your doctor can determine whether it is safe for you to continue taking Medrol.

■ *Side effects may include:*

Abdominal swelling, allergic reactions, bone fractures, bruising, congestive heart failure, cataracts, convulsions, Cushingoid symptoms (moon face, weight gain, high blood pressure, emotional disturbances, growth of facial hair in women), facial redness, fluid and salt retention, headache, high blood pressure, increased eye pressure, increased sweating, increase in amounts of insulin or hypoglycemic medications needed, inflammation of the pancreas, irregular menstruation, muscle wasting and weakness, osteoporosis, poor healing of wounds, protruding eyes, stomach ulcer, suppression of growth in children, symptoms of diabetes, thin, fragile skin, tiny red or purplish spots on the skin, vertigo

Why should this drug not be prescribed?

Medrol should not be used if you have a fungal infection or if you are sensitive to or allergic to steroids (corticosteroids).

Special warnings about this medication

The 24-milligram Medrol tablet contains FD&C Yellow No. 5 (tartrazine), which has caused allergic reactions (including asthma) in some people. Although this is rare, it is more common in people who are sensitive to aspirin.

Medrol can alter the way your body responds to unusual stress. If you are injured, need surgery, or develop an acute illness, inform your doctor. Your dosage may need to be increased.

You should avoid immunization shots with live or live, attenuated vaccines while taking high doses of Medrol, because Medrol can suppress the immune system. Immunization with killed or inactivated vaccines is safe, but may have diminished effect.

Long-term use of Medrol may cause cataracts, glaucoma (increased eye pressure), and eye infections.

Large doses of Medrol may cause high blood pressure, salt and water retention, and potassium and calcium loss. It may be necessary to restrict your salt intake and take a potassium supplement.

Medrol may reactivate dormant cases of tuberculosis. If you have inactive tuberculosis and must take Medrol for an extended period of time, your doctor will prescribe anti-TB medication as well.

Medrol should be used cautiously if you have an underactive thyroid, liver cirrhosis, or herpes simplex (virus) infection of the eye.

This medication may aggravate existing emotional problems or cause new ones. You may experience euphoria (an exaggerated sense of well-being) and difficulty sleeping, mood swings, or mental problems. If you have any changes in mood, contact your doctor.

People taking corticosteroids, such as Medrol, have developed Kaposi's sarcoma, a form of cancer.

Medrol should also be taken with caution if you have any of the following conditions:

Diverticulitis or other inflammatory conditions of the intestine
High blood pressure
Certain kidney diseases
Active or dormant peptic ulcer
Myasthenia gravis (a muscle weakness disorder)
Osteoporosis (brittle bones)
Threadworm
Ulcerative colitis with impending danger of infection

Long-term use of Medrol can slow the growth and development of infants and children.

Use aspirin cautiously with Medrol if you have a blood-clotting disorder.

Avoid exposure to chickenpox and measles.

Possible food and drug interactions when taking this medication

If Medrol is taken with certain other drugs, the effects of either drug could be increased, decreased, or altered. It is especially important to check with your doctor before combining Medrol with the following:

Aspirin
Barbiturates such as phenobarbital
Blood thinners such as Coumadin
Carbamazepine (Tegretol)
Cyclosporine (Sandimmune, Neoral)
Estrogen medications such as Premarin
Insulin
Ketoconazole (Nizoral)
Nonsteroidal anti-inflammatory medications such as Indocin
Oral diabetes drugs such as Glucotrol
Phenytoin (Dilantin)
Rifampin (Rifadin)
Troleandomycin (Tao)
Water pills such as Lasix and HydroDIURIL

Special information if you are pregnant or breastfeeding

If you are pregnant or plan to become pregnant, tell your doctor immediately. There is no information about the safety of Medrol during pregnancy. Babies born to mothers who have taken doses of Medrol (corticosteroids) during pregnancy should be carefully watched for adrenal problems. Medrol may appear in breast milk and could affect a nursing infant. If Medrol is essential to your health, your doctor may advise you to stop breastfeeding until your treatment with Medrol is finished.

Recommended dosage

The starting dose of Medrol tablets may vary from 4 to 48 milligrams per day, depending on the specific problem being treated.

Once you've shown a satisfactory response, the doctor will gradually lower the dosage to the smallest effective amount. If you are taking Medrol for an extended period, the doctor may instruct you to take the drug only every other day, at twice your daily dosage.

For a worsening of multiple sclerosis, the dosage is 160 milligrams a day for one week, then 64 milligrams every other day for a month.

Overdosage

Any medication taken in excess can have serious consequences. If you suspect an overdose of Medrol, seek medical treatment immediately.

Medroxyprogesterone for contraception

See Depo-Provera, page 414.

Medroxyprogesterone for menstrual problems

See Provera, page 1189.

Mefenamic acid See Ponstel, page 1114.

MELLARIL

Pronounced: MEL-ah-rill
Generic name: Thioridazine hydrochloride

Why is this drug prescribed?

Mellaril combats the crippling mental disorder known as schizophrenia (a severe loss of contact with reality). Because Mellaril has been known to cause dangerous heartbeat irregularities, it is usually prescribed only when at least two other medications have failed.

Most important fact about this drug

The danger of potentially fatal cardiac irregularities increases when Mellaril is combined with any medication that prolongs a part of the heartbeat known as the QTc interval. Many of the drugs prescribed for heartbeat irregularities (including Cordarone, Inderal, Quinaglute, Quinidex, and Rythmol) prolong the QTc interval and should never be combined with Mellaril. Other drugs to avoid when taking Mellaril include fluvoxamine, Norvir, Paxil, Pindolol, Prozac, Rescriptor, and Tagamet. Make sure the doctor knows you are taking Mellaril whenever a new drug is prescribed.

How should you take this medication?

If you are taking Mellaril in a liquid concentrate form, you can dilute it with a liquid such as distilled water, soft tap water, or juice just before taking it.

Do not change from one brand of thioridazine to another without consulting your doctor.

■ *If you miss a dose...*
If you take 1 dose a day and remember later in the day, take the dose immediately. If you don't remember until the next day, skip the dose and go back to your regular schedule.

If you take more than 1 dose a day and remember the forgotten dose within an hour or so after its scheduled time, take it immediately. If you don't remember until later, skip the dose and go back to your regular schedule.

Never try to catch up by doubling a dose.

■ *Storage instructions...*
Store at room temperature, tightly closed, in the container the medication came in.

What side effects may occur?

Side effects cannot be anticipated. If any develop or change in intensity, inform your doctor as soon as possible. Only your doctor can determine if it is safe for you to continue taking Mellaril.

■ *Side effects may include:*
Blurred vision, breast development in men, breast milk secretion, constipation, diarrhea, drowsiness, dry mouth, impotence, nausea, swelling in the arms and legs (edema), tardive dyskinesia (see *Special warnings about this medication*), vomiting

Why should this drug not be prescribed?

Due to the danger of cardiac irregularities, Mellaril must never be combined with drugs that increase its effects or prolong the part of the heartbeat known as the QTc interval (see *Most important fact about this drug*). It is also important to avoid combining Mellaril with excessive amounts of central nervous system depressants such as alcohol, barbiturates, or narcotics. Do not take Mellaril if you have heart disease accompanied by severe high or low blood pressure.

Special warnings about this medication

Mellaril may cause tardive dyskinesia—a condition marked by involuntary muscle spasms and twitches in the face and body. This condition may be permanent, and appears to be most common among the elderly, especially women. Ask your doctor for information about this possible risk.

Drugs such as Mellaril are also known to cause a potentially fatal condition known as Neuroleptic Malignant Syndrome. Symptoms of this problem include high fever, rigid muscles, altered mental status, sweating, fast or irregular heartbeat, and changes in blood pressure. If you develop these symptoms, see your doctor immediately. Mellaril therapy may have to be permanently discontinued.

Animal studies suggest that antipsychotics such as Mellaril may increase the risk of breast cancer, although human studies have not confirmed such a risk. If you have a history of breast cancer, be sure to see your doctor regularly for checkups.

In rare cases, Mellaril has been known to trigger blood disorders and seizures. It can cause dizziness or faintness when you first stand up. High doses can also cause vision problems, including blurring, brownish coloring of vision, and poor night vision.

This drug may impair your ability to drive a car or operate potentially dangerous machinery. Do not participate in any activities that require full alertness until you are certain the drug will not interfere.

Possible food and drug interactions when taking this medication

Remember that combining Mellaril with certain drugs can increase the danger of potentially fatal heartbeat irregularities. Among the drugs to avoid are the following:

Amiodarone (Cordarone)
Cimetidine (Tagamet)
Delavirdine (Rescriptor)
Fluoxetine (Prozac)
Fluvoxamine
Paroxetine (Paxil)
Pindolol
Propafenone (Rythmol)
Propranolol (Inderal)
Quinidine (Quinaglute, Quinidex)
Ritonavir (Norvir)

Check with your doctor before adding any new drug to your regimen. Remember, too, that extreme drowsiness and other potentially serious effects can result if Mellaril is combined with alcohol or other central nervous system depressants such as narcotics, painkillers, and sleeping medications.

Special information if you are pregnant or breastfeeding

Pregnant women should use Mellaril only if clearly needed. If you are pregnant or plan to become pregnant, inform your doctor immediately.

There is no information on the effects of Mellaril during breastfeeding. The doctor may advise you to stop breastfeeding until your treatment with this medication is finished.

Recommended dosage

Your doctor will tailor your dose to your needs, using the smallest effective amount.

ADULTS

The starting dose ranges from 50 to 100 milligrams 3 times a day. Your doctor may gradually increase your dosage to as much as 800 milligrams a day, taken in 2 to 4 doses. Once your symptoms improve, your doctor will decrease the dosage to the lowest effective amount.

CHILDREN

The usual starting dose for schizophrenic children is 0.5 milligram per 2.2 pounds of body weight per day, divided into smaller doses. The dose may be gradually increased to a maximum of 3 milligrams per 2.2 pounds per day.

Overdosage

Any medication taken in excess can have serious consequences. An overdose of Mellaril can be fatal. If you suspect an overdose, seek medical help immediately.

■ *Symptoms of Mellaril overdose may include:*
Agitation, blurred vision, coma, confusion, constipation, difficulty breathing, dilated or constricted pupils, diminished flow of urine, dry mouth, dry skin, excessively high or low body temperature, extremely low blood pressure, fluid in the lungs, heart abnormalities, inability to urinate, intestinal blockage, nasal congestion, restlessness, sedation, seizures, shock

Meloxicam *See Mobic, page 879.*

Memantine *See Namenda, page 910.*

Meperidine *See Demerol, page 402.*

Meprobamate *See Miltown, page 862.*

MERIDIA
Pronounced: mer-ID-dee-uh
Generic name: Sibutramine hydrochloride

Why is this drug prescribed?

Meridia helps the seriously overweight shed pounds and keep them off. It is especially recommended for those who in addition to being overweight have other health problems such as high blood pressure, diabetes, or high cholesterol. It is used in conjunction with a low-calorie diet.

Meridia works by boosting levels of certain chemical messengers in the nervous system, including serotonin, dopamine, and norepinephrine.

Most important fact about this drug

Make a point of keeping follow-up appointments with your doctor. Meridia can increase your blood pressure, so it's important to have your blood pressure and pulse monitored at the beginning of therapy and regularly thereafter.

How should you take this medication?

Meridia can be taken with or without food.

■ *If you miss a dose...*
Take it as soon as you remember. If it is almost time for your next dose, skip the one you missed and go back to your regular schedule. Do not take 2 doses at once.

■ *Storage instructions...*
Store at room temperature away from heat and moisture in a tight, light-resistant container.

What side effects may occur?

Side effects cannot be anticipated. If any develop or change in intensity, inform your doctor as soon as possible. Only your doctor can determine if it is safe for you to continue taking Meridia.

■ *Side effects may include:*
Abdominal pain, acid indigestion, anxiety, back pain, constipation, cough increase, depression, dizziness, dry mouth, flu symptoms, headache, increased appetite, insomnia, joint pain, loss of appetite, loss of strength, nasal inflammation, nausea, nervousness, painful menstruation, rash, sinus inflammation, stomachache, sore throat

Why should this drug not be prescribed?

If Meridia gives you an allergic reaction, you won't be able to use it. You should also avoid Meridia (and certainly don't need it) if you suffer from the compulsive dieting disorder known as anorexia nervosa. Do not combine Meridia with other drugs used to suppress appetite, and do not use it within 2 weeks of taking a drug classified as an MAO inhibitor, including the antidepressant medications Marplan, Nardil, and Parnate.

Special warnings about this medication

Use Meridia with caution if you have uncontrolled high blood pressure or are predisposed to bleeding; the drug could make the problem worse. Avoid Meridia completely if you've had a stroke or suffer from heart disease, heart failure, or irregular heartbeat. Also avoid it if you have severe kidney or liver problems; the drug has not been tested under these conditions. Seizures are a rare, but possible, side effect. If you've had seizures in the past, use Meridia with caution. If you have a seizure while taking the drug, stop using it and call your doctor immediately.

Any drug that acts on the nervous system can theoretically impair judgment, thinking, and motor skills. Meridia does not seem to have this effect, but caution is still in order until you know how the drug affects you.

If you have narrow-angle glaucoma or thyroid problems, make sure the doctor knows; Meridia should be used with caution in these circumstances. If you are prone to gallstones, be aware that weight loss can cause more of them to form. Meridia has not been tested in people under 16 years old. It should be used with caution in those over 65. Although it has been classified as a controlled substance (potentially subject to abuse), the possibility of developing physical or psychological dependence is low.

Possible food and drug interactions when taking this medication

Remember that Meridia must never be taken within 2 weeks of using an MAO inhibitor such as Marplan, Nardil, or Parnate. The combination could lead to serious, even fatal, overstimulation.

Meridia may also interact with a wide variety of other prescription and over-the-counter drugs, especially weight-reducing agents, decongestants, antidepressants, allergy medications, and cough and cold remedies that contain ephedrine or pseudoephedrine. Among the many drugs that pose a potential problem are the following:

Alcohol (excessive amounts)
Blood thinners such as warfarin (Coumadin)
Dextromethorphan (found in many over-the-counter cough preparations)
Dihydroergotamine (D.H.E. Injection, Migranal Nasal Spray)
Drugs that affect platelet function
Erythromycin (Eryc, Ery-Tab, PCE)
Fentanyl (Duragesic)
Fluoxetine (Prozac)
Fluvoxamine (Luvox)
Ketoconazole (Nizoral)
Lithium (Eskalith, Lithobid)
Meperidine (Demerol)
Naratriptan (Amerge)
Paroxetine (Paxil)
Pentazocine (Talwin NX, Talacen)
Sertraline (Zoloft)
Stimulants such as Adderall, amphetamines, Dexedrine, Desoxyn, Didrex, and Ionamin
Sumatriptan (Imitrex)
Tryptophan (L-Tryptophan)
Venlafaxine (Effexor)
Zolmitriptan (Zomig)

If you have any doubt about the safety of a combination, be sure to check with your doctor.

Special information if you are pregnant or breastfeeding

The use of Meridia during pregnancy is not recommended. If you are in your childbearing years, take reliable contraceptive measures while using this drug. If you do become pregnant, or plan on becoming pregnant, tell your doctor immediately. It is not known whether Meridia appears in breast milk; its use while breastfeeding is not recommended.

Recommended dosage

ADULTS

The starting dose is 10 milligrams once daily. If you have not lost at least 4 pounds after 4 weeks, the doctor may increase the dose to 15 milligrams daily. This is the maximum; if weight loss still fails to occur, Meridia will be discontinued.

For those who experience side effects at the 10-milligram level, a 5-milligram dose may prove sufficient.

Use of Meridia for longer than 1 year has not been studied.

Overdosage

Although doctors have had little experience with overdoses of Meridia, increased heart rate and blood pressure are possible results. Since any medication taken in excess can have serious consequences, seek medical attention immediately if you suspect an overdose.

Mesalamine *See Rowasa, page 1280.*

Mesoridazine *See Serentil, page 1297.*

Metadate *See Ritalin, page 1270.*

METAGLIP

Pronounced: MET-ah-glip
Generic ingredients: Glipizide, Metformin hydrochloride

Why is this drug prescribed?

Metaglip is an oral medication used to control blood sugar levels in people with type 2 (non-insulin-dependent) diabetes. It contains two drugs commonly used to lower blood sugar, glipizide (Glucotrol) and metformin (Glucophage). Metaglip replaces the need to take these two drugs separately. It is prescribed when diet and exercise alone do not control blood sugar levels, or when treatment with another antidiabetic medication does not work.

Blood sugar levels are ordinarily controlled by the body's natural supply of insulin, which helps sugar move out of the bloodstream and into the cells to be used for energy. People who have type 2 diabetes do not make enough insulin or do not respond normally to the insulin their bodies make, causing a buildup of unused sugar in the bloodstream. Metaglip helps remedy this problem in two ways: by causing your body to release more insulin and by helping your body use insulin more effectively.

Most important fact about this drug

Metaglip could cause a very rare—but potentially fatal—side effect known as lactic acidosis. It is caused by a buildup of lactic acid in the blood. The problem is most likely to occur in people whose liver or kidneys are not working well, and in those who have multiple medical problems, take several medications, or have congestive heart failure. The risk also is higher if you are an older adult or drink alcohol. Lactic acidosis is a medical emergency that must be treated in a hospital. Notify your doctor immediately if you experience any of the following:

■ *Symptoms of lactic acidosis may include:*
Dizziness, extreme weakness or tiredness, light-headedness, low blood pressure, low body temperature, slow or irregular heartbeat, rapid breathing or trouble breathing, sleepiness, unexpected or unusual stomach discomfort, unusual muscle pain

How should you take this medication?

Do not take more or less of this medication than directed by your doctor. Metaglip should be taken in divided doses with meals to reduce the possibility of nausea or diarrhea, especially during the first few weeks of therapy.

■ *If you miss a dose...*
Take the forgotten dose as soon as you remember. However, if it is almost time for your next dose, skip the one you missed and return to your regular schedule. Never take 2 doses at once.
■ *Storage instructions...*
Store at room temperature.

What side effects may occur?

Side effects cannot be anticipated. If any develop or change in intensity, tell your doctor as soon as possible. Only your doctor can determine if it is safe for you to continue using Metaglip.

■ *Side effects may include:*
Abdominal pain, diarrhea, dizziness, headache, high blood pressure, hypoglycemia (low blood sugar), muscle pain, upper respiratory infection

Why should this drug not be prescribed?

Metaglip is processed primarily by the kidneys, and can build up to excessive levels in the body if the kidneys aren't working properly. It should be avoided if you have kidney disease or your kidney function has been impaired by a condition such as shock, blood poisoning, or a heart attack.

You should not use Metaglip if you need to take medicine for congestive heart failure.

Do not take Metaglip if you have ever had an allergic reaction to glipizide or metformin.

Do not take Metaglip if you have metabolic or diabetic ketoacidosis (a life-threatening medical emergency caused by insufficient insulin and marked by excessive thirst, nausea, fatigue, pain below the breastbone, and fruity breath).

Special warnings about this medication

Some studies suggest that the glipizide component of Metaglip may lead to more heart problems than treatment with diet alone, or diet plus insulin. In a long-term trial of a similar drug, researchers noted an increase in heart-related deaths (though the overall mortality rate remained unchanged). If you have a heart condition or you're at risk for heart disease, you should discuss this potential danger with your doctor.

Because Metaglip can cause hypoglycemia (low blood sugar), it's very important to follow your doctor's instructions carefully. Low blood sugar is more likely to happen if you're older, weak, or undernourished, or if you have kidney, liver, adrenal, or pituitary gland problems. Your risk also increases if you miss meals or fail to eat after doing strenuous exercise. Combining Metaglip with other diabetes medications can also cause blood sugar to drop. Symptoms of a mild case include cold sweats, dizziness, shakiness, a light-headed feeling, and hunger. Check with your doctor immediately if you notice any of these warning signs, since severe low blood sugar can occasionally lead to seizures or coma.

Before you start therapy with Metaglip, and at least once a year thereafter, your doctor will do a complete assessment of your kidney function. If you develop kidney problems while on Metaglip, your doctor will discontinue this medication. If you are an older person, you will need to have your kidney function monitored more frequently, and your doctor may want to start you at a lower dosage.

You should temporarily stop taking Metaglip for 2 days before and after having an X-ray procedure (such as an angiogram) that uses an injectable dye. Also, if you are going to have surgery, except minor surgery, you should stop taking Metaglip. Once you have resumed normal food and fluid intake, your doctor will tell you when you can start drug therapy again.

Avoid drinking too much alcohol while taking Metaglip. Heavy drinking increases the danger of lactic acidosis and can also trigger an attack of low blood sugar.

Because poor liver function could increase the risk of lactic acidosis, your doctor may decide to check your liver function before prescribing Metaglip and periodically thereafter. If you develop liver problems, your doctor may stop treatment with Metaglip.

Metaglip occasionally causes a mild deficiency of vitamin B_{12}. Your doctor will check for this with yearly blood tests and may prescribe a supplement if necessary.

You should stop taking Metaglip if you become seriously dehydrated, since this increases the likelihood of developing lactic acidosis. Tell your doctor if you lose a significant amount of fluid due to vomiting, diarrhea, fever, or some other condition.

While taking Metaglip, you should check your blood or urine periodically for abnormal sugar levels. If you notice sudden changes after you've been stabilized for a while, tell your doctor immediately. It could be a sign you're developing lactic acidosis or ketoacidosis.

Possible food and drug interactions when taking this medication

If Metaglip is taken with certain other drugs, the effects of either could be increased, decreased, or altered. It is especially important to check with your doctor before combining Metaglip with the following:

Amiloride (Moduretic)
Antibiotics known as sulfonamides, including Bactrim, Cotrim, and Septra
Antidepressants known as MAO inhibitors, including Nardil and Parnate
Antifungal drugs that are taken orally, such as fluconazole (Diflucan) and miconazole
Anti-inflammatories that contain salicylates, such as aspirin, Dolobid, and Rowasa
Beta-blocking blood pressure medicines such as Inderal, Lopressor, and Tenormin
Calcium channel blockers (heart medications) such as Calan, Isoptin, and Procardia
Chloramphenicol (Chloromycetin)
Cimetidine (Tagamet)
Decongestant, airway-opening drugs such as Sudafed and Ventolin
Digoxin (Lanoxin)
Estrogens such as Premarin
Furosemide (Lasix)
Isoniazid (Rifamate), a drug used for tuberculosis
Morphine
Niacin (Niaspan)
Nifedipine (Adalat, Procardia)
Nonsteroidal anti-inflammatory drugs such as Aleve, Motrin, and Naprosyn
Oral contraceptives
Phenytoin (Dilantin)
Probenecid (Benemid)
Procainamide (Procanbid, Pronestyl)
Quinidine (Quinidex)

Quinine
Ranitidine (Zantac)
Steroids such as prednisone (Deltasone)
Thyroid hormones such as Synthroid
Tranquilizers such as Thorazine
Triamterene (Dyazide, Dyrenium)
Trimethoprim (Bactrim, Septra)
Vancomycin (Vancocin)
Warfarin sodium (Coumadin)
Water pills (diuretics) such as Dyazide, HydroDIURIL, and Moduretic

Do not drink too much alcohol, since excessive alcohol consumption can cause low blood sugar and increase the risk of developing lactic acidosis.

Special information if you are pregnant or breastfeeding

If you are pregnant or plan to become pregnant, tell your doctor immediately. Metaglip has not been adequately studied in pregnant women and should not be taken during pregnancy unless the potential benefit outweighs the potential risk. Since studies suggest the importance of maintaining normal blood sugar levels during pregnancy, your doctor may prescribe insulin injections instead.

It is not known whether Metaglip appears in human breast milk. Therefore, you should discuss with your doctor whether to discontinue the medication or to stop breastfeeding. If the medication is discontinued and if diet alone does not control blood sugar levels, your doctor may prescribe insulin injections.

Recommended dosage

ADULTS

Your doctor will start therapy at a low dose and increase it until your blood sugar levels are under control.

Patients Not Previously Treated with Diabetes Medications
The recommended starting dose is 2.5 milligrams of glipizide with 250 milligrams of metformin once a day. If your fasting blood sugar levels are particularly high, you doctor may have you take 2.5 milligrams of glipizide with 500 milligrams of metformin twice a day.

The daily dosage can be increased by 1 tablet every 2 weeks until blood sugar levels are controlled. The maximum daily dose is 10 milligrams of glipizide with 2,000 milligrams of metformin.

Patients Previously Treated with Glipizide (or a Similar Drug) or Metformin
The recommended starting dose of Metaglip is either 2.5 or 5 milligrams of glipizide with 500 milligrams of metformin twice a day. If this regimen doesn't control your blood sugar, the daily dose can be increased in increments of up to 5 milligrams (glipizide)/500 milligrams (metformin).

The maximum daily dose is 20 milligrams of glipizide with 2,000 milligrams of metformin.

Patients on Combination Therapy Taking Separate Doses of Glipizide and Metformin
The maximum daily dose should not exceed your current doses of glipizide and metformin. The usual daily starting dose is either 2.5 or 5 milligrams of glipizide with 500 milligrams of metformin. If this regimen doesn't control your blood sugar, the daily dose can be increased in increments of up to 5 milligrams (glipizide)/500 milligrams (metformin). The maximum daily dose is 20 milligrams of glipizide with 2,000 milligrams of metformin.

CHILDREN

Children should not take Metaglip, since the safety and effectiveness of the drug have not been studied in this group.

Overdosage

An overdose of Metaglip can cause an attack of low blood sugar requiring immediate treatment. If you experience any of the symptoms listed in *Special warnings about this medication,* see a doctor immediately.

An excessive dose of Metaglip can also trigger lactic acidosis. If you begin to notice the warning signs listed in *Most important fact about this drug,* seek emergency treatment.

Metaproterenol See Alupent, page 83.

Metaxalone See Skelaxin, page 1318.

Metformin See Glucophage, page 620.

Methamphetamine See Desoxyn, page 418.

Methazolamide See Neptazane, page 929.

Methenamine See Urised, page 1532.

METHERGINE

Pronounced: METH-er-jin
Generic name: Methylergonovine maleate

Why is this drug prescribed?

Methergine, a blood vessel constrictor, is given to prevent or control excessive bleeding following childbirth. It works by causing the uterine muscles to contract, thereby reducing the mother's blood loss.

Methergine comes in tablet and injectable forms.

Most important fact about this drug

Some blood vessel disorders and certain infections make the use of Methergine dangerous. Make sure your doctor is aware of any medical conditions you may have.

How should you take this medication?

Take Methergine tablets exactly as prescribed.

■ *If you miss a dose...*
Do not take the missed dose at all and do not double the next one. Instead, go back to your regular schedule.

■ *Storage instructions...*
Store at room temperature in a tightly closed container, away from light.

What side effects may occur?

Side effects cannot be anticipated. If any develop or change in intensity, inform your doctor as soon as possible. Only your doctor can determine if it is safe for you to continue taking Methergine.

The most common side effect is high blood pressure, which may cause a headache or even a seizure. In some people, however, Methergine may cause low blood pressure.

Why should this drug not be prescribed?

You should not take Methergine if you are allergic to it, if you are pregnant, or if you have high blood pressure or toxemia (poisons circulating in the blood).

Special warnings about this medication

It may be dangerous to take Methergine if you have an infection, certain blood vessel disorders, or a liver or kidney problem. Inform your doctor if you think you have any such condition.

Your doctor will use intravenous Methergine only when necessary, because of the possibility of a sudden rise in blood pressure or a stroke.

Possible food and drug interactions when taking this medication

If Methergine is taken with certain other drugs, the effects of either may be increased, decreased, or altered. It is especially important to check with your doctor before combining Methergine with the following:

Other blood vessel constrictors such as EpiPen
Other ergot-derived medications such as Ergotrate

Special information if you are pregnant or breastfeeding

Methergine should not be taken during pregnancy. Methergine appears in breast milk. Although no specific information is available about possible effects of Methergine on a nursing baby, the general rule is that a mother who is breastfeeding should not take any drug unless it is clearly needed.

Recommended dosage
The usual dose is 1 tablet (0.2 milligram) 3 or 4 times daily after childbirth for a maximum of 1 week.

Overdosage
Any medication taken in excess can have serious consequences. If you suspect symptoms of a Methergine overdose, seek medical attention immediately.

■ *Symptoms of Methergine overdose may include:*
Abdominal pain, coma, convulsions, elevated blood pressure, hypothermia (drop in body temperature), lowered blood pressure, nausea, numbness, slowed breathing, tingling of the arms and legs, vomiting

Methocarbamol *See Robaxin, page 1274.*

METHOTREXATE
Pronounced: meth-oh-TREX-ate
Brand names: Rheumatrex, Trexall

Why is this drug prescribed?
Methotrexate is an anticancer drug used in the treatment of lymphoma (cancer of the lymph nodes) and certain forms of leukemia. It is also given to treat some forms of cancers of the uterus, breast, lung, head, neck, and ovary. Methotrexate is also given to treat rheumatoid arthritis when other treatments have proved ineffective, and is sometimes used to treat very severe and disabling psoriasis (a skin disease characterized by thickened patches of red, inflamed skin often covered by silver scales).

Most important fact about this drug
Be certain to remember that in the treatment of psoriasis and rheumatoid arthritis, methotrexate is taken once a *week*, not once a day. Accidentally taking the recommended weekly dosage on a daily basis can lead to fatal overdosage. Be sure to read the patient instructions that come with the package.

How should you take this medication?
Take methotrexate exactly as prescribed, and promptly report to your doctor any new symptoms that may develop.

Methotrexate is given at a higher dosage for cancer than for psoriasis or rheumatoid arthritis. After high-dose methotrexate treatment, a drug called leucovorin may be given to limit the toxic effects.

■ *If you miss a dose...*
Skip it and go back to your regular schedule. Do not take 2 doses at once.

■ *Storage instructions...*
Store at room temperature, away from light.

What side effects may occur?

Side effects cannot be anticipated. If any develop or change in intensity, inform your doctor as soon as possible. Only your doctor can determine whether it is safe for you to continue taking methotrexate.

■ *Side effects may include:*
Abdominal pain and upset, chills and fever, decreased resistance to infection, dizziness, fatigue, general feeling of illness, mouth ulcers, nausea

If you are taking methotrexate for psoriasis, you may also experience hair loss and/or sun sensitivity, and your patches of psoriasis may give a burning sensation.

Methotrexate can sometimes cause serious lung damage that makes it necessary to limit the treatment. If you experience a dry cough, fever, or breathing difficulties while taking methotrexate, be sure to tell your doctor right away.

During and immediately after treatment with methotrexate, fertility may be impaired. Men may have an abnormally low sperm count; women may have menstrual irregularities.

People on high doses of methotrexate may develop a brain condition signaled by confusion, partial paralysis, seizures, or coma.

Why should this drug not be prescribed?

Do not take this medication if you are sensitive to it or it has given you an allergic reaction.

Do not take this medication if you are pregnant.

Methotrexate treatment is not suitable for you if you suffer from psoriasis or rheumatoid arthritis and also have one of the following conditions:

Abnormal blood cell count
Alcoholic liver disease or other chronic liver disease
Alcoholism
Anemia
Immune system deficiency

Special warnings about this medication

Before you start taking methotrexate, your doctor will do a chest X-ray plus blood tests to determine your blood cell counts, liver enzyme levels, and the efficiency of your kidney function. While you are taking methotrexate, the blood tests will be repeated at regular intervals; if you develop a cough or chest pain, the chest X-ray will be repeated.

If you are being treated for psoriasis or rheumatoid arthritis, your doctor will test your liver function at regular intervals. You should avoid alcoholic beverages while taking this drug.

You may develop an opportunistic infection—one that takes advantage of your altered body chemistry—while you are taking methotrexate. Before receiving an immunization or vaccination, be sure to inform health care workers that you are taking this drug.

Older or physically debilitated people are particularly vulnerable to toxic effects from methotrexate. Your doctor will prescribe methotrexate with great caution if you have any of the following:

Active infection
Liver disease
Peptic ulcer
Ulcerative colitis

Possible food and drug interactions when taking this medication

If you are being given methotrexate for the treatment of cancer or psoriasis, you should not take aspirin or other nonsteroidal painkillers such as Advil or Naprosyn; this combination could increase the toxic effects of methotrexate. If you are taking methotrexate for rheumatoid arthritis, you may be able to continue taking aspirin or a nonsteroidal painkiller, but your doctor should monitor you carefully.

Other drugs that may increase the toxic effects of methotrexate include:

Cisplatin (Platinol)
Penicillins
Phenylbutazone
Phenytoin (Dilantin)
Probenecid
Retinoid drugs such as Retin-A and Renova
Sulfa drugs such as Bactrim and Gantrisin

Sulfa drugs may increase methotrexate's toxic effect on the bone marrow, where new blood cells are made.

Certain antibiotics, including tetracycline (Sumycin) and chloramphenicol (Chloromycetin), may reduce the effectiveness of methotrexate. This is also true of vitamin preparations that contain folic acid.

In addition, methotrexate can alter the effect of theophylline (Quibron, Theo-Dur).

Special information if you are pregnant or breastfeeding

A woman should not start methotrexate therapy until the doctor is sure she is not pregnant. Because methotrexate causes birth defects and miscarriages, it must not be taken during pregnancy by women with psoriasis or rheumatoid arthritis. It should be taken by women being treated for cancer only if the potential benefit outweighs the risk to the developing baby. In fact, a couple should avoid pregnancy if either the man or the woman is taking methotrexate. After the end of methotrexate treatment, a man should wait at least 3 months, and a woman should wait for the completion of at least one menstrual cycle, before attempting to conceive a child.

Methotrexate should not be taken by a woman who is breastfeeding; it does pass into breast milk and may harm a nursing baby.

Recommended dosage

Treatment with methotrexate is highly individualized. Your doctor will carefully tailor your dosage of methotrexate in order to avoid serious side effects and possible under- or overdosing.

Overdosage

Taken in excess, methotrexate can cause serious and even fatal damage to the liver, kidneys, bone marrow, lungs, or other parts of the body. Symptoms of overdosage may include lung or breathing problems, mouth ulcers, or diarrhea. Initially, however, serious damage caused by methotrexate may be apparent only in the results of blood tests. For this reason, careful, regular monitoring by your doctor is necessary. If for any reason you suspect symptoms of an overdose of this drug, seek medical attention immediately.

Methyldopa See Aldomet, page 67.

Methylergonovine See Methergine, page 832.

Methylin See Ritalin, page 1270.

Methylphenidate See Ritalin, page 1270.

Methylprednisolone See Medrol, page 817.

Metoclopramide See Reglan, page 1222.

Metolazone See Zaroxolyn, page 1613.

Metoprolol See Lopressor, page 775.

MetroCream See MetroGel, below.

METROGEL

Pronounced: MET-roh-jell
Generic name: Metronidazole
Other brand names: MetroCream, MetroLotion

Why is this drug prescribed?

MetroGel is a preparation of the drug metronidazole used for the treatment of a skin condition called rosacea (red eruptions, usually on the face). The cream and lotion forms of metronidazole are used for the same problem. All are for external (topical) use only.

Most important fact about this drug

Metronidazole may irritate the skin. If local irritation occurs, consult your doctor. You may need to use the medication less frequently or to discontinue use.

How should you take this medication?

After washing the affected area, apply a thin film of the preparation and rub in. Topical metronidazole should be applied twice daily, in the morning and evening. Cosmetics may be used after the drug is applied. (If using the lotion, wait 5 minutes for it to dry.)

Be sure to wash your hands after applying the medication so as not to irritate the eyes.

■ *If you miss a dose...*
Apply it as soon as you remember. If it is almost time for your next dose, skip the one you missed and go back to your regular schedule.
■ *Storage instructions...*
Store at room temperature. Protect the lotion from freezing.

What side effects may occur?

Side effects cannot be anticipated. If any develop or change in intensity, inform your doctor as soon as possible. Only your doctor can determine if it is safe for you to continue using topical metronidazole.

■ *Side effects may include:*
Burning or stinging, dryness, itching, metallic taste, nausea, redness, skin irritation, tingling or numbness of hands and feet, worsening of rosacea

Why should this drug not be prescribed?

Do not use topical metronidazole if you have ever had an allergic reaction to Flagyl or any other metronidazole product, or if you have been told that you are sensitive to chemicals called parabens.

Special warnings about this medication

This medication may cause tearing of the eye. Avoid contact with the eyes.

Be sure to tell your doctor if you have ever had any diseases or abnormalities of the blood.

Possible food and drug interactions when taking this medication

Oral metronidazole strengthens the activity of blood thinners such as Coumadin. It's not known whether topical preparations have the same effect.

Special information if you are pregnant or breastfeeding

There is no evidence that metronidazole can harm a developing baby. Nevertheless, it should be used during pregnancy only if clearly needed. If you are pregnant or plan to become pregnant, tell your doctor immediately.

Topical metronidazole does find its way into breast milk. You'll need to choose between breastfeeding your baby and continuing treatment with the drug.

Recommended dosage

ADULTS

Apply a thin layer to the affected area twice a day.

Overdosage

There is no information on overdose with topical forms of metronidazole, but any medication taken in excess can have serious consequences. If you suspect an overdose, seek medical attention immediately.

MetroLotion *See MetroGel, page 837.*

Metronidazole *See Flagyl, page 574.*

Metronidazole cream, gel, and lotion *See MetroGel, page 837.*

MEVACOR

Pronounced: MEV-uh-core
Generic name: Lovastatin

Why is this drug prescribed?

Mevacor is used, along with diet, to lower cholesterol levels in people with primary hypercholesterolemia (too much cholesterol in the bloodstream). High cholesterol levels foster the buildup of artery-clogging plaque, which can be especially dangerous when it collects in the vessels serving the muscles of the heart. Mevacor is prescribed to prevent this problem—called coronary heart disease—or to slow its advance if the arteries are already clogging up.

Most important fact about this drug

Mevacor is usually prescribed only if diet, exercise, and weight loss fail to bring your cholesterol levels under control. It's important to remember that Mevacor is a supplement to—not a substitute for—these other measures. To get the full benefit of the medication, you need to stick to the diet and exercise program prescribed by your doctor.

How should you take this medication?

Mevacor should be taken with meals.

■ *If you miss a dose...*
Take it as soon as you remember. If it is almost time for your next dose, skip the one you missed and go back to your regular schedule. Never take 2 doses at the same time.

■ *Storage instructions...*
Protect Mevacor from light. Store at room temperature. Keep container tightly closed.

What side effects may occur?

Mevacor is generally well tolerated. Any side effects that have occurred have usually been mild and short-lived. If any side effects develop or change in intensity, inform your doctor as soon as possible. Only your doctor can determine if it is safe for you to continue taking Mevacor.

■ *Side effects may include:*
Abdominal pain/cramps, altered sense of taste, blurred vision, constipation, diarrhea, dizziness, gas, headache, heartburn, indigestion, itching, muscle cramps, muscle pain, muscle weakness with rash, nausea, rash, weakness

Why should this drug not be prescribed?

If you are sensitive to or have ever had an allergic reaction to Mevacor or similar anticholesterol drugs, you should not take this medication. Make sure that your doctor is aware of any drug reactions that you have experienced.

Unless you are directed to do so by your doctor, do not take this medication if you are being treated for liver disease.

Do not take this drug if you are pregnant or nursing.

Special warnings about this medication

If you are being treated for any disease that contributes to increased blood cholesterol, such as hypothyroidism, diabetes, nephrotic syndrome (kidney and blood vessel disorder), dysproteinemia (an excess of protein in the blood), or liver disease, your doctor will closely monitor your reaction to Mevacor.

Drugs like Mevacor have occasionally been known to damage muscle tissue, so be sure to tell your doctor immediately if you notice any unexplained muscle tenderness, weakness, or pain, especially if you also have a fever or feel sick. Your doctor may want to do a blood test to check for signs of muscle damage.

It is recommended that liver function tests be performed by your doctor before treatment with Mevacor begins, at 6 and 12 weeks after your treatment has started or your dosage has been raised, and periodically (about 6-month intervals) thereafter.

If you are planning to have elective surgery, Mevacor should be discontinued a few days before the operation. This drug should be used with caution if you consume substantial quantities of alcohol or have a past history of liver disease.

Possible food and drug interactions when taking this medication

Mevacor tends to enhance the blood-thinning effect of Coumadin. In rare instances, it can also cause muscle pain and potential kidney damage when combined with the following:

Amiodarone (Cordarone)
Clarithromycin (Biaxin)
Clofibrate (Atromid-S)
Cyclosporine (Sandimmune, Neoral)
Erythromycin (E.E.S., PCE, others)
Fenofibrate (Tricor)
Fluconazole (DiFlucan)
Gemfibrozil (Lopid)
Itraconazole (Sporanox)
Ketoconazole (Nizoral)
Nefazodone (Serzone)
Nicotinic acid or niacin (Niaspan)
Protease inhibitors (a type of drug for HIV) such as Agenerase,
  Crixivan, Fortovase, Invirase, Norvir, and Viracept
Verapamil (Calan)

If you are taking Mevacor with any of these drugs (or with large quantities of grapefruit juice), alert your doctor immediately at the first sign of muscle pain, tenderness, or weakness, especially if accompanied by fever or general body discomfort. If you need to take erythromycin, Biaxin, Nizoral, or Sporanox, the doctor may temporarily take you off Mevacor.

Special information if you are pregnant or breastfeeding

You should take Mevacor only if pregnancy is highly unlikely. If you become pregnant while taking this drug, discontinue using it and notify your physician immediately. There may be a potential hazard to the developing baby. This medication may appear in breast milk and may have an effect on nursing infants. If this medication is essential to your health, you should discontinue breastfeeding until your treatment with this medication is finished.

Recommended dosage

ADULTS

The recommended starting dose is 20 milligrams once a day, taken with the evening meal. Your doctor may start you at 10 milligrams a day if you need only a small reduction in cholesterol. The maximum recommended dose is 80 milligrams per day, taken as a single dose or divided into smaller doses, as determined by your doctor. Adjustments to any dose, as determined by your doctor, should be made at intervals of 4 weeks or more.

If you are taking cyclosporine, Lopid, Atromid-S, Tricor, or nicotinic acid in combination with Mevacor, your dose of Mevacor should not exceed 20 milligrams per day. If you are taking amiodarone (Cordarone) or verapamil (Calan), your dose of Mevacor should not exceed 40 milligrams a day.

Cholesterol levels should be monitored periodically by your doctor, who may decide to reduce the dose if your cholesterol level falls below the targeted range.

If you have reduced kidney function, your doctor will be cautious about increasing your dosage.

CHILDREN 10 TO 17 YEARS OLD

The recommended dosage is 10 to 40 milligrams per day, taken with meals. Adjustments to any dose, as determined by the doctor, should be made at intervals of 4 weeks or more. Girls must have been menstruating for at least 1 year before starting therapy with Mevacor.

The safety and effectiveness of Mevacor in children under 10 years old or in doses greater than 40 milligrams a day have not been studied.

Overdosage
There have been no reported cases of overdose with Mevacor. However, if you suspect an overdose, seek medical attention immediately.

Mexiletine *See Mexitil, below.*

MEXITIL
Pronounced: MEX-ih-till
Generic name: Mexiletine hydrochloride

Why is this drug prescribed?
Mexitil is used to treat severe irregular heartbeat (arrhythmia). Irregular heart rhythms are generally divided into two main types: heartbeats that are faster than normal (tachycardia) and heartbeats that are slower than normal (bradycardia). Arrhythmias are often caused by drugs or disease but can occur in otherwise healthy people with no history of heart disease or other illness.

Most important fact about this drug
While you are taking Mexitil, your doctor should carefully monitor your heartbeat to make sure the drug is working properly.

How should you take this medication?
Take Mexitil with food or an antacid. Take it exactly as prescribed.

■ *If you miss a dose…*
If you remember within 4 hours, take it immediately. If more than 4 hours have passed, skip the missed dose and return to your regular schedule. Never take 2 doses at the same time.
■ *Storage instructions…*
Store at room temperature.

What side effects may occur?
Side effects cannot be anticipated. If any develop or change in intensity, inform your doctor as soon as possible. Only your doctor can determine if it is safe for you to continue taking Mexitil.

■ *Side effects may include:*
Blurred vision, changes in sleep habits, chest pain, constipation, depression, diarrhea, difficult or labored breathing, dizziness, headache, heartburn, light-headedness, nausea, nervousness, numbness, poor coordination, rash, swelling due to fluid retention, throbbing heartbeat, tingling or pins and needles, tremors, upset stomach, vision changes, vomiting

Why should this drug not be prescribed?
This drug should not be used if you have heart failure, a heartbeat irregularity called heart block that has not been corrected by a pacemaker, or structural heart disease, or if you have recently had a heart attack.

Special warnings about this medication
If you have heart block and a pacemaker, Mexitil may be prescribed, but you should be continuously monitored while taking it.

Mexitil can aggravate low blood pressure and severe congestive heart failure, so it will be prescribed cautiously for people with these conditions.

You should be monitored carefully if you have liver disease or abnormal liver function as a result of congestive heart failure.

Diets that change the pH (acid/alkaline content) of your urine can alter the excretion of Mexitil from your body. Talk to your doctor or pharmacist about proper diet.

Blood disorders have occurred with Mexitil use. Make sure your doctor performs periodic blood tests while you are using this medication.

If you have a seizure disorder, use Mexitil with caution.

Possible food and drug interactions when taking this medication
If Mexitil is taken with certain other drugs, the effects of either may be increased, decreased, or altered. It is especially important that you consult with your doctor before taking any of the following:

Antacids such as Maalox
Caffeine products such as Nō-Dōz
Cimetidine (Tagamet)
Other antiarrhythmic drugs such as Norpace and Quinidex
Phenobarbital
Phenytoin (Dilantin)
Rifampin (Rifadin)
Theophylline products such as Theo-Dur

Special information if you are pregnant or breastfeeding

The effects of Mexitil during pregnancy have not been adequately studied. If you are pregnant or plan to become pregnant, inform your doctor immediately. Mexitil appears in breast milk and could affect a nursing infant. If this medication is essential to your health, your doctor may advise you to discontinue breastfeeding until your treatment is finished.

Recommended dosage

Treatment is usually begun in the hospital.

ADULTS

The dosage of Mexitil will be adjusted to your individual needs on the basis of your response to the drug.

The usual starting dose is 200 milligrams every 8 hours when quick control of an irregular heartbeat is not necessary. Your doctor may adjust the dose by 50 or 100 milligrams up or down every 2 to 3 days.

Most people will do well on 200 to 300 milligrams taken every 8 hours with food or antacids. If you do not, your doctor may raise your dose to 400 milligrams every 8 hours. You should not take more than 1,200 milligrams in a day.

When fast relief is needed, your doctor may start you on 400 milligrams of Mexitil, followed by 200 milligrams in 8 hours. You should see the effects of this drug within 30 minutes to 2 hours.

In general, people with reduced kidney function are prescribed the usual doses of Mexitil, but those with severe liver disease may require lower doses and will be monitored closely.

Some people who handle this drug well may be transferred to a 12-hour dosage schedule that will make it easier and more convenient to take Mexitil. If you do well on a Mexitil dose of 300 milligrams or less every 8 hours, your doctor may decide to divide the daily total into 2 doses taken every 12 hours.

CHILDREN

The safety and efficacy of Mexitil have not been established in children.

OLDER ADULTS

Dosages will be adjusted according to the individual's needs.

Overdosage

Any medication taken in excess can have serious consequences. There have been deaths from Mexitil overdose. If you suspect an overdose, seek medical attention immediately.

■ *The symptoms of Mexitil overdose may include:*
Coma, low blood pressure, nausea, seizures, slow heartbeat or other heart problems, tingling or pins and needles

MIACALCIN

Pronounced: my-ah-CAL-sin
Generic name: Calcitonin-salmon

Why is this drug prescribed?

Miacalcin is a synthetic form of calcitonin, a naturally occurring hormone produced by the thyroid gland. Miacalcin reduces the rate of calcium loss from bones. Since less calcium passes from the bones to the blood, Miacalcin also helps control blood calcium levels.

Miacalcin Nasal Spray is used to treat postmenopausal osteoporosis (bone loss occurring after menopause) in women who cannot or will not take estrogen.

Most important fact about this drug

Although no allergic reactions have been reported with Miacalcin Nasal Spray, calcitonin-salmon has been reported to cause serious allergic reactions (such as shock, difficulty breathing, wheezing, and swelling of the throat or tongue) in a few people. The possibility exists for such a reaction with the nasal spray. Your doctor may give you a skin test to see if you are allergic to calcitonin-salmon.

How should you take this medication?

Spray Miacalcin into one nostril one day, the other the next.

Follow the manufacturer's instructions for activating the pump before the first dose.

Keep your head upright. Put the nozzle into your nostril and depress the pump toward the bottle.

Be sure your diet provides enough calcium and vitamin D. Foods that are good sources of calcium include dairy products (such as milk and cheese) and fish. Good sources of vitamin D include fish (such as salmon, sardines, and tuna), liver, and dairy products. Sunlight is an indirect source of vitamin D.

■ *If you miss a dose...*
Take it as soon as you remember. Never take 2 doses at once.
■ *Storage instructions...*
Store the unopened medication in the refrigerator. Protect from freezing. Before you prime the pump and open a new bottle, let it come to

room temperature. You can keep the bottle at room temperature for 30 days; be sure it stays upright.

What side effects may occur?
Side effects cannot be anticipated. If any develop or change in intensity, inform your doctor as soon as possible. Only your doctor can determine if it is safe for you to continue using Miacalcin Nasal Spray.

■ *Side effects may include:*
Back pain, headache, joint pain, nasal inflammation, nasal symptoms (crusts, dryness, redness, sores, irritation, itching, thick feeling, soreness, paleness, infection, narrowing of passages, runny or blocked nose, small wounds, bleeding wound, uncomfortable feeling), nosebleed

Why should this drug not be prescribed?
You should not be using Miacalcin if you are allergic to calcitonin-salmon.

Special warnings about this medication
Your doctor will examine your nose before you use Miacalcin Nasal Spray and periodically while you are using it.
If your nose becomes very irritated, notify your doctor.
Miacalcin may cause small wounds or ulcers in your nose.

Possible food and drug interactions when taking this medication
There are no interactions listed for this drug. However, people with Paget's disease of bone who have taken certain drugs such as Didronel may find that Miacalcin Nasal Spray is not working as well as it should.

Special information if you are pregnant or breastfeeding
The effects of calcitonin-salmon in pregnancy have not been adequately studied, but use of Miacalcin Nasal Spray if you are pregnant is not recommended.
It is not known whether Miacalcin appears in breast milk. Women are usually advised not to use Miacalcin while breastfeeding an infant.

Recommended dosage
The usual dose is 1 spray (200 I.U.) a day, sprayed into the nose. Alternate nostrils. Ask your doctor about taking supplemental vitamin D and calcium.
Miacalcin Nasal Spray should not be used by children.

Overdosage
Any medication taken in excess can have serious consequences. If you suspect an overdose, seek medical help immediately.

■ *Symptoms of Miacalcin overdose may include:*
Spasms

MICARDIS

Pronounced: my-CAR-diss
Generic name: Telmisartan

Why is this drug prescribed?

Micardis controls high blood pressure. It works by blocking the effects of a hormone called angiotensin II. Unopposed, this substance tends to constrict the blood vessels while promoting retention of salt and water—actions that tend to raise blood pressure. Micardis prevents these effects and thus keeps blood pressure lower. It can be prescribed alone or with other high blood pressure medications, such as diuretics that help rid the body of excess water.

Most important fact about this drug

Micardis should reduce your blood pressure within a couple of weeks, although it may take a month to achieve its maximum effect. You need to continue taking this drug regularly, even if you feel well. Micardis does not cure high blood pressure; it merely keeps it under control.

How should you take this medication?

You can take Micardis with or without food. To avoid forgetting a dose, make a habit of taking it at the same time each day.

■ *If you miss a dose...*
   Take it as soon as you remember. If it is almost time for your next dose, skip the one you missed and go back to your regular schedule. Do not take 2 doses at once.
■ *Storage instructions...*
   Store at room temperature. Leave each tablet in its blister pack until you're ready to take it.

What side effects may occur?

Side effects cannot be anticipated. If any develop or change in intensity, inform your doctor as soon as possible. Only your doctor can determine if it is safe for you to continue taking Micardis.

■ *Side effects may include:*
   Back pain, diarrhea, respiratory tract infection, sinus inflammation

Why should this drug not be prescribed?

If Micardis gives you an allergic reaction, you cannot continue using it.

Special warnings about this medication

Micardis can cause a severe drop in blood pressure, especially when you first start taking the drug. The problem is more likely to occur if your body's supply of water has been depleted by diuretics (water pills).

Symptoms include light-headedness, dizziness, and faintness. Call your doctor if they occur. You may need to have your dose adjusted.

If you have liver or kidney disease, Micardis must be used with caution. Be sure your doctor is aware of either problem.

Possible food and drug interactions when taking this medication

If Micardis is taken with certain other drugs, the effects of either could be increased, decreased, or altered. It is especially important to check with your doctor before combining Micardis with the following:

Digoxin (Lanoxin)
Warfarin (Coumadin)

Special information if you are pregnant or breastfeeding

When used in the second or third trimester of pregnancy, Micardis can cause injury or even death to the unborn child. Stop taking Micardis as soon as you know that you are pregnant.

It is not known whether Micardis appears in breast milk. However, for safety's sake it's considered best to either avoid breastfeeding or give up the drug.

Recommended dosage

ADULTS

The usual starting dose is 40 milligrams once a day. If necessary, the dose can be increased to a maximum of 80 milligrams daily.

Overdosage

Any medication taken in excess can have serious consequences. If you suspect an overdose, seek medical attention immediately.

■ *Symptoms of Micardis overdose may include:*
Abnormally rapid or slow heartbeat, dizziness, low blood pressure

MICARDIS HCT

Pronounced: my-CAR-diss
Generic name: Telmisartan, Hydrochlorothiazide

Why is this drug prescribed?

Micardis HCT is a combination medication used in the treatment of high blood pressure. One component, telmisartan, belongs to a class of blood pressure medications that work by preventing the hormone angiotensin II from constricting the blood vessels. This allows the blood to flow more freely and helps keep blood pressure down. The other component of Micardis HCT, hydrochlorothiazide, is a diuretic that increases the output of urine. This removes excess fluid from the body and helps lower blood pressure. Doctors usually prescribe Micardis HCT in place of its individual components. It can also be prescribed along with other blood pressure medications.

Most important fact about this drug
Micardis HCT should reduce your blood pressure within a couple of weeks. You need to continue taking this drug regularly, even if you feel well. Micardis HCT does not cure high blood pressure; it merely keeps it under control.

How should you take this medication?
Micardis HCT may be taken with or without food. Take Micardis HCT exactly as directed. Try to take it at the same time each day so that it is easier to remember.

■ *If you miss a dose...*
Take it as soon as you remember. If it is almost time for your next dose, skip the one you missed and go back to your regular schedule. Do not take 2 doses at once.

■ *Storage instructions...*
Store at room temperature. Leave each tablet in its blister pack until you're ready to take it.

What side effects may occur?
Side effects cannot be anticipated. If any develop or change in intensity, inform your doctor as soon as possible. Only your doctor can determine if it is safe for you to continue taking Micardis HCT.

■ *Side effects may include:*
Diarrhea, dizziness, fatigue, sinus inflammation, upper respiratory infection

Why should this drug not be prescribed?
Do not take this drug if you are allergic to telmisartan, hydrochlorothiazide, or any sulfa drugs.

Special warnings about this medication
Micardis HCT can cause low blood pressure, especially if you are also taking another diuretic. This may make you feel light-headed or faint, especially during the first days of therapy. If these symptoms occur, contact your doctor. Your dosage may need to be adjusted. If you actually faint, stop taking this medication until you have talked to your doctor.

If you have congestive heart failure, liver or kidney disease, lupus, gout, or diabetes, Micardis HCT should be used with caution. This drug may bring out hidden diabetes. If you are already taking insulin or oral diabetes drugs, your medication may have to be adjusted. The hydrochlorothiazide component of Micardis HCT also has a tendency to raise cholesterol levels.

If you have bronchial asthma or a history of allergies, you may be at greater risk for an allergic reaction to this medication.

The diuretic in Micardis HCT can cause a chemical imbalance in the body, especially if vomiting has depleted your fluids. Your doctor will perform blood tests periodically to check for this imbalance. Signs include dry mouth, thirst, weakness, sluggishness, drowsiness, restlessness, confusion, seizures, muscle pain or cramps, muscle fatigue, low blood pressure, decreased urination, rapid heartbeat, nausea, and vomiting. Call your doctor if you experience any of these symptoms.

Diuretics also can cause your body to lose too much potassium (hypokalemia). Signs of an excessively low potassium level include muscle weakness and rapid or irregular heartbeat. To boost your potassium level, your doctor may recommend eating potassium-rich foods or taking a potassium supplement. If you think you need a supplement, check with your doctor; do not start taking one on your own. Likewise, check with your doctor before using a potassium-containing salt substitute.

Dehydration, excessive sweating, severe diarrhea, or vomiting could deplete your body's fluids and cause your blood pressure to become too low. Be careful when exercising and during hot weather.

Micardis HCT has not been evaluated for use in children.

Possible food and drug interactions when taking this medication

If Micardis HCT is taken with certain other drugs, the effects of either could be increased, decreased, or altered. It is especially important to check with your doctor before combining Micardis HCT with the following:

Alcohol
Barbiturates such as phenobarbital and Seconal
Cholestyramine (Questran)
Colestipol (Colestid)
Digoxin
Insulin
Lithium (Eskalith)
Muscle relaxants such as tubocurarine
Narcotic painkillers such as Percocet
Nonsteroidal anti-inflammatory drugs such as Advil, Motrin, and Naprosyn
Norepinephrine (Levophed)
Oral diabetes drugs such as Diabinese, Diabeta, and Glucotrol
Other blood pressure–lowering drugs
Steroid medications such as prednisone

Special information if you are pregnant or breastfeeding
Micardis HCT can cause injury or even death to an unborn child when used during the last 6 months of pregnancy. As soon as you learn that you are pregnant, stop taking Micardis HCT and call your doctor. Micardis HCT appears in breast milk and can affect a nursing infant. You'll need to choose between breastfeeding and using Micardis HCT.

Recommended dosage

ADULTS

Micardis HCT is available in tablets containing either 40 or 80 milligrams of telmisartan and 12.5 or 25 milligrams of hydrochlorothiazide. The usual starting dose is one 40/12.5 tablet per day. If your blood pressure does not respond to this dose, after 2 to 4 weeks your doctor may increase your dose up to a maximum of two 80/12.5 tablets once daily. If the diuretic (hydrochlorothiazide) in Micardis HCT causes hypokalemia (see *Special warnings about this medication*), your doctor may switch you to a once-daily dosage that contains a lower dose of the diuretic.

Overdosage
Any medication taken in excess can have serious consequences. If you suspect an overdose, seek medical help immediately.

■ *Symptoms of Micardis HCT overdose may include:*
Dizziness, dry mouth, excessive thirst, irregular heartbeat, low blood pressure, muscle pain or cramps, nausea, rapid or slow heartbeat, vomiting, weakness

Miconazole See Monistat, page 885.

MICRO-K
Pronounced: MY-kroe-kay
Generic name: Potassium chloride
Other brand names: Klor-Con, K-Dur, K-Tab, Kaon-CL, Slow-K

Why is this drug prescribed?
Micro-K is used to treat or prevent low potassium levels in people who may face potassium loss caused by digitalis (Lanoxin), non-potassium-sparing diuretics (such as Diuril and Dyazide), and certain diseases.

Potassium plays an essential role in the proper functioning of a wide range of systems in the body, including the kidneys, muscles, and nerves. As a result, a potassium deficiency may have a wide range of effects, including dry mouth, thirst, reduced urination, weakness, fatigue, drowsiness, low blood pressure, restlessness, muscle cramps, abnormal heart rate, nausea, and vomiting.

Micro-K and the other products discussed here are slow-release potassium formulations.

Most important fact about this drug

There have been reports of intestinal and gastric ulcers and bleeding associated with use of slow-release potassium chloride medications. Micro-K should be used only by people who cannot take potassium chloride in liquid or effervescent forms.

Do not change from one brand of potassium chloride to another without consulting your doctor or pharmacist.

How should you take this medication?

Take Micro-K with meals and with a full glass of water or some other liquid.

Tell your doctor if you have difficulty swallowing Micro-K. You may sprinkle the contents of the capsule onto a spoonful of soft food. Capsules and tablets should not be crushed, chewed, or sucked.

■ *If you miss a dose…*
If it is within 2 hours of the scheduled time, take it as soon as you remember. If you do not remember until later, skip the dose you missed and go back to your regular schedule. Do not take 2 doses at once.

■ *Storage instructions…*
Store at room temperature in a tightly closed container.

What side effects may occur?

Side effects cannot be anticipated. If any develop or change in intensity, inform your doctor as soon as possible. Only your doctor can determine if it is safe for you to continue taking Micro-K.

■ *Side effects may include:*
Abdominal pain or discomfort, diarrhea, gas, nausea, stomach and intestinal ulcers and bleeding, blockage, or perforation, vomiting

Why should this drug not be prescribed?

You should not use Micro-K in a solid form if you are taking any drug or have any condition that could stop or slow Micro-K as it goes through the gastrointestinal tract.

If you have high potassium levels, you should not use Micro-K.

You should not use these products if you are allergic to any of their ingredients.

People with certain heart conditions should not use slow-release forms of potassium.

Special warnings about this medication

Before taking Micro-K, tell your doctor if you have ever had acute dehydration, heat cramps, adrenal insufficiency, diabetes, heart disease, kidney disease, liver disease, ulcers, or severe burns.

Tell your doctor immediately if you notice that your stools are black or tarry.

Possible food and drug interactions when taking this medication

If Micro-K is taken with certain other drugs, the effects of either could be increased, decreased, or altered. It is important to check with your doctor before combining Micro-K with the following:

Antispasmodic drugs such as Bentyl
Blood pressure medications classified as ACE inhibitors, such as
    Vasotec and Capoten
Digitalis (Lanoxin)
Potassium-sparing diuretics such as Midamor and Aldactone

Also tell your doctor if you use salt substitutes.

Special information if you are pregnant or breastfeeding

Micro-K is generally considered safe for pregnant women or women who breastfeed their babies.

Recommended dosage

Dosages must be adjusted for each individual. Safety and effectiveness in children have not been established. The following are typical dosages for Micro-K and other leading slow-release potassium supplements.

TO TREAT LOW POTASSIUM LEVELS

Micro-K, Klor-Con 8, Slow-K
The usual dosage is 5 to 12 tablets or capsules per day.

Micro-K 10, Klor-Con 10, Klor-Con M10, K-Dur 10, K-Tab, Kaon-CL 10
The usual dose is 4 to 10 tablets or capsules per day.

K-Dur 20, Klor-Con M15, Klor-Con M20
The usual dose is 2 to 5 tablets per day.

TO PREVENT LOW POTASSIUM LEVELS

Micro-K, Klor-Con 8, Slow-K, Kaon-CL 10
The usual dosage is 2 or 3 tablets or capsules per day.

K-Tab, Micro-K 10, K-Dur 10, Klor-Con 10, Klor-Con M10
The usual dose is 2 tablets or capsules per day.

K-Dur 20, Klor-Con M15, Klor-Con M20
The usual dose is 1 tablet per day.

If you are taking more than 2 tablets or capsules per day, your total daily dose will be divided into smaller doses.

Overdosage

Any medication taken in excess can have serious consequences. Overdoses of these supplements can result in potentially fatal levels of potassium. Overdose symptoms may not be noticeable in their early stages. Therefore, if you have any reason to suspect an overdose, seek medical help immediately.

■ *Symptoms of potassium overdose may include:*
Blood in stools, cardiac arrest, irregular heartbeat, muscle paralysis, muscle weakness

MICRONASE

Pronounced: MIKE-roh-naze
Generic name: Glyburide
Other brand names: DiaBeta, Glynase

Why is this drug prescribed?

Micronase is an oral antidiabetic medication used to treat type 2 diabetes, the kind that occurs when the body either does not make enough insulin or fails to use insulin properly. Insulin transfers sugar from the bloodstream to the body's cells, where it is then used for energy.

There are two forms of diabetes: type 1 and type 2. Type 1 diabetes results from a complete shutdown of normal insulin production and usually requires insulin injections for life, while type 2 diabetes can usually be treated by dietary changes, exercise, and/or oral antidiabetic medications such as Micronase. This medication controls diabetes by stimulating the pancreas to produce more insulin and by helping insulin to work better. Type 2 diabetics may need insulin injections, sometimes only temporarily during stressful periods such as illness, or on a long-term basis if an oral antidiabetic medication fails to control blood sugar.

Micronase can be used alone or along with a drug called metformin (Glucophage) if diet plus either drug alone fails to control sugar levels.

Most important fact about this drug

Always remember that Micronase is an aid to, not a substitute for, good diet and exercise. Failure to follow a sound diet and exercise plan can lead to serious complications, such as dangerously high or low blood sugar levels. Remember, too, that Micronase is *not* an oral form of insulin, and cannot be used in place of insulin.

How should you take this medication?
In general, Micronase should be taken with breakfast or the first main meal of the day.

■ *If you miss a dose...*
Take it as soon as you remember. If it is almost time for your next dose, skip the one you missed and go back to your regular schedule. Never take 2 doses at the same time.

■ *Storage instructions...*
Keep this medication in the container it came in, tightly closed. Store it at room temperature.

What side effects may occur?
Side effects cannot be anticipated. If any develop or change in intensity, inform your doctor as soon as possible. Only your doctor can determine if it is safe for you to continue taking Micronase.

Side effects of Micronase are rare and seldom require discontinuation of the medication.

■ *Side effects may include:*
Bloating, heartburn, nausea

Micronase, like all oral antidiabetics, may cause hypoglycemia (low blood sugar) especially in elderly, weak, and undernourished people, and those with kidney, liver, adrenal, or pituitary gland problems. The risk of hypoglycemia can be increased by missed meals, alcohol, other medications, fever, trauma, infection, surgery, or excessive exercise. To avoid hypoglycemia, you should closely follow the dietary and exercise plan suggested by your physician.

■ *Symptoms of mild hypoglycemia may include:*
Cold sweat, drowsiness, fast heartbeat, headache, nausea, nervousness

■ *Symptoms of more severe hypoglycemia may include:*
Coma, pale skin, seizures, shallow breathing

Eating sugar or a sugar-based product will often correct mild hypoglycemia.

Severe hypoglycemia should be considered a medical emergency, and prompt medical attention is essential.

Why should this drug not be prescribed?
You should not take Micronase if you have had an allergic reaction to it or to similar drugs such as Glucotrol or Diabinese.

Micronase should not be taken if you are suffering from diabetic ketoacidosis (a life-threatening medical emergency caused by insufficient insulin and marked by excessive thirst, nausea, fatigue, pain below the breastbone, and fruity breath).

Special warnings about this medication

It's possible that drugs such as Micronase may lead to more heart problems than diet treatment alone, or diet plus insulin. If you have a heart condition, you may want to discuss this with your doctor.

If you are taking Micronase, you should check your blood or urine periodically for abnormal sugar (glucose) levels.

It is important that you closely follow the diet and exercise plan recommended by your doctor.

The effectiveness of any oral antidiabetic, including Micronase, may decrease with time. This may occur either because of a diminished responsiveness to the medication or a worsening of the diabetes.

Possible food and drug interactions when taking this medication

If Micronase is taken with certain other drugs, the effects of either could be increased, decreased, or altered. It is especially important to check with your doctor before combining Micronase with the following:

Airway-opening drugs such as Proventil and Ventolin
Anabolic steroids such as testosterone and Danazol
Antacids such as Mylanta
Aspirin
Beta-blockers such as the blood pressure medications Inderal and
    Tenormin
Blood thinners such as Coumadin
Calcium channel blockers such as the blood pressure medications
    Cardizem and Procardia
Certain antibiotics such as Cipro
Chloramphenicol (Chloromycetin)
Cimetidine (Tagamet)
Clofibrate (Atromid-S)
Estrogens such as Premarin
Fluconazole (Diflucan)
Furosemide (Lasix)
Gemfibrozil (Lopid)
Isoniazid (Nydrazid)
Itraconazole (Sporanox)
Major tranquilizers such as Stelazine and Mellaril
MAO inhibitors such as the antidepressants Nardil and Parnate
Metformin (Glucophage)
Niacin (Niacor, Niaspan)
Nonsteroidal anti-inflammatory drugs such as Advil, Motrin,
    Naprosyn, and Voltaren
Oral contraceptives
Phenytoin (Dilantin)
Probenecid (Benemid)
Steroids such as prednisone

Sulfa drugs such as Bactrim and Septra
Thiazide diuretics such as the water pills Diuril and HydroDIURIL
Thyroid medications such as Synthroid

Be careful about drinking alcohol, since excessive alcohol consumption can cause low blood sugar.

Special information if you are pregnant or breastfeeding

The effects of Micronase during pregnancy have not been adequately studied in humans. This drug should be used during pregnancy only if the benefit outweighs the potential risk to the unborn baby. Since studies suggest the importance of maintaining normal blood sugar (glucose) levels during pregnancy, your physician may prescribe insulin injections during pregnancy.

While it is not known if Micronase appears in breast milk, other oral diabetes medications do. Therefore, women should discuss with their doctors whether to discontinue the medication or to stop breastfeeding. If the medication is discontinued, and if diet alone does not control glucose levels, then your doctor may consider insulin injections.

Recommended dosage

Your doctor will tailor your dosage to your individual needs.

ADULTS

Usually the doctor will prescribe an initial daily dose of 2.5 to 5 milligrams. Maintenance therapy usually ranges from 1.25 to 20 milligrams daily. Daily doses greater than 20 milligrams are not recommended. In most cases, Micronase is taken once a day; however, people taking more than 10 milligrams a day may respond better to twice-a-day dosing.

CHILDREN

The safety and effectiveness of Micronase have not been established in children.

OLDER ADULTS

Older, malnourished, or debilitated individuals, or those with impaired kidney and liver function, usually receive lower initial and maintenance doses to minimize the risk of low blood sugar (hypoglycemia).

Overdosage

An overdose of Micronase can cause low blood sugar (hypoglycemia).

■ *Symptoms of severe hypoglycemia include:*
Coma, pale skin, seizure, shallow breathing

If you suspect a Micronase overdose, seek medical attention immediately.

Micronor *See Oral Contraceptives, page 1000.*

MIDRIN
Pronounced: MID-rin
Generic ingredients: Isometheptene mucate,
  Dichloralphenazone, Acetaminophen

Why is this drug prescribed?
Midrin is prescribed for the treatment of tension headaches. It is also used to treat vascular headaches such as migraine.

Most important fact about this drug
Midrin can be used only after the headache starts. It does not prevent headaches.

How should you take this medication?
You should start taking Midrin at the first sign of a migraine attack.
  Do not take more than the maximum dose of Midrin.
  Take this medication exactly as prescribed by your doctor.

■ *If you miss a dose...*
  Take this medication only as needed.
■ *Storage instructions...*
  Store at room temperature in a dry place.

What side effects may occur?
Side effects cannot be anticipated. If any develop or change in intensity, tell your doctor immediately. Only your doctor can determine whether it is safe for you to continue taking Midrin.

■ *Side effects may include:*
  Short periods of dizziness, skin rash

Why should this drug not be prescribed?
Unless directed to do so by your doctor, do not take Midrin if you have the eye condition called glaucoma or severe kidney disease, high blood pressure, a physical defect of the heart, or liver disease, or if you are currently taking antidepressant drugs known as MAO inhibitors, including Nardil and Parnate.

Special warnings about this medication
Take Midrin cautiously if you have high blood pressure or any abnormal condition of the blood vessels outside the heart, or have recently had a cardiovascular attack such as a heart attack or stroke.

Possible food and drug interactions when taking this medication
Avoid alcoholic beverages.

If Midrin is taken with certain other drugs, the effects of either drug could be increased, decreased, or altered. It is especially important to check with your doctor before combining Midrin with the following:

Acetaminophen-containing pain relievers such as Tylenol
Antidepressants classified as MAO inhibitors, including Nardil and Parnate
Antihistamines such as Benadryl
Central nervous system depressants such as Halcion, Valium, and Xanax

Special information if you are pregnant or breastfeeding
If you are pregnant, plan to become pregnant, or are breastfeeding your baby, check with your doctor before taking Midrin.

Recommended dosage

ADULTS

Relief of Migraine Headache
The usual dosage is 2 capsules at once, followed by 1 capsule every hour until the headache is relieved; do not take more than 5 capsules within a 12-hour period.

Relief of Tension Headache
The usual dosage is 1 or 2 capsules every 4 hours up to a maximum of 8 capsules a day.

Overdosage
Any medication taken in excess can have serious consequences. If you suspect a Midrin overdose, seek emergency medical treatment immediately.

MIGRANAL

Pronounced: MY-grah-nal
Generic name: Dihydroergotamine mesylate

Why is this drug prescribed?
Migranal Nasal Spray is used for relief of migraine headache attacks, whether or not preceded by an aura (visual disturbances, usually including sensations of halos or flickering lights).

This nasally administered remedy contains the same active ingredient as D.H.E. 45, an injectable form of the drug. It constricts the blood vessels, and may defeat migraine through this action.

Most important fact about this drug

Migranal Nasal Spray is for use only during a genuine attack of classic migraine. Do not attempt to prevent migraines with this drug, and do not use it for tension headaches, cluster headaches, or unusual types of migraine such as hemiplegic or basilar migraine.

How should you take this medication?

Migranal comes in single-dose ampuls, each with an accompanying nasal sprayer. Do not open an ampul until needed. Once opened, the drug must be used within 8 hours to be fully effective.

Take this medication at the first sign of a developing migraine. Assemble the ampul and sprayer according to package directions, pump the sprayer 4 times to prime it with medication, then spray once in each nostril. While spraying, do *not* tilt your head back or inhale through your nose. Wait 15 minutes, then spray once in each nostril again. After the second spray, discard the sprayer and the ampul's cap. To be prepared for the next attack, remember to load a new ampul and sprayer into the assembly case that comes with the medication.

Migranal will be effective even if you have a stuffy nose, a cold, or allergies.

■ *If you miss a dose...*
   Migranal Nasal Spray is not for regular use. Use it only during a migraine attack.
■ *Storage instructions...*
   Store at room temperature away from heat and light. Do not refrigerate or freeze.

What side effects may occur?

Side effects cannot be anticipated. If any develop or change in intensity, inform your doctor as soon as possible. Only your doctor can determine if it is safe for you to continue using Migranal Nasal Spray.

■ *Side effects may include:*
   Altered sense of taste, dizziness, drowsiness, nasal inflammation, nausea, sore throat, vomiting

Why should this drug not be prescribed?

Do not take Migranal if you have ever had an allergic reaction to an ergotamine-based drug such as the migraine remedies Cafergot, Ergostat, and D.H.E. 45 Injection, or the senility drug Hydergine.

You should avoid Migranal if you have certain types of heart or blood vessel disease, including angina (crushing chest pain) or a history of heart attack, or if you suffer from uncontrolled high blood pressure, severe kidney or liver disease, or a severe blood infection. Avoid it, too, if you have recently had blood vessel surgery.

Do not use Migranal within 24 hours of taking another ergotamine-based drug, another migraine remedy such as Amerge, Imitrex, Maxalt, or Zomig, or the migraine-preventing drug Sansert. Also avoid combining Migranal with other drugs that constrict the blood vessels, such as the decongestants pseudoephedrine and phenylpropanolamine, found in many over-the-counter cold products.

Do not use Migranal Nasal Spray while pregnant or nursing.

Special warnings about this medication

If you have heart disease, Migranal could trigger a serious problem. Risk factors for this disorder include high blood pressure, high cholesterol, diabetes, a family history of heart disease, smoking, and passing menopause. Your doctor will probably want to observe your reaction to the first dose of Migranal if any of these factors applies.

Because Migranal constricts blood vessels, you should use it with caution if you have circulation problems in your arms, legs, fingers, or toes. Use it cautiously, too, if you are being treated for high blood pressure; it occasionally aggravates the problem.

Alert your doctor immediately if you have any of the following side effects: pain in the arms and legs, numbness or tingling in your fingers or toes, coldness, pallor, weakness in the legs, chest pain, temporary speeding or slowing of the heart rate, swelling, itching, or a bluish color in your fingers and toes.

Possible food and drug interactions when taking this medication

If Migranal is taken with certain other drugs, the effects of either can be increased, decreased, or altered. Completely avoid other migraine remedies and ergotamine-based drugs, and check with your doctor before combining Migranal with the following:

Azithromycin (Zithromax)
Clarithromycin (Biaxin)
Erythromycin (Ery-Tab, Eryc)
Nicotine (from any source, including cigarettes, patches, and
    inhalers)
Phenylpropanolamine (Propagest)
Propranolol (Inderal)
Pseudoephedrine (Afrin, Sudafed)
Troleandomycin (Tao)

Special information if you are pregnant or breastfeeding

Migranal can harm a developing baby; do not use it during pregnancy. Also avoid it while breastfeeding. It appears in breast milk and may cause diarrhea, vomiting, weak pulse, and unstable blood pressure in a nursing infant.

Recommended dosage

ADULTS

Use one spray (0.5 milligram) in each nostril followed by another spray in each nostril 15 minutes later for a total of 4 sprays (2 milligrams).

Do not use more than 3 milligrams (6 sprays) in 24 hours or 4 milligrams (8 sprays) in 7 days.

Overdosage

Any medication taken in excess can have serious consequences. If you suspect an overdose, seek medical attention immediately.

■ *Symptoms of Migranal overdose may include:*
Abdominal pain, abnormal speech, coma, confusion, convulsions, hallucinations, increase and/or decrease in blood pressure, nausea, numbness, tingling, pain in and a bluish color of your fingers and toes, slowed breathing, vomiting

MILTOWN

Pronounced: MILL-town
Generic name: Meprobamate

Why is this drug prescribed?

Miltown is a tranquilizer used in the treatment of anxiety disorders and for short-term relief of the symptoms of anxiety.

Most important fact about this drug

Miltown can be habit-forming. You can develop tolerance and dependence, and you may experience withdrawal symptoms if you stop using this drug abruptly. Discontinue this drug or change your dose only on your doctor's advice.

How should you take this medication?

Take Miltown exactly as prescribed.

■ *If you miss a dose...*
Take it as soon as you remember if it is within an hour of your scheduled time. If you do not remember until later, skip the dose you missed and go back to your regular schedule. Never take 2 doses at the same time.
■ *Storage instructions...*
Store at room temperature in a tightly closed container.

What side effects may occur?

Side effects cannot be anticipated. If any develop or change in intensity, inform your doctor as soon as possible. Only your doctor can determine if it is safe for you to continue taking Miltown.

- *Side effects may include:*
  Broken capillary blood vessels, diarrhea, drowsiness, impaired coordination, irregular or rapid heartbeat, low red blood cell count, nausea, rash, slurred speech, vertigo, vomiting, weakness
- *Side effects due to rapid decrease in dose or abrupt withdrawal from Miltown:*
  Anxiety, confusion, convulsions, hallucinations, inability to fall or stay asleep, loss of appetite, loss of coordination, muscle twitching, tremors, vomiting

Withdrawal symptoms usually become apparent within 12 to 48 hours after discontinuation of this medication and should disappear in another 12 to 48 hours.

Why should this drug not be prescribed?

If you are sensitive to or have ever had an allergic reaction to Miltown or related drugs such as carisoprodol (Soma), you should not take this medication.

You should not take Miltown if you have acute intermittent porphyria, an inherited disease of the body's metabolism. It can make your symptoms worse.

Anxiety or tension related to everyday stress usually does not require treatment with Miltown. Discuss your symptoms thoroughly with your doctor.

Special warnings about this medication

If you develop a skin rash, sore throat, fever, or shortness of breath, contact your doctor immediately. You may be having an allergic reaction to the drug.

Miltown may cause you to become drowsy or less alert; therefore, you should not drive or operate dangerous machinery, or participate in any hazardous activity that requires full mental alertness, until you know how this drug affects you.

Long-term use of this drug should be evaluated by your doctor periodically for its usefulness.

If you have liver or kidney disorders, make sure your doctor is aware of these conditions before you begin using this medication.

If you have epilepsy, use of this drug may bring on seizures. Consult your doctor before taking it.

Possible food and drug interactions when taking this medication

Miltown may intensify the effects of alcohol. Do not drink alcohol while taking this medication.

If Miltown is taken with certain other drugs, the effects of either could be increased, decreased, or altered. It is especially important to check with your doctor before combining Miltown with mood-altering drugs and central nervous system depressants such as the following:

Antidepressant drugs such as Elavil, Nardil, and Tofranil
Antipsychotics such as chlorpromazine and thioridazine (Mellaril)
Barbiturates such as Seconal and phenobarbital
Narcotics such as Percocet or Demerol
Tranquilizers such as Halcion, Restoril, and Valium

Special information if you are pregnant or breastfeeding

Do not take Miltown if you are pregnant or planning to become pregnant.
There is an increased risk of birth defects. Miltown appears in breast milk
and could affect a nursing infant. If this medication is essential to your
health, your doctor may advise you to discontinue breastfeeding until
your treatment is finished.

Recommended dosage

ADULTS

The usual dosage is 1,200 milligrams to 1,600 milligrams per day divided
into 3 or 4 doses. You should not take more than 2,400 milligrams a day.

CHILDREN

The usual dose for children 6 to 12 years of age is 200 to 600 milligrams
per day divided into 2 or 3 doses.
    Miltown is not recommended for children under age 6.

OLDER ADULTS

Your doctor will limit your dose to the smallest effective amount to avoid
oversedation.

Overdosage

Any medication taken in excess can have serious consequences. If you
suspect an overdose, seek emergency medical attention immediately.

■ *The symptoms of Miltown overdose may include:*
    Coma, drowsiness, loss of muscle control, severely impaired breath-
    ing, shock, sluggishness, and unresponsiveness

MINIPRESS

Pronounced: MIN-ee-press
Generic name: Prazosin hydrochloride

Why is this drug prescribed?

Minipress is used to treat high blood pressure. It is effective used alone
or with other high blood pressure medications such as diuretics or beta-
blocking medications (drugs that ease heart contractions) such as Tenormin.

Minipress is also prescribed for the treatment of benign prostatic hyperplasia (BPH), an abnormal enlargement of the prostate gland.

Most important fact about this drug
If you have high blood pressure, you must take Minipress regularly for it to be effective. Since blood pressure declines gradually, it may be several weeks before you get the full benefit of Minipress; and you must continue taking it even if you are feeling well. Minipress does not cure high blood pressure; it merely keeps it under control.

How should you take this medication?
Minipress can be taken with or without food.

This medication should be taken exactly as prescribed by your doctor even if your symptoms have disappeared. Try not to miss any doses. If this medication is not taken regularly, your blood pressure will increase.

■ *If you miss a dose...*
Take it as soon as you remember. If it is almost time for your next dose, skip the one you missed and go back to your regular schedule. Never take 2 doses at the same time.
■ *Storage instructions...*
Protect from heat, light, and moisture.

What side effects may occur?
Side effects cannot be anticipated. If any develop or change in intensity, inform your doctor as soon as possible. Only your doctor can determine if it is safe for you to continue taking Minipress.

■ *Side effects may include:*
Dizziness, drowsiness, headache, lack of energy, nausea, palpitations (pounding heartbeat), weakness

Why should this drug not be prescribed?
Avoid Minipress if it, or similar drugs such as Cardura and Hytrin, gives you an allergic reaction.

Special warnings about this medication
Minipress can cause low blood pressure, especially when you first start taking the medication. This can cause you to become faint, dizzy, or light-headed, particularly on standing up. You should avoid driving or any hazardous tasks where injury could occur for 24 hours after taking the first dose or after your dose has been increased. Dizziness, fainting, or light-headedness may also occur in hot weather, when exercising, or when standing for long periods of time. Ask your doctor what precautions you should take.

Possible food and drug interactions when taking this medication
Minipress can intensify the effects of alcohol. Be careful of the amount you drink.

If Minipress is taken with certain other drugs, the effects of either could be increased, decreased, or altered. It is especially important that you check with your doctor before combining Minipress with the following:

Beta-blockers such as Inderal
Dextroamphetamine (Dexedrine)
Diuretics such as Dyazide
Ibuprofen (Motrin, Advil, others)
Other high blood pressure medications
Verapamil (Calan, Verelan)

Special information if you are pregnant or breastfeeding
The effects of Minipress during pregnancy have not been adequately studied. If you are pregnant or plan to become pregnant, notify your doctor immediately. Minipress appears in breast milk and can affect a nursing infant. If this medication is essential to your health, your doctor may advise you to discontinue breastfeeding until your treatment is finished.

Recommended dosage

ADULTS

Dosages of this drug should be adjusted by your doctor according to your response.

The usual starting dose is 1 milligram, 2 or 3 times per day.

The doctor may slowly increase the amount to as much as 20 milligrams per day, divided into smaller doses. The typical dose is 6 to 15 milligrams per day, divided into smaller doses. Although doses higher than 20 milligrams per day usually have no extra effect, some people may benefit from a daily dose of 40 milligrams, divided into smaller doses.

If Minipress is used with a diuretic or other high blood pressure drug, the dose can be reduced to 1 to 2 milligrams, 3 times a day.

CHILDREN

The safety and effectiveness of Minipress have not been established in children.

Overdosage
Any medication taken in excess can have serious consequences. If you suspect a Minipress overdose, seek medical treatment immediately.

■ *The symptoms of Minipress overdose may include:*
Extreme drowsiness, low blood pressure

MINOCIN

Pronounced: MIN-o-sin
Generic name: Minocycline hydrochloride
Other brand name: Dynacin

Why is this drug prescribed?

Minocin is a form of the antibiotic tetracycline. It is given to help treat many different kinds of infection, including:

Acne
Amebic dysentery
Anthrax
Cholera
Gonorrhea (when penicillin cannot be given)
Plague
Respiratory infections such as pneumonia
Rocky Mountain spotted fever
Syphilis (when penicillin cannot be given)
Urinary tract infections, rectal infections, and infections of the cervix
    caused by certain microbes

Most important fact about this drug

To help clear up your infection completely, keep taking Minocin for the full time of treatment, even if you begin to feel better after a few days. Minocin, like other antibiotics, works best when there is a constant amount in the body. To help keep the level constant, take the doses at evenly spaced times around the clock.

It's important to take Minocin exactly as your doctor prescribes. Skipping doses or not completing the full dosage schedule may decrease the drug's effectiveness and increase the chances of bacterial resistance to Minocin and similar antibiotics.

How should you take this medication?

You should take Minocin at least 1 hour before or 2 hours after meals. Take Minocin exactly as directed. Your doctor will prescribe it for a specific number of days according to the type of infection being treated; keep taking the medication until you have used it all up.

To reduce the risk of throat irritation, take the capsule and tablet forms of Minocin with plenty of fluids. Swallow the pellet-filled capsules whole.

You should avoid use of antacids that contain aluminum, calcium, or magnesium, such as Maalox and Mylanta, and iron preparations such as Feosol. If you must take these medicines, take them 2 to 3 hours before or after taking Minocin.

■ *If you miss a dose...*
Take it as soon as you remember, then space out evenly any remaining doses for that day. Never take 2 doses at the same time.

■ *Storage instructions...*
Store capsules, tablets, or liquid at room temperature. Keep capsules and tablets away from moist places and direct light. Do not freeze the liquid.

What side effects may occur?

Side effects cannot be anticipated. If any develop or change in intensity, inform your doctor as soon as possible. Only your doctor can determine if it is safe for you to continue taking Minocin.

■ *Side effects may include:*
Abdominal cramping, blisters, blood disorders, bruising, colitis, cough, diarrhea, difficulty swallowing, discolored skin or tooth enamel, dizziness, drowsiness, headache, heart inflammation, hives, indigestion, inflamed mouth or tongue, itching, hives, joint stiffness or swelling, kidney disorders, liver disorders, loss of appetite, muscle pain, nausea, pancreatitis, peeling skin, rash, ringing in the ears, seizures, sensitivity to light, severe allergic reactions, shortness of breath, swelling of face and neck, swollen lymph nodes, swollen mouth and throat, vaginal inflammation, vertigo, vomiting, wheezing

Why should this drug not be prescribed?

Do not take Minocin if you have ever had an allergic reaction to it or to any other tetracycline antibiotic.

Although Minocin may be given to kill meningococcal (spinal) bacteria in people who are carriers, it should not be given to treat actual meningococcal meningitis (inflammation in the spinal canal).

Minocin is not a first-choice drug for treating any staphylococcal (staph) infection.

Special warnings about this medication

If you have a kidney problem, a normal dose of Minocin may amount to an overdose for you and could cause liver damage. Use caution if you have a liver condition. Expect a lower than average dosage if you have a kidney problem. If you need to take Minocin for an extended period of time, your doctor may order frequent blood tests to make sure you are not getting too much of the drug.

Because Minocin may make you dizzy or light-headed or cause a whirling feeling, do not drive, climb, or perform hazardous tasks until you know how the medication affects you.

Minocin should not be given to children 8 years old or younger, since it may cause discoloration of the teeth. Occasionally, Minocin has also caused tooth discoloration in adults.

Like other tetracycline antibiotics, Minocin may cause a sensitivity to light, and you may sunburn very easily. Be careful in sun and under sunlamps. If your skin turns red and hot, stop taking Minocin immediately.

While taking Minocin you may be especially susceptible to infections, including fungus infections such as vaginal yeast infection. If you do get an infection, check with your doctor immediately.

If you get a headache and blurry vision while taking Minocin, or if an infant receiving Minocin develops bulging of the soft spots (fontanels) on the head, this could mean that the drug is causing a buildup of fluid within the skull. It is important to stop taking Minocin and see a doctor immediately.

Minocin liquid contains a sulfite that can cause severe allergic reactions in susceptible people.

Possible food and drug interactions when taking this medication

If Minocin is taken with certain other drugs, the effects of either could be increased, decreased, or altered. It is especially important to check with your doctor before combining Minocin with the following:

Antacids containing aluminum, calcium, or magnesium, such as
    Mylanta
Blood thinners such as Coumadin
Iron-containing preparations such as Feosol
Isotretinoin (Accutane)
Oral contraceptives
Penicillin (Pen-Vee K)

Special information if you are pregnant or breastfeeding

If you are pregnant or plan to become pregnant, inform your doctor immediately. If you take Minocin during the second half of pregnancy, it may cause permanent yellow, gray, or brown discoloration of your baby's teeth.

There is reason to believe that taking Minocin during pregnancy could also harm the baby in other ways. Therefore, Minocin should be taken during pregnancy only as a last resort. Because Minocin appears in breast milk and could harm the baby, it should not be taken by a woman who is breastfeeding. If this drug is essential to your health, your doctor may advise you to discontinue breastfeeding until treatment is finished.

Recommended dosage

ADULTS

The usual dosage of Minocin is 200 milligrams to start with, followed by 100 milligrams every 12 hours. If you need to take more frequent doses, your doctor may prescribe two or four 50-milligram capsules initially, and then one 50-milligram capsule 4 times daily.

The dosage and the length of time you take the drug can vary according to your condition and the specific infection.

CHILDREN ABOVE 8 YEARS OF AGE

The usual dosage of Minocin is 4 milligrams per 2.2 pounds of body weight to start, followed by 2 milligrams per 2.2 pounds every 12 hours, up to the usual adult dose.

Overdosage

Any medication taken in excess can have serious consequences. If you suspect symptoms of an overdose of Minocin, seek medical attention immediately.

■ *Symptoms of Minocin overdose may include:*
  Dizziness, nausea, vomiting

Minocycline See Minocin, page 867.

MIRADON

Pronounced: MIR-a-don
Generic name: Anisindione

Why is this drug prescribed?

Miradon is a blood thinner (an anticoagulant). It is used to prevent and treat blood clots in the veins. It is also used in the prevention and treatment of pulmonary embolism (a clot lodged in an artery serving the lungs), and in the treatment of certain serious heart conditions.

Miradon is prescribed only if you cannot take coumarin-type anticoagulants such as Coumadin.

Most important fact about this drug

Miradon is a powerful drug with serious potential side effects. The benefits of taking it must be weighed against the risks.

The worst potential side effects of Miradon include severe bleeding (hemorrhage) and destruction of skin tissue (necrosis) or gangrene. In occasional cases, hemorrhage and necrosis have led to death or permanent disability. Severe necrosis can result in removal of damaged tissue or amputation of a limb. Necrosis usually occurs within a few days of starting Miradon therapy. If it develops, the doctor will have to switch to a different type of blood thinner.

How should you take this medication?

The purpose of treatment with a blood thinner is to prevent abnormal clots from forming and cutting off the blood supply necessary for normal body function. To achieve this, treatment must maintain a delicate balance between too much clotting and too little, since a failure to clot could lead to uncontrolled bleeding and even death. It is very important, therefore, that you take this medication exactly as prescribed and that your doctor monitor your condition on a regular basis. Be especially careful to stick to the exact dosage schedule and to follow your doctor's directions for periodic blood tests.

Effective treatment with minimal complications depends on your co-operation and communication with your doctor. Many foods and drugs can significantly change the effectiveness of Miradon, so check with the doctor before starting or discontinuing any other medication or making any change in your diet, and do not stop taking this medication suddenly.

■ *If you miss a dose...*
Take it as soon as possible. If it is almost time for your next dose, skip the one you missed and go back to your regular schedule. Do not take 2 doses at once.

■ *Storage instructions...*
Store at room temperature.

What side effects may occur?

Side effects cannot be anticipated. If any develop or change in intensity, inform your doctor as soon as possible. Only your doctor can determine if it is safe for you to continue taking Miradon.

■ *Side effects may include:*
Abdominal cramps, abnormal healing of broken bones, anemia, blood disorders, blurred vision, diarrhea, fever, greasy stools, hair loss, headache, hemorrhage, hepatitis, hives, inability to urinate, kidney damage, liver damage, loss of appetite, lung inflammation, minor bleeding, mouth or throat ulcers, nausea, necrosis (gangrene), prolonged, painful erection, paralyzed eye muscle, purple toes, rash, red or peeling skin, sore mouth, sore throat, vomiting, yellowed skin and whites of eyes

Why should this drug not be prescribed?

You should not take Miradon if you have any condition that may increase the danger of hemorrhage, including:

A bleeding disorder or a tendency to hemorrhage, such as hemophilia, bleeding under the skin, or leukemia
A recent cerebral hemorrhage (bleeding stroke)
Aneurysm (balloon-like swelling of a blood vessel)
Bleeding, ulcers, or inflammation in the stomach or intestines
Continuous tube drainage of the small intestine
Eclampsia, a serious pregnancy disorder producing life-threatening convulsions, or preeclampsia, a toxic condition marked by high blood pressure that can lead to eclampsia

Infection or inflammation of the heart
Malnutrition or excessive loss of weight
Open wounds
Polyarthritis
Recent or planned brain, eye, prostate, or spinal surgery
Severely high blood pressure
Severe kidney or liver disease
Spinal puncture from regional or lumbar block anesthesia
Threatened miscarriage
Tumors
Vitamin C or K deficiency

This drug can damage a developing baby and should not be used during pregnancy.

Special warnings about this medication

Treatment with blood thinners may increase the risk that part of a blood clot will break away from the wall of an artery and lodge at another point, causing a blockage of the blood vessel. Tell your doctor if you or anyone in your family has a history of blood clots moving and causing blockages.

Notify your doctor immediately if you have any symptoms of abnormal bleeding, such as blood in urine; blood in stools or black, tarry stools; bleeding from gums or nose; patches of discoloration or bruises on the arms, legs, or toes; or excessive bleeding from minor cuts. Also tell the doctor about any other symptoms that may develop, such as fatigue, chills, or fever.

If you are taking Miradon, your doctor should periodically check the time it takes for your blood to start the clotting process (prothrombin time). Carefully follow your doctor's directions for taking the periodic clotting test. Your doctor also should do periodic urine and stool tests to monitor the side effects of this drug.

A number of things may affect your response to this drug, including your environment and your mental, medical, and nutritional state. Factors that may affect your sensitivity to this medication include hot weather, increased age, poor nutrition, vitamin K deficiency, intestinal disorders, high cholesterol levels, congestive heart failure or heart damage, diabetes, liver disorders, thyroid disorders, pregnancy, bowel sterilization, recent surgery, X-ray therapy, heredity, and the length of time you have been taking this medication.

Possible food and drug interactions when taking this medication

Starting or stopping any medication while taking Miradon may affect your body's response to the drug, requiring an adjustment in dosage. Check with your doctor before making any change in the drugs you take, whether prescription or nonprescription.

Certain foods also affect your body's response to Miradon, so get your doctor's approval for any change in your typical diet while taking Miradon, and for any vitamins or nutritional supplements you'd like to take.

Special information if you are pregnant or breastfeeding

Miradon must not be taken during pregnancy because it may cause a fatal hemorrhage or birth defects in the developing baby. If you become pregnant while taking Miradon, inform your doctor immediately.

Miradon appears in breast milk and could affect a nursing infant. Do not breastfeed while on Miradon therapy.

Recommended dosage

ADULTS

The usual doses at the start of therapy are 300 milligrams on the first day, 200 milligrams on the second day, and 100 milligrams on the third day. After the initial doses, you'll be maintained at a level of 25 to 250 milligrams a day. Your doctor will individualize the dosage of Miradon according to your sensitivity to the drug.

Overdosage

An overdose of Miradon is likely to cause abnormal bleeding.

■ *Symptoms of abnormal bleeding include:*
Bleeding from gums or nose, blood in urine or stools, excessive bleeding from minor cuts, patches of discoloration or bruises on the skin

If you suspect an overdose of Miradon, seek emergency medical attention immediately.

MIRALAX

Pronounced: MEER-uh-lacks
Generic name: Polyethylene glycol

Why is this drug prescribed?

MiraLax is a remedy for constipation. It works by retaining water in the stool, softening it and increasing the frequency of bowel movements. It may take up to 2 to 4 days to work.

Most important fact about this drug

Unless your doctor directs otherwise, do not use MiraLax for more than 2 weeks. Sustained, frequent, or excessive use can upset the body's chemical balance, and can lead to dependence on laxatives.

How should you take this medication?

Dissolve 1 capful or packet of MiraLax powder (17 grams) in 8 ounces of water, juice, soda, coffee, or tea.

■ *If you miss a dose...*
Take the forgotten dose as soon as you remember. However, if it is almost time for your next dose, skip the one you missed and return to your regular schedule. Do not take two doses at once.

■ *Storage instructions...*
Store at room temperature.

What side effects may occur?

Side effects cannot be anticipated. If any develop or change in intensity, tell your doctor as soon as possible. Only your doctor can determine if it is safe to continue using MiraLax.

■ *Side effects may include:*
Bloating, cramps, gas, nausea

High doses may cause diarrhea and excessive frequency.

Why should this drug not be prescribed?

Do not take MiraLax if there's any chance that you have a bowel obstruction. Symptoms suggesting an obstruction include abdominal pain or distention, nausea, and vomiting.

Also avoid MiraLax if you are allergic to its active ingredient, polyethylene glycol.

Special warnings about this medication

Remember that MiraLax is not for prolonged use. To promote regularity, make sure your diet includes plenty of fiber and fluids, and get regular exercise.

Possible food and drug interactions when taking this medication

No interactions have been reported.

Special information if you are pregnant or breastfeeding

Nothing is known about the effects of MiraLax during pregnancy. If you are pregnant or plan to become pregnant, inform your doctor immediately. MiraLax should be used only if clearly needed.

There is no information on the use of MiraLax while nursing. Check with your doctor if you plan to breastfeed.

Recommended dosage

ADULTS

The usual dose is 17 grams daily.

Overdosage

Any medication taken in excess can have serious consequences. If you suspect an overdose, seek medical attention immediately.

■ *Symptoms of MiraLax overdose may include:*
Dehydration, diarrhea

MIRAPEX

Pronounced: MERE-a-pecks
Generic name: Pramipexole dihydrochloride

Why is this drug prescribed?

Although it is not a cure, Mirapex eases the symptoms of Parkinson's disease—a progressive disorder marked by muscle rigidity, weakness, shaking, tremor, and eventually difficulty with walking and talking. Parkinson's disease results from a shortage of the chemical messenger dopamine in certain areas of the brain. Mirapex is believed to work by boosting the action of whatever dopamine is available. The drug can be used with other Parkinson's medications such as Eldepryl, Sinemet, and Larodopa.

Most important fact about this drug

If you are taking Sinemet or Larodopa, Mirapex may allow a reduction in your dosage. And if you suffer from the "on-off" effect that often develops during Parkinson's therapy (symptom-free periods alternating with severe attacks), Mirapex may extend the good "on" times and shorten your "off" periods.

How should you take this medication?

Take Mirapex exactly as prescribed. If it makes you nauseous, try taking it with food.

When discontinuing Mirapex therapy, it's best to do it gradually. Your doctor will tell you how to taper your dose over a week's time.

■ *If you miss a dose...*
Take it as soon as you remember. If it is almost time for your next dose, skip the one you missed and go back to your regular schedule. Do not take 2 doses at the same time.

■ *Storage instructions...*
Store at room temperature; protect from light.

What side effects may occur?

Side effects cannot be anticipated. If any develop or change in intensity, inform your doctor as soon as possible. Only your doctor can determine if it is safe for you to continue taking Mirapex.

■ *Side effects may include:*
Abnormal dreams, arthritis, chest pain, confusion, constipation, decreased sensitivity to touch, difficulty breathing, difficulty walking, dizziness, dizziness upon standing, drowsiness, dry mouth, hallucina-

tions, increased muscle tone, increased urination, insomnia, involuntary movement (jerky motions), lack of appetite, memory loss, nasal inflammation, nausea, swelling, urinary tract infections, vision abnormalities, weakness

Why should this drug not be prescribed?
If Mirapex gives you an allergic reaction, you'll be unable to use it.

Special warnings about this drug
Mirapex can cause your blood pressure to drop when you first stand up, resulting in symptoms such as dizziness, nausea, fainting, blackouts, and sometimes sweating. To avoid or reduce these symptoms, try to stand up slowly, especially at the beginning of treatment with Mirapex.

Mirapex can cause drowsiness and may trigger hallucinations, especially if you are over 65 or have an advanced case of Parkinson's. You may even fall asleep—without warning and without feeling drowsy—while performing everyday activities. Check with your doctor immediately if you find that you're getting drowsy or falling asleep while eating, talking, or watching television. Do not drive a car or undertake other dangerous activities until you've spoken with the doctor. Be especially cautious when taking other drugs that cause sleepiness.

If you have a kidney condition, make sure the doctor is aware of it. You'll probably need regular blood tests to check your kidney function, and your dosage of Mirapex may have to be reduced.

In very rare cases, Mirapex may cause muscle wasting. If you develop muscle aches or soreness after you start Mirapex, be sure to tell your doctor. Also alert your doctor if you notice any changes in your eyesight.

Possible food and drug interactions when taking this medication
If Mirapex is taken with certain other drugs, the effects of either could be increased, decreased, or altered. It is especially important to check with your doctor before combining Mirapex with the following:

Carbidopa/levodopa (Sinemet)
Cimetidine (Tagamet)
Diltiazem (Cardizem, Dilacor XR)
Major tranquilizers such as Compazine, Haldol, Mellaril, Navane, Prolixin, Stelazine, and Thorazine
Metoclopramide (Reglan)
Quinidine (Quinidex, Quinaglute)
Quinine
Ranitidine (Zantac)
Sedatives and tranquilizers such as chloral hydrate, codeine products, Dalmane, Halcion, and phenobarbital
Triamterene (Dyrenium)
Verapamil (Calan, Isoptin)

Combining Mirapex with Sinemet or Larodopa sometimes triggers twitching and jerky movements. If this happens, tell your doctor. A reduction in your dose of Sinemet or Larodopa may solve the problem.

Special information if you are pregnant or breastfeeding

The effects of Mirapex during pregnancy have not been adequately studied, so it's best to avoid it if you're expecting. If you are pregnant or plan to become pregnant, inform your doctor immediately.

It is not known whether Mirapex appears in breast milk. If the drug is considered essential to your health, your doctor may advise you to stop breastfeeding while taking the medication.

Recommended dosage

ADULTS

The usual starting dose is 0.125 milligram 3 times a day. If necessary, your doctor may increase the dose every 5 to 7 days until the maximum dose of 4.5 milligrams a day is reached. Dosage is usually increased gradually to minimize the drug's potential side effects. If you have kidney disease, the doctor will keep the dosage quite low.

CHILDREN

The safety and effectiveness of Mirapex in children have not been established.

Overdosage

Although there is no information on Mirapex overdose, any medication taken in excess can have dangerous consequences. If you suspect an overdose, seek medical attention immediately.

Mircette *See Oral Contraceptives, page 1000.*

Mirtazapine *See Remeron, page 1232.*

Misoprostol *See Cytotec, page 377.*

MOBAN

Pronounced: MOW-ban
Generic name: Molindone hydrochloride

Why is this drug prescribed?

Moban is used in the treatment of schizophrenia, the crippling psychological disorder that causes its victims to lose touch with reality, often triggering hallucinations, delusions, and disorganized thought.

Most important fact about this drug

Moban can cause tardive dyskinesia, a condition marked by involuntary movements in the face and body, including chewing movements, puckering, puffing the cheeks, and sticking out the tongue. This condition may be permanent and appears to be most common among the elderly, especially elderly women. Ask your doctor for more information about this possible risk.

How should you take this medication?

Take Moban exactly as prescribed. Do not take with alcohol.

■ *If you miss a dose...*
Take it as soon as you remember. If it is almost time for your next dose, skip the one you missed and go back to your regular schedule. Do not take 2 doses at once.

■ *Storage instructions...*
Store at room temperature. Protect from light.

What side effects may occur?

Side effects cannot be anticipated. If any develop or change in intensity, inform your doctor as soon as possible. Only your doctor can determine if it is safe for you to continue taking Moban.

■ *Side effects may include:*
Blurred vision, depression, drowsiness (especially at the start of therapy), dry mouth, euphoria, hyperactivity, nausea, Parkinson's-like movements, restlessness

Why should this drug not be prescribed?

Moban should not be combined with alcohol, barbiturates (sleep aids), narcotics (painkillers), or other substances that slow down the nervous system, nor should it be given to anyone in a comatose state. Moban cannot be used by anyone who is hypersensitive to the drug. The concentrate form of Moban contains a sulfite that may cause life-threatening allergic reactions in some people, especially in those with asthma.

Special warnings about this medication

Drugs such as Moban can cause a potentially fatal condition called Neuroleptic Malignant Syndrome (NMS). Symptoms include high fever, rigid muscles, irregular pulse or blood pressure, rapid heartbeat, excessive perspiration, and changes in heart rhythm. If you develop these symptoms, contact your doctor immediately. Moban should be discontinued.

Moban should be used with caution if you have ever had breast cancer. The drug stimulates production of a hormone that promotes the growth of certain types of tumors.

Because this drug may cause drowsiness, do not participate in activities that require full alertness, such as driving or operating machinery, until you are sure how this medicine affects you.

Moban may mask signs of a brain tumor or intestinal blockage. It causes increased activity in some people. On rare occasions, it causes seizures.

Possible food and drug interactions when taking this medication

Remember that Moban must never be combined with alcohol, barbiturates, or narcotics. In addition, Moban tablets contain calcium, which may interfere with the absorption of tetracycline antibiotics (Achromycin V, Sumycin) and phenytoin (Dilantin).

Special information if you are pregnant or breastfeeding

The safety and effectiveness of Moban during pregnancy have not been adequately studied. If you are pregnant or planning to become pregnant, tell your doctor immediately. Moban should be used during pregnancy only if the benefits outweigh the potential risks.

It is not known whether Moban appears in breast milk. Check with your doctor before deciding to breastfeed.

Recommended dosage

ADULTS

The usual starting dose is 50 to 75 milligrams a day. Your doctor may increase the dose to 100 milligrams a day after 3 or 4 days of treatment.

The long-term maintenance dose depends on your body's response to the medication. The usual maintenance dose for treatment of mild symptoms is 5 to 15 milligrams taken 3 or 4 times a day. For moderate symptoms, it is 10 to 25 milligrams taken 3 or 4 times a day. For severe symptoms, up to 225 milligrams a day may be prescribed. Older adults generally take lower dosages of Moban.

CHILDREN

The safety and effectiveness of Moban in children under age 12 have not been established.

Overdosage

Any medication taken in excess can have serious consequences. If you suspect an overdose, seek medical help immediately.

MOBIC

Pronounced: MOH-bik
Generic name: Meloxicam

Why is this drug prescribed?

Mobic is a nonsteroidal anti-inflammatory drug (NSAID) in prescription form. It is used to relieve the pain and stiffness of osteoarthritis.

Most important fact about this drug

You should have frequent checkups by your doctor if you take Mobic regularly. Like other nonsteroidal anti-inflammatory drugs, Mobic can cause ulcers or internal bleeding that occurs without warning.

How should you take this medication?

Mobic may be taken with or without food.

■ *If you miss a dose...*
Take it as soon as you remember. If it is almost time for your next dose, skip the one you missed and go back to your regular schedule. Never take 2 doses at once.

■ *Storage instructions...*
Store at room temperature in a tightly closed container. Keep away from moisture.

What side effects may occur?

Side effects cannot be anticipated. If any develop or change in intensity, inform your doctor as soon as possible. Only your doctor can determine if it is safe for you to continue taking Mobic.

■ *Side effects may include:*
Diarrhea, flu-like symptoms, indigestion, nausea

Why should this drug not be prescribed?

Do not take Mobic if you have ever had an allergic reaction to another NSAID such as aspirin, ibuprofen (Advil, Motrin), or naproxen (Aleve, Naprosyn), or have had asthma attacks or skin eruptions caused by drugs of this type. Make sure that your doctor is aware of any drug reactions that you may have experienced.

Special warnings about this medication

Serious, potentially fatal allergic reactions are possible if you are sensitive to aspirin or other NSAIDs, especially if you have asthma. Seek medical help immediately if you experience difficulty breathing or develop hives while taking this medication.

NSAIDs may trigger ulcers, inflammation, bleeding, and perforation of the stomach or intestines, especially if you're an older adult or you've had such problems in the past. The risk increases if you're also taking steroid medications or a blood-thinning drug, or smoke tobacco or drink alcohol. The chances of a problem also increase the longer you take the drug. Check with your doctor immediately if you develop any stomach or intestinal problems.

Because Mobic can cause liver or kidney problems in some people, it should be used with great caution if you already have severe liver or kidney disease, or are suffering from dehydration. Stop taking the drug and call your doctor immediately if you notice these warning signs of liver trouble: nausea, fatigue, drowsiness, itching, yellowish skin, flu-like symptoms, and pain in the upper right abdomen.

Mobic may cause anemia. It can also cause water retention, so you should use it with caution if you have high blood pressure or heart disease. Alert your doctor if you develop swelling or weight gain. Mobic also tends to slow the clotting process. If you have a clotting disorder or are taking blood thinners, your doctor should monitor you carefully.

Mobic's safety in children under 18 has not been verified.

Possible food and drug interactions when taking this medication

If Mobic is taken with certain other drugs, the effects of either could be increased, decreased, or altered. It is especially important to check with your doctor before combining Mobic with the following:

Aspirin
Blood pressure and heart medications called ACE inhibitors,
   including Accupril, Aceon, Altace, Prinivil, Univasc, and Zestril
Blood-thinning drugs such as Coumadin
Furosemide (Lasix)
Lithium (Lithonate)

Special information if you are pregnant or breastfeeding

It is possible that Mobic could cause harm during pregnancy, and it is best to avoid it. Under no circumstances should you take it late in a pregnancy.

Mobic may appear in breast milk and could cause serious side effects in the infant. Do not take Mobic while nursing; discontinue the drug or stop breastfeeding.

Recommended dosage

ADULTS

The usual dosage is 7.5 milligrams once a day. If necessary, your doctor may increase the dose to 15 milligrams a day. Due to the risk of side effects, he should limit dosage to the lowest effective amount, and prescribe it for the shortest possible time.

Overdosage

Any medication taken in excess can have serious consequences. If you suspect an overdose, seek medical attention immediately.

■ *Typical symptoms of Mobic overdose include:*
   Drowsiness, nausea, stomach pain and bleeding, vomiting
■ *Symptoms of massive Mobic overdose include:*
   Breathing difficulties, coma, convulsions, heart attack

Modafinil *See Provigil, page 1192.*

Modicon *See Oral Contraceptives, page 1000.*

MODURETIC
Pronounced: mod-your-ET-ik
Generic ingredients: Amiloride, Hydrochlorothiazide

Why is this drug prescribed?
Moduretic is a diuretic combination used in the treatment of high blood pressure and congestive heart failure, conditions which require the elimination of excess fluid (water) from the body. When used for high blood pressure, Moduretic can be used alone or with other high blood pressure medications. Diuretics help your body produce and eliminate more urine, which helps lower blood pressure. Amiloride, one of the ingredients, helps minimize the potassium loss that can be caused by the other component, hydrochlorothiazide.

Most important fact about this drug
If you have high blood pressure, you must take Moduretic regularly for it to be effective. Since blood pressure declines gradually, it may be several weeks before you get the full benefit of Moduretic; and you must continue taking it even if you are feeling well. Moduretic does not cure high blood pressure; it merely keeps it under control.

How should you take this medication?
Take this medication with food.

Take Moduretic exactly as prescribed by your doctor. Stopping Moduretic suddenly could cause your condition to worsen.

■ *If you miss a dose...*
Take the forgotten dose as soon as you remember. If it is almost time for your next does, skip the one you missed and go back to your regular schedule. Never take a double dose.

■ *Storage instructions...*
Store at room temperature. Keep this medication in the container it came in, tightly closed, and protected from moisture, light, and freezing.

What side effects may occur?
Side effects cannot be anticipated. If any develop or change in intensity, inform your doctor as soon as possible. Only your doctor can determine if it is safe for you to continue taking Moduretic.

■ *Side effects may include:*
Diarrhea, dizziness, elevated potassium levels, fatigue, headache, irregular heartbeat, itching, leg pain, loss of appetite, nausea, rash, shortness of breath, stomach and intestinal pain, weakness

Why should this drug not be prescribed?

If you are unable to urinate or have serious kidney disease, or if you have high potassium levels in your blood, you should not take this medication.

If you are sensitive to or have ever had an allergic reaction to amiloride, hydrochlorothiazide or similar drugs, or if you are sensitive to other sulfonamide-derived drugs, you should not take this medication. Make sure your doctor is aware of any drug reactions you may have experienced.

Special warnings about this medication

Potassium supplements, potassium-containing salt substitutes, and other diuretics (such as Dyazide) that minimize loss of potassium should not be used while you are taking Moduretic unless your doctor specifically says otherwise. You should also limit your consumption of potassium-rich foods such as bananas, prunes, raisins, orange juice, and whole and skim milk. Ask your doctor for advice on how much of these foods to consume.

If you are taking Moduretic, a complete assessment of your kidney function should be done; kidney function should continue to be monitored.

If you are taking an ACE-inhibitor type of blood pressure medication such as Vasotec, this drug should be used with extreme caution.

If you have liver disease, diabetes, gout, or collagen vascular disease (lupus erythematosus), Moduretic should be used with caution.

If you have bronchial asthma or a history of allergies, you may be at risk for an allergic reaction to this medication.

Dehydration, excessive sweating, severe diarrhea, or vomiting could deplete your fluids and cause your blood pressure to become too low. Be careful when exercising and in hot weather.

Notify your doctor or dentist that you are taking Moduretic if you have a medical emergency or before you have surgery.

Possible food and drug interactions when taking this medication

Moduretic may increase the effects of alcohol. Avoid alcohol while taking this medication.

If Moduretic is taken with certain other drugs, the effects of either could be increased, decreased, or altered. It is especially important to check with your doctor before combining Moduretic with the following:

ACE inhibitors such as Vasotec
Barbiturates such as phenobarbital
Cholestyramine (Questran)
Colestipol (Colestid)
Corticosteroids such as prednisone
Cyclosporine (Sandimmune, Neoral)
Insulin

Lithium (Eskalith, Lithobid)
Muscle relaxants such as tubocurarine
Narcotics such as Percocet
Nonsteroidal anti-inflammatory drugs such as Naprosyn
Norepinephrine (Levophed)
Oral drugs for treating diabetes such as Micronase, DiaBeta
Other high blood pressure medications
Tacrolimus (Prograf)

Special information if you are pregnant or breastfeeding

The effects of Moduretic during pregnancy have not been adequately studied. If you are pregnant or plan to become pregnant, inform your doctor immediately. Moduretic appears in breast milk and could affect a nursing infant. If this medication is essential to your health, your doctor may advise you to discontinue breastfeeding until your treatment is finished.

Recommended dosage

Your doctor will tailor the dosage to meet your individual requirements, taking into consideration other medical conditions you may have and other medications you may be taking.

ADULTS

The usual starting dose is 1 tablet per day, which may be increased to 2 tablets per day taken at the same time or separately.

CHILDREN

The safety and effectiveness of Moduretic have not been established in children.

Overdosage

Any medication taken in excess can cause symptoms of overdose. If you suspect an overdose, seek medical attention immediately.

No specific information on symptoms of Moduretic overdose is available, but dehydration might be expected.

Moexipril *See Univasc, page 1529.*

Moexipril with Hydrochlorothiazide *See Uniretic, page 1526.*

Molindone *See Moban, page 877.*

Mometasone furoate *See Elocon, page 509.*

Mometasone furoate monohydrate *See Nasonex, page 921.*

MONISTAT

Pronounced: MON-ih-stat
Generic name: Miconazole nitrate

Why is this drug prescribed?

Monistat is available in several formulations, including Monistat 3 vaginal suppositories, Monistat 7 vaginal cream and suppositories, and Monistat-Derm skin cream. Monistat's active ingredient, miconazole, fights fungal infections.

Monistat 3 and Monistat 7 are used for vaginal yeast infections. Monistat-Derm is used for skin infections such as athlete's foot, ringworm, jock itch, yeast infection on the skin (cutaneous candidiasis), and tinea versicolor (a common skin condition that produces patches of white, tan, or brown finely flaking skin over the neck and trunk).

Most important fact about this drug

Keep using this medicine regularly for the full time of the treatment, even if the infection seems to have disappeared. If you stop too soon, the infections could return. You should continue using the vaginal forms of the medicine even during your menstrual period.

How should you use this medication?

Use this medication exactly as prescribed.

Keep all forms of this medicine away from your eyes.

Before applying Monistat-Derm to your skin, be sure to wash your hands. Massage the medication gently into the affected area and the surrounding skin.

To administer the vaginal cream or suppository:

1. Load the applicator to the fill line with cream or unwrap a tablet, wet it with warm water, and place it in the applicator as shown in the instructions you received with the product.
2. Lie on your back with your knees drawn up.
3. Gently insert the application high into the vagina and push the plunger.
4. Withdraw the applicator and discard it if disposable, or wash it with soap and water.

To keep the vaginal medication from getting on your clothing, wear a sanitary napkin. Do not use tampons because they will absorb the medicine. Wear cotton underwear—avoid synthetic fabrics such as rayon or nylon. Do not douche unless your doctor tells you to do so.

Dry the genital area thoroughly after a shower, bath, or swim. Change out of a wet bathing suit or damp workout clothes as soon as possible. Yeast is less likely to flourish in a dry environment.

Do not scratch if you can help it. Scratching can cause more irritation and can spread the infection.

■ *If you miss a dose...*
Make up for it as soon as you remember. However, if it is almost time for your next dose, skip the one you missed and go back to your regular schedule.

■ *Storage instructions...*
Store at room temperature.

What side effects may occur?

Side effects cannot be anticipated. If any develop or change in intensity, inform your doctor. Only your doctor can determine whether it is safe for you to continue taking Monistat.

■ *Side effects may include:*
Burning sensation, cramping, headaches, hives, irritation, rash, vulval or vaginal itching

Why should this drug not be prescribed?

If you have ever had an allergic reaction to or are sensitive to miconazole nitrate, you should not use this medication. Make sure your doctor is aware of any drug reactions you have experienced.

Special warnings about this medication

If symptoms persist, or if an irritation or allergic reaction develops while you are using Monistat, notify your doctor.

The hydrogenated vegetable oil base of Monistat 3 may interact with the latex in vaginal diaphragms, so concurrent use of these two products is not recommended.

Your doctor may recommend Monistat 7 vaginal cream if you are using a diaphragm. However, you should be aware that the mineral oil in the vaginal cream can weaken the latex in condoms and diaphragms, making them less reliable for prevention of pregnancy or sexually transmitted disease.

If you are using Monistat 3 or Monistat 7 suppositories, you should either avoid sexual intercourse or make sure your partner uses a condom.

Do not give Monistat 7 to girls less than 12 years of age. Also avoid using Monistat 7 if you have any of the following symptoms:

Fever above 100 degrees Fahrenheit orally
Foul-smelling vaginal discharge
Pain in the lower abdomen, back, or either shoulder

If these symptoms develop while you are using Monistat 7, stop treatment and contact your doctor right away. You may have a more serious infection.

If the infection fails to improve or worsens within 3 days, you do not obtain complete relief within 7 days, or symptoms return within 2 months, you may have something other than a yeast infection.

Possible food and drug interactions when taking this medication
No interactions have been reported.

Special information if you are pregnant or breastfeeding
Unless you are directed to do so by your doctor, do not use Monistat during the first trimester (three months) of pregnancy because it is absorbed in small amounts from the vagina. It is not known whether miconazole appears in breast milk. If Monistat is essential to your health, your doctor may advise you to discontinue breastfeeding until your treatment with this medication is finished.

Recommended dosage

MONISTAT 7 VAGINAL CREAM

The usual daily dose is 1 applicatorful inserted into the vagina at bedtime for 7 consecutive days.

MONISTAT 7 VAGINAL SUPPOSITORIES

The usual daily dose is 1 suppository inserted into the vagina at bedtime for 7 consecutive days.

MONISTAT-DERM

For jock itch, ringworm, athlete's foot, or yeast infection of the skin, apply a thin layer of Monistat-Derm over the affected area morning and night. For tinea versicolor, apply a thin layer over the affected area once daily.

Overdosage
Overdose of Monistat has not been reported. However any medication used in excess can have serious consequences. If you suspect an overdose, seek medical attention immediately.

Monoket *See Imdur, page 667.*

MONOPRIL
Pronounced: MON-oh-prill
Generic name: Fosinopril sodium

Why is this drug prescribed?
Monopril is a high blood pressure medication known as an ACE inhibitor. It is effective when used alone or in combination with other medications for the treatment of high blood pressure. Monopril is also prescribed for heart failure.

Monopril works by preventing the conversion of a chemical in your blood called angiotensin I into a more potent substance that increases salt and water retention in your body. Monopril also enhances blood flow in your circulatory system.

Most important fact about this drug
You must take Monopril regularly for it to be effective. Since blood pressure declines gradually, it may be several weeks before you get the full benefit of Monopril; and you must continue taking it even if you are feeling well. Monopril does not cure high blood pressure; it merely keeps it under control.

How should you take this medication?
Monopril is best taken 1 hour before meals; but it can be taken with food if it upsets your stomach.
   Take this medication exactly as prescribed by your doctor.

■ *If you miss a dose…*
   Suddenly stopping Monopril could cause your blood pressure to increase. If you forget to take a dose, take it as soon as you remember. If it is almost time for your next dose, skip the one you missed and go back to your regular schedule. Never take 2 doses at the same time.
■ *Storage instructions…*
   Store Monopril at room temperature in a tightly closed container to protect the medication from moisture.

What side effects may occur?
Side effects cannot be anticipated. If any develop or change in intensity, inform your doctor as soon as possible. Only your doctor can determine if it is safe for you to continue taking Monopril.

WHEN TAKEN FOR HIGH BLOOD PRESSURE

■ *Side effects may include:*
   Cough, dizziness, nausea, vomiting

WHEN TAKEN FOR HEART FAILURE

■ *Side effects may include:*
   Chest pain, cough, dizziness, low blood pressure, muscle and bone pain

Why should this drug not be prescribed?
If you are sensitive to or have ever had an allergic reaction to Monopril or other ACE inhibitors such as Accupril or Zestril, you should not take this medication. Make sure that your doctor is aware of any drug reactions that you have experienced.

Special warnings about this medication

If you develop a sore throat or fever, you should contact your doctor immediately. It could indicate a more serious illness.

If you develop swelling of your face, lips, tongue, or throat, or arms and legs, or have difficulty swallowing, you should stop taking Monopril and contact your doctor immediately. You may need emergency treatment.

Make sure your doctor knows about any kidney or liver problems you may have. If you notice your skin or the whites of your eyes turning yellow, stop taking Monopril and contact your doctor immediately.

Your kidney function should be monitored while you are taking Monopril for either high blood pressure or heart failure. If you have heart failure and your kidneys are not functioning properly, you may develop low blood pressure. Also, certain blood tests may be needed if you have a disease of the connective tissue.

If you are taking high doses of a diuretic along with Monopril, you may develop excessively low blood pressure.

You may experience light-headedness while taking Monopril, especially during the first few days of therapy. If this occurs, notify your doctor. If you actually faint, discontinue the use of this medication and notify your doctor immediately.

Do not use potassium-containing salt substitutes or potassium supplements without consulting your doctor.

If you have heart failure, this drug should be started under close medical supervision. Your doctor should continue to monitor your progress for the first 2 weeks of treatment and whenever your dosage is increased.

Excessive sweating, dehydration, severe diarrhea, or vomiting could lead to excessive loss of water and cause your blood pressure to drop dangerously. Take precautions to avoid excessive water loss while exercising.

This drug should be used with caution if you are on dialysis. There have been reports of extreme allergic reactions during dialysis in people taking ACE inhibitors such as Monopril. There have also been reports of severe allergic reactions in people given bee or wasp venom to protect against stings.

Possible food and drug interactions when taking this medication

If Monopril is taken with certain other drugs, the effects of either could be increased, decreased, or altered. It is especially important to check with your doctor before combining Monopril with the following:

Antacids such as Mylanta and Maalox
Lithium (Eskalith, Lithobid)
Potassium preparations such as K+10 and K-Lyte
Potassium-sparing diuretics such as Moduretic and Aldactone
Thiazide diuretics such as Diucardin and Diuril

Special information if you are pregnant or breastfeeding

ACE inhibitors such as Monopril have been shown to cause injury and even death in the developing baby when used in pregnancy during the second or third trimesters. If you are pregnant your doctor should discontinue the use of this medication as soon as possible. If you plan to become pregnant and are taking Monopril, contact your doctor immediately to discuss the potential hazard to your unborn child. Monopril appears in breast milk and could affect a nursing infant. If this medication is essential to your health, your doctor may advise you to discontinue breastfeeding until your treatment with this medication is finished.

Recommended dosage

ADULTS

High Blood Pressure

The usual initial dose is 10 milligrams taken once a day, either alone or added to a diuretic. Dosage, after blood pressure is adjusted, should be 20 to 40 milligrams a day in a single dose. For some patients, the doctor may divide the daily total into several smaller doses.

Diuretic use should, if possible, be stopped before using Monopril. If not, your physician may give an initial dose of 10 milligrams under his supervision before any further medication is prescribed.

Heart Failure

The usual starting dose is 10 milligrams once a day, with diuretics and possibly digitalis. Your doctor will gradually increase the dose to one that works for you—usually between 20 milligrams daily and the maximum dose of 40 milligrams per day. If your kidneys are impaired you will probably start with a dose of 5 milligrams.

CHILDREN

The safety and effectiveness of Monopril have not been established in children.

Overdosage

Any medication taken in excess can have serious consequences. If you suspect an overdose, seek medical attention immediately.

The primary effect of a Monopril overdose is likely to be a sudden drop in blood pressure.

MONOPRIL-HCT

Pronounced: MON-oh-prill
Generic ingredients: Fosinopril sodium, Hydrochlorothiazide

Why is this drug prescribed?

Monopril-HCT is used to treat high blood pressure. It usually is prescribed after other blood pressure medications have failed to do the job. Monopril-HCT combines two types of blood pressure medicine. The first, fosinopril sodium, is an ACE (angiotensin-converting enzyme) inhibitor. It works by preventing a chemical in your blood called angiotensin I from converting into a more potent form (angiotensin II) that increases salt and water retention in your body and causes blood vessels to constrict—two actions that tend to increase blood pressure. To aid in clearing water from the body, Monopril-HCT also contains hydrochlorothiazide, a diuretic that promotes the production of urine.

Most important fact about this drug

You must take Monopril-HCT regularly for it to be effective, and you must continue taking it even if you are feeling well. Like other blood pressure medications, Monopril-HCT does not cure high blood pressure; it merely keeps it under control.

How should you take this medication?

Take this medication exactly as prescribed. Do not take it within 2 hours of taking an antacid.

■ *If you miss a dose...*
Take it as soon as you remember. If it is almost time for your next dose, skip the one you missed and go back to your regular schedule. Do not take 2 doses at once.

■ *Storage instructions...*
Store Monopril-HCT at room temperature in a tightly closed container and protect from moisture.

What side effects may occur?

Side effects cannot be anticipated. If any develop or change in intensity, inform your doctor as soon as possible. Only your doctor can determine if it is safe for you to continue taking.

■ *Side effects may include:*
Dizziness, dry cough, fatigue, headache

Why should this drug not be prescribed?

You should not take Monopril-HCT if you have difficulty urinating. You'll also need to avoid this medication if you are allergic to fosinopril, to any other ACE inhibitor, to hydrochlorothiazide, or to sulfa drugs.

Special warnings about this medication

If you develop swelling of your face, lips, tongue, or throat, or have difficulty breathing, stop taking Monopril-HCT and contact your doctor immediately. You may need emergency treatment.

Excessive sweating, inadequate fluid intake, severe diarrhea, or vomiting could cause you to lose too much water, resulting in a dangerous drop in blood pressure. Be careful in hot weather and whenever exercising.

If you develop a sore throat or fever, you should contact your doctor immediately. It could be a sign of a serious side effect—a decline in the number of infection-fighting white blood cells in your system.

Contact your doctor if you develop dry mouth, thirst, weakness, drowsiness, muscle pain or tiredness, rapid heartbeat, reduced urination, or nausea and vomiting. These side effects could be symptoms of a serious chemical imbalance.

You may experience light-headedness while taking Monopril-HCT, especially during the first few days of therapy. If this occurs, notify your doctor. If you actually faint, stop taking this medication and contact your doctor immediately.

If you have kidney disease or severe congestive heart failure, Monopril-HCT may interfere with your kidney function. The doctor will monitor your kidneys under these conditions. If you have congestive heart failure, you'll also be watched for excessively low blood pressure, especially during the first 2 weeks of treatment and when the dosage is increased.

Monopril-HCT should be used with caution if you have a history of liver disorders. If you notice your skin or the whites of your eyes turning yellow, contact your doctor immediately.

Monopril-HCT occasionally may trigger diabetes, lupus, or gout. Use it with caution if you have any of these conditions.

If you are taking bee or wasp venom to desensitize yourself to stings, you may have a severe allergic reaction to Monopril-HCT. This medication is more likely to cause an allergic reaction if you have a history of allergy or bronchial asthma. ACE inhibitors such as Monopril-HCT have also been known to cause extreme allergic reactions during kidney dialysis.

The safety and effectiveness of Monopril-HCT in children have not been established.

Possible food and drug interactions when taking this medication

If Monopril-HCT is taken with certain other drugs, the effects of either could be increased, decreased, or altered. It is especially important to check with your doctor before combining Monopril-HCT with the following:

Antacids such as Mylanta and Maalox
Cholestyramine (Questran)
Colestipol (Colestid)
Insulin

Lithium (Eskalith, Lithobid)
Methenamine (Urised)
Nonsteroidal anti-inflammatory drugs such as Naprosyn, Advil, and
  Motrin
Other blood pressure medications
Potassium supplements such as K-Lyte and K-Tab
Salt substitutes containing potassium
Tubocurarine

Special information if you are pregnant or breastfeeding

ACE inhibitors such as Monopril-HCT have been shown to cause injury
and even death in the developing baby when used during the second or
third trimesters of pregnancy. If you become pregnant, Monopril-HCT
should be discontinued as soon as possible. If you plan to become pregnant, discuss the situation with your doctor.

Monopril-HCT appears in breast milk and could affect a nursing infant.
You'll need to make a choice between breastfeeding your baby and continuing your therapy with Monopril-HCT.

Recommended dosage

ADULTS

Monopril-HCT tablets are available in two strengths. Based on your previous response to blood pressure medication, your doctor will prescribe
the dosage that brings your blood pressure into the desired range.

Overdosage

Any medication taken in excess can have serious consequences. If you
suspect an overdose, seek medical help immediately.

■ *Symptoms of Monopril-HCT overdose may include:*
  Dehydration, irregular heartbeat, low blood pressure

Montelukast See Singulair, page 1315.

MONUROL
Pronounced: MON-your-all
Generic name: Fosfomycin tromethamine

Why is this drug prescribed?

Monurol is an antibiotic used to treat bladder infections (cystitis) in women.

Most important fact about this drug

You need take only one dose of Monurol. Additional doses won't speed a
cure, but will make side effects more likely. If your symptoms do not improve in 2 to 3 days, contact your physician.

How should you take this medication?

Monurol is packaged in a sachet, which contains granules of the drug. Open the sachet and pour the contents into 3 or 4 ounces (half a cup) of cold water, stir to dissolve, and drink immediately. Do not use hot water. Do not take the drug in its dry form. The solution can be taken with or without food.

■ *If you miss a dose...*
Only 1 dose is needed.
■ *Storage instructions...*
Store at room temperature.

What side effects may occur?

Side effects cannot be anticipated. If any develop or change in intensity, inform your doctor as soon as possible. Only your doctor can determine if it is safe for you to continue taking Monurol.

■ *More common side effects may include:*
Diarrhea, dizziness, headache, indigestion, nausea, vaginal inflammation, weakness

Why should this drug not be prescribed?

If you have an allergic reaction to Monurol, avoid it in the future. The drug is used only for bladder infections, not for infections of the kidney (pyelonephritis).

Special warnings about this medication

Call your doctor if symptoms fail to improve within 2 to 3 days. You may need a different prescription.

Possible food and drug interactions when taking this medication

Check with your doctor before combining Monurol with Reglan, a drug that speeds digestion. Reglan and similar drugs will reduce Monurol's effectiveness.

Special information if you are pregnant or breastfeeding

There have been no adequate studies in pregnant women; and it is not known whether Monurol appears in breast milk. If you are pregnant or plan to become pregnant, make sure the doctor is aware of it.

Recommended dosage

ADULTS

The usual dose for women 18 years and older is 1 sachet (3 grams) dissolved in water.

CHILDREN

The safety and effectiveness of Monurol have not been established in children 12 and under.

Overdosage

No Monurol overdoses have been reported. However, any medication taken in excess can have serious consequences. If you suspect an overdose, seek medical treatment immediately.

Morphine See MS Contin, page 898.

MOTRIN

Generic name: Ibuprofen
Other brand name: Advil

Why is this drug prescribed?

Motrin is a nonsteroidal anti-inflammatory drug available in both prescription and nonprescription forms. Prescription Motrin is used in adults for relief of the symptoms of rheumatoid arthritis and osteoarthritis, treatment of menstrual pain, and relief of mild to moderate pain. In children aged 6 months and older it can be given to reduce fever and relieve mild to moderate pain. It is also used to relieve the symptoms of juvenile arthritis.

Motrin IB tablets, caplets, and gelcaps; Children's Motrin Suspension; and Advil tablets and caplets are available without a prescription. Check the packages for uses, dosage, and other information on these products.

Most important fact about this drug

You should have frequent checkups with your doctor if you take Motrin regularly. Ulcers or internal bleeding can occur without warning.

How should you take this medication?

Your doctor may ask you to take Motrin with food or an antacid to avoid stomach upset. The suspension can be given with meals or milk if it upsets the stomach.

A drink of water or other fluid after taking a chewable tablet can help your body absorb the drug.

If you are using Motrin for arthritis, you should take it regularly, exactly as prescribed.

■ *If you miss a dose...*
  Take it as soon as you remember. If it is almost time for your next dose, skip the one you missed and go back to your regular schedule. Never take 2 doses at the same time.

■ *Storage instructions...*
Store at room temperature.

What side effects may occur?
Side effects cannot be anticipated. If any develop or change in intensity, inform your doctor as soon as possible. Only your doctor can determine if it is safe for you to continue taking Motrin.

■ *Side effects may include:*
Abdominal cramps or pain, abdominal discomfort, bloating and gas, constipation, diarrhea, dizziness, fluid retention and swelling, headache, heartburn, indigestion, itching, loss of appetite, nausea, nervousness, rash, ringing in ears, stomach pain, vomiting

Why should this drug not be prescribed?
If you are sensitive to or have ever had an allergic reaction to ibuprofen, aspirin, or similar drugs, such as Aleve and Naprosyn, or if you have had asthma attacks caused by aspirin or other drugs of this type, or if you have angioedema, a condition whose symptoms are skin eruptions, you should not take this medication.

Make sure that your doctor is aware of any drug reactions that you have experienced.

Special warnings about this medication
Peptic ulcers and bleeding can occur without warning. Tell your doctor if you have bleeding or any other problems.

This drug should be used with caution if you have kidney or liver disease, or are severely dehydrated; it can cause liver or kidney inflammation or other problems in some people.

Do not take aspirin or any other anti-inflammatory medications while taking Motrin unless your doctor tells you to do so.

If you have a severe allergic reaction, seek medical help immediately.

Motrin may cause vision problems. If you experience any changes in your vision, inform your doctor.

Motrin may prolong bleeding time. If you are taking blood-thinning medication, this drug should be taken with caution.

This drug can cause water retention. It should be used with caution if you have high blood pressure or poor heart function.

Avoid the use of alcohol while taking this medication.

Motrin may mask the usual signs of infection or other diseases. Use with care in the presence of an existing infection.

If you have diabetes, remember that the suspension contains 1.5 grams of sucrose and 8 calories per teaspoonful.

Motrin chewable tablets contain phenylalanine. If you have a hereditary disease called phenylketonuria, you should be aware of this.

Possible food and drug interactions when taking this medication

If Motrin is taken with certain other drugs, the effects of either could be increased, decreased, or altered. It is especially important to check with your doctor before combining Motrin with the following:

Aspirin
Blood pressure medications known as ACE inhibitors, including
    Vasotec and Capoten
Blood-thinning drugs such as Coumadin
Diuretics such as Lasix and HydroDIURIL
Lithium (Lithonate)
Methotrexate (Rheumatrex)

Special information if you are pregnant or breastfeeding

The effects of ibuprofen during pregnancy have not been adequately studied. If you are pregnant or plan to become pregnant, inform your doctor immediately. Ibuprofen may appear in breast milk and could affect a nursing infant. If this medication is essential to your health, your doctor may advise you to discontinue breastfeeding until your treatment with this medication is finished.

Recommended dosage

ADULTS

Rheumatoid Arthritis and Osteoarthritis
The usual dosage is 1,200 to 3,200 milligrams per day divided into 3 or 4 doses. Your doctor will tailor the dose to your individual needs. Symptoms should be reduced within 2 weeks. Daily dosage should not be greater than 3,200 milligrams.

Mild to Moderate Pain
The usual dose is 400 milligrams every 4 to 6 hours as necessary.

Menstrual Pain
The usual dose is 400 milligrams every 4 hours as necessary. Begin treatment when symptoms first appear.

CHILDREN 6 MONTHS TO 12 YEARS OF AGE

Fever Reduction
The recommended dose is 5 milligrams per 2.2 pounds of body weight if temperature is less than 102.5 degrees Fahrenheit or 10 milligrams per 2.2 pounds of body weight if temperature is 102.5 degrees Fahrenheit or greater. The fever should go down for 6 to 8 hours. Do not give the child more than 40 milligrams per 2.2 pounds of body weight in one day.

Mild to Moderate Pain
The usual dose is 10 milligrams per 2.2 pounds of body weight every 6 to 8 hours. Do not give the child more than 4 such doses per day.

Juvenile Arthritis
The usual dose is 30 to 40 milligrams daily per 2.2 pounds of body weight, divided into 3 or 4 doses. Some children may need only 20 milligrams daily per 2.2 pounds.

Overdosage

Any medication taken in excess can have serious consequences. An overdose of Motrin can be fatal. If you suspect an overdose, seek medical attention immediately.

■ *Symptoms of Motrin overdose may include:*
Abdominal pain, breathing difficulties, coma, drowsiness, headache, irregular heartbeat, kidney failure, low blood pressure, nausea, ringing in the ears, seizures, sluggishness, vomiting

Moxifloxacin *See Avelox, page 166.*

MS CONTIN
Pronounced: em-ess KON-tin
Generic name: Morphine sulfate
Other brand name: Kadian

Why is this drug prescribed?

MS Contin, a controlled-release tablet containing morphine, is used to relieve moderate to severe pain. While regular morphine is usually given every 4 hours, MS Contin is typically taken every 12 hours—only twice a day. The Kadian brand may be taken once or twice a day. The drugs are intended for people who need a morphine painkiller for more than just a few days.

Most important fact about this drug

Like other narcotics, MS Contin is potentially addictive. If you take MS Contin for some time and then stop abruptly, you could experience withdrawal symptoms. For this reason, do not make dosage changes on your own; always consult your doctor.

How should you take this medication?

Take MS Contin exactly as prescribed by your doctor—typically one tablet every 12 hours. Swallow the tablets whole. If you crush or chew the tablets, a dangerously large amount of morphine could enter your bloodstream all at once.

Kadian capsules and the pellets they contain should not be dissolved or mixed with food, either.

Do not increase the dose or take the drug more frequently than prescribed. It will take a little time for the drug to begin working.

Do not drink alcoholic beverages while using MS Contin.

■ *If you miss a dose...*
Take the forgotten dose as soon as you remember. If it is almost time for your next dose, skip the one you missed and go back to your regular schedule. Do not take 2 doses at once.

■ *Storage instructions...*
Store at room temperature in a tightly closed container, away from light and moisture.

What side effects may occur?

Side effects cannot be anticipated. If any develop or change in intensity, tell your doctor immediately. Only your doctor can determine whether it is safe for you to continue taking MS Contin.

As with other narcotics, the most hazardous potential side effect of MS Contin is respiratory depression (dangerously slow breathing). If you are older or in a weakened condition, you are particularly vulnerable to respiratory depression; you may be at special risk at any age if you have a lung or breathing problem.

■ *Side effects may include:*
Anxiety, constipation, depressed or irritable mood, dizziness, drowsiness, exaggerated sense of well-being, light-headedness, nausea, sedation, sweating, vomiting

You may be able to lessen some of these side effects by lying down.

If you stop taking MS Contin after a long period of use, you will probably experience some degree of narcotic withdrawal syndrome. During the first 24 hours, you may have: dilated pupils, goose bumps, restlessness, restless sleep, runny nose, sweating, tearing, or yawning.

■ *Over the next 72 hours, the following may be added:*
Abdominal and leg pains, abdominal and muscle cramps, anxiety, diarrhea, hot and cold flashes, inability to fall or stay asleep, increase in body temperature, blood pressure, and breathing and heart rate, kicking movements, loss of appetite, nasal discharge, nausea, severe backache, sneezing, twitching and spasm of muscles, vomiting, weakness

Even without treatment, your withdrawal symptoms will probably disappear within a week or two. However, you could experience a second phase of withdrawal, involving aching muscles, irritability, and insomnia, which might last for 2 to 6 months.

Why should this drug not be prescribed?

Do not take MS Contin if you have ever had an allergic reaction to morphine or are sensitive to it, or if you have bronchial asthma.

If your breathing is abnormally slow, you should not take MS Contin unless there is resuscitation equipment nearby.

MS Contin should not be prescribed if you are suffering an intestinal blockage.

Special warnings about this medication

MS Contin should not be used by anyone who might have a brain injury, or the beginnings of an abdominal problem requiring surgery; the drug could mask the symptoms, making correct diagnosis difficult or impossible. For people facing biliary tract surgery, there is a chance that the drug could make their condition worse. Your doctor will also prescribe MS Contin with extreme caution if you have any of the following conditions:

Alcoholism
Coma
Curvature of the spine
Delirium tremens (severe alcohol withdrawal)
Drug-related psychosis
Enlarged prostate or constricted urinary canal
Kidney disorder
Liver disorder
Low adrenalin levels
Low thyroid levels
Lung disorder
Swallowing difficulty

If taken by an epileptic person, MS Contin could increase the likelihood of a seizure.

Since MS Contin can impair judgment and coordination, do not drive, climb, or operate hazardous equipment while taking this drug. If you become overly calm or lethargic, call your doctor.

MS Contin can lower blood pressure; you may feel dizzy or light-headed, especially when you first stand up.

Possible food and drug interactions when taking this medication

If MS Contin is taken with certain other drugs, the effects of either could be increased, decreased, or altered. It is especially important to check with your doctor before combining MS Contin with the following:

Alcohol
Certain analgesics such as Talwin, Nubain, Stadol, and Buprenex
Drugs classified as MAO inhibitors, such as the antidepressants
    Nardil and Parnate
Drugs that control vomiting, such as Compazine and Tigan
Major tranquilizers such as Thorazine and Haldol
Muscle relaxants such as Flexeril and Valium

Sedatives such as Dalmane and Halcion
Tranquilizers such as Librium and Xanax
Water pills such as Diuril and Lasix

Special information if you are pregnant or breastfeeding

If you are pregnant or plan to become pregnant, inform your doctor immediately. Although there is no evidence so far that a pregnant woman's short-term use of MS Contin can harm her unborn baby, this drug should be taken during pregnancy only if the benefit to the mother outweighs a possible risk to the child.

MS Contin is not recommended for use as a painkiller during childbirth. If a woman takes this drug shortly before giving birth, her baby may have trouble breathing. Babies born to mothers who use morphine chronically may suffer from drug withdrawal symptoms.

Since some of the morphine from MS Contin appears in breast milk, do not take this medication while breastfeeding. If you do nurse while using MS Contin, your baby could experience withdrawal symptoms once you stop taking this medication.

Recommended dosage

ADULTS

Because MS Contin and Kadian are so potent, the doctor will set the dosage schedule and amount to meet your individual needs.

Overdosage

Any medication taken in excess can have serious consequences. An overdose of MS Contin can be fatal. If you suspect an overdose, seek medical attention immediately.

■ *Symptoms of MS Contin overdose may include:*
  Cold, clammy skin, flaccid muscles, fluid in the lungs, lowered blood pressure, pinpoint or dilated pupils, sleepiness leading to stupor and coma, slowed breathing, slow pulse rate

MULTIVITAMINS
Brand names: Centrum, Theragran, Vi-Daylin

Why is this supplement prescribed?

Multivitamins are nutritional supplements for people whose diet may be deficient in certain vitamins and minerals. You may need a supplement if you are on a special diet, or don't eat the right foods. A supplement may also be necessary if you are a strict vegetarian, take medications that prevent the body from using certain nutrients, or have an illness that affects your appetite. In addition, special formulas are available for use during pregnancy.

Vitamin/mineral supplements come in a wide range of formulations. Three of the most widely used are Centrum, Theragran, and Vi-Daylin. Each of these brands offers a variety of formulas tailored to the needs of different groups.

Centrum is a multivitamin/multimineral supplement that includes all antioxidants, the vitamins that strengthen the body's natural defenses against cell damage. *Centrum Silver* contains higher strengths of the vitamins that people 50 years of age or older need the most.

Centrum, Jr., formulations are geared to children's needs.

Theragran is a multivitamin supplement.

Theragran-M adds minerals to the formulation. *Theragran Stress Formula* contains higher strengths of the B vitamins that may be needed for people under stress, plus extra vitamin C.

Vi-Daylin is a multivitamin supplement; *Vi-Daylin + Iron* is a multivitamin plus iron, which may be needed by women who have heavy menstrual periods. Some Vi-Daylin formulations also contain fluoride.

Vi-Daylin drops are given to infants and young children.

Most important fact about this supplement

Do not use supplements as a replacement for a diet rich in essential vitamins and minerals. Food contains many important ingredients not available in supplements.

How should you take this supplement?

Follow the dosing instructions on the bottle, or use as directed by your doctor.

Do not take more than suggested.

■ *If you miss a dose...*
If you forget to take your multivitamin for a day, don't be concerned. Resume your regular schedule the following day.

■ *Storage instructions...*
Keep out of the reach of children. Store at room temperature, and keep tightly closed.

Why should this supplement not be used?

If you have any serious chronic medical conditions, check with your doctor before starting on a multivitamin supplement. You may have special requirements.

If your multivitamin supplement contains fluoride, check with your doctor. You should not use it if your drinking water contains more than 0.7 part per million of fluoride.

Special warnings about this supplement

Do not take more of a multivitamin supplement than suggested on the packaging or directed by your doctor. Very high doses of some vitamins and minerals can be harmful or even dangerous.

Possible food and drug interactions when taking this supplement

When taken as suggested on the packaging, there are no known supplement interactions.

Special information if you are pregnant or breastfeeding

Ask your doctor whether you should take a multivitamin supplement while you are pregnant or breastfeeding. Taking too much of any supplement may be harmful to you or your unborn child.

Recommended dosage

ADULTS

The usual dose is 1 tablet, teaspoonful, or tablespoonful daily according to package instructions, or as directed by your doctor.

CHILDREN

The usual dose of children's formulations is 1 tablet, teaspoonful, or dropperful daily or as directed by your doctor. Younger children may require only half this dose. Check the instructions on the package.

Overdosage

Megadoses of some vitamins and minerals can be harmful when taken for extended periods. If you have unexplained symptoms and suspect an overdose, check with your doctor.

Mupirocin *See Bactroban, page 192.*

Muse *See Caverject, page 257.*

Mycelex *See Gyne-Lotrimin, page 640.*

MYCELEX-3

Pronounced: MI-seh-lecks
Generic name: Butoconazole nitrate

Why is this drug prescribed?

Mycelex-3 Vaginal Cream cures yeast-like fungal infections of the vulva and vagina.

Most important fact about this drug

To obtain maximum benefit, it is important that you continue to use Mycelex-3 for 3 consecutive days, even if your symptoms have disappeared.

How should you use this medication?

To keep this medication from getting on your clothing, wear a sanitary napkin. Do not use a tampon; it will absorb the drug. Do not douche unless your doctor tells you to do so.

1. Following the instructions, fill the applicator that comes with the vaginal cream to the level indicated; the cream also comes in a prefilled applicator.
2. Lie on your back with your knees drawn up.
3. Gently insert the applicator high into the vagina and push the plunger.
4. Withdraw the applicator and discard it.

■ *If you miss a dose...*
Insert it as soon as you remember. If it is almost time for your next dose, skip the one you missed and go back to your regular schedule.
■ *Storage instructions...*
Store at room temperature, away from heat. Do not freeze.

What side effects may occur?

Side effects cannot be anticipated. If any develop or change in intensity, inform your doctor as soon as possible. Only your doctor can determine if it is safe for you to continue using Mycelex-3.

■ *Side effects may include:*
Itching of the fingers, soreness, swelling, vaginal discharge, vulvar itching, vulvar or vaginal burning

Why should this drug not be prescribed?

If you are sensitive to or have ever had an allergic reaction to butoconazole nitrate or any other ingredients in this product, you should not use this medication. Make sure your doctor is aware of any drug reactions you have experienced.

Special warnings about this medication

If your symptoms persist, or if you become irritated or have an allergic reaction while using this medication, notify your doctor.

If this is the first time you have had vaginal itching and discomfort, see your doctor before using Mycelex-3 to be sure it is the right medication to use.

Do not use this medication if you have abdominal pain, a fever, or a vaginal discharge with a foul odor; instead, see your doctor.

If your infection doesn't clear up in 3 days, call your doctor. The problem may not be a yeast infection.

If your symptoms come back within 2 months, call your doctor. They could be a sign of pregnancy or a condition such as AIDS or diabetes.

Do not use this product if you have diabetes, have tested positive for HIV, or have AIDS.

Mycelex-3 may damage condoms and diaphragms. Employ another method of birth control while you are using this product.

This product is for vaginal use only. Avoid getting it in your eyes or mouth.

Possible food and drug interactions when taking this medication

No interactions with other drugs have been reported.

Special information if you are pregnant or breastfeeding

You should not use Mycelex-3 if you are pregnant or think you may be pregnant. It is not known whether this drug appears in breast milk. If this medication is essential to your health, your doctor may advise you to discontinue breastfeeding until your treatment is finished.

Recommended dosage

ADULTS

The recommended dose is 1 applicatorful of cream inserted into the vagina at bedtime for 3 days.

CHILDREN

Not for use by girls under 12 years of age.

Overdosage

No overdosage has been reported.

MYCOLOG-II

Pronounced: MY-koe-log too
Generic ingredients: Nystatin, Triamcinolone acetonide
Other brand names: Myco-Triacet II, Mytrex

Why is this drug prescribed?

Mycolog-II Cream and Ointment are prescribed for the treatment of candidiasis (a yeast-like fungal infection) of the skin. The combination of an antifungal (nystatin) and a steroid (triamcinolone acetonide) provides greater benefit than nystatin alone during the first few days of treatment. Nystatin kills the fungus or prevents its growth; triamcinolone helps relieve the redness, swelling, itching, and other discomfort that can accompany a skin infection.

Most important fact about this drug

Absorption of this drug through the skin can affect the whole body instead of just the surface of the skin being treated. Although unusual, it is possible that you could experience symptoms of steroid excess such as weight gain, reddening and rounding of the face and neck, growth of excess body and facial hair, high blood pressure, emotional disturbances, increased blood sugar, and urinary excretion of glucose (marked by an increase in frequency of urination).

Use of this medication over large surface areas, for prolonged periods, or with airtight dressings or bandages could cause these problems Your doctor will watch your condition and periodically check for symptoms.

How should you use this medication?

Use this medicine for the full course of treatment, even if your symptoms are gone. Apply a thin layer to the affected area and gently rub it in. Do not bandage or wrap the area being treated, unless your doctor tells you to. Keep the area cool and dry.

Use this medication exactly as prescribed by your doctor. Do not use it more often or for a longer time. It is for external use only. Avoid contact with the eyes.

■ *If you miss a dose…*
Apply it as soon as you remember. If it is almost time for your next dose, skip the one you missed and go back to your regular schedule.
■ *Storage instructions…*
Store away from heat and light. Do not freeze.

What side effects may occur?

Side effects cannot be anticipated. If any develop or change in intensity, inform your doctor as soon as possible. Only your doctor can determine if it is safe for you to continue taking Mycolog-II.

■ *Side effects may include:*
Blistering, burning, dryness, eruptions resembling acne, excessive discoloring of the skin, excessive growth of hair (especially on the face), hair loss (especially on the scalp), inflammation around the mouth, inflammation of hair follicles, irritation, itching, peeling, prickly heat, reddish purple lines on skin, secondary infection, severe inflammation of the skin, softening of the skin, stretch marks, stretching or thinning of the skin

Why should this drug not be prescribed?

If you are sensitive to or have ever had an allergic reaction to nystatin, triamcinolone acetonide, or other antifungals or steroids, you should not take this medication. Make sure your doctor is aware of any drug reactions you have experienced.

Special warnings about this medication

Do not use this drug for any disorder other than the one for which it was prescribed.

Remember to avoid wrapping or bandaging the affected area. The use of tight-fitting diapers or plastic pants is not recommended for a child being treated in the diaper area with Mycolog-II. These garments may act in the same way as airtight dressings or bandages.

If an irritation or allergic reaction develops while using Mycolog-II, notify your doctor.

If used in the groin area, apply Mycolog-II sparingly and wear loose-fitting clothing.

If your condition does not show improvement after 2 to 3 weeks, or if it gets worse, consult your doctor.

Possible food and drug interactions when taking this medication
No interactions have been reported.

Special information if you are pregnant or breastfeeding
The effects of Mycolog-II in pregnancy have not been adequately studied. If you are pregnant or plan to become pregnant, inform your doctor before using Mycolog-II.

It is not known whether this medication appears in breast milk. If this drug is essential to your health, your doctor may advise you to discontinue breastfeeding until your treatment with this medication is finished.

Recommended dosage

ADULTS

Mycolog-II Cream
Mycolog-II Cream is usually applied to the affected areas 2 times a day, in the morning and evening, by gently and thoroughly massaging the preparation into the skin. Your doctor will have you stop using the cream if your symptoms persist after 25 days of treatment.

Mycolog-II Ointment
A thin film of Mycolog-II Ointment is usually applied to the affected areas 2 times a day, in the morning and the evening. Your doctor will have you stop using the ointment if your symptoms persist after 25 days of treatment.

CHILDREN

Your doctor will limit use of Mycolog-II for children to the least amount that is effective. Long-term treatment may interfere with the growth and development of children.

Overdosage
An acute overdosage is unlikely with the use of Mycolog-II; however, long-term or prolonged use can produce reactions throughout the body. See *Most important fact about this drug.*

Myco-Triacet II *See Mycolog-II, page 905.*

Mykrox *See Zaroxolyn, page 1613.*

Mylanta *See Antacids, page 114.*

MYSOLINE
Pronounced: MY-soh-leen
Generic name: Primidone

Why is this drug prescribed?
Mysoline is used to treat epileptic and other seizures. It can be used alone or with other anticonvulsant drugs. It is chemically similar to barbiturates.

Most important fact about this drug
Mysoline should not be stopped suddenly; this could cause you to have seizures. If you no longer need the medication, your doctor will reduce the dosage gradually.

How should you take this medication?
Take Mysoline exactly as prescribed. Do not change from one manufacturer's product to another without consulting your doctor.

If using Mysoline Suspension, shake well before using.

■ *If you miss a dose...*
Take it as soon as you remember. If it is within an hour of your next dose, skip the one you missed and go back to your regular schedule. Never take 2 doses at the same time.

■ *Storage instructions...*
Store at room temperature in a tightly closed container, away from light.

What side effects may occur?
Side effects cannot be anticipated. If any develop or change in intensity, inform your doctor as soon as possible. Only your doctor can determine if it is safe for you to continue taking Mysoline.

■ *Side effects may include:*
Lack of muscle coordination, vertigo or severe dizziness

Why should this drug not be prescribed?
You should not take Mysoline if you have porphyria (an inherited metabolic disorder) or if you are allergic to phenobarbital.

Special warnings about this medication
Remember that you must not stop taking Mysoline suddenly.

It can take several weeks for the full effectiveness of Mysoline to be seen.

Since Mysoline is generally given for long periods of time, your doctor will check your blood count every 6 months.

Possible food and drug interactions when taking this medication

If Mysoline is taken with certain other drugs, the effects of either could be increased, decreased, or altered. It is especially important to check with your doctor before combining Mysoline with the following:

Antidepressants called MAO inhibitors, such as Parnate and Nardil
Blood-thinning drugs such as Coumadin
Doxycycline (Doryx, Vibramycin)
Estrogen-containing oral contraceptives such as Ortho-Novum and Triphasil
Griseofulvin (Fulvicin-U/F, Grifulvin V)
Steroid drugs such as Decadron

Avoid alcoholic beverages while you are taking Mysoline.

Special information if you are pregnant or breastfeeding

Although the effects of Mysoline in pregnancy and nursing infants are not known, recent studies show an increase in birth defects in infants born to epileptic women taking anticonvulsant medications (particularly Dilantin and phenobarbital). Although most pregnant women taking anticonvulsant medication give birth to normal, healthy babies, this possibility may also exist with Mysoline. If you are pregnant or plan to become pregnant, inform your doctor immediately. Mysoline appears in breast milk and can affect a nursing infant, causing excessive sleepiness and drowsiness. If this medication is essential to your health, your doctor may advise you to stop breastfeeding.

Recommended dosage

ADULTS

For people 8 years of age and older who have not been treated before, the doctor will start Mysoline as follows, using either 50-milligram or scored 250-milligram Mysoline tablets:

Days 1 to 3: 100 to 125 milligrams at bedtime
Days 4 to 6: 100 to 125 milligrams 2 times a day
Days 7 to 9: 100 to 125 milligrams 3 times a day
Day 10 to maintenance: 250 milligrams 3 times a day

For most adults and children 8 years of age and over, the usual maintenance dosage is 250 milligrams 3 or 4 times a day. If you need more, your doctor may increase the dose to five or six 250-milligram tablets. You should not take more than 500 milligrams 4 times a day (2,000 milligrams, or 2 grams).

In patients already receiving other anticonvulsants, the usual starting dose of Mysoline is 100 to 125 milligrams at bedtime; your doctor will gradually increase this dose to a maintenance level as the other drug is gradually decreased. Your doctor will either find a working level for the combination or withdraw the other medication completely. When Mysoline is to be used as a single drug, it will take at least 2 weeks to make the transition from 2 drugs to 1.

CHILDREN UNDER AGE 8

Days 1 to 3: 50 milligrams at bedtime
Days 4 to 6: 50 milligrams 2 times a day
Days 7 to 9: 100 milligrams 2 times a day
Day 10 to maintenance: 125 milligrams 3 times a day to 250 milligrams 3 times day

The usual maintenance dosage is 125 to 250 milligrams 3 times daily or 10 to 25 milligrams per 2.2 pounds of body weight per day, divided into smaller doses.

Overdosage
Any medication taken in excess can have serious consequences. If you suspect a Mysoline overdose, seek medical attention immediately.

Mytrex See Mycolog-II, page 905.

Nabumetone See Relafen, page 1225.

Nadolol See Corgard, page 338.

Nadolol with Bendroflumethiazide See Corzide, page 345.

Nafarelin See Synarel, page 1372.

Naltrexone See ReVia, page 1249.

NAMENDA
Pronounced: nah-MEN-dah
Generic name: Memantine

Why is this drug prescribed?
Namenda is a new kind of medication used for treating moderate to severe Alzheimer's disease. While other Alzheimer's drugs work to prevent the breakdown of the brain chemical acetylcholine, Namenda works by targeting glutamate. Both chemicals are associated with memory and learning. Studies show that Namenda can help improve the mental state and daily functioning of some people with Alzheimer's disease.

Most important fact about this drug

Remember that Namenda does not cure or slow the progression of Alzheimer's disease; it merely treats the symptoms.

How should you take this medication?

Namenda should be taken exactly as prescribed. The dose of Namenda is increased gradually at 1-week intervals. Be sure to wait at least 1 week before increasing the dose. Using doses that are higher than recommended provides no additional benefit. Namenda may be taken with or without food.

■ *If you miss a dose...*
Give the forgotten dose as soon as you remember. However, if it is almost time for the next dose, skip the one you missed and return to the regular schedule. Do not give 2 doses at once.

■ *Storage instructions...*
Store at room temperature.

What side effects may occur?

Side effects cannot be anticipated. If any develop or change in intensity, tell your doctor as soon as possible. Only your doctor can determine if it is safe to continue using Namenda.

■ *Side effects may include:*
Confusion, constipation, coughing, dizziness, hallucinations, headache, high blood pressure, pain, sleepiness, vomiting

Why should this drug not be prescribed?

People who have ever had an allergic reaction to Namenda should not take this medication.

Special warnings about this medication

Namenda is not recommended for use in patients who have severe kidney impairment.

Certain conditions can alter the alkaline balance of the urine, which may cause a buildup of Namenda in the body. Be sure to tell the doctor about any major dietary changes, kidney problems such as renal acidosis, or urinary tract infections.

Make sure the doctor knows about any history of seizures. Namenda has not been formally studied in people with seizure disorders.

Possible food and drug interactions when taking this medication

If Namenda is taken with certain other drugs, the effects of either could be increased, decreased, or altered. It is especially important to check with the doctor before combining Namenda with the following:

Amantadine (Symmetrel)
Cimetidine (Tagamet, Tagamet HB)
Cough suppressants that contain dextromethorphan (usually
    denoted as "DM")
Glaucoma drugs such as Diamox and Neptazane
Hydrochlorothiazide (HydroDIURIL)
Ketamine (Ketalar)
Nicotine (Nicoderm patch, Nicorette gum)
Quinidine (Quinidex)
Ranitidine (Zantac)
Sodium bicarbonate (baking soda, Alka-Seltzer)
Triamterene (Dyrenium)

Special information if you are pregnant or breastfeeding

Namenda is not usually prescribed for women of childbearing age. There
are no adequate and well-controlled studies in pregnant women. It should
be used in pregnant women only if the potential benefit to the mother outweighs the risk to the fetus.

It is not known whether Namenda appears in human breast milk. If this
drug is essential to your health, the doctor may advise you to stop nursing until your treatment is finished.

Recommended dosage

ADULTS

The recommended dosage is 10 milligrams twice a day. The doctor will
start treatment at 5 milligrams once a day for 7 days, and gradually increase the dose by 5 milligrams every 7 days, up to a maximum total daily
dose of 20 milligrams.

If Namenda causes side effects, the doctor may wait more than 1 week
to increase the dose. People who have impaired kidney function may require lower doses.

Overdosage

Any medication taken in excess can have serious consequences. If you
suspect an overdose, seek emergency treatment immediately.

■ *Symptoms of overdose may include:*
    Hallucinations, loss of consciousness, psychosis, restlessness, sleep-
    iness, stupor

Naphazoline with Pheniramine *See Naphcon-A, page 913.*

NAPHCON-A

Pronounced: NAFF-kon ay
Generic ingredients: Naphazoline hydrochloride,
  Pheniramine maleate
Other brand name: Opcon-A

Why is this drug prescribed?

Naphcon-A, an eyedrop containing both a decongestant and an antihistamine, is used to relieve itchy, red eyes caused by ragweed, pollen, and animal hair.

Most important fact about this drug

If this medication causes changes in your vision, be careful when driving or performing other tasks that could be hazardous.

How should you use this medication?

Remove contact lenses before administering this medication. Do not use the solution if it becomes cloudy or changes color.

To administer the eyedrops, follow these steps:
1. Wash your hands thoroughly.
2. Gently pull your lower eyelid down to form a pocket between your eye and the lid.
3. Hold the eyedrop bottle on your forehead or the bridge of your nose.
4. Do not touch the applicator tip to your eye or any other surface.
5. Tilt your head back and squeeze the medication into your eye.
6. Close your eyes gently and keep them closed for a minute or two.
7. Do not rinse the dropper.

■ *If you miss a dose...*
Use this medication only as needed.
■ *Storage instructions...*
Store at room temperature in a tightly closed bottle. Protect from light.

What side effects may occur?

Aside from temporarily enlarging your pupils, Naphcon is unlikely to cause side effects. However, overuse can cause reddening of the eyes.

Why should this drug not be prescribed?

Do not take Naphcon-A if you have ever had an allergic reaction to it or are sensitive to any of its ingredients.

Do not use Naphcon-A if you have heart disease, high blood pressure, or trouble urinating because of enlargement of the prostate gland.

Do not use this medication if you have glaucoma.

Special warnings about this medication

Contact your doctor before giving Naphcon-A to infants or children under 6 years of age. Swallowing this medication can cause stupor or coma and a serious drop in body temperature in an infant or child.

If your eyes hurt or continue to be red or irritated, if you experience changes in vision, if your eyes get worse, or if the itching and redness last more than 72 hours, stop using Naphcon-A and call your doctor.

Recommended dosage

ADULTS

Place 1 or 2 drops in the affected eyes, up to 4 times a day.

Overdosage

Overdose from accidental oral use can have serious consequences, especially in young children. If you suspect an overdose, seek medical attention immediately.

Naprelan *See Anaprox, page 105.*

NAPROSYN

Pronounced: NA-proh-sinn
Generic name: Naproxen
Other brand name: EC-Naprosyn

Why is this drug prescribed?

Naprosyn, a nonsteroidal anti-inflammatory drug, is used to relieve the inflammation, swelling, stiffness, and joint pain associated with rheumatoid arthritis, osteoarthritis (the most common form of arthritis), juvenile arthritis, ankylosing spondylitis (spinal arthritis), tendinitis, bursitis, and acute gout; it is also used to relieve menstrual cramps and other types of mild to moderate pain.

Most important fact about this drug

You should have frequent checkups with your doctor if you take Naprosyn regularly. Ulcers or internal bleeding can occur without warning.

How should you take this medication?

Naprosyn may be taken with food or an antacid, and with a full glass of water to avoid stomach upset. Avoid taking it on an empty stomach.

If you are using Naprosyn for arthritis, it should be taken regularly; take it exactly as prescribed.

Do not break, crush, or chew an EC-Naprosyn tablet.

■ *If you miss a dose...*
And you take the drug on a regular schedule, take the dose as soon as you remember. If it is almost time for your next dose, skip the one you missed and go back to your regular schedule. Do not take 2 doses at once.

■ *Storage instructions...*
Store at room temperature in a well-closed container. Protect from light and extreme heat.

What side effects may occur?
Side effects cannot be anticipated. If any develop or change in intensity, inform your doctor as soon as possible. Only your doctor can determine if it is safe for you to continue taking Naprosyn.

■ *Side effects may include:*
Abdominal pain, bruising, constipation, difficult or labored breathing, dizziness, drowsiness, headache, heartburn, itching, nausea, ringing in ears, skin eruptions, swelling due to fluid retention

Why should this drug not be prescribed?
If you are sensitive to or have ever had an allergic reaction to Naprosyn, EC-Naprosyn, Anaprox, Anaprox DS, or Aleve, you should not take this drug. Also, if aspirin or other nonsteroidal anti-inflammatory drugs have ever given you asthma or nasal inflammation or tumors, you should not take this medication. Make sure your doctor is aware of any drug reactions you have experienced.

Special warnings about this medication
Remember that peptic ulcers and bleeding can occur without warning. Call your doctor immediately if you suspect a problem.

Use this drug with caution if you have kidney or liver disease; it can cause liver or kidney problems in some people.

Naprosyn may prolong bleeding time. If you are taking blood-thinning medication, your doctor will prescribe Naprosyn with caution.

By reducing fever and inflammation, Naprosyn may hide an underlying condition.

This medication may cause vision problems. If you experience any changes in your vision, inform your doctor.

This drug can increase water retention. It will be prescribed with caution if you have heart disease or high blood pressure. Naprosyn suspension contains a significant amount of sodium. If you are on a low-sodium diet, discuss this with your doctor.

Naprosyn may cause you to become drowsy or less alert; therefore, avoid driving, operating dangerous machinery, or participating in any hazardous activity that requires full mental alertness until you are sure of the drug's effect on you.

Possible food and drug interactions when taking this medication

If Naprosyn is taken with certain other drugs, the effects of either could be increased, decreased, or altered. It is especially important to check with your doctor before combining Naprosyn with the following:

ACE inhibitors such as the blood pressure drug Zestril
Aspirin
Beta-blockers such as the blood pressure drug Tenormin
Blood-thinning drugs such as Coumadin
Furosemide (Lasix)
Lithium (Eskalith, Lithobid)
Methotrexate
Naproxen sodium (Aleve, Anaprox)
Oral diabetes drugs such as Diabinese and Micronase
Phenytoin (Dilantin)
Probenecid (Benemid)
Sulfa drugs such as the antibiotics Bactrim and Septra

EC-Naprosyn should not be used with antacids, H_2 blockers such as Tagamet, or sucralfate (Carafate).

Special information if you are pregnant or breastfeeding

The effects of Naprosyn during pregnancy have not been adequately studied. If you are pregnant or plan to become pregnant, inform your doctor immediately. Naprosyn appears in breast milk and could affect a nursing infant. If this medication is essential to your health, your doctor may advise you to discontinue breastfeeding until your treatment with this medication is finished.

Recommended dosage

Naprosyn is available in tablet and liquid form. When taking the liquid, use a teaspoon or the measuring cup, marked in ½ teaspoon and 2.5 milliliter increments, that comes with Naprosyn suspension.

ADULTS

Rheumatoid Arthritis, Osteoarthritis, and Ankylosing Spondylitis

The usual dose of Naprosyn is 250 milligrams (10 milliliters or 2 teaspoons of suspension), 375 milligrams (15 milliliters or 3 teaspoons), or 500 milligrams (20 milliliters or 4 teaspoons) 2 times a day (morning and evening). EC-Naprosyn is taken in doses of 375 or 500 milligrams twice a day. Your dose may be adjusted by your doctor over your period of treatment. Improvement of symptoms should be seen in 2 to 4 weeks.

Acute Gout

The starting dose of Naprosyn is 750 milligrams (30 milliliters or 6 teaspoons), followed by 250 milligrams (10 milliliters or 2 teaspoons) every

8 hours until the symptoms are relieved. EC-Naprosyn should not be used to treat gout.

Mild to Moderate Pain, Menstrual Cramps, Acute Tendinitis, and Bursitis
The starting dose is 500 milligrams (20 milliliters or 4 teaspoons of suspension), followed by 250 milligrams (10 milliliters or 2 teaspoons) every 6 to 8 hours as needed. The most you should take in a day is 1,250 milligrams (50 milliliters or 10 teaspoons). Do not take EC-Naprosyn for these problems.

CHILDREN

Juvenile Arthritis
The usual daily dose is 10 milligrams per 2.2 pounds of body weight, divided into 2 doses. Follow your doctor's directions carefully when giving a child this medicine.

The safety and effectiveness of Naprosyn have not been established in children under 2 years of age.

OLDER ADULTS

Your doctor will probably have you take a reduced dose.

Overdosage
Any medication taken in excess can have serious consequences. If you suspect an overdose, seek medical attention immediately.

■ *Symptoms of Naprosyn overdose may include:*
   Drowsiness, heartburn, indigestion, nausea, vomiting

Naproxen *See Naprosyn, page 914.*

Naproxen sodium *See Anaprox, page 105.*

Naratriptan *See Amerge, page 92.*

NARDIL
Pronounced: NAHR-dill
Generic name: Phenelzine sulfate

Why is this drug prescribed?
Nardil is a monoamine oxidase (MAO) inhibitor used to treat depression as well as anxiety or phobias mixed with depression. MAO is an enzyme responsible for breaking down certain neurotransmitters (chemical messengers) in the brain. By inhibiting MAO, Nardil helps restore more normal mood states. Unfortunately, MAO inhibitors such as Nardil also block MAO activity throughout the body, an action that can have serious, even

fatal, side effects—especially if MAO inhibitors are combined with other foods or drugs containing a substance called tyramine.

Most important fact about this drug

Avoid the following foods, beverages, and medications while taking Nardil and for 2 weeks after stopping it:

Beer (including alcohol-free or reduced-alcohol beer)
Caffeine (in excessive amounts)
Cheese (except for cottage cheese and cream cheese)
Chocolate (in excessive amounts)
Dry sausage (including Genoa salami, hard salami, pepperoni, and Lebanon bologna)
Fava bean pods
Liver
Meat extract
Pickled, fermented, aged, or smoked meat, fish, or dairy products
Pickled herring
Sauerkraut
Spoiled or improperly stored meat, fish, or dairy products
Wine (including alcohol-free or reduced-alcohol wine)
Yeast extract (including large amounts of brewer's yeast)
Yogurt

Medications to avoid:
Amphetamines
Appetite suppressants such as Redux and Tenuate
Antidepressants and related medications such as Celexa, Effexor, Elavil, Flexeril, fluvoxamine, Paxil, Prozac, Remeron, Serzone, Tegretol, Triavil, Wellbutrin, Zoloft
Asthma inhalants such as Proventil and Ventolin
Cold and cough preparations including those with dextromethorphan, such as Robitussin DM
Hay fever medications such as Contac and Dristan
L-tryptophan-containing products
Nasal decongestants in tablet, drop, or spray form such as Sudafed
Sinus medications such as Sinutab
Stimulants such as Ritalin and epinephrine (EpiPen)

Taking Nardil with any of the above foods, beverages, or medications can cause serious, potentially fatal high blood pressure. Therefore, when taking Nardil you should immediately report the occurrence of a headache, heart palpitations, or any other unusual symptom. In addition, make certain that you inform any other physician or dentist you see that you are currently taking Nardil or have taken Nardil within the last 2 weeks.

How should you take this medication?
Nardil may be taken with or without food. Take it exactly as prescribed. It can take up to 4 weeks for the drug to begin working.

Use of Nardil may complicate other medical treatment. Always carry a card that says you take Nardil, or wear a Medic Alert bracelet.

■ *If you miss a dose...*
Take it as soon as you remember. If it is within 2 hours of your next dose, skip the one you missed and go back to your regular schedule. Do not take 2 doses at once.

■ *Storage instructions...*
Store at room temperature.

What side effects may occur?
Side effects cannot be anticipated. If any develop or change in intensity, inform your doctor as soon as possible. Only your doctor can determine if it is safe for you to continue taking Nardil.

■ *Side effects may include:*
Constipation, dizziness, drowsiness, dry mouth, headache, liver problems, low blood pressure upon standing, sexual problems, sleep disturbances, stomach and intestinal problems, water retention, weight gain

Why should this drug not be prescribed?
You should not take this drug if you have pheochromocytoma (a tumor of the adrenal gland), congestive heart failure, or a history of liver disease, or if you have had an allergic reaction to it.

You should not take Nardil if you are taking medications that may increase blood pressure (such as amphetamines, cocaine, allergy and cold medications, or Ritalin), other MAO inhibitors, L-dopa, methyldopa (Aldomet), phenylalanine, L-tryptophan, L-tyrosine, fluoxetine (Prozac), buspirone (BuSpar), bupropion (Wellbutrin), guanethidine (Ismelin), meperidine (Demerol), dextromethorphan, or substances that slow the central nervous system such as alcohol and narcotics; or if you must consume the foods, beverages, or medications listed above in the *Most important fact about this drug* section.

Special warnings about this medication
In clinical studies, antidepressants increased the risk of suicidal thinking and behavior in children and adolescents with depression and other psychiatric disorders. Anyone considering the use of Nardil or any other antidepressant in a child or adolescent must balance this risk with the clinical need. Nardil is not approved for treating children.

Additionally, the progression of major depression is associated with a worsening of symptoms and/or the emergence of suicidal thinking or behavior in both adults and children, whether or not they are taking antidepressants. Individuals being treated with Nardil and their caregivers should watch for any change in symptoms or any new symptoms that appear suddenly—especially agitation, anxiety, hostility, panic, restlessness, extreme hyperactivity, and suicidal thinking or behavior—and report them to the doctor immediately. Be especially observant at the beginning of treatment or whenever there is a change in dose.

You must follow the food and drug limitations established by your physician; failure to do so may lead to potentially fatal side effects. While taking Nardil, you should promptly report the occurrence of a headache or any other unusual symptoms.

If you are diabetic, your doctor will prescribe Nardil with caution, since it is not clear how MAO inhibitors affect blood sugar levels.

If you are taking Nardil, talk to your doctor before you decide to have elective surgery.

If you stop taking Nardil abruptly, you may have withdrawal symptoms. They may include nightmares, agitation, strange behavior, and convulsions.

Possible food and drug interactions when taking this medication

If Nardil is taken with certain other drugs, the effects of either could be increased, decreased, or altered. It is important that you closely follow your doctor's dietary and medication limitations when taking Nardil. Consult the *Most important fact about this drug* and *Why should this drug not be prescribed?* sections for lists of the foods, beverages, and medications that should be avoided while taking Nardil.

In addition, you should use blood pressure medications (including water pills and beta-blockers) with caution when taking Nardil, since excessively low blood pressure may result. Symptoms of low blood pressure include dizziness when rising from a lying or sitting position, fainting, and tingling in the hands or feet.

Special information if you are pregnant or breastfeeding

The effects of Nardil during pregnancy have not been adequately studied. Nardil should be used during pregnancy only if the benefits of therapy clearly outweigh the potential risks to the fetus. If you are pregnant or plan to become pregnant, inform your doctor immediately. Breastfeeding mothers should use Nardil only after consulting their physician, since it is not known whether Nardil appears in human milk.

Recommended dosage

ADULTS

The usual starting dose is 15 milligrams (1 tablet) 3 times a day. Your doctor may increase the dosage to 90 milligrams per day.

It may be 4 weeks before the drug starts to work.

Once you have had good results, your doctor may gradually reduce the dose, possibly to as low as 15 milligrams daily or every 2 days.

OLDER ADULTS

Because older people are more likely to have poor liver, kidney, or heart function, or other diseases that could increase the likelihood of side effects, a relatively low dose of Nardil is usually recommended at the start.

CHILDREN

Nardil is not recommended, since its safety and efficacy in children have not been determined.

Overdosage

Any medication taken in excess can have serious consequences. An overdose of Nardil can be fatal. If you suspect an overdose, seek medical help immediately.

■ *Symptoms of overdose may include:*
Agitation, backward arching of the head, neck, and back, cool, clammy skin, coma, convulsions, difficulty breathing, dizziness, drowsiness, faintness, hallucinations, high blood pressure, high fever, hyperactivity, irritability, jaw muscle spasms, low blood pressure, pain in the heart area, rapid and irregular pulse, rigidity, severe headache, sweating

Nasacort *See Azmacort, page 180.*

Nasalcrom *See Intal, page 694.*

Nasalide *See AeroBid, page 49.*

NASONEX
Pronounced: NAZE-oh-necks
Generic name: Mometasone furoate monohydrate

Why is this drug prescribed?

Nasonex nasal spray prevents and relieves the runny, stuffy nose that accompanies hay fever and year-round allergies. It contains a steroid medication that fights inflammation.

Most important fact about this drug

A long-term treatment for allergies, Nasonex does not provide immediate relief. To be effective, it must be used regularly once a day. It starts working within 2 days after the first dose, but takes 1 to 2 weeks to yield its maximum benefits. If you suffer from hay fever, you should begin taking it 2 to 4 weeks before the start of pollen season.

How should you take this medication?

Take Nasonex regularly at the same time each day. Do not use more than the prescribed amount, and do not take it more than once a day.

Shake the bottle thoroughly before each use. Before the first use, prime the pump by pressing it repeatedly until a fine mist appears. If more than a week passes between uses, you'll need to prime the pump again. Avoid spraying the mist into your eyes.

Administer the spray as follows:

1. Gently blow your nose to clear the nostrils.
2. Press one nostril closed, tilt your head slightly forward, and insert the nasal applicator into the other nostril.
3. For each spray, press once on the shoulders of the applicator with your forefinger and middle finger, while supporting the base of the bottle with your thumb.
4. Breathe inward through the nostril, then breathe outward through your mouth.
5. Repeat in the other nostril.

Discard the bottle after 120 sprays. Any medication remaining in it will not be dispensed at the correct dosage.

■ *If you miss a dose...*
Take it as soon as you remember. If it is time for your next dose, skip the one you missed and go back to your regular schedule. Do not take 2 doses at the same time.

■ *Storage instructions...*
Store at room temperature away from direct light.

What side effects may occur?

Side effects cannot be anticipated. If any develop or change in intensity, inform your doctor as soon as possible. Only your doctor can determine if it is safe for you to continue taking this medication.

■ *Side effects may include:*
Coughing, flu-like symptoms, headache, muscle and bone pain, nosebleed, painful menstruation, sinus inflammation, sore throat, upper respiratory tract infection, viral infection

Why should this drug not be prescribed?

If Nasonex gives you an allergic reaction, you cannot continue using it.

Special warnings about this medication

If your allergy symptoms fail to improve—or get worse—while you are using Nasonex, inform your doctor.

When switching from steroid tablets to Nasonex nasal spray, some people develop withdrawal symptoms such as fatigue, depression, and joint or muscle pain. If you notice any of these symptoms, tell your doctor.

In rare cases, a hypersensitivity to steroids or excessive use of Nasonex leads to menstrual irregularities, acne, obesity, and muscle weakness. If these symptoms occur, you should tell your doctor immediately. You may have to gradually discontinue use of this product under your doctor's supervision.

Steroids can slow down growth in children, so your doctor will monitor the situation carefully if your child is using this drug.

Steroids can suppress your immune system, leaving you more vulnerable to infection. Take extra care to avoid exposure to measles or chickenpox if you have never had them. If you are exposed, seek medical advice immediately.

For the same reason, if you develop a throat or nose infection while using Nasonex, stop taking it and call your doctor. Use Nasonex with caution—if at all—if you suffer from tuberculosis, herpes simplex infection of the eye, or an untreated fungal, bacterial, or viral infection.

Steroid nasal sprays have, on rare occasions, caused perforations in the wall between the nostrils. If you have sores in this area, or have recently had nose surgery or trauma to the nose, do not use Nasonex until the problem has healed.

In rare instances, steroid nasal sprays have also been known to raise pressure within the eyes and promote the development of cataracts. Use Nasonex with caution if you have either problem. If you notice any changes in your vision, report them to your doctor.

Possible food and drug interactions when taking this medication
No interactions have been reported.

Special information if you are pregnant or breastfeeding
The effects of Nasonex during pregnancy have not been adequately studied. If you are pregnant or plan to become pregnant, alert your doctor immediately.

It is not known whether Nasonex appears in breast milk. However, other steroids do appear in breast milk and can harm a nursing infant. Your doctor may therefore suggest discontinuing Nasonex if you intend to breastfeed.

Recommended dosage

ADULTS

The recommended dose for adults and children 12 years of age and older is 2 sprays into each nostril once a day.

CHILDREN

For children 3 to 11 years of age, the recommended dose is one spray in each nostril once a day. The safety and effectiveness of Nasonex have not been established in children under 3.

Overdosage
A single overdose of Nasonex is unlikely to cause any harm. However, habitual overuse of the product can cause symptoms of steroid overload, including menstrual irregularities, acne, obesity, and muscle weakness. Check with your doctor immediately if you develop such symptoms.

Natalins See Prenatal Vitamins, page 1141.

Nateglinide See Starlix, page 1345.

NAVANE
Pronounced: NA-vain
Generic name: Thiothixene

Why is this drug prescribed?
Navane is used in the treatment of schizophrenia (a disruption of thought and the understanding of reality). Researchers theorize that antipsychotic medications such as Navane work by lowering levels of dopamine, a neurotransmitter (or chemical messenger) in the brain. Excessive levels of dopamine are believed to be related to psychotic behavior.

Most important fact about this drug
Navane may cause tardive dyskinesia—a condition marked by involuntary muscle spasms and twitches in the face and body. This condition can be permanent and appears to be most common among the elderly, especially women. Ask your doctor for information about this possible risk.

How should you take this medication?
Navane may be taken in liquid or capsule form. With the liquid form, a dropper is supplied.

■ If you miss a dose...
Take it as soon as you remember. If it is within 2 hours of your next dose, skip the one you missed and go back to your regular schedule. Do not take 2 doses at once.

■ Storage instructions...
Store at room temperature away from heat, light, and moisture. Keep the liquid form from freezing.

What side effects may occur?
Side effects cannot be anticipated. If any develop or change in intensity, inform your doctor as soon as possible. Only your doctor can determine if it is safe for you to continue taking Navane.

■ Side effects may include:
Agitation, blood disorders, blurred vision, drowsiness, dry mouth, exaggerated reflexes, fainting, high blood pressure, insomnia, light-

headedness, low blood pressure, Parkinson's-like movements, profuse sweating, rapid or irregular heartbeat, rash, sensitivity to sunlight, skin color changes

Why should this drug not be prescribed?

Do not give Navane to comatose individuals. Do not take Navane if you are known to be hypersensitive to it. Also, you should not use Navane if the activity of your central nervous system is slowed down for any reason—for example, by a sleeping medication, if you have had circulatory system collapse, or if you have an abnormal bone marrow or blood condition.

Special warnings about this medication

Navane may hide symptoms of brain tumor and intestinal obstruction. Your doctor will prescribe Navane cautiously if you have or have ever had a brain tumor, breast cancer, convulsive disorders, the eye condition called glaucoma, intestinal blockage, or heart disease; or if you are exposed to extreme heat or are recovering from alcohol addiction.

This drug may impair your ability to drive a car or operate potentially dangerous machinery. Do not participate in any activities that require full alertness if you are unsure of your ability.

Possible food and drug interactions when taking this medication

If Navane is taken with certain other drugs, the effects of either could be increased, decreased, or altered. It is especially important to check with your doctor before combining Navane with the following:

Antihistamines such as Benadryl
Barbiturates such as phenobarbital
Drugs that contain atropine, such as Donnatal

Extreme drowsiness and other potentially serious effects can result if Navane is combined with alcohol or other central nervous system depressants such as painkillers, narcotics, or sleeping medications.

Special information if you are pregnant or breastfeeding

If you are pregnant or plan to become pregnant, inform your doctor immediately; pregnant women should use Navane only if clearly needed. Consult your doctor if you are breastfeeding; he or she may have you stop while you are taking Navane.

Recommended dosage

Dosages of Navane are tailored to the individual. Usually treatment begins with a small dose, which is increased if needed.

ADULTS

For Milder Conditions

The usual starting dosage is a daily total of 6 milligrams, divided into doses of 2 milligrams and taken 3 times a day. Your doctor may increase the dose to a total of 15 milligrams a day.

For More Severe Conditions

The usual starting dosage is a daily total of 10 milligrams, taken in 2 doses of 5 milligrams each. Your doctor may increase this dose to a total of 60 milligrams a day.

Taking more than 60 milligrams a day rarely increases the benefits of Navane.

Some people are able to take Navane once a day. Check with your doctor to see whether you can follow this schedule.

CHILDREN

Navane is not recommended for children younger than 12 years old.

OLDER ADULTS

In general, older adults are prescribed dosages of Navane in the lower ranges. Because older adults may develop low blood pressure while taking Navane, their doctors will monitor them closely. Older adults (especially women) may be more susceptible to such side effects as involuntary muscle spasms and twitches in the face and body. Check with your doctor for more information about these potential risks.

Overdosage

Any medication taken in excess can have serious consequences If you suspect an overdose, seek medical help immediately.

■ *Symptoms of Navane overdose may include:*
Central nervous system depression, coma, difficulty swallowing, dizziness, drowsiness, head tilted to the side, low blood pressure, muscle twitching, rigid muscles, salivation, tremors, walking disturbances, weakness

Necon *See Oral Contraceptives, page 1000.*

Nedocromil *See Tilade, page 1438.*

Nelfinavir *See Viracept, page 1567.*

NEODECADRON OPHTHALMIC OINTMENT AND SOLUTION

Pronounced: Nee-oh-DECK-uh-drohn
Generic ingredients: Dexamethasone sodium phosphate,
* Neomycin sulfate*

Why is this drug prescribed?

Neodecadron is a steroid and antibiotic combination that is used to treat inflammatory eye conditions in which there is also a bacterial infection or the possibility of a bacterial infection. Dexamethasone (the steroid) decreases inflammation. Neomycin, the antibiotic, kills some of the more common bacteria.

Most important fact about this drug

Prolonged use of Neodecadron may increase the possibility of developing additional eye infections. It could also cause vision problems, raise the pressure inside your eyes, and even lead to glaucoma and cataracts. If you take this medication for 10 days or longer, your doctor will routinely check your eye pressure.

How should you use this medication?

Neodecadron Ophthalmic Solution
1. Wash your hands thoroughly before use.
2. Tilt your head backward or lie down and gaze upward.
3. Gently pull the lower eyelid away from the eye to form a pouch.
4. Drop the medicine in the pouch and gently close your eyes. Try not to blink.
5. Keep your eye closed for a couple of minutes. Do not rub the eye.
6. Do not touch the applicator tip or dropper to any surface (including the eye).

Neodecadron Ophthalmic Ointment
1. Wash your hands thoroughly before use.
2. Hold the ointment tube in your hand for a few minutes to warm the ointment and make it flow more smoothly.
3. Tilt your head backward or lie down and gaze upward.
4. Gently pull the lower eyelid away from the eye to form a pouch.
5. Squeeze the tube gently, and with a sweeping motion along the inside of the lower lid, apply 0.25 to 0.5 inch of ointment.
6. Close your eyes for a couple of minutes and roll them in all directions.

■ *If you miss a dose…*
  Take the forgotten dose as soon as you remember. If it is almost time for the next dose, skip the one you missed and go back to your regular schedule. Never try to catch up by doubling the dose.

■ *Storage instructions…*
Store at room temperature. Protect solution from light.

What side effects may occur?
Side effects cannot be anticipated. If any develop or change in intensity, notify your doctor as soon as possible. Only your doctor can determine whether it is safe to continue using Neodecadron.

■ *Side effects may include:*
Allergic skin reactions, cataracts, delay in healing of wounds, development of additional eye infections, increased eye pressure with possible glaucoma and optic nerve damage

Why should this drug not be prescribed?
Neodecadron should be avoided if you have an inflammation of the cornea (the transparent surface of the eye); chickenpox; or other bacterial, fungal, or viral eye infections. Do not use Neodecadron if you have ever had an allergic reaction or are sensitive to any of its ingredients.

Neodecadron solution contains a sulfite that can cause an allergic reaction in susceptible people.

Special warnings about this medication
Neodecadron is absorbed into your bloodstream when applied to your eye. Its steroid component can lower your resistance to infection, and it can prolong or worsen the severity of many viral infections of the eye. Diseases such as measles and chickenpox can be serious and even fatal in adults. If you are using Neodecadron and are exposed to chickenpox or measles, notify your doctor immediately.

Remember that using Neodecadron for a long time may result in increased pressure in the eye, including glaucoma, as well as vision changes and cataracts. Long-term use also increases the chances of developing an additional eye infection. If you use Neodecadron for 10 days or longer, your doctor should check your eye pressure regularly.

If you undergo eye surgery, sustain an eye injury, or develop an eye infection, check with your doctor immediately.

Eye medications can become contaminated if they are not used properly, causing dangerous infections. Do not let the tip of the container touch anything. If your eyes continue to be red, irritated, swollen, or painful, or if they get worse, notify your doctor immediately.

A preservative in Neodecadron solution can be absorbed by soft contact lenses. If you wear contacts, wait at least 15 minutes after using the solution before you insert your lenses.

If you develop a skin rash or any other allergic reaction, stop using the medication and contact your doctor.

If you have had cataract surgery, Neodecadron may delay healing. Neodecadron may cause temporary blurring of vision or stinging.

This prescription should not be renewed unless your doctor has re-examined your eyes.

If your signs and symptoms have not improved after two days, your doctor will reconsider your treatment.

Possible food and drug interactions when taking this medication
No interactions have been reported.

Special information if you are pregnant or breastfeeding
Neodecadron has not been adequately studied during pregnancy. If you are pregnant or plan to become pregnant, inform your doctor immediately. Steroids can appear in breast milk. Your doctor may advise you not to breastfeed while you are using Neodecadron.

Recommended dosage
The length of treatment varies with the type of condition being treated. Treatment can take a few days or several weeks.

NEODECADRON OPHTHALMIC OINTMENT

Apply a thin coating of Neodecadron Ophthalmic Ointment 3 or 4 times a day. When the condition gets better, daily applications should be reduced to 2 and later to 1 if a maintenance dose is required to control the symptoms.

NEODECADRON OPHTHALMIC SOLUTION

The recommended initial dose is to place 1 or 2 drops into the conjunctival sac every hour during the day and every 2 hours during the night. When your condition improves, the doctor will lower the dose to 1 drop every 4 hours, and then to 1 drop 3 or 4 times a day.

Overdosage
Any medication taken in excess can have serious consequences. If you suspect a Neodecadron overdose, seek medical treatment immediately.

Neoral *See Sandimmune, page 1287.*

NEPTAZANE
Pronounced: NEP-tuh-zayne
Generic name: Methazolamide

Why is this drug prescribed?
Neptazane anhydrase is used to treat the eye condition called chronic open-angle glaucoma. This type of glaucoma is caused by a gradual blockage of the outflow of fluid in the front compartment of the eye over

a period of years, causing a slow rise in pressure. It rarely occurs before the age of 40. Neptazane is also used in the type called acute angle-closure glaucoma when pressure within the eye must be lowered before surgery.

Most important fact about this drug

This medication is related to sulfa drugs and can cause allergic reactions, including fever, rash, redness and peeling of the skin, hives, difficulty breathing, serious skin and blood disorders, and even death. Make sure your doctor is aware of any drug reactions you have experienced. He or she should monitor your blood while you are taking this drug. Call your doctor immediately if you experience any allergic symptoms.

How should you take this medication?

Take Neptazane exactly as prescribed. Your doctor may have you use it with other eye medications.

■ *If you miss a dose...*
Take it as soon as you remember. If it is almost time for your next dose, skip the one you missed and go back to your regular schedule. Do not take 2 doses at once.

■ *Storage instructions...*
Store at room temperature.

What side effects may occur?

Side effects cannot be anticipated. If any occur or change in intensity, inform your doctor as soon as possible. Only your doctor can determine if it is safe for you to continue taking Neptazane. Most reactions to Neptazane have been mild and disappear when the medication is stopped or the dosage is adjusted.

■ *Side effects may include:*
Confusion, depression, diarrhea, dizziness, drowsiness, excessive urination, fatigue, fever, general feeling of not being well, headache, hearing problems, loss of appetite, nausea and vomiting, rash, ringing in the ears, severe allergic reaction, taste changes, temporary nearsightedness, tingling in fingers, toes, hands, or feet

Why should this drug not be prescribed?

Neptazane is not for use against all types of glaucoma—only the ones mentioned in *Why is this drug prescribed?* Also, you should not use Neptazane if you have kidney or liver disease, adrenal gland disorders, or low sodium or potassium levels.

Special warnings about this medication

Neptazane can aggravate acidosis, a condition in which the blood is too acidic.

If you have emphysema or a lung blockage, this drug will be prescribed cautiously.

Possible food and drug interactions when taking this medication

If Neptazane is taken with certain other drugs, the effects of either could be increased, decreased, or altered.

Neptazane and high-dose aspirin taken at the same time can cause loss of appetite, rapid breathing, lethargy, coma, and even death.

The use of Neptazane with steroids may lower your potassium level.

Special information if you are pregnant or breastfeeding

The effects of Neptazane in pregnancy have not been adequately studied. Neptazane should be used by a pregnant woman only if the potential benefit outweighs the potential risk to the developing baby. If you are pregnant or plan to become pregnant, inform your doctor immediately. Neptazane may appear in breast milk and could affect a nursing infant. If this medication is essential to your health, your doctor may advise you to stop breastfeeding until your treatment with Neptazane is finished.

Recommended dosage

ADULTS

The usual dosage is 50 to 100 milligrams taken 2 to 3 times a day.

Overdosage

Any drug taken in excess can have serious consequences. If you suspect an overdose of Neptazane, seek medical attention immediately.

NEURONTIN

Pronounced: NUHR-on-tin
Generic name: Gabapentin

Why is this drug prescribed?

Neurontin has two uses. First, it may be prescribed with other medications to treat partial seizures (the type in which symptoms are limited). It can be used whether or not the seizures eventually become general and result in loss of consciousness.

Second, it can be used to relieve the burning nerve pain that sometimes persists for months or even years after an attack of shingles (herpes zoster).

Most important fact about this drug

Take Neurontin exactly as directed by your doctor. To effectively control your seizures, it is important that you take Neurontin 3 times a day, approximately every 8 hours. You should not go longer than 12 hours without a dose of medication.

How should you take this medication?

Do not increase or decrease the dosage of this medication without your doctor's approval; and do not suddenly stop taking it, as this may cause an increase in the frequency of your seizures. If you are taking an antacid such as Maalox, take Neurontin at least 2 hours after the antacid.

You may take Neurontin with or without food.

■ *If you miss a dose...*
Try not to allow more than 12 hours to pass between doses. Do not double doses.
■ *Storage instructions...*
Store capsules and tablets at room temperature. Keep the oral solution refrigerated.

What side effects may occur?

Side effects cannot be anticipated. If any develop or change in intensity, inform your doctor as soon as possible. Only your doctor can determine if it is safe for you to continue taking Neurontin.

■ *When taken for epilepsy, more common side effects may include:*
Blurred, dimmed, or double vision, bronchitis (in children), dizziness, drowsiness, fatigue, fever (in children), involuntary eye movements, itchy, runny nose, lack of muscular coordination, nausea, tremor, viral infection (in children), vomiting, weight increase (in children)
■ *When taken for nerve pain, more common side effects may include:*
Accidental injury, constipation, diarrhea, dizziness, drowsiness, dry mouth, headache, infection, lack of muscular coordination, nausea, swelling in arms and legs, vomiting, weakness

A wide variety of uncommon and rare side effects have also been reported. If you develop any new or unusual symptoms while taking Neurontin, be sure to let your doctor know.

Why should this drug not be prescribed?

You should not take Neurontin if you have ever had an allergic reaction to it.

Special warnings about this medication

Neurontin causes some people to become drowsy and less alert. Combining it with morphine makes this more likely. Do not drive or operate dangerous machinery or participate in any hazardous activity that requires full mental alertness until you are certain Neurontin does not have this effect on you.

In children, Neurontin occasionally triggers behavioral problems such as unstable emotions, hostility, aggression, hyperactivity, and lack of concentration. However, such problems (if they occur) are usually mild.

Be sure to tell your doctor if you have any kidney problems or are on hemodialysis, as your doctor will need to adjust your dosage of Neurontin.

Tell your doctor about any medications you are taking, including over-the-counter drugs.

Possible food and drug interactions when taking this medication

If Neurontin is taken with certain other drugs, the effects of either can be increased, decreased, or altered. It is especially important to check with your doctor before combining Neurontin with the following:

Antacids such as Maalox
Hydrocodone (Lortab, Vicodin)
Morphine (Kadian, MS Contin)
Naproxen (Naprosyn)

Special information if you are pregnant or breastfeeding

The effects of Neurontin on pregnant women have not been adequately studied, although birth defects have occurred in babies whose mothers took an antiepileptic medication while they were pregnant. The drug should be used during pregnancy only if clearly needed. If you are pregnant or plan to become pregnant, tell your doctor immediately. This medication may appear in breast milk and could affect a nursing infant. It should be used by mothers who nurse their babies only if its benefits clearly outweigh the risks.

Recommended dosage

EPILEPSY

Adults and Children 12 Years and Over
The recommended starting dose is 300 milligrams three times a day. After that, the usual daily dosage ranges from 900 to 1,800 milligrams divided into 3 doses.

Children 3 to 12 Years of Age
Daily dosage is calculated according to the child's weight. The usual starting dosage is 10 to 15 milligrams per 2.2 pounds. Dosage is then increased over a period of three days to 40 milligrams per 2.2 pounds for children aged 3 and 4, and 25 to 35 milligrams per 2.2 pounds for children aged 5 and over. The total daily dosage is taken as 3 smaller doses throughout the day.

PAIN FOLLOWING A SHINGLES ATTACK

Treatment typically starts with a single 300-milligram dose on the first day, two 300-milligram doses on the second day, and three 300-milligram doses on the third day. If necessary, the doctor may increase the daily total to as much as 1,800 milligrams, divided into 3 doses. Whether you are taking Neurontin for epilepsy or pain, the doctor will lower the dose if you have poor kidney function. Also, if Neurontin is discontinued or another drug is added to therapy, your doctor will do this gradually, over a 1-week period.

Overdosage

Any medication taken in excess can have serious consequences. If you suspect an overdose, seek medical treatment immediately.

■ *Symptoms of Neurontin overdose may include:*
  Diarrhea, double vision, drowsiness, lethargy, slurred speech

Nevirapine See Viramune, page 1570.

NEXIUM

Pronounced: NECKS-ee-um
Generic name: Esomeprazole magnesium

Why is this drug prescribed?

Nexium relieves heartburn and other symptoms caused by the backflow of stomach acid into the canal to the stomach (the esophagus)—a condition known as gastroesophageal reflux disease. It is also prescribed to heal the damage (erosive esophagitis) that reflux disease can cause.

Prescribed in combination with the antibiotics Biaxin and Amoxil, Nexium is also used to treat the infection that causes most duodenal ulcers (ulcers occurring just beyond the exit from the stomach).

Like its sister drug Prilosec, Nexium works by reducing the production of stomach acid.

Most important fact about this drug

Nexium comes in delayed-release capsules that should be swallowed whole. Be sure to avoid crushing or chewing the capsules.

How should you take this medication?

Take Nexium at least one hour before meals. Be careful to swallow it whole. If you have trouble swallowing capsules, you can open the capsule and carefully pour the pellets onto one tablespoon of applesauce. The applesauce should not be hot. Mix in the pellets, then swallow the applesauce immediately, without chewing.

■ *If you miss a dose...*
Take it as soon as you remember. If it is almost time for your next dose, skip the one you missed and go back to your regular schedule. Never take 2 doses at the same time.

■ *Storage instructions...*
Store at room temperature in a tightly closed container.

What side effects may occur?
Side effects cannot be anticipated. If any develop or change in intensity, inform your doctor as soon as possible. Only your doctor can determine if it is safe for you to continue taking Nexium.

■ *Side effects may include:*
Abdominal pain, diarrhea, headache

Why should this drug not be prescribed?
If Nexium gives you an allergic reaction, or you've ever had an allergic reaction to Prilosec, you will not be able to use this medication.

Special warnings about this medication
The antibiotics prescribed in conjunction with Nexium for the treatment of ulcers have occasionally been known to cause severe side effects and life-threatening allergic reactions. If you've been prescribed this combination, be sure to check the entries on Amoxil and Biaxin for more information.

Possible food and drug interactions when taking this medication
If Nexium is taken with certain other drugs, the effects of either could be increased, decreased, or altered. It is especially important to check with your doctor before combining Nexium with the following:

Diazepam (Valium)
Digoxin (Lanoxin)
Iron salts (Ferro-Sequels)
Ketoconazole (Nizoral)
Warfarin (Coumadin)

There's no problem, however, with combining antacids and Nexium; no unwanted interaction will result.

Special information if you are pregnant or breastfeeding
The effects of Nexium during pregnancy have not been adequately studied. If you are pregnant or plan to become pregnant, check with your doctor.

Because Nexium is likely to appear in breast milk and could harm a nursing infant, you'll need to choose between taking Nexium and breast-feeding your baby

Recommended dosage

ADULTS

Gastroesophageal Reflux Disease (GERD)
For relief of symptoms, the usual dosage is one 20-milligram capsule daily for 4 weeks. If symptoms persist, your doctor may prescribe an additional 4 weeks of therapy.

Erosive Esophagitis
To heal damage, the dosage is 20 or 40 milligrams of Nexium once daily for 4 to 8 weeks. If you haven't fully healed after 8 weeks, your doctor may prescribe an additional 4 to 8 weeks of therapy. To maintain healing, the dosage is 20 milligrams once daily.

Duodenal Ulcers
As part of a three-drug treatment to rid the body of ulcer-causing *H. pylori* bacteria, Nexium is prescribed at a dosage of 40 milligrams once daily for 10 days.

If you have severe liver problems, you should take no more than 20 milligrams of Nexium per day.

Overdosage

Any medication taken in excess can have serious consequences. There have been some reports of Nexium overdoses. If you suspect an overdose, seek medical attention immediately.

■ *Symptoms of Nexium overdose may include:*
Blurred vision, confusion, drowsiness, dry mouth, flushing, headache, nausea, rapid heartbeat, sweating

Niacin *See Niaspan, below.*

NIASPAN

Pronounced: NYE-uh-span
Generic name: Niacin

Why is this drug prescribed?

Although the niacin in Niaspan is one of the B-complex vitamins, this drug isn't taken to prevent deficiencies. In large doses, niacin also lowers cholesterol, and Niaspan extended-release tablets are designed specifically for this purpose.

Excessive levels of cholesterol in the blood can lead to clogged arteries and increased risk of heart attack. Niaspan is prescribed, along with a low-fat, low-cholesterol diet, to reduce blood cholesterol levels, combat clogged arteries, and lower the chance of repeated heart attacks. It is used only when diet alone fails to do the job, and is often taken along with another type of cholesterol-lowering drug known as a bile acid sequestrant (Colestid, Questran, WelChol). It can also be combined with any of the cholesterol-lowering statin drugs (Lescol, Lipitor, Mevacor, Pravachol, Zocor).

Niaspan is also used to reduce very high levels of the blood fats known as triglycerides, a condition that can cause painful inflammation of the pancreas.

Most important fact about this drug

Before starting therapy with Niaspan, your doctor will try to control your cholesterol and triglyceride (fat) levels with a diet low in cholesterol and saturated fat, as well as a program of exercise and, if necessary, weight reduction. It's important to remember that Niaspan (like other cholesterol-lowering drugs) is a supplement to—not a substitute for—these measures. To get the most from Niaspan, you need to continue the diet and exercise program prescribed by your doctor.

How should you take this medication?

Take this medication exactly as prescribed by your doctor. To minimize the flushing effect of Niaspan, your doctor may ask you to take aspirin or a nonsteroidal anti-inflammatory medication (NSAID) such as Motrin or Aleve 30 minutes before taking Niaspan.

Niaspan is taken once a day at bedtime after a low-fat snack. Do not take Niaspan on an empty stomach. If flushing wakes you up during the night, get up slowly, especially if you feel dizzy or faint, or if you are also taking blood pressure medicine.

Niaspan tablets should be swallowed whole, never crushed or chewed.

■ *If you miss a dose...*
Take it as soon as you remember. If it is almost time for your next dose, skip the one you missed and go back to your regular schedule. Do not take 2 doses at once.

■ *Storage instructions...*
Store at room temperature.

What side effects may occur?

Side effects cannot be anticipated. If any develop or change in intensity, inform your doctor as soon as possible. Only your doctor can determine if it is safe for you to continue taking Niaspan.

■ *Side effects may include:*
Abdominal pain, chills, diarrhea, dizziness, fainting, flushing, headache, indigestion, itching, nasal inflammation, nausea, pain, rapid heartbeat, rash, shortness of breath, sweating, swelling due to fluid retention, vomiting

Why should this drug not be prescribed?

Do not take Niaspan if you have significant liver disease, an active ulcer, or arterial bleeding. You'll also have to avoid Niaspan if it gives you an allergic reaction.

Special warnings about this medication

Niaspan is an extended-released form of niacin. It is not interchangeable with immediate-release or sustained-release forms of niacin.

Niaspan can cause problems if your liver is weak. Before you start taking this medication, your doctor may order a blood test to check your liver. Blood tests will probably be repeated 6 and 12 weeks after you start taking Niaspan and periodically after that. While you are taking Niaspan, your doctor will monitor you very closely if you have ever had liver disease or if you are or have ever been a heavy drinker.

Do not drink alcohol or hot beverages with Niaspan because they may intensify the flushing and itching effect of the medication.

Niaspan should be used with caution if you have diabetes, a heart condition, or problems with gout. If you have diabetes, tell your doctor if you have a change in blood sugar levels while taking Niaspan. Also use Niaspan with caution if you have kidney problems.

Before undergoing surgery, make sure the doctor is aware that you are taking Niaspan. This medication tends to slow the clotting process, and could prolong bleeding.

To reduce the chance of side effects, Niaspan therapy is usually started at a low dosage and gradually increased. If you stop taking Niaspan for an extended period, contact your doctor. You'll probably need to build up to your old dose over a period of several months.

Tell your doctor if you experience any dizziness while taking Niaspan.

Possible food and drug interactions when taking this medication

There have been occasional cases of muscle damage when Niaspan is combined with a statin drug such as Lescol, Lipitor, Mevacor, Pravachol, or Zocor. Tell your doctor if you experience any muscle pain, tenderness, or weakness, especially when starting either Niaspan or one of these drugs, or when increasing the dosage.

The cholesterol-lowering drugs known as bile acid sequestrants can cancel Niaspan's effect when taken at the same time. Try to space doses of the two types of drug at least 4 to 6 hours apart.

Multivitamins containing large doses of niacin and related compounds increase the chance of side effects from Niaspan. Tell your doctor about any nutritional supplements you may be taking.

Combining Niaspan with certain blood pressure medications can lead to excessively low blood pressure. Make sure the doctor is aware of any blood pressure drugs that you're taking.

Niaspan has not been tested in children under 21 years of age.

Special information if you are pregnant or breastfeeding
The high doses of niacin needed to lower cholesterol and triglycerides have not been proven safe in pregnancy. If you are taking Niaspan to lower cholesterol, you should discontinue the drug while pregnant. If you need it to control triglyceride levels, your doctor will weigh the benefits of treatment against the potential risk to the baby.

Niacin appears in breast milk, and high doses could cause side effects in the nursing infant. You'll need to choose between breastfeeding your baby and continuing Niaspan therapy.

Recommended dosage

ADULTS

The usual starting dose is one 500-milligram tablet taken at bedtime after a low-fat snack. Every 4 weeks, your doctor may increase your dosage by 500 milligrams, up to a maximum dosage of 2,000 milligrams taken once a day, depending on your response to the drug. Women generally respond to lower doses than men do.

Overdosage
Excessive doses of niacin—more than 2,000 milligrams a day—taken for a long period of time can damage the liver or cause a stomach ulcer to flare up. Nausea, vomiting, abdominal cramps, faintness, and yellowish skin and eyes can be warning signs of long-term overdose. If you develop any of these symptoms, check with your doctor without delay.

Nicardipine See Cardene, page 246.

NicoDerm CQ See Nicotine Patches, below.

Nicotine inhalation system See Nicotrol Inhaler, page 944.

Nicotine nasal spray See Nicotrol NS, page 946.

NICOTINE PATCHES
Brand names: Habitrol, NicoDerm CQ, Nicotrol

Why is this drug prescribed?
Nicotine patches, which are available under several brand names, are designed to help you quit smoking by reducing your craving for tobacco. Each adhesive patch contains a specific amount of nicotine embedded in a pad or gel.

Nicotine, the habit-forming ingredient in tobacco, is a stimulant and a mood lifter. When you give up smoking, lack of nicotine makes you crave cigarettes and may also cause anger, anxiety, concentration problems, irritability, frustration, or restlessness.

When you wear a nicotine patch, a specific amount of nicotine steadily travels out of the patch, through your skin, and into your bloodstream, keeping a constant low level of nicotine in your body. Although the resulting level of nicotine is less than you would get from smoking, it may be enough to keep you from craving cigarettes or experiencing other withdrawal symptoms.

Habitrol patches are round and come in three strengths: 21, 14, or 7 milligrams of nicotine per patch. You wear a Habitrol patch 24 hours a day.

NicoDerm CQ patches are rectangular and come in three strengths: 21, 14, or 7 milligrams of nicotine per patch. You wear a NicoDerm CQ patch 24 hours a day.

Nicotrol patches are rectangular and deliver 15 milligrams of nicotine per patch. You put on a Nicotrol patch in the morning, wear it all day, and remove it at bedtime. You do not use it when you sleep. Nicotrol is available over the counter.

Most important fact about this drug
Nicotine patch therapy should be part of an overall stop-smoking program that also includes behavior modification, counseling, and support. The goal of the therapy should be complete cessation of smoking, not just cutting down.

How should you use this medication?
Use nicotine patches exactly as prescribed. The general procedure is as follows:

- Take a fresh patch out of its packaging and remove the protective liner from the adhesive. Save the wrapper for later disposal of the used patch.
- Stick the patch onto your outer upper arm or any clean, dry, non-hairy part of your trunk.
- Press the patch firmly onto your skin for about 10 seconds, making sure that the edges are sticking well.
- Wash your hands. Any nicotine sticking to your hands could get into your eyes or nose, causing irritation.
- After 16 or 24 hours (depending on the brand), remove that patch and apply a fresh patch to a different spot on your body. To reduce the chances of irritation, do not return to a previously used spot for at least a week.
- Fold the used patch in half, place it back in its own wrapper, and throw it in a trash container that cannot be reached by children or pets.

Water will not harm the nicotine patch. You may keep wearing your patch while bathing, showering, swimming, or using a hot tub.

If your patch does fall off, dispose of it carefully and apply a new patch. As a memory aid, pick a specific time of day and always apply a fresh patch at that time. You may change the schedule if you need to. Just remember not to wear any single patch for more than the recommended time (16 or 24 hours), since after that time the patch will begin to lose strength and may begin to irritate your skin.

Do not change brands without consulting your doctor, and do not attempt to adjust your dosage by cutting a patch into pieces.

If you are unable to stop smoking after 4 to 10 weeks of wearing nicotine patches, it is likely that patch treatment will not work for you.

■ *If you miss a dose...*
Apply the patch as soon as you remember. Never use 2 patches at once.

■ *Storage instructions...*
Do not remove a patch from its wrapping until you are ready to use it. Store your supply of patches at temperatures no higher than 86 degrees Fahrenheit; remember that in warm weather the inside of a car can get much hotter than this.

What side effects may occur?
Side effects cannot be anticipated. If any develop or change in intensity, inform your doctor as soon as possible. Only your doctor can determine if it is safe for you to continue using nicotine patches.

■ *Side effects may include:*
Dizziness, high blood pressure, itching and burning at the application site, nausea, redness of the skin

Why should this drug not be prescribed?
Do not take this medication if you are sensitive to or have ever had an allergic reaction to nicotine. Be cautious if you have ever had a bad reaction to a different brand of nicotine patch or to adhesive tape or other adhesive material.

Special warnings about this medication
Do not smoke, chew, or sniff any form of tobacco while wearing a patch; doing so could give you an overdose of nicotine. Be aware that for several hours after you remove a patch, nicotine from the patch is still in your skin and passing into your bloodstream, so you should not smoke even when the patch is off.

The use of nicotine patches may aggravate certain medical conditions. Before you use any brand of nicotine patch, make sure your doctor knows if you have, or have ever had, any of the following conditions:

Allergies to drugs, adhesive tape, or bandages
Chest pain from a heart condition (angina)
Diabetes requiring insulin injections
Heart attack or heart disease

High blood pressure (severe)
Irregular heartbeat (heart arrhythmia)
Kidney disease
Liver disease
Overactive thyroid
Skin disease
Stomach ulcer

Nicotine, from any source, can be toxic and addictive. Do not use nicotine patches any longer than your doctor prescribes or the product instructions recommend. Thoroughly discuss with your doctor the benefits and risks of nicotine replacement therapy.

If your heartbeat becomes irregular or you have heart palpitations, stop using the patch and call your doctor. Do the same if redness caused by the patch doesn't go away in 4 days or if your skin swells or develops a rash.

Nicotine patches sometimes can cause vivid dreams or other sleep disturbances. If this happens, take the patch off at bedtime.

Do not use a patch if its pouch is unsealed.

The safety and effectiveness of nicotine patches have not been tested in children. Over-the-counter Nicotrol is not for use by children under age 18.

Because a used nicotine patch still contains enough nicotine to poison a child or a pet, you must dispose of used patches with special care. Wrap each patch in the opened pouch or aluminum foil in which it came and throw it in a trash receptacle that is out of the reach of youngsters and animals.

Possible food and drug interactions when taking this medication
If nicotine patches are used with certain other drugs, the effects of either could be increased, decreased, or altered. It is especially important to check with your doctor before combining nicotine patches with the following:

Acetaminophen-containing drugs such as Tylenol
Caffeine-containing drugs such as No Doz
Certain airway-opening drugs such as Isuprel, Dristan, and Neo-Synephrine
Certain blood pressure medicines such as Minipress, Trandate, and Normodyne
Cimetidine (Tagamet)
Haloperidol (Haldol)
Imipramine (Tofranil)
Insulin
Lithium (Eskalith, Lithobid)
Non-nicotine quit-smoking drugs such as Zyban
Oxazepam

Pentazocine (Talwin)
Propranolol (Inderal)
Theophylline (Theo-Dur)

Special information if you are pregnant or breastfeeding

If you are pregnant or plan to become pregnant, inform your doctor immediately. Ideally, a pregnant woman should not take nicotine in any form. Do your best to quit smoking with the aid of counseling and support and without drug therapy. If you are unable to quit, you and your doctor should discuss which is more likely to harm your unborn baby: continued smoking or use of nicotine patches to help you quit smoking. Because nicotine passes very readily into breast milk, ideally it should not be taken in any form during breastfeeding. If you are breastfeeding and are unable to quit smoking, discuss with your doctor the pros and cons of using nicotine patches.

Remember that if you smoke while wearing a patch, you are giving your body a double dose of nicotine; if you are pregnant or breastfeeding, your baby will get the double dose, too.

Recommended dosage

Nicotine patches come in one, two, or three strengths, depending on the brand; larger patches contain higher doses of nicotine. The usual starting dose is 1 high-strength patch per day. If you weigh less than 100 pounds, however, or if you smoke less than half a pack of cigarettes a day or have heart disease, your doctor may start you on a lower-dose patch.

Your doctor will work closely with you to determine the best product and the most effective cessation program.

Overdosage

Any medication used in excess, including nicotine patches, can have serious consequences. If you suspect symptoms of an overdose of nicotine, either from a patch or from smoking while wearing a patch, seek medical attention immediately.

■ *Symptoms of nicotine overdose may include:*
Abdominal pain, blurred vision, breathing abnormalities, cold sweat, confusion, diarrhea, dizziness, drooling, fainting, hearing difficulties, heart palpitations, low blood pressure, nausea, pallor, rapid heartbeat, salivation, severe headaches, sweating, tremor, upset stomach, vision problems, vomiting, weakness

Nicotrol *See Nicotine Patches, page 939.*

NICOTROL INHALER

Pronounced: NICK-o-trole
Generic name: Nicotine inhalation system

Why is this drug prescribed?

A quit-smoking aid, the Nicotrol Inhaler provides a substitute source of nicotine when you first give up cigarettes. A sudden decline in nicotine levels can cause such withdrawal symptoms as nervousness, restlessness, irritability, anxiety, depression, dizziness, drowsiness, concentration problems, sleep disturbances, increased appetite, weight gain, headache, constipation, fatigue, muscle aches, and a craving for tobacco. Nicotrol Inhaler prevents these symptoms and, through a familiar hand-to-mouth ritual, acts as a replacement for cigarettes. (Most of the nicotine in the product is, however, deposited in the mouth instead of the lungs.)

Most important fact about this drug

To get the most from this system, you must be genuinely committed to quitting, and should give up smoking completely before you begin using the inhaler. It should be employed as part of an overall stop-smoking program that includes behavior modification, counseling, and support. The goal is to become a total non-smoker. If you find that you are still smoking after 4 weeks with the inhaler, you should probably stop treatment and try again when you are really ready to quit.

How should you take this medication?

Each Nicotrol Inhaler package includes a mouthpiece and 42 cartridges of nicotine. Treatment takes place in two stages. During the first stage (up to 12 weeks), you should use as many Nicotrol cartridges as needed (at least 6 but no more than 16 daily) to quell the craving for cigarettes. During the second stage (6 to 12 weeks), you should gradually reduce your daily consumption until you are nicotine-free.

For best effect, puff frequently on each cartridge for about 20 minutes. Remember to clean the mouthpiece regularly with soap and water.

■ *If you miss a dose...*
Use the inhaler no more than needed to control the urge to smoke.
■ *Storage instructions...*
Store at room temperature away from light. Keep the mouthpiece in its plastic storage case.

What side effects may occur?

Side effects cannot be anticipated. If any develop or change in intensity, inform your doctor as soon as possible. Only your doctor can determine if it is safe for you to continue using the Nicotrol Inhaler.

■ *Side effects may include:*
Acid indigestion, allergies, back pain, coughing, diarrhea, fever, flu-like symptoms, gas, headache, hiccups, jaw and neck pain, mouth and throat irritation, nasal inflammation, nausea, pain, sinus inflammation, taste disturbances, tingling skin sensation, tooth disorders

Why should this drug not be prescribed?

Nicotrol Inhaler should not be used by anyone allergic to nicotine or menthol.

Special warnings about this medication

Nicotine from any source can be toxic and addictive, and you can become dependent on the Nicotrol Inhaler. To minimize this risk, it's important to gradually cut back on use of the inhaler after the first 3 months. Its use for more than 6 months is not recommended.

Do not smoke while using the inhaler. The added nicotine will increase your risk of developing nicotine toxicity.

Nicotrol Inhaler may not be your best quit-smoking option if you have angina, heartbeat irregularities, Raynaud's phenomenon (periodic loss of circulation in the fingers), Buerger's disease (a dangerous decline in circulation in the hands and feet), or a history of heart attack. If you develop an irregular heartbeat or palpitations, stop using the product and call your doctor immediately.

Nicotrol Inhaler should also be used with caution if you have a respiratory disease, an overactive thyroid, pheochromocytoma (adrenal tumors), insulin-dependent diabetes, an ulcer, severe high blood pressure, or advanced kidney disease.

The nicotine in Nicotrol cartridges can be fatal if inhaled or swallowed by children or pets. Keep used and unused cartridges in a safe place.

Possible food and drug interactions when taking this medication

If you have been taking certain medications regularly, their effects may increase, decrease, or change when you stop smoking. It is especially important to check with your doctor if you have been taking the following drugs:

Antidepressants such as Anafranil
Elavil
Norpramin
Pamelor
Sinequan, and Tofranil
Theophylline (Theo-Dur, Theo-24, Slo-bid)

Special information if you are pregnant or breastfeeding

Cigarette smoking during pregnancy is associated with low birth weight, an increased risk of stillbirth, and a greater chance of miscarriage, so it's extremely important to quit. The Nicotrol Inhaler system may be less harmful than cigarettes, since it does not contain the hydrogen cyanide and carbon monoxide present in cigarette smoke. Nevertheless, nicotine alone can cause fetal harm in lab animals, and your best course is to avoid nicotine in any form. Quitting with the aid of a nicotine replacement system such as Nicotrol Inhaler should be considered only if all other quit-smoking strategies fail. Discuss the problem thoroughly with your doctor.

Nicotine passes into breast milk and ideally should not be taken in any form during breastfeeding. However, use of the Nicotrol Inhaler system could be preferable to smoking, since it may reduce the level of nicotine in your system. If you are breastfeeding, discuss with your doctor the relative pros and cons of quitting with the Nicotrol Inhaler.

Recommended dosage

ADULTS

Dosage varies with the stage of treatment.

Initial Treatment (Up to 12 Weeks)

Use at least 6 cartridges a day for the first 3 to 6 weeks. Additional doses may be needed to control the urge to smoke, up to a maximum of 16 cartridges a day. The average number of doses falls between these extremes.

Gradual Reduction of Dose (Up to 12 Weeks)

Start using Nicotrol Inhaler less frequently. You may find it helpful to keep a tally of daily usage, set a steadily diminishing target, or plan a fixed quit date. Some people find that they can stop abruptly with success.

Overdosage

Excessive doses of nicotine can cause severe symptoms, and may even be fatal. If you suspect an overdose, seek medical attention immediately.

■ *Symptoms of nicotine overdose may include:*
Abdominal pain, breathing abnormalities, cold sweat, confusion, diarrhea, dizziness, exhaustion, headaches, hearing difficulties, increased salivation, low blood pressure, nausea, pallor, tremor, vision problems, vomiting, weakness

NICOTROL NS

Pronounced: NIK-oh-troll
Generic name: Nicotine nasal spray

Why is this drug prescribed?

Nicotrol NS is used to relieve withdrawal symptoms in people who are attempting to give up smoking. It should be used as part of a comprehensive smoking cessation program.

Most important fact about this drug

If you continue to smoke and take Nicotrol NS at the same time, you may experience side effects due to high nicotine levels in your body.

How should you take this medication?

You should stop smoking completely before you begin using Nicotrol NS. Tilt your head back slightly when administering the spray and be careful not to sniff, swallow, or inhale through the nose.

The amount of Nicotrol NS you require depends on your individual needs. One dose is made up of 1 spray in each nostril. The recommended starting regimen is 1 or 2 doses per hour. This may be increased to a maximum of 40 doses (80 sprays) per day if you've been a heavy smoker. Take at least 8 doses (16 sprays) per day; anything less is unlikely to be effective.

■ *If you miss a dose...*
Take it as soon as you remember. If it is almost time for your next dose, skip the one you missed and go back to your regular schedule. Never take 2 doses at the same time.

■ *Storage instructions...*
Store at room temperature, away from children and pets.

What side effects may occur?

Problems experienced by people using Nicotrol NS include nicotine withdrawal symptoms, common complaints of smokers, and local effects of the spray. Most people report some nasal irritation, which usually diminishes with continued use of the product. Other side effects are unpredictable. If any develop or change in intensity, inform your doctor as soon as possible. Only your doctor can determine if it is safe for you to continue taking Nicotrol NS.

■ *More common side effects may include:*
Abdominal pain, acne, back pain, confusion, cough, dental problems, difficulty breathing, gas, gum problems, headache, itching, joint pain, menstrual pain or disorders, muscle aches, nasal irritation, nausea, palpitations, runny nose, sneezing, throat irritation, watering eyes

■ *Rare side effects may include:*
Abnormal vision, allergy, amnesia, asthma, bronchitis, bruises, burning of the nose or eyes, change in sense of smell, diarrhea, dry mouth, earache, eye irritation, facial flushing, hiccups, hoarseness, inability to comprehend words, increased sputum, migraine, nasal congestion, nasal ulcer or blister, nosebleeds, numbness, numbness of the nose or mouth, pain, rash, sinus irritation, sore throat, swelling due to fluid retention, taste alteration

Why should this drug not be prescribed?

Do not use Nicotrol NS if you are allergic to nicotine or if you have ever had a hypersensitivity reaction to it.

Special warnings about this medication

Stop smoking completely when you start using Nicotrol NS. The extra nicotine it delivers could lead to a toxic overdose. If you're still smoking after 4 weeks of Nicotrol NS therapy, check with your doctor. You should probably stop using the product.

It is possible to become dependent on Nicotrol NS. The product is less addictive than cigarettes, but nearly a third of the people using it report some feelings of dependence, and 15 to 20 percent use the product for longer than the recommended period. Remember, though, that Nicotrol NS has not been studied for more than 6 months and long-term use is not recommended.

Use Nicotrol NS with caution if you have a heart condition or a circulation problem. Avoid it completely if you're recovering from a heart attack or have severe angina or serious heartbeat irregularities.

Nicotrol NS is not recommended for people with asthma. It can make the condition worse. You should also avoid Nicotrol NS if you have a chronic nasal disorder such as allergy, nasal polyps, nasal inflammation, or sinusitis. Use Nicotrol NS with caution if you have a glandular problem such as hyperthyroidism, pheochromocytoma, or insulin-dependent diabetes. Nicotine affects the glands. Caution is also warranted if you have an ulcer. Nicotine delays healing of ulcers.

Use Nicotrol NS cautiously, too, if you have serious high blood pressure. The product can make this condition worse.

Possible food and drug interactions when taking this medication

When you quit smoking, the dosage of certain drugs may have to be changed. It is especially important to check with your doctor if you are taking one of the following:

Acetaminophen-containing products such as Tylenol
Caffeine-containing products such as No Doz
Certain airway-opening products such as Isuprel, Afrin,
    and Neo-Synephrine
Drugs classified as beta-blockers, such as Inderal, Sectral,
    and Tenormin
Imipramine (Tofranil)
Insulin
Labetalol (Normodyne, Trandate)
Oxazepam (Serax)
Pentazocine (Talwin)
Prazosin (Minipress)
Theophylline (Theo-Dur)

Special information if you are pregnant or breastfeeding

Nicotine from any source can harm a developing baby. If you're pregnant, it's best to quit without a nicotine replacement product. Use Nicotrol NS only if you think it will speed the moment when you're nicotine-free.

Nicotine makes its way into breast milk. A nursing infant may be exposed to less nicotine from Nicotrol NS than from cigarette smoking, but the best course is to avoid nicotine entirely.

Recommended dosage

ADULTS

A dose is defined as 1 spray in each nostril. When you start Nicotrol NS, 1 or 2 doses per hour is recommended. Take no more than 5 doses per hour, or 40 doses per day. During the treatment period, a minimum of 8 doses per day is usually needed for the drug to be effective.

If you succeed in avoiding cigarettes for 8 weeks of Nicotrol NS therapy, your doctor will instruct you to discontinue the spray over the next 4 to 6 weeks. Recommended strategies for discontinuation include:

Stop "cold turkey."
Cut each dose in half (1 spray instead of 2).
Use the spray less frequently.
Keep a tally of daily usage and try to decrease the amount used each day.
Skip doses by not medicating every hour.
Set a quit date for stopping use of the spray.

Overdosage

Nicotine can be especially toxic to children and pets. Even the residual nicotine in a used container of Nicotrol NS can be harmful. Keep all bottles of Nicotrol NS, used and unused, out of the reach of children.

If a bottle of Nicotrol NS breaks, the spill should be cleaned up immediately with an absorbent cloth or paper towel. Avoid contact with the skin. The area of the spill should be washed several times. If even a small amount of Nicotrol NS comes into contact with the skin, lips, mouth, eyes, or ears, rinse the affected area with water. Keep pets and children away from the area of the spill.

■ *Symptoms of Nicotrol NS overdose may include:*
Abdominal pain, cold sweats, convulsions, diarrhea, disturbed hearing and vision, dizziness, headache, heart failure, nausea, pallor, prostration, hypotension, respiratory failure, salivation, tremor, mental confusion, vomiting, weakness

If you suspect an overdose, seek medical attention immediately.

Nifedipine *See Procardia, page 1162.*

NILANDRON

Pronounced: nigh-LAND-ron
Generic name: Nilutamide

Why is this drug prescribed?

Nilandron is used for advanced prostate cancer—cancer that has begun to spread beyond the prostate gland. An antiandrogen drug, it blocks the effects of the male hormone testosterone, which is known to encourage prostate cancer. The drug is part of a treatment program that begins with removal of the testes, a major—but not the only—source of testosterone.

Most important fact about this drug

Nilandron treatment must begin on the same day as, or on the day after, surgical removal of the testes. You should not interrupt the doses or stop taking Nilandron without consulting your doctor.

How should you take this medication?

Take Nilandron exactly as prescribed. You may take Nilandron with or without food.

■ *If you miss a dose...*
Take the forgotten dose as soon as you remember. If it is almost time for your next dose, skip the one you missed and go back to your regular schedule. Never take 2 doses at the same time.

■ *Storage instructions...*
Store at room temperature away from light.

What side effects may occur?

Side effects cannot be anticipated. If any develop or change in intensity, inform your doctor immediately. Only your doctor can determine if it is safe for you to continue taking Nilandron.

■ *Side effects may include:*
Abnormal vision, alcohol intolerance, constipation, decreased sex drive, difficulty breathing, dizziness, heart failure, hot flashes, impotence, increase in blood pressure, lung problems, nausea, poor adaptation to the dark, tingling feeling, urinary tract infection

Why should this drug not be prescribed?

Do not take Nilandron if you have ever had an allergic reaction to it or to any of its ingredients. If you have severe liver disease or severe breathing problems, you should not take this medication. Make sure your doctor is aware of these conditions.

Special warnings about this medication

Nilandron occasionally causes inflammation of the lungs; and if a problem does develop, you may have to stop taking the drug. Report any symptoms that might suggest a lung problem to your doctor right away. Warning signs include difficulty breathing upon exertion or worsening of a pre-existing problem, cough, chest pain, and fever. This lung condition almost always goes away when Nilandron treatment is stopped.

Nilandron may also cause liver damage in some people. Your doctor will do blood tests to check your liver function before you start treatment at regular intervals for the first 4 months of treatment, and periodically thereafter. If a liver problem does develop, you may have to stop taking Nilandron. Report any symptoms of liver damage to your doctor immediately. Warning signs include dark urine, jaundice (a yellowing of the skin and eyes), fatigue, abdominal pain, tenderness in the upper right part of the stomach, loss of appetite, nausea, or vomiting.

While taking Nilandron, you may also find that your eyes are slow to adapt to the dark when you leave a lighted area. Be careful when driving at night or through tunnels. Tinted glasses will help this problem.

Possible food and drug interactions when taking this medication

Nilandron can cause a reaction to alcohol. If you develop a facial flush, flu-like symptoms, and a decrease in blood pressure after drinking alcohol, you'll need to give up alcoholic beverages while taking this drug.

If Nilandron is taken with certain drugs, the effects of either could be increased, decreased, or altered. It is especially important to check with your doctor before combining Nilandron with the following:

Phenytoin (Dilantin)
Theophylline (Theo-Dur)
Vitamin K antagonists (Coumadin)

If you are already taking Coumadin, you will need to be monitored especially closely after treatment with Nilandron begins. Your doctor may need to lower your dosage of Coumadin.

Special information if you are pregnant or breastfeeding

Nilandron is for use only by men.

Recommended dosage

The recommended adult dosage is 300 milligrams once a day for 30 days. The dosage is then reduced to 150 milligrams once a day.

Overdosage

Any medication taken in excess can have serious consequences. If you suspect an overdose, seek medical attention immediately.

■ *Symptoms of Nilandron overdose may include:*
Dizziness, general discomfort, headache, nausea, vomiting

Nilutamide *See Nilandron, page 950.*

Nisoldipine *See Sular, page 1353.*

Nitazoxanide *See Alinia, 70.*

Nitro-Bid *See Nitroglycerin, below.*

Nitro-Dur *See Nitroglycerin, below.*

Nitrofurantoin *See Macrodantin, page 806.*

NITROGLYCERIN
Pronounced: NIGHT-row-GLISS-err-in
Brand names: Nitro-Bid, Nitro-Dur, Nitrolingual Spray,
Nitrostat Tablets, Transderm-Nitro

Why is this drug prescribed?
Nitroglycerin is prescribed to prevent and treat angina pectoris (suffocating chest pain). This condition occurs when the coronary arteries become constricted and are not able to carry sufficient oxygen to the heart muscle. Nitroglycerin is thought to improve oxygen flow by relaxing the walls of arteries and veins, thus allowing them to dilate.

Nitroglycerin is used in different forms. As a patch or ointment, nitroglycerin may be applied to the skin. The patch and the ointment are for *prevention* of chest pain.

Swallowing nitroglycerin in capsule or tablet form also helps to *prevent* chest pain from occurring.

In the form of sublingual (held under the tongue) or buccal (held in the cheek) tablets, or in oral spray (sprayed on or under the tongue), nitroglycerin helps relieve chest pain that has *already occurred*. The spray can also prevent anginal pain. The type of nitroglycerin you use will depend on your condition.

Most important fact about this drug
Nitroglycerin may cause severely low blood pressure (possibly marked by dizziness or light-headedness), especially if you are in an upright position or have just gotten up from sitting or lying down. You may also find your heart rate slowing and your chest pain increasing. People taking diuretic medication, or who have low systolic blood pressure (less than 90 mm Hg) should use nitroglycerin with caution.

How should you take this medication?
Since nitroglycerin is available in many forms, it is crucial for you to follow your doctor's directions for taking the type of nitroglycerin prescribed for you. Never interchange brands.

Ideally, you should take nitroglycerin while sitting down—especially if you feel dizzy or light-headed—so as to avoid a fall.

■ *If you miss a dose…*
If you are using a skin patch or ointment:
Apply it as soon as you remember. If it is almost time for your regular dose, skip the one you missed and go back to your regular schedule. Never apply 2 skin patches at the same time. If you are taking oral tablets or capsules: Take the forgotten dose as soon as you remember. However, if it is within 2 hours of your next dose, skip the one you missed and go back to your regular schedule. Never take 2 doses at the same time.

■ *Storage instructions…*
Keep this medication in the container it came in, tightly closed. Store it at room temperature. Do not refrigerate.

Avoid puncturing the spray container, and keep it away from excess heat.

Do not open the container of sublingual tablets until you need a dose. Close the container tightly immediately after each use. Do not put other medications, a cotton plug, or anything else in the container. Keep the sublingual tablets handy at all times. Keep the patches in the protective pouches they come in until use.

What side effects may occur?
Side effects cannot be anticipated. If any develop or change in intensity, inform your doctor as soon as possible. Only your doctor can determine if it is safe for you to continue taking nitroglycerin.

■ *Side effects may include:*
Dizziness, flushed skin (neck and face), headache, light-headedness, worsened angina pain

Why should this drug not be prescribed?
You should not be using nitroglycerin if you are allergic to it or to the adhesive in the patch, if you have a head injury, or if you have any condition caused by increased fluid pressure in your head. Nitroglycerin should not be taken if you have severe anemia or if you have recently had a heart attack. The capsule form should not be used if you have closed-angle glaucoma (pressure in the eye) or suffer from postural hypotension (dizziness upon standing up). Do not take the tablets if you are using the impotence drug Viagra.

Special warnings about this medication
If your vision becomes blurry or your mouth becomes dry while taking nitroglycerin, it should be discontinued. Contact your doctor immediately if these symptoms develop.

You may develop acute headaches if you take nitroglycerin excessively. Also, some people may develop a tolerance to nitroglycerin, and it may become less beneficial over time, especially if used in excess.

Nitroglycerin tablets lose their effectiveness when exposed to air. If you are taking sublingual nitroglycerin, you may notice a burning or tingling sensation. This does not necessarily mean that tablets that have been exposed to air for a long period of time are still good.

Take no more than the smallest possible amount needed to relieve pain.

Daily headaches may be an indicator of the drug's activity. Do not change your dose to avoid the headache, because you may reduce the drug's effectiveness at the same time.

Before taking nitroglycerin, tell your doctor if you have had a recent heart attack, head injury, or stroke; or if you have anemia, glaucoma (pressure in the eye), or heart, kidney, liver, or thyroid disease.

If you use a patch, dispose of it carefully. There is enough drug left in a used patch to be harmful to children and pets.

Since nitroglycerin can cause dizziness, you should observe caution while driving, operating machinery, or performing other tasks that demand concentration.

The benefits of applying nitroglycerin to the skin of people experiencing heart attacks or congestive heart failure have not been established. If you are using the medication for these conditions, your doctor will monitor you to prevent low blood pressure and pounding heartbeat.

Possible food and drug interactions when taking this medication

If nitroglycerin is taken with certain other drugs, the effects of either could be increased, decreased, or altered.

Taken with many high blood pressure drugs, nitroglycerin may cause extremely low blood pressure (dizziness, fainting, numbness). Take particular care with calcium channel blockers such as Calan and Procardia XL, as well as isosorbide dinitrate (Sorbitrate, Isordil, others), isosorbide mononitrate (Ismo, others), blood vessel dilators such as Loniten, and beta-blocker medications such as Tenormin. Nitroglycerin may also cause a severe drop in blood pressure when taken with the impotence drug Viagra.

Aspirin can increase the effects of nitroglycerin.

Alcohol may interact with nitroglycerin and cause a swift decrease in blood pressure, possibly causing dizziness and fainting.

Also be alert for an interaction with dihydroergotamine (D.H.E.). Check with your doctor if you are uncertain about any combination you plan to take.

Special information if you are pregnant or breastfeeding

It has not been determined whether nitroglycerin might harm a fetus or a pregnant woman. As a result, nitroglycerin should be used only when the benefits of therapy clearly outweigh the potential risks to the fetus and woman. It is not known if nitroglycerin appears in breast milk; therefore, a nursing mother should use nitroglycerin only on advice of her doctor.

Recommended dosage
The following section is intended to provide guidelines for taking nitroglycerin. Follow your doctor's instructions carefully for using nitroglycerin in the form prescribed for you.

ADULTS

Sublingual or Buccal Tablets
At the first sign of chest pain, 1 tablet should be dissolved under the tongue or inside the cheek. You may repeat the dose every 5 minutes until the pain is relieved. If your pain continues after you have taken 3 tablets in a 15-minute period, notify your doctor or seek medical attention immediately.

You may take sublingual or buccal nitroglycerin from 5 to 10 minutes before starting activities that may cause chest pain.

Patch Form
A patch is applied to the skin for 12 to 14 hours. After this time, the patch is removed; it is not applied again for 10 to 12 hours (a "patch-off" period). Apply the patch as soon as you remove it from its protective pouch.

Spray Form
At the first sign of chest pain, spray 1 or 2 pre-measured doses onto or under the tongue. You should not use more than 3 doses within a 15-minute period. If your chest pain continues, you should contact your doctor or seek medical attention immediately.

The spray can be used 5 to 10 minutes before activity that might precipitate an attack.

Ointment Form
Your initial dose may be a daily total of 1 inch of ointment. Apply one-half inch on rising in the morning, and the remaining one-half inch 6 hours later. If needed, follow your doctor's instructions for increasing your dosage. Apply in a thin, uniform layer, regardless of the amount of your dosage. There should be a daily period where no ointment is applied. Usually, the "ointment-off" period will last from 10 to 12 hours.

Absorption varies with site of application—more is absorbed through the chest.

Sustained-Release Capsules or Tablets
The smallest effective amount should be taken 2 or 3 times a day at 8- to 12-hour intervals.

CHILDREN

The safety and effectiveness of nitroglycerin have not been established for children.

OLDER ADULTS

In general, dosages less than the above adult dosages are recommended, since the elderly may be more susceptible to low blood pressure and headaches.

Overdosage

Any medication taken in excess can have serious consequences. Severe overdosage of nitroglycerin may result in death. If you suspect an overdose, seek medical attention immediately.

■ *Symptoms of overdose may include:*
Bluish skin, clammy skin, colic, coma, confusion, diarrhea (may be bloody), difficult and/or slow breathing, dizziness, fainting, fever, flushed skin, headache (persistent, throbbing), increased pressure within the skull, irregular pulse, loss of appetite, nausea, palpitations (an abnormally rapid throbbing or fluttering of the heart), paralysis, rapid decrease in blood pressure, seizures, slow or fast pulse/heartbeat, sweating, vertigo, visual disturbances, vomiting

Nitrolingual Spray *See Nitroglycerin, page 952.*

Nitrostat Tablets *See Nitroglycerin, page 952.*

Nizatidine *See Axid, page 174.*

NIZORAL
Pronounced: NYE-zore-al
Generic name: Ketoconazole

Why is this drug prescribed?

Nizoral, a broad-spectrum antifungal drug available in tablet form, may be given to treat several fungal infections within the body, including oral thrush and candidiasis.

It may also be given to treat severe, hard-to-treat fungal skin infections that have not cleared up after treatment with creams or ointments, or the oral drug griseofulvin (Fulvicin, Grisactin).

Most important fact about this drug

In some people, Nizoral may cause serious or even fatal damage to the liver. Before starting to take Nizoral, and at frequent intervals while you are taking it, you should have blood tests to evaluate your liver function. Tell your doctor immediately if you experience any signs or symptoms that could mean liver damage: these include unusual fatigue, loss of appetite, nausea or vomiting, jaundice, dark urine, or pale stools.

How should you take this medication?

Take Nizoral exactly as prescribed.

You should keep taking the drug until tests show that your fungal infection has subsided. If you stop too soon, the infection might return.

You may want to take Nizoral Tablets with meals to avoid stomach upset.

Avoid alcohol and do not take with antacids. If antacids are necessary, you should wait 2 to 3 hours before taking them.

■ *If you miss a dose...*
Take the forgotten dose as soon as you remember. This will help to keep the proper amount of medicine in the body. However, if it is almost time for your next dose, skip the one you missed and go back to your regular schedule. Do not take double doses.

■ *Storage instructions...*
Nizoral should be stored at room temperature.

What side effects may occur?

Side effects from Nizoral cannot be anticipated. If any develop or change in intensity, inform your doctor as soon as possible. Only your doctor can determine if it is safe for you to continue taking Nizoral.

■ *Side effects may include:*
Nausea, vomiting

Why should this drug not be prescribed?

Do not take Nizoral if you are sensitive to it or have ever had an allergic reaction to it. Never take Nizoral together with Seldane, Hismanal, Halcion, or Propulsid. Rare, but sometimes fatal, reactions have been reported when these drugs are combined.

Special warnings about this medication

In rare cases, people have had anaphylaxis (a life-threatening allergic reaction) after taking their first dose of Nizoral.

Observe caution when driving or performing other tasks requiring alertness, due to potential side effects of headache, dizziness, and drowsiness.

Possible food and drug interactions when taking this medication

If Nizoral is taken with certain other drugs, the effects of either could be increased, decreased, or altered. It is especially important to check with your doctor before combining Nizoral with the following:

Alcoholic beverages
Antacids such as Di-Gel, Maalox, Mylanta, and others
Anticoagulants such as Coumadin, Dicumarol, and others

Antiulcer medications such as Axid, Pepcid, Tagamet, and Zantac
Astemizole (Hismanal)
Cisapride (Propulsid)
Cyclosporine (Sandimmune, Neoral)
Digoxin (Lanoxin)
Drugs that relieve spasms, such as Donnatal
Isoniazid (Nydrazid)
Methylprednisolone (Medrol)
Midazolam (Versed)
Oral diabetes drugs such as Diabinese and Micronase
Phenytoin (Dilantin)
Rifampin (Rifadin, Rifamate, and Rimactane)
Tacrolimus (Prograf)
Terfenadine (Seldane)
Theophyllines (Slo-Phyllin, Theo-Dur, others)
Triazolam (Halcion)

Special information if you are pregnant or breastfeeding

If you are pregnant or plan to become pregnant, inform your doctor immediately. Nizoral should be taken during pregnancy only if the benefit outweighs the possible harm to your unborn child.

Since Nizoral can probably make its way into breast milk, it should not be taken during breastfeeding. If you are a new mother, check with your doctor. You may need to stop breastfeeding while you are taking Nizoral.

Recommended dosage

ADULTS

The recommended starting dose of Nizoral is a single daily dose of 200 milligrams (1 tablet).

In very serious infections, or if the problem does not clear up within the expected time, the dose of Nizoral may be increased to 400 milligrams (2 tablets) once daily. Treatment lasts at least 1 to 2 weeks, and for some infections much longer.

CHILDREN

In small numbers of children over 2 years of age, a single daily dose of 3.3 to 6.6 milligrams per 2.2 pounds of body weight has been used.

Nizoral has not been studied in children under 2 years of age.

Overdosage

Although no specific information is available, any medication taken in excess can have serious consequences. If you suspect an overdose of Nizoral, seek medical attention immediately.

NOLVADEX

Pronounced: NOLL-vah-decks
Generic name: Tamoxifen citrate

Why is this drug prescribed?

Nolvadex, an anticancer drug, is given to treat breast cancer. It also has proved effective when cancer has spread to other parts of the body. Nolvadex is most effective in stopping the kind of breast cancer that thrives on estrogen.

Nolvadex is also prescribed to reduce the risk of invasive breast cancer following surgery and radiation therapy for ductal carcinoma in situ. The drug can also be used to reduce the odds of breast cancer in women at high risk of developing the disease. It does not completely eliminate your chances, but in a five-year study of over 1,500 high-risk women, it slashed the number of cases by 44 percent.

Most important fact about this drug

Although Nolvadex reduces the risk of breast cancer, it *increases* the possibility of developing endometrial (uterine) cancer. Women taking Nolvadex should have routine gynecological examinations and report any abnormal vaginal bleeding, changes in menstrual periods, change in vaginal discharge, or pelvic pain or pressure to the doctor immediately. Even after Nolvadex therapy has stopped, any abnormal vaginal bleeding should be reported at once.

How should you take this medication?

Take Nolvadex exactly as prescribed. Do not stop taking this medication without first consulting your doctor. It may be necessary to continue taking the drug for several years.

■ *If you miss a dose...*
 Do not try to make it up. Go back to your regular schedule with the next dose.
■ *Storage instructions...*
 Nolvadex may be stored at room temperature.

What side effects may occur?

Side effects from Nolvadex are usually mild and rarely require the drug to be stopped. If any develop or change in intensity, inform your doctor as soon as possible. Only your doctor can determine if it is safe for you to continue taking Nolvadex.

■ *Side effects may include:*
 Hot flashes, nausea, vomiting

Why should this drug not be prescribed?

Do not take Nolvadex if you are sensitive to it or have ever had an allergic reaction to it.

If you are taking the blood-thinning drug Coumadin or have had problems with clots in your veins or your lungs, you should not take Nolvadex to reduce the risk of breast cancer, and when taking it to treat an actual case of the disease, you should use it with caution.

Special warnings about this medication

In addition to increasing the risk of uterine cancer, Nolvadex also raises the odds of developing endometriosis (the spread of endometrial tissue outside the uterus), uterine fibroids, uterine polyps, and ovarian cysts. Women who take Nolvadex also face a greater risk of stroke and blood clots lodging in their lungs. The risk increases further when Nolvadex is combined with toxic cancer drugs. Nolvadex can also cause liver damage, and should be used with caution if you already have liver problems.

If you experience visual problems while taking Nolvadex, notify your doctor immediately.

In a few women Nolvadex may raise the level of cholesterol and other fats in the blood. Your doctor may periodically do blood tests to check your cholesterol and triglyceride levels.

Nolvadex may produce an abnormally high level of calcium in the blood. Symptoms include muscle pain and weakness, loss of appetite, and, if severe, kidney failure. If you experience any of these symptoms, notify your doctor as soon as possible.

If tests show that your blood contains too few white blood cells or platelets while you are taking Nolvadex, your doctor should monitor you with special care. These problems have sometimes been found in women taking Nolvadex; whether the drug caused the blood cell abnormalities is uncertain.

Possible food and drug interactions when taking this medication

If Nolvadex is taken with certain other drugs, the effects of either could be increased, decreased, or altered. It is especially important to check with your doctor before combining Nolvadex with the following:

Aminoglutethimide (Cytadren)
Blood-thinning drugs such as Coumadin
Bromocriptine (Parlodel)
Cancer drugs such as Cytoxan
Letrozole (Femara)
Phenobarbital
Rifampin (Rifadin)

Special information if you are pregnant or breastfeeding

It is important to avoid pregnancy while taking Nolvadex, because the drug could harm the unborn child. Since Nolvadex is an antiestrogen drug, you will need to use a non-hormonal form of contraception, such as a condom and/or diaphragm, and not birth control pills. If you accidentally become pregnant while taking Nolvadex, or within 2 months after you have stopped taking it, discuss this with your doctor immediately.

Because Nolvadex might cause serious harm to a nursing infant, you should not breastfeed your baby while taking this drug. If this medication is essential to your health, your doctor may advise you to discontinue breastfeeding until your treatment is finished.

Recommended dosage

ADULTS

Breast Cancer Treatment
The daily dosage ranges from 20 to 40 milligrams. If you are taking more than 20 milligrams a day, your doctor will have you divide the total into 2 smaller doses taken in the morning and evening. Nolvadex comes in 10- and 20-milligram tablets.

Ductal Carcinoma in Situ
The recommended dose is 20 milligrams once daily for 5 years.

Breast Cancer Prevention
The recommended dose is 20 milligrams once a day for up to 5 years.

CHILDREN

The safety and efficacy of Novadex in children have not been established.

Overdosage

Any medication taken in excess can have serious consequences. If you suspect an overdose of Nolvadex, seek medical attention immediately.

■ *Symptoms of Nolvadex overdose may include:*
  Dizziness, overactive reflexes, tremor, unsteady gait

Norco *See Vicodin, page 1557.*

Nordette *See Oral Contraceptives, page 1000.*

Norethindrone acetate *See Aygestin, page 176.*

Norfloxacin *See Noroxin, page 966.*

NORGESIC

Pronounced: nor-JEE-zic
Generic ingredients: Orphenadrine citrate, Aspirin, Caffeine
Other brand name: Norgesic Forte

Why is this drug prescribed?

Norgesic is prescribed, along with rest, physical therapy, and other measures, for the relief of mild to moderate pain of severe muscle disorders.

Most important fact about this drug

Norgesic may impair your ability to drive a car or operate dangerous machinery. Do not participate in potentially hazardous activities until you know how you react to this medication.

How should you take this medication?

If aspirin upsets your stomach, you may take Norgesic with food. Take it exactly as prescribed.

■ *If you miss a dose…*
 If it is within an hour of your scheduled time, take it as soon as you remember. If you do not remember until later, skip the dose you missed and go back to your regular schedule. Do not take 2 doses at once.
■ *Storage instructions…*
 Store at room temperature.

What side effects may occur?

Side effects cannot be anticipated. If any develop or change in intensity, inform your doctor as soon as possible. Only your doctor can determine if it is safe for you to continue taking Norgesic.

■ *Side effects may include:*
 Blurred vision, confusion (in the elderly), constipation, difficulty urinating, dilation of the pupils, dizziness, drowsiness, dry mouth, fainting, hallucinations, headache, hives, light-headedness, nausea, palpitations, rapid heart rate, skin diseases, stomach and intestinal bleeding, vomiting, weakness

Why should this drug not be prescribed?

If you are sensitive to or have ever had an allergic reaction to the ingredients of Norgesic—orphenadrine, aspirin, and caffeine—you should not take this medication. Make sure your doctor is aware of any drug reactions you have experienced.

You should not take Norgesic if you have the eye condition called glaucoma, a stomach or intestinal blockage, an enlarged prostate gland, a bladder obstruction, achalasia (failure of stomach or intestinal muscles to relax), or myasthenia gravis (muscle weakness and fatigue).

Because taking aspirin while you have chickenpox or flu may cause a rare but serious condition called Reye's syndrome, do not give Norgesic to anyone with these diseases. Call your doctor if fever or swelling develops.

Special warnings about this medication

Because the safety of continuous, long-term therapy with Norgesic has not been established, your doctor should monitor your blood, urine, and liver function if you use this drug for a prolonged period of time.

Because Norgesic contains aspirin, you should be careful taking it if you have a peptic ulcer or problems with blood clotting.

Possible food and drug interactions when taking this medication

If Norgesic is taken with certain other drugs, the effects of either could be increased, decreased, or altered. It is especially important to check with your doctor before combining Norgesic with propoxyphene (Darvon). The combination can cause confusion, anxiety, and tremors.

Special information if you are pregnant or breastfeeding

The effects of Norgesic during pregnancy have not been adequately studied. If you are pregnant or plan to become pregnant, inform your doctor immediately. This drug may appear in breast milk and could affect a nursing infant. If this medication is essential to your health, your doctor may advise you to discontinue breastfeeding until your treatment is finished.

Recommended dosage

ADULTS

The usual dose of Norgesic is 1 to 2 tablets taken 3 or 4 times a day.

The usual dosage of Norgesic Forte, which is exactly twice the strength of Norgesic, is one-half to 1 tablet, taken 3 or 4 times per day.

CHILDREN

The safety and effectiveness of Norgesic have not been established in children.

OLDER ADULTS

Some older adults have experienced confusion when taking this drug. Your doctor may adjust the dosage accordingly.

Overdosage

Any medication taken in excess can have serious consequences. If you suspect an overdose of Norgesic, seek emergency medical treatment immediately.

Norinyl *See Oral Contraceptives, page 1000.*

NORMODYNE

Pronounced: NORM-oh-dine
Generic name: Labetalol hydrochloride
Other brand name: Trandate

Why is this drug prescribed?

Normodyne is used in the treatment of high blood pressure. It is effective when used alone or in combination with other high blood pressure medications, especially thiazide diuretics such as HydroDIURIL and loop diuretics such as Lasix.

Most important fact about this drug

You must take Normodyne regularly for it to be effective. Since blood pressure declines gradually, it may be several weeks before you get the full benefit of Normodyne; and you must continue taking it even if you are feeling well. Normodyne does not cure high blood pressure; it merely keeps it under control.

How should you take this medication?

Normodyne can be taken with or without food. The amount of Normodyne absorbed into your bloodstream is actually increased by food.

This medication should be taken exactly as prescribed by your doctor, even if your symptoms have disappeared.

Try not to miss any doses. If Normodyne is not taken regularly, your condition may worsen.

- *If you miss a dose...*
  Take it as soon as you remember. If it is almost time for your next dose, skip the one you missed and go back to your regular schedule. Never take 2 doses at the same time.
- *Storage instructions...*
  Store at room temperature.

What side effects may occur?

Side effects cannot be anticipated. If any develop or change in intensity, inform your doctor as soon as possible. Only your doctor can determine if it is safe for you to continue taking Normodyne.

- *Side effects may include:*
  Dizziness, fatigue, indigestion, nausea, stuffy nose

Why should this drug not be prescribed?

You should not take Normodyne if you suffer from an obstructive airway disease such as bronchial asthma, congestive heart failure, heart block (a heart irregularity), inadequate blood supply to the circulatory system (cardiogenic shock), a severely slow heartbeat, or any other condition that causes severe and continued low blood pressure.

If you are sensitive to or have ever had an allergic reaction to Normodyne or any of its ingredients you should not take this medication.

Special warnings about this medication

Normodyne has caused severe liver damage in some people. Although this is a rare occurrence, if you develop any symptoms of abnormal liver function—itching, dark urine, continuing loss of appetite, yellow eyes and skin, or unexplained flu-like symptoms—contact your doctor immediately.

If you have a history of congestive heart failure, or kidney or liver disease, Normodyne should be used with caution.

Normodyne should not be stopped suddenly. This can cause chest pain and heart attack. Dosage should be gradually reduced.

If you suffer from asthma, chronic bronchitis, emphysema, or other bronchial diseases, Normodyne should be used cautiously.

This medication may mask the symptoms of low blood sugar or alter blood sugar levels. If you are diabetic, discuss this with your doctor.

Notify your doctor or dentist that you are taking Normodyne if you have a medical emergency, and before you have surgery or dental treatment.

Possible food and drug interactions when taking this medication

If Normodyne is taken with certain other drugs, the effects of either could be increased, decreased, or altered. It is especially important to check with your doctor before taking Normodyne with the following:

Airway-opening drugs such as Proventil and Ventolin
Antidepressant medications such as Elavil
Cimetidine (Tagamet)
Diabetes drugs such as Micronase
Epinephrine (EpiPen)
Insulin
Nitroglycerin products such as Transderm-Nitro
Nonsteroidal anti-inflammatory drugs such as Advil and Motrin
Ritodrine (Yutopar)
Verapamil (Calan)

Special information if you are pregnant or breastfeeding

The effects of Normodyne during pregnancy have not been adequately studied. If you are pregnant or plan to become pregnant, inform your doctor immediately. Normodyne appears in breast milk and could affect a nursing infant. If this medication is essential to your health, your doctor may advise you to discontinue breastfeeding until your treatment is finished.

Recommended dosage

ADULTS

Your doctor will adjust the dosages to fit your needs. Your doctor may observe the drug's effect in his or her office over a 1- to 3-hour period after you begin taking it, and then check your pressure again at regular office visits (12 hours after a dose) to make sure that the medicine is effective.

The usual starting dose is 100 milligrams 2 times per day, alone or with a diuretic drug. After 2 to 3 days of checking your blood pressure, your doctor may begin increasing your dose by 100 milligrams 2 times per day, at intervals of 2 to 3 days.

The regular dose ranges from 200 to 400 milligrams 2 times per day. Some people may require total daily dosage of as much as 1,200 to 2,400 milligrams, either alone or with a thiazide diuretic. In these cases, your doctor will observe the drug's effect and adjust your dose accordingly.

CHILDREN

The safety and effectiveness of Normodyne in children have not been established.

OLDER ADULTS

The usual starting dose is the same as younger people's—100 milligrams twice a day. Your doctor may increase the dose, but usually to no more than 200 milligrams twice a day.

Overdosage

Any medication taken in excess can have serious consequences. If you suspect an overdose, seek medical treatment immediately.

■ *Symptoms of Normodyne overdose may include:*
Dizziness when standing up, severely low blood pressure, severely slow heartbeat

NOROXIN

Pronounced: Nor-OX-in
Generic name: Norfloxacin

Why is this drug prescribed?

Noroxin is an antibacterial medication used to treat infections of the urinary tract, including cystitis (inflammation of the inner lining of the bladder caused by a bacterial infection), prostatitis (inflammation of the prostate gland), and certain sexually transmitted diseases, such as gonorrhea.

Most important fact about this drug

Noroxin is not given for the treatment of syphilis. When used in high doses for a short period of time to treat gonorrhea, it may actually mask or delay the symptoms of syphilis. Your doctor may perform certain tests for syphilis at the time of diagnosing gonorrhea, and after treatment with Noroxin.

How should you take this medication?

Noroxin should be taken, with a glass of water, either 1 hour *before* or 2 hours *after* eating a meal or drinking milk. Do not take more than the dosage prescribed by your doctor.

Your doctor will prescribe Noroxin only to treat a bacterial infection; it will not cure a viral infection, such as the common cold. It's important to take the full dosage schedule of this medication, even if you're feeling better in a few days. Not completing the full dosage schedule may decrease the drug's effectiveness and increase the chances that the bacteria may become resistant to Noroxin and similar antibiotics.

It is important to drink plenty of fluids while taking Noroxin.

■ *If you miss a dose...*
Be sure to take it as soon as possible. This will help to keep a constant amount of Noroxin in your body. However, if it is almost time for your next dose, skip the one you missed and go back to your regular schedule. Do not take 2 doses at the same time.

■ *Storage instructions...*
Store at room temperature. Keep container tightly closed. Store out of reach of children.

What side effects may occur?

Side effects cannot be anticipated. If any develop or change in intensity, inform your doctor as soon as possible. Only your doctor can determine whether it is safe for you to continue taking Noroxin.

■ *Side effects may include:*
Abdominal cramping, dizziness, headache, nausea, weakness

Why should this drug not be prescribed?

You should not use Noroxin if you are sensitive to it or to other drugs of the same type, such as Cipro, or if you have suffered tendon inflammation or tearing due to the use of such drugs. See the *Special warnings about this medication* section.

Special warnings about this medication

Noroxin is not recommended for:

Children (under the age of 18)
Nursing mothers
Pregnant women

People with disorders such as epilepsy, severe cerebral arteriosclerosis, and other conditions that might lead to seizures should use Noroxin cautiously. There have been reports of convulsions in some people taking Noroxin.

Use Noroxin with caution if you suffer from the disease Myasthenia gravis. Noroxin may cause life-threatening respiratory problems under these circumstances.

If you develop diarrhea, tell your doctor. It could be a symptom of a potentially serious intestinal inflammation.

Some people taking drugs chemically similar to Noroxin have experienced severe, sometimes fatal reactions, occasionally after only one dose. These reactions may include: confusion, convulsions, difficulty breathing, hallucinations, heart collapse, hives, increased pressure in the head, itching, light-headedness, loss of consciousness, psychosis, rash, restlessness, shock, swelling in the face or throat, tingling, tremors.

If you experience any of these reactions you should immediately stop taking Noroxin and seek medical help.

There is a small chance that Noroxin may weaken the muscle tendons in your shoulder, hand, or heel, causing them to tear. Should this happen, surgery or at least a long period of disability would be in store. If you feel any pain, inflammation, or tearing, stop taking this drug immediately and call your doctor. Rest and avoid exercise until the doctor is certain the tendons are intact.

In rare cases, people taking Noroxin have developed an irregular heartbeat. Although it is unknown if Noroxin was definitely the cause, you should still use the drug with caution if you have low potassium levels, a slow heartbeat, or take drugs to control your heartbeat.

Some people find needle-shaped crystals in their urine after taking Noroxin. Drink plenty of fluids while taking Noroxin. This will increase urine output and reduce crystallization.

Noroxin may cause dizziness or light-headedness and might impair your ability to drive a car or operate potentially dangerous machinery. Use caution when undertaking any activities that require full alertness if you are unsure of your ability.

You should avoid excessive exposure to direct sunlight while taking Noroxin. Stop taking Noroxin and contact your doctor immediately if you have a severe reaction to sunlight, such as a skin rash.

Possible food and drug interactions when taking this medication
If Noroxin is taken with certain other drugs, the effects of either could be increased, decreased, or altered. It is especially important to check with your doctor before combining Noroxin with the following:

Antacids such as Maalox and Tums
Caffeine (including coffee, tea, and some soft drinks)
Calcium supplements
Cyclosporine (Sandimmune, Neoral)
Didanosine (Videx)

Glyburide (Micronase)
Multivitamins and other products containing iron or zinc
Nitrofurantoin (Macrodantin, Macrobid)
Oral blood thinners such as warfarin (Coumadin)
Probenecid (Benemid)
Sucralfate (Carafate)
Theophylline (Theo-Dur)

Special information if you are pregnant or breastfeeding

The effects of Noroxin during pregnancy have not been adequately studied. Inform your doctor if you are pregnant or planning a pregnancy.

Do not take Noroxin while breastfeeding. There is a possibility of harm to the infant.

Recommended dosage

Take Noroxin with a full glass of water 1 hour before, or 2 hours after, eating a meal or drinking milk. Drink plenty of liquids while taking Noroxin.

The elderly and people with kidney problems may need to use a reduced dosage or have their kidney function monitored.

Uncomplicated Urinary Tract Infections

The suggested dose is 800 milligrams per day; 400 milligrams should be taken twice a day for 3 to 10 days, depending upon the kind of bacteria causing the infection. People with impaired kidney function may take 400 milligrams once a day for 3 to 10 days.

Complicated Urinary Tract Infections

The suggested dose is 800 milligrams per day; 400 milligrams should be taken twice a day for 10 to 21 days.

Prostatitis

The usual daily dose is 800 milligrams, divided into 2 doses of 400 milligrams each, taken for 28 days.

Sexually Transmitted Diseases (Gonorrhea)

The usual recommended dose is one single dose of 800 milligrams for 1 day.

The total daily dosage of Noroxin should not be more than 800 milligrams.

Overdosage

The symptoms of overdose with Noroxin are not known. However, any medication taken in excess can have serious consequences. If you suspect a Noroxin overdose, seek medical help immediately.

NORPACE

Pronounced: NOR-pace
Generic name: Disopyramide phosphate
Other brand name: Norpace CR

Why is this drug prescribed?

Norpace is used to treat severe irregular heartbeat. It relaxes an overactive heart and improves the efficiency of the heart's pumping action.

Most important fact about this drug

Do not stop taking Norpace without first consulting your doctor. Stopping suddenly can cause serious changes in heart function.

How should you take this medication?

Be sure to take this medication exactly as prescribed.

Norpace may cause dry mouth. For temporary relief suck on a hard candy, chew gum, or melt ice chips in your mouth.

■ *If you miss a dose...*
Take it as soon as you remember, if the next dose is 4 or more hours away. If you do not remember until later, skip the dose you missed and go back to your regular schedule. Do not take 2 doses at once.
■ *Storage instructions...*
Store at room temperature.

What side effects may occur?

Side effects cannot be anticipated. If any develop or change in intensity, inform your doctor as soon as possible. Only your doctor can determine if it is safe for you to continue taking Norpace.

■ *Side effects may include:*
Abdominal pain, aches and pains, bloating and gas, blurred vision, constipation, dizziness, dry eyes, nose, and throat, dry mouth, fatigue, headache, inability to urinate, increased urinary frequency and urgency, muscle weakness, nausea, vague feeling of bodily discomfort

Why should this drug not be prescribed?

This drug should not be used if the output of your heart is inadequate (cardiogenic shock) or if you are sensitive to or have ever had an allergic reaction to Norpace.

Norpace can be used for only certain types of irregular heartbeat, and must not be used for others.

Special warnings about this medication

If you have structural heart disease, inflammation of the heart muscle, or other heart disorders, use this medication with extreme caution.

Norpace may cause or worsen congestive heart failure and can cause severely low blood pressure. If you have a history of heart failure, your doctor will carefully monitor your heart function while you are taking this medication.

Norpace can cause low blood sugar (hypoglycemia), especially if you have congestive heart failure; poor nutrition; or kidney, liver, or other diseases; or if you are taking beta-blocking blood pressure drugs such as Tenormin or drinking alcohol.

Your doctor will prescribe Norpace along with other heart-regulating drugs, such as quinidine, procainamide, encainide, flecainide, propafenone, and propranolol, only if the irregular rhythm is considered life-threatening and other antiarrhythmic medication has not worked.

If you have the eye condition called glaucoma, myasthenia gravis, or difficulty urinating (particularly if you have a prostate condition), use this drug cautiously.

You will take lower dosages if you have liver or kidney disease.

Your doctor should check your potassium levels before starting you on Norpace. Low potassium levels may make this drug ineffective; high levels may increase its toxic effects.

Possible food and drug interactions when taking this medication

Avoid alcoholic beverages while taking Norpace.

If Norpace is taken with certain other drugs, the effects of either could be increased, decreased, or altered. It is especially important to check with your doctor before combining Norpace with the following:

Clarithromycin (Biaxin)
Drugs that inhibit the breakdown of other drugs by the liver, including Tagamet
Erythromycin (Eryc, Ery-Tab, PCE)
Other heart-regulating drugs such as lidocaine (Xylocaine), procainamide (Procan SR), propranolol (Inderal), quinidine (Quinidex), and Verapamil (Calan)
Phenytoin (Dilantin)
Troleandomycin (Tao)

Special information if you are pregnant or breastfeeding

The effects of Norpace during pregnancy have not been adequately studied. If you are pregnant or plan to become pregnant, inform your doctor immediately. Norpace appears in breast milk and may affect a nursing infant. If this medication is essential to your health, your doctor may advise you to discontinue breastfeeding until your treatment with this medication is finished.

Recommended dosage

Treatment with Norpace should be started in the hospital.

ADULTS

Your doctor will adjust your dosage according to your own response to, and tolerance of, Norpace or Norpace CR.

The usual dosage range of Norpace and Norpace CR is 400 milligrams to 800 milligrams per day, divided into smaller doses.

The recommended dosage for most adults is 600 milligrams per day, divided into smaller doses (either 150 milligrams every 6 hours for immediate-release Norpace or 300 milligrams every 12 hours for Norpace CR).

For those who weigh less than 110 pounds, the recommended dosage is 400 milligrams per day, divided into smaller doses (either 100 milligrams every 6 hours for immediate-release Norpace or 200 milligrams every 12 hours for Norpace CR).

For people with severe heart disease, the starting dose will be 100 milligrams of immediate-release Norpace every 6 to 8 hours. Your doctor will adjust the dosage gradually and watch you closely for any signs of low blood pressure or heart failure.

For people with moderately reduced kidney or liver function, the dosage is 400 milligrams per day, divided into smaller doses (either 100 milligrams every 6 hours for immediate-release Norpace or 200 milligrams every 12 hours for Norpace CR). This dosage is also recommended for people with glaucoma (high pressure in the eye), urinary retention, or an enlarged prostate gland, in the event they develop side effects.

For those who have severe kidney impairment, the dosage of immediate-release Norpace is 100 milligrams; the times will vary with the individual as determined by your doctor.

Norpace CR is not recommended for people with severe kidney disease.

CHILDREN

Dosage in children to age 18 is based on body weight. The total daily dosage should be divided into equal doses taken orally every 6 hours or at intervals that are best for the individual.

Overdosage

Any medication taken in excess can have serious consequences. An overdose of Norpace can be fatal. If you suspect an overdose, seek medical treatment immediately.

■ *The symptoms of Norpace overdose may include:*
Cessation of breathing, irregular heartbeat, loss of consciousness, low blood pressure, slow heartbeat, worsening of congestive heart failure

NORPRAMIN

Pronounced: NOR-pram-in
Generic name: Desipramine hydrochloride

Why is this drug prescribed?

Norpramin is used in the treatment of depression. It is one of a family of drugs called tricyclic antidepressants. Drugs in this class are thought to work by affecting the levels of the brain's natural chemical messengers (called neurotransmitters), and adjusting the brain's response to them.

Norpramin has also been used to treat bulimia and attention deficit disorders, and to help with cocaine withdrawal.

Most important fact about this drug

Serious, sometimes fatal, reactions have been known to occur when drugs such as Norpramin are taken with another type of antidepressant called an MAO inhibitor. Drugs in this category include Nardil and Parnate. Do not take Norpramin within 2 weeks of taking one of these drugs. Make sure your doctor and pharmacist know of all the medications you are taking.

How should you take this medication?

Norpramin should be taken exactly as prescribed.

Do not stop taking Norpramin if you feel no immediate effect. It can take up to 2 or 3 weeks for improvement to begin.

Norpramin can cause dry mouth. Sucking hard candy or chewing gum can help this problem.

■ *If you miss a dose...*
If you take several doses per day, take the forgotten dose as soon as you remember, then take any remaining doses for the day at evenly spaced intervals. If you take Norpramin once a day at bedtime and don't remember until morning, skip the missed dose. Never try to catch up by doubling the dose.

■ *Storage instructions...*
Norpramin can be stored at room temperature. Protect it from excessive heat.

What side effects may occur?

Side effects cannot be anticipated. If any develop or change in intensity, inform your doctor as soon as possible. Only your doctor can determine if it is safe for you to continue taking Norpramin.

■ *Side effects may include:*
Anxiety, confusion, dizziness, dry mouth, frequent urination or problems urinating, hallucinations, high blood pressure, hives, impaired coordination, irregular heartbeat, low blood pressure, numbness,

rapid heartbeat, sensitivity to sunlight, sex drive changes, tingling, tremors

Why should this drug not be prescribed?
Norpramin should not be used if you are known to be hypersensitive to it, or if you have had a recent heart attack.

People who take antidepressant drugs known as MAO inhibitors (including Nardil and Parnate) should not take Norpramin.

Special warnings about this medication
In clinical studies, antidepressants increased the risk of suicidal thinking and behavior in children and adolescents with depression and other psychiatric disorders. Anyone considering the use of Norpramin or any other antidepressant in a child or adolescent must balance this risk with the clinical need. Norpramin has not been studied in children.

Additionally, the progression of major depression is associated with a worsening of symptoms and/or the emergence of suicidal thinking or behavior in both adults and children, whether or not they are taking antidepressants. Individuals being treated with Norpramin and their caregivers should watch for any change in symptoms or any new symptoms that appear suddenly—especially agitation, anxiety, hostility, panic, restlessness, extreme hyperactivity, and suicidal thinking or behavior—and report them to the doctor immediately. Be especially observant at the beginning of treatment or whenever there is a change in dose.

Before using Norpramin, tell your doctor if you have heart or thyroid disease, a seizure disorder, a history of being unable to urinate, or glaucoma.

Nausea, headache, and uneasiness can result if you suddenly stop taking Norpramin. Consult your doctor and follow instructions closely when discontinuing Norpramin.

This drug may impair your ability to drive a car or operate potentially dangerous machinery. Do not participate in any activities that require full alertness if you are unsure about your ability.

Norpramin may increase your skin's sensitivity to sunlight. Overexposure could cause rash, itching, redness, or sunburn. Avoid direct sunlight or wear protective clothing.

If you are planning to have elective surgery, make sure that your doctor is aware that you are taking Norpramin. It should be discontinued as soon as possible prior to surgery.

Tell your doctor if you develop a fever and sore throat while you are taking Norpramin. He may want to do some blood tests.

Possible food and drug interactions when taking this medication
People who take antidepressant drugs known as MAO inhibitors (including Nardil and Parnate) should not take Norpramin.

If Norpramin is taken with certain other drugs, the effects of either could be increased, decreased, or altered. It is especially important to check with your doctor before combining Norpramin with the following:

Cimetidine (Tagamet)
Drugs that improve breathing, such as Proventil
Drugs that relax certain muscles, such as Bentyl
Fluoxetine (Prozac)
Guanethidine (Ismelin)
Paroxetine (Paxil)
Sedatives/hypnotics (Halcion, Valium)
Sertraline (Zoloft)
Thyroid medications (Synthroid)

Extreme drowsiness and other potentially serious effects can result if Norpramin is combined with alcohol or other depressants, including narcotic painkillers such as Percocet and Demerol, sleeping medications such as Halcion and Nembutal, and tranquilizers such as Valium and Xanax.

Special information if you are pregnant or breastfeeding
Pregnant women or mothers who are breastfeeding an infant should use Norpramin only when the potential benefits clearly outweigh the potential risks. If you are pregnant or planning to become pregnant, inform your doctor immediately.

Recommended dosage
Your doctor will tailor the dose to your individual needs.

ADULTS

The usual dose ranges from 100 to 200 milligrams per day, taken in 1 dose or divided into smaller doses. If needed, dosages may gradually be increased to 300 milligrams a day. Dosages above 300 milligrams per day are not recommended.

CHILDREN

Norpramin is not recommended for children.

OLDER ADULTS AND ADOLESCENTS

The usual dose ranges from 25 to 100 milligrams per day. If needed, dosages may gradually be increased to 150 milligrams a day. Doses above 150 milligrams per day are not recommended.

Overdosage
Any medication taken in excess can have serious consequences. An overdosage of Norpramin can be fatal. If you suspect an overdose, seek medical help immediately.

■ *Symptoms of overdose may include:*
Agitation, coma, confusion, convulsions, dilated pupils, disturbed concentration, drowsiness, extremely low blood pressure, hallucinations, high fever, irregular heart rate, low body temperature, overactive reflexes, rigid muscles, stupor, vomiting

Nor-QD *See Oral Contraceptives, page 1000.*

Nortriptyline *See Pamelor, page 1026.*

NORVASC

Pronounced: NOR-vask
Generic name: Amlodipine besylate

Why is this drug prescribed?

Norvasc is prescribed for angina, a condition characterized by episodes of crushing chest pain that usually results from a lack of oxygen in the heart muscle due to clogged arteries. Norvasc is also prescribed for high blood pressure. It is a type of medication called a calcium channel blocker. These drugs dilate blood vessels and slow the heart to reduce blood pressure and the pain of angina.

Most important fact about this drug

If you have high blood pressure, you must take Norvasc regularly for it to be effective. Since blood pressure declines gradually, it may be several weeks before you get the full benefit of Norvasc; and you must continue taking it even if you are feeling well. Norvasc does not cure high blood pressure; it merely keeps it under control.

How should you take this medication?

Norvasc may be taken with or without food. A once-a-day medication, Norvasc may be used alone or in combination with other drugs for high blood pressure or angina.

You should take this medication exactly as prescribed, even if your symptoms have disappeared. You will begin to see a drop in your blood pressure 24 hours after you start the medication.

■ *If you miss a dose...*
If you forget to take a dose, take it as soon as you remember. If it is almost time for your next dose, skip the one you missed and go back to your regular schedule. Never take 2 doses at the same time.

■ *Storage instructions...*
Store at room temperature in a tightly closed container, away from light.

What side effects may occur?

Side effects cannot be anticipated. If any develop or change in intensity, tell your doctor as soon as possible. Only your doctor can determine if it is safe for you to continue taking Norvasc.

■ *Side effects may include:*
Dizziness, fatigue, flushing, fluid retention and swelling, headache, palpitations (fluttery or throbbing heartbeat)

Why should this drug not be prescribed?

If you are sensitive to or have ever had an allergic reaction to Norvasc, do not take this medication.

Special warnings about this medication

Check with your doctor before you stop taking Norvasc, as a slow reduction in the dose may be needed.

Your doctor will prescribe Norvasc with caution if you have certain heart conditions or liver disease. Make sure the doctor is aware of all your medical problems before you start therapy with Norvasc.

Although very rare, if you have severe heart disease, you may experience an increase in frequency and duration of angina attacks, or even have a heart attack, when you are starting on Norvasc or your dosage is increased.

The safety and effectiveness of Norvasc in children less than 6 years old have not been established.

Possible food and drug interactions

There are no known food or drug interactions with this medication.

Special information if you are pregnant or breastfeeding

The effects of Norvasc during pregnancy have not been adequately studied. If you are pregnant or planning to become pregnant, tell your doctor immediately. Norvasc should be used during pregnancy only if clearly needed. Norvasc may appear in breast milk. If this medication is essential to your health, your doctor may tell you to discontinue breastfeeding your baby until your treatment with Norvasc is finished.

Recommended dosage

HIGH BLOOD PRESSURE

Adults
The usual starting dose is 5 milligrams taken once a day. The most you should take in a day is 10 milligrams. If your doctor is adding Norvasc to other high blood pressure medications, the dose is 2.5 milligrams once daily. The lower 2.5-milligram starting dose also applies if you have liver disease.

Children 6 to 17 Years
The usual dose is 2.5 to 5 milligrams once a day. Doses exceeding 5 milligrams have not been studied in children.

Older Adults
You will be prescribed a lower starting dose of 2.5 milligrams.

ANGINA

Adults
The usual starting dose is 5 to 10 milligrams once daily. If you have liver disease, the lower 5-milligram dose will be used at the start.

Older Adults
The usual starting dose is 5 milligrams. Your doctor may adjust the dose based on your response to the drug.

Overdosage
Experience with Norvasc is limited; but if you suspect an overdose, seek medical attention immediately. The most likely symptoms are a drop in blood pressure and a faster heartbeat.

NORVIR
Pronounced: NOR-veer
Generic name: Ritonavir

Why is this drug prescribed?
Norvir is prescribed to slow the progress of HIV (human immunodeficiency virus) infection. HIV causes the immune system to break down so that it can no longer respond effectively to infection, leading to the fatal disease known as acquired immune deficiency syndrome (AIDS). Without treatment, HIV takes over certain human cells, especially white blood cells, and uses the inner workings of the infected cell to make additional copies of itself. Norvir belongs to a class of HIV drugs called protease inhibitors, which work by interfering with an important step in this process. Although Norvir cannot get rid of HIV already present in the body, it can reduce the amount of virus available to infect other cells.

Norvir is used in combination with other HIV drugs called nucleoside analogues (Retrovir, Hivid, and others). These two types of drugs act against HIV in different ways thus improving the odds of success.

Most important fact about this drug
Do not take Norvir with the following medications. The combination could cause serious, even life-threatening, effects.

Amiodarone (Cordarone)
Astemizole

Bepridil (Vascor)
Dihydroergotamine (D.H.E.)
Ergonovine
Ergotamine (Wigraine)
Flecainide (Tambocor)
Methylergonovine (Methergine)
Midazolam (Versed)
Pimozide (Orap)
Propafenone (Rythmol)
Quinidine (Quinidex)
Terfenadine
Triazolam (Halcion)

Be sure to tell your doctor and pharmacist what medications you are taking, both prescription and over-the-counter, and let them know when you *stop* taking any medication.

How should you take this medication?

Take Norvir every day, exactly as prescribed by your doctor. Do not share this medication with anyone and do not take more than your recommended dosage.

Take Norvir with food, if possible, or the medication may not work properly.

Norvir is available in soft gelatin capsule and oral solution forms. If you are taking Norvir oral solution and want to improve the taste, you can mix the liquid with chocolate milk or a liquid nutritional product (Ensure or Advera) within 1 hour of taking the dose. Use a measuring cup or spoon to measure each dose of the oral solution accurately. A household teaspoon may not hold the correct amount of oral solution.

■ *If you miss a dose...*
Take it as soon as possible. If it is almost time for the next dose, skip the one you missed and go back to your regular schedule. Never double the dose.

■ *Storage instructions...*
Capsules are best kept in the refrigerator, although they do not require refrigeration if used within 30 days and stored below 77 degrees Fahrenheit. Protect from light and heat.

Do not refrigerate the oral solution. Store at room temperature. Shake before each use. Avoid exposure to extreme heat, and keep cap tightly closed.

Keep Norvir in its original container, and use by the expiration date.

What side effects may occur?

Side effects cannot be anticipated. If any develop or change in intensity, tell your doctor as soon as possible. Only your doctor can determine if it is safe for you to continue taking Norvir.

■ *Side effects may include:*
Abdominal pain, anxiety, bedwetting, confusion, diarrhea, dizziness, drowsiness, fatigue, fever, general feeling of illness, headache, indigestion, insomnia, loss of appetite, muscle aches, nausea, numbness or tingling sensation around the face or mouth, pins and needles sensation in the arms and legs, rash, sore or irritated throat, sweating, taste alteration, vomiting, weakness

Why should this drug not be prescribed?

If you have ever had an allergic reaction to Norvir or any of its ingredients, do not take the drug. Never combine Norvir with the drugs listed under *Most important fact about this drug.*

Special warnings about this medication

Norvir has been studied for only a limited period of time. Its long-term effects are still unknown.

Norvir is not a cure for AIDS or HIV infection. You may continue to experience symptoms and develop complications, including opportunistic infections (rare diseases that attack when the immune system falters, such as certain types of pneumonia, tuberculosis, and fungal infections).

Norvir does not reduce the danger of transmission of HIV to others through sexual contact or blood contamination. Therefore, you should continue to avoid practices that could give HIV to others.

If you have liver disease, take this medication with caution; it has caused liver damage in some patients. It has also been known to trigger or aggravate cases of diabetes. It may increase your cholesterol levels. And it can also cause a serious problem called pancreatitis. If you develop warning signs such as nausea, vomiting, and abdominal pain, be sure to tell your doctor. You may have to stop taking the drug.

Some patients undergo an accumulation or redistribution of body fat while taking Norvir. It's not known whether this has any ill effects on health over the long term.

Possible food and drug interactions when taking this medication

Combining Norvir with certain drugs (see *Most important fact about this drug*) may cause serious or life-threatening effects. Other drugs may cause less dangerous—but still worrisome—effects. It is especially important to check with your doctor before combining Norvir with the following:

Anticonvulsants such as Depakote, Dilantin, Klonopin, Lamictal, Tegretol, and Zarontin
Antidepressants such as Norpramin, Prozac, Serzone, and Wellbutrin
Anti-nausea drugs such as Marinol
Atovaquone (Mepron)
Calcium channel blockers (another type of heart and blood pressure medications) such as Calan, Cardizem, and Procardia
Cholesterol-lowering drugs such as Lipitor, Mevacor, and Zocor

Clarithromycin (Biaxin)
Didanosine (Videx)
Disulfiram (Antabuse)
Heart medications such as lidocaine, Mexitil, and Norpace
Immunosuppressants such as Neoral, ProGraf, Rapamune, and
   Sandimmune
Indinavir (Crixivan)
Itraconazole (Sporanox)
Ketoconazole (Nizoral)
Medications for mental illness such as Mellaril, Risperdal, and
   Trilafon
Methadone
Methamphetamine
Metoprolol (Lopressor)
Metronidazole (Flagyl)
Oral contraceptives
Painkillers such as Demerol, Darvon, and Ultram
Quinine
Rifabutin (Mycobutin)
Rifampin (Rifadin)
Saquinavir (Invirase)
Sedatives such as Ambien, Dalmane, ProSom, Tranxene, and Valium
Sildenafil (Viagra)
Steroids such as dexamethasone, fluticasone, and prednisone
St. John's wort *(hypericum perforatum)*
Timolol (Timoptic)
Theophylline (Theo-Dur)

Less significant interactions may occur with many other drugs. Your wisest course is to check with your doctor before combining *any* drug with Norvir.

Tobacco use decreases the effects of Norvir. The effects of antacids taken with Norvir have not been studied.

Special information if you are pregnant or breastfeeding

The effects of Norvir during pregnancy have not been adequately studied. If you are pregnant or plan to become pregnant, tell your doctor immediately.

To avoid transmitting HIV to a newborn baby, HIV-positive women should not breastfeed.

Recommended dosage

ADULTS

The recommended dose of Norvir is 600 milligrams twice a day with food.

Should you experience nausea when first starting on Norvir, your doctor may lower your starting dosage to 300 milligrams twice a day for 1 day, then increase it to 400 milligrams twice a day for 2 days, 500 milligrams twice a day for 1 day, and then 600 milligrams twice a day thereafter.

Your doctor may suggest taking Norvir alone at first and adding a second drug later in the first 2 weeks of therapy. This approach may cause fewer stomach problems.

If you are taking Norvir along with saquinavir, the dosage of both drugs may be reduced to 400 milligrams twice daily.

CHILDREN AGE 2 TO 16 YEARS

The dosage of Norvir in children is based on the child's size, and should not exceed 600 milligrams twice a day. Use of a special spoon or dosing syringe with measurements on it will help ensure that the child receives the proper dose.

Overdosage

Information on acute overdose with Norvir is limited. However, any medication taken in excess can have serious consequences. If you suspect an overdose, seek emergency medical treatment immediately.

■ *Symptoms of Norvir overdose may include:*
Numbness, tingling, or a pins and needles sensation, particularly in the arms and legs

Because Norvir oral solution is 43 percent alcohol, severe alcohol toxicity can follow its ingestion by a young child.

NOVASAL
Pronounced: NO-vah-sawl
Generic name: Magnesium salicylate tetrahydrate

Why is this drug prescribed?
Novasal is an aspirin-like drug used to relieve symptoms of rheumatoid arthritis and osteoarthritis.

Most important fact about this drug
As with all aspirin-like drugs, Novasal should be avoided if you have liver damage, blood clotting problems, or vitamin K deficiency, or if you're scheduled to have surgery.

How should you take this medication?
Take Novasal tablets exactly as prescribed. Do not take more without first checking with your doctor, even if higher doses make you feel better. Taking too much Novasal can cause serious side effects.

■ *If you miss a dose...*
Take it as soon as you remember. If it is almost time for your next dose, skip the one you missed and go back to your regular schedule.

■ *Storage instructions...*
Store at room temperature.

What side effects may occur?

Side effects cannot be anticipated. If any develop or change in intensity, tell your doctor as soon as possible. Only your doctor can determine if it is safe for you to continue using Novasal.

■ *Side effects may include:*
Blood in the stool, blood clotting problems, low blood sugar, ringing in the ears, stomach bleeding, stomach pain

Why should this drug not be prescribed?

If you are especially sensitive to Novasal or to any of its ingredients, you should not take Novasal. Make sure that your doctor knows about any drug reactions you have experienced.

You should not use Novasal if you have advanced or chronic kidney disease or take antigout drugs such as probenecid (Benemid).

If you are 65 or older, you should not take Novasal if you have chronic liver disease, carditis (inflammation of the heart muscle), or have ever had a stomach ulcer or severe stomach inflammation. Also avoid the drug if you are sensitive to aspirin or similar drugs, if you've taken aspirin regularly in the past, or if you take drugs that prevent blood clotting.

Special warnings about this medication

Novasal can interfere with blood clotting. Make sure your doctor knows if you have blood clotting problems or vitamin K deficiency, or if you're scheduled to have surgery. Also let the doctor know if you have liver problems.

Be aware that if you have diabetes or you're receiving hemodialysis, Novasal may lower your blood sugar.

If you're over 65 and take high doses of Novasal, your doctor will monitor your blood levels of magnesium to make sure they do not become too high. In addition, your doctor may want you to stop taking other drugs that contain magnesium. This also applies if you have kidney problems.

Possible food and drug interactions when taking this medication

If Novasal is taken with certain other drugs, the effects of either may be increased, decreased, or altered. It is especially important to check with your doctor before combining Novasal with the following:

Antigout medications such as probenecid (Benemid)
Aspirin

Barbiturates such as secobarbital (Seconal)
Blood thinners such as warfarin (Coumadin)
Diabetes medications known as sulfonylureas, such as glyburide
   (Micronase)
Diuretics such as spironolactone (Aldactone)
Magnesium-containing drugs
Methotrexate (Rheumatrex)
Nonsteroidal anti-inflammatory drugs or other pain relievers
Phenytoin (Dilantin)

Special information if you are pregnant or breastfeeding

You should not use Novasal if you are pregnant. Novasal is similar to aspirin, and studies show that aspirin increases the risk of stillbirth and
death shortly after birth. Aspirin can also lengthen pregnancy and prolong labor. Taking Novasal in the last 3 months of pregnancy could cause
fatal lung damage to the baby. If you are pregnant or plan to become
pregnant, inform your doctor immediately.

   Drugs such as Novasal can enter breast milk and affect a nursing baby.
If this medication is essential to your health, your doctor may advise you
not to breastfeed until your treatment is finished.

Recommended dosage

ADULTS

The starting dose is one 600-milligram tablet taken 3 or 4 times a day. Depending on your response, the doctor may tell you to take as many as 6
to 8 tablets daily.

CHILDREN

Novasal is not recommend for use in children.

OLDER ADULTS

If you are 65 or older, your doctor will prescribe the lowest dose that relieves your symptoms to prevent possible side effects or overdose.

Overdosage

If you suspect an overdose, seek emergency treatment immediately. Even
a single overdose of Novasal can be fatal.

■ *Early symptoms of overdose may include:*
   Confusion, diarrhea, difficulty hearing, dim vision, dizziness, drowsiness, excessive thirst, exhaustion, headache, nausea, rapid breathing,
   ringing in the ears, sweating, vomiting

If you are 65 or older, you are less likely to notice the early warning signs
of an overdose. Be especially watchful for any of the above symptoms, as
prompt treatment is important.

Novolin *See Insulin, page 689.*

NuLev *See Levsin, page 742.*

Nutracort *See Hydrocortisone Skin Preparations, page 656.*

NUVARING
Pronounced: NEW-va-ring
Generic name: Etonogestrel and Ethinyl estradiol vaginal ring

Why is this drug prescribed?
NuvaRing is a contraceptive device. Like oral contraceptives, it prevents pregnancy by providing a steady level of the female hormones estrogen and progestin. This eliminates the hormonal surge that ordinarily triggers the release of an egg. Hormonal contraceptives such as NuvaRing are extremely reliable when used exactly as directed.

Most important fact about this drug
To make sure NuvaRing works properly, you must follow a strict schedule for insertion and removal. Each ring should be inserted and left in place for exactly 3 weeks, then removed. Exactly 1 week after removal, a new ring should be inserted for the following 3 weeks. Always insert and remove NuvaRing on the same day of the week, at approximately the same time of day.

How should you take this medication?
Wash and dry your hands and remove NuvaRing from its foil pouch. Choose the position that is most comfortable for you, such as lying down, squatting, or standing with one leg up. Hold NuvaRing between your thumb and index finger and press the opposite sides of the ring together. Gently push the folded ring into your vagina. The exact position of the ring is not important for it to work. If you feel discomfort, use your finger to gently push NuvaRing further into the vagina. Most women do not feel the ring once it is in place, although some are aware of it.

Leave the ring in place for exactly 3 weeks, then remove it. Hook your index finger under the forward rim or hold the rim between your index finger and middle finger and pull the ring out. Place the used ring in the foil pouch it came in and dispose of it in the garbage, away from children and pets. Do not discard in the toilet.

Your menstrual period will usually start 2 to 3 days after the ring is removed and may not have finished before it's time to insert the next ring. For continued pregnancy protection, you need to insert the new ring exactly 1 week after the old one was removed, even if your period has not stopped.

■ *If you miss a dose...*
If NuvaRing slips out, you'll still be protected against pregnancy provided the ring is replaced within 3 hours. You can use the old ring (after rinsing it with cool or lukewarm water) or insert a new ring. Remove the ring according to your original schedule.

If you're unable to replace the ring within 3 hours, insert it as soon as possible and use an additional method of birth control for 7 days.

If you forget and leave the ring in place for an extra week, remove it, take a 1-week break, and reinsert a new one on day 7. If you leave the ring in place for more than 4 weeks, you may not be adequately protected against pregnancy.

If you miss a menstrual period, you should check to be sure you are not pregnant if any of the following circumstances apply:

If NuvaRing was out of the vagina for more than 3 hours during the 3 weeks of ring use

If you waited longer than 1 week to insert a new ring after removing the old one

If you followed the instructions but miss 2 periods in a row

If you have left NuvaRing in place for longer than 4 weeks.

■ *Storage instructions...*
Store at room temperature and avoid sunlight. Discard unused rings after the expiration date marked on the label.

What side effects may occur?

Side effects cannot be anticipated. If any develop or change in intensity, inform your doctor as soon as possible. Only your doctor can determine if it is safe for you to continue using NuvaRing.

■ *Side effects may include:*
Abdominal cramps, allergic rash, bloating, blood clots, breakthrough bleeding and spotting, breast secretions, change in menstrual flow, changes in the breast such as tenderness or enlargement, dark pigmentation of the skin, decreased milk production in nursing mothers, depression, emotional instability, gallbladder disease, headaches, heart attack, high blood pressure, intolerance to contact lenses, liver disease, liver tumors, migraine headaches, missed periods, nausea, problems with the ring, sinus inflammation, stroke, swelling, temporary infertility after discontinuing NuvaRing, upper respiratory tract infections, vaginal inflammation or discharge, vision problems, vomiting, weight gain or loss, yeast infections, yellow tint to the skin

Why should this drug not be prescribed?

Do not use NuvaRing if you have any of the following conditions:

A clotting disorder (past or present)
A tendency to strokes or mini-strokes (past or present)

Heart disease (past or present)
A heart valve disorder
Severe high blood pressure
Diabetes with impaired circulation
Certain types of headaches
Breast cancer (past or present)
Endometrial cancer or any other estrogen-dependent cancer
Unexplained vaginal bleeding
Liver disease or liver tumors
Jaundice during pregnancy or from prior hormonal
    contraceptive use
Pregnancy
Smoking 15 or more cigarettes per day past age 35
Planned surgery that will keep you immobilized
Allergy to any component of NuvaRing

Special warnings about this medication

Hormonal contraceptives pose a slightly increased risk of blood clots and related disorders such as phlebitis, heart disease, heart attack, vision loss, and stroke. Smoking and advancing age increase this risk.

The estrogen in hormonal contraceptives also appears to cause a slight increase in the risk of breast cancer while the contraceptives are in use. This increase subsides after the contraceptives are stopped.

The risk of developing dangerous liver tumors also goes up very slightly. If you develop signs of liver problems, such as yellowing of the skin or whites of the eyes, you should stop using NuvaRing. Hormonal contraceptives can also hasten the development of gallbladder disease in susceptible women.

If you have diabetes, hormonal contraceptives may worsen the problem. In a few women, they cause an increase in triglyceride (blood fat) levels as well.

Especially in older women, hormonal contraceptives may foster an increase in blood pressure. If you already suffer from high blood pressure or kidney disease, it's best to avoid these drugs. If you do decide to use them and sustain an increase in blood pressure, you'll have to discontinue their use.

Similarly, if NuvaRing triggers migraine headaches or makes them worse, you'll need to stop using this product.

Hormonal contraceptives sometimes leave the user depressed. If you've suffered from depression in the past, use NuvaRing with caution. If you become depressed, alert your doctor immediately; you may need to discontinue use of NuvaRing.

Remember that NuvaRing, like other forms of hormonal contraception, does not protect against HIV infection (AIDS) and other sexually transmitted diseases.

Possible food and drug interactions when taking this medication
If NuvaRing is used with certain other drugs, the effects of either could be increased, decreased, or altered. It is especially important to check with your doctor before combining NuvaRing with the following:

Acetaminophen (Tylenol)
Antibiotics such as ampicillin and tetracycline
Anticonvulsants such as Dilantin, Felbatol, Phenobarbital, Tegretol, Topamax, and Trileptal
Antifungals such as Gris-PEG, Nizoral, and Sporanox
Atorvastatin (Lipitor)
Clofibrate (Atromid-S)
Cyclosporine (Neoral, Sandimmune)
HIV drugs classified as protease inhibitors (Agenerase, Crixivan, Fortovase, Invirase, Kaletra, Norvir, Viracept)
Morphine (Astramorph, Kadian, MS Contin)
Phenylbutazone
Prednisolone (Prelone)
Rifadin (rifampin)
St. John's wort
Temazepam
Theophylline (Theo-Dur)
Vitamin C

Special information if you are pregnant or breastfeeding
NuvaRing should not be used during pregnancy or while nursing.

Recommended dosage

ADULTS

NuvaRing is inserted in the vagina once a month. It stays in the vagina continuously for three weeks. It must be removed exactly 21 days after insertion. A new ring is inserted precisely 7 days later.

The time to start use of NuvaRing depends on your previous contraceptive program:

If you did not use a hormonal contraceptive in the past month
Count the first day of your menstrual period as day 1. Insert the first ring between day 1 and day 5 of the cycle, even if you are still bleeding on day 5. During the first cycle, use an extra method of birth control such as male condoms or spermicide for the first 7 days of ring use.

If you are switching from a combination birth control pill
Insert NuvaRing any time during the first 7 days after the last tablet and no later than the day you would have started a new pill cycle. No extra birth control method is needed.

If you are switching from a progestin-only contraceptive
When you are switching from a progestin-only contraceptive, use an extra method of birth control, such as male condoms or spermicide, for the first 7 days after inserting NuvaRing.

■ If you are switching from the mini-pill, you can start using NuvaRing on any day of the month. Do not skip days between your last pill and first day of NuvaRing use.
■ If you are switching from a progestin implant (Norplant), start using NuvaRing on the same day you have your implant removed.
■ If you are switching from an injectable contraceptive (Depo-Provera), start using NuvaRing on the day when your next injection is due.
■ If you are switching from a progestin-containing IUD, start using NuvaRing on the same day you have your IUD removed.

Following a first trimester abortion or miscarriage
If you start using NuvaRing within 5 days after a complete first-trimester abortion or miscarriage, you do not need to use an extra method of contraception. If more than 5 days have passed, proceed as you would if you had not used a hormonal contraceptive for the past month.

Overdosage
Given the design of NuvaRing, it is unlikely that overdosage will occur. Symptoms of overdose with other hormonal contraceptives include nausea, vomiting, vaginal bleeding, and other menstrual irregularities.

Nystatin with Triamcinolone *See Mycolog-II, page 905.*

OCUFLOX
Pronounced: OK-yew-flocks
Generic name: Ofloxacin

Why is this drug prescribed?
Ocuflox is an antibiotic used in the treatment of eye infections. It is prescribed for eye inflammations and for ulcers or sores on the cornea (the transparent covering over the pupil). Ofloxacin, the active ingredient, is a member of the quinolone family of antibiotics.

Most important fact about this drug
Other forms of ofloxacin have been known to cause allergic reactions in a few patients. These reactions can be extremely serious, leading to loss of consciousness and cardiovascular collapse. Early warning signs include a skin rash, hives, and itching. Other symptoms may include swelling of the face or throat, shortness of breath, and a tingling feeling. One patient

using Ocuflox developed severe blisters and skin peeling. If you develop any of these symptoms, stop using Ocuflox and seek emergency help immediately.

How should you take this medication?
Ocuflox is administered with an eyedropper. Be careful to avoid touching the tip to the eye or any other surface. This could contaminate the solution.

■ *If you miss a dose...*
Take the forgotten dose as soon as you remember. However, if it is almost time for your next dose, skip the one you missed and return to your regular schedule. Do not take two doses at once.

■ *Storage instructions...*
Store at room temperature.

What side effects may occur?
Side effects cannot be anticipated. If any develop or change in intensity, tell your doctor as soon as possible. Only your doctor can determine if it is safe to continue using Ocuflox.

■ *Side effects may includes:*
Allergic reaction, blurred vision, dizziness, dry eye, eye pain, feeling of a foreign body in the eye, inflammation, itching, local burning or discomfort, nausea, redness, sensitivity to light, stinging, swelling of the eye or face, tearing

Why should this drug not be prescribed?
If you've ever had an allergic reaction to a quinolone antibiotic such as Cipro, Floxin, Levaquin, Noroxin, Avelox, or Tequin, you should not use this medication.

Special warnings about this medication
Prolonged use of Ocuflox sometimes promotes the growth of germs that are unaffected by the medication. The doctor will examine your eyes for signs of this development, and discontinue the drug if it appears.

Safety and effectiveness have not been established in children under 1 year of age.

Possible food and drug interactions when using this medication
There is no information on interactions with Ocuflox. When taken internally, however, the similar quinolone antibiotic ciprofloxacin is known to interact with the following:

Caffeine
Cyclosporine (Neoral, Sandimmune)
Theophylline (Theo-Dur)
Warfarin (Coumadin)

Special information if you are pregnant or breastfeeding

The effects of Ocuflox during pregnancy have not been adequately studied. If you are pregnant or plan to become pregnant, alert your doctor immediately.

Researchers do not know whether Ocuflox makes its way into breast milk; but when ciprofloxacin is taken internally, it definitely appears. You'll need to choose between breastfeeding your baby and undergoing treatment with Ocuflox.

Recommended dosage

EYE INFLAMMATION

Apply 1 or 2 drops every 2 to 4 hours for the first 2 days, then 4 times daily for the next 5 days.

CORNEAL ULCERS

For the first 2 days, apply 1 or 2 drops to the affected eye every 30 minutes while awake; also get up 4 to 6 hours after retiring and apply 1 or 2 drops. On days 3 through 7 to 9, apply 1 or 2 drops hourly while awake. From days 7 to 9 onward, apply 1 or 2 drops 4 times a day.

Overdosage

The results of long-term overdosing of Ocuflox are unknown. If you suspect a problem, check with your doctor.

Ofloxacin See Floxin, page 581.

Ofloxacin, ocular See Ocuflox, page 989.

OGEN

Pronounced: OH-jen
Generic name: Estropipate
Other brand name: Ortho-Est

Why is this drug prescribed?

Ogen and Ortho-Est are estrogen replacement drugs. The tablets are used to reduce symptoms of menopause, including feelings of warmth in the face, neck, and chest, and the sudden intense episodes of heat and sweating known as hot flashes. They also may be prescribed for teenagers who fail to mature at the usual rate.

In addition, either the tablets or Ogen vaginal cream can be used for other conditions caused by lack of estrogen, such as dry, itchy external genitals and vaginal irritation.

Along with diet, calcium supplements, and exercise, Ogen and Ortho-

Est tablets are also prescribed to prevent osteoporosis, a condition in which the bones become brittle and easily broken.

Some doctors also prescribe these drugs to treat breast cancer and cancer of the prostate.

Most important fact about this drug

Because estrogens have been linked with increased risk of endometrial cancer (cancer in the lining of the uterus) in women who have had their menopause, it is essential to have regular checkups and to report any unusual vaginal bleeding to your doctor immediately.

How should you take this medication?

Be careful to follow the cycle of administration your doctor establishes for you. Take the medication exactly as prescribed.

When using Ogen Vaginal Cream, follow the instructions printed on the carton. It is for short-term use only. Remove the cap from the tube and make sure the plunger of the applicator is all the way into the barrel. Screw the nozzle of the applicator onto the tube and squeeze the cream into the applicator. The number on the plunger, which indicates the dose you should take, should be level with the top of the barrel. Unscrew the applicator and replace the cap on the tube. Insert the applicator into the vagina and push the plunger all the way down. Between uses, take the plunger out of the barrel and wash the applicator with warm, soapy water. Never use hot or boiling water.

■ *If you miss a dose...*
Take the forgotten dose as soon as you remember. If it is almost time for the next dose, skip the one you missed and go back to your regular schedule. Never try to catch up by doubling the dose.

■ *Storage instructions...*
Store at room temperature.

What side effects may occur?

Side effects cannot be anticipated. If any develop or change in intensity, notify your doctor as soon as possible. Only your doctor can determine if it is safe for you to continue taking estrogen.

■ *Side effects may include:*
Abdominal cramps, bloating, breakthrough bleeding, breast enlargement, breast tenderness and secretions, change in amount of cervical secretion, changes in sex drive, changes in vaginal bleeding patterns, chorea (irregular, rapid, jerky movements, usually affecting the face and limbs), depression, dizziness, enlargement of benign tumors (fibroids), excessive hairiness, fluid retention, hair loss, headache, inability to use contact lenses, menstrual changes, migraine, nausea, reduced ability to tolerate carbohydrates, spotting, spotty darkening of

the skin, especially around the face, skin eruptions (especially on the legs and arms) with bleeding, skin irritation, skin redness and scaling, vaginal yeast infection, vision problems, vomiting, weight gain or loss, yellow eyes and skin

Why should this drug not be prescribed?

Estrogens should not be used if you know or suspect you have breast cancer or other cancers promoted by estrogen. Do not use estrogen if you are pregnant or think you may be pregnant. Also avoid estrogen if you have abnormal, undiagnosed genital bleeding, or if you have blood clots or a blood clotting disorder or a history of blood clotting disorders associated with previous estrogen use.

Ogen Vaginal Cream should not be used if you are sensitive to or have ever had an allergic reaction to any of its components.

Special warnings about this medication

The risk of cancer of the uterus increases when estrogen is used for a long time or taken in large doses. There also may be increased risk of breast cancer in women who take estrogen for an extended period of time.

Women who take estrogen after menopause are more likely to develop gallbladder disease.

Ogen also increases the risk of blood clots. These blood clots can cause stroke, heart attack, or other serious disorders.

Your doctor will check your blood pressure regularly. It could go up or down.

While taking estrogen, get in touch with your doctor right away if you notice any of the following:

Abdominal pain, tenderness, or swelling
Abnormal bleeding from the vagina
Breast lumps
Coughing up blood
Pain in your chest or calves
Severe headache, dizziness, or faintness
Speech changes
Sudden shortness of breath
Vision changes
Vomiting
Weakness or numbness in an arm or leg
Yellowing of the skin

Ogen may cause fluid retention in some people. If you have asthma, epilepsy, migraine, or heart or kidney disease, use this medication with care.

Estrogen therapy may cause uterine bleeding or breast pain.

Possible food and drug interactions when taking this medication

If Ogen is taken with certain other drugs, the effects of either could be increased, decreased, or altered. It is especially important to check with your doctor before combining Ogen with the following:

Barbiturates such as phenobarbital
Blood thinners such as Coumadin
Epilepsy drugs (Tegretol, Dilantin, others)
Insulin
Tricyclic antidepressants (Elavil, Tofranil, others)
Rifampin (Rifadin)

Special information if you are pregnant or breastfeeding

Estrogens should not be used during pregnancy. If you are pregnant or plan to become pregnant, notify your doctor immediately. These drugs may appear in breast milk and could affect a nursing infant. If this medication is essential to your health, your doctor may advise you to discontinue breastfeeding until your treatment is finished.

Recommended dosage

HOT FLASHES AND NIGHT SWEATS

Ogen Tablets
The usual dose ranges from one .625-milligram tablet to two 2.5-milligram tablets per day. Tablets should be taken in cycles, according to your doctor's instructions.

Ortho-Est Tablets
The usual dose ranges from half a tablet to 4 tablets per day of Ortho-Est 1.25 or 1 to 8 tablets of Ortho-Est .625. Tablets should be taken in cycles, according to your doctor's instructions.

VAGINAL INFLAMMATION AND DRYNESS

Ogen Tablets
The usual dose ranges from one .625-milligram tablet to two 2.5-milligram tablets per day. Tablets should be taken in cycles, according to your doctor's instructions.

Ortho-Est Tablets
The usual dose ranges from half a tablet to 4 tablets per day of Ortho-Est 1.25 or 1 to 8 tablets of Ortho-Est .625. Tablets should be taken in cycles, according to your doctor's instructions.

Ogen Vaginal Cream
The usual dose is 2 to 4 grams daily. Cream should be used in cycles, and only for limited periods of time.

ESTROGEN HORMONE DEFICIENCY

Ogen Tablets
The usual dose ranges from one 1.25-milligram tablet to three 2.5-milligram tablets per day, taken for 3 weeks, followed by a rest period of 8 to 10 days.

Ortho-Est Tablets
The usual dose ranges from 1 to 6 tablets per day of Ortho-Est 1.25 or 2 to 12 tablets of Ortho-Est .625, given for 3 weeks, followed by a rest period of 8 to 10 days.

OVARIAN FAILURE

Ogen Tablets
The usual dose ranges from one 1.25-milligram tablet to three 2.5-milligram tablets per day for 3 weeks, followed by a rest period of 8 to 10 days. Your doctor may increase or decrease your dosage according to your response.

Ortho-Est Tablets
The usual dose ranges from 1 to 6 tablets per day of Ortho-Est 1.25 or 2 to 12 tablets of Ortho-Est .625 for 3 weeks, followed by a rest period of 8 to 10 days. Your doctor may increase or decrease your dosage according to your response.

PREVENTION OF OSTEOPOROSIS

Ogen and Ortho-Est Tablets
The usual dose is one .625-milligram tablet per day for 25 days of a 31-day monthly cycle.

Overdosage
Any medication taken in excess can have serious consequences. If you suspect an overdose, seek emergency medical treatment immediately

■ *Symptoms of Ogen overdose may include:*
  Nausea, vomiting, withdrawal bleeding

Ogestrel *See Oral Contraceptives, page 1000.*

Olanzapine *See Zyprexa, page 1670.*

Olanzapine and Fluoxetine *See Symbyax, page 1365.*

Olmesartan *See Benicar, page 198.*

Olopatadine *See Patanol, page 1041.*

Olsalazine *See Dipentum, page 454.*

Omeprazole *See Prilosec, page 1155.*

OMNICEF
Pronounced: OM-knee-seff
Generic name: Cefdinir

Why is this drug prescribed?

Omnicef is a member of the family of antibiotics known as cephalosporins. It is used to treat mild to moderate infections, including:

Acute flare-ups of chronic bronchitis
Middle ear infections (otitis media)
Throat and tonsil infections (pharyngitis/tonsillitis)
Pneumonia
Sinus infections
Skin infections

Most important fact about this drug

Omnicef, like other antibiotics, works best when there is a constant amount in the blood. To maintain effective blood levels, be sure to take every dose on schedule.

How should you take this medication?

Omnicef is available in capsules (for individuals aged 13 years and up) and an oral suspension (for children aged 6 months to 12 years). Shake the oral suspension thoroughly before each use. The drug can be taken with or without food.

Be sure to finish your entire prescription, even if you begin to feel better. If you stop taking the drug too soon, some germs may survive and cause a relapse.

If you use antacids, iron supplements, or multivitamins containing iron, allow at least 2 hours between a dose of these products and a dose of Omnicef. Antacids and iron tend to reduce the amount of Omnicef in the bloodstream. It's okay, however, to combine iron-fortified infant formula with Omnicef suspension.

■ *If you miss a dose...*
Take it as soon as you remember. If it is almost time for your next dose, skip the one you missed and go back to your regular schedule. Do not take 2 doses at once.
■ *Storage instructions...*
Both the capsules and the oral suspension can be stored at room temperature. The suspension will keep for 10 days, after which any unused portion must be thrown away.

What side effects may occur?

Side effects cannot be anticipated. If any develop or change in intensity, inform your doctor as soon as possible. Only your doctor can determine if it is safe for you to continue taking Omnicef.

CAPSULES

■ *Side effects may include:*
Diarrhea, nausea, vaginal infection

SUSPENSION

■ *Side effects may include:*
Diarrhea, rash

Why should this drug not be prescribed?

If you've ever had an allergic reaction to a cephalosporin antibiotic, you should not take this medication. Note, too, that if you are allergic to penicillin, you may also be allergic to cephalosporins. The reaction can be extremely severe. Be sure to let the doctor know about any allergies you may have.

Special warnings about this medication

Use Omnicef with caution if you suffer from colitis (inflammation of the bowel). Omnicef has been known to cause colitis. If you develop symptoms such as diarrhea while taking this medication, notify your doctor.

The use of an antibiotic to kill one type of germ can sometimes promote the growth of other germs that are resistant to the drug. If a new infection (called a superinfection) occurs, alert your doctor. You may need to take a different antibiotic.

If you suffer from seizures, use Omnicef with caution. If you have a seizure while using Omnicef, stop taking it and call your doctor immediately.

Omnicef suspension contains 2.86 grams of sugar per teaspoonful. If a child is diabetic, this could cause an increase in blood sugar levels.

Possible food and drug interactions when taking this medication

If Omnicef is taken with certain other drugs, the effects of either could be increased, decreased, or altered. It is especially important to check with your doctor before combining Omnicef with the following:

Antacids such as Maalox and Mylanta
Iron supplements
Multivitamins containing iron
Probenecid (Benemid)

The combination of iron and Omnicef sometimes turns the stool red. This is not a cause for concern.

Special information if you are pregnant or breastfeeding
The effects of Omnicef during pregnancy have not been adequately studied. If you are pregnant, inform your doctor. Omnicef does not appear in breast milk.

Recommended dosage

ADULTS

For adults and adolescents 13 years and over, the maximum daily dose is 600 milligrams, regardless of the infection under treatment.

Flare-ups of Chronic Bronchitis
300 milligrams every 12 hours for 5 to 10 days or 600 milligrams once a day for 10 days.

Throat and Tonsil Infections
300 milligrams every 12 hours for 5 to 10 days or 600 milligrams once a day for 10 days.

Pneumonia
300 milligrams every 12 hours for 10 days.

Sinus Infections
300 milligrams every 12 hours or 600 milligrams once a day for 10 days.

Skin Infections
300 milligrams every 12 hours for 10 days.

CHILDREN

For children 6 months through 12 years old, the dose of Omnicef Suspension is based on body weight. The suspension contains 125 milligrams per teaspoonful. Dosage should never exceed 600 milligrams daily.

Middle Ear Infections
7 milligrams per 2.2 pounds every 12 hours for 5 to 10 days or 14 milligrams per 2.2 pounds once a day for 10 days.

Throat and Tonsil Infections
7 milligrams per 2.2 pounds every 12 hours for 5 to 10 days or 14 milligrams per 2.2 pounds once a day for 10 days.

Sinus Infections
7 milligrams per 2.2 pounds every 12 hours or 14 milligrams per 2.2 pounds once a day for 10 days.

Skin Infections
7 milligrams per 2.2 pounds every 12 hours for 10 days.

If you have kidney problems, your doctor will lower the dosage.

Overdosage

The effects of an Omnicef overdose are unknown, but overdoses of similar antibiotics produce abdominal pain, convulsions, diarrhea, nausea, and vomiting. If you suspect an overdose, seek medical attention immediately.

Ondansetron *See Zofran, page 1641.*

Opcon-A *See Naphcon-A, page 913.*

OPTIVAR

Pronounced: OP-tee-var
Generic name: Azelastine hydrochloride

Why is this drug prescribed?

Optivar is taken to relieve and prevent the itchy eyes brought on by seasonal allergies. The drug usually starts to work within 3 minutes of placing the drops in the eye, and its effects usually last for about 8 hours.

Most important fact about this drug

Do not use Optivar to treat eye irritation that isn't caused by seasonal allergies.

How should you take this medication?

Use Optivar solution only in the eyes; never swallow it. Optivar is packaged in a bottle with a dropper tip. To prevent contamination of the solution, do not touch the dropper tip to any surface, to your eyelids, or to the surrounding area of the eye.

If you wear soft contact lenses and your eyes are not red, wait at least 10 minutes after using Optivar before inserting your lenses. This will prevent them from absorbing the preservative in Optivar. You should not wear contact lenses if your eyes are red.

■ *If you miss a dose...*
Take it as soon as you remember. If it is almost time for your next dose, skip the one you missed and go back to your regular schedule. Never take 2 doses at the same time.

■ *Storage instructions...*
Store upright at room temperature. Keep the bottle tightly closed.

What side effects may occur?

Side effects cannot be anticipated. If any develop or change in intensity, tell your doctor as soon as possible. Only your doctor can determine if it is safe for you to continue using Optivar.

■ *Side effects may include:*
Bitter taste, headache, temporary eye burning or stinging

Why should this drug not be prescribed?
Do not use Optivar if you have ever had an allergic reaction to it.

Special warnings about this medication
If you wear contact lenses, remember that Optivar should not be used to treat eye irritation caused by your lenses.

Optivar is not recommended for use in children younger than 3 years old.

Possible food and drug interactions when taking this medication
No interactions with Optivar have been reported.

Special information if you are pregnant or breastfeeding
The possibility of harm to a developing baby has not been completely ruled out. Before using Optivar, let your doctor know if you are pregnant or plan to become pregnant.

It is not known whether Optivar appears in breast milk. If you plan to breastfeed, discuss your medication options with your doctor.

Recommended dosage
The usual dose is one drop in each affected eye twice a day.

Overdosage
There is no information on Optivar overdose. However, any medication taken in excess can have serious consequences. If you suspect an overdose, seek medical attention immediately.

ORAL CONTRACEPTIVES
Brand names: Alesse, Apri, Brevicon, Cyclessa, Demulen,
Desogen, Estrostep, Levlen, Levlite, Levora, Loestrin,
Lo/Ovral, Low-Ogestrel, Micronor, Mircette, Modicon,
Necon, Nordette, Norinyl, Nor-QD, Ogestrel, Ortho-Cept,
Ortho-Cyclen, Ortho-Novum, Ortho Tri-Cyclen, Ovcon,
Ovral, Ovrette, Tri-Levlen, Tri-Norinyl, Triphasil, Trivora,
Yasmin, Zovia

Why is this drug prescribed?
Oral contraceptives are highly effective means of preventing pregnancy. Oral contraceptives consist of synthetic forms of two hormones produced naturally in the body: either progestin alone or estrogen and progestin. Estrogen and progestin regulate a woman's menstrual cycle,

and the fluctuating levels of these hormones play an essential role in fertility.

To reduce side effects, oral contraceptives are available in a wide range of estrogen and progestin concentrations. Progestin-only products (such as Micronor) are usually prescribed for women who should avoid estrogens; however, they may not be as effective as estrogen/progestin contraceptives.

One variety of the Pill—the Ortho Tri-Cyclen 28-day Dialpak—is also used in the treatment of moderate acne in women aged 15 and older. It is taken just as it would be for contraception.

Most important fact about this drug

Cigarette smoking increases the risk of serious heart-related side effects (stroke, heart attack, blood clots, etc.) in women who use oral contraceptives. This risk increases with heavy smoking (15 or more cigarettes per day) and with age. There is an especially significant increase in heart disease risk in women over 35 years old who smoke and use oral contraceptives.

How should you take this medication?

Oral contraceptives should be taken daily, no more than 24 hours apart, for the duration of the prescribed cycle of 21 or 28 days. Start the cycle according to package directions. Ideally, you should take your pill at the same time every day to reduce the chance of forgetting a dose; with progestin-only contraceptives, taking the pill at the same time each day is essential.

■ *If you miss a dose...*
If you neglect to take only one estrogen/progestin pill, take it as soon as you remember, take the next pill at your regular time, and continue taking the rest of the medication cycle. The risk of pregnancy is small if you miss only 1 combination pill per cycle. If you miss more than 1 tablet, check your product's patient information for instructions.

Missing a single progestin-only tablet increases the chance of pregnancy. Consult your doctor immediately if you miss a single dose or if you take it 3 or more hours late, and use another method of birth control until your next period begins or pregnancy is ruled out.

■ *Storage instructions...*
To help keep track of your doses, use the original container. Store at room temperature.

What side effects may occur?

Side effects cannot be anticipated. If any develop or change in intensity, inform your doctor as soon as possible. Only your doctor can determine if it is safe for you to continue taking an oral contraceptive.

■ *Side effects may include:*

Breakthrough bleeding between menstrual periods (spotting), depression, loss of menstrual periods, migraine, nausea, vomiting, water retention, weight gain, yeast infection

Why should this drug not be prescribed?

You should not take oral contraceptives if you have had an allergic reaction to them or if you are pregnant (or think you might be). Avoid them, too, if you suffer from migraine headaches preceded by an aura (visual disturbances such as pulsing lights and blind spots, temporary numbness, and similar symptoms).

If you have ever had breast cancer or cancer in the reproductive organs or liver tumors, you should not take oral contraceptives.

If you have or have ever had a stroke, heart disease, liver disease, angina (severe chest pain), or blood clots, you should not take oral contraceptives. They are not recommended for women with significantly high blood pressure. Women who have had pregnancy-related jaundice or jaundice stemming from previous use of oral contraceptives should not take them.

If you have undiagnosed and/or unexplained abnormal vaginal bleeding, do not take oral contraceptives.

In addition, if you have liver, kidney, or adrenal disease, you should avoid the Yasmin brand of oral contraceptive. It contains an ingredient that can increase potassium levels in the body, leading to serious problems if you have one of these diseases.

Finally, you should not take oral contraceptives if you are having major surgery with a prolonged period of being immobile.

Special warnings about this medication

Oral contraceptives should be used with caution if you are over 40 years old; smoke tobacco; have liver, heart, gallbladder, kidney, or thyroid disease; have high blood pressure, high cholesterol, diabetes, epilepsy, asthma, or porphyria (a blood disorder); or are seriously overweight. Caution is also advised if you have blood circulation problems or have had a heart attack or stroke in the past. Be cautious, too, if you have problems with depression, migraine or other headaches, irregular menstrual periods, or visual disturbances.

Because oral contraceptives may speed up development of gallbladder disease, see your doctor right away if you develop symptoms such as sharp stomach pains, fever, or nausea and vomiting.

If you have a family history of breast cancer or other cancers, you might want to consider using a progestin-only product. The estrogen in combination oral contraceptives has been linked with an increase in the risk of breast cancer during use of the pill, though this added risk appears to decrease once you stop taking it. If you do use a combination, choose one with a relatively low amount of estrogen. Take high-estrogen pills (0.05 milligram of estrogen) only if your doctor feels it's necessary.

You should also be aware that some studies link oral contraceptives with an increased risk of cervical cancer. However, some experts think other factors besides the pill are to blame.

Since the blood's clotting ability may be affected by oral contraceptives, your doctor may take you off them prior to surgery. If bleeding lasts more than 8 days while you are on a progestin-only oral contraceptive, or if you have no period at all, be sure to let your doctor know. The risk of blood clots is greater with oral contraceptives that contain desogestrel, such as Ortho-Cept. This risk is also higher during the first year you take a combined oral contraceptive.

Oral contraceptives do not protect against HIV infection (AIDS) or any other sexually transmitted disease. If there is a danger of infection, use a latex condom and spermicide in addition to the pill.

If you develop a migraine or severe headache that does not let up or keeps recurring while you are taking a progestin-only oral contraceptive, check with your doctor. You may need to switch to a different type of pill.

If you miss a menstrual period but have taken your pills regularly, contact your doctor but do not stop taking your pills. If you miss a period and have not taken your pills regularly, or if you miss two consecutive periods, you may be pregnant; stop taking your pills and check with your doctor immediately to see if you are pregnant. Use another form of birth control while you are not taking your pills.

If you are taking a progestin-only oral contraceptive and you have sudden or severe abdominal pain, call your doctor immediately. There is a higher risk of ectopic (outside the womb) pregnancy or ovarian cysts with this type of contraceptive.

You should also be aware that oral contraceptives have been known to cause rare cases of noncancerous—but dangerous—liver tumors. In people prone to high cholesterol and similar problems, oral contraceptives have been known to raise triglyceride levels, leading to pancreatitis.

If you use a combination oral contraceptive, be aware that it may take a couple of months to get pregnant after you stop using it.

Possible food and drug interactions when taking this medication

If oral contraceptives are taken with certain other drugs, the effects of either could be increased, decreased, or altered. It is especially important to check with your doctor before combining oral contraceptives with the following:

Acetaminophen (Tylenol)
Amitriptyline (Elavil)
Ampicillin (Principen)
Aspirin
Atorvastatin (Lipitor)
Barbiturates (phenobarbital, Seconal)
Carbamazepine (Tegretol)

Chloramphenicol (Chloromycetin)
Clofibrate (Questran)
Clomipramine (Anafranil)
Cyclosporine (Neoral, Sandimmune)
Dexamethasone
Diazepam (Valium)
Doxepin (Sinequan)
Felbamate (Felbatol)
Fluconazole (Diflucan)
Glipizide (Glucotrol)
Griseofulvin (Fulvicin, Gris-PEG)
HIV protease inhibitor drugs such as Crixivan (indinavir)
Imipramine (Tofranil)
Itraconazole (Sporanox)
Ketoconazole (Nizoral)
Lorazepam (Ativan)
Metoprolol (Lopressor)
Modafinil (Provigil)
Morphine (MS Contin)
Oxazepam (Serax)
Oxcarbazepine (Trileptal)
Penicillin (Veetids, Pen-Vee K)
Phenylbutazone
Phenytoin (Dilantin)
Prednisolone (Prelone, Pediapred)
Prednisone (Deltasone)
Primidone (Mysoline)
Propranolol (Inderal)
Rifabutin (Mycobutin)
Rifampin (Rifadin, Rimactane)
St. John's wort
Sulfonamides (Bactrim, Septra)
Temazepam (Restoril)
Tetracycline (Sumycin)
Theophylline (Theo-Dur)
Topiramate (Topamax)
Troleandomycin (Tao)
Vitamin C
Warfarin (Coumadin)

In addition, before using the Yasmin brand of oral contraceptive check with your doctor if you regularly take nonsteroidal anti-inflammatory drugs such as Motrin and Aleve, potassium supplements such as Micro-K, certain water pills such as Aldactone, and certain high blood pressure medications, including Avapro, Capoten, Cozaar, Diovan, Vasotec, and Zestril.

Remember, too, that oral contraceptives may affect tests for blood sugar levels and thyroid function and may cause an increase in blood cholesterol levels.

Special information if you are pregnant or breastfeeding

If you are pregnant (or think you might be), you should not use oral contraceptives, since they are not safe during pregnancy. For safety's sake, switch to a nonhormonal method of contraception if you miss a period after forgetting a scheduled dose of the Pill. In addition, wait at least 4 weeks after delivery before starting an oral contraceptive.

Nursing mothers should not use most oral contraceptives, since these drugs can appear in breast milk and may cause jaundice and enlarged breasts in nursing infants. In this situation, your doctor may advise you to use a different form of contraception while you are breastfeeding your baby. However, progestin-only oral contraceptives should not affect your milk or your baby's health.

Recommended dosage

If you have any questions about how you should take oral contraceptives, consult your doctor or the patient instructions that come in the drug package. The following is a partial list of instructions for taking oral contraceptives; it should not be used as a substitute for consultation with your doctor.

Some brands can be started on the first day of your menstrual cycle or on the first Sunday afterwards. Others must be started on the fifth day of the cycle or the first Sunday afterwards. The instructions below are for the first-Sunday schedule.

Oral contraceptives are supplied in 21-day and 28-day packages.

FOR A 21-DAY SCHEDULE

Oral contraceptives are taken every day for a 3-week period, followed by 1 week of no oral contraceptives; this cycle is repeated each month.

1. Starting on the first Sunday after the beginning of your menstrual period, take one tablet daily (at the same time each day) for the next 21 days. Note: If your period begins on Sunday, take the first tablet that day.
2. Wait 1 week before taking any more tablets. Your menstrual period should occur during this time.
3. Following this 1-week waiting time, begin taking a daily tablet again for the next 21 days.

FOR A 28-DAY SCHEDULE

Starting on the first Sunday after the beginning of your menstrual period, take one tablet daily (at the same time each day) for the next 28 days. Continue taking the oral contraceptives according to your physician's instructions. Note: If your period begins on Sunday, take the first tablet that day.

FOR BOTH 21- AND 28-DAY REGIMENS

When following a regimen with a Sunday or Day 5 start, use an additional method of birth control for the first 7 days of the cycle.

Progestin-only tablets should be taken at the same time of day every day of the year.

Overdosage

While any medication taken in excess can cause overdose, the risk associated with oral contraceptives is minimal. Even young children who have taken large amounts of oral contraceptives have not experienced serious adverse effects. However, if you suspect an overdose, seek medical help immediately.

■ *Symptoms of overdose may include:*
Drowsiness, fatigue, nausea, vomiting, withdrawal bleeding in females

ORINASE

Pronounced: OR-in-aze
Generic name: Tolbutamide

Why is this drug prescribed?

Orinase is an oral antidiabetic medication used to treat type 2 (non-insulin-dependent) diabetes. Diabetes occurs when the body does not make enough insulin, or when the insulin that is produced no longer works properly. Insulin works by helping sugar get inside the body's cells, where it is then used for energy.

There are two forms of diabetes: type 1 (insulin-dependent) and type 2 (non-insulin-dependent). Type 1 diabetes usually requires taking insulin injections for life, while type 2 diabetes can usually be treated by dietary changes, exercise, and/or oral antidiabetic medications such as Orinase. Orinase controls diabetes by stimulating the pancreas to secrete more insulin and by helping insulin work better.

Occasionally, type 2 diabetics must take insulin injections temporarily during stressful periods or times of illness. When diet, exercise, and an oral antidiabetic medication fail to reduce symptoms and/or blood sugar levels, a person with type 2 diabetes may require long-term insulin injections.

Most important fact about this drug

Always remember that Orinase is an aid to, not a substitute for, good diet and exercise. Failure to follow a sound diet and exercise plan can lead to serious complications, such as dangerously high or low blood sugar levels. Remember, too, that Orinase is *not* an oral form of insulin, and cannot be used in place of insulin.

How should you take this medication?

In general, Orinase should be taken 30 minutes before a meal to achieve the best control over blood sugar levels. However, the exact dosing schedule, as well as the dosage amount, must be determined by your physician. Ask your doctor when it is best for you to take this medication.

To help prevent low blood sugar levels (hypoglycemia) you should:

Understand the symptoms of hypoglycemia.
Know how exercise affects your blood sugar levels.
Maintain an adequate diet.
Keep a product containing quick-acting sugar with you at all times.
Limit alcohol intake. If you drink alcohol, it may cause
 breathlessness and facial flushing.

■ *If you miss a dose...*
Take it as soon as you remember. If it is almost time for the next dose, skip the one you missed and go back to your regular schedule. Do not take 2 doses at the same time.

■ *Storage instructions...*
Store at room temperature.

What side effects may occur?

Side effects cannot be anticipated. If any develop or change in intensity, inform your doctor as soon as possible. Only your doctor can determine if it is safe for you to continue taking Orinase.

Side effects from Orinase are rare and seldom require discontinuation of the medication.

■ *Side effects may include:*
Bloating, heartburn, nausea
Orinase, like all oral antidiabetics, may cause hypoglycemia (low blood sugar). The risk of hypoglycemia can be increased by missed meals, alcohol, other medications, fever, trauma, infection, surgery, or excessive exercise. To avoid hypoglycemia, you should closely follow the dietary and exercise plan suggested by your physician.

■ *Symptoms of mild hypoglycemia may include:*
Cold sweat, drowsiness, fast heartbeat, headache, nausea, nervousness.

■ *Symptoms of more severe hypoglycemia may include:*
Coma, pale skin, seizures, shallow breathing.

Contact your doctor immediately if these symptoms of severely low blood sugar occur.

Ask your doctor what you should do if you experience mild hypoglycemia. Severe hypoglycemia should be considered a medical emergency, and prompt medical attention is essential.

Why should this drug not be prescribed?

You should not take Orinase if you have had an allergic reaction to it.

Orinase should not be taken if you are suffering from diabetic ketoacidosis (a life-threatening medical emergency caused by insufficient insulin and marked by excessive thirst, nausea, fatigue, pain below the breastbone, and fruity breath).

In addition, Orinase should not be used as the sole therapy in treating type 1 (insulin-dependent) diabetes.

Special warnings about this medication

It's possible that drugs such as Orinase may lead to more heart problems than diet treatment alone, or diet plus insulin. If you have a heart condition, you may want to discuss this with your doctor.

If you are taking Orinase, you should check your blood or urine periodically for abnormal sugar (glucose) levels.

It is important that you closely follow the diet and exercise plan recommended by your doctor.

Even people with well-controlled diabetes may find that stress, illness, surgery, or fever results in a loss of control over their diabetes. In these cases, your physician may recommend that you temporarily stop taking Orinase and use injected insulin instead.

In addition, the effectiveness of any oral antidiabetic, including Orinase, may decrease with time. This may occur because of either a diminished responsiveness to the medication or a worsening of the diabetes.

Like other antidiabetic drugs, Orinase may produce severe low blood sugar if the dosage is wrong. While taking Orinase, you are particularly susceptible to episodes of low blood sugar if:

You suffer from a kidney or liver problem;

You have a lack of adrenal or pituitary hormone;

You are elderly, run-down, malnourished, hungry, exercising heavily, drinking alcohol, or using more than one glucose-lowering drug.

Possible food and drug interactions when taking this medication

If Orinase is taken with certain other drugs, the effects of either could be increased, decreased, or altered. It is especially important to check with your doctor before combining Orinase with the following:

Adrenal corticosteroids such as prednisone (Deltasone) and cortisone (Cortone)
Airway-opening drugs such as Proventil and Ventolin
Anabolic steroids such as testosterone

Barbiturates such as Amytal, Seconal, and phenobarbital
Beta-blockers such as Inderal and Tenormin
Blood-thinning drugs such as Coumadin
Calcium channel blockers such as Cardizem and Procardia
Chloramphenicol (Chloromycetin)
Cimetidine (Tagamet)
Clofibrate (Atromid-S)
Colestipol (Colestid)
Epinephrine (EpiPen)
Estrogens (Premarin)
Fluconazole (Diflucan)
Furosemide (Lasix)
Isoniazid (Nydrazid)
Itraconazole (Sporanox)
Major tranquilizers such as Stelazine and Mellaril
MAO inhibitors such as Nardil and Parnate
Methyldopa (Aldomet)
Miconazole (Monistat)
Niacin (Nicobid, Nicolar)
Nonsteroidal anti-inflammatory agents such as Advil, aspirin, Motrin, Naprosyn, and Voltaren
Oral contraceptives
Phenytoin (Dilantin)
Probenecid (Benemid)
Rifampin (Rifadin)
Sulfa drugs such as Bactrim and Septra
Thiazide and other diuretics such as Diuril and HydroDIURIL
Thyroid medications such as Synthroid

Be cautious about drinking alcohol, since excessive alcohol can cause low blood sugar.

Special information if you are pregnant or breastfeeding
The effects of Orinase during pregnancy have not been adequately established in humans. Since Orinase has caused birth defects in rats, it is not recommended for use by pregnant women. Therefore, if you are pregnant or planning to become pregnant, you should take Orinase only on the advice of your physician. Since studies suggest the importance of maintaining normal blood sugar (glucose) levels during pregnancy, your physician may prescribe injected insulin during your pregnancy. While it is not known if Orinase enters breast milk, other similar medications do. Therefore, you should discuss with your doctor whether to discontinue the medication or to stop breastfeeding. If the medication is discontinued, and if diet alone does not control glucose levels, your doctor will consider giving you insulin injections.

Recommended dosage
Dosage levels are based on individual needs.

ADULTS
Usually an initial daily dose of 1 to 2 grams is recommended. Maintenance therapy usually ranges from 0.25 to 3 grams daily. Daily doses greater than 3 grams are not recommended.

CHILDREN
Safety and effectiveness have not been established in children.

OLDER ADULTS
Older, malnourished, or debilitated people, or those with impaired kidney or liver function, are usually prescribed lower initial and maintenance doses to minimize the risk of low blood sugar (hypoglycemia).

Overdosage
Any medication taken in excess can have serious consequences. An overdose of Orinase can cause low blood sugar (see *Special warnings about this medication*). Eating sugar or a sugar-based product will often correct mild hypoglycemia. If you suspect an overdose, seek medical attention immediately.

Orlistat *See Xenical, page 1598.*

Orphenadrine, Aspirin, and Caffeine *See Norgesic, page 962.*

Ortho-Cept *See Oral Contraceptives, page 1000.*

Ortho-Cyclen *See Oral Contraceptives, page 1000.*

Ortho-Est *See Ogen, page 991.*

ORTHO EVRA
Pronounced: OR-thoe EV-rah
Generic ingredients: Ethinyl estradiol, Norelgestromin

Why is this drug prescribed?
Ortho Evra is a contraceptive skin patch. It contains estrogen and progestin, the same hormones found in many birth control pills. Fertility depends on regular fluctuations in the levels of these hormones. Contraceptives such as Ortho Evra reduce fertility by eliminating the fluctuations. Once applied to the skin, the Ortho Evra patch releases a steady supply of estrogen and progestin through the skin and into the bloodstream.

Most important fact about this drug

Cigarette smoking increases the risk of serious heart-related side effects (stroke, heart attack, blood clots, etc.) in women who use hormonal contraceptives. This risk increases with heavy smoking (15 or more cigarettes per day) and with age. There is an especially significant increase in heart disease risk in women over 35 years old who smoke and use hormonal birth control. Therefore, women who use Ortho Evra are strongly advised not to smoke.

How should you take this medication?

You should use 3 separate Ortho Evra patches during each 4-week menstrual cycle. Wear 1 patch a week for the first 3 weeks, then spend the fourth week patch-free. Your menstrual period should start during the fourth week.

■ *If you miss a dose...*
If your patch becomes loose or falls off for less than 1 day, try to stick it back on, or apply a new patch immediately. If it's been missing for more than 1 day, or you're not sure how long it's been off, there's a chance you could become pregnant and you should use a backup method of birth control. Check the Ortho Evra patient information for instructions.

If you forget to change your patch at any time during the 4-week cycle, check the Ortho Evra patient information for instructions.

■ *Storage instructions...*
Keep patches in their protective pouches until you're ready to wear them. Store at room temperature. Do not store in the refrigerator or freezer.

Used patches still contain some active hormones. Fold each patch so that it sticks to itself before throwing it away. Do not flush the used patch down the toilet.

What side effects may occur?

Side effects cannot be anticipated. If any develop or change in intensity, inform your doctor as soon as possible. Only your doctor can determine if it is safe for you to continue using Ortho Evra.

■ *Side effects may include:*
Abdominal pain, application site reaction, breast tenderness or enlargement, headache, menstrual cramps, mood swings, nausea and/or vomiting, upper respiratory infection

In addition, side effects associated with birth control pills may also apply to Ortho Evra. See the list of side effects in the profile "Oral Contraceptives."

Why should this drug not be prescribed?

Do not use Ortho Evra if you are pregnant (or think you might be). Also avoid it if the ingredients give you an allergic reaction or you suffer from headaches with neurological symptoms such as visual disturbances (pulsing lights and blind spots) and temporary numbness.

If you have ever had breast cancer or cancer in the reproductive organs or liver tumors, you should not take Ortho Evra. Avoid it, too, if you have or have ever had a stroke, heart disease, liver disease, angina (severe chest pain), or blood clots. It is also not recommended for women with significantly high blood pressure or diabetes-related complications of the kidneys, eyes, nerves, or blood vessels.

Women who have had pregnancy-related jaundice (yellowing of the skin or whites of eyes) or jaundice stemming from previous use of hormonal contraceptives should not take Ortho Evra. You should also avoid it if you have undiagnosed and/or unexplained abnormal vaginal bleeding, or if you need prolonged bed rest after major surgery.

Do not use Ortho Evra if you are already taking birth control pills. Avoid the drug, too, if you are breastfeeding.

Special warnings about this medication

Hormonal contraceptives, including Ortho Evra, should be used with caution if you are over 40 years old; smoke tobacco; have liver, heart, gallbladder, or kidney disease; have high blood pressure, high cholesterol, diabetes, or epilepsy; or tend to be seriously overweight. Caution is also advised if you have blood circulation problems or have had a heart attack or stroke in the past. Be cautious, too, if you have problems with depression, migraine or other headaches, irregular menstrual periods, or visual disturbances.

There have been conflicting reports on whether using hormonal contraceptives increases the risk of breast cancer. It appears that using hormonal contraceptives may slightly increase the chance of breast cancer, particularly if they're used before age 20. After hormonal contraceptives are stopped, the risk begins to go back down. If you use Ortho Evra, you should examine your breasts monthly and have yearly breast exams by a doctor. Also tell your doctor if you have a family history of breast cancer or if you have had breast nodules, fibrocystic breast disease, or an abnormal mammogram.

You should also be aware that some experts think hormonal contraceptives may increase the risk of cervical cancer. This remains controversial, however. Many doctors think other factors are to blame.

Since the blood's clotting ability may be affected by hormonal contraceptives, your doctor may take you off Ortho Evra prior to surgery or during a period of prolonged bed rest. You should wait at least 4 weeks after having a baby before starting Ortho Evra; and if you're breastfeeding, wait until the child is weaned before starting the drug. If you are recovering from a second-trimester miscarriage or abortion, talk to your doctor before using Ortho Evra.

If you develop a migraine or severe headache that does not let up or keeps recurring while you are taking Ortho Evra, check with your doctor. You may need to switch to a different form of birth control.

You should also be aware that hormonal contraceptives have been know to cause rare cases of noncancerous—but dangerous—liver tumors. In people prone to high cholesterol and similar problems, hormonal contraceptives have been known to raise triglyceride levels, leading to pancreatitis.

If you miss a menstrual period but have followed the Ortho Evra regimen correctly, contact your doctor but do not stop using the patches. If you miss a period and have not followed the regimen correctly, or if you miss two consecutive periods, you may be pregnant; stop using the patches and check with your doctor immediately to see if you are pregnant. Use another form of birth control while you're off the patch.

Ortho Evra may be less effective in women who weigh more than 198 pounds; if you fall into this category, ask your doctor which form of birth control is best for you.

Hormonal contraceptives do not protect against HIV infection (AIDS) or any other sexually transmitted disease. If there is a danger of infection, use a latex condom in addition to Ortho Evra.

Be sure to tell the doctor that you are taking Ortho Evra before having lab tests done, since certain blood tests may be affected by hormonal contraceptives.

Possible food and drug interactions when taking this medication

If hormonal contraceptives are taken with certain other drugs, the effects of either could be increased, decreased, or altered. It is especially important to check with your doctor before combining Ortho Evra with the following:

Acetaminophen (Tylenol)
Antibiotics such as ampicillin and rifampin
Anticonvulsants such as Dilantin, Felbatol, Tegretol, Trileptal, and
    Topamax
Aspirin
Atorvastatin (Lipitor)
Barbiturates (phenobarbital, Seconal)
Clofibrate (Questran)
Cyclosporine (Neoral, Sandimmune)
Diabetes drugs such as Glucotrol
Folic acid
Griseofulvin (Fulvicin, Grisactin)
Itraconazole (Sporanox)

Ketoconazole (Nizoral)
Morphine (MS Contin)
Phenylbutazone (Butazolidin)
Prednisolone (Prelone, Pediapred)
Protease inhibitors (HIV drugs such as Crixivan and Viracept)
St. John's wort
Temazepam (Restoril)
Theophylline (Theo-Dur, Slo-bid)
Vitamin C

Remember, too, that hormonal contraceptives may affect tests for blood sugar levels and thyroid function and may cause an increase in blood triglyceride levels.

Special information if you are pregnant or breastfeeding

If you are pregnant (or think you might be), you should not use hormonal contraceptives, since they are not safe during pregnancy. For safety's sake, switch to a non-hormonal method of contraception if you miss a period and have not followed your patch schedule correctly. In addition, wait at least 4 weeks after delivery before starting Ortho Evra.

Nursing mothers should not use most hormonal contraceptives, since these drugs can appear in breast milk and may cause jaundice and enlarged breasts in nursing infants. In this situation, your doctor may advise you to use a different form of contraception while you are nursing your baby.

Recommended dosage

If you have any questions about how you should use Ortho Evra, consult your doctor or the patient instructions that come in the drug package. The following is a partial list of instructions for using Ortho Evra; it should not be used as a substitute for consultation with your doctor.

You should use 3 Ortho Evra patches during each 28-day cycle. You should apply a new patch each week for 3 weeks (21 total days). Do not apply a patch during the fourth week. Your menstrual period should start during this patch-free week.

Apply each new patch on the same day of the week. This will be your "patch change day." The patch can be applied on the first day of your menstrual cycle or on the first Sunday afterwards. The instructions below are for the first-Sunday schedule.

FOR A SUNDAY PATCH CHANGE SCHEDULE

1. Apply your first patch on the first Sunday after your menstrual period starts. *You must use backup contraception for the first week of your cycle when starting Ortho Evra for the first time.*
2. Choose a place on your body to put the patch where it won't be rubbed by tight clothing. You can apply the patch to your buttock, ab-

domen, upper outer arm, or upper back. *Never put the patch on your breasts.* To avoid irritation, apply each new patch to a different place on your skin.

3. Open the foil pouch that contains the patch by tearing along the top edge and one side edge. Peel the foil pouch apart and open it flat.

4. You will see that the patch is covered by a layer of clear plastic. It is important to remove the patch and the plastic together from the pouch. Using your fingernail, lift one corner of the patch and peel the patch and plastic off the foil liner. Sometimes a patch can stick to the inside of the pouch; be careful not to accidentally remove the clear liner as you remove the patch.

5. Peel away half of the clear plastic liner. Be careful not to touch the exposed sticky surface of the patch with your fingers.

6. Apply the sticky side of the patch to clean, dry skin, then remove the other half of the clear plastic. Press firmly on the patch with the palm of your hand for 10 seconds, making sure the edges stick well. Run your finger around the edge of the patch to make sure it is sticking properly. Check your patch every day to make sure all the edges are sticking.

7. Wear the patch for 7 days. On the next Sunday (day 8), remove the used patch. Apply a new patch immediately. The used patch still contains some medicine; carefully fold it in half so that it sticks to itself before throwing it away. Do not flush the used patch down the toilet.

8. Apply a new patch on the following Sunday (day 15). After 7 days, throw away the patch.

9. Do not wear a patch during the fourth week (day 22 through day 28). Your period should start during this week.

10. Begin your next 4-week cycle by applying a new patch on the Sunday after day 28, even if your period hasn't ended yet.

Overdosage

While any medication taken in excess can cause unwanted effects, the risk associated with Ortho Evra is minimal because the patch is designed to release a small amount of hormones at a slow, steady rate. Furthermore, even when young children have swallowed large amounts of oral hormonal contraceptives, they've suffered no ill effects. Nevertheless, if you suspect an overdose, seek medical help immediately.

■ *Symptoms of Ortho Evra overdose may include:*
Nausea, vomiting, vaginal bleeding

Ortho-Novum *See Oral Contraceptives, page 1000.*

Ortho Tri-Cyclen *See Oral Contraceptives, page 1000.*

ORUDIS

Pronounced: Oh-ROO-dis
Generic name: Ketoprofen
Other brand names: Actron, Orudis KT, Oruvail

Why is this drug prescribed?

Orudis, a nonsteroidal anti-inflammatory drug, is used to relieve the inflammation, swelling, stiffness, and joint pain associated with rheumatoid arthritis and osteoarthritis (the most common form of arthritis). It is also used to relieve mild to moderate pain, as well as menstrual pain.

Oruvail, an extended-release form of the drug, is used to treat the signs and symptoms of rheumatoid arthritis and osteoarthritis over the long term, not severe attacks that come on suddenly.

Actron and Orudis KT are over-the-counter forms of the drug. They are used to relieve minor aches and pains associated with the common cold, headache, toothache, muscle aches, backache, minor arthritis, and menstrual cramps. They are also used to reduce fever.

Most important fact about this drug?

You should have frequent checkups by your doctor if you take Orudis regularly. Ulcers or internal bleeding can occur without warning.

How should you take this medication?

To minimize side effects, your doctor may recommend that you take Orudis with food, an antacid, or milk.

If you are using Orudis for arthritis, it should be taken regularly.

Orudis and Oruvail should not be taken together.

Actron and Orudis KT should be taken with a full glass of water or other fluid. Do not use them for more than 3 days for fever or 10 days for pain.

■ *If you miss a dose...*
If you take Orudis on a regular schedule, take the forgotten dose as soon as you remember. If it is almost time for your next dose, skip the one you missed and go back to your regular schedule. Do not take 2 doses at once.

■ *Storage instructions...*
Store at room temperature in a tightly closed container. Protect Oruvail capsules from direct light and excessive heat and humidity.

What side effects may occur?

Side effects cannot be anticipated. If any develop or change in intensity, inform your doctor as soon as possible. Only your doctor can determine if it is safe for you to continue taking Orudis.

■ *Side effects may include:*
Abdominal pain, changes in kidney function, constipation, diarrhea, dreams, fluid retention, gas, headache, inability to sleep, indigestion, nausea, nervousness

Why should this drug not be prescribed?

If you are sensitive to or have ever had an allergic reaction to Orudis, or if you have had asthma attacks, hives, or other allergic reactions caused by aspirin or other nonsteroidal anti-inflammatory drugs, you should not take this medication. Make sure your doctor is aware of any drug reactions you have experienced.

Special warnings about this medication

Remember that stomach ulcers and bleeding can occur without warning.

This drug should be used with caution if you have kidney or liver disease.

If you are taking Orudis for an extended period of time, your doctor will check your blood for anemia.

This drug can increase water retention. Use with caution if you have heart disease or high blood pressure.

Make sure your doctor knows what other conditions you have and what other drugs you are taking.

Check with your doctor before taking Actron if the painful area is red or swollen. Also check with your doctor if, after you have started taking Actron, your symptoms continue or get worse, new symptoms appear, or you have stomach pain.

Possible food and drug interactions when taking this medication

If Orudis is taken with certain other drugs, the effects of either could be increased, decreased, or altered. It is especially important to check with your doctor before combining Orudis with the following:

Aspirin
Blood thinners such as Coumadin
Diuretics such as hydrochlorothiazide (HydroDIURIL)
Lithium (Lithonate)
Methotrexate
Probenecid (the gout medication Benemid)

Orudis can prolong bleeding time. If you are taking blood-thinning medication, use this drug cautiously.

Do not combine pain relievers without asking your doctor.

If you usually have 3 or more alcoholic drinks a day, ask your doctor about taking pain relievers.

Special information if you are pregnant or breastfeeding

The effects of Orudis during pregnancy have not been adequately studied. If you are pregnant or plan to become pregnant, inform your doctor immediately. It is particularly important not to use this product during the last 3 months of pregnancy unless your doctor has told you to; its use may cause problems in your baby or during delivery. Orudis may appear in breast milk and could affect a nursing infant. If this medication is essential to your health, your doctor may advise you to discontinue breast-feeding until your treatment with this medication is finished.

Recommended dosage

ADULTS

Rheumatoid Arthritis and Osteoarthritis
The starting dose of Orudis is 75 milligrams 3 times a day or 50 milligrams 4 times a day; for Oruvail, 200 milligrams taken once a day. The most you should take in a day is 300 milligrams of Orudis or 200 milligrams of Oruvail. Some side effects, such as headache and upset stomach, increase in severity as the dose gets higher.

Mild to Moderate Pain and Menstrual Pain
The usual dose of Orudis is 25 to 50 milligrams every 6 to 8 hours as needed.

Smaller people, older people, and those with kidney or liver disease need smaller doses of Orudis. Doses above 75 milligrams have no additional effect.

The usual dose of Actron or Orudis KT is 1 tablet or caplet (12.5 milligrams) every 4 to 6 hours. If you get no relief in 1 hour, you may take another tablet or caplet. Do not take more than 2 tablets or caplets in a 4- to 6-hour period. Do not take more than 6 tablets or caplets each 24 hours.

CHILDREN

Not for use in children under 16 years of age, unless recommended by a doctor.

OLDER ADULTS

Dosage may be lower.

Overdosage

Any medication taken in excess can have serious consequences. If you suspect an overdose of Orudis, seek medical attention immediately.

■ *Symptoms of Orudis overdose may include:*
Breathing difficulty, coma, convulsions, drowsiness, high blood pressure, kidney failure, low blood pressure, nausea, sluggishness, stomach and intestinal bleeding, stomach pain, vomiting

Oruvail *See Orudis, page 1016.*

Oseltamivir *See Tamiflu, page 1385.*

Ovcon *See Oral Contraceptives, page 1000.*

Ovral *See Oral Contraceptives, page 1000.*

Ovrette *See Oral Contraceptives, page 1000.*

Oxaprozin *See Daypro, page 388.*

OXAZEPAM

Pronounced: oks-AS-eh-pam
Brand name: Serax

Why is this drug prescribed?

Oxazepam is used in the treatment of anxiety disorders, including anxiety associated with depression.

This drug seems to be particularly effective for anxiety, tension, agitation, and irritability in older people. It is also prescribed to relieve symptoms of acute alcohol withdrawal.

Oxazepam belongs to a class of drugs known as benzodiazepines.

Most important fact about this drug

Oxazepam can be habit-forming or addicting and can lose its effectiveness over time, as you develop a tolerance for it. You may experience withdrawal symptoms if you stop using the drug abruptly. When discontinuing the drug, your doctor will reduce the dose gradually.

How should you take this medication?

Take Oxazepam exactly as prescribed.

- *If you miss a dose...*
  If you remember within an hour or so, take the dose immediately. If you do not remember until later, skip the dose you missed and go back to your regular schedule. Do not take 2 doses at once.
- *Storage instructions...*
  Store at room temperature in a tightly closed container.

What side effects may occur?

Side effects cannot be anticipated. If any develop or change in intensity, inform your doctor as soon as possible. Only your doctor can determine if it is safe for you to continue taking Oxazepam. Your doctor should periodically reassess the need for this drug.

- *Side effects may include:*
  Dizziness, drowsiness, headache, memory impairment, paradoxical excitement, transient amnesia, vertigo

■ *Side effects due to rapid decrease in dose or abrupt withdrawal from oxazepam may include:*
Abdominal and muscle cramps, convulsions, depression, inability to fall asleep or stay asleep, sweating, tremors, vomiting

Why should this drug not be prescribed?

If you are sensitive to or have ever had an allergic reaction to oxazepam or other tranquilizers such as Valium, you should not take this medication. Make sure your doctor is aware of any drug reactions you have experienced.

Anxiety or tension related to everyday stress usually does not require treatment with oxazepam. Discuss your symptoms thoroughly with your doctor.

Oxazepam should not be prescribed if you are being treated for mental disorders more serious than anxiety.

Special warnings about this medication

Oxazepam may cause you to become drowsy or less alert; therefore, you should not drive or operate dangerous machinery or participate in any hazardous activity that requires full mental alertness until you know how this drug affects you.

This medication may cause your blood pressure to drop. If you have any heart problems, consult your doctor before taking this medication.

Possible food and drug interactions when taking this medication

Oxazepam may intensify the effects of alcohol. It may be best to avoid alcohol while taking this medication.

If oxazepam is taken with certain other drugs, the effects of either could be increased, decreased, or altered. It is especially important to check with your doctor before combining oxazepam with the following:

Antihistamines such as Benadryl
Narcotic painkillers such as Percocet and Demerol
Sedatives such as Seconal and Halcion
Tranquilizers such as Valium and Xanax

Special information if you are pregnant or breastfeeding

Do not take oxazepam if you are pregnant or planning to become pregnant. There is an increased risk of birth defects. Oxazepam may appear in breast milk and could affect a nursing infant. If this drug is essential to your health, your doctor may advise you to stop breastfeeding until your treatment with this medication is finished.

Recommended dosage

ADULTS

Mild to Moderate Anxiety with Tension, Irritability, Agitation
The usual dose is 10 to 15 milligrams 3 or 4 times per day.

Severe Anxiety, Depression with Anxiety, or Alcohol Withdrawal
The usual dose is 15 to 30 milligrams, 3 or 4 times per day.

CHILDREN

The safety and effectiveness of oxazepam have not been established for children under 6 years of age, nor have dosage guidelines been established for children 6 to 12 years. The doctor will adjust the dosage to fit your child's needs.

OLDER ADULTS

The usual starting dose is 10 milligrams, 3 times a day. Your doctor may increase the dose to 15 milligrams 3 or 4 times a day, if needed.

Overdosage

An overdose of oxazepam can be fatal. If you suspect an overdose, seek medical attention immediately.

- *Symptoms of mild oxazepam overdose may include:*
  Confusion, drowsiness, lethargy
- *Symptoms of more serious overdose may include:*
  Coma, hypnotic state, lack of coordination, limp muscles, low blood pressure

Oxcarbazepine *See Trileptal, page 1496.*

Oxiconazole *See Oxistat, below.*

OXISTAT

Pronounced: OX-ee-stat
Generic name: Oxiconazole nitrate

Why is this drug prescribed?

Oxistat is used to treat fungal skin diseases commonly called ringworm (tinea). Oxistat is prescribed for athlete's foot (tinea pedis), jock itch (tinea cruris), ringworm of the entire body (tinea corporis), and tinea versicolor, which appears as patches on the skin. It is available as a cream or lotion.

Most important fact about this drug

Oxistat should not be used in, on, or near the eyes, or applied to the vagina.

How should you use this medication?

Use Oxistat exactly as prescribed.

Wash and dry the area to be treated before applying Oxistat and then apply the cream or lotion so that it covers the entire affected area and the area right around it.

Be careful when applying to raw, blistered, or oozing skin.

■ *If you miss a dose...*
Apply the cream or lotion when you remember, then return to your regular schedule.
■ *Storage instructions...*
Store Oxistat at room temperature.

What side effects may occur?

Side effects cannot be anticipated. If any develop or change in intensity, notify your doctor as soon as possible. Only your doctor can determine whether it is safe for you to continue using Oxistat.

■ *Side effects may include:*
Allergic skin inflammation, burning, cracks in the skin, eczema, irritation, itching, pain, rash, scaling, skin redness, skin softening, small, firm, raised skin eruptions similar to those of chickenpox, stinging, tingling

Why should this drug not be prescribed?

Do not use Oxistat if you have ever had an allergic reaction or are sensitive to oxiconazole or any other ingredients in the cream.

Special warnings about this medication

If you develop an irritation or sensitivity to the medication, notify your doctor.

Possible food and drug interactions when taking this medication

No interactions have been reported.

Special information if you are pregnant or breastfeeding

Oxistat has not been proved safe during pregnancy. If you are pregnant or plan to become pregnant, inform your doctor immediately.

Oxistat appears in breast milk and could affect a nursing infant. If Oxistat is essential to your health, your doctor may advise you to stop breastfeeding until your treatment is finished.

Recommended dosage

ADULTS AND CHILDREN

For athlete's foot, jock itch, or ringworm of the body, use Oxistat cream or lotion once or twice a day. Athlete's foot is treated for 1 month. Jock itch and ringworm of the body are treated for 2 weeks.

For tinea versicolor, apply Oxistat cream once a day for 2 weeks.

Overdosage

Overdose of Oxistat has not been reported. However, if you suspect an overdose, seek medical attention immediately.

Oxybutynin See Ditropan, page 460.

Oxycodone See OxyContin, below.

Oxycodone with Aspirin See Percodan, page 1076.

OXYCONTIN

Pronounced: oks-ee-CON-tin
Generic name: Oxycodone hydrochloride

Why is this drug prescribed?

OxyContin is a controlled-release form of the narcotic painkiller oxycodone. It is prescribed for moderate to severe pain when continuous, around-the-clock relief is needed for an extended period of time.

Most important fact about this drug

Be sure to swallow OxyContin tablets whole. If broken, crushed, or chewed, the tablets quickly release a potentially fatal overdose of oxycodone. Abusing OxyContin by chewing the tablets, snorting crushed tablets, or dissolving and injecting their contents can slow down or stop breathing and lead to death. Injecting OxyContin can also kill the tissue around the injection site and trigger heart and lung problems.

How should you take this medication?

It is important to take OxyContin on a regular basis, every 12 hours, in exactly the dose prescribed. This drug is not intended for occasional as-needed use, and should never be taken more often than directed. If you suffer episodes of increased pain, check with your doctor; do not change the dosage on your own.

■ *If you miss a dose...*
    Take it as soon as you remember. However, if it is almost time for your next dose, skip the one you missed and return to your regular schedule. Do not take 2 doses at once.

■ *Storage instructions...*
Store at room temperature in a secure place out of reach of children. Protect from light. Dispose of unused tablets by flushing them down the toilet.

What side effects may occur?

Side effects cannot be anticipated. If any develop or change in intensity, tell your doctor as soon as possible. Only your doctor can determine if it is safe to continue using OxyContin.

■ *Side effects may include:*
Constipation, dizziness, drowsiness, dry mouth, headache, itching, nausea, sweating, vomiting, weakness

This side effects list is not complete. If you have any questions about side effects, you should consult your doctor. Report any new or continuing symptoms to your doctor right away.

Why should this drug not be prescribed?

Do not take OxyContin if you have asthma or any other serious breathing problem; the drug can further diminish respiration. Also avoid OxyContin if you have an intestinal blockage or an allergy to hydrocodone.

OxyContin is not intended for the relief of postoperative pain unless you've already been taking the drug or the pain is expected to last for an extended period. OxyContin is not prescribed for brief periods or for mild pain.

Special warnings about this medication

The two highest-strength OxyContin tablets—80 and 160 milligrams—are dangerous for anyone who has not already developed a tolerance to narcotics. If you have been prescribed one of these strengths, do not give the tablets to anyone else; they could impair respiration and lead to death.

Follow your doctor's dosage instructions carefully. Misuse of OxyContin promotes physical dependence, abuse, and addiction. When OxyContin therapy is no longer necessary, the doctor will taper your dosage down gradually in order to prevent withdrawal symptoms. Abruptly discontinuing the drug can cause such symptoms as restlessness, enlarged pupils, watery eyes, runny nose, yawning, sweating, chills, and muscle aches. More severe symptoms may include irritability, anxiety, joint pain, weakness, cramps, insomnia, nausea, vomiting, diarrhea, rapid breathing, and a fast pulse.

OxyContin should be used cautiously by anyone with a respiratory condition. The drug is especially prone to cause breathing problems in older adults, people in poor health, and those with disorders such as chronic obstructive pulmonary disease. Doctors generally try to use non-narcotic painkillers for patients such as these.

OxyContin should be used with caution by people with head injuries, brain tumors, and other conditions that increase pressure on the brain. Caution is also warranted for people who are semi-conscious or in a coma, and those who suffer from acute alcoholism, adrenal or thyroid problems, spinal deformities that impair breathing, an enlarged prostate, difficulty urinating, drug-induced psychosis, pancreatitis and related disorders, or severe kidney or liver disease.

OxyContin has been known to trigger seizures or make them worse. Use it with caution if you have a seizure disorder.

Like other narcotic painkillers, OxyContin can slow your reactions and make you drowsy. Do not drive, operate dangerous machinery, or undertake other hazardous activities until you know how the drug affects you.

OxyContin can cause a severe drop in blood pressure, leading to dizziness and light-headedness, especially when you first stand up.

The empty shell of the OxyContin tablet sometimes appears in the stool. This is not a reason for concern.

OxyContin is not for use in children.

Possible food and drug interactions when taking this medication

While using OxyContin, check with your doctor before taking any other drugs that slow the nervous system. The combined effect can impair breathing, reduce blood pressure, and lead to coma. Drugs in this category include the following:

Alcoholic beverages
Antipsychotic drugs such as Compazine, Mellaril, Stelazine, and Thorazine
Muscle relaxants such as Flexeril, Robaxin, and Skelaxin
Narcotic painkillers such as Demerol, Percodan, and Vicodin
Sleep aids such as Ambien, Halcion, and Sonata
Sleep-inducing antihistamines such as Benadryl and Phenergan.
Tranquilizers such as Ativan, Librium, Valium, and Xanax

If you are already taking such drugs, your starting dose of OxyContin will be reduced by at least half.

Certain other painkillers can reduce OxyContin's effect, or even cause withdrawal symptoms. Caution is necessary when combining OxyContin with drugs such as the following:

Butorphanol (Stadol)
Nalbuphine (Nubain)
Pentazocine (Talacen, Talwin NX)

Special Information if you are pregnant or breastfeeding

OxyContin should be used during pregnancy only if clearly needed. If you are pregnant or plan to become pregnant, inform your doctor immediately.

OxyContin makes its way into breast milk. Breastfeeding is not recommended if you are taking this drug.

Recommended dosage

ADULTS

OxyContin is taken every 12 hours. The tablets come in strengths of 10, 20, 40, 80, and 160 milligrams. The starting dose of OxyContin is determined by your physical condition, the type of painkillers you've been taking, and your tolerance for narcotics. The doctor will adjust the dose until you have little or no pain when OxyContin is supplemented with no more than 2 doses of a second painkiller. The dose of OxyContin can be increased every 1 or 2 days. If a higher dose has excessive side effects, the doctor will adjust it downward and increase the dosage of supplemental painkillers.

Overdosage

An overdose of OxyContin can be fatal. If you suspect an overdose, seek emergency treatment immediately.

■ *Symptoms of OxyContin overdose may include:*
Cold and clammy skin, diminished breathing, drowsiness progressing to stupor or coma, flaccid muscles, pinpoint pupils, slow heart rate

PAMELOR

Pronounced: PAM-eh-lore
Generic name: Nortriptyline hydrochloride
Other brand name: Aventyl

Why is this drug prescribed?

Pamelor is prescribed for the relief of symptoms of depression. It is one of the drugs known as tricyclic antidepressants.

Some doctors also prescribe Pamelor to treat chronic hives, premenstrual depression, attention deficit hyperactivity disorder in children, and bedwetting.

Most important fact about this drug

Pamelor must be taken regularly to be effective and it may be several weeks before you begin to feel better. Do not skip doses, even if they seem to make no difference.

How should you take this medication?

Take Pamelor exactly as prescribed. Pamelor may make your mouth dry. Sucking on hard candy, chewing gum, or melting ice chips in your mouth can provide relief.

■ *If you miss a dose…*
Take it as soon as you remember. If it is almost time for the next dose, skip the one you missed and go back to your regular schedule. If you

take Pamelor once a day at bedtime and you miss a dose, do not take it in the morning, since disturbing side effects could occur. Never take 2 doses at once.

■ *Storage instructions...*
Keep Pamelor in the container it came in, tightly closed and away from light. Be sure to keep this drug out of reach of children; an overdose is particularly dangerous in the young. Store at room temperature.

What side effects may occur?

Side effects cannot be anticipated. If any develop or change in intensity, inform your doctor as soon as possible. Only your doctor can determine if it is safe for you to continue taking Pamelor.

■ *Side effects may include:*
Anxiety, blurred vision, confusion, dry mouth, hallucinations, heart attack or vascular heart blockage, heartbeat irregularities, high blood pressure, insomnia, loss of muscle coordination, low blood pressure, rapid heartbeat, sensitivity to sunlight, skin rash, stroke, tremors, weight loss

■ *Side effects due to rapid decrease in dose or abrupt withdrawal from Pamelor after prolonged treatment include:*
Headache, nausea, vague feeling of bodily discomfort

These side effects do not indicate addiction to this drug.

Why should this drug not be prescribed?

If you are sensitive to or have ever had an allergic reaction to Pamelor or similar drugs, you should not take this medication. Make sure your doctor is aware of any drug reactions you have experienced.

Do not take Pamelor if you are taking—or have taken within the past 14 days—a drug classified as an MAO inhibitor. Drugs in this category include the antidepressants Nardil and Parnate. Combining these drugs with Pamelor can cause fever and convulsions, and could even be fatal.

Unless you are directed to do so by your doctor, do not take this medication if you are recovering from a heart attack or are taking any other antidepressant drugs.

If you have been taking Prozac, you may have to wait at least 5 weeks before beginning therapy with Pamelor. A drug interaction could result.

Special warnings about this medication

In clinical studies, antidepressants increased the risk of suicidal thinking and behavior in children and adolescents with depression and other psychiatric disorders. Anyone considering the use of Pamelor or any other antidepressant in a child or adolescent must balance this risk with the clinical need. Pamelor is not approved for use in children.

Additionally, the progression of major depression is associated with a worsening of symptoms and/or the emergence of suicidal thinking or behavior in both adults and children, whether or not they are taking antidepressants. Individuals being treated with Pamelor and their caregivers should watch for any change in symptoms or any new symptoms that appear suddenly—especially agitation, anxiety, hostility, panic, restlessness, extreme hyperactivity, and suicidal thinking or behavior—and report them to the doctor immediately. Be especially observant at the beginning of treatment or whenever there is a change in dose.

Pamelor may cause you to become drowsy or less alert; therefore, you should not drive or operate dangerous machinery or participate in any hazardous activity that requires full mental alertness until you know how this drug affects you.

Use Pamelor with caution if you have a history of seizures, difficulty urinating, diabetes, or chronic eye conditions such as glaucoma. Be careful, also, if you have heart disease, high blood pressure, or an overactive thyroid, or are receiving thyroid medication. You should discuss all of your medical problems with your doctor before taking this medication.

If you are being treated for a severe mental disorder (schizophrenia or manic depression), tell your doctor before taking Pamelor.

Pamelor may make your skin more sensitive to sunlight. Try to stay out of the sun, wear protective clothing, and apply a sunblock.

Before having surgery, dental treatment, or any diagnostic procedure, tell your doctor that you are taking Pamelor. Certain drugs used during these procedures, such as anesthetics and muscle relaxants, may interact with Pamelor.

Possible food and drug interactions when taking this medication
Combining Pamelor and MAO inhibitors can be fatal.

Pamelor may intensify the effects of alcohol. Do not drink alcohol while taking this medication.

If Pamelor is taken with certain other drugs, the effects of either can be increased, decreased, or altered. It is especially important to check with your doctor before combining Pamelor with the following:

Airway-opening drugs such as Ventolin and Proventil
Antidepressants such as Wellbutrin and Desyrel
Antidepressants that act on serotonin, such as Prozac, Paxil, and Zoloft
Blood pressure medications such as Catapres and Esimil
Chlorpropamide (Diabinese)
Cimetidine (Tagamet)
Drugs for heart irregularities, such as Tambocor and Rythmol
Drugs that control spasms, such as Donnatal and Bentyl
Levodopa (Larodopa)
Major tranquilizers such as Thorazine and Mellaril

Quinidine (Quinidex)
Reserpine (Diupres)
Stimulants such as Dexedrine
Thyroid medication such as Synthroid
Warfarin (Coumadin)

Special information if you are pregnant or breastfeeding

The effects of Pamelor during pregnancy have not been adequately studied. If you are pregnant or planning to become pregnant, inform your doctor immediately. Also consult your doctor before breastfeeding.

Recommended dosage

This medication is available in tablet and liquid form. Only tablet dosages are listed. Consult your doctor if you cannot take the tablet form of this medication.

ADULTS

Your doctor will monitor your response to this medication carefully and will gradually increase or decrease the dose to suit your needs.

The usual starting dosage is 25 milligrams 3 or 4 times per day.

Alternatively, your doctor may prescribe that the total daily dose be taken once a day.

Doses above 150 milligrams per day are not recommended.

Your doctor may want to perform a blood test to help in deciding the best dose you should receive.

CHILDREN

The safety and effectiveness of Pamelor have not been established for children and its use is not recommended. However, adolescents may be given 30 to 50 milligrams per day, either in a single dose or divided into smaller doses, as determined by your doctor.

OLDER ADULTS

The usual dose is 30 to 50 milligrams taken in a single dose or divided into smaller doses, as determined by your doctor.

Overdosage

An overdose of this type of antidepressant can be fatal. If you suspect an overdose, seek medical help immediately.

■ *Symptoms of Pamelor overdose may include:*
Agitation, coma, confusion, congestive heart failure, convulsions, dilated pupils, disturbed concentration, drowsiness, excessive reflexes, extremely high fever, fluid in the lungs, hallucinations, irregular heartbeat, low body temperature, restlessness, rigid muscles, severely low blood pressure, shock, stupor, vomiting

PANCREASE

Pronounced: PAN-kree-ace
Generic name: Pancrelipase
Other brand names: Creon, Pancrease MT, Viokase, Ultrase

Why is this drug prescribed?

Pancrease is used to treat pancreatic enzyme deficiency. It is often prescribed for people with cystic fibrosis, chronic inflammation of the pancreas, or blockages of the pancreas or common bile duct caused by cancer. It is also taken by people who have had their pancreas removed or who have had gastrointestinal bypass surgery. Pancrease is taken to help with digestion of proteins, starches, and fats.

Most important fact about this drug

Pancrease capsules should not be chewed or crushed.

How should you take this medication?

Take this medication exactly as prescribed. If you are taking Pancrease for cystic fibrosis, your doctor may also prescribe a special diet for you. Be sure to follow the diet closely, as well as taking Pancrease.

Pancrelipase is available in capsule, tablet, and powder forms. Do not change brands or dosage forms of this medication without first checking with your doctor.

If swallowing the Pancrease capsule is difficult, open the capsule and shake the contents (microspheres) onto a small amount of soft food, such as applesauce or gelatin, that does not require chewing, then swallow it immediately. Avoid mixing it with alkaline foods, such as ice cream or milk. They can reduce the medication's effect.

Pancrease should be taken with meals and snacks. Drink plenty of fluids while you are taking Pancrease. Do not hold the medication in your mouth; it may irritate the lining. Be careful to avoid inhaling dust from the powdered form; it may irritate the nose, throat, and lungs, and has been known to cause asthma attacks.

■ *If you miss a dose...*
Resume taking the medication with your next meal or snack.
■ *Storage instructions...*
Store at room temperature in a tightly closed container away from moisture. Do not refrigerate.

What side effects may occur?

Side effects cannot be anticipated. If any develop or change in intensity, inform your doctor as soon as possible. Only your doctor can determine if it is safe for you to continue taking Pancrease.

■ *Side effects may include:*
Stomach and intestinal upset

Why should this drug not be prescribed?

Pancrease should not be used if you are sensitive to or have ever had an allergic reaction to pork protein, if you have recently had an inflamed pancreas, or if you have a disease of the pancreas that gets worse.

Special warnings about this medication

If you develop an allergic reaction to Pancrease, stop taking the medication and inform your doctor immediately. If you have cystic fibrosis and develop any signs of an intestinal blockage, call your doctor.

Possible food and drug interactions when taking this medication

If Pancrease is taken with certain other drugs, the effects of either can be increased, decreased, or altered. It is especially important that you check with your doctor before combining Pancrease with the following:

Certain antacids such as Tums and Milk of Magnesia
Certain acid-blocking ulcer medications such as Pepcid and Zantac

Special information if you are pregnant or breastfeeding

The effects of Pancrease during pregnancy have not been adequately studied. If you are pregnant or plan to become pregnant, inform your doctor immediately.

It is not known whether Pancrease appears in breast milk. Your doctor may advise you not to nurse while you are taking this drug.

Recommended dosage

ADULTS

The doctor will set your dosage according to your weight and your response to the enzymes, gradually increasing your dose until your digestion is adequate. Doses above 2,500 units per 2.2 pounds of body weight per meal are generally not recommended.

CHILDREN

Your doctor will determine the best dosage of Pancrease based on the child's individual needs.

Overdosage

Although no specific information is available, any medication taken in excess can have serious consequences. If you suspect an overdose of Pancrease, seek medical treatment immediately.

Pancrelipase See Pancrease, page 1030.

Pantoprazole *See Protonix, page 1182.*

PARAFON FORTE DSC

Pronounced: PAIR-a-fahn FOR-tay DEE-ESS-SEE
Generic name: Chlorzoxazone

Why is this drug prescribed?

Parafon Forte DSC is prescribed, along with rest and physical therapy, for the relief of discomfort associated with severe, painful muscle spasms.

Most important fact about this drug

Although rare, serious, sometimes fatal liver problems have been reported in people using Parafon Forte DSC. You should stop taking this medication and notify your doctor immediately if you develop any of the following signs of liver toxicity: fever, rash, loss of appetite, nausea, vomiting, fatigue, pain in the upper right part of your abdomen, dark urine, or yellow skin or eyes.

How should you take this medication?

Take Parafon Forte DSC exactly as prescribed by your doctor. Do not increase the dose or take it more often than prescribed.

Parafon Forte DSC occasionally discolors urine orange or purple-red.

■ *If you miss a dose...*
Take it as soon as you remember, if it is within an hour or so of the missed time. Otherwise, skip the dose and go back to your regular schedule. Do not take 2 doses a once.
■ *Storage instructions...*
Store at room temperature in a tightly closed container.

What side effects may occur?

Parafon Forte DSC rarely produces undesirable side effects. However, if any develop or change in intensity, inform your doctor as soon as possible. Only your doctor can determine if it is safe for you to continue taking Parafon Forte DSC.

Why should this drug not be prescribed?

If you have had any reaction to this drug, notify your doctor. Make sure he or she is aware of any drug reactions you have experienced.

Special warnings about this medication

Be careful using this drug if you have allergies or have ever had an allergic reaction to a drug. If you have a sensitivity reaction such as hives, redness, or itching of skin while you are taking Parafon Forte DSC, notify your doctor immediately.

Possible food and drug interactions when taking this medication
Parafon Forte DSC may intensify the effects of alcohol. Be cautious about drinking alcohol while taking this medication.

If Parafon Forte DSC is taken with certain other drugs, the effects of either could be increased, decreased, or altered. It is especially important to check with your doctor before combining Parafon Forte DSC with drugs that slow the action of the central nervous system, such as Percocet, Valium, and Xanax.

Special information if you are pregnant or breastfeeding
The effects of Parafon Forte DSC during pregnancy have not been adequately studied. If you are pregnant or plan to become pregnant, inform your doctor immediately. This drug may appear in breast milk and could affect a nursing infant. If this medication is essential to your health, your doctor may advise you to discontinue breastfeeding until your treatment is finished.

Recommended dosage

ADULTS

The usual dosage of Parafon Forte DSC is 1 caplet taken 3 or 4 times per day. If you do not respond to this dosage, your doctor may increase it to one and a half caplets (750 milligrams) taken 3 or 4 times per day.

Overdosage
Any medication taken in excess can have serious consequences. If you suspect an overdose, seek medical treatment immediately.

- *Symptoms of Parafon Forte DSC overdose may include:*
  Diarrhea, dizziness, drowsiness, headache, light-headedness, nausea, vomiting
- *Symptoms that may develop after a period of time include:*
  Feeling of illness, loss of muscle strength, lowered blood pressure, sluggishness, troubled or rapid breathing

PARLODEL
Pronounced: PAR-luh-del
Generic name: Bromocriptine mesylate

Why is this drug prescribed?
Parlodel inhibits the secretion of the hormone prolactin from the pituitary gland. It also mimics the action of dopamine, a chemical lacking in the brain of someone with Parkinson's disease. It is used to treat a variety of medical conditions, including:

Infertility in some women

Menstrual problems such as the abnormal stoppage or absence of flow, with or without excessive production of milk

Growth hormone overproduction leading to acromegaly, a condition characterized by an abnormally large skull, jaw, hands, and feet

Parkinson's disease

Pituitary gland tumors

Some doctors also prescribe Parlodel to treat cocaine addiction, the eye condition known as glaucoma, erection problems in certain men, restless leg syndrome, and a dangerous reaction to major tranquilizers called neuroleptic malignant syndrome.

Most important fact about this drug

Notify your doctor immediately if you develop a severe headache that does not let up or continues to get worse. It could be a warning of the possibility of other dangerous reactions, including seizure, stroke, or heart attack.

How should you take this medication?

Parlodel should be taken with food. Take the first dose while lying down. You may faint or become dizzy due to lower blood pressure, especially following the first dose.

You may not feel the full effect of this medication for a few weeks. Do not stop taking Parlodel without first checking with your doctor.

■ *If you miss a dose...*
Take it as soon as you remember if it is within 4 hours of the scheduled time. Otherwise, skip the dose you missed and go back to your regular schedule. Do not take 2 doses at once.

■ *Storage instructions...*
Store at room temperature in a tightly closed, light-resistant container.

What side effects may occur?

The number and severity of side effects depend on many factors, including the condition being treated, dosage, and duration of treatment. Side effects cannot be anticipated. If any develop or change in intensity, inform your doctor as soon as possible. Only your doctor can determine if it is safe for you to continue taking Parlodel.

■ *Side effects may include:*
Abdominal cramps or discomfort, confusion, constipation, depression, diarrhea, dizziness, drop in blood pressure, drowsiness, dry mouth, fainting, fatigue, hallucinations (particularly in Parkinson's patients), headache, inability to sleep, indigestion, light-headedness, loss of appetite, loss of coordination, nasal congestion, nausea, shortness of breath, uncontrolled body movement, vertigo, visual disturbance, vomiting, weakness

Some of the above side effects are also symptoms of Parkinson's disease.

Why should this drug not be prescribed?
You should not be using Parlodel if you have high blood pressure that is not under control or if you are pregnant (unless your doctor finds it medically necessary). You should also not take Parlodel if you are allergic to it or to any other drugs containing ergot alkaloids, such as Bellergal-S and Cafergot.

Women who have severe heart conditions should not use Parlodel after they have had a baby unless it is medically necessary.

Special warnings about this medication
Your doctor will check your pituitary gland thoroughly before you are treated with Parlodel.

Since Parlodel can restore fertility and pregnancy can result, women who do not want to become pregnant should use a barrier method of contraception during treatment with this medication. Do not use oral contraceptives, as they may prevent Parlodel from working properly.

Notify your doctor immediately if you become pregnant while you are being treated with Parlodel.

If you have kidney or liver disease, consult your doctor before taking Parlodel.

If you are being treated with Parlodel for endocrine problems related to a tumor and stop taking this medication, the tumor may grow back rapidly.

Use Parlodel with caution if you have had mental problems, any disease of the heart and circulatory system, peptic ulcer, or bleeding in the stomach and intestines.

If you are being treated for Parkinson's disease, the use of Parlodel alone or Parlodel with levodopa may cause hallucinations, confusion, and low blood pressure. If this happens, notify your doctor immediately.

If you have an abnormal heartbeat rhythm caused by a previous heart attack, consult your doctor before taking Parlodel.

If you experience a persistent watery nasal discharge while taking Parlodel, notify your doctor.

This drug may impair your ability to drive a car or operate potentially dangerous machinery. Do not participate in any activities that require full alertness if you are unsure about your ability to do so.

Your first dose of Parlodel may cause dizziness. If so, check with your doctor.

Possible food and drug interactions when taking this medication
Combining alcohol with Parlodel can cause blurred vision, chest pain, pounding heartbeat, throbbing headache, confusion, and other problems. Do not drink alcoholic beverages while taking this medication.

Certain drugs used for psychotic conditions, including Thorazine and Haldol, inhibit the action of Parlodel. It is important that you consult your doctor before taking these drugs while on Parlodel therapy.

Other drugs that may interact with Parlodel include:
Blood pressure–lowering drugs such as Aldomet and Catapres
Metoclopramide (Reglan)
Oral contraceptives
Other ergot derivatives such as Hydergine
Pimozide (Orap)

Special information if you are pregnant or breastfeeding

The use of Parlodel during pregnancy should be discussed thoroughly with your doctor. If Parlodel is essential to your treatment, your doctor will carefully monitor you throughout your pregnancy.

You should not take Parlodel while breastfeeding.

Recommended dosage

ADULTS

Parlodel is available as 2.5-milligram tablets and 5-milligram capsules. Dosage information given is for 2.5-milligram tablets.

Excess Prolactin Hormone

If you are being treated for conditions associated with excess prolactin, such as menstrual problems, with or without excessive milk production, infertility, or pituitary gland tumors, the usual starting dose is ½ to 1 tablet daily. Your doctor may add a tablet every 3 to 7 days, until the treatment works. The usual longer-term dose is 5 to 7.5 milligrams per day and ranges from 2.5 to 15 milligrams per day.

Growth Hormone Overproduction

Treatment for the overproduction of growth hormones is usually ½ to 1 tablet with food at bedtime for 3 days. Your doctor may add ½ to 1 tablet every 3 to 7 days. The usual treatment dose varies from 20 to 30 milligrams per day. The dose should not exceed 100 milligrams per day. Your doctor will do a monthly re-evaluation.

Parkinson's Disease

Parlodel taken in combination with levodopa may provide additional treatment benefits if you are currently taking high doses of levodopa or developing a tolerance to the drug, or if the benefits of levodopa wear off before the next dose.

The usual starting dose of Parlodel is ½ tablet twice a day with meals. Your dose will be monitored by your doctor at 2-week intervals. If necessary, your doctor may increase the dose every 14 to 28 days by 1 tablet per day.

CHILDREN

The safety and effectiveness of Parlodel have not been established in children.

Overdosage

Any medication taken in excess can have serious consequences. If you suspect an overdose of Parlodel, contact your doctor immediately or seek other medical attention.

■ *Symptoms of Parlodel overdose may include:*
Confusion, constipation, delusions, dizziness, drowsiness, feeling unwell, hallucinations, lethargy, nausea, pallor, severely low blood pressure, sweating, vomiting, yawning repeatedly

PARNATE

Pronounced: PAR-nate
Generic name: Tranylcypromine sulfate

Why is this drug prescribed?

Parnate is prescribed for the treatment of major depression—that is, a depressed mood that lasts for at least 2 weeks and interferes with daily functioning. Major depression is marked by at least 4 of the following 8 symptoms: changes in appetite, changes in sleep patterns, agitation or listlessness, loss of interest in usual activities or a decrease in sex drive, fatigue, feelings of guilt or worthlessness, slowed thinking or difficulty concentrating, and thoughts of suicide.

Parnate is a member of the class of drugs known as monoamine oxidase (MAO) inhibitors. It works by increasing concentrations of the brain chemicals epinephrine, norepinephrine, and serotonin.

Most important fact about this drug

Parnate is a potent drug with the capability of producing serious side effects. It is typically prescribed only if other antidepressants fail, and then only for adults who are under close medical supervision. It is considered especially risky because it can interact with a long list of drugs and foods to produce life-threatening side effects (see *Possible food and drug interactions when taking this medication*).

How should you take this medication?

Your doctor will adjust the dosage of Parnate according to your individual needs and response. The drug usually produces improvement within 48 hours to 3 weeks after starting therapy.

■ *If you miss a dose...*
Take it as soon as you remember. If it is within 2 hours of your next dose, skip the one you missed and go back to your regular schedule. Never take 2 doses at once.

■ *Storage instructions...*
Store at room temperature.

What side effects may occur?
Side effects cannot be anticipated. If any develop or change in intensity, inform your doctor as soon as possible. Only your doctor can determine if it is safe for you to continue taking Parnate.

■ *Side effects may include:*
Blood disorders, diarrhea, dizziness, drowsiness, dry mouth, insomnia, muscle spasm, nausea, overstimulation, rapid or irregular heartbeat, restlessness, ringing in the ears, water retention, weakness, weight loss

Why should this drug not be prescribed?
Do not take Parnate if you are in danger of a stroke, if you have heart or liver disease, high blood pressure, or a history of headaches, if you have a type of tumor known as pheochromocytoma, or if you will be undergoing elective surgery requiring general anesthesia.

Special warnings about this medication
In clinical studies, antidepressants increased the risk of suicidal thinking and behavior in children and adolescents with depression and other psychiatric disorders. Anyone considering the use of Parnate or any other antidepressant in a child or adolescent must balance this risk with the clinical need. Parnate is not approved for use in children.

Additionally, the progression of major depression is associated with a worsening of symptoms and/or the emergence of suicidal thinking or behavior in both adults and children, whether or not they are taking antidepressants. Individuals being treated with Parnate and their caregivers should watch for any change in symptoms or any new symptoms that appear suddenly—especially agitation, anxiety, hostility, panic, restlessness, extreme hyperactivity, and suicidal thinking or behavior—and report them to the doctor immediately. Be especially observant at the beginning of treatment and whenever there is a change in dose.

The most dangerous reaction to Parnate is a surge in blood pressure, which has sometimes been fatal. For this reason, report promptly to your doctor any of the following symptoms: constriction or pain in the throat or chest, dizziness, fever, headache, irregular heartbeat, light sensitivity, nausea, neck stiffness or soreness, palpitations, pupil dilation, sweating, or vomiting.

A number of people who take Parnate experience low blood pressure, faintness, or drowsiness, so exercise great care when performing potentially hazardous tasks, such as driving a car or operating machinery.

Some people become physically dependent on Parnate and experience withdrawal symptoms when the drug is stopped, including restlessness, anxiety, depression, confusion, hallucinations, headache, weakness, and diarrhea.

If you have kidney problems, make sure the doctor is aware of this. The doctor may need to reduce your dosage of Parnate to avoid a buildup of the drug. Parnate should also be used with caution if you have an overactive thyroid gland.

MAO inhibitors can suppress heart pain that would otherwise serve as a warning sign of a heart attack. For this reason and others, it should be used with caution by older adults. Also, it should be used with caution by diabetics and people with epilepsy or other convulsive disorders because it can alter the level of drugs used to treat these conditions. Tell every doctor or dentist whom you see that you are taking Parnate.

Possible food and drug interactions when taking this medication
Never take Parnate with the following drugs; the combination can trigger seizures or a dangerous spike in blood pressure:

Other MAO inhibitors such as Nardil
Antidepressant drugs classified as tricyclics, such as Anafranil, Elavil, and Tofranil
Carbamazepine (Tegretol)
Cyclobenzaprine (Flexeril)

When switching from one of these drugs to Parnate, or vice versa, allow an interval of at least 1 week between medications.

Also avoid combining Parnate with any of the following:

Antidepressant drugs classified as selective serotonin reuptake inhibitors, such as Paxil, Prozac, and Zoloft
Amphetamines such as Adderall and Dexedrine
Anesthetics
Antihistamines such as Allegra, Benadryl, and Clarinex
Blood pressure medications such as Accupril, Lotensin, and Prinivil
Bupropion (Wellbutrin)
Buspirone (BuSpar)
Cold and hay fever remedies that constrict blood vessels
Cough remedies containing dextromethorphan
Demerol and other narcotic painkillers such as Percodan, OxyContin, and Vicodin
Disulfiram (Antabuse)
Guanethidine
Methyldopa
Over-the-counter weight reduction aids
Parkinson's disease medications such as Parlodel, Requip, and Sinemet

Reserpine
Sedatives such as Halcion, Nembutal, and Seconal
Tryptophan
Water pills such as HydroDIURIL

While taking Parnate, you should also avoid foods that contain a high amount of a substance called tyramine, including:

Anchovies
Avocados
Bananas
Beer (including non-alcoholic beer)
Caviar
Cheese (especially strong and aged varieties)
Chianti wine
Chocolate
Dried fruits (including raisins, prunes, and figs)
Liqueurs
Liver
Meat extracts and meat prepared with tenderizers
Overripe fruit
Pickled herring
Pods of broad beans such as fava beans
Raspberries
Sauerkraut
Sherry
Sour cream
Soy sauce
Yeast extracts
Yogurt

Likewise, avoid alcohol and large amounts of caffeine.

Special information if you are pregnant or breastfeeding

If you are pregnant or plan to become pregnant, inform your doctor immediately. Parnate should be used during pregnancy only if its benefits outweigh the potential risks.

Parnate makes its way into breast milk. If the drug is essential to your health, your doctor may advise you to stop nursing until your treatment is finished.

Recommended dosage

ADULTS

The usual dosage is 30 milligrams per day, divided into smaller doses. If ineffective, the dosage may be slowly increased under your doctor's supervision to a maximum of 60 milligrams per day.

Overdosage

Any medication taken in excess can have serious consequences. If you suspect an overdose of Parnate, seek medical help immediately.

■ *Symptoms of Parnate overdose may include:*
Agitation, confusion, coma, dizziness, drowsiness, high fever, incoherence, rigid muscles, severe headache, twitching, weakness

Paroxetine See Paxil, page 1042.

PATANOL

Pronounced: PAT-ah-nol
Generic name: Olopatadine hydrochloride

Why is this drug prescribed?

Patanol is an antihistamine that relieves the red, itchy eyes often caused by allergies.

Most important fact about this drug

Patanol should be used only for allergic conditions. It is not a remedy for irritation from contact lenses.

How should you take this medication?

When applying the eyedrops, be careful to avoid touching the eyelids with the dropper tip. This could contaminate the solution.

Do not wear soft contact lenses while the eyes are red. At other times, wait at least 10 minutes after applying Patanol before inserting the lenses.

■ *If you miss a dose…*
Take the forgotten dose as soon as you remember. However, if it is almost time for your next dose, skip the one you missed and return to your regular schedule. Do not take 2 doses at once.
■ *Storage instructions…*
Keep bottle tightly closed. Store at room temperature.

What side effects may occur?

Side effects cannot be anticipated. If any develop or change in intensity, tell your doctor as soon as possible. Only your doctor can determine if it is safe to continue using Patanol.

■ *Side effects may includes:*
Allergic reactions, bloodshot eyes, blurred vision, burning or stinging, changes in taste, cold-like symptoms, dry eye, headache (occurs in 7 percent of patients), inflammation of the cornea, itching, nausea, runny nose, sensation of a foreign body in the eye, sinus inflammation, sore throat, swollen eyelids, weakness

Why should this drug not be prescribed?
You'll need to avoid this drug if it causes an allergic reaction.

Special warnings about this medication
Use only in the eyes. Patanol should not be taken orally or by injection. Safety and effectiveness have not been established in children under 3.

Possible food and drug interactions when using this medication
There is no information on potential interactions.

Special information if you are pregnant or breastfeeding
The effects of Patanol during pregnancy have not been adequately studied. If you are pregnant or plan to become pregnant, alert your doctor immediately.

Researchers do not know how much of the eyedrops can make their way into breast milk. Be cautious if using Patanol while breastfeeding.

Recommended dosage
The usual dose is 1 drop in each affected eye 2 times a day. Allow 6 to 8 hours between doses.

Overdosage
There is no information on Patanol overdose. However, excessive use of any medication can have serious consequences. If you suspect an overdose, seek medical attention without delay.

PAXIL
Pronounced: PACKS-ill
Generic name: Paroxetine hydrochloride
Other brand name: Paxil CR

Why is this drug prescribed?
Paxil relieves a variety of emotional problems. It can be prescribed for serious, continuing depression that interferes with your ability to function. Symptoms of this type of depression often include changes in appetite and sleep patterns, a persistent low mood, loss of interest in people and activities, decreased sex drive, feelings of guilt or worthlessness, suicidal thoughts, difficulty concentrating, and slowed thinking.

Paxil is also used to treat obsessive-compulsive disorder (OCD), a disease marked by unwanted but stubbornly persistent thoughts, or unreasonable rituals you feel compelled to repeat.

In addition, Paxil is prescribed for panic disorder, a crippling emotional problem characterized by sudden attacks of at least 4 of the following symptoms: palpitations, sweating, shaking, numbness, chills or hot flashes, shortness of breath, a feeling of choking, chest pain, nausea or abdominal distress, dizziness or faintness, feelings of unreality or de- tachment, fear of losing control, or fear of dying.

Paxil can be prescribed for generalized anxiety disorder, a disease marked by excessive anxiety and worry that persists for at least 6 months and can't be easily controlled. True cases of generalized anxiety disorder are accompanied by at least 3 of the following symptoms: restlessness or a keyed-up or on-edge feeling, a tendency to tire easily, difficulty concen- trating or spells when the mind goes blank, irritability, muscle tension, or sleep disturbance.

Paxil can be used in the treatment of social anxiety disorder (also known as social phobia), a condition marked by shyness or stage fright so intense that it interferes with an individual's work and social life.

Paxil is also prescribed for post-traumatic stress disorder, a crippling condition that sometimes develops in reaction to a disastrous or horrify- ing experience. Symptoms, which stubbornly refuse to abate, include un- wanted memories and dreams, intense distress when confronted with reminders of the event, a general numbing of interest and enjoyment, jumpiness, irritability, poor sleep, and loss of concentration.

Paxil CR, the controlled-release version, is prescribed for major de- pression, panic disorder, social anxiety disorder, and severe premen- strual symptoms classified as premenstrual dysphoric disorder.

Paxil belongs to the class of drugs known as selective serotonin reup- take inhibitors (SSRIs). Serotonin is one of the chemical messengers believed to govern moods. Ordinarily, it is quickly reabsorbed after its re- lease at the junctures between nerves. Reuptake inhibitors such as Paxil slow this process, thereby boosting the levels of serotonin available in the brain.

Most important fact about this drug

Your symptoms may seem to improve within 1 to 4 weeks after beginning treatment with Paxil. Even if you feel better, continue to take the medica- tion as long as your doctor tells you to do so.

How should you take this medication?

Paxil is taken once a day, with or without food, usually in the morning. In- form your doctor if you are taking or plan to take any prescription or over- the-counter drugs, since they may interact unfavorably with Paxil. Shake the oral suspension well before using. Paxil CR should be swallowed whole; it should not be chewed or crushed.

■ *If you miss a dose...*
Skip the forgotten dose and go back to your regular schedule with the next dose. Do not take a double dose to make up for the one you missed.

■ *Storage instructions...*
Paxil tablets and suspension can be stored at room temperature.

What side effects may occur?

Side effects cannot be anticipated. If any develop or change in intensity, inform your doctor as soon as possible. Only your doctor can determine whether it is safe for you to continue taking this medication.

During the first 4 to 6 weeks, you may find some side effects less troublesome (nausea and dizziness, for example) than others (dry mouth, drowsiness, and weakness).

■ *Side effects may include:*
Abnormal ejaculation, abnormal orgasm, constipation, decreased appetite, decreased sex drive, diarrhea, dizziness, drowsiness, dry mouth, gas, impotence, male and female genital disorders, nausea, nervousness, sleeplessness, sweating, tremor, weakness, vertigo

Why should this drug not be prescribed?

Dangerous and even fatal reactions are possible when Paxil is combined with thioridazine (Mellaril) or drugs classified as monoamine oxidase (MAO) inhibitors, such as the antidepressants Nardil and Parnate. Never take Paxil with any of these medications, or within 2 weeks of starting or stopping use of an MAO inhibitor. You'll also need to avoid Paxil if it gives you an allergic reaction.

Special warnings about this medication

In clinical studies, antidepressants increased the risk of suicidal thinking and behavior in children and adolescents with depression and other psychiatric disorders. Anyone considering the use of Paxil or any other antidepressant in a child or adolescent must balance this risk with the clinical need. Paxil has not been studied in children or adolescents and is not approved for treating anyone less than 18 years old.

Additionally, the progression of major depression is associated with a worsening of symptoms and/or the emergence of suicidal thinking or behavior in both adults and children, whether or not they are taking antidepressants. Individuals being treated with Paxil and their caregivers should watch for any change in symptoms or any new symptoms that appear suddenly—especially agitation, anxiety, hostility, panic, restlessness, extreme hyperactivity, and suicidal thinking or behavior—and report them to the doctor immediately. Be especially observant at the beginning of treatment or whenever there is a change in dose.

Paxil should be used cautiously by people with a history of manic disorders and those with high pressure in the eyes (glaucoma).

If you have a history of seizures, make sure your doctor knows about it. Paxil should be used with caution in this situation. If you develop seizures once therapy has begun, the drug should be discontinued.

If you have a disease or condition that affects your metabolism or blood circulation, make sure your doctor is aware of it. Paxil should be used cautiously in this situation.

Paxil may impair your judgment, thinking, or motor skills. Do not drive, operate dangerous machinery, or participate in any hazardous activity that requires full mental alertness until you are sure the medication is not affecting you in this way.

Antidepressants such as Paxil could potentially cause stomach bleeding, especially when combined with nonsteroidal anti-inflammatory drugs (NSAIDs) such as aspirin, ibuprofen (Advil, Motrin), naproxen (Aleve), and ketoprofen (Orudis KT). Consult your doctor before combining Paxil with NSAIDs or blood-thinning drugs.

It's best to avoid an abrupt discontinuation of Paxil therapy. It can lead to symptoms such as dizziness, abnormal dreams, and tingling sensations. To prevent such problems, your doctor will reduce your dose gradually.

Possible food and drug interactions when taking this medication

Remember that Paxil must never be combined with Mellaril or MAO inhibitors such as Nardil and Parnate, or taken within 2 weeks of starting or stopping an MAO inhibitor.

If Paxil is taken with certain other drugs, the effects of either could be increased, decreased, or altered. It is especially important to check with your doctor before combining Paxil with any of the following:

Alcohol
Antidepressants such as Elavil, Tofranil, Norpramin, Pamelor, Prozac
Aspirin
Cimetidine (Tagamet)
Diazepam (Valium)
Digoxin (Lanoxin)
Flecainide (Tambocor)
Lithium (Eskalith)
Nonsteroidal anti-inflammatory drugs (NSAIDs) such as aspirin,
    ibuprofen (Advil, Motrin), naproxen (Aleve), and ketoprofen
    (Orudis KT)
Phenobarbital
Phenytoin (Dilantin)
Procyclidine (Kemadrin)
Propafenone (Rythmol)
Propranolol (Inderal, Inderide)
Quinidine (Quinaglute)
Sumatriptan (Imitrex)
Theophylline (Theo-24, Uniphyl)
Tryptophan
Warfarin (Coumadin)

Special information if you are pregnant or breastfeeding

The effects of Paxil during pregnancy have not been adequately studied. There have been reports of serious complications in newborns who were exposed to Paxil late in the last 3 months of pregnancy. If you are pregnant or plan to become pregnant, inform your doctor immediately.

Paxil appears in breast milk and could affect a nursing infant. If this medication is essential to your health, your doctor may advise you to discontinue breastfeeding until your treatment with Paxil is finished.

Recommended dosage

The following dosages are for adults. The safety and effectiveness of Paxil have not been studied in children or adolescents.

DEPRESSION

Paxil
The usual starting dose is 20 milligrams a day taken as a single dose, usually in the morning. At intervals of at least 1 week, your physician may increase your dosage by 10 milligrams a day, up to a maximum of 50 milligrams a day.

Paxil CR
The recommended starting dose is 25 milligrams a day, usually taken in the morning. At intervals of at least 1 week, the dosage may be increased by 12.5 milligrams a day, up to a maximum of 62.5 milligrams a day.

OBSESSIVE-COMPULSIVE DISORDER

The usual starting dose is 20 milligrams a day, typically taken in the morning. At intervals of at least 1 week, your doctor may increase the dosage by 10 milligrams a day. The recommended long-term dosage is 40 milligrams daily. The maximum is 60 milligrams a day.

PANIC DISORDER

Paxil
The usual starting dose is 10 milligrams a day taken in the morning. At intervals of 1 week or more, the doctor may increase the dose by 10 milligrams a day. The target dose is 40 milligrams daily; dosage should never exceed 60 milligrams.

Paxil CR
The recommended starting dose is 12.5 milligrams a day, usually taken in the morning. At intervals of at least 1 week, the dosage may be increased by 12.5 milligrams a day, up to a maximum of 75 milligrams a day.

GENERALIZED ANXIETY DISORDER

The recommended dose is 20 milligrams taken once a day, usually in the morning.

SOCIAL ANXIETY DISORDER

Paxil
The recommended dose is 20 milligrams taken once a day, usually in the morning.

Paxil CR
The recommended starting dose is 12.5 milligrams a day, usually taken in the morning. At intervals of at least 1 week, the dosage may be increased by 12.5 milligrams a day, up to a maximum of 37.5 milligrams a day.

POST-TRAUMATIC STRESS DISORDER

The recommended dose is 20 milligrams taken once a day, usually in the morning.

PREMENSTRUAL DYSPHORIC DISORDER

Paxil CR
The recommended starting dose is 12.5 milligrams a day, usually taken in the morning. The doctor will instruct the patient to take the dose either every day of the month or only during the 2 weeks before menstruation begins (the luteal phase of her cycle). If needed, the dose can be increased to 25 milligrams a day.

DOSAGE ADJUSTMENT

For older adults, the weak, and those with severe kidney or liver disease, starting doses are reduced to 10 milligrams daily, and later doses are limited to no more than 40 milligrams a day. Starting doses of Paxil CR are limited to 12.5 milligrams daily, and later doses are limited to no more than 50 milligrams a day.

Overdosage
Any medication taken in excess can have serious consequences. If you suspect an overdose, seek medical attention immediately.

■ *The symptoms of Paxil overdose may include:*
  Coma, dizziness, drowsiness, facial flushing, nausea, sweating, tremor, vomiting

PCE *See Erythromycin, Oral, page 520.*

PEDIAPRED

Pronounced: PEE-dee-uh-pred
Generic name: Prednisolone sodium phosphate

Why is this drug prescribed?

Pediapred, a steroid drug, is used to reduce inflammation and improve symptoms in a variety of disorders, including rheumatoid arthritis, acute gouty arthritis, and severe cases of asthma. It may be given to people to treat primary or secondary adrenal cortex insufficiency (lack of or insufficient adrenal cortical hormone in the body). It is also given to help treat the following disorders:

Blood disorders such as leukemia and various anemias
Certain cancers (along with other drugs)
Connective tissue diseases such as systemic lupus erythematosus
Digestive tract diseases such as ulcerative colitis
Eye diseases of various kinds
Fluid retention due to nephrotic syndrome (a condition in which
    damage to the kidneys causes a loss of protein in the urine)
High blood levels of calcium associated with cancer
Lung diseases such as tuberculosis
Severe allergic conditions such as drug-induced allergic reactions
Severe skin eruptions

Studies have shown that high doses of Pediapred are effective in controlling severe symptoms of multiple sclerosis, although they do not affect the ultimate outcome or natural history of the disease.

Most important fact about this drug

Pediapred decreases your resistance to infection. It may also mask some of the signs and symptoms of an infection, which makes it difficult for a doctor to diagnose the actual problem.

How should you take this medication?

Pediapred may cause stomach upset and should be taken with food. Take this medication exactly as prescribed.

■ *If you miss a dose...*
Take it as soon as you remember. If it is almost time for your next dose, skip the one you missed and go back to your regular schedule. Never take 2 doses at the same time.

■ *Storage instructions...*
Store Pediapred in a cool place, and keep the bottle tightly closed. This medication may be refrigerated.

What side effects may occur?

Side effects cannot be anticipated. If any develop or change in intensity, inform your doctor as soon as possible. Only your doctor can determine if it is safe for you to continue taking Pediapred.

■ *Side effects may include:*

Abnormal loss of bony tissue causing fragile bones, abnormal redness of the face, backbone break that collapses the spinal column, bruising, cataracts, convulsions, dizziness, excess growth of body or facial hair, feeling of illness, fluid retention (edema), fracture of long bones, glaucoma (increased eye pressure), headache, high blood pressure, hives, increased appetite, increased sweating, loss of muscle mass, menstrual irregularities, mental capacity changes, muscle disease, muscle weakness, nausea, peptic ulcer (stomach ulcer with possible bleeding), protrusion of eyeball, psychotic disorders, ruptured tendons, salt retention, slow growth in children, slow wound healing, sugar diabetes, swelling of the abdomen, thinning of the skin, vertigo, weight gain

Why should this drug not be prescribed?

This drug should not be used for fungal infections within the body. Avoid it if it gives you an allergic reaction.

Special warnings about this medication

You should not be vaccinated against smallpox while being treated with Pediapred. Avoid other immunizations as well, especially if you are taking Pediapred in high doses, because of the possible hazards of nervous system complications and a lack of natural immune response.

Because Pediapred reduces resistance to infection, people who have never had measles or chickenpox—or been vaccinated against them—should be careful to avoid exposure. These diseases can be severe, or even fatal, in people with lowered resistance.

Likewise, an ordinary case of threadworm or other intestinal parasites can grow into a grave emergency when the immune system is weak. Symptoms of threadworm include stomach pain, vomiting, and diarrhea. If you suspect an infection, call your doctor immediately.

If you are taking Pediapred and are subjected to unusual stress, notify your doctor. The drug reduces the function of your adrenal glands, and they may be unable to cope. Your doctor may therefore increase your dosage of this rapidly acting steroid before, during, and after the stressful situation.

Prolonged use of steroids may produce posterior subcapsular cataracts (a disorder under the envelope-like structure at the back of the eye that causes the lens to become less transparent) or the eye disease glaucoma, and may intensify additional eye infections due to fungi or viruses.

Average and high doses of this medication may cause an increase in blood pressure, salt and water retention, and an increased loss of potassium. Your doctor may have you decrease your salt intake and increase your potassium intake.

The effects of Pediapred may be intensified if you have an underactive thyroid or long-term liver disease.

If you have ocular herpes simplex (painful blisters of the eye), you should be careful using this drug because of the possibility of corneal perforation (puncture of the outer, transparent part of the eye).

The use of Pediapred may cause mood swings, feelings of elation, insomnia, personality changes, severe depression, or even severe mental disorders.

If you are being treated for a blood clotting factor deficiency, use aspirin with caution when taking Pediapred. Do not use this drug for any disorder other than that for which it was prescribed.

Your doctor will prescribe this medication very cautiously if you have ulcerative colitis (inflammation of the colon and rectum) where there is a possibility of a puncture, abscess, or other infection; diverticulitis (inflammation of a sac formed at weak points of the colon); recent intestinal anastomoses (a surgical connection between two separate parts of the colon); active or inactive peptic (stomach) ulcers; unsatisfactory kidney function; high blood pressure; osteoporosis (brittle bones that may fracture); and myasthenia gravis (a long-term disease characterized by abnormal fatigue and weakness of certain muscles).

Do not discontinue the use of Pediapred abruptly or without medical supervision.

If you should develop a fever or other signs of infection while taking Pediapred, notify your doctor immediately.

Possible food and drug interactions when taking this medication
If Pediapred is taken with certain other drugs, the effects of either could be increased, decreased, or altered. It is especially important to check with your doctor before combining Pediapred with the following:

Amphotericin B
Aspirin
Barbiturates such as phenobarbital and Seconal
Cyclosporine (Sandimmune and Neoral)
Diabetes drugs such as Glucotrol
Ephedrine (in products such as Marax and Rynatuss)
Estrogens such as Premarin
Isoniazid (Nydrazid)
Ketoconazole (Nizoral)
Nonsteroidal anti-inflammatory drugs such as Motrin
Oral contraceptives
Phenytoin (Dilantin)

Rifampin (Rifadin)
Warfarin (Coumadin)
Water pills such as Lasix

Special information if you are pregnant or breastfeeding

The effects of Pediapred during pregnancy have not been adequately studied. If you are pregnant or plan to become pregnant, inform your doctor immediately. This medication may appear in breast milk and could affect a nursing infant. If this drug is essential to your health, your doctor may advise you to discontinue breastfeeding until your treatment is finished.

Recommended dosage

ADULTS

The starting dosage of Pediapred may vary from 5 to 60 milliliters, depending on the specific disease being treated.

Your doctor will adjust the dose until the results are satisfactory. If your condition does not improve after a reasonable period of time, the doctor may switch you to another medication.

Once you've shown a favorable response, your doctor will gradually decrease the dosage to the minimum that maintains the effect.

If you stop taking Pediapred after long-term therapy, your doctor will have you withdraw slowly, rather than abruptly.

For acute flare-ups of multiple sclerosis (MS), the usual dose is 200 milligrams per day of Pediapred for one week followed by 80 milligrams every other day or 4 to 8 milligrams of dexamethasone every other day for 1 month.

CHILDREN

The starting dosage for children ranges from 0.14 to 2 milligrams per 2.2 pounds of body weight per day, divided into 3 or 4 smaller doses. For asthma, the recommended dosage is 1 to 2 milligrams per 2.2 pounds of body weight per day, taken in a single or several smaller doses.

Overdosage

Although no specific information is available, any medication taken in excess can have serious consequences. If you suspect an overdose of Pediapred, seek medical treatment immediately.

PEDIAZOLE

Pronounced: PEE-dee-uh-zole
Generic ingredients: Erythromycin ethylsuccinate,
   Sulfisoxazole acetyl
Other brand name: Eryzole

Why is this drug prescribed?

Pediazole is prescribed for the treatment of severe middle ear infections in children.

Most important fact about this drug

Sulfisoxazole is one of a group of drugs called sulfonamides, which prevent the growth of certain bacteria in the body. However, sulfonamides have been known to cause rare but sometimes fatal reactions such as Stevens-Johnson syndrome (a skin condition characterized by severe blisters and bleeding in the mucous membranes of the lips, mouth, nose, and eyes), sudden and severe liver damage, a severe blood disorder (agranulocytosis), and a lack of red and white blood cells because of a bone marrow disorder.

Notify your doctor at the first sign of a side effect such as skin rash, sore throat, fever, abnormal skin paleness, reddish or purplish skin spots, or yellowing of the skin or whites of the eyes.

How should you take this medication?

Be sure to keep giving Pediazole for the full time prescribed, even if your child begins to feel better after the first few days. Keep to a regular schedule; the medication works best when there is a constant amount in the blood.

Pediazole can be given with or without food. However, you should not give this medication with or immediately after carbonated beverages, fruit juice, or tea. If the child develops an upset stomach, give the medicine with crackers or a light snack.

To prevent sediment in the urine and the formation of stones, make sure that the child drinks plenty of fluids during treatment with Pediazole.

This medication increases the skin's sensitivity to sunlight. Overexposure can cause a rash, itching, redness, or sunburn. Keep the child out of direct sunlight, or provide protective clothing.

Shake well before using.

■ *If you miss a dose...*
   Give the forgotten dose as soon as you remember, then give the rest of the day's doses at evenly spaced intervals.
■ *Storage instructions...*
   Store Pediazole in the refrigerator. Keep tightly closed. Do not allow it to freeze. Use within 14 days; discard unused portion.

What side effects may occur?

Side effects cannot be anticipated. If any develop or change in intensity, inform your doctor as soon as possible. Only your doctor can determine if it is safe to continue giving Pediazole.

■ *Side effects may include:*
  Abdominal pain and discomfort, diarrhea, lack or loss of appetite, nausea, vomiting

Why should this drug not be prescribed?

If your child is sensitive to or has ever had an allergic reaction to erythromycin, sulfonamides, or other drugs of this type, do not use this medication. Make sure that your doctor is aware of any drug reactions that your child has experienced.

Pediazole should not be used if the child is taking Seldane or Hismanal.

This medication should not be prescribed for infants under 2 months of age.

Pediazole should not be taken by pregnant women at the end of their pregnancy or by mothers nursing infants under 2 months of age.

Special warnings about this medication

If your child has impaired kidney or liver function or a history of severe allergies or bronchial asthma, Pediazole may not be the best drug to use. Check with your doctor.

Prolonged or repeated use of Pediazole may cause new infections. If your child develops a new infection (called a superinfection), talk to your doctor. A different antibiotic may be needed.

If your child develops a cough or becomes short of breath, call your doctor. Also seek care immediately if the child develops diarrhea; it could signal a serious intestinal disorder.

If your child has the muscle-weakening disorder myasthenia gravis, Pediazole could make the condition worse.

Your doctor may recommend frequent urine tests while your child is taking Pediazole.

Possible food and drug interactions when taking this medication

If Pediazole is taken with certain other drugs, the effects of either could be increased, decreased, or altered. It is especially important to check with your doctor before combining Pediazole with the following:

Blood thinners such as warfarin (Coumadin)
Bromocriptine (Parlodel)
Carbamazepine (Tegretol)
Cyclosporine (Sandimmune)
Digoxin (Lanoxin)
Disopyramide (Norpace)
Ergotamine (Cafergot, Ergostat)

Lovastatin (Mevacor)
Methotrexate (Rheumatrex)
Oral antidiabetic drugs such as Micronase
Phenytoin (Dilantin)
Theophylline (Theo-Dur)
Triazolam (Halcion)

Special information if you are pregnant or breastfeeding

This drug is not prescribed for adults, and should never be taken at term of pregnancy or when breastfeeding.

Recommended dosage

CHILDREN

The recommended dose for children 2 months of age or older is determined by weight. The total daily amount is divided into several smaller doses given 3 or 4 times a day for 10 days.

Four-times-a-day schedule
Less than 18 pounds: Determined by doctor
18 pounds: ½ teaspoonful
35 pounds: 1 teaspoonful
53 pounds: 1½ teaspoonfuls
Over 70 pounds: 2 teaspoonfuls

Three-times-a-day schedule
Less than 13 pounds: Determined by doctor
13 pounds: ½ teaspoonful
26 pounds: 1 teaspoonful
40 pounds: 1½ teaspoonfuls
53 pounds: 2 teaspoonfuls
Over 66 pounds: 2½ teaspoonfuls

Overdosage

Any medication taken in excess can have serious consequences. If you suspect an overdose, seek medical treatment immediately.

■ *Symptoms of Pediazole overdose may include:*
Blood in the urine, colic, dizziness, drowsiness, fever, headache, loss of appetite, nausea, unconsciousness, vomiting, yellowed eyes and skin

PEGANONE

Pronounced: PEG-ah-known
Generic name: Ethotoin

Why is this drug prescribed?

Peganone is an antiepileptic drug prescribed to control tonic-clonic seizures (also known as grand mal seizures), a type of seizure in which the individual experiences a sudden loss of consciousness immediately followed by generalized convulsions. It is also used to treat complex partial seizures (also called psychomotor or temporal lobe seizures), which occur in only certain parts of the brain and are characterized by blank staring and repetitive movements.

Most important fact about this drug

If you have been taking Peganone regularly to prevent major seizures, do not stop abruptly. This may precipitate prolonged or repeated epileptic seizures without any recovery of consciousness between attacks—a condition called status epilepticus—that can be fatal if not treated promptly.

How should you take this medication?

Take Peganone with food to avoid stomach upset. Depending on the type of seizure disorder, your doctor may give you another drug to take with Peganone.

It is important that you strictly follow the prescribed dosage regimen and tell your doctor about any condition that makes it impossible for you to take Peganone as prescribed.

■ *If you miss a dose…*
Take the missed dose as soon as possible. However, if it is within 4 hours of your next dose, skip the one you missed and go back to your regular schedule. Never take 2 doses at once.

If you forget to take your medication 2 or more days in a row, check with your doctor.

■ *Storage instructions…*
Store at room temperature, but not above 77 degrees Fahrenheit.

What side effects may occur?

Side effects cannot be anticipated. If any develop or change in intensity, inform your doctor as soon as possible. Only your doctor can determine whether it is safe for you to continue taking Peganone.

■ *Side effects of Peganone may include:*
Chest pain, diarrhea, dizziness, double vision, fatigue, fever, gum overgrowth or thickening, headache, insomnia, involuntary or rapid eye movement, loss of or impaired muscle coordination, lymph node disease, nausea, numbness, skin rash, vomiting

Why should this drug not be prescribed?

Do not take Peganone if you have liver problems or blood disorders.

Special warnings about this medication

Blood abnormalities have occurred in some patients taking Peganone, although it is unknown whether the drug was the cause. Your doctor will do monthly blood tests when you first start therapy to guard against any such problems. Call your doctor immediately if you have symptoms such as sore throat, fever, malaise (marked by bodily discomfort, fatigue, or a general feeling of illness), easy bruising, small purple skin spots, nosebleeds, or any sign of infection or bleeding tendency.

The doctor may also check your liver function if he or she suspects a problem.

There is some evidence that Peganone may interfere with the body's metabolism of folic acid, which could lead to anemia. Talk to your doctor about taking supplements, especially if you're planning to become pregnant.

If you have systemic lupus erythematosus, you should be aware that Peganone could make the symptoms worse.

Because Peganone may cause gum hypertrophy (excessive formation of the gums over the teeth), it's important to practice good dental hygiene while taking this drug.

Possible food and drug interactions when taking this medication

If Peganone is taken with certain other drugs, the effects of either could be increased, decreased, or altered. It is especially important to check with your doctor before combining Peganone with the following:

Blood-thinning drugs such as Coumadin
Drugs used to treat blood disorders
Phenacemide (Phenurone)

Although no specific problems with alcohol have been reported, it's still a good idea to watch your alcohol intake while taking this drug.

Special information if you are pregnant or breastfeeding

If you are pregnant or plan to become pregnant, inform your doctor immediately. Because of the possibility of birth defects with antiepileptic drugs such as Peganone, you may need to discontinue the drug. Do not, however, stop taking it without first consulting your doctor. Because Peganone appears in breast milk, you should not breastfeed during treatment with the drug.

Recommended dosage

Dosage is tailored to each individual's needs. Your doctor will monitor blood levels of the drug closely. If you're switching from another antiepileptic drug, the doctor will have you slowly taper off the dosage while increasing the dose of Peganone.

ADULTS

The recommended starting dose is 1,000 milligrams or less a day, taken in 4 to 6 divided doses spaced as evenly as possible. Depending on your response, the doctor may raise your dose. The usual effective maintenance dose is 2,000 to 3,000 milligrams a day.

CHILDREN

Dosage depends on the child's age and weight. The initial starting dose should not exceed 750 milligrams a day, taken in 4 to 6 divided doses spaced as evenly as possible. The usual maintenance dose is 500 to 1,000 milligrams a day, although occasionally doses as high as 3,000 milligrams a day may be necessary.

Overdosage

Any medication taken in excess can have serious consequences. If you suspect an overdose of Peganone, seek medical attention immediately.

■ *Symptoms of Peganone overdose may include:*
Drowsiness, loss of or impaired muscle coordination, nausea, visual disturbance, and, at very high doses, coma

PEGASYS

Pronounced: PEG-ah-sis
Generic name: Peginterferon alfa-2a

Why is this drug prescribed?

Pegasys is used to treat adults who have chronic hepatitis C infection, including those who are also infected with HIV and are clinically stable. Additionally, the drug is used to treat hepatitis B. Pegasys is an injection prescribed for people who show signs of liver damage and have not been previously treated with alpha interferon.

Pegasys is a synthetic (man-made) version of interferon, a substance normally produced in the body to fight various infections, including the virus that causes hepatitis C. Pegasys can be taken alone or in combination with Copegus (ribavirin), which works with interferon to help your body get rid of the virus and prevent it from coming back. Treatment with Copegus alone, however, is not effective against hepatitis C.

Most important fact about this drug

Pegasys, taken alone or combined with Copegus, can have serious side effects that may cause death in rare cases (see *Special warnings about this medication*). Combining Pegasys with Copegus can induce anemia severe enough to cause a heart attack, especially in people who already have heart disease. Before using Pegasys, you should talk with your doctor about the possible benefits and side effects of treatment. Once you start taking Pegasys, you will need to see your doctor regularly for exams and blood tests to make sure the treatment is working and to check for side effects.

In addition, combination treatment with Pegasys and Copegus can cause death, serious birth defects, or other harm to an unborn baby. Female patients and female partners of male patients being treated with Pegasys and Copegus must have a pregnancy test before treatment begins and then monthly during treatment to prove they are not pregnant. Both women and men must use two effective forms of birth control during combination therapy and for 6 months after stopping the drugs. Men should use a condom with spermicide as one of the two forms.

How should you take this medication?

Pegasys is given by injection under the skin. It should be taken once a week, on the same day each week and around the same time. Your doctor will train you or your caregiver on the best way to give the injection.

Pegasys comes in two forms: a liquid in a single-use vial and a liquid in a prefilled syringe. Your doctor will determine which is best for you. Be sure to inspect the medication before injecting it. If you see floating particles or the medication is discolored, do not use it.

Your doctor will also decide whether you should take Pegasys with Copegus, which comes in tablet form. If the doctor prescribes Copegus, you should take it twice a day with food (breakfast and dinner).

Drink plenty of fluids and avoid dehydration while taking Pegasys, especially during the beginning of treatment.

■ *If you miss a dose...*
If it is within 2 days of when you should have taken Pegasys, give the injection as soon as you remember. Take your next dose on the day you would usually take it. If more than 2 days have passed, ask your doctor what to do.

If you miss a dose of Copegus, take the forgotten dose as soon as you remember. However, if it is almost time for your next dose, skip the one you missed and return to your regular schedule. Do not take 2 doses at once.

■ *Storage instructions...*
Store Pegasys in the refrigerator at a temperature of 36 to 46 degrees Fahrenheit. Keeping Pegasys at temperatures outside the recommended range can destroy the medicine. Do not leave Pegasys outside the refrigerator for more than 24 hours.

Do not freeze or shake the medication; protect it from light.

What side effects may occur?

Side effects cannot be anticipated. If any develop or change in intensity, tell your doctor as soon as possible. Only your doctor can determine if it is safe to continue using Pegasys.

■ *Side effects may include:*

Anxiety, depression, diarrhea, flu-like symptoms (chills, fatigue, fever, headache, muscle pain), hair thinning, insomnia, irritability, itchy spots, joint pain, loss of appetite, nausea and vomiting, skin reactions (especially at the injection site), weight loss

Why should this drug not be prescribed?

Do not take Pegasys if you:

■ Have ever had an allergic reaction to another alpha interferon drug or to any of the ingredients in Pegasys
■ Have hepatitis caused by your immune system attacking your liver (autoimmune hepatitis)
■ Have unstable or severe liver disease

Do not take Pegasys combined with Copegus if you:

■ Have ever had an allergic reaction to Copegus or to any of the ingredients in the drug
■ Are pregnant or planning to become pregnant during treatment or during the 6 months after treatment has ended, or if you're breastfeeding. If you're a man and have a female partner who fits these criteria, you must also avoid combination therapy.
■ Have a disorder that affects the red blood cells, such as sickle-cell anemia or thalassemia major

Special warnings about this medication

Pegasys should be used with extreme caution in people who have a history of severe mental illness, especially depression or anxiety, or those with a history of drug or alcohol addiction. Possible side effects of the drug include irritability, aggressive behavior, anxiety, depression, and suicidal thoughts. A few individuals have committed suicide while using this drug. In addition, people formerly addicted to drugs or alcohol could have a relapse while taking Pegasys.

Other serious—and possibly life-threatening—side effects of treatment include:

Blood disorders that could increase the risk of serious infection or bleeding
Infections, including ones that have caused death
Lung problems, such as difficulty breathing or pneumonia
Eye problems, including blurred vision or loss of vision

Autoimmune disorders, including psoriasis, systemic lupus erythematosus, and thyroid problems

Heart problems, including chest pain and, very rarely, heart attack

Liver problems

Colitis (inflammation of the bowel). Symptoms include abdominal pain, bloody diarrhea, and fever.

Severe allergic reactions, including rash, hives, and difficulty breathing

Combination treatment with Copegus can also cause severe side effects, including:

Birth defects or death of an unborn baby

Decrease in red blood cells (anemia). This is especially dangerous in people who already have heart disease or circulatory problems.

Pancreatitis (inflammation of the pancreas). Symptoms include severe pain in the upper abdomen, diarrhea, weight loss, nausea and vomiting, and fever.

Before taking Pegasys (with or without Copegus), tell your doctor if you've ever had any of the following: history of heart disease or heart attack; history of cancer; autoimmune disorders such as psoriasis, systemic lupus erythematosus, or rheumatoid arthritis; kidney problems; blood disorders; diabetes; thyroid problems; liver problems other than hepatitis C; hepatitis B infection; an organ transplant; or colitis (inflammation of the bowel).

Contact your doctor immediately if you develop any of these symptoms while taking Pegasys: depression or suicidal thoughts, severe chest pain, difficulty breathing, vision changes, unusual bleeding or bruising, high or persistent fever, severe stomach or lower back pain, or bloody diarrhea. Also alert the doctor if you have psoriasis that gets worse while taking this drug.

It is not known whether Pegasys, either alone or combined with Copegus, can permanently eliminate the hepatitis C virus or prevent liver cancer or liver failure caused by hepatitis C infection. It is also not known whether treatment can prevent you from infecting another person with the virus.

Pegasys may cause dizziness, confusion, sleepiness, or fatigue. Avoid driving or operating dangerous machinery until you know how this drug affects you.

Possible food and drug interactions when taking this medication
If you are taking didanosine (Videx), combination treatment with Pegasys and Copegus is not recommended. Serious and even fatal reactions have occurred.

If Pegasys is taken with certain other drugs, the effects of either could be increased, decreased, or altered. It is especially important to check with your doctor before combining Pegasys (either alone or combined with Copegus) with the following:

> HIV drugs known as nucleoside analogues, such as Combivir, Epivir, Retrovir, and Zerit
> Methadone
> Theophylline

In addition, tell the doctor if you are taking or planning to take other prescription medicines, over-the-counter medicines, or vitamin, mineral, or herbal supplements.

Special information if you are pregnant or breastfeeding

You must **not** become pregnant or breastfeed a baby during combination treatment with Pegasys and Copegus (see *Most important fact about this drug*). This also applies to female partners of men who are taking the drugs.

Recommended dosage

ADULTS 18 YEARS AND OLDER

Your doctor will determine the best dose based on your condition and how your body responds to the drug. If you develop severe side effects, your dosage may need to be reduced or stopped altogether.

The safety and effectiveness of long-term treatment with Pegasys (more than a year) have not been studied.

Overdosage

If you take more than the prescribed amount of Pegasys, call your doctor immediately. You may need to have an exam or blood test to check for adverse reactions.

■ *Symptoms of overdose may include:*
Blood disorders, fatigue, liver problems

Peginterferon alfa-2a See *Pegasys, page 1057.*

Peginterferon alfa-2b See *PEG-Intron, below.*

PEG-INTRON
Pronounced: PEG-in-tron
Generic name: Peginterferon alfa-2b

Why is this drug prescribed?

PEG-Intron is used to treat adults who have chronic hepatitis C infection. PEG-Intron is an injection prescribed for people who show signs of liver damage and have not been previously treated with alpha interferon.

PEG-Intron is a synthetic (man-made) version of interferon, a substance normally produced in the body to fight various infections, including the virus that causes hepatitis C. PEG-Intron can be taken alone or in combination with Rebetol (ribavirin), which works with interferon to help your body get rid of the virus and prevent it from coming back. Treatment with Rebetol alone, however, is not effective against hepatitis C.

Most important fact about this drug

PEG-Intron, taken alone or combined with Rebetol, can have serious side effects that may cause death in rare cases (see *Special warnings about this medication*). Combining PEG-Intron with Rebetol can induce anemia severe enough to cause a heart attack, especially in people who already have heart disease. Before using PEG-Intron, you should talk with your doctor about the possible benefits and side effects of treatment. Once you start taking PEG-Intron, you will need to see your doctor regularly for exams and blood tests to make sure the treatment is working and to check for side effects.

In addition, combination treatment with PEG-Intron and Rebetol can cause death, serious birth defects, or other harm to an unborn baby. Female patients and female partners of male patients being treated with PEG-Intron and Rebetol must have a pregnancy test before treatment begins and then monthly during treatment to prove they are not pregnant. Both women and men must use two effective forms of birth control during combination therapy and for 6 months after stopping the drugs.

How should you take this medication?

PEG-Intron is taken by injection, either using a special pen (Redipen) or a traditional syringe. It should be taken once a week, on the same day each week and around the same time.

Your doctor will train you or your caregiver on the best way to give the injection. Be sure to inspect the medication before injecting it. If you see floating particles or the medication is discolored, do not use it.

Your doctor will also decide whether you should take PEG-Intron with Rebetol, which comes in capsule and oral solution forms. If the doctor prescribes Rebetol, you should take it twice a day with food (breakfast and dinner).

Drink plenty of fluids and avoid dehydration while taking PEG-Intron, especially during the beginning of treatment.

■ *If you miss a dose...*
Take the forgotten dose as soon as possible during the same day or the next day, then continue on your regular dosing schedule. If several days go by after you miss a dose, check with your doctor about what to do. Do not double the next dose or take more than 1 dose a week without talking to your doctor.

■ *Storage instructions…*
Store the Redipen in the refrigerator at a temperature of 36 to 46 degrees Fahrenheit. The vials of the medication can be stored at room temperature. Do not freeze the Redipen or vials.

What side effects may occur?

Side effects cannot be anticipated. If any develop or change in intensity, tell your doctor as soon as possible. Only your doctor can determine if it is safe to continue using PEG-Intron.

■ *Side effects may include:*
Anxiety, depression, diarrhea, flu-like symptoms (chills, fatigue, fever, headache, muscle pain), hair thinning, insomnia, irritability, itchy spots, joint pain, loss appetite, nausea, skin reactions (especially at the injection site), weight loss

Why should this drug not be prescribed?

Do not take PEG-Intron if you:

■ Have ever had an allergic reaction to another alpha interferon drug or to any of the ingredients in PEG-Intron
■ Have hepatitis caused by your immune system attacking your liver (autoimmune hepatitis)
■ Have unstable or severe liver disease

Do not take PEG-Intron combined with Rebetol if you:

■ Have ever had an allergic reaction to Rebetol or to any of the ingredients in the drug
■ Are pregnant or planning to become pregnant during treatment or during the 6 months after treatment has ended, or if you're breastfeeding. If you're a man and have a female partner who fits these criteria, you must also avoid combination therapy.
■ Have a disorder that affects the red blood cells, such as sickle-cell anemia or thalassemia major
■ Have severe kidney dysfunction

Special warnings about this medication

PEG-Intron should be used with extreme caution by people who have a history of severe mental illness, especially depression or anxiety, or those with a history of drug or alcohol addiction. Possible side effects of the drug include irritability, aggressive behavior, anxiety, depression, and suicidal thoughts. A few individuals have committed suicide while using this drug. In addition, people formerly addicted to drugs or alcohol could have a relapse while taking PEG-Intron.

Other serious—and possibly life-threatening—side effects of treatment include:

Blood disorders that could increase the risk of serious infection or bleeding

Infections, including ones that have caused death

Lung problems, such as difficulty breathing or pneumonia

Eye problems, including blurred vision or loss of vision

Autoimmune disorders, including psoriasis, systemic lupus erythematosus, and thyroid problems

Heart problems, including chest pain and, very rarely, heart attack

Pancreas or liver problems

Colitis (inflammation of the bowel); symptoms include abdominal pain, bloody diarrhea, and fever.

Blood sugar problems, including diabetes

Severe allergic reactions, including rash, hives, and difficulty breathing

Combination treatment with Rebetol can also cause severe side effects, including:

Birth defects or death of an unborn baby

Decrease in red blood cells (anemia). This is especially dangerous in people who already have heart disease or circulatory problems.

Before taking PEG-Intron (with or without Rebetol), tell your doctor if you've ever had any of the following: history of heart disease or heart attack; history of cancer; autoimmune disorders such as psoriasis, systemic lupus erythematosus, or rheumatoid arthritis; kidney problems; blood disorders; diabetes; high triglyceride levels; thyroid problems; liver problems other than hepatitis C; hepatitis B infection; HIV infection; an organ transplant; or colitis (inflammation of the bowel).

Contact your doctor immediately if you develop any of these symptoms while taking PEG-Intron: depression or suicidal thoughts, severe chest pain, difficulty breathing, vision changes, unusual bleeding or bruising, high or persistent fever, severe stomach or lower back pain, or bloody diarrhea. Also alert the doctor if you have psoriasis that gets worse while taking this drug.

It is not known whether PEG-Intron, either alone or combined with Rebetol, can permanently eliminate the hepatitis C virus or prevent liver cancer or liver failure caused by hepatitis C infection. It is also not known whether treatment can prevent you from infecting another person with the virus.

Possible food and drug interactions when taking this medication

If you are taking didanosine (Videx), combination treatment with PEG-Intron and Rebetol is not recommended. Serious and even fatal reactions have occurred.

If PEG-Intron is taken with certain other drugs, the effects of either could be increased, decreased, or altered. It is especially important to check with your doctor before combining PEG-Intron (either alone or combined with Rebetol) with methadone.

In addition, tell the doctor if you are taking or planning to take other prescription medicines, over-the-counter medicines, or vitamin, mineral, or herbal supplements.

Special information if you are pregnant or breastfeeding

You must *not* become pregnant or breastfeed a baby during combination treatment with PEG-Intron and Rebetol (see *Most important fact about this drug*). This also applies to female partners of men who are taking the drugs.

Recommended dosage

ADULTS 18 YEARS AND OLDER

Your doctor will determine the best dose based on your condition and how your body responds to the drug. If you develop severe side effects, your dosage may need to be reduced or stopped altogether.

The safety and effectiveness of long-term treatment with PEG-Intron (more than a year) have not been studied.

Overdosage

If you take more than the prescribed amount of PEG-Intron, call your doctor immediately. You may need to have an exam or blood test to check for adverse reactions.

Pemirolast See *Alamast, page 59.*

Penciclovir See *Denavir, page 405.*

Penicillin VK See *Penicillin V Potassium, below.*

PENICILLIN V POTASSIUM
Brand names: Penicillin VK, Veetids

Why is this drug prescribed?

■ *Penicillin V potassium is used to treat infections, including:*
   Dental infection, infections in the heart, middle ear infections, rheumatic fever, scarlet fever, skin infections, upper and lower respiratory tract infections

Penicillin V works against only certain types of bacteria—it is ineffective against fungi, viruses, and parasites.

Most important fact about this drug

If you are allergic to either penicillin or cephalosporin antibiotics in any form, consult your doctor before taking penicillin V. There is a possibility that you are allergic to both types of medication; and if a reaction occurs, it could be extremely severe. If you take the drug and feel signs of a reaction, seek medical attention immediately.

How should you take this medication?

Penicillin V may be taken on a full or empty stomach, though it is better absorbed when the stomach is empty. Be sure to take it for the full time of treatment.

Doses of the oral solution of penicillin V should be measured with a calibrated measuring spoon. Shake the solution well before using.

■ *If you miss a dose…*
Take it as soon as you remember. If it is almost time for the next dose, and you take 2 doses a day, take the one you missed and the next dose 5 to 6 hours later. If you take 3 or more doses a day, take the one you missed and the next dose 2 to 4 hours later, or double the next dose. Then go back to your regular schedule.

■ *Storage instructions…*
Store in a tightly closed container. The reconstituted oral solution must be refrigerated; discard any unused solution after 14 days.

Tablets and powder for oral solution may be stored at room temperature.

What side effects may occur?

Side effects cannot be anticipated. If any develop or change in intensity, inform your doctor as soon as possible. Only your doctor can determine if it is safe for you to continue taking this medication.

■ *Side effects may include:*
Anemia, black, hairy tongue, diarrhea, fever, hives, nausea, skin eruptions, stomach upset or pain, swelling in throat, vomiting

Why should this drug not be prescribed?

You should not use penicillin V if you have had an allergic reaction to penicillin or cephalosporin antibiotics.

Special warnings about this medication

If any allergic reactions occur, stop taking penicillin V and contact your doctor immediately.

If new infections (called superinfections) occur, consult your doctor.

If you have ever had allergic reactions such as rashes, hives, or hay fever, consult with your doctor before taking penicillin V.

Before taking penicillin V, tell your doctor if you have ever had asthma, colitis (inflammatory bowel disease), diabetes, or kidney or liver disease.

For infections such as strep throat, it is important to take penicillin V for the entire amount of time your doctor has prescribed. Even if you feel better, you need to continue taking this medication. If you stop taking this medication before your treatment time is complete, your infection may recur.

Possible food and drug interactions when taking this medication

If penicillin V is taken with certain other drugs, the effects of either could be increased, decreased, or altered. It is especially important to check with your doctor before combining penicillin V with the following:

Chloramphenicol (Chloromycetin)
Oral contraceptives
Tetracyclines such as Achromycin V and Sumycin

Special information if you are pregnant or breastfeeding

The effects of penicillin V in pregnancy have not been adequately studied. If you are pregnant or planning to become pregnant, inform your doctor immediately. Penicillin V should be used during pregnancy only if your doctor determines that the potential benefit justifies the potential risk to the fetus. Since penicillin V appears in breast milk, you should consult with your doctor if you plan to breastfeed your baby. If this medication is essential to your health, your doctor may advise you to discontinue breastfeeding until your treatment is finished.

Recommended dosage

ADULTS AND CHILDREN 12 YEARS AND OLDER

Continue taking penicillin V for the full time of treatment, even if you begin to feel better after a few days. Failure to take a full course of therapy may prevent complete elimination of the infection. It is best to take the doses at evenly spaced times, around the clock.

For mild to moderately severe strep infections of the upper respiratory tract and skin, and scarlet fever
The usual dosage is 125 to 250 milligrams every 6 to 8 hours for 10 days.

For mild to moderately severe pneumococcal infections of the respiratory tract, including middle ear infections
The usual dosage is 250 milligrams to 500 milligrams every 6 hours until you have been without a fever for at least 2 days.

For mild staph infections of skin
The usual dosage is 250 milligrams to 500 milligrams every 6 to 8 hours.

For mild to moderately severe gum infections known as Vincent's gingivitis
The usual dosage is 250 milligrams to 500 milligrams every 6 to 8 hours.

To prevent recurring rheumatic fever and/or chorea (infective disorder of the nervous system)

The usual dosage is 125 milligrams to 250 milligrams 2 times a day on a continuing basis.

Prevention of bacterial endocarditis (inflammation of the heart membrane) in people with heart disease who are undergoing dental or surgical procedures

For oral therapy, the usual dose is 2 grams of penicillin V taken one-half to 1 hour before the procedure, then 1 gram 6 hours later.

Overdosage

Any medication taken in excess can have serious consequences. If you suspect an overdose, seek medical attention immediately.

■ *Symptoms of penicillin V overdose may include:*
  Diarrhea, nausea, vomiting

PENLAC

Pronounced: PEN-lak
Generic name: Ciclopirox

Why is this drug prescribed?

Penlac is a nail lacquer used in the treatment of nail infections caused by the fungus *Trichophyton rubrum* (ringworm of the nails). It is prescribed only if the pale semicircle at the base of the nail is free of infection. It is part of a comprehensive treatment plan that includes professional removal of the unattached infected nails as frequently as monthly.

Most important fact about this drug

Patience is the watchword with Penlac therapy. It can take 6 months of daily Penlac application and periodic nail removal before symptoms begin to abate. Treatment typically lasts up to 48 weeks, and the infected nails may not be completely clear when treatment is finished.

How should you take this medication?

Before starting treatment, remove any loose nail material with clippers or a file. Brush Penlac evenly over the entire surface of all affected nails once daily, preferably at bedtime. Where possible, also apply the lacquer to the underside of the nail and the skin beneath. Allow the lacquer to dry for 30 seconds before putting on socks or stockings. Wait 8 hours before taking a bath or shower. Once a week, remove the lacquer with alcohol and trim away as much of the damaged nail as possible before applying a new coat. Do not apply Penlac near an open flame.

■ *If you miss a dose...*
Apply the forgotten dose as soon as you remember. However, if it is almost time for your next dose, skip the one you missed and return to your regular schedule.

■ *Storage instructions...*
Store at room temperature. After each use, close the bottle tightly and replace it in its carton to protect the medication from light.

What side effects may occur?

Side effects cannot be anticipated. Be sure to tell the doctor immediately if the area of application shows any signs of increased irritation, such as redness, itching, burning, blistering, swelling, or oozing. Only your doctor can determine if it is safe to continue using Penlac.

■ *Side effects may include:*
Rash or redness around the nail

Why should this drug not be prescribed?

If you find that you're allergic to Penlac, you won't be able to use it.

Special warnings about this medication

Keep Penlac away from the eyes and mucous membranes. Avoid contact with any skin outside the immediate area of the nail. For external use only.

If you have foot problems due to diabetes, trimming and removal of infected nails should be undertaken with caution.

Do not use nail polish or other cosmetic nail products on the treated nails.

Let the doctor know if your immune system has been weakened by HIV infection, transplant treatments, therapy with steroids, or any other cause, or if you take epilepsy medication. Penlac has not been tested in patients with these problems.

Possible food and drug interactions when using this medication

The manufacturer does not recommend use of Penlac in conjunction with oral antifungal medications such as griseofulvin (GrisPEG), terbinafine (Lamisil Tablets), and itraconazole (Sporanox).

Special information if you are pregnant or breastfeeding

The possibility of harm to a developing baby has not been entirely ruled out. If you are pregnant or planning to become pregnant, let the doctor know immediately.

It is not known whether Penlac appears in breast milk. Use it with caution when breastfeeding.

Recommended dosage

ADULTS

Apply once daily at bedtime to the entire surface of all infected nails.

Overdosage

There is no information on overdosage. If the lacquer is accidentally swallowed, seek medical attention immediately.

Pentasa *See Rowasa, page 1280.*

Pentoxifylline *See Trental, page 1475.*

PEPCID

Pronounced: PEP-sid
Generic name: Famotidine
Other brand name: Pepcid AC

Why is this drug prescribed?

Pepcid is prescribed for the short-term treatment of active duodenal ulcer (in the upper intestine) for 4 to 8 weeks and for active, benign gastric ulcer (in the stomach) for 6 to 8 weeks. It is prescribed for maintenance therapy, at reduced dosage, after a duodenal ulcer has healed. It is also used for short-term treatment of GERD, a condition in which the acid contents of the stomach flow back into the food canal (esophagus), and for resulting inflammation of the esophagus. And it is prescribed for certain diseases that cause the stomach to produce excessive quantities of acid, such as Zollinger-Ellison syndrome. Pepcid belongs to a class of drugs known as histamine H_2 blockers.

An over-the-counter formulation, Pepcid AC, is used to relieve and prevent heartburn, acid indigestion, and sour stomach.

Most important fact about this drug

To cure your ulcer, you need to take Pepcid for the full time of treatment your doctor prescribes. Keep taking the drug even if you begin to feel better.

How should you take this medication?

It may take several days for Pepcid to begin relieving stomach pain. You can use antacids for the pain at the same time you take Pepcid.

If you are taking Pepcid suspension, shake it vigorously for 5 to 10 seconds before use.

Take Pepcid AC with water. To prevent symptoms, take it 1 hour before a meal you expect will cause trouble.

■ *If you miss a dose...*
Take it as soon as you remember. If it is almost time for your next dose, skip the one you missed and go back to your regular schedule. Do not take 2 doses at once.

■ *Storage instructions...*
Store at room temperature in a dry place. Protect the suspension from freezing, and discard any unused portion after 30 days.

What side effects may occur?

Side effects cannot be anticipated. If any develop or change in intensity, inform your doctor as soon as possible. Only your doctor can determine if it is safe for you to continue taking Pepcid.

■ *Side effects may include:*
Headache

Why should this drug not be prescribed?

If you are sensitive to or have ever had an allergic reaction to Pepcid, or a comparable H₂ blocker such as Tagamet, Zantac, or Axid, you should not take this medication. Make sure your doctor is aware of any drug reactions you have experienced.

Special warnings about this medication

If you have stomach cancer, Pepcid may relieve the symptoms without curing the disease. Your doctor will be careful to rule out this possibility.

Use Pepcid with caution if you have severe kidney disease.

Although heartburn and acid indigestion are common, see your doctor if you have trouble swallowing or abdominal pain that does not let up.

Do not take 2 tablets of Pepcid AC a day continuously for more than 2 weeks unless your doctor tells you to.

You can help avoid heartburn and acid indigestion by:

Avoiding or limiting caffeine, chocolate, fatty foods, and alcohol
Keeping your weight down
Not eating just before bedtime
Not lying down soon after eating
Stopping smoking, or at least cutting down

Possible food and drug interactions when taking this medication

If Pepcid is taken with certain other drugs, the effects of either can be increased, decreased, or altered. It is especially important that you check with your doctor before combining Pepcid with the following:

Itraconazole (Sporanox)
Ketoconazole (Nizoral)

Special information if you are pregnant or breastfeeding
The effects of Pepcid during pregnancy have not been adequately studied. If you are pregnant or plan to become pregnant, inform your doctor immediately. Pepcid may appear in breast milk and could affect a nursing infant. If this medication is essential to your health, your doctor may advise you to discontinue breastfeeding until your treatment with this medication is finished.

Recommended dosage

ADULTS

Duodenal Ulcer
The usual starting dose is 40 milligrams or 5 milliliters (1 teaspoonful) once a day at bedtime. Results should be seen within 4 weeks, and this medication should not be used at full dosage longer than 6 to 8 weeks. Your doctor may have you take 20 milligrams or 2.5 milliliters (half a teaspoonful) twice a day. The normal maintenance dose after your ulcer has healed is 20 milligrams or 2.5 milliliters (½ teaspoonful) once a day at bedtime.

Benign Gastric Ulcer
The usual dose is 40 milligrams or 5 milliliters (1 teaspoonful) once a day at bedtime.

Gastroesophageal Reflux Disease (GERD)
The usual dose is 20 milligrams or 2.5 milliliters (½ teaspoonful) twice a day for up to 6 weeks. For inflammation of the esophagus due to GERD, the dose is 20 or 40 milligrams or 2.5 to 5 milliliters twice a day for up to 12 weeks.

Excess Acid Conditions (such as Zollinger-Ellison Syndrome)
The usual starting dose is 20 milligrams every 6 hours, although some people need a higher dose. Doses of up to 160 milligrams every 6 hours have been given in severe cases.

   If your kidneys are not functioning properly, your doctor will adjust the dosage.

CHILDREN 1 TO 16 YEARS OLD

Peptic Ulcer
The usual daily dose is 0.5 milligram per 2.2 pounds of body weight. The entire dose may be given at bedtime, or divided and given in 2 smaller doses. Do not give more than 40 milligrams per day.

   If your child's kidneys are not functioning properly, your doctor will adjust the dosage.

Gastroesophageal Reflux Disease (GERD)
The usual daily dose is 1 milligram per 2.2 pounds of body weight, divided and given in 2 smaller doses. Do not exceed 40 milligrams daily.

If your child's kidneys are not functioning properly, your doctor will adjust the dosage.

INFANTS UNDER 12 MONTHS OLD

Gastroesophageal Reflux Disease (GERD)
The usual starting dose of the oral suspension is 0.5 milligram per 2.2 pounds of body weight once a day for infants under 3 months and twice a day for infants 3 to 11 months. The dosage can be given for up to 8 weeks. Your doctor may also recommend additional measures to relieve the symptoms, such as thickening the child's food.

If your child's kidneys are not functioning properly, your doctor will adjust the dosage.

PEPCID AC

Do not give Pepcid AC to children under 12 years old unless your doctor approves. Swallow tablets or gelcaps with a glass of water. Chew the chewable tablets completely; do not swallow them whole. Do not take more than 2 pills a day or take them for longer than 2 weeks unless your doctor approves.

For Prevention
Take 1 tablet, gelcap, or chewable tablet 15 minutes or more before eating a meal that could cause heartburn.

For Relief
Take 1 tablet, gelcap, or chewable tablet.

Overdosage

Any medication taken in excess can have serious consequences. If you suspect an overdose, seek medical attention immediately.

PERCOCET

Pronounced: PERK-o-set
Generic ingredients: Acetaminophen, Oxycodone hydrochloride
Other brand names: Endocet, Roxicet, Tylox

Why is this drug prescribed?

Percocet, a narcotic analgesic, is used to treat moderate to moderately severe pain. It contains two drugs—acetaminophen and oxycodone. Acetaminophen is used to reduce both pain and fever. Oxycodone, a narcotic analgesic, is used for its calming effect and for pain.

Most important fact about this drug

Percocet contains a narcotic and, even if taken only in prescribed amounts, can cause physical and psychological dependence when taken for a long time.

How should you take this medication?

Percocet may be taken with meals or with milk.

■ *If you miss a dose...*
If you take Percocet on a regular schedule, take it as soon as you remember. If it is almost time for the next dose, skip the one you missed and go back to your regular schedule. Never take 2 doses at once.

■ *Storage instructions...*
Store at room temperature.

What side effects may occur?

Side effects cannot be anticipated. If any develop or change in intensity, inform your doctor as soon as possible. Only your doctor can determine if it is safe for you to continue taking Percocet.

■ *Side effects may include:*
Dizziness, light-headedness, nausea, sedation, vomiting

You may be able to alleviate some of these side effects by lying down.

Why should this drug not be prescribed?

You should not use Percocet if you are sensitive to either acetaminophen or oxycodone.

Special warnings about this medication

You should take Percocet cautiously and according to your doctor's instructions, as you would take any medication containing a narcotic. If you have ever had a problem with alcohol addiction, make sure your doctor is aware of it.

If you have experienced a head injury, consult your doctor before taking Percocet. The effects of Percocet may be stronger for people with head injuries, and using it may delay recovery.

If you have stomach problems, such as an ulcer, check with your doctor before taking Percocet. Percocet may hide the symptoms of stomach problems, making them difficult to diagnose and treat.

If you have ever had liver, kidney, thyroid gland, or Addison's disease (a disease of the adrenal glands), difficulty urinating, or an enlarged prostate, consult your doctor before taking Percocet.

Elderly people or those in a weakened condition should take Percocet cautiously.

This drug may impair your ability to drive a car or operate potentially dangerous machinery. Do not participate in any activities that require full alertness if you are unsure about the drug's effect on you.

Possible food and drug interactions when taking this medication

Alcohol may increase the sedative effects of Percocet. You should not take Percocet with alcohol.

If Percocet is taken with certain other drugs, the effects of either could be increased, decreased, or altered. It is especially important to check with your doctor before combining Percocet with the following:

Antispasmodic drugs such as Bentyl, Cogentin, and Donnatal
Major tranquilizers such as Mellaril and Thorazine
Other narcotic painkillers such as Darvon and Demerol
Sedatives such as phenobarbital and Seconal
Tranquilizers such as Valium and Xanax

Special information if you are pregnant or breastfeeding

It is not known whether Percocet can injure a developing baby or affect a woman's reproductive capacity. Using any medication that contains a narcotic during pregnancy may cause physical addiction for your newborn baby. If you are pregnant or plan to become pregnant, inform your doctor immediately. As with other narcotic painkillers, taking Percocet shortly before delivery (especially at higher dosages) may cause some degree of impaired breathing in the mother and newborn. It is not known whether Percocet appears in breast milk, possibly harming a nursing infant. If you are breastfeeding, use Percocet only under a doctor's directions.

Recommended dosage

ADULTS

The usual dose is 1 to 2 tablets of the lowest strength (2.5 milligrams oxycodone/325 milligrams acetaminophen) every 6 hours. Doctors sometimes prescribe a higher dose if necessary. The total daily dose of acetaminophen should not exceed 4 grams. The maximum daily dose recommended for each strength of Percocet (oxycodone/acetaminophen) is as follows:

2.5 milligrams/325 milligrams: 12 tablets
5 milligrams/325 milligrams: 12 tablets
7.5 milligrams/500 milligrams: 8 tablets
10 milligrams/650 milligrams: 6 tablets

CHILDREN

The safety and effectiveness of Percocet have not been established in children.

Overdosage

A severe overdose of Percocet can be fatal. If you suspect an overdose, seek medical help immediately.

■ *Symptoms of Percocet overdose may include:*
Bluish skin, eyes or skin with yellow tone, cold and clammy skin, decreased or irregular breathing (ceasing in severe overdose), extreme sleepiness progressing to stupor or coma, heart attack, low blood pressure, muscle weakness, nausea, slow heartbeat, sweating, vague bodily discomfort, vomiting

PERCODAN

Pronounced: PERK-o-dan
Generic ingredients: Oxycodone, Aspirin

Why is this drug prescribed?

Percodan combines two pain-killing drugs: the narcotic analgesic oxycodone, and the common pain reliever aspirin. It is prescribed for moderate to moderately severe pain.

Most important fact about this drug

The oxycodone in Percodan can cause physical and psychological dependence. Use this product with caution.

How should you take this medication?

Take no more of this drug than your doctor directs.

■ *If you miss a dose...*
Take it as soon as you remember. If it is almost time for your next dose, skip the one you missed and go back to your regular schedule. Never take 2 doses at the same time.
■ *Storage instructions...*
Store at room temperature. Protect from light.

What side effects may occur?

Side effects cannot be anticipated. If any develop or change in intensity, inform your doctor as soon as possible. Only your doctor can determine if it is safe for you to continue taking Percodan. Many of the side effects associated with Percodan go away if you lie down.

■ *Side effects may include:*
Constipation, dizziness, exaggerated feelings of well-being or sadness, itching, light-headedness, nausea, sedation, vomiting

Why should this drug not be prescribed?

If you are allergic to either aspirin or oxycodone, you will not be able to use this product.

Special warnings about this medication

Percodan can impair the skills needed to drive a car or operate machinery safely. Do not attempt to drive if you are not fully alert.

In children and teenagers who have a viral infection, the aspirin in Percodan can trigger a severe and even fatal disorder called Reye's syndrome. Do not give Percodan to any child with an illness such as flu or chickenpox.

Percodan's effects may be severely exaggerated in people who have suffered a head injury. The drug should also be used with caution if you have a history of peptic ulcer disease or a clotting disorder.

Make sure your doctor knows if you have any of the following medical conditions: abdominal disorders, a thyroid condition, Addison's disease, kidney problems, liver problems, an enlarged prostate, or difficulty urinating. Percodan should be used with extra caution under these circumstances.

Possible food and drug interactions when taking this medication

If Percodan is taken with certain other drugs, the effects of either could be increased, decreased, or altered. It is especially important to check with your doctor before combining Percodan with the following:

Alcohol
Antidepressants such as Elavil, Nardil, Pamelor, and Parnate
Blood-thinning drugs such as Coumadin
Gout medications such as probenecid
Major tranquilizers such as Compazine, Stelazine, and Thorazine
Other narcotic pain killers such as Demerol and OxyContin
Promethazine (Phenergan)
Sleep aids such as Halcion and Seconal
Tranquilizers such as Valium and Xanax

Special information if you are pregnant or breastfeeding

It is not known whether Percodan can harm a developing baby. The drug is not recommended for pregnant women under ordinary circumstances, and you should inform your doctor immediately if you become pregnant. Also consult your doctor before using this drug while breastfeeding.

Recommended dosage

ADULTS

The usual dose is one tablet every 6 hours as needed for pain. Your doctor may adjust the dosage according to the severity of pain and your response to the drug. The maximum dose is 12 tablets per day.

CHILDREN

A special formulation of Percodan called Percodan Demi is available for children. Do not give full-strength Percodan to a child.

Overdosage

An overdose of Percodan can be fatal. If you suspect an overdose, seek medical attention immediately.

■ *Warning signs of Percodan overdose may include:*
Bluish skin, cold and clammy skin, decreased breathing, limp muscles, sleepiness progressing to stupor or coma, slow heartbeat

Untreated, a severe overdose can shut down breathing and stop the heart.

PERIACTIN

Pronounced: pair-ee-AK-tin
Generic name: Cyproheptadine hydrochloride

Why is this drug prescribed?

Periactin is an antihistamine given to help relieve cold- and allergy-related symptoms such as hay fever, nasal inflammation, stuffy nose, red and inflamed eyes, hives, and swelling. Periactin may also be given after epinephrine to help treat anaphylaxis, a life-threatening allergic reaction.

Some doctors prescribe Periactin to treat cluster headache and to stimulate appetite in underweight people.

Most important fact about this drug

Like other antihistamines, Periactin may make you feel sleepy and sluggish. However, some people, particularly children, may have the opposite reaction and become excited.

How should you take this medication?

Take Periactin exactly as prescribed by your doctor.

■ *If you miss a dose...*
Take it as soon as you remember. If it is almost time for your next dose, skip the one you missed and go back to your regular schedule. Do not take 2 doses at once.
■ *Storage instructions...*
Store at room temperature in a tightly closed container.

What side effects may occur?

Side effects cannot be anticipated. If any develop or change in intensity, tell your doctor immediately. Only your doctor can determine whether it is safe for you to continue taking Periactin.

■ *Side effects may include:*
Anaphylaxis (life-threatening allergic reaction), anemia, appetite loss, chest congestion or tightness, chills, confusion, constipation, con-

vulsions, diarrhea, difficulty urinating, dizziness, dry mouth, nose, or throat, earlier-than-expected menstrual period, exaggerated feeling of well-being, excessive perspiration, excitement, faintness, fatigue, fluttery or throbbing heartbeat, frequent urination, hallucinations, headache, hives, hysteria, inability to urinate, increased appetite and weight gain, insomnia, irritability, lack of coordination, light sensitivity, liver problems, low blood pressure, nausea, nervousness, rapid heartbeat, rash and swelling, restlessness, ringing in the ears, sleepiness, stomach pain, stuffy nose, tingling or pins and needles, tremor, vertigo, vision problems (double vision, blurred vision), vomiting, weight gain, wheezing, yellow eyes and skin

Older people, in particular, are likely to become dizzy or drowsy, or develop low blood pressure in response to Periactin.

Why should this drug not be prescribed?
Do not take Periactin if you are sensitive to it, or have ever had an allergic reaction to it or to a similar antihistamine.

Do not take Periactin if you are taking an antidepressant drug known as an MAO inhibitor. Drugs in this category include Nardil and Parnate.

Do not take Periactin if you have the eye condition called angle-closure glaucoma, a peptic ulcer, an enlarged prostate, obstruction of the neck of the bladder, or obstruction of the outlet of the stomach.

Newborn or premature infants should not be given this drug, nor should it be used by women who are breastfeeding an infant.

The elderly and those in a weakened condition should not take this drug.

Special warnings about this medication
Like other antihistamines, Periactin may make you drowsy or impair your coordination. Be very careful about driving, climbing, or operating machinery, or doing hazardous tasks, until you know how you react to this medication.

Be cautious about taking Periactin if you have bronchial asthma, the eye condition called glaucoma, an overactive thyroid gland, high blood pressure, heart disease, or circulatory problems.

Possible food and drug interactions when taking this medication
Avoid alcoholic beverages while taking Periactin.

If Periactin is taken with certain other drugs, the effects of either could be increased, decreased, or altered. It is especially important to check with your doctor before combining Periactin with the following:

Antidepressant drugs classified as MAO inhibitors, including Nardil and Parnate
Sedatives such as Nembutal and Seconal
Tranquilizers such as Librium and Valium

Special information if you are pregnant or breastfeeding

Because of possible harm to the unborn baby, Periactin should not be used during pregnancy unless it is clearly needed. Periactin should not be taken by a woman who is breastfeeding. If you have just given birth, you will need to choose between breastfeeding and taking Periactin.

Recommended dosage

ADULTS

The usual initial dose is 4 milligrams (1 tablet) 3 times daily. Dosage may range from 4 to 20 milligrams a day, but most people will take between 12 and 16 milligrams. Some may need as much as 32 milligrams a day. If you are over 65, the doctor will probably keep the dosage relatively low.

CHILDREN

Ages 2 to 6 Years
The usual dose is 2 milligrams (one-half tablet) 2 or 3 times a day; your doctor may adjust the dose if necessary. A child this age should not take more than 12 milligrams a day.

Ages 7 to 14 Years
The usual dose is 4 milligrams (1 tablet) 2 or 3 times a day; your doctor may adjust the dose if needed. A child this age should not take more than 16 milligrams a day.

Overdosage

Any drug taken in excess may have serious consequences. An overdose of Periactin can be fatal. If you suspect an overdose, seek medical attention immediately.

■ *Symptoms of Periactin overdose may include:*
   Dilated pupils, dry mouth, extreme excitement and agitation, fever, flushing, stomach or bowel distress, stupor or coma

Overdosage in children may produce hallucinations and convulsions.

PERIDEX

Pronounced: PAIR-i-decks
Generic name: Chlorhexidine gluconate

Why is this drug prescribed?

Peridex is an oral rinse used to treat gingivitis, a condition in which the gums become red and swollen. Peridex is also used to control gum bleeding caused by gingivitis.

Most important fact about this drug
Peridex may stain front-tooth fillings, especially those with a rough surface. These stains have no adverse effect on the gums, and usually can be removed by a professional cleaning.

How should you take this medication?
You should get a thorough dental cleaning and examination before beginning treatment with Peridex.

After brushing, thoroughly rinsing, and flossing your teeth, rinse with Peridex by swishing one-half fluid ounce (marked in the cap) around in your mouth for 30 seconds, then spit it out. Do not dilute Peridex and do not rinse with water or mouthwash, eat, brush your teeth, or drink immediately after using this medication.

■ *If you miss a dose…*
Resume your regular schedule the next time you brush.
■ *Storage instructions…*
Protect from freezing.

What side effects may occur?
Side effects cannot be anticipated. If any develop or change in intensity, inform your doctor as soon as possible. Only your doctor can determine if it is safe for you to continue using Peridex.

■ *Side effects may include:*
Change in taste, increase in plaque, staining of teeth, mouth, tooth fillings, dentures, or other appliances in the mouth

Why should this drug not be prescribed?
Unless you are directed to do so by your doctor, do not use Peridex if you have shown a sensitivity to or are allergic to Peridex.

Special warnings about this medication
If you have both gingivitis and periodontitis (disease of the tissue that supports and attaches the teeth), remember that Peridex is used only for gingivitis. Periodontitis may require additional treatment by your doctor or dentist.

The use of Peridex may leave a bitter aftertaste. Rinsing your mouth with or drinking water after using Peridex may increase the bitterness.

In addition to staining, Peridex can also cause an excess of tartar build-up on your teeth. It is recommended that you have your teeth cleaned at least every 6 months.

Foods may taste different to you for several hours after rinsing with Peridex. In most cases, this effect becomes less noticeable after continued use. Taste should return to normal when treatment with Peridex is finished.

Possible food and drug interactions when taking this medication
No interactions with other drugs have been reported.

Special information if you are pregnant or breastfeeding
The effects of Peridex during pregnancy have not been adequately studied. If you are pregnant or plan to become pregnant, inform your doctor immediately. It is not known whether this medication appears in breast milk. If it is essential for you to use Peridex, your doctor may advise you to stop breastfeeding until your treatment is finished.

Recommended dosage

ADULTS

The usual dose of undiluted Peridex is one-half fluid ounce. Rinse for 30 seconds twice a day, morning and evening, after brushing. Peridex should be spit out after rinsing and never swallowed.

CHILDREN

The effectiveness and safety of Peridex have not been established in children under 18 years of age.

Overdosage
If you suspect that a child of 22 pounds or less has swallowed 4 or more ounces of Peridex, seek medical attention immediately.

Also seek immediate medical attention if any child shows signs of alcohol intoxication such as slurred speech, staggering, or sleepiness, and you suspect he or she has swallowed Peridex.

If a small child swallows 1 or 2 ounces of Peridex, he or she may have an upset stomach and nausea.

Perindopril See Aceon, page 16.

Perphenazine See Trilafon, page 1493.

PERSANTINE
Pronounced: per-SAN-teen
Generic name: Dipyridamole

Why is this drug prescribed?
Persantine helps reduce the formation of blood clots in people who have had heart valve surgery. It is used in combination with blood thinners such as Coumadin.

Some doctors also prescribe Persantine in combination with other drugs, such as aspirin, to reduce the damage from a heart attack and prevent a recurrence, to treat angina, and to prevent complications during heart bypass surgery.

Most important fact about this drug

Persantine is sometimes used with aspirin to provide better protection against the formation of blood clots. However, the risk of bleeding may also be increased. To reduce this risk, take *only* the amount of aspirin prescribed by the *same* doctor who directed you to take Persantine. If you need a medication for pain or a fever, do not take extra aspirin without first consulting your doctor.

How should you take this medication?

Persantine must be taken exactly as your doctor prescribes, at regularly scheduled times.

It is best to take Persantine on an empty stomach, with a full glass of water. However, if this upsets your stomach, you can take the drug with food or milk.

Do not change from one brand of dipyridamole to another without consulting your doctor or pharmacist. Products manufactured by different companies may not be equally effective.

■ *If you miss a dose...*
Take it as soon as you remember. If it is within 4 hours of your next scheduled dose, skip the dose you missed and go back to your regular schedule. Never take 2 doses at the same time.

■ *Storage instructions...*
Store at room temperature. Protect from excessive heat.

What side effects may occur?

Side effects cannot be anticipated. If any develop or change in intensity, inform your doctor as soon as possible. Only your doctor can determine if it is safe for you to continue taking Persantine.

■ *Side effects may include:*
Abdominal distress, dizziness

Why should this drug not be prescribed?

If you are sensitive to or have ever had an allergic reaction to Persantine or any of its ingredients, you should not use this medication. Make sure your doctor is aware of any drug reactions you have experienced.

Special warnings about this medication

Use this medication carefully if you have low blood pressure.

Persantine has been known to cause liver problems, including liver failure. Contact your doctor immediately if you notice any of the following signs of liver trouble: nausea, fatigue, drowsiness, itching, yellowish skin, flu-like symptoms, and pain in the upper right abdomen.

Persantine should be used with caution if you have any heart problems, including angina or recent heart attack. Notify your doctor immediately if you experience any unusual chest pain.

Tell the doctor that you are taking Persantine if you have a medical emergency, and before you have surgery or dental treatment.

Possible food and drug interactions when taking this medication

If Persantine is taken with certain other drugs, the effects of either could be increased, decreased, or altered. It is especially important to check with your doctor before combining Persantine with the following:

Alzheimer's drugs such as Aricept, Cognex, and Exelon
Aspirin
Blood thinners such as Coumadin
Heart medications such as adenosine
Indomethacin (Indocin)
Ticlopidine (Ticlid)
Valproic acid (Depakene)

Special information if you are pregnant or breastfeeding

The effects of Persantine during pregnancy have not been adequately studied. If you are pregnant or plan to become pregnant, inform your doctor immediately. This drug appears in breast milk and may affect a nursing infant. If this medication is essential to your health, your doctor may advise you to discontinue breastfeeding until your treatment with this medication is finished.

Recommended dosage

ADULTS

The usual recommended dose is 75 to 100 milligrams 4 times a day.

CHILDREN

The safety and effectiveness of this medication have not been established in children under 12 years of age.

Overdosage

Any medication taken in excess can have serious consequences. If you suspect an overdose of Persantine, seek medical attention immediately.

■ *Symptoms of Persantine overdose may include:*
Dizziness, feeling of warmth, flushing, low blood pressure, rapid heartbeat, restlessness, sweating, weakness

Phenaphen with Codeine *See Tylenol with Codeine, page 1516.*

Phenazopyridine *See Pyridium, page 1210.*

Phenelzine *See Nardil, page 917.*

PHENERGAN

Pronounced: FEN-er-gan
Generic name: Promethazine hydrochloride

Why is this drug prescribed?

Phenergan is an antihistamine that relieves nasal stuffiness and inflammation and red, inflamed eyes caused by hay fever and other allergies. It is also used to treat itching, swelling, and redness from hives and other rashes; allergic reactions to blood transfusions; and, with other medications, anaphylactic shock (severe allergic reaction).

Phenergan is also used as a sedative and sleep aid for both children and adults, and is prescribed to prevent and control nausea and vomiting before and after surgery and to prevent and treat motion sickness. It is also used, with other medications, for pain after surgery.

Antihistamines work by decreasing the effects of histamine, a chemical the body releases in response to certain irritants. Histamine narrows air passages in the lungs and contributes to inflammation. Antihistamines reduce itching and swelling and dry up secretions from the nose, eyes, and throat.

Most important fact about this drug

Phenergan may cause considerable drowsiness. You should not drive or operate dangerous machinery or participate in any hazardous activity that requires full mental alertness until you know how you react to Phenergan. Children should be carefully supervised while they are bike riding, roller-skating, or playing until the drug's effect on them is established.

How should you take this medication?

Take Phenergan exactly as prescribed.

- *If you miss a dose...*
  If you are taking Phenergan on a regular schedule, take the forgotten dose as soon as you remember. If it is almost time for your next dose, skip the one you missed and go back to your regular schedule. Never take 2 doses at once.
- *Storage instructions...*
  Tablets should be stored at room temperature, away from light. Suppositories should be stored in the refrigerator, in a tightly closed container.

What side effects may occur?

Side effects cannot be anticipated. If any develop or change in intensity, inform your doctor as soon as possible. Only your doctor can determine if it is safe for you to continue taking Phenergan.

■ *Side effects may include:*
Blurred vision, dizziness, drowsiness, dry mouth, increased or decreased blood pressure, nausea, rash, sedation, vomiting

Why should this drug not be prescribed?

Do not take Phenergan if you have ever had an allergic reaction to it or to related medications, such as Thorazine, Mellaril, Stelazine, or Prolixin. Phenergan is not for use in comatose patients, and should not be used to treat asthma or other breathing problems.

Special warnings about this medication

If you are taking other medications that cause sedation, your doctor may reduce the dosage of these medications or eliminate them while you are using Phenergan.

If you have a seizure disorder, Phenergan may cause your seizures to occur more often.

Phenergan can cause a serious—even fatal—decline in the breathing function. Avoid this medication if you have chronic breathing problems such as emphysema, or if you suffer from sleep apnea (periods during sleep when breathing stops).

Phenergan can also cause a potentially fatal condition called Neuroleptic Malignant Syndrome. Symptoms include high fever, rigid muscles, sweating, and a rapid or irregular heartbeat. If you develop these symptoms, stop taking Phenergan and see your doctor immediately.

Use Phenergan cautiously if you have heart disease, high blood pressure or circulatory problems, liver problems, the eye condition called narrow-angle glaucoma, peptic ulcer or other abdominal obstructions, or urinary bladder obstruction due to an enlarged prostate.

Phenergan may affect the results of pregnancy tests and can raise your blood sugar.

Some people have developed jaundice (yellow eyes and skin) while on this medication.

Tell your doctor if you have any uncontrolled movements or seem to be unusually sensitive to sunlight.

Remember that Phenergan can cause drowsiness.

Phenergan should not be given to children under 2 years of age, and should be used with caution in older children, due to the danger of impaired breathing. Large doses have been known to cause hallucinations, seizures, and sudden death, especially in children who are dehydrated. Drugs such as Phenergan are not recommended for the treatment of vomiting in children unless the problem is severe. Phenergan should also be avoided if the child has the serious neurological disease known as Reye's syndrome or any disease of the liver.

Possible food and drug interactions when taking this medication
Phenergan may increase the effects of alcohol. Do not drink alcohol, or at least substantially reduce the amount you drink, while taking this medication.

If Phenergan is taken with certain other drugs, the effects of either could be increased, decreased, or altered. It is especially important to check with your doctor before combining Phenergan with the following:

Certain antidepressant drugs, including Elavil and Tofranil
Drugs that control spasms, such as Cogentin
Drugs that reduce bone marrow function (certain cancer drugs)
MAO inhibitors such as the antidepressants Nardil and Parnate
Narcotic pain relievers such as Demerol and Dilaudid
Sedatives such as Dalmane, Halcion, and Seconal
Tranquilizers such as Valium and Xanax

Special information if you are pregnant or breastfeeding
The effects of Phenergan during pregnancy have not been adequately studied. If you are pregnant or plan to become pregnant, inform your doctor immediately. Although it is not known whether Phenergan appears in breast milk, there is a chance that it could cause a nursing infant serious harm. The use of Phenergan is not recommended during breastfeeding.

Recommended dosage
Phenergan is available in tablet, syrup, and suppository form. The suppositories are for rectal use only. Phenergan tablets and suppositories are not recommended for children under 2 years of age.

ALLERGY

Adults
The average oral dose is 25 milligrams taken before bed; however, your doctor may have you take 12.5 milligrams before meals and before bed.

Children
The usual dose is a single 25-milligram dose at bedtime, or 6.25 to 12.5 milligrams 3 times daily.

MOTION SICKNESS

Adults
The average adult dose is 25 milligrams taken twice daily. The first dose should be taken one-half to 1 hour before you plan to travel, and the second dose 8 to 12 hours later, if necessary. On travel days after that, the

recommended dose is 25 milligrams when you get up and again before the evening meal.

Children
The usual dose of Phenergan tablets, syrup, or rectal suppositories is 12.5 to 25 milligrams taken twice a day.

NAUSEA AND VOMITING

The average dose of Phenergan for nausea and vomiting in children or adults is 25 milligrams. When oral medication cannot be tolerated, use the rectal suppository. Your doctor may have you take 12.5 to 25 milligrams every 4 to 6 hours, if necessary.

For nausea and vomiting in children, the dose is usually calculated at 0.5 milligram per pound of body weight and will also be based on the age of the child and the severity of the condition being treated. Phenergan and other antivomiting drugs should not be given to children if the cause of the problem is unknown.

INSOMNIA

Adults
The usual dose is 25 to 50 milligrams for nighttime sedation.

Children
The usual dose is 12.5 to 25 milligrams by tablets or rectal suppository at bedtime.

Older Adults
The dosage is usually reduced for people over 60.

Overdosage
Any medication taken in excess can have serious consequences. An overdose of Phenergan can be fatal. If you suspect an overdose, seek medical treatment immediately.

■ *Symptoms of Phenergan overdose may include:*
Difficulty breathing, dry mouth, fixed and dilated pupils, flushing, heightened reflexes, loss of consciousness, muscle tension, poor coordination, seizures, slowdown in brain activity, slowed heartbeat, stomach and intestinal problems, very low blood pressure, writhing movements

Children may become overstimulated and have nightmares. Older adults may also become overstimulated.

PHENERGAN WITH CODEINE

Pronounced: FEN-er-gan
Generic ingredients: Promethazine hydrochloride,
  Codeine phosphate

Why is this drug prescribed?

Phenergan with Codeine is used to relieve coughs and other symptoms of allergies and the common cold. Promethazine, an antihistamine, helps reduce itching and swelling and dries up secretions from the nose, eyes, and throat. It also has sedative effects and helps control nausea and vomiting. Codeine, a narcotic analgesic, helps relieve pain and stops coughing.

Most important fact about this drug

Phenergan with Codeine may cause considerable drowsiness. You should not drive or operate dangerous machinery or participate in any hazardous activity that requires full mental alertness until you know how you react to this medication. Children should be carefully supervised while they are bike riding, roller-skating, or playing until the drug's effect on them is established.

How should you take this medication?

Take this medication exactly as prescribed.

■ *If you miss a dose...*
If you take Phenergan with Codeine on a regular schedule, take the forgotten dose as soon as you remember. If it is almost time for your next dose, skip the one you missed and go back to your regular schedule. Never take 2 doses at once.

■ *Storage instructions...*
Store at room temperature, away from light.

What side effects may occur?

Side effects cannot be anticipated. If any develop or change in intensity, inform your doctor as soon as possible. Only your doctor can determine if it is safe for you to continue taking Phenergan with Codeine.

■ *Side effects may include:*
Anxiety, blurred vision, constipation, convulsions, decreased amount of urine, depressed feeling, difficulty breathing, disorientation, dizziness, dizziness on standing, dry mouth, exaggerated sense of well-being, fainting, faintness, fast, fluttery heartbeat, flushing, headache, hives, inability to urinate, increased/decreased blood pressure, itching, light-headedness, nausea, passing hallucinations, rapid heartbeat, rash, restlessness, sedation (extreme calm), sleepiness, slow heart-

beat, sweating, swelling due to fluid retention (including the throat), vision changes, vomiting, weakness, yellowed skin or whites of eyes

Why should this drug not be prescribed?

Phenergan with Codeine should not be used if you have asthma or other breathing difficulties or if you are sensitive to or have ever had an allergic reaction to codeine, promethazine, or related medications, such as Thorazine, Mellaril, Stelazine, or Prolixin.

Special warnings about this medication

It is possible to develop psychological and physical dependence on codeine. Although the likelihood of this is quite low with oral codeine, be cautious if you have a history of drug abuse or dependence.

Never take more cough syrup than has been prescribed. If your cough does not seem better within 5 days, check back with your doctor.

Codeine can cause or worsen constipation.

Phenergan with Codeine should be used with extreme caution in young children.

Use this medication very carefully if you have a head injury, the eye condition called narrow-angle glaucoma, peptic ulcer or other abdominal obstruction, urinary bladder obstruction due to an enlarged prostate, heart disease, high blood pressure or circulatory problems, liver or kidney disease, fever, seizures, an underactive thyroid gland, intestinal inflammation, or Addison's disease (a disorder of the adrenal glands). Be cautious, too, if you have had recent stomach/intestinal or urinary tract surgery. The very young, the elderly, and people in a weakened condition may have problems taking Phenergan with Codeine.

This medication may make you dizzy when you first stand up. Getting up slowly can help prevent this problem.

If you are taking other medications with sedative effects, your doctor may reduce their dosage or eliminate them altogether while you are using Phenergan with Codeine.

If you have a seizure disorder, this medication may cause your seizures to occur more often.

Avoid using Phenergan with Codeine if you have sleep apnea (periods during sleep when breathing stops).

Phenergan with Codeine may affect the results of pregnancy tests; and it can raise your blood sugar.

Tell your doctor if you have any involuntary muscle movements or seem to be unusually sensitive to sunlight.

Possible food and drug interactions when taking this medication

Phenergan with Codeine may increase the effects of alcohol. Do not drink alcohol, or at least substantially reduce the amount you drink, while taking this medication.

If Phenergan with Codeine is taken with certain other drugs, the effects of either could be increased, decreased, or altered. It is especially important to check with your doctor before combining Phenergan with Codeine with the following:

All antidepressant drugs, including Elavil, Marplan, Nardil, and Prozac
Narcotic pain relievers such as Demerol and Dilaudid
Sedatives such as Dalmane, Halcion, and Seconal
Tranquilizers such as Valium and Xanax

Special information if you are pregnant or breastfeeding

The effects of Phenergan with Codeine during pregnancy have not been adequately studied. If you are pregnant or plan to become pregnant, inform your doctor immediately. Phenergan with Codeine may appear in breast milk and may affect a nursing infant. If this medication is essential to your health, your doctor may advise you to discontinue breastfeeding until your treatment is finished.

Recommended dosage

ADULTS

The usual dosage is 1 teaspoon (5 milliliters) every 4 to 6 hours, not to exceed 6 teaspoons, or 30 milliliters, in 24 hours.

CHILDREN 6 YEARS TO UNDER 12 YEARS

The usual dose is one-half to 1 teaspoon (2.5 to 5 milliliters) every 4 to 6 hours, not to exceed 6 teaspoons, or 30 milliliters, in 24 hours.

CHILDREN UNDER 6 YEARS

The usual dose is one-quarter to one-half teaspoon (1.25 to 2.5 milliliters) every 4 to 6 hours. The total daily dose should not exceed 9 milliliters for children weighing 40 pounds, 8 milliliters for 35 pounds, 7 milliliters for 30 pounds, and 6 milliliters for 25 pounds.

Phenergan with Codeine is not recommended for children under 2 years of age.

Overdosage

Any medication taken in excess can have serious consequences. An overdose of codeine can be fatal. If you suspect an overdose, seek medical treatment immediately.

■ *Symptoms of an overdose of Phenergan with Codeine may include:*
Bluish skin, cold, clammy skin, coma, convulsions, difficulty breathing, dilated pupils, dry mouth, extreme sleepiness, flushing, low blood pressure, muscle softness, nightmares, overexcitability, slow heartbeat, small pupils, stomach and intestinal problems, stupor, unconsciousness

PHENOBARBITAL

Pronounced: fee-noe-BAR-bi-tal

Why is this drug prescribed?

Phenobarbital, a barbiturate, is used as a sleep aid and in the treatment of certain types of epilepsy, including generalized or grand mal seizures and partial seizures.

Most important fact about this drug

Phenobarbital can be habit-forming. You may become tolerant (needing more and more of the drug to achieve the same effect) and physically and psychologically dependent with continued use. Never increase the amount of phenobarbital you take without checking with your doctor.

How should you take this medication?

Take this medication exactly as prescribed.

If you are taking phenobarbital for seizures, do not discontinue it abruptly.

- *If you miss a dose...*
  Take it as soon as you remember. If it is almost time for your next dose, skip the one you missed and go back to your regular schedule. Never take 2 doses at once.
- *Storage instructions...*
  Store at room temperature in a tightly closed container.

What side effects may occur?

Side effects cannot be anticipated. If any develop or change in intensity, notify your doctor as soon as possible. Only your doctor can determine whether it is safe for you to continue taking phenobarbital.

- *Side effects may include:*
  Allergic reaction, drowsiness, headache, lethargy, nausea, oversedation, sleepiness, slowed or delayed breathing, vertigo, vomiting

Why should this drug not be prescribed?

Phenobarbital should not be used if you suffer from porphyria (an inherited metabolic disorder), liver disease, or a lung disease that causes blockages or breathing difficulties, or if you have ever had an allergic reaction to or are sensitive to phenobarbital or other barbiturates.

Special warnings about this medication

Remember that phenobarbital may be habit-forming. Make sure you take the medication exactly as prescribed.

Phenobarbital should be used with extreme caution, or not at all, by people who are depressed or have a history of drug abuse.

Be sure to tell your doctor if you are in pain, or if you have constant pain, before you take phenobarbital.

Phenobarbital may cause excitement, depression, or confusion in elderly or weakened individuals, and excitement in children.

If you have been diagnosed with liver disease or your adrenal glands are not functioning properly, make sure the doctor knows about it. Phenobarbital should be prescribed with caution.

Barbiturates such as phenobarbital may cause you to become tired or less alert. Be careful driving, operating machinery, or doing any activity that requires full mental alertness until you know how you react to this medication.

Possible food and drug interactions when taking this medication

Phenobarbital may increase the effects of alcohol. Avoid alcoholic beverages while taking phenobarbital.

If phenobarbital is taken with certain other drugs, the effects of either could be increased, decreased, or altered. It is especially important to check with your doctor before combining phenobarbital with the following:

Antidepressant drugs known as MAO inhibitors, including Nardil and
    Parnate
Antihistamines such as Benadryl
Blood-thinning medications such as Coumadin
Doxycycline (Doryx, Vibramycin)
Griseofulvin (Fulvicin-P/G, Grifulvin V)
Narcotic pain relievers such as Percocet
Oral contraceptives
Other epilepsy drugs such as Depakene, Depakote, and Dilantin
Other sedatives such as Nembutal and Seconal
Steroids such as Deltasone and Medrol
Tranquilizers such as Valium and Xanax

Special information if you are pregnant or breastfeeding

Barbiturates such as phenobarbital may cause damage to the developing baby during pregnancy. Withdrawal symptoms may occur in an infant whose mother took barbiturates during the last 3 months of pregnancy. If you are pregnant or plan to become pregnant, inform your doctor immediately.

Phenobarbital appears in breast milk and could affect a nursing infant. If phenobarbital is essential to your health, your doctor may advise you to stop breastfeeding until your treatment is finished.

Recommended dosage

ADULTS

Sedation
The usual initial dose of phenobarbital is a single dose of 30 to 120 milligrams. Your doctor may repeat this dose at intervals, depending on how you respond to this medication.

You should not take more than 400 milligrams during a 24-hour period.

Daytime Sedation
The usual dose is 30 to 120 milligrams a day, divided into 2 to 3 doses.

To Induce Sleep
The usual dose is 100 to 200 milligrams.

Anticonvulsant Use
Phenobarbital dosage must be individualized on the basis of specific laboratory tests. Your doctor will determine the exact dose best for you. The usual dose is 60 to 200 milligrams daily.

CHILDREN

Anticonvulsant Use
The phenobarbital dosage must be individualized on the basis of specific laboratory tests. Your doctor will determine the exact dose best for your child.

The usual dose is 3 to 6 milligrams per 2.2 pounds of body weight per day.

DOSAGE ADJUSTMENT

People who are elderly or weak may be prescribed a lower dose. People who have liver or kidney disease may also require a lower dose of phenobarbital.

Overdosage

Barbiturate overdose can be fatal. If you suspect an overdose, seek medical treatment immediately.

■ *Symptoms of phenobarbital overdose may include:*
Congestive heart failure, diminished breathing, extremely low body temperature, fluid in lungs, involuntary eyeball movements, irregular heartbeat, kidney failure, lack of muscle coordination, low blood pressure, poor reflexes, skin reddening or bloody blisters, slowdown of the central nervous system

Phenobarbital, Hyoscyamine, Atropine, and Scopolamine
See Donnatal, page 469.

Phentermine *See Adipex-P, page 40.*

Phenytoin *See Dilantin, page 443.*

Phillips' Liqui-Gels *See Colace, page 317.*

PHOSPHOLINE IODIDE
Pronounced: FOS-foh-lin I-o-dide
Generic name: Echothiophate iodide

Why is this drug prescribed?
Phospholine Iodide is used to treat chronic open-angle glaucoma, a partial loss of vision or blindness resulting from a gradual increase in pressure of fluid in the eye. Because the vision loss occurs slowly, people often do not experience any symptoms and do not realize that their vision has declined. By the time the loss is noticed, it may be irreversible. Phospholine Iodide helps by reducing fluid pressure in the eye.

Phospholine Iodide is also used to treat secondary glaucoma (such as glaucoma following surgery to remove cataracts), for subacute or chronic angle-closure glaucoma after iridectomy (surgical removal of a portion of the iris) or when someone cannot have surgery or refuses it. The drug is also prescribed for children with accommodative esotropia (cross-eye).

Most important fact about this drug
Avoid exposure to certain pesticides or insecticides such as Sevin and Trolene. They can boost the side effects of Phospholine Iodide. If you work with these chemicals, wear a mask over your nose and mouth, wash and change your clothing frequently, and wash your hands often.

How should you use this medication?

To use Phospholine Iodide:
1. To minimize drainage of Phospholine Iodide into your nose, your doctor may instruct you to apply pressure with the middle finger to the inside corner of the eye for 1 to 2 minutes after placing the drops in your eyes.
2. Wipe off any excess Phospholine Iodide around the eye with a tissue.
3. Wash off any Phospholine Iodide that may get onto your hands.

■ *If you miss a dose…*
If you use 1 dose every other day: Apply the dose you missed as soon as you remember, if it is still the scheduled day. If you do not remember until the next day, apply it as soon as you remember, then skip a day and start your schedule again.

If you use 1 dose a day: Apply the dose you missed as soon as you remember. If you do not remember until the next day, skip the dose you missed and go back to your regular schedule.

If you use 2 doses a day: Apply the dose you missed as soon as you remember. If it is almost time for your next dose, skip the one you missed and go back to your regular schedule.

Never apply 2 doses at once.

■ *Storage instructions...*
You may keep the eyedrops at room temperature for up to 4 weeks.

What side effects may occur?

Side effects cannot be anticipated. If any develop or change in intensity, tell your doctor immediately. Only your doctor can determine whether it is safe to continue taking Phospholine Iodide.

■ *Side effects may include:*
Ache above the eyes, blurred vision, burning, clouded eye lens, cyst formation, decreased pupil size, decreased visual sharpness, excess tears, eye pain, heart irregularities, increased eye pressure, inflamed iris, lid muscle twitching, nearsightedness, red eyes, stinging

Why should this drug not be prescribed?

You should not use Phospholine Iodide if you have an inflammation in the eye.

Most people with angle-closure glaucoma (a condition in which there is a sudden increase in pressure of fluid in the eye) should not use Phospholine Iodide.

If you have ever had an allergic reaction to or are sensitive to Phospholine Iodide or any of its ingredients, you should not use this medication.

Special warnings about this medication

Drugs such as Phospholine Iodide should be used cautiously (if at all) if you have or have ever had:

Bronchial asthma
Detached retina
Epilepsy
Extremely low blood pressure
Parkinson's disease
Peptic ulcer
Recent heart attack
Slow heartbeat
Stomach or intestinal problems

If you notice any problems with your heart, notify your doctor immediately.

Stop taking the drug and notify your doctor immediately if you experience any of the following: breathing difficulties, diarrhea, inability to hold urine, muscle weakness, profuse sweating, or salivation.

If you will be using Phospholine Iodide for a long time, your doctor should schedule regular examinations to make sure that it is not causing unwanted effects.

Phospholine Iodide may cause vision problems. Be careful when driving at night or performing tasks in dim or poor light.

Possible food and drug interactions when taking this medication

If Phospholine Iodide is taken with certain other drugs, the effects of either could be increased, decreased, or altered. It is especially important to check with your doctor before combining Phospholine Iodide with drugs such as Enlon, Mestinon, or Tensilon, used to treat myasthenia gravis, a condition of muscle weakness that usually affects muscles in the eyes, face, limbs, and throat.

Special information if you are pregnant or breastfeeding

If you are pregnant or plan to become pregnant, inform your doctor immediately. No information is available about the safety of Phospholine Iodide during pregnancy.

Phospholine Iodide should not be used by women who are breastfeeding.

Recommended dosage

ADULTS

Glaucoma
A dose of 0.03 percent should be used 2 times a day, in the morning and at bedtime. Your doctor may increase the dose if necessary. Your doctor may have you take 1 dose a day or 1 dose every other day, instead.

CHILDREN

Accommodative Esotropia
Place 1 drop of 0.125 percent solution in both eyes at bedtime for 2 or 3 weeks to diagnose the condition.

Your doctor may then change the schedule to 0.125 percent every other day or reduce the dose to 0.06 percent every day.

The maximum dose usually recommended is 0.125 percent solution once daily.

If the eye drops are slowly withdrawn after a year or two of treatment, and the eye problem returns, your doctor may want you to consider surgery.

Overdosage

Any medication used in excess can have serious consequences. If you suspect an overdose of Phospholine Iodide, seek medical help immediately.

PILOCAR

Pronounced: PYE-low-car
Generic name: Pilocarpine hydrochloride
Other brand names: Isopto Carpine, Pilopine HS Gel

Why is this drug prescribed?

Pilocar causes constriction of the pupils (miosis) and reduces pressure within the eye. It is used to treat the increased pressure of open-angle glaucoma and to lower eye pressure before surgery for acute angle-closure glaucoma. It can be used alone or in combination with other medications. Glaucoma, one of the leading causes of blindness in the United States, is characterized by increased pressure in the eye that can damage the optic nerve and cause loss of vision.

Most important fact about this drug

There is no cure for glaucoma. Pilocar and similar drugs can keep ocular pressure under control, but only as long as you take them. You will probably need to continue treatment for life; and you must be sure to take the medication regularly.

How should you use this medication?

Follow these steps to administer Pilocar:
1. Wash your hands thoroughly.
2. Gently pull your lower eyelid down to form a pocket next to your eye.
3. Brace the eyedrop bottle on the bridge of your nose or your forehead.
4. Tilt your head back and squeeze the medication into your eye.
5. Close your eyes gently. Keep them closed for 1 to 2 minutes.
6. Do not rinse the dropper.
7. Wait for 5 to 10 minutes before using a second eye medication.

To avoid contaminating the dropper and solution, do not touch the eyelids or surrounding areas with the tip of the dropper.
  Do not use if the solution is discolored.

■ *If you miss a dose...*
  Apply it as soon as you remember. If it is almost time for your next dose, skip the one you missed and go back to your regular schedule. Do not take 2 doses at once.
■ *Storage instructions...*
  Store away from heat and light. Do not freeze.
  Keep the bottle tightly closed when it is not being used.

What side effects may occur?

Side effects cannot be anticipated. If any develop or change in intensity, inform your doctor as soon as possible. Only your doctor can determine if it is safe for you to continue using Pilocar.

■ *Side effects may include:*
Cloudy vision, detached retina, headache over your eye, nearsightedness, reduced vision in poor light, spasms of the eyelids, tearing eyes

Why should this drug not be prescribed?
Pilocar should not be used if you are sensitive to or have ever had an allergic reaction to any of the components of this solution. Your doctor will not prescribe it for you if you have an eye condition in which your pupils should not be constricted.

Special warnings about this medication
Pilocar may make it difficult for you to see in the dark. Be careful driving at night, or doing any hazardous activity in dim light.

Possible food and drug interactions when using this medication
No interactions have been reported.

Special information if you are pregnant or breastfeeding
The effects of Pilocar during pregnancy have not been adequately studied. If you are pregnant or plan to become pregnant, inform your doctor immediately. Pilocar may appear in breast milk and could affect a nursing infant. If this medication is essential to your health, your doctor may advise you to stop breastfeeding until your treatment with Pilocar is finished.

Recommended dosage

ADULTS

The usual starting dose is 1 or 2 drops up to 6 times a day, depending on the severity of the glaucoma and your response. During a severe attack, your doctor will tell you to put drops into the unaffected eye as well.

Overdosage
Any medication taken in excess can have serious consequences. If you suspect an overdose, seek medical attention immediately.

Pilocarpine See Pilocar, page 1098.

Pilopine HS Gel See Pilocar, page 1098.

Pimecrolimus See Elidel, page 507.

PINDOLOL

Pronounced: PIN-doh-loll

Why is this drug prescribed?

Pindolol, a type of medication known as a beta-blocker, is used in the treatment of high blood pressure. It is effective alone or combined with other high blood pressure medications, particularly with a thiazide-type diuretic. Beta-blockers decrease the force and rate of heart contractions.

Most important fact about this drug

You must take pindolol regularly for it to be effective. Since blood pressure declines gradually, it may be several weeks before you get the full benefit of pindolol; and you must continue taking it even if you are feeling well. Pindolol does not cure high blood pressure; it merely keeps it under control.

How should you take this medication?

Pindolol can be taken with or without food.

Take this medication exactly as prescribed, even if your symptoms have disappeared. Try not to miss any doses. If this medication is not taken regularly, your condition may worsen.

■ *If you miss a dose...*
Take it as soon as you remember. If it's within 4 hours of your next scheduled dose, skip the one you missed and go back to your regular schedule. Never take 2 doses at the same time.

■ *Storage instructions...*
Store at room temperature in a tightly closed, light-resistant container.

What side effects may occur?

Side effects cannot be anticipated. If any develop or change in intensity, inform your doctor as soon as possible. Only your doctor can determine if it is safe for you to continue taking pindolol.

■ *Side effects may include:*
Abdominal discomfort, chest pain, difficult or labored breathing, dizziness, fatigue, joint pain, muscle pain or cramps, nausea, nervousness, strange dreams, swelling due to fluid retention, tingling or pins and needles, trouble sleeping, weakness

Why should this drug not be prescribed?

If you have bronchial asthma, severe congestive heart failure, inadequate blood supply to the circulatory system (cardiogenic shock), heart block (a heart irregularity), or a severely slow heartbeat, you should not take this medication.

Special warnings about this medication

If you have had severe congestive heart failure in the past, pindolol should be used with caution.

Pindolol should not be stopped suddenly. It can cause increased chest pain and heart attack. Dosage should be gradually reduced.

If you suffer from asthma, chronic bronchitis, emphysema, seasonal allergies or other bronchial conditions, coronary artery disease, or kidney or liver disease, this medication should be used with caution.

Ask your doctor if you should check your pulse while taking pindolol. This medication can cause your heartbeat to become too slow.

This medication may mask the symptoms of low blood sugar in diabetics or alter blood sugar levels. If you are diabetic, discuss this with your doctor.

Pindolol may cause you to become disoriented. If it has this effect on you, driving or operating dangerous machinery or participating in any hazardous activity that requires full mental alertness is not recommended.

If you have a history of severe allergic reactions, inform your doctor before taking pindolol.

Notify your doctor or dentist that you are taking pindolol if you have a medical emergency and before you have surgery or dental treatment.

Possible food and drug interactions when taking this medication

If pindolol is taken with certain other drugs, the effects of either could be increased, decreased, or altered. It is especially important to check with your doctor before combining pindolol with the following:

Airway-opening drugs such as Proventil and Ventolin
Blood pressure drugs such as reserpine
Digoxin (Lanoxin)
Epinephrine (EpiPen)
Hydrochlorothiazide (HydroDIURIL)
Insulin or oral antidiabetic agents such as Micronase
Nonsteroidal anti-inflammatory drugs such as Motrin
Ritodrine (Yutopar)
Theophylline (Theo-Dur, others)
Thioridazine (Mellaril)
Verapamil (Calan, Verelan)

Special information if you are pregnant or breastfeeding

The effects of pindolol during pregnancy have not been adequately studied. If you are pregnant or plan to become pregnant, inform your doctor immediately. Pindolol appears in breast milk and could affect a nursing infant. If this medication is essential to your health, your doctor may advise you to discontinue breastfeeding until your treatment with this medication is finished.

Recommended dosage

ADULTS

Your doctor will determine the dosage according to your specific needs.

The usual starting dose is 5 milligrams 2 times per day, alone or with other high blood pressure medication. Your blood pressure should be lower in 1 to 2 weeks. If blood pressure is not reduced sufficiently within 3 to 4 weeks, your doctor may increase your total daily dosage by 10 milligrams at a time, at 3- to 4-week intervals, up to a maximum of 60 milligrams a day.

CHILDREN

The safety and effectiveness of pindolol have not been established in children.

OLDER ADULTS

The doctor will determine dosage for an elderly individual based on his or her particular needs.

Overdosage

Any medication taken in excess can have serious consequences. If you suspect an overdose, seek medical attention immediately.

■ *Symptoms of pindolol overdose may include:*
Bronchospasm (spasm of the air passages), excessively slow heartbeat, heart failure, low blood pressure

Pioglitazone *See Actos, page 32.*

Piroxicam *See Feldene, page 558.*

PLAN B
Generic name: Levonorgestrel

Why is this drug prescribed?

Plan B is intended as "morning after" birth control to prevent pregnancy after known or suspected contraceptive failure (for instance, a broken condom) or unprotected sex. Plan B treatment must begin within 72 hours after having sex.

Plan B contains only one hormone, a progestin. It may prevent a pregnancy but will not end one that has already begun. It is believed to work mainly by inhibiting ovulation (release of an egg) and fertilization. It may block implantation of the egg in the lining of the uterus. It is not effective once the process of implantation has begun.

Most important fact about this drug

Plan B is meant for emergency use only and not as a regular method of birth control. It is not as reliable as regular birth control. Using Plan B correctly after a single act of unprotected sex reduces the average chance of pregnancy to about 1 percent.

How should you take this medication?

Plan B comes in a package with two tablets. Take the first tablet as soon as possible after having sex, within 72 hours at the latest. Take the second tablet 12 hours after the first one. You can take Plan B at any time during your menstrual cycle.

- *If you miss a dose…*
  Call your doctor immediately. Your chances of pregnancy increase when you do not take the pills as prescribed.
- *Storage instructions…*
  Store at room temperature.

What side effects may occur?

Side effects cannot be anticipated. If any develop or change in intensity, tell your doctor as soon as possible. Only your doctor can determine if it is safe to continue using Plan B.

- *Side effects may include:*
  Abdominal pain, breast tenderness, diarrhea, dizziness, fatigue, headache, menstrual changes, nausea, vomiting

Why should this drug not be prescribed?

Do not take Plan B if you have had an allergic reaction to progestin, the type of hormone found in the drug. You should also avoid this medication if you have any unexplained vaginal bleeding.

Special warnings about this medication

Remember that Plan B should not be used as a regular form of birth control, and it will not work if you are already pregnant.

Plan B may affect your next menstrual cycle by delaying it or making it much heavier or lighter than normal. It could also cause spotting between cycles. If your next period is delayed by more than a week, you should consider the possibility that you may be pregnant.

Let your doctor know right away if you become pregnant or develop abdominal pain after taking Plan B. There is a slight chance that progestin, the hormone in Plan B, could cause an ectopic pregnancy, which occurs when a fertilized egg becomes implanted outside the uterus, usually in the fallopian tube.

Plan B could slightly raise blood sugar levels. If you have diabetes, your doctor may want to monitor you during treatment.

Emergency contraceptive pills, like other oral contraceptives, do not protect against infection with HIV (the virus that causes AIDS) and other sexually transmitted diseases.

Possible food and drug interactions when taking this medication
When Plan B is taken together with other medications, the effectiveness of Plan B may be altered or reduced. Notify your doctor if you are taking the following:

Barbiturates such as Amytal and Nembutal, among others
Carbamazepine (Tegretol)
Phenytoin (Dilantin)
Rifampin (Rifadin, Rimactane)

Special information if you are pregnant or breastfeeding
Contraceptives like Plan B that contain the hormone progestin do not appear to harm a developing baby. However, if you're pregnant or suspect that you're pregnant, you should not take Plan B, since it's not effective after pregnancy has begun.

Although small amounts of progestin can pass into breast milk, no side effects have been identified. Still, it's always best to check with your doctor before breastfeeding during treatment with any medication.

Recommended dosage

ADULTS AND ADOLESCENTS

Plan B comes in a package with two tablets. Take the first pill as soon as possible after unprotected sex, within 72 hours at the latest. Take the second pill 12 hours after the first one.

If you vomit within 1 hour after taking either pill, contact your doctor right away to see if you should take another dose.

Overdosage
If you suspect an overdose, seek medical attention immediately.

■ *Symptoms of overdose may include:*
Nausea, vomiting

PLAQUENIL
Pronounced: PLAK-en-ill
Generic name: Hydroxychloroquine sulfate

Why is this drug prescribed?
Plaquenil is prescribed for the prevention and treatment of certain forms of malaria.

Plaquenil is also used to treat the symptoms of rheumatoid arthritis such as swelling, inflammation, stiffness, and joint pain. It is also prescribed for lupus erythematosus, a chronic inflammation of the connective tissue.

Most important fact about this drug

Children are especially sensitive to Plaquenil. Relatively small doses of this medication have caused fatalities. Keep this drug in a childproof container and out of the reach of children.

How should you take this medication?

Take Plaquenil exactly as prescribed for the full course of therapy.

If you have been prescribed Plaquenil for rheumatoid arthritis, it will take several weeks for beneficial effects to appear. Take each dose with a meal or a glass of milk.

■ *If you miss a dose...*
And you take 1 dose every 7 days, take it as soon as you remember, then go back to your regular schedule.

If you take 1 dose a day and you miss your dose, take it as soon as you remember. If you do not remember until the next day, skip the one you missed and go back to your regular schedule.

If you take more than 1 dose a day, take it as soon as you remember if it is within an hour or so of the missed time. If you do not remember until later on, skip the missed dose and go back to your regular schedule. Do not take 2 doses at once.

■ *Storage information...*
Store at room temperature, away from heat, light, and moisture.

What side effects may occur?

Side effects cannot be anticipated. If any develop or change in intensity, inform your doctor as soon as possible. Only your doctor can determine if it is safe for you to continue taking Plaquenil.

■ *Side effects of treatment for an acute malarial attack may include:*
Abdominal cramps, diarrhea, dizziness, heart problems, lack or loss of appetite, mild headache, nausea, vomiting

■ *Side effects of treatment for lupus erythematosus and rheumatoid arthritis may include:*
Abdominal cramps, abnormal eye pigmentation, acne, anemia, bleaching of hair, blind spots, blisters in mouth and eyes, blood disorders, blurred vision, convulsions, decreased vision, diarrhea, difficulty focusing the eyes, diminished reflexes, dizziness, emotional changes, excessive coloring of the skin, eye muscle paralysis, foggy vision, halos around lights, headache, hearing loss, heart problems, hives, involuntary eyeball movement, irritability, itching, light flashes and streaks, light intolerance, liver problems or failure, loss of hair, loss or

lack of appetite, muscle paralysis, muscle weakness and wasting, nausea, nervousness, nightmares, psoriasis (dry, scaly, red skin patches), reading difficulties, ringing in the ears, skin eruptions, skin inflammation and scaling, skin rash, vertigo, vomiting, weariness, weight loss

Why should this drug not be prescribed?

If you are sensitive to or have ever had an allergic reaction to Plaquenil or similar drugs such as Aralen and Chloroquine, you should not take this medication. Make sure your doctor is aware of any drug reactions you have experienced.

Plaquenil should not be prescribed if you have suffered partial or complete loss of vision in small areas while taking this medication or similar drugs. Notify your doctor of any past or present visual changes you have experienced.

This drug should not be used for long-term therapy in children.

Special warnings about this medication

Unless you are directed to do so by your doctor, do not take this medication if you have psoriasis (a recurrent skin disorder characterized by patches of red, dry, scaly skin) or porphyria (an inherited metabolic disorder affecting the liver or bone marrow). The use of Plaquenil may cause a severe attack of psoriasis and may increase the severity of porphyria.

Disorders of the retina causing impairment or loss of vision may be related to the length of time and the dose of Plaquenil given for lupus and rheumatoid arthritis. Problems have occurred several months to several years after beginning daily therapy. When you are on prolonged therapy, your doctor will perform eye examinations at the beginning of treatment and every 3 months after that. Visual disturbances may progress, even after you have stopped taking this drug. If you have any problem with your vision or your eyes, notify your doctor immediately.

All people on long-term therapy with this drug should have a physical examination periodically, including testing of knee and ankle reflexes, to detect any evidence of muscular weakness.

Consult your doctor if you experience ringing in the ears, or other hearing problems.

If you are being treated for rheumatoid arthritis and have shown no improvement (such as reduced joint swelling or increased mobility) within 6 months, your doctor may decide to discontinue this drug.

Plaquenil should be used with caution by alcoholics and those who have liver disease or kidney problems.

Your doctor should conduct periodic blood cell counts if you are on prolonged therapy with this medication. If any severe blood disorder develops that is not attributed to the disease you are being treated for, your doctor may discontinue use of this drug.

Consult your doctor if you are taking a drug that has a tendency to produce dermatitis (inflammation of the skin), because you may have some skin reactions while taking Plaquenil.

Possible food and drug interactions when taking this medication

If Plaquenil is taken with certain other drugs, the effects of either could be increased, decreased, or altered. It is especially important to check with your doctor before combining Plaquenil with the following:

Any medication that may cause liver damage
Aurothioglucose (Solganal)
Cimetidine (Tagamet)
Digoxin (Lanoxin)

Special information if you are pregnant or breastfeeding

Use of this drug during pregnancy should be avoided except in the suppression or treatment of malaria when, in the judgment of your doctor, the benefit outweighs the possible hazard. This drug may appear in breast milk and could affect a nursing infant. If this medication is essential to your health, your doctor may advise you to discontinue breastfeeding until your treatment is finished.

Recommended dosage

ADULTS

Restraint or Prevention of Malaria

The usual dose is 400 milligrams taken once every 7 days on exactly the same day of each week. If circumstances permit, preventive therapy should begin 2 weeks prior to exposure. If this is not possible, your doctor will have you take a starting dose of 800 milligrams, which may be divided into 2 doses taken 6 hours apart. You should continue this suppressive therapy for 8 weeks after leaving the area where malaria occurs.

Acute Attack of Malaria

The usual starting dose is 800 milligrams, to be followed by 400 milligrams in 6 to 8 hours and 400 milligrams on each of 2 consecutive days.

Alternatively, your doctor may prescribe a single dose of 800 milligrams.

Lupus Erythematosus

The usual starting dose for adults is 400 milligrams once or twice daily. You will continue to take this dose for several weeks or months, depending on your response. For longer-term maintenance therapy, your doctor may reduce the dose to 200 to 400 milligrams per day.

Rheumatoid Arthritis

The usual starting dose for adults is 400 to 600 milligrams a day taken with a meal or a glass of milk. If your condition improves, usually within

4 to 12 weeks, your doctor will reduce the dose to a maintenance level of 200 to 400 milligrams daily.

CHILDREN

For the treatment of malaria, your doctor will calculate the dosage on the basis of your child's weight.

This drug has not been proved safe for treatment of juvenile arthritis.

Overdosage

Any medication taken in excess can have serious consequences. If you suspect an overdose, seek emergency medical treatment immediately.

■ *Symptoms of an overdose of Plaquenil may occur within 30 minutes. They include:*
Convulsions, drowsiness, headache, heart problems and failure, inability to breathe, visual problems

PLAVIX

Pronounced: PLA-vicks
Generic name: Clopidogrel bisulfate

Why is this drug prescribed?

Plavix keeps blood platelets slippery and discourages formation of clots, thereby improving blood flow to your heart, brain, and body. The drug is prescribed to reduce the risk of heart attack, stroke, and serious circulation problems in people with hardening of the arteries or unstable angina (dangerous chest pain), and in people who've already suffered a heart attack or stroke.

Most important fact about this drug

Because Plavix slows clotting, it will take longer than usual to stop bleeding. Be sure to report any unusual bleeding to your doctor immediately, and tell any doctor or dentist planning a procedure that you have been taking Plavix. You should discontinue the drug 5 days before any kind of surgery.

How should you take this medication?

Plavix can be taken with or without food.

■ *If you miss a dose...*
Take it as soon as you remember. If it is almost time for your next dose, skip the one you missed and go back to your regular schedule. Do not take 2 doses at the same time.
■ *Storage instructions...*
Store at room temperature.

What side effects may occur?

Side effects cannot be anticipated. If any develop or change in intensity, inform your doctor as soon as possible. Only your doctor can determine if it is safe for you to continue using Plavix.

■ *Side effects may include:*

Abdominal pain, back pain, bronchitis, bruising and bleeding under the skin, chest pain, coughing, depression, diarrhea, difficulty breathing, dizziness, fatigue, fluid retention and swelling, flu symptoms, headache, high blood pressure, high cholesterol, indigestion, inflammation of the nasal passages, itching, joint pain, nausea, pain, purple discoloration of the skin, rash, upper respiratory tract infection, urinary tract infection

Why should this drug not be prescribed?

Do not take Plavix if you have a bleeding stomach ulcer or bleeding in the area around the brain. Also avoid this medication if it gives you an allergic reaction.

Special warnings about this medication

If you've ever had a stomach ulcer or bleeding in the digestive tract, make sure the doctor is aware of it; Plavix should be used with caution. The drug should also be used carefully if you suffer from problems inside the eyes, have bleeding problems due to severe liver disease, or expect to be at risk of bleeding from any other cause.

In extremely rare cases (about 4 in a million), a dangerous bleeding problem called thrombotic thrombocytopenic purpura has been known to develop in patients taking Plavix. Signs include fever and bleeding under the skin. Call your doctor immediately if you develop these symptoms.

Possible food and drug interactions when taking this medication

Plavix increases the clot-fighting effect of aspirin. The two drugs are often taken together, and combined treatment has lasted for up to one year.

If Plavix is taken with certain other drugs, the effects of either could be increased, decreased, or altered. Ask your doctor before starting any new drug; and be doubly careful before combining Plavix with the following:

Aspirin
Fluvastatin (Lescol)
Nonsteroidal anti-inflammatory drugs such as Advil, Aleve, Motrin, and Naprosyn
Phenytoin (Dilantin)
Tamoxifen (Nolvadex)
Tolbutamide (Orinase)
Torsemide (Demadex)
Warfarin (Coumadin)

Special Information if you are pregnant or breastfeeding

The effects of Plavix during pregnancy have not been adequately studied. If you are pregnant or plan to become pregnant, inform your doctor immediately. Use Plavix during pregnancy only if absolutely necessary. Do not breastfeed while taking Plavix, since the drug may appear in breast milk.

Recommended dosage

ADULTS

The usual dose is 75 milligrams once a day. To give people with unstable angina an extra boost, their first dose is usually increased to 300 milligrams.

CHILDREN

The safety and effectiveness of Plavix have not been established in children.

Overdosage

Any medication taken in excess can have serious consequences. If you suspect an overdose of Plavix, seek medical attention immediately.

■ *Potential symptoms of Plavix overdose may include:*
   Difficulty breathing, exhaustion, stomach or intestinal bleeding, vomiting

PLENDIL

Pronounced: PLEN-dill
Generic name: Felodipine

Why is this drug prescribed?

Plendil is prescribed for the treatment of high blood pressure. It is effective alone or in combination with other high blood pressure medications. A type of medication called a calcium channel blocker, Plendil eases the workload of the heart by slowing down its muscle contractions and the passage of nerve impulses through it. This improves blood flow through the heart and throughout the body, reduces blood pressure, and helps prevent angina pain (chest pain, often accompanied by a feeling of choking, usually caused by lack of oxygen in the heart due to clogged arteries).

Most important fact about this drug

If you have high blood pressure, you must take Plendil regularly for it to be effective. Since blood pressure declines gradually, it may be several weeks before you get the full benefit of Plendil; you must continue taking it even if you are feeling well. Plendil does not cure high blood pressure; it merely keeps it under control.

How should you take this medication?

Plendil can be taken with a light meal or without food. The tablets should be swallowed whole, not crushed or chewed.

Try not to miss any doses. If Plendil is not taken regularly, your blood pressure may increase.

■ *If you miss a dose...*
   Take the forgotten dose as soon as you remember. If it is almost time for the next dose, skip the one you missed and go back to your regular schedule. Never try to catch up by doubling the dose.

■ *Storage instructions...*
   Store at room temperature. Protect from light.

What side effects may occur?

Side effects cannot be anticipated. If any develop or change in intensity, inform your doctor as soon as possible. Only your doctor can determine if it is safe for you to continue taking Plendil.

■ *Side effects may include:*
   Flushing, headache, swelling of the legs and feet

Why should this drug not be prescribed?

If you are sensitive to or have ever had an allergic reaction to Plendil or other calcium channel blockers, such as Calan and Procardia, you should not take this medication. Make sure your doctor is aware of any drug reactions you have experienced.

Special warnings about this medication

Plendil can cause your blood pressure to become too low. If you feel light-headed or faint, or if you feel your heart racing or you experience chest pain, contact your doctor immediately.

If you have congestive heart failure, Plendil should be used with caution, especially if you are also taking one of the beta-blocker family of drugs, such as Inderal or Tenormin.

Your legs and feet may swell when you start taking Plendil, usually within the first 2 to 3 weeks of treatment.

If you have liver disease or are over age 65, your doctor should monitor your blood pressure carefully while adjusting your dosage of Plendil.

Your gums may become swollen and sore while you are taking Plendil. Good dental hygiene will help control this problem.

Possible food and drug interactions when taking this medication

If Plendil is taken with certain other drugs, the effects of either could be increased, decreased, or altered. It is especially important to check with your doctor before combining Plendil with the following:

Beta-blocking blood pressure medicines such as Inderal, Lopressor, and Tenormin

Cimetidine (Tagamet)
Digoxin (Lanoxin)
Epilepsy medications such as Tegretol and Dilantin
Erythromycin (PCE, ERYC, others)
Itraconazole (Sporanox)
Ketoconazole (Nizoral)
Phenobarbital
Theophylline (Theo-Dur)

Taking Plendil with grapefruit juice can more than double the blood level of the drug.

Special information if you are pregnant or breastfeeding

Although the effects of Plendil during pregnancy have not been adequately studied in humans, birth defects have occurred in animal studies. If you are pregnant or plan to become pregnant, inform your doctor immediately. Plendil may appear in breast milk and may affect a nursing infant. If this medication is essential to your health, your doctor may advise you to discontinue breastfeeding until your treatment is finished.

Recommended dosage

ADULTS

Your doctor will adjust the dosage according to your response to the drug.

The usual starting dose is 5 milligrams once a day; your doctor will adjust the dose at intervals of not less than 2 weeks.

The usual dosage range is 2.5 to 10 milligrams once daily.

CHILDREN

The safety and effectiveness of Plendil in children have not been established.

OLDER ADULTS

If you are over 65 years of age, your doctor will start treatment with a dosage of 2.5 milligrams once a day and will monitor your blood pressure closely during dosage adjustment.

People with liver problems usually require lower doses of Plendil and are carefully monitored while the dose is adjusted.

Overdosage

Any medication taken in excess can have serious consequences. If you suspect an overdose, seek medical treatment immediately.

■ *Symptoms of Plendil overdose may include:*
Severely low blood pressure, slow heartbeat

Polyethylene glycol See MiraLax, page 873.

Polymyxin B, Neomycin, and Hydrocortisone
See Cortisporin Ophthalmic Suspension, page 341.

POLY-VI-FLOR
Pronounced: pol-ee-VIE-floor
Generic ingredients: Vitamins, Fluoride

Why is this drug prescribed?
Poly-Vi-Flor is a multivitamin and fluoride supplement. The drops have 9 essential vitamins; the chewable tablets have 10. Poly-Vi-Flor is prescribed for children aged 2 and older to provide fluoride where the drinking water contains less than the amount recommended by the American Dental Association to build strong teeth and prevent cavities. Poly-Vi-Flor also supplies significant amounts of vitamins to help prevent deficiencies. The American Academy of Pediatrics recommends that children up to age 16 take a fluoride supplement if they live in areas where the drinking water contains less than the recommended amount of fluoride.

Most important fact about this drug
Do not give your child more than the recommended dose. Too much fluoride can cause discoloration and pitting of teeth.

How should you take this medication?
Do not give your child more than your doctor prescribes.

Poly-Vi-Flor chewable tablets should be chewed or crushed before swallowing. You can put Poly-Vi-Flor drops directly into a child's mouth with the dropper provided or mix them into cereal, juice, or other food.

■ *If you miss a dose…*
Give it as soon as you remember. If it is almost time for the next dose, skip the one you missed and go back to your regular schedule. Do not give 2 doses at once.

■ *Storage instructions…*
Store away from heat, light, and moisture.

What side effects may occur?
Rarely, an allergic rash has occurred.

Why should this drug not be prescribed?
Children should not take Poly-Vi-Flor if they are getting significant amounts of fluoride from other medications or sources.

Special warnings about this medication
Do not give your child more than the recommended dosage. Your child's teeth should be checked periodically for discoloration or pitting. Notify your doctor if white, brown, or black spots appear on your child's teeth.

The fluoride level of your drinking water should be determined before Poly-Vi-Flor is prescribed.

Let your doctor know if you change drinking water or filtering systems.

Fluoride does not replace proper dental habits, such as brushing, flossing, and having dental checkups.

Recommended dosage

The usual dose is 1 tablet or 1 milliliter every day as prescribed by the doctor; your doctor will choose the strength according to your child's age and the amount of fluoride in the drinking water.

Overdosage

Although overdose is unlikely, any medication taken in excess can have serious consequences. If you suspect an overdose, seek medical treatment immediately.

PONSTEL

Pronounced: PON-stel
Generic name: Mefenamic acid

Why is this drug prescribed?

Ponstel, a nonsteroidal anti-inflammatory drug, is used for the relief of moderate pain (when treatment will not last for more than 7 days) and for the treatment of menstrual pain.

Most important fact about this drug

You should have frequent checkups by your doctor if you take Ponstel regularly. Ulcers or internal bleeding can occur without warning.

How should you take this medication?

Take Ponstel with food if possible. If it upsets your stomach, be sure to take it with food or an antacid or with a full glass of milk.

Take Ponstel exactly as prescribed by your doctor.

■ *If you miss a dose...*
If you take Ponstel on a regular schedule, take the forgotten dose as soon as you remember. If it is almost time for your next dose, skip the one you missed and go back to your regular schedule. Do not take 2 doses at once.

■ *Storage instructions...*
Store away from heat, light, and moisture.

What side effects may occur?

Side effects cannot be anticipated. If any develop or change in intensity, inform your doctor as soon as possible. Only your doctor can determine if it is safe for you to continue taking Ponstel.

■ *Side effects may include:*
Abdominal pain, diarrhea, nausea, stomach and intestinal upset, vomiting

Why should this drug not be prescribed?

Do not take Ponstel if you are sensitive to or have ever had an allergic reaction to it. You should not take it, either, if you have had asthma attacks, hay fever, or hives caused by aspirin or other nonsteroidal anti-inflammatory drugs, such as Motrin and Nuprin. Make sure your doctor is aware of any drug reactions you have experienced.

Do not take Ponstel if you have ulcerations or frequently recurring inflammation of your stomach or intestines.

Avoid this drug if you have serious kidney disease.

Special warnings about this medication

Use Ponstel with extreme caution if you've suffered from stomach ulcers or bleeding in the past. If you develop a rash, diarrhea, or other stomach problems, contact your doctor.

If you are an older adult; have kidney problems, liver disease, or heart failure; take drugs such as diuretics or ACE inhibitors; or suffer from dehydration, Ponstel could damage your kidneys and should be used with caution.

Ponstel occasionally causes liver damage. If you develop warning signs such as nausea, fatigue, yellowing of the skin and eyes, itching, flu-like symptoms, and upper abdominal pain, stop taking Ponstel and seek medical attention immediately.

Ponstel can also aggravate high blood pressure, asthma, and heart failure. Use it with caution if you have any of these conditions. Use it cautiously, too, if you smoke or are in poor health.

Possible food and drug interactions when taking this medication

If Ponstel is taken with certain other drugs, the effects of either can be increased, decreased, or altered. It is especially important to check with your doctor before combining Ponstel with the following:

ACE inhibitors (drugs for high blood pressure) such as Capoten and Vasotec
Alcohol
Aspirin
Blood-thinning medications such as Coumadin
Diuretics such as Lasix and HydroDIURIL
Fluconazole (DiFlucan)
Lithium (Lithonate)
Lovastatin (Mevacor)
Methotrexate (Rheumatrex)
Steroids such as prednisone and hydrocortisone
Trimethoprim (Proloprim, Bactrim, Septra)

Special information if you are pregnant or breastfeeding

The effects of Ponstel during pregnancy have not been adequately studied. If you are pregnant or plan to become pregnant, inform your doctor immediately. You should not use Ponstel in late pregnancy because nonsteroidal anti-inflammatory drugs affect the heart and blood vessels of the developing baby. Ponstel may appear in breast milk and could affect a nursing infant. If this medication is essential to your health, your doctor may advise you to discontinue breastfeeding until your treatment is finished.

Recommended dosage

ADULTS AND CHILDREN OVER 14

Moderate Pain

The usual starting dose is 500 milligrams, followed by 250 milligrams every 6 hours, if needed, for 1 week.

Menstrual Pain

The usual starting dose, once symptoms appear, is 500 milligrams, followed by 250 milligrams every 6 hours for 2 to 3 days.

CHILDREN

The safety and effectiveness of Ponstel have not been established in children under 14.

Overdosage

If you suspect an overdose of Ponstel, seek medical attention immediately.

■ *Symptoms of Ponstel overdose may include:*
Drowsiness, lack of energy, nausea, stomach or abdominal pain, vomiting

In severe cases, breathing problems and coma can develop.

Potassium chloride *See Micro-K, page 851.*

Pramipexole *See Mirapex, page 875.*

PRANDIN

Pronounced: PRAN-din
Generic name: Repaglinide

Why is this drug prescribed?

Prandin is used to reduce blood sugar levels in people with type 2 diabetes (the kind that does not require insulin shots). It's prescribed when diet and exercise alone fail to correct the problem. A combination of Prandin and a second diabetes drug called Glucophage can be prescribed if either drug alone proves insufficient.

Most important fact about this drug

Chronically high glucose levels have been implicated in the kidney failure, blindness, and loss of sensation that plague many people with long-standing diabetes. A low-calorie diet, weight loss, and exercise are your first line of defense against these problems. Medications such as Prandin are prescribed only as a backup when these other measures still leave sugar too high. If diet, exercise, and a combination of Prandin and Glucophage all fail to do the job, your doctor may have to start you on insulin.

How should you take this medication?

Prandin should be taken shortly before each meal. You can take it 30 minutes ahead of time or wait until just before starting; a 15-minute period is typical. You can take Prandin 2, 3, or 4 times a day, depending on the number of meals you have. If you skip a meal (or add an extra meal), skip (or add) a dose accordingly.

■ *If you miss a dose...*
Wait until your next meal, then take your regular dose. Do not take 2 doses at once.
■ *Storage instructions...*
Store at room temperature away from moisture in a tightly closed container.

What side effects may occur?

Side effects cannot be anticipated. If any develop or change in intensity, inform your doctor as soon as possible. Only your doctor can determine if it is safe for you to continue taking Prandin.

■ *More common side effects may include:*
Back pain, bronchitis, chest pain, constipation, diarrhea, headache, indigestion, joint pain, low blood sugar, nasal inflammation, nausea, sinus inflammation, skin tingling, upper respiratory tract infection, urinary tract infection, vomiting

Why should this drug not be prescribed?

If you have type 1 (insulin-dependent) diabetes, you cannot use Prandin. The drug also cannot be used for diabetic ketoacidosis (a life-threatening emergency first signaled by excessive thirst, nausea, fatigue, and fruity-smelling breath). This condition must be treated with insulin.

If you find that Prandin gives you an allergic reaction, you'll be unable to continue using it.

Special warnings about this medication

While taking Prandin, you should check your blood sugar regularly. Your doctor will also watch it; and to measure long-term glucose control, he will probably give you a glycosylated hemoglobin (HbA1C) test as well.

Too much Prandin can cause low blood sugar (hypoglycemia), marked by shaking, sweating, and cold, clammy skin. If you develop these symptoms, drink some orange juice or suck on a hard candy. The problem is more likely to surface if you are elderly, debilitated, or malnourished, have liver problems, or suffer from poor adrenal or pituitary function.

Possible food and drug interactions when taking this medication

If Prandin is taken with certain other drugs, the effects of either could be increased, decreased, or altered. It is especially important to check with your doctor before combining Prandin with the following:

Airway-opening medications such as Alupent, Proventil, and Ventolin
Alcohol (excessive amounts can cause low blood sugar)
Aspirin
Barbiturates such as the sedatives Seconal and Nembutal
Beta-blockers such as the blood pressure medications Inderal and
    Tenormin
Blood thinners such as Dicumarol and Miradon
Calcium channel blockers such as the blood pressure medications
    Cardizem and Procardia
Carbamazepine (Tegretol)
Chloramphenicol (Chloromycetin)
Clarithromycin (Biaxin)
Erythromycin (Eryc, Ery-Tab, PCE)
Estrogens such as Premarin
Furosemide (Lasix)
Glucose-lowering agents such as Glucotrol and Micronase
Isoniazid
Ketoconazole (Nizoral)
Major tranquilizers such as Mellaril and Stelazine
MAO inhibitors such as the antidepressants Marplan, Nardil, and
    Parnate
Niacin (Nicobid)
Nonsteroidal anti-inflammatory drugs such as Advil, Motrin,
    Naprosyn, and Voltaren
Oral contraceptives
Phenytoin (Dilantin)
Probenecid (Benemid, ColBENEMID)
Rifampin (Rifadin, Rimactane)
Steroids such as prednisone
Sulfa drugs such as Gantanol

Thyroid medications such as Synthroid
Water pills such as the thiazide diuretics Dyazide and HydroDIURIL

Additionally, you should not start taking Prandin if you are already taking the triglyceride-lowering medication Lopid. Conversely, you should not start taking Lopid if you are already using Prandin. Combining the two drugs could lead to a dangerous drop in blood sugar. However, if you're already taking both drugs, the doctor will monitor your blood sugar levels closely and adjust the dosages as needed.

Special information if you are pregnant or breastfeeding

Because abnormal blood sugar during pregnancy can cause fetal defects, your doctor will probably prescribe insulin injections until the baby is born. The effects of Prandin during pregnancy have not been adequately studied.

It is not known whether Prandin appears in breast milk. Discuss with your doctor whether to discontinue breastfeeding or give up Prandin. If the medication is discontinued, and diet alone does not control your blood sugar levels, your doctor may recommend insulin injections.

Recommended dosage

ADULTS

Take Prandin before each meal. The recommended dose ranges from 0.5 milligram to 4 milligrams. If you have never taken a glucose-lowering medication before, you should start with the 0.5-milligram dose. If you have taken these drugs in the past, the starting dose is 1 or 2 milligrams. Take no more than 16 milligrams a day.

Dose Adjustment

Your dose of Prandin will be adjusted according to your fasting blood sugar levels. If your pre-meal glucose level appears normal and you are still experiencing glucose control problems, your doctor may test your glucose level after you have eaten a meal. Your doctor will wait at least a week after each change in dose to check your response.

Switching to Prandin

When Prandin replaces another oral glucose-lowering medicine, you should start taking it the day after your final dose of the previous drug. Be alert for signs of low blood sugar; effects of the drugs may overlap.

Combination Therapy:

If Prandin is being added to Glucophage therapy, you should begin with a 0.5-milligram dose. Dosage will then be adjusted according to your blood glucose levels.

Overdosage

An overdose of Prandin taken without food can cause low blood sugar (hypoglycemia).

- *Symptoms of mild hypoglycemia may include:*
  Cold sweat, confusion, depression, dizziness, drowsiness, fatigue, headache, hunger, nausea, nervousness, rapid heartbeat, shaking
- *Symptoms of severe hypoglycemia may include:*
  Coma, pale skin, seizure, shallow breathing

Consuming some sugar will usually correct the problem. If symptoms persist or worsen, contact your doctor.

PRAVACHOL
Pronounced: PRAV-a-coll
Generic name: Pravastatin sodium

Why is this drug prescribed?
Pravachol is a cholesterol-lowering drug. Your doctor may prescribe it along with a cholesterol-lowering diet if your blood cholesterol level is dangerously high and you have not been able to lower it by diet alone.

High cholesterol can lead to heart problems. By lowering your cholesterol, Pravachol improves your chances of avoiding a heart attack, heart surgery, and death from heart disease. In people who already have hardening of the arteries, it slows progression of the disease and cuts the risk of acute attacks.

The drug works by helping to clear harmful low-density lipoprotein (LDL) cholesterol out of the blood and by limiting the body's ability to form new LDL cholesterol. For people at high risk of heart disease, current guidelines call for considering drug therapy when LDL levels reach 130. For people at lower risk, the cutoff is 160. For those at little or no risk, it's 190.

Pravachol can also be prescribed for children ages 8 and older when diet alone fails to lower their cholesterol levels.

Most important fact about this drug
Pravachol is usually prescribed only if diet, exercise, and weight loss fail to bring your cholesterol levels under control. It's important to remember that Pravachol is a supplement to—not a substitute for—those other measures. To get the full benefit of the medication, you need to stick to the diet and exercise program prescribed by your doctor. All these efforts to keep your cholesterol levels normal are important because together they may lower your risk of heart disease.

How should you take this medication?
For an even greater cholesterol-lowering effect, your doctor may prescribe Pravachol along with a different kind of lipid-lowering drug such as Questran or Colestid. However, you must not take Pravachol at the same time of day as the other cholesterol-lowering drug. Take Pravachol at least 1 hour before or 4 hours after taking the other drug.

Pravachol should be taken once daily. You may take it anytime, with or without food.

Your doctor will probably do blood tests for cholesterol levels every 4 weeks to determine the effectiveness of the dose.

■ *If you miss a dose...*
Take the forgotten dose as soon as you remember. If it is almost time for your next dose, skip the one you missed and go back to your regular schedule. Do not take a double dose.

■ *Storage instructions...*
Store at room temperature, in a tightly closed container, away from moisture and light.

What side effects may occur?

Side effects from Pravachol cannot be anticipated. If any develop or change in intensity, inform your doctor as soon as possible. Only your doctor can determine if it is safe for you to continue taking Pravachol.

■ *Side effects may include:*
Abdominal pain, chest pain, constipation, cough, diarrhea, dizziness, fatigue, gas, headache, heartburn, inflammation of nasal passages, muscle aching or weakness, nausea, rash, stomach or intestinal discomfort, urinary problems, vomiting

Why should this drug not be prescribed?

Do not take Pravachol if you are sensitive or have ever had an allergic reaction to it.

Do not take Pravachol if you have liver disease.

Special warnings about this medication

Pravachol should not be used to try to lower high cholesterol that stems from a medical condition such as alcoholism, poorly controlled diabetes, an underactive thyroid gland, or a kidney or liver problem.

Because Pravachol may cause damage to the liver, your doctor will probably do blood tests before you start taking the drug and whenever he plans a dosage increase. The doctor should monitor you especially carefully if you've recently had liver disease, if you have any symptoms that might mean liver disease, or if you're a heavy drinker.

Since Pravachol may cause damage to muscle tissue, promptly report to your doctor any unexplained muscle pain, tenderness, or weakness, especially if you also have a fever or you just generally do not feel well.

Possible food and drug interactions when taking this medication

If Pravachol is taken with certain other drugs, the effects of either could be increased, decreased, or altered. It is especially important to check with your doctor before combining Pravachol with the following:

Cholestyramine (Questran)
Cimetidine (Tagamet)
Colestipol (Colestid)
Diltiazem (Cardizem, Dilacor, Tiazac)
Drugs that suppress the immune system, such as Sandimmune
and Neoral
Erythromycin (E.E.S., Erythrocin, others)
Gemfibrozil (Lopid)
Itraconazole (Sporanox)
Niacin (Niacor, Niaspan)
Warfarin (Coumadin)

Special information if you are pregnant or breastfeeding

You must not become pregnant while taking Pravachol. Because this drug lowers cholesterol, and cholesterol is necessary for the proper development of an unborn baby, there is some suspicion that Pravachol might cause birth defects. Your doctor will prescribe Pravachol only if you are highly unlikely to become pregnant while taking the drug. If you do become pregnant while taking Pravachol, inform your doctor immediately.

Because Pravachol appears in breast milk, and because its cholesterol-lowering effects might prove harmful to a nursing baby, you should not take Pravachol while you are breastfeeding.

Recommended dosage

ADULTS

The usual starting dose is 40 milligrams once a day. If this doesn't reduce LDL levels sufficiently, your doctor may increase the dose to 80 milligrams once daily.

CHILDREN 8 TO 13 YEARS OLD

The recommended starting dose is 20 milligrams once a day. Doses greater than 20 milligrams have not been studied in this age group.

CHILDREN 14 TO 18 YEARS OLD

The recommended starting dose is 40 milligrams once a day. Doses greater than 40 milligrams have not been studied in this age group.

For people with kidney or liver problems and those taking a medication that suppresses the immune system, the starting dose is 10 milligrams. People on immunosuppressive drugs generally take no more than 20 milligrams of Pravachol daily.

Overdosage

Although no specific information is available, any medication taken in excess can have serious consequences. If you suspect an overdose of Pravachol, seek medical attention immediately.

Pravastatin *See Pravachol, page 1120.*

Pravastatin with Aspirin *See Pravigard PAC, below.*

PRAVIGARD PAC
Pronounced: PRAV-ih-guard Pack
Generic name: Pavastatin sodium with Buffered aspirin

Why is this drug prescribed?
Each Pravigard PAC contains a single dose of two medications—one tablet of aspirin and one tablet of the cholesterol-lowering drug Pravachol (pravastatin sodium). Both Pravachol and aspirin are prescribed for people with heart disease to help reduce the risk of heart attack and stroke, as well as reduce the risk of dying from heart disease. They're also used to improve the chances of avoiding heart surgery and procedures such as angioplasty.

In addition, Pravachol is used to lower cholesterol levels and slow the buildup of fatty deposits in the arteries. It's important to remember, however, that Pravigard PAC is not a substitute for diet, exercise, and weight loss. To get the full benefit of the medication, you need to stick to the diet and exercise program prescribed by your doctor.

Most important fact about this drug
On rare occasions, Pravachol (one of the medications in Pravigard PAC) has caused severe muscle damage. It's important to tell your doctor right away about any unexplained muscle pain, tenderness, or weakness, especially if you also have a fever or you just generally do not feel well.

How should you take this medication?
Pravigard PAC comes in individual blister cards that contain aspirin and Pravachol tablets packaged side by side. You should take both tablets at the same time.

The daily dose of Pravigard PAC can be taken at any time of the day, with or without food. Unless your doctor tells you to restrict fluids, you should take the medication with a full glass of water.

■ *If you miss a dose...*
Take it as soon as you remember. If it is almost time for your next dose, skip the one you missed and go back to your regular schedule. Do not take 2 doses at once.
■ *Storage instructions...*
Store at room temperature.

What side effects may occur?
Side effects cannot be anticipated. If any develop or change in intensity, tell your doctor as soon as possible. Only your doctor can determine if it is safe to continue using Pravigard PAC.

■ *Side effects may include:*
Abdominal pain, chest pain, constipation, cough, diarrhea, dizziness, fatigue, flu-like symptoms, gas, headache, heartburn, inflammation of nasal passages, muscle aching or weakness, nausea, possible involvement in formation of stomach ulcers and bleeding (aspirin component), rash, small amounts of blood in stool (aspirin component), stomach or intestinal discomfort, urinary problems, vomiting

Why should this drug not be prescribed?

Do not take Pravigard PAC if you have ever had an allergic reaction to Pravachol, aspirin, or other nonsteroidal anti-inflammatory drugs. Also, you may be more likely to have an allergic reaction to this drug if you have asthma or asthma-related conditions such as rhinitis and nasal polyps.

Because Pravigard PAC contains aspirin, children and teenagers should not use this product because of the risk of Reye's syndrome, a dangerous disorder characterized by disorientation, lethargy, and eventually coma.

In addition, you should not use Pravigard PAC if you have liver disease, ulcers, or ulcer symptoms, or if you are taking a medication that affects the clotting of your blood, unless specifically told to do so by your doctor.

Because the aspirin component of Pravigard PAC contains salt, you should not use this drug if you have a condition that causes you to retain salt, such as congestive heart failure or kidney disease.

You should not use Pravigard PAC if you are pregnant or breastfeeding.

Special warnings about this medication

The drug manufacturer of Pravigard PAC recommends liver function testing before using this drug. In addition, the doctor will need to monitor you closely if you have kidney problems.

Be sure to report any muscle aches or weakness to your doctor immediately (see *Most important fact about this drug*).

If you have more than 3 alcoholic drinks per day, check with your doctor before using Pravigard PAC, since this could increase the chance of internal bleeding.

Be aware that the aspirin component of Pravigard PAC could raise your risk of developing ulcers or internal bleeding, especially if you also have an inherited bleeding disorder such as hemophilia. Call your doctor immediately if you develop stomach pain, chronic heartburn, nausea, or vomiting.

Possible food and drug interactions when taking this medication

If Pravigard PAC is taken with certain other drugs, the effects of either could be increased, decreased, or altered. It is especially important to check with your doctor before combining Pravigard PAC with any of the drugs listed below. Also check the interactions listed in the individual Pravachol and aspirin drug profiles.

Possible interactions with Pravachol include:

Cholestyramine (Questran)
Colestipol (Colestid)
Diltiazem (Cardizem, Dilacor, Tiazac)
Erythromycin (E.E.S., Erythrocin, others)
Gemfibrozil (Lopid)
Itraconazole (Sporanox)
Ketoconazole (Nizoral)
Mibefradil

Possible interactions with aspirin include:

Acetazolamide (Diamox)
Alcohol (three or more drinks a day)
Blood pressure and heart medications that are ACE inhibitors,
     such as Capoten
Blood pressure and heart medications that are beta-blockers,
     such as Tenormin and Lopressor
Blood thinners such as heparin and warfarin (Coumadin)
Diabetes medications such as DiaBeta and Micronase
Diuretics such as Lasix
Methotrexate (Rheumatrex, Trexall)
Nonsteroidal anti-inflammatory drugs such as Aleve, Dolobid,
     and Motrin
Probenecid (Benemid)
Seizure medications such as Dilantin, Depakene, and Depakote
Sulfinpyrazone

Special information if you are pregnant or breastfeeding
You should not use Pravigard PAC if you are pregnant or breastfeeding.

Recommended dosage

ADULTS

The recommended daily dose is 40 milligrams of Pravachol with either 81
milligrams or 325 milligrams of aspirin. Depending on your response,
your doctor may increase the dose of Pravachol to 80 milligrams.

Some people, especially those with kidney or liver problems, may require lower doses.

CHILDREN

Pravigard PAC should not be used in children.

Overdosage
Although no specific information on Pravachol overdose is available, any
medication taken in excess can have serious consequences. If you suspect an overdose of Pravigard PAC, seek medical attention immediately.

Theoretically, an extremely large dose of aspirin could cause death.

Symptoms of aspirin overdose include abnormally fast breathing, dehydration, high body temperature, and ringing in the ears.

Prazosin *See Minipress, page 864.*

PRECOSE
Pronounced: PREE-cohs
Generic name: Acarbose

Why is this drug prescribed?
Precose is an oral medication used to treat type 2 (non-insulin-dependent) diabetes when high blood sugar levels cannot be controlled by diet alone. Precose works by slowing the body's digestion of carbohydrates so that blood sugar levels won't surge upward after a meal. Precose may be taken alone or in combination with certain other diabetes medications such as Diabinese, Micronase, Glucophage, and insulin.

Most important fact about this drug
Always remember that Precose is an aid to, not a substitute for, good diet and exercise. Failure to follow the diet and exercise plan recommended by your doctor can lead to serious complications such as dangerously high or low blood sugar levels. If you are overweight, losing pounds and exercising are critically important in controlling your diabetes. Remember, too, that Precose is not an oral form of insulin and cannot be used in place of insulin.

How should you take this medication?
Do not take more or less of this medication than directed by your doctor. Precose is usually taken 3 times a day with the first bite of each main meal.

■ *If you miss a dose...*
Take it as soon as you remember. If it is almost time for your next dose, skip the one you missed and go back to your regular schedule. Never take 2 doses at the same time. Taking Precose with your 3 main meals will help you to remember your medication schedule.

■ *Storage instructions...*
Keep the container tightly closed. Protect from temperatures above 77 degrees Fahrenheit. Store away from moisture.

What side effects may occur?
Side effects cannot be anticipated. If any develop or change in intensity, tell your doctor as soon as possible. Only your doctor can determine if it is safe for you to continue taking Precose.

If side effects do occur, they usually appear during the first few weeks of therapy and generally become less intense and less frequent over time. They are rarely severe.

■ *More common side effects may include:*
Abdominal pain, diarrhea, gas

Why should this drug not be prescribed?

Do not take Precose when suffering diabetic ketoacidosis (a life-threatening medical emergency caused by insufficient insulin and marked by mental confusion, excessive thirst, nausea, vomiting, headache, fatigue, and a sweet fruity smell to the breath).

You should not take Precose if you have cirrhosis (chronic degenerative liver disease). Also avoid Precose therapy if you have inflammatory bowel disease, ulcers in the colon, any intestinal obstruction or chronic intestinal disease associated with digestion, or any condition that could become worse as a result of gas in the intestine.

Special warnings about this medication

Every 3 months during your first year of treatment, your doctor will give you a blood test to check your liver and see how it is reacting to Precose. While you are taking Precose, you should check your blood and urine periodically for the presence of abnormal sugar (glucose) levels.

Even people with well-controlled diabetes may find that stress such as injury, infection, surgery, or fever results in a loss of control over their blood sugar. If this happens to you, your doctor may recommend that Precose be discontinued temporarily and injected insulin used instead.

When taken alone, Precose does not cause hypoglycemia (low blood sugar), but when you take it in combination with other medications such as Diabinese or Glucotrol, or with insulin, your blood sugar may fall too low. If you have any questions about combining Precose with other medications, be sure to discuss them with your doctor.

If you are taking Precose along with other diabetes medications, be sure to have some source of glucose, such as Glutose tablets, available in case you experience any symptoms of mild or moderate low blood sugar. (Table sugar won't work because Precose inhibits its absorption.)

■ *Symptoms of mild hypoglycemia may include:*
Cold sweat, fast heartbeat, fatigue, headache, nausea, and nervousness
■ *Symptoms of more severe hypoglycemia may include:*
Coma, pale skin, and shallow breathing

Severe hypoglycemia is an emergency. Contact your doctor immediately if the symptoms occur.

Possible food and drug interactions when taking this medication

When you take Precose with certain other drugs, the effects of either could be increased, decreased, or altered. It is especially important to check with your doctor before taking Precose with the following:

Airway-opening drugs such as Proventil

Calcium channel blockers (heart and blood pressure medications such as Cardizem and Procardia)

Charcoal tablets

Digestive enzyme preparations such as Creon 20 and Donnazyme

Digoxin (Lanoxin)

Estrogens such as Premarin

Isoniazid (Rifamate)

Major tranquilizers such as Compazine and Mellaril

Nicotinic acid (Nicobid, Nicolar)

Oral contraceptives

Phenytoin (Dilantin)

Steroid medications such as Deltasone and Prelone

Thyroid medications such as Synthroid and Thyrolar

Water pills (diuretics) such as Enduron, HydroDIURIL, and Moduretic

Special information if you are pregnant or breastfeeding

The effects of Precose during pregnancy have not been adequately studied. If you are pregnant or plan to become pregnant, tell your doctor immediately. Since studies suggest the importance of maintaining normal blood sugar levels during pregnancy, your doctor may prescribe injected insulin. It is not known whether Precose appears in breast milk. Because many drugs do appear in breast milk, you should not take Precose while breastfeeding.

Recommended dosage

ADULTS

The recommended starting dose of Precose is 25 milligrams (half of a 50-milligram tablet) 3 times a day, taken with the first bite of each main meal. Some people need to work up to this dose gradually and start with 25 milligrams only once a day. Your doctor will adjust your dosage at 4- to 8-week intervals, based on blood tests and your individual response to Precose. The doctor may increase the medication to 50 milligrams 3 times a day or, if needed, 100 milligrams 3 times a day. You should not take more than this amount. If you weigh less than 132 pounds, the maximum dosage is 50 milligrams 3 times a day.

If you are also taking another oral antidiabetic medication or insulin and you show signs of low blood sugar, your doctor will adjust the dosage of both medications.

CHILDREN

The safety and effectiveness of Precose in children have not been established.

Overdosage

An overdose of Precose alone will not cause low blood sugar. However, it may cause a temporary increase in gas, diarrhea, and abdominal discomfort. The symptoms will disappear quickly.

PRED FORTE

Pronounced: PRED FORT
Generic name: Prednisolone acetate

Why is this drug prescribed?

Pred Forte contains a steroid medication that eases redness, irritation, and swelling due to inflammation of the eye.

Most important fact about this drug

Do not use Pred Forte more often or for a longer period than your doctor orders. Overuse can increase the risk of side effects and can lead to eye damage. If your eye problems return, do not use any leftover Pred Forte without first consulting your doctor.

How should you use this medication?

Keep using Pred Forte for the full time prescribed.

To avoid spreading infection, do not let anyone else use your prescription.

Pred Forte may increase the chance of infection from contact lenses. Your doctor may advise you to stop wearing your contacts while using this medication.

Follow these steps to administer Pred Forte:

1. Wash your hands thoroughly.
2. Vigorously shake the dropper bottle.
3. Gently pull your lower eyelid down to form a pocket next to your eye.
4. Do not touch the applicator tip to any surface including your eye.
5. Brace the bottle against the bridge of your nose or your forehead.
6. Tilt your head back and squeeze the medication into your eye.
7. Close your eyes gently. Keep them closed for 1 to 2 minutes.
8. Do not rinse the dropper.
9. Wait for 5 to 10 minutes before using a second eye medication.

■ *If you miss a dose...*
Apply it as soon as you remember. If it is almost time for your next dose, skip the one you missed and go back to your regular schedule.

■ *Storage instructions...*
Store away from heat and direct light. Keep the bottle tightly closed and protect from freezing.

What side effects may occur?

Side effects cannot be anticipated. If any develop or change in intensity, inform your doctor as soon as possible. Only your doctor can determine if it is safe for you to continue taking Pred Forte.

■ *Side effects may include:*

Allergic reactions, blurred vision, burning/stinging, cataract formation, delayed wound healing, dilated pupils, drooping eyelid, increased pressure inside the eyeball, inflamed eyes, perforation of the eyeball, secondary infection, ulcers of the cornea

Since many of these developments could affect your vision temporarily or permanently, it is important to keep in close contact with your doctor while using Pred Forte eyedrops, and to use the drops only as directed.

Occasionally, long-term use of Pred Forte eyedrops may cause body-wide side effects due to an overload of steroid hormone. Such side effects may include a *moon-faced* appearance, obese trunk, humped upper back, wasted limbs, and purple stretch marks on the skin. These effects are likely to disappear once the medication is withdrawn. If bodywide side effects occur, you will need to stop using the eyedrops gradually rather than all at once.

Why should this drug not be prescribed?

You should not use Pred Forte if you have herpes or other viral diseases of the eye, or certain bacterial or fungal diseases of the eye.

Do not use Pred Forte if you are allergic to prednisolone or other steroids.

Special warnings about this medication

You must stay in close touch with your doctor while using this medication, for the following reasons:

If you use Pred Forte eyedrops extensively and/or for an extended period of time, you may be at increased risk for cataracts or vision problems. Prolonged use also increases the risk of another infection.

If you have had cataract surgery, this medication can delay healing.

Some eye diseases, together with long-term use of steroids, can cause thinning of the cornea; you may be at increased risk for perforation of the eyeball.

If you have a persistent ulceration of the cornea of your eye while using Pred Forte eyedrops, the problem may be a secondary fungus infection which Pred Forte cannot cure. An eye doctor should evaluate this possibility.

If you use Pred Forte eyedrops for 10 days or longer, an eye doctor should check your intraocular pressure (pressure inside the eyeball) frequently, since prolonged use of steroids may increase this pressure. If you already have glaucoma, use this medication cautiously. If increased pressure is allowed to continue, it may cause loss of vision.

Corticosteroids can mask, or worsen, pus-forming eye infections. If your eye inflammation or pain lasts longer than 48 hours or becomes worse, stop using Pred Forte and call your doctor.

Pred Forte contains sodium bisulfite, which can cause allergic-type reactions, including severe or even life-threatening asthma attacks. You are more likely to be sensitive to sulfites if you suffer from asthma.

Possible food and drug interactions when using this medication
Prednisolone acetate, the active ingredient in Pred Forte eyedrops, is also available in tablet and injectable forms for the treatment of other disorders. It's known that when these other forms of prednisolone acetate are taken with certain drugs, the effects of either medication can be increased, decreased, or altered. Therefore, it's wise to check with your doctor before combining Pred Forte eyedrops with other medications.

Special information if you are pregnant or breastfeeding
If you are pregnant or plan to become pregnant, inform your doctor immediately. Pred Forte eyedrops should be used during pregnancy only if the potential benefit outweighs the potential risk to the developing baby.

It is not known whether the hormone in Pred Forte eyedrops appears in breast milk. If it does, the small quantity involved would be unlikely to harm a breastfeeding baby. Nevertheless, caution is advised when using Pred Forte eyedrops while breastfeeding.

Recommended dosage

ADULTS

Put 1 to 2 drops under the eyelid 2 to 4 times daily. During the first 24 to 48 hours, your doctor may want you to use more frequent doses.

Overdosage
A one time accidental overdose of Pred Forte eyedrops ordinarily will not cause acute problems. Over time, however, overdosage may have serious consequences (see *What side effects may occur?*). If you suspect symptoms of a chronic overdose with Pred Forte eyedrops, seek medical attention immediately.

If you accidentally swallow Pred Forte eyedrops, drink fluids to dilute the medication. Call your local poison center or your doctor for assistance.

Prednisolone acetate *See Pred Forte, page 1129.*

Prednisolone sodium phosphate *See Pediapred, page 1048.*

PREDNISONE
Pronounced: PRED-nih-sohn

Why is this drug prescribed?

Prednisone, a steroid drug, is used to reduce inflammation and alleviate symptoms in a variety of disorders, including rheumatoid arthritis and severe cases of asthma. It may be given to treat primary or secondary adrenal cortex insufficiency (lack of sufficient adrenal hormone in the body). It is used in treating all of the following:

Abnormal adrenal gland development
Allergic conditions (severe)
Blood disorders
Certain cancers (along with other drugs)
Diseases of the connective tissue including systemic lupus
    erythematosus
Eye diseases of various kinds
Flare-ups of multiple sclerosis
Fluid retention due to nephrotic syndrome (a condition in which
    damage to the kidneys causes protein to be lost in the urine)
Lung diseases, including tuberculosis
Meningitis (inflamed membranes around the brain)
Prevention of organ rejection
Rheumatoid arthritis and related disorders
Severe flare-ups of ulcerative colitis or enteritis (inflammation of the
    intestines)
Skin diseases
Thyroid gland inflammation
Trichinosis (with complications)

Most important fact about this drug

Prednisone lowers your resistance to infections and can make them harder to treat. Prednisone may also mask some of the signs of an infection, making it difficult for your doctor to diagnose the actual problem.

How should you take this medication?

Take prednisone exactly as prescribed. Dosages are kept to an absolute minimum.

If you need long-term prednisone treatment, your doctor may prescribe alternate day therapy, in which you take the medication only every other morning. The "resting day" gives your adrenal glands a chance to produce some hormone naturally so they will not lose the ability to do so.

If you have been taking prednisone for a period of time, you will probably need an increased dosage of the medication before, during, and after any stressful situation. Always consult your doctor if you are anticipating stress and think you may need a temporary dosage increase.

When stopping prednisone treatment, tapering off is better than quitting abruptly. Your doctor will probably have you decrease the dosage very gradually over a period of days or weeks.

You should take prednisone with food to avoid stomach upset.

If you are on alternate day therapy or have been prescribed a single daily dose, take prednisone in the morning with breakfast (about 8 A.M.). If you have been prescribed several doses per day, take them at evenly spaced intervals around the clock.

Patients on long-term prednisone therapy should wear or carry identification.

■ *If you miss a dose...*
If you take your dose once a day, take it as soon as you remember. If you don't remember until the next day, skip the one you missed.

If you take several doses a day, take the forgotten dose as soon as you remember and then go back to your regular schedule. If you don't remember until your next dose, double the dose you take.

If you take your dose every other day, and you remember it the same morning, take it as soon as you remember, then go back to your regular schedule. If you don't remember until the afternoon, do not take a dose until the following morning, then skip a day.

■ *Storage instructions...*
Store at room temperature.

What side effects may occur?

Side effects cannot be anticipated. If any develop or change in intensity, inform your doctor as soon as possible. Only your doctor can determine if it is safe for you to continue taking prednisone.

Prednisone may cause euphoria, insomnia, mood changes, personality changes, psychotic behavior, or severe depression. It may worsen any existing emotional instability.

At a high dosage, prednisone may cause fluid retention and high blood pressure. If this happens, you may need a low-salt diet and a potassium supplement.

With prolonged prednisone treatment, eye problems (e.g., a viral or fungal eye infection, cataracts, or glaucoma) may develop.

If you take prednisone over the long term, the buildup of adrenal hormones in your body may cause a condition called Cushing's syndrome, marked by weight gain, a "moon-faced" appearance, thin, fragile skin, muscle weakness, brittle bones, and purplish stripe marks on the skin. Women are more vulnerable to this problem than men. Alternate day therapy may help prevent its development.

Why should this drug not be prescribed?

Do not take prednisone if you have ever had an allergic reaction to it.

You should not be treated with prednisone if you have a body-wide fungus infection, such as candidiasis or cryptococcosis.

Special warnings about this medication

Do not get a smallpox vaccination or any other immunization while you are taking prednisone. The vaccination might not take, and could do harm to the nervous system.

Prednisone may reactivate a dormant case of tuberculosis. If you have inactive TB and must take prednisone for an extended time, you should be given anti-TB medication as well.

If you have an underactive thyroid gland or cirrhosis of the liver, your doctor will probably need to prescribe prednisone for you at a lower than average dosage.

If you have an eye infection caused by the herpes simplex virus, prednisone should be used with great caution; there is a potential danger that the cornea will become perforated.

A few people taking prednisone develop Kaposi's sarcoma, a form of cancer; it may disappear when the drug is stopped.

Prednisone should also be taken with caution if you have any of the following conditions:

Diverticulitis or other disorder of the intestine
High blood pressure
Kidney disorder
Myasthenia gravis (a muscle weakness disorder)
Osteoporosis (brittle bones)
Peptic ulcer
Ulcerative colitis (inflammation of the bowel)

Long-term treatment with prednisone may stunt growth. If this medication is given to a child, the youngster's growth should be monitored carefully.

Diseases such as chickenpox or measles can be very serious or even fatal in both children and adults who are taking this drug. Try to avoid exposure to these diseases.

Possible food and drug interactions when taking this medication

Prednisone may decrease your carbohydrate tolerance or activate a latent case of diabetes. If you are already taking insulin or oral medication for diabetes, make sure your doctor knows this; you may need an increased dosage while you are being treated with prednisone.

If you have a blood-clotting disorder caused by a vitamin K deficiency and are taking prednisone, check with your doctor before you use aspirin.

You may be at risk of convulsions if you take the immunosuppressant drug cyclosporine (Sandimmune) while being treated with prednisone.

If prednisone is taken with certain other drugs, the effects of either could be increased, decreased, or altered. Check with your doctor before combining prednisone with any of the following:

Amphotericin B (Fungizone)
Blood thinners such as Coumadin
Carbamazepine (Tegretol)
Estrogen drugs such as Premarin
Ketoconazole (Nizoral)
Oral contraceptives
Phenobarbital (Donnatal, others)
Phenytoin (Dilantin)
Potent diuretics such as Lasix
Rifampin (Rifadin)
Troleandomycin (Tao)

Special information if you are pregnant or breastfeeding

If you are pregnant or plan to become pregnant, inform your doctor immediately. Prednisone should be taken during pregnancy or while breastfeeding only if clearly needed and only if the benefit outweighs the potential risks to the child.

Recommended dosage

Dosage is determined by the condition being treated and your response to the drug. Typical starting doses can range from 5 to 60 milligrams a day. Once you respond to the drug, your doctor will lower the dose gradually to the minimum effective amount. For treatment of acute attacks of multiple sclerosis, doses of as much as 200 milligrams per day may be given for a week, followed by 80 milligrams every other day for a month.

Overdosage

Long-term high doses of prednisone may produce Cushing's syndrome (see *What side effects may occur?*). Although no specific information is available regarding short-term overdosage, any medication taken in excess can have serious consequences. If you suspect an overdose of prednisone, seek medical attention immediately.

Prefest *See Activella and femhrt, page 26.*

PREMARIN

Pronounced: PREM-uh-rin
Generic name: Conjugated estrogens
Other brand names: Cenestin, Premphase, Prempro

Why is this drug prescribed?

Premarin is an estrogen replacement drug. The tablets are used to reduce moderate to severe symptoms of menopause, including feelings of warmth in the face, neck, and chest, and the sudden intense episodes of heat and sweating known as hot flashes. Cenestin tablets, containing a synthetic form of conjugated estrogens, may also be prescribed for these symptoms.

In addition to the symptoms of menopause, Premarin tablets are prescribed for teenagers who fail to mature at the usual rate, and to relieve the symptoms of certain types of cancer, including some forms of breast and prostate cancer.

In addition, either the tablets or Premarin vaginal cream can be used for other conditions caused by lack of estrogen, such as dry, itchy external genitals and vaginal irritation.

Along with diet, calcium supplements, and exercise, Premarin tablets are also prescribed to prevent postmenopausal osteoporosis, a condition in which the bones become brittle and easily broken. Before taking Premarin solely for this purpose, you should carefully consider using alternative, non-estrogen therapies.

The addition of progesterone to estrogen replacement therapy has been shown to reduce the risk of uterine cancer. Prempro combines estrogen and progesterone in a single tablet taken once daily. Premphase is a 28-day supply of tablets. The first 14 contain only estrogen. The second 14 supply both estrogen and progesterone. Both Prempro and Premphase are prescribed to reduce the symptoms of menopause, including vaginal problems, and to prevent osteoporosis.

Most important fact about this drug
Because estrogens have been linked with an increased risk of uterine and endometrial cancer (cancer in the lining of the uterus), it is essential to have regular checkups and to report any unusual vaginal bleeding to your doctor immediately.

Premarin and other estrogen drugs, with or without progesterone, should not be used to prevent heart disease. Recent studies have confirmed an increased rate of heart attack, stroke, and dangerous blood clots among women taking estrogen or estrogen combinations for 5 years. Blood clots can lead to phlebitis, stroke, heart attack, a loss of blood supply to the lungs, a blockage in the blood vessels serving the eye, and other serious disorders.

How should you take this medication?
Take Premarin exactly as prescribed. Do not share it with anyone else.

If you are taking calcium supplements as a part of the treatment to help prevent brittle bones, check with your doctor about how much to take.

You should take a few moments to read the patient package insert provided with your prescription.

To apply Premarin vaginal cream:
1. Remove cap from tube.
2. Screw nozzle end of applicator onto tube.

3. Gently squeeze tube from the bottom to force sufficient cream into the barrel to provide the prescribed dose. Use the marked stopping points on the applicator as a guide.
4. Unscrew applicator from tube.
5. Lie on back with knees drawn up. Gently insert applicator deeply into the vagina and press plunger downward to its original position.

To cleanse the applicator, pull the plunger to remove it from the barrel, then wash with mild soap and warm water. Do not boil or use hot water.

■ *If you miss a dose...*
Take the forgotten dose as soon as you remember. If it is almost time for the next dose, skip the one you missed and go back to your regular schedule. Never try to catch up by doubling the dose.
■ *Storage instructions...*
Store at room temperature.

What side effects may occur?
Side effects cannot be anticipated. If any develop or change in intensity, inform your doctor immediately. Only your doctor can determine whether it is safe to continue taking Premarin.

■ *Side effects of conjugated estrogens may include:*
Abdominal/stomach cramps, bloating, breast pain, enlargement of benign tumors of the uterus (also called fibroids), fluid retention, hair loss, headache, high blood pressure, high blood sugar, irregular vaginal bleeding or spotting, liver problems, nausea and vomiting, vaginal yeast infections
■ *Other possible side effects of Cenestin may include:*
Constipation, increased heart rate, joint pain, skin tingling

Why should this drug not be prescribed?
Do not take Premarin if you have ever had a bad reaction to it, or have undiagnosed abnormal vaginal bleeding.

Except in certain special circumstances, you should not be given Premarin if you have ever had breast cancer, uterine cancer, or any other estrogen-dependent cancer.

Do not take Premarin if you have had any circulation problem involving blood clots, or have had a stroke or heart attack in the past year.

Do not take Premarin if you have liver disease or your liver is not working properly.

Do not use Premarin if you are pregnant or trying to become pregnant.

Special warnings about this medication
For women who have not had a hysterectomy, the risk of endometrial and uterine cancer increases when estrogen-only drugs are used for a long time or taken in large doses. Estrogen therapy can also worsen endo-

metriosis (uterine tissue growing outside the uterus). If you've ever had endometriosis, make sure the doctor is aware of it. If you've had a hysterectomy but still have residual endometriosis, your doctor may want you to use an estrogen/progesterone combination.

Certain studies have shown that women taking estrogen for prolonged periods of time (4 years or more) face an increased risk of breast cancer, and a study by the National Heart, Lung, and Blood Institute (NHLBI) has confirmed an increased risk among women taking estrogen/progesterone combinations. Use combination products (and estrogen-only preparations, too) with special caution if you have a family history of breast cancer or have ever had an abnormal mammogram. Be sure to get an annual breast exam from your doctor, and do your own self-examination each month.

The NHLBI study also found an increased risk of dementia for women taking estrogen or estrogen/progesterone combinations.

Because Premarin can increase the risk of heart attack, stroke, blood clots, and certain estrogen-dependent cancers, contact your doctor right away if you notice any of the following:

Abdominal pain, tenderness, or swelling
Abnormal bleeding from the vagina
Breast lumps
Coughing up blood
Pain in your chest or calves
Severe headache, dizziness, or faintness
Sudden shortness of breath
Vision changes

Women who take Premarin after menopause are more likely to develop gallbladder disease.

Estrogens such as Premarin can cause hypercalcemia, a severe increase of calcium levels in the blood. Women with breast or bone cancer are especially at risk and should stop taking Premarin immediately if they develop hypercalcemia. In addition, women with the opposite problem—hypocalcemia, or a severe *decrease* of calcium in the blood—should use Premarin with caution.

Women who have not had a hysterectomy and take estrogen along with progesterone have a lower risk of precancerous endometrial changes. However, you should be aware that estrogen/progesterone combinations could increase "bad" LDL cholesterol and blood sugar levels as well as increase the risk of breast cancer.

There is a slight chance that estrogen therapy could cause an increase in blood pressure. Ask your doctor to check your blood pressure regularly.

If you have high levels of fat in your blood, specifically a high triglyceride level, conjugated estrogens such as Premarin are likely to cause side effects in the pancreas.

Use Premarin with caution if you have a history of liver problems, including jaundice. Call your doctor right away if you develop abdominal pain or yellowing of the skin.

Premarin can alter thyroid function. If you're taking thyroid medication, you may need your dosage adjusted.

Premarin can also cause fluid retention. Use the drug with caution if you have heart or kidney problems, or any other condition that's affected by excess fluid in the body.

Some studies have shown that using estrogen-only drugs, especially for 10 years or more, could increase the risk of ovarian cancer. It's unknown whether this also applies to estrogen/progesterone combinations.

Estrogens such as Premarin have been known to make certain conditions worse, including asthma, diabetes, epilepsy, migraine, porphyria (a genetic enzyme deficiency), lupus, and liver tumors.

If you are using Premarin vaginal cream, you should be aware that this product can weaken latex condoms, diaphragms, and cervical caps.

Possible food and drug interactions when taking this medication

If Premarin is taken with certain other drugs, the effects of either could be increased, decreased, or altered. It is especially important to check with your doctor before combining Premarin with the following:

Barbiturates such as phenobarbital
Blood thinners such as Coumadin
Carbamazepine (Tegretol)
Clarithromycin (Biaxin)
Drugs used for epilepsy, such as Dilantin
Erythromycin
Grapefruit juice
Itraconazole (Sporanox)
Ketoconazole (Nizoral)
Major tranquilizers such as Thorazine
Oral diabetes drugs such as Micronase
Rifampin (Rifadin)
Ritonavir (Norvir)
Steroid medications such as Deltasone
St. John's wort
Thyroid preparations such as Synthroid
Tricyclic antidepressants such as Elavil and Tofranil
Vitamin C

Special Information if you are pregnant or breastfeeding

If you are pregnant or plan to become pregnant, notify your doctor immediately. Premarin and conjugated estrogens should not be taken during pregnancy because of the possibility of harm to the unborn child. Premarin cannot prevent a miscarriage. Estrogens can decrease the quantity and quality of breast milk, and progestins appear in breast milk. Your doctor may advise you not to breastfeed while you are taking this drug.

Recommended dosage

Your doctor will start therapy with this medication at a low dose and adjust the dosage according to your response. He or she will want to check you periodically at 3- to 6-month intervals to determine the need for continued therapy.

PREMARIN TABLETS

Hot Flashes Associated with Menopause
The usual starting dosage is 0.3 milligram daily, taken continuously or in cycles such as 25 days on Premarin and 5 days off.

Tissue Degeneration in the Vagina
The usual starting dosage is 0.3 milligram daily, taken continuously or in cycles.

Low Estrogen Levels Due to Reduced Ovary Function
The usual dosage is 0.3 to 0.625 milligram daily, taken cyclically.

Ovary Removal or Ovarian Failure
The usual dosage is 1.25 milligrams daily, taken cyclically.

Prevention of Osteoporosis (Loss of Bone Mass)
The usual starting dosage is 0.3 milligram daily, taken continuously or in cycles.

Advanced Androgen-Dependent Cancer of the Prostate,
for Relief of Symptoms Only
The usual dosage is 1.25 to 2.5 milligrams 3 times daily.

Breast Cancer (for Relief of Symptoms Only) in Appropriately
Selected Women and Men with Metastatic Disease
The suggested dosage is 10 milligrams 3 times daily for a period of at least 3 months. Tell your doctor if you have any unusual bleeding.

PREMARIN VAGINAL CREAM

Given cyclically for short-term use only.

Degeneration of Genital Tissue or Severe Itching in the
Genital Area
The recommended dosage is one-half to 2 grams daily, inserted into the vagina, depending on the severity of the condition. You will use the cream for 3 weeks, then stop for 1 week. Tell your doctor if you notice any unusual bleeding.

PREMPRO TABLETS/PREMPHASE THERAPY

Symptoms Associated with Menopause (Hot Flashes, Night Sweats, and Vaginal Tissue Degeneration) or for the Prevention of Osteoporosis (Loss of Bone Mass)
The usual starting dose for Prempro is one 0.3-milligram/1.5-milligram tablet once a day. If this dose proves insufficient, your doctor may increase the dose to one 0.625-milligram/0.25- or 0.5-milligram tablet once a day.

For Premphase therapy, follow a 28-day cycle. Take 1 maroon Premarin tablet (equal to 0.625 milligram estrogen) every day for the first 14 days; on the 15th day, begin taking 1 light blue tablet (equal to 0.625 milligram estrogen/5 milligrams progesterone) daily.

CENESTIN TABLETS

The usual starting dose is 0.45 milligram a day. If this proves insufficient, the doctor may gradually increase the dose to a maximum of 1.25 milligrams daily.

Overdosage
Any medication taken in excess can have serious consequences. If you suspect an overdose of Premarin, seek medical attention immediately.

■ *Symptoms of conjugated estrogen overdose may include:*
Nausea, vomiting, withdrawal bleeding

Premphase *See Premarin, page 1135.*
Prempro *See Premarin, page 1135.*

PRENATAL VITAMINS
Brand names: Advanced Natalcare, Materna, Natalins, Prenate Advance

Why is this drug prescribed?
These prenatal products contain vitamins and minerals including iron, calcium, zinc, and folic acid. The tablets are given during pregnancy and after childbirth to ensure an adequate supply of these critical nutrients. They may also be prescribed to improve a woman's nutritional status before she becomes pregnant.

Most important fact about this drug
Nutritional supplementation is especially important during pregnancy. Be sure to take the pills regularly as prescribed.

How should you take this medication?

Take these products exactly as prescribed, with or without food. Do not take more than the recommended dose.

- *If you miss a dose…*
  Take it as soon as you remember, then return to your regular schedule.
- *Storage instructions…*
  Store at room temperature in a tightly closed container, away from excessive heat.

Why should this drug not be prescribed?

Certain rare diseases allow copper or iron to accumulate in the body. If you've been diagnosed with such a disease, you should avoid vitamin and mineral supplements such as these.

Special warnings about this medication

Your doctor will test you for pernicious anemia before you take this drug, since folic acid can cover up the symptoms.

If you have kidney stones, you need to limit your calcium intake. Your doctor should take this into account when prescribing a vitamin and mineral supplement.

Keep this product out of children's reach. An overdose could be fatal.

Special information if you are pregnant or breastfeeding

Pregnancy and breastfeeding impose special nutritional demands on the mother. A vitamin and mineral supplement can help ensure that there are enough nutrients for both you and your baby.

Recommended dosage

ADULTS

Follow your doctor's recommendation.

Overdosage

Although no specific overdose information is available, even a nutritional supplement can have serious consequences when taken in extremely large amounts. In children, an overdose of the iron in vitamin supplements could be dangerous or even fatal. If you suspect an overdose, seek medical attention immediately.

Prenate Advance *See Prenatal Vitamins, page 1141.*

PREVACID

Pronounced: PREH-va-sid
Generic name: Lansoprazole

Why is this drug prescribed?

Prevacid blocks the production of stomach acid. It is prescribed for the short-term (4 to 8 weeks) treatment of the following:

Stomach ulcer
Duodenal ulcer (near the exit from the stomach)
Erosive esophagitis (inflammation of the esophagus)
Heartburn and other symptoms of gastroesophageal reflux disease
(also known as GERD), which occurs when stomach acid backs
up into the tube connecting the throat to the stomach.

Once a duodenal ulcer or case of esophagitis has cleared up, the doctor may continue prescribing Prevacid to prevent a relapse. Prevacid is also prescribed to reduce the risk of stomach ulcers in people who develop this problem while taking nonsteroidal anti-inflammatory drugs such as Advil, Motrin, and Naprosyn. The drug is also used for long-term treatment of certain diseases marked by excessive acid production, such as Zollinger-Ellison syndrome.

Prevacid is also prescribed as part of a combination treatment to eliminate the *H. pylori* infection that causes most cases of duodenal ulcer.

Most important fact about this drug

To relieve your symptoms and to heal your ulcer, you need to take Prevacid for the full time of treatment your doctor prescribes. Keep taking the drug even if you begin to feel better, and be sure to keep your appointments with your doctor.

How should you take this medication?

Prevacid should be taken before meals. If you're using the regular delayed-release capsules and you're having trouble swallowing them, you can sprinkle the contents on a tablespoon of applesauce; swallow immediately without chewing or crushing the granules. You can also mix the granules with 2 ounces of orange juice or tomato juice. (Rinse the glass with an additional 4 ounces of juice to make sure you get the entire dose.)

You can also use delayed-release Prevacid SoluTabs, which are orally disintegrating tablets. Each tablet should be placed on the tongue, where it will dissolve in about 1 minute. The dissolved particles can be swallowed with or without water. The SoluTabs should not be chewed or swallowed whole. If you or your child has trouble swallowing the SoluTabs, you have the option of dissolving the tablet in water and administering the solution with an oral syringe or through a nasogastric tube. For specific instructions, talk to your doctor.

The general steps for administration are as follows:
1. Place the tablet in an oral syringe. Follow your doctor's directions on the amount of water you need to draw up into the syringe.
2. Gently shake the syringe to dissolve the tablet.
3. Administer the solution within 15 minutes. This can be done directly, with the oral syringe, or by injecting the syringe into a nasogastric tube.
4. To be sure you have taken all of the drug, rinse out any remaining residue by refilling the syringe with water and shaking gently; then administer the remaining contents.

Alternatively, you can use Prevacid for Delayed-Release Oral Suspension. Empty the packet into 2 tablespoonfuls of water, stir well, and swallow immediately. Do not use any other liquid, and avoid chewing or crushing the granules. If any material remains in the glass, add more water, stir, and drink immediately.

If you are taking antacids for pain, you may continue to do so. You also may continue to take sucralfate (Carafate), but take your dose of Prevacid at least 30 minutes prior to the Carafate.

■ *If you miss a dose...*
Take it as soon as you remember. If it is almost time for your next dose, skip the one you missed and go back to your regular schedule. Do not take 2 doses at once.

■ *Storage instructions...*
Store at room temperature in a tightly closed container. Keep away from moisture.

What side effects may occur?
Side effects cannot be anticipated. If any develop or change in intensity, tell your doctor as soon as possible. Only your doctor can determine if it is safe for you to continue taking Prevacid.

■ *Side effects may include:*
Abdominal pain, constipation, diarrhea, dizziness or headache (more common in children), nausea

Why should this drug not be prescribed?
Do not take Prevacid if you've ever had an allergic reaction to it, or if you've ever had an allergic reaction to penicillin or macrolide antibiotics, such as clarithromycin (Biaxin) or erythromycin (E.E.S., E-Mycin, ERYC, Ery-Tab, Erythrocin, PCE).

You must also avoid Prevacid if you're taking cisapride, pimozide, astemizole, or terfenadine. Combining Prevacid with these drugs could cause dangerous—and even fatal—heartbeat irregularities.

Special warnings about this medication

Do not take Prevacid any longer than your doctor has prescribed; this medication should not be used for long-term therapy of duodenal ulcer or erosive esophagitis.

If you have liver disease, be sure your doctor knows about it. Prevacid should be used cautiously.

If you do not begin to feel better on Prevacid therapy, or if your symptoms become worse, be sure to call your doctor.

Prevacid has no effect on stomach cancer. It could be present even if Prevacid relieves your symptoms.

Be sure to tell your doctor if you have phenylketonuria and must avoid the amino acid phenylalanine, since Prevacid contains this substance.

Possible food and drug interactions when taking this medication

If Prevacid is taken with certain other drugs, the effects of either could be increased, decreased, or altered. It is especially important to check with your doctor before combining Prevacid with the following:

Ampicillin
Digoxin (Lanoxin)
Iron salts (Ferro-Sequels, Ferro-Sulfate)
Ketoconazole (Nizoral)
Sucralfate (Carafate)
Theophylline (Theo-Dur)
Warfarin (Coumadin)

Special information if you are pregnant or breastfeeding

The effects of Prevacid in pregnant women have not been adequately studied. If you are pregnant or plan to become pregnant, tell your doctor. It is not known whether Prevacid appears in human breast milk. If this medication is essential to your health, your doctor may have you stop breastfeeding your baby while you are taking it.

Recommended dosage

ADULTS

If you have severe liver disease, your doctor will adjust the dosage as needed.

For Short-Term Treatment of Duodenal Ulcer
The usual dose is 15 milligrams once daily, before eating, for 4 weeks.

To Prevent Relapse of Duodenal Ulcer
Take 15 milligrams once a day.

To Eradicate Ulcer-causing Bacteria
To eliminate the *H. pylori* bacteria that cause most duodenal ulcers, Prevacid is taken with amoxicillin alone or amoxicillin and Biaxin. When com-

bined with amoxicillin only, the usual dosage is 30 milligrams of Prevacid and 1 gram of amoxicillin 3 times daily for 14 days. If all three drugs are used, the usual dosage is 30 milligrams of Prevacid, 1 gram of amoxicillin, and 500 milligrams of Biaxin twice daily for 10 to 14 days.

For Short-Term Treatment of Stomach Ulcer
The usual dose is 30 milligrams once a day for up to 8 weeks.

To Prevent Stomach Ulcer due to Nonsteroidal
Anti-inflammatory Drugs
The usual dose is 15 milligrams once a day for up to 12 weeks.

For Short-Term Treatment of Gastroesophageal Reflux
Disease (GERD)
The usual dose is 15 milligrams once a day for up to 8 weeks.

For Short-Term Treatment of Erosive Esophagitis
The usual dose is 30 milligrams daily, before eating, for up to 8 weeks. Depending on your response to the medication, your doctor may suggest another 8-week treatment regimen.

For Other Excess Acid Conditions (such as Zollinger-Ellison syndrome)
The usual starting dose is 60 milligrams once daily. This dose can be adjusted upward by your doctor, depending on your response. Dosages totaling more than 120 milligrams a day should be divided into smaller doses.

CHILDREN 12 TO 17 YEARS OLD

For Short-Term Treatment of Gastroesophageal Reflux
Disease (GERD)
The usual dose is 15 milligrams once a day for up to 8 weeks.

For Short-Term Treatment of Erosive Esophagitis
The usual dose is 30 milligrams once a day for up to 8 weeks.

CHILDREN 1 TO 11 YEARS OLD

For Short-Term Treatment of Gastroesophageal Reflux Disease (GERD) or Erosive Esophagitis
Dosage is based on the child's weight. For children weighing 66 pounds or less, the usual dose is 15 milligrams once a day for up to 12 weeks. For children weighing more than 66 pounds, the usual dose is 30 milligrams once a day for up to 12 weeks. If the child's symptoms don't improve after 2 or more weeks, the doctor may increase the dose up to a maximum of 30 milligrams twice a day. Children with severe liver problems will need their dosage adjusted.

The safety and effectiveness of Prevacid have not been studied in children less than 1 year old.

Overdosage

Overdoses of Prevacid are not known to cause any problems. Nevertheless, no medication should be taken in excess. If you suspect an overdose, seek medical attention immediately.

PREVACID NAPRAPAC

Pronounced: PREH-va-sid NAP-rah-pack
Generic ingredients: Lansoprazole and Naproxen

Why is this drug prescribed?

Prevacid NapraPAC is prescribed to relieve arthritis symptoms in people who also have a history of stomach ulcers. It's used to treat pain caused by osteoarthritis, rheumatoid arthritis, and ankylosing spondylitis (spinal arthritis).

Prevacid NapraPAC is a combination package containing two drugs: lansoprazole (Prevacid) and naproxen (Naprosyn). Prevacid is used to prevent or treat stomach ulcers, among other conditions. Naprosyn is a nonsteroidal anti-inflammatory drug (NSAID) used to treat various types of pain. Using an NSAID for a long time may increase the risk of stomach ulcers. The medications in Prevacid NapraPAC were combined to help reduce this risk while also providing pain relief.

Most important fact about this drug

Other prescription or over-the-counter products may also contain naproxen (Aleve, Anaprox, and Naprelan), aspirin and other NSAIDs, or Prevacid and other acid-reducing medications. Combining these other medicines with Prevacid NapraPAC may increase the risk of serious side effects. Do not take any other prescription or over-the-counter medicines—especially ones for a cold, pain, or heartburn—without first talking to your doctor.

How should you take this medication?

Prevacid NapraPAC contains four blister cards. Each blister card contains enough medication for 1 week (seven Prevacid capsules and 14 Naprosyn tablets). Take one Prevacid capsule and one Naprosyn tablet in the morning, before eating, with a glass of water. Take a second Naprosyn tablet in the evening with a glass of water.

Swallow the Prevacid capsule whole. Do not chew or crush it.

■ *If you miss a dose…*
Take it as soon as you remember. If it is almost time for your next dose, skip the one you missed and go back to your regular schedule. Do not take 2 doses at once.

■ *Storage instructions…*
Store at room temperature.

What side effects may occur?

Side effects cannot be anticipated. If any develop or change in intensity, tell your doctor as soon as possible. Only your doctor can determine if it is safe to continue using Prevacid NapraPAC.

■ *Side effects may include:*

Abdominal pain, bruising, constipation, diarrhea, dizziness, drowsiness, heartburn, headache, itching, nausea, ringing in the ear, skin eruptions, shortness of breath, swelling due to fluid retention

Why should this drug not be prescribed?

You should not use Prevacid NapraPAC if you have ever had an allergic reaction to Prevacid, Naprosyn, or any other medication containing naproxen, such as Aleve or Anaprox. If aspirin or other NSAIDs have ever given you asthma, nasal inflammation, or nasal polyps, you should not take this medication. Be sure to tell your doctor about any drug reactions you've had.

Special warnings about this medication

When taking NSAIDs such as Naprosyn, serious ulcers and internal bleeding can occur without warning. Ask your doctor about the warning signs of stomach problems, and what to do if they appear. Notify your doctor immediately if you have any stomach or abdominal pain. Your doctor may want to monitor you closely while you are being treated with Prevacid NapraPAC.

Naprosyn can cause kidney or liver problems in some people. Use Prevacid NapraPAC with caution if you have kidney or liver disease.

The symptom relief provided by Prevacid NapraPAC could mask certain medical problems. By reducing fever and inflammation, Naprosyn may hide an underlying infection or inflammatory condition. Prevacid could hide an underlying stomach cancer by providing relief from stomach pain.

Naprosyn may cause vision problems. Tell your doctor if you experience any change in your vision while taking Prevacid NapraPAC.

Naprosyn may cause you to become drowsy or less alert. Avoid driving, operating dangerous machinery, or participating in any hazardous activity until you know how this drug affects you.

Possible food and drug interactions when taking this medication

Always check with your doctor before combining Prevacid NapraPAC with other NSAIDs, ulcer medication, or similar drugs (see *Most important fact about this drug*).

If Prevacid NapraPAC is taken with certain other drugs, the effects of either could be increased, decreased, or altered. It is especially important to check with your doctor before taking the following:

Acid-reducing drugs such as Tagamet, Zantac, and Pepcid
Ampicillin (Principen)

Aspirin
Beta-blockers such as the blood pressure drugs Inderal and
   Tenormin
Blood-thinning drugs such as warfarin (Coumadin)
Digoxin (Lanoxin)
Fosphenytoin (Cerebyx)
Furosemide (Lasix)
Hydantoin (Peganone and others)
Lithium (Eskalith, Lithobid)
Mephenytoin (Mesantoin)
Iron supplements (the most common is ferrous sulfate)
Ketoconazole (Nizoral)
Methotrexate (Rheumatrex, Trexall)
Phenytoin (Dilantin)
Probenecid (Benemid)
Sucralfate (Carafate)
Sulfonamides and other sulfa drugs (Gantrisin, Sulten, and others)
Sulfonylurea
Theophylline (Theo-Dur and others)

Special information if you are pregnant or breastfeeding

You should not use Prevacid NapraPAC during the last 3 months of pregnancy. The risk during the first 6 months has not been fully determined. Notify your doctor if you are pregnant or plan to become pregnant. This drug should be used during pregnancy only if clearly needed.

Prevacid NapraPAC is not recommended for breastfeeding mothers. If this drug is essential to your health, the doctor may have you stop breastfeeding until your treatment is finished.

Recommended dosage

ADULTS

The recommended daily dose is one Prevacid capsule (15 milligrams) and two Naprosyn tablets (either 375 or 500 milligrams). The maximum daily dose of Naprosyn is 1,000 milligrams.

The dose of Naprosyn may need to be reduced in people who are elderly or have liver or kidney problems.

Prevacid NapraPAC has not been studied in children.

Overdosage

Any medication taken in excess can have serious consequences. If you suspect an overdose, seek emergency treatment immediately. At this time, the symptoms of Prevacid overdose are unknown.

■ *Symptoms of Naprosyn overdose may include:*
Drowsiness, heartburn, indigestion, nausea, vomiting

PREVEN

Pronounced: PREH-vin
Generic name: Levonorgestrel and Ethinyl Estradiol

Why is this drug prescribed?

The Preven Emergency Contraception Kit provides "morning after" birth control following a contraceptive failure (for instance, a broken condom) or unprotected intercourse.

The hormone pills in the Preven kit can prevent a pregnancy, but will not end one that's already begun. They work primarily by inhibiting ovulation (release of an egg) and possibly by blocking fertilization and implantation of the egg in the lining of the uterus.

Most important fact about this drug

Preven is meant for emergency use only and not as a regular method of birth control. When taken within 72 hours after unprotected intercourse, the pills in the Preven kit reduce the chance of pregnancy by 75 percent. In contrast, regular use of oral contraceptives slashes the odds of a pregnancy to 0.5 percent or less.

How should you take this medication?

Before you take the pills, you must first take the pregnancy test provided in the kit. You should take the pills only if the test indicates that you are not pregnant.

Take the first dose as soon as possible after intercourse, within 72 hours at the latest. The second dose must be taken exactly 12 hours after the first. Do not take any extra pills. They won't improve your odds of avoiding pregnancy, but they will increase the likelihood of side effects such as nausea and vomiting.

■ *If you miss a dose...*
Call your doctor immediately. Your chances of pregnancy increase when you do not take the pills as prescribed.
■ *Storage instructions...*
Store at room temperature.

What side effects may occur?

About half of the women who use Preven experience temporary nausea, and one woman in five actually vomits. One woman in four suffers temporary menstrual irregularities; 10 to 20 percent develop breast tenderness, and 10 percent have headaches. Less common complaints include abdominal pain and dizziness. Side effects usually disappear within a day or two after taking the pills.

Why should this drug not be prescribed?

The pills in the Preven kit are combination oral contraceptive tablets. Regular use of such pills is not recommended for women with the following conditions:

Blood clots in the deep veins of the legs
Blood clot in the lungs
Diabetes with blood vessel problems
Heart attack
Heart disease
Liver tumors or liver disease
Pregnancy
Severe headaches such as migraines
Severe high blood pressure
A history of stroke
Heavy smoking (more than 15 cigarettes a day) past age 35
An allergy to the pills

If you meet any of these criteria, consult with your doctor about the advisability of using Preven.

Special warnings about this medication

You may notice temporary changes in your menstrual cycle after you use Preven. If your period lasts longer than normal, or fails to start within 21 days after taking the pills, call your doctor. In any event, a follow-up visit with your doctor is recommended after 3 weeks.

If you miss your period after using Preven, do call your doctor as soon as possible, but don't be alarmed. Women who unknowingly take combination oral contraceptives while pregnant do not face any increased risk of harm to the baby.

Preven may not prevent an ectopic pregnancy (pregnancy outside of the womb). This type of pregnancy is a medical emergency. Warning signs include spotting and cramping pain shortly after the first menstrual period following use of Preven. Call your doctor immediately if these symptoms appear.

Although it's not known whether occasional use of Preven has the same effect, regular use of combination oral contraceptives poses a slight risk of blood clots and liver problems. If you develop any of the following warning signs while using (or shortly after using) Preven, call your doctor immediately:

Sharp chest pain, coughing up blood, or sudden shortness of breath (indicates a possible blood clot in the lung)
Pain in the calf (indicates a possible blood clot in the leg)
Crushing chest pain or heaviness in the chest (indicates a possible heart attack)

Sudden severe headache, weakness or numbness in an arm or leg, disturbances of vision or speech, dizziness, confusion, or loss of consciousness (indicates a possible stroke)

Sudden partial or complete loss of vision (indicates a possible blood clot in the eye)

Severe pain or tenderness in the stomach area (indicates liver problems or ectopic pregnancy) in the calf (indicates a possible blood clot in the leg)

Emergency contraception pills, like all oral contraceptives, do not protect against infection with HIV, the virus that causes AIDS, or other sexually transmitted diseases.

Possible food and drug interactions when taking this medication

If Preven is taken with certain other drugs, the effects of either could be increased, decreased, or altered. It is especially important to check with your doctor before combining Preven with the following:

Alcohol
Amitriptyline (Elavil)
Ampicillin (Omnipen, Principen)
Cisapride (Propulsid)
Cyclosporine (Neoral, Sandimmune)
Griseofulvin (Fulvicin, Gris-PEG)
Imipramine (Tofranil)
Metoclopramide (Maxolon and Reglan)
Rifampin (Rifadin, Rimactane)
Seizure medications such as barbiturates, Celontin, Dilantin, Mysoline, Tegretol, and Zarontin
Tetracycline (Achromycin V, Sumycin)
Theophylline (Theo-Dur, Slo-bid)
Vitamin C supplements

Special information if you are pregnant or breastfeeding

If taken by mistake during early pregnancy, Preven is unlikely to cause any harm to the developing baby. The hormones in Preven do appear in breast milk, but do not seem to cause any harm to a nursing infant.

Recommended dosage

ADULTS

There are 4 pills in the Preven Emergency Contraception Kit. The first dose of 2 pills must be taken within 72 hours of unprotected intercourse. The second dose of 2 pills must be taken 12 hours later. If you vomit within 1 hour of taking either dose, check your doctor for further instructions.

Overdosage

An overdose of oral contraceptives poses no danger, though it may cause nausea and vomiting, and, in females, vaginal bleeding. If you suspect an overdose, seek medical attention immediately.

PREVPAC

Pronounced: PREV-pack
Generic name: Amoxicillin, Clarithromycin,
*   and Lansoprazole*

Why is this drug prescribed?

Prevpac is a prepackaged combination of drugs designed to cure duodenal ulcers caused by *H. pylori* bacteria, the most common source of ulcers. With two antibiotics and an acid-blocking agent, Prevpac will eradicate the *H. pylori* infection and improve your odds of remaining ulcer-free. This type of therapy is usually reserved for people with an active ulcer and those who've had one for at least a year.

Most important fact about this drug

Prevpac will work only if you take all the medications as prescribed and finish your entire course of therapy. If you stop too soon, the ulcer may not heal completely and your symptoms may return.

How should you take this medication?

Each pack contains a full day's supply of medication, consisting of two 30-milligram capsules of lansoprazole (Prevacid), four 500-milligram capsules of amoxicillin, and two 500-milligram tablets of clarithromycin (Biaxin). Take half the supply in the morning and the remainder at night. Prevpac can be taken with or without food. Swallow each pill whole; do not crush or chew.

■ *If you miss a dose...*
    Take it as soon as you remember. If it is almost time for your next dose, skip the one you missed and go back to your regular schedule. Do not take 2 doses at the same time.
■ *Storage instructions...*
    Store at room temperature, away from light and moisture.

What side effects may occur?

Side effects cannot be anticipated. If any develop or change in intensity, inform your doctor as soon as possible. Only your doctor can determine if it is safe for you to continue taking Prevpac.

■ *Side effects may include:*
    Diarrhea, headache, taste disturbances

Why should this drug not be prescribed?

You cannot use Prevpac if you've ever had an allergic reaction to antibiotics such as amoxicillin, clarithromycin, erythromycin, penicillin, or Biaxin. Also avoid Prevpac if you've had a reaction to a cephalosporin-type antibiotic such as Ceclor, Duricef, and Keflex.

While on Prevpac therapy, be sure to avoid taking cisapride, pimozide, astemizole, and terfenadine. Combining any of these drugs with Prevpac could cause serious heart irregularities.

Special warnings about this medication

Serious and occasionally fatal allergic reactions have occurred in people taking antibiotics similar to the ones in Prevpac. Seek emergency medical treatment if you develop symptoms such as hives, swelling, itching, fainting, breathing difficulties, or chest pain.

If you develop severe diarrhea after taking Prevpac, call your doctor. Prevpac therapy is not recommended if you have severe kidney disease. Use Prevpac with caution if you are over 65 years old.

Possible food and drug interactions when taking this medication

If Prevpac is taken with certain other drugs, the effects of either could be increased, decreased, or altered. It is especially important to check with your doctor before combining Prevpac with the following:

Alfentanil (Alfenta)
Alprazolam (Xanax)
Ampicillin
Antiarrhythmic heart medications such as quinidine (Quinidex)
   and disopyramide (Norpace)
Astemizole
Blood-thinning pills such as warfarin (Coumadin)
Bromocriptine (Parlodel)
Carbamazepine (Tegretol)
Cholesterol-lowering drugs such as lovastatin (Mevacor) and
   simvastatin (Zocor)
Cilostazol (Pletal)
Cisapride
Cyclosporine (Neoral, Sandimmune)
Digoxin (Lanoxin)
Disopyramide (Norpace)
Ergotamine-based drugs for migraine such as Cafergot, D.H.E. 45
   Injection, Ergostat, and Migranal Nasal Spray
Ketoconazole (Nizoral)
Hexobarbital
Iron supplements
Lovastatin (Mevacor)
Methylprednisolone (Medrol)

Midazolam (Versed)
Phenytoin (Dilantin)
Pimozide
Probenecid
Rifabutin (Mycobutin)
Sildenafil (Viagra)
Sucralfate (Carafate)
Tacrolimus (Prograf)
Terfenadine
Theophylline (Theo-Dur, Theolair)
Triazolam (Halcion)
Valproic acid (Depakene, Depakote)

You should also check with your doctor before combining Prevpac with any drugs used to treat HIV infection.

Special information if you are pregnant or breastfeeding

Do not use Prevpac during pregnancy. The Biaxin component can harm the developing baby. You should also avoid Prevpac while breastfeeding.

Recommended dosage

ADULTS

The recommended dosage is 1 capsule of lansoprazole (Prevacid), 2 capsules of amoxicillin, and 1 tablet of clarithromycin (Biaxin) taken together twice a day (morning and evening) for 10 or 14 days.

Your doctor will adjust your dose if you have kidney problems.

Overdosage

Any medication taken in excess can have serious consequences. If you suspect an overdose of Prevpac, seek medical attention immediately.

PRILOSEC

Pronounced: PRY-low-sek
Generic name: Omeprazole

Why is this drug prescribed?

Prilosec is prescribed for the short-term (4 to 8 weeks) treatment of the following:

Stomach ulcer
Duodenal ulcer (near the exit from the stomach)
Erosive esophagitis (inflammation of the esophagus)
Heartburn and other symptoms of gastroesophageal reflux disease
(also known as GERD), which occurs when stomach acid backs
up into the tube connecting the throat to the stomach.

It is also used to maintain healing of erosive esophagitis and for the long-term treatment of conditions in which too much stomach acid is secreted, including Zollinger-Ellison syndrome, multiple endocrine adenomas (benign tumors), and systemic mastocytosis (cancerous cells).

Combined with the antibiotic clarithromycin (Biaxin) (and sometimes with the antibiotic amoxicillin as well), Prilosec is also used to cure patients whose ulcers are caused by infection with the germ *H. pylori.*

In addition, Prilosec is available as an over-the-counter (OTC) product. However, Prilosec OTC is approved only for frequent heartburn (occurs two or more days a week). The prescription version is still needed for treatment of ulcers, esophagitis, GERD, and other conditions that require monitoring by a doctor.

Most important fact about this drug
Prilosec's healing effect can mask the signs of stomach cancer. Your doctor should be careful to rule out this possibility.

How should you take this medication?
Prilosec works best when taken before meals. It can be taken with an antacid.

The capsule should be swallowed whole. It should not be opened, chewed, or crushed.

If you have difficulty swallowing capsules, you can empty the contents of the Prilosec capsule onto a tablespoonful of applesauce, mix, and swallow with a glass of cool water. Use cool, soft applesauce and do not chew or crush the pellets. Use the mixture immediately. Do not store it for future use.

Avoid excessive amounts of caffeine while taking this drug.

It may take several days for Prilosec to begin relieving stomach pain. Be sure to continue taking the drug exactly as prescribed even if it seems to have no effect.

■ *If you miss a dose...*
Take it as soon as you remember. If it is almost time for your next dose, skip the one you missed and go back to your regular schedule. Do not take 2 doses at once.

■ *Storage information...*
Store at room temperature in a tightly closed container, away from light and moisture.

What side effects may occur?
Side effects cannot be anticipated. If any develop or change in intensity, inform your doctor as soon as possible. Only your doctor can determine if it is safe for you to continue taking Prilosec.

■ *Side effects may include:*
Abdominal pain, diarrhea, headache, nausea, vomiting

Why should this drug not be prescribed?

If you are sensitive to or have ever had an allergic reaction to Prilosec or any of its ingredients, you should not take this medication. Make sure your doctor is aware of any drug reactions you have experienced.

You should avoid the Prilosec/Biaxin combination treatment if you are allergic to certain antibiotics called macrolides or if you are taking Orap.

Special warnings about this medication

Long-term use of this drug can cause severe stomach inflammation.

Possible food and drug interactions when taking this medication

If Prilosec is taken with certain other drugs, the effects of either could be increased, decreased, or altered. It is especially important to check with your doctor before combining Prilosec with the following:

Ampicillin-containing drugs such as Unasyn
Cyclosporine (Sandimmune, Neoral)
Diazepam (Valium)
Disulfiram (Antabuse)
Iron
Ketoconazole (Nizoral)
Phenytoin (Dilantin)
Warfarin (Coumadin)

Special information if you are pregnant or breastfeeding

The effects of Prilosec during pregnancy have not been adequately studied. If you are pregnant or plan to become pregnant, inform your doctor immediately. Avoid combined therapy with Biaxin unless there is no alternative. Prilosec (and Biaxin) may appear in breast milk and could affect a nursing infant. If this medication is essential to your health, your doctor may advise you to discontinue breastfeeding until your treatment with this medication is finished.

Recommended dosage

ADULTS

Short-term Treatment of Active Duodenal Ulcer
The usual dose is 20 milligrams once a day. Most people heal within 4 weeks, although some require an additional 4 weeks of Prilosec therapy.

Treatment of Duodenal Ulcers Caused by H. Pylori
In combination therapy with Biaxin alone, the usual dosage is 40 milligrams of Prilosec once daily and 500 milligrams of Biaxin 3 times a day for 14 days, followed by 20 milligrams of Prilosec once daily for an additional 14 days.

If amoxicillin is included in the treatment, the recommended dosage is

20 milligrams of Prilosec, 500 milligrams of Biaxin, and 1,000 milligrams of amoxicillin twice a day for 10 days, followed by 20 milligrams of Prilosec once daily for an additional 18 days.

Gastric Ulcer
The usual dose is 40 milligrams once a day for 4 to 8 weeks.

Gastroesophageal Reflux Disease (GERD)
The usual dose for people with symptoms of GERD is 20 milligrams daily for up to 4 weeks. For erosive esophagitis accompanied by GERD symptoms, the usual dose is 20 milligrams a day for 4 to 8 weeks.
   The dose may be continued to maintain healing.

Pathological Hypersecretory Conditions
The usual starting dose is 60 milligrams once a day. If you take more than 80 milligrams a day, your doctor will divide the total into smaller doses. The dosing will be based on your needs.

CHILDREN 2 TO 16 YEARS OLD

Gastroesophageal Reflux Disease (GERD) and Acid-Related Disorders
For children weighing less than 44 pounds, the usual dose is 10 milligrams a day. For those weighing 44 pounds or more, the usual dose is 20 milligrams a day. For children with erosive esophagitis, your doctor will determine the correct dose based on the child's weight.

The safety and effectiveness of Prilosec have not been studied in children under 2 years old.

Overdosage
Overdose with Prilosec has been rare, but any medication taken in excess can have serious consequences. If you suspect an overdose, seek medical attention immediately.

■ *Symptoms of Prilosec overdose may include:*
   Blurred vision, confusion, drowsiness, dry mouth, flushing, headache, nausea, rapid heartbeat, sweating, vomiting

Primidone *See Mysoline, page 908.*

Principen *See Ampicillin, page 98.*

Prinivil *See Zestril, page 1624.*

Prinzide *See Zestoretic, page 1621.*

Procainamide *See Procanbid, page 1159.*

PROCANBID

Pronounced: PROH-can-bid
Generic name: Procainamide hydrochloride
Other brand names: Pronestyl, Pronestyl-SR

Why is this drug prescribed?

Procanbid is used to treat severe irregular heartbeats (arrhythmias). Arrhythmias are generally divided into two main types: heartbeats that are faster than normal (tachycardia), and heartbeats that are slower than normal (bradycardia). Irregular heartbeats are often caused by drugs or disease but can occur in otherwise healthy people with no history of heart disease or other illness.

Most important fact about this drug

Procanbid can cause serious blood disorders, especially during the first 3 months of treatment. Be sure to notify your doctor if you notice any of the following: joint or muscle pain, dark urine, yellowing of skin or eyes, muscular weakness, chest or abdominal pain, appetite loss, diarrhea, hallucinations, dizziness, depression, wheezing, cough, easy bruising or bleeding, tremors, palpitations, rash, soreness or ulcers in the mouth, sore throat, nausea, vomiting, fever, and chills.

How should you take this medication?

Take only your prescribed doses of Procanbid; never take more.

Procanbid should be swallowed whole. Do not break or chew the tablet. You may see remnants of the tablet in your stool, since it does not disintegrate following release of procainamide.

Try not to miss any doses. Skipping doses, changing the intervals between doses, or making up missed doses by doubling up later may cause your condition to worsen and could be dangerous.

- *If you miss a dose...*
  Take it as soon as you remember. If it is almost time for your next dose, skip the one you missed and go back to your regular schedule. Never take 2 doses at the same time.
- *Storage instructions...*
  Store at room temperature in a tightly closed container, away from heat, light, and moisture.

What side effects may occur?

Side effects cannot be anticipated. If any develop or change in intensity, inform your doctor as soon as possible. Only your doctor can determine if it is safe for you to continue taking Procanbid.

- *Side effects may include:*
  Abdominal pain, bitter taste, blood disorders, chest pain, chills, diarrhea, dizziness, fever, flushing, giddiness, hallucinations, hives, itch-

ing, joint pain or inflammation, loss of appetite, low blood pressure, mental depression, muscle pain, nausea, rash, skin lesions, swelling, vague feeling of illness, vomiting, weakness

Why should this drug not be prescribed?

Procanbid should not be taken if you have the heart irregularity known as complete heart block or incomplete heart block without a pacemaker, or if you have ever had an allergic reaction to procaine or similar local anesthetics.

Your doctor will not prescribe this drug if you have been diagnosed with the connective tissue disease lupus erythematosus or the heartbeat irregularity known as torsades de pointes.

Special warnings about this medication

To check for the serious blood disorders that can develop during Procanbid therapy, your doctor will do a complete blood count weekly for the first 12 weeks and will continue to monitor your blood count carefully after that.

If you develop a fever, chills, sore throat or mouth, bruising or bleeding, infections, chest or abdominal pain, loss of appetite, weakness, muscle or joint pain, skin rash, nausea, fluttery heartbeat, vomiting, diarrhea, hallucinations, dizziness, depression, wheezing, yellow eyes and skin, or dark urine, contact your doctor immediately. It could indicate a serious illness.

Be sure your doctor knows if you have ever had congestive heart failure or other types of heart disease.

Your doctor will prescribe Procanbid along with other antiarrhythmic drugs, such as quinidine or disopyramide, only if they have been tried and have not worked when used alone.

If you have ever had kidney disease, liver disease, or myasthenia gravis (a disease that causes muscle weakness, especially in the face and neck), your doctor will watch you carefully while you are taking Procanbid.

Make sure your doctor is aware of any drug reactions you have experienced, especially to procaine, other local anesthetics, or aspirin.

Procanbid has been known to trigger a disorder similar to lupus erythematosus. Notify your doctor if you develop any of the following lupus-like symptoms: joint pain or inflammation, abdominal or chest pain, fever, chills, muscle pain, skin lesions.

Doses of this medication must be very precise. Different brands of procainamide have different dosing instructions. If your prescription looks different in any way, ask your doctor or pharmacist to check it and make sure it was dispensed correctly.

Possible food and drug interactions when taking this medication

If Procanbid is taken with certain other drugs, the effects of either could be increased, decreased, or altered. It is especially important to check with your doctor before combining Procanbid with the following:

Alcohol
Amiodarone (Cordarone)
Antiarrhythmic drugs such as quinidine (Quinidex) and mexiletine
  (Mexitil)
Cimetidine (Tagamet)
Drugs that ease muscle spasms, such as Cogentin and Artane
Lidocaine
Ranitidine (Zantac)
Trimethoprim (Proloprim)

Special information if you are pregnant or breastfeeding

The effects of Procanbid during pregnancy have not been adequately studied. If you are pregnant or plan to become pregnant, inform your doctor immediately. Procanbid appears in breast milk and may affect a nursing infant. If this medication is essential to your health, your doctor may advise you to discontinue breastfeeding until your treatment is finished.

Recommended dosage

ADULTS

Your dosage will be based on your doctor's assessment of the degree of underlying heart disease, your age, your weight, and the way your kidneys are functioning. The following is a general guide for determining the dose of Procanbid by body weight. (The dose of other brands will be different.) Your dose may be higher or lower, depending on your individual circumstances. Doses are usually taken every 12 hours.

88–110 pounds—1,000 milligrams
132–154 pounds—1,500 milligrams
176–198 pounds—2,000 milligrams
More than 220 pounds—2,500 milligrams

CHILDREN

The safety and effectiveness of this drug have not been established in children.

OLDER ADULTS

Older people, especially those over 50 years of age, or those with reduced kidney, liver, or heart function, get lower doses or wait a longer time between doses.

Overdosage

Any medication taken in excess can have serious consequences. If you suspect an overdose, seek medical treatment immediately.

■ *Symptoms of Procanbid overdose may include:*
Changes in heart function and heartbeat

PROCARDIA

Pronounced: pro-CAR-dee-uh
Generic name: Nifedipine
Other brand names: Procardia XL, Adalat, Adalat CC

Why is this drug prescribed?

Procardia and Procardia XL are used to treat angina (chest pain caused by lack of oxygen to the heart due to clogged arteries or spasm of the arteries). Procardia XL is also used to treat high blood pressure. Procardia and Procardia XL are calcium channel blockers. They ease the workload of the heart by relaxing the muscles in the walls of the arteries, allowing them to dilate. This improves blood flow through the heart and throughout the body, reduces blood pressure, and helps prevent angina. Procardia XL is taken once a day and provides a steady rate of medication over a 24-hour period.

Most important fact about this drug

If you have high blood pressure, you must take Procardia XL regularly for it to be effective. Since blood pressure declines gradually, it may be several weeks before you get the full benefit of Procardia XL; and you must continue taking it even if you are feeling well. Procardia XL does not cure high blood pressure; it merely keeps it under control.

How should you take this medication?

Procardia and Procardia XL should be taken exactly as prescribed by your doctor, even if your symptoms have disappeared.

Procardia XL tablets are specially designed to release the medication into your bloodstream slowly. As a result, something that looks like a tablet may occasionally appear in your stool. This is normal and simply means that the medication has been released, and the shell that contained the medication has been eliminated from your body.

Procardia and Procardia XL tablets should be swallowed whole. Do not break, crush, or chew.

Procardia and Procardia XL can be taken with or without food. Adalat CC should be taken on an empty stomach.

Do not substitute another brand of nifedipine for Procardia or Procardia XL unless your doctor directs.

Procardia XL should be taken once a day. You can take it in the morning or evening, but should hold to the same time each day.

■ *If you miss a dose...*
Take the forgotten dose as soon as you remember. If it is almost time for your next dose, skip the one you missed. Never take 2 doses at the same time.

MEDROL

(methylprednisolone)
PHARMACIA & UPJOHN

2 mg

4 mg

8 mg

16 mg

MERIDIA

(sibutramine HCl monohydrate)
ABBOTT

5 mg

10 mg

15 mg

METAGLIP

(glipizide/metformin HCl)
BRISTOL-MYERS SQUIBB

2.5 mg/250 mg

2.5 mg/500 mg

5 mg/500 mg

MEVACOR

(lovastatin)
MERCK & CO., INC.

10 mg

20 mg

40 mg

MICARDIS

(telmisartan)
BOEHRINGER INGELHEIM

40 mg

80 mg

MICARDIS HCT

(telmisartan/
hydrochlorothiazide)
BOEHRINGER INGELHEIM

40 mg/12.5 mg

80 mg/12.5 mg

80 mg/12.5 mg

MIDRIN

(isometheptene mucate/
dichloralphenazone/
acetaminophen)
WOMEN'S FIRST HEALTHCARE

65 mg/100 mg/325 mg

MINOCIN

(minocycline HCl)
WYETH

50 mg

100 mg

MIRAPEX

(pramipexole dihydrochloride)
PHARMACIA & UPJOHN

0.125 mg

0.25 mg

0.5 mg

1 mg

1.5 mg

MOBAN

(molindone HCl)
ENDO PHARMACEUTICALS

5 mg

10 mg

25 mg

50 mg

100 mg

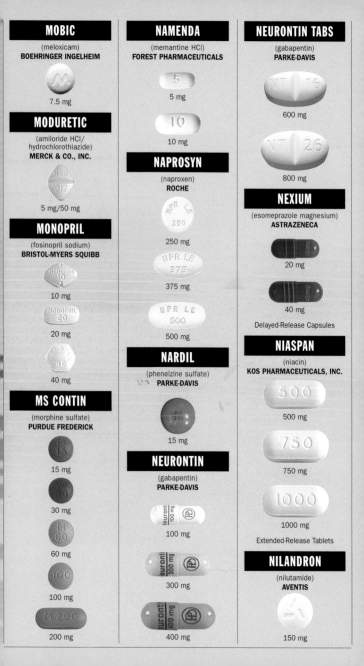

MOBIC
(meloxicam)
BOEHRINGER INGELHEIM

7.5 mg

MODURETIC
(amiloride HCl/
hydrochlorothiazide)
MERCK & CO., INC.

5 mg/50 mg

MONOPRIL
(fosinopril sodium)
BRISTOL-MYERS SQUIBB

10 mg

20 mg

40 mg

MS CONTIN
(morphine sulfate)
PURDUE FREDERICK

15 mg

30 mg

60 mg

100 mg

200 mg

NAMENDA
(memantine HCl)
FOREST PHARMACEUTICALS

5 mg

10 mg

NAPROSYN
(naproxen)
ROCHE

250 mg

375 mg

500 mg

NARDIL
(phenelzine sulfate)
PARKE-DAVIS

15 mg

NEURONTIN
(gabapentin)
PARKE-DAVIS

100 mg

300 mg

400 mg

NEURONTIN TABS
(gabapentin)
PARKE-DAVIS

600 mg

800 mg

NEXIUM
(esomeprazole magnesium)
ASTRAZENECA

20 mg

40 mg

Delayed-Release Capsules

NIASPAN
(niacin)
KOS PHARMACEUTICALS, INC.

500 mg

750 mg

1000 mg

Extended-Release Tablets

NILANDRON
(nilutamide)
AVENTIS

150 mg

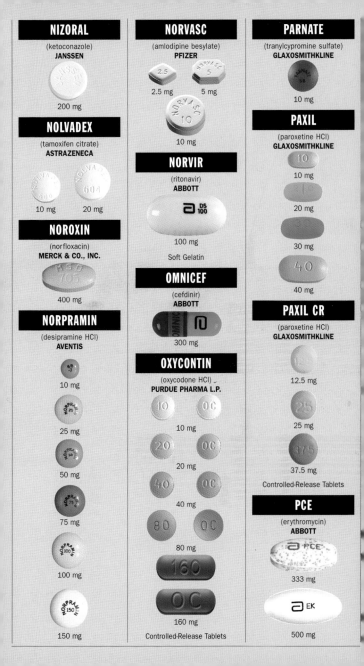

NIZORAL

(ketoconazole)
JANSSEN

200 mg

NOLVADEX

(tamoxifen citrate)
ASTRAZENECA

10 mg   20 mg

NOROXIN

(norfloxacin)
MERCK & CO., INC.

400 mg

NORPRAMIN

(desipramine HCl)
AVENTIS

10 mg

25 mg

50 mg

75 mg

100 mg

150 mg

NORVASC

(amlodipine besylate)
PFIZER

2.5 mg   5 mg

10 mg

NORVIR

(ritonavir)
ABBOTT

100 mg

Soft Gelatin

OMNICEF

(cefdinir)
ABBOTT

300 mg

OXYCONTIN

(oxycodone HCl)
PURDUE PHARMA L.P.

10 mg

20 mg

40 mg

80 mg

160 mg

Controlled-Release Tablets

PARNATE

(tranylcypromine sulfate)
GLAXOSMITHKLINE

10 mg

PAXIL

(paroxetine HCl)
GLAXOSMITHKLINE

10 mg

20 mg

30 mg

40 mg

PAXIL CR

(paroxetine HCl)
GLAXOSMITHKLINE

12.5 mg

25 mg

37.5 mg

Controlled-Release Tablets

PCE

(erythromycin)
ABBOTT

333 mg

500 mg

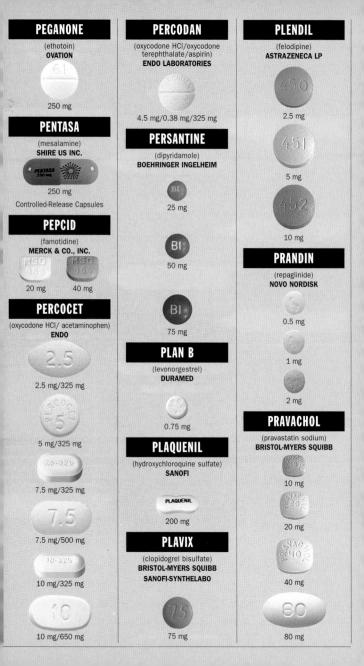

PEGANONE

(ethotoin)
OVATION

250 mg

PENTASA

(mesalamine)
SHIRE US INC.

250 mg

Controlled-Release Capsules

PEPCID

(famotidine)
MERCK & CO., INC.

20 mg   40 mg

PERCOCET

(oxycodone HCl/ acetaminophen)
ENDO

2.5 mg/325 mg

5 mg/325 mg

7.5 mg/325 mg

7.5 mg/500 mg

10 mg/325 mg

10 mg/650 mg

PERCODAN

(oxycodone HCl/oxycodone
terephthalate/aspirin)
ENDO LABORATORIES

4.5 mg/0.38 mg/325 mg

PERSANTINE

(dipyridamole)
BOEHRINGER INGELHEIM

25 mg

50 mg

75 mg

PLAN B

(levonorgestrel)
DURAMED

0.75 mg

PLAQUENIL

(hydroxychloroquine sulfate)
SANOFI

PLAQUENIL

200 mg

PLAVIX

(clopidogrel bisulfate)
BRISTOL-MYERS SQUIBB
SANOFI-SYNTHELABO

75 mg

PLENDIL

(felodipine)
ASTRAZENECA LP

2.5 mg

5 mg

10 mg

PRANDIN

(repaglinide)
NOVO NORDISK

0.5 mg

1 mg

2 mg

PRAVACHOL

(pravastatin sodium)
BRISTOL-MYERS SQUIBB

10 mg

20 mg

40 mg

80 mg

PRECOSE

(acarbose)
BAYER

25 mg

50 mg

100 mg

PREMARIN

(conjugated estrogens)
WYETH

0.3 mg

0.45 mg

0.625 mg

0.9 mg

1.25 mg

PREMPHASE

(conjugated estrogens/
medroxyprogesterone acetate)
WYETH

0.625 mg | 5 mg

PREVACID

(lansoprazole)
TAP

15 mg

30 mg

Delayed-Release Capsules

PRILOSEC

(omeprazole)
ASTRAZENECA LP

10 mg

20 mg

40 mg

PRINIVIL

(lisinopril)
MERCK & CO., INC.

2.5 mg

5 mg

10 mg

20 mg

40 mg

PRINZIDE

(lisinopril/hydrochlorothiazide)
MERCK & CO., INC.

10 mg/12.5 mg

20 mg/12.5 mg

20 mg/25 mg

PROMETRIUM

(progesterone, USP)
SOLVAY PHARMACEUTICALS,

100 mg

200 mg

PROPECIA

(finasteride)
MERCK & CO., INC.

1 mg

PROSCAR

(finasteride)
MERCK & CO., INC.

5 mg

PROTONIX

(pantoprazole sodium)
WYETH

20 mg

40 mg

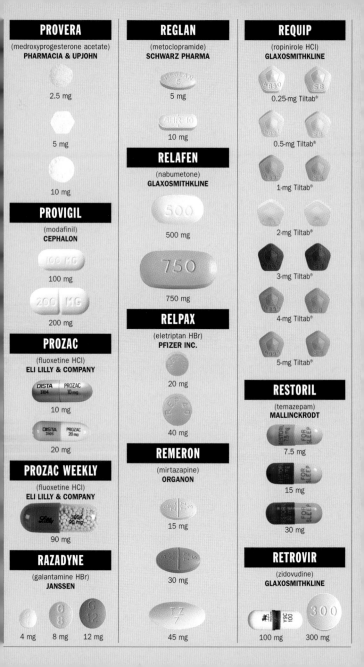

PROVERA
(medroxyprogesterone acetate)
PHARMACIA & UPJOHN

2.5 mg

5 mg

10 mg

PROVIGIL
(modafinil)
CEPHALON

100 mg

200 mg

PROZAC
(fluoxetine HCl)
ELI LILLY & COMPANY

DISTA 3104 | PROZAC 10 mg
10 mg

DISTA 3105 | PROZAC 20 mg
20 mg

PROZAC WEEKLY
(fluoxetine HCl)
ELI LILLY & COMPANY

Lilly 3004 90 mg
90 mg

RAZADYNE
(galantamine HBr)
JANSSEN

4 mg 8 mg 12 mg

REGLAN
(metoclopramide)
SCHWARZ PHARMA

5 mg

10 mg

RELAFEN
(nabumetone)
GLAXOSMITHKLINE

500 mg

750 mg

RELPAX
(eletriptan HBr)
PFIZER INC.

20 mg

40 mg

REMERON
(mirtazapine)
ORGANON

15 mg

30 mg

45 mg

REQUIP
(ropinirole HCl)
GLAXOSMITHKLINE

0.25-mg Tiltab®

0.5-mg Tiltab®

1-mg Tiltab®

2-mg Tiltab®

3-mg Tiltab®

4-mg Tiltab®

5-mg Tiltab®

RESTORIL
(temazepam)
MALLINCKRODT

7.5 mg

15 mg

30 mg

RETROVIR
(zidovudine)
GLAXOSMITHKLINE

100 mg 300 mg

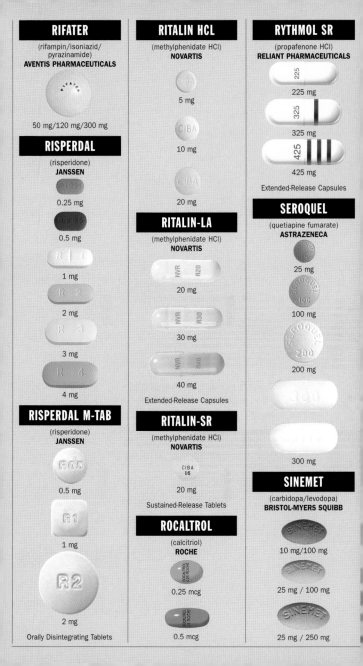

RIFATER

(rifampin/isoniazid/
pyrazinamide)
AVENTIS PHARMACEUTICALS

50 mg/120 mg/300 mg

RISPERDAL

(risperidone)
JANSSEN

0.25 mg

0.5 mg

1 mg

2 mg

3 mg

4 mg

RISPERDAL M-TAB

(risperidone)
JANSSEN

0.5 mg

1 mg

2 mg

Orally Disintegrating Tablets

RITALIN HCL

(methylphenidate HCl)
NOVARTIS

5 mg

10 mg

20 mg

RITALIN-LA

(methylphenidate HCl)
NOVARTIS

20 mg

30 mg

40 mg

Extended-Release Capsules

RITALIN-SR

(methylphenidate HCl)
NOVARTIS

20 mg

Sustained-Release Tablets

ROCALTROL

(calcitriol)
ROCHE

0.25 mcg

0.5 mcg

RYTHMOL SR

(propafenone HCl)
RELIANT PHARMACEUTICALS

225 mg

325 mg

425 mg

Extended-Release Capsules

SEROQUEL

(quetiapine fumarate)
ASTRAZENECA

25 mg

100 mg

200 mg

300 mg

SINEMET

(carbidopa/levodopa)
BRISTOL-MYERS SQUIBB

10 mg/100 mg

25 mg / 100 mg

25 mg / 250 mg

SINEMET CR

(carbidopa/levodopa)
BRISTOL-MYERS SQUIBB

25 mg / 100 mg

50 mg / 200 mg

Sustained-Release Tablets

SINGULAIR

(montelukast sodium)
MERCK & CO., INC.

4 mg
Chewable

5 mg
Chewable

10 mg

SKELAXIN

(metaxalone)
KING PHARMACEUTICALS

800 mg

SOMA

(carisoprodol)
WALLACE

350 mg

SONATA

(zaleplon)
KING PHARMACEUTICALS

5 mg

10 mg

SORIATANE

(acitretin)
CONNECTICS

10 mg

25 mg

SPECTRACEF

(cefditoren/pivoxil)
PURDUE

Purdue
200 mg

200 mg

SPORANOX

(itraconazole)
JANSSEN

100 mg

STALEVO

(carbidopa/levodopa/
entacapone)
NOVARTIS

12.5 mg/50 mg/200 mg

25 mg/100 mg/200 mg

37.5 mg/150 mg/200 mg

STARLIX

(nateglinide)
NOVARTIS

60 mg

120 mg

STRATTERA

(atomoxetine HCl)
ELI LILLY & COMPANY

10 mg

18 mg

25 mg

40 mg

60 mg

STRIANT

(testosterone buccal system)
COLUMBIA

30 mg

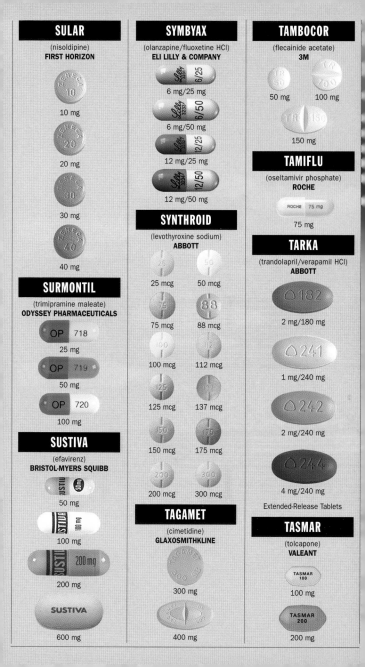

SULAR
(nisoldipine)
FIRST HORIZON

10 mg

20 mg

30 mg

40 mg

SURMONTIL
(trimipramine maleate)
ODYSSEY PHARMACEUTICALS

OP 718
25 mg

OP 719
50 mg

OP 720
100 mg

SUSTIVA
(efavirenz)
BRISTOL-MYERS SQUIBB

50 mg

100 mg

200 mg

SUSTIVA
600 mg

SYMBYAX
(olanzapine/fluoxetine HCl)
ELI LILLY & COMPANY

Lilly 6/25
6 mg/25 mg

Lilly 6/50
6 mg/50 mg

Lilly 12/25
12 mg/25 mg

Lilly 12/50
12 mg/50 mg

SYNTHROID
(levothyroxine sodium)
ABBOTT

25
25 mcg

50
50 mcg

75
75 mcg

88
88 mcg

100
100 mcg

112 mcg

125
125 mcg

137 mcg

150
150 mcg

175
175 mcg

200
200 mcg

300
300 mcg

TAGAMET
(cimetidine)
GLAXOSMITHKLINE

300 mg

400 mg

TAMBOCOR
(flecainide acetate)
3M

TR 50
50 mg

TR 100
100 mg

TR 150
150 mg

TAMIFLU
(oseltamivir phosphate)
ROCHE

ROCHE 75 mg
75 mg

TARKA
(trandolapril/verapamil HCl)
ABBOTT

182
2 mg/180 mg

241
1 mg/240 mg

242
2 mg/240 mg

244
4 mg/240 mg

Extended-Release Tablets

TASMAR
(tolcapone)
VALEANT

TASMAR 100
100 mg

TASMAR 200
200 mg

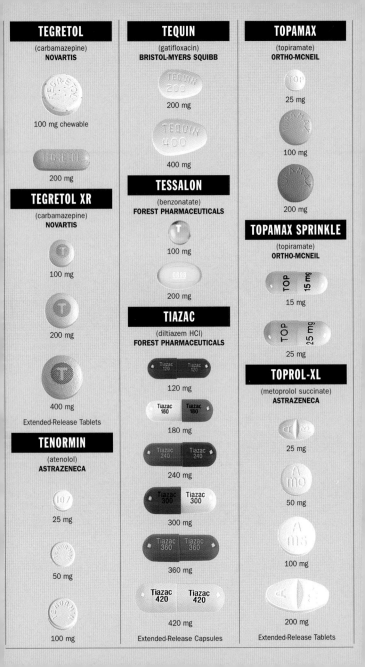

TEGRETOL
(carbamazepine)
NOVARTIS

100 mg chewable

200 mg

TEGRETOL XR
(carbamazepine)
NOVARTIS

100 mg

200 mg

400 mg

Extended-Release Tablets

TENORMIN
(atenolol)
ASTRAZENECA

25 mg

50 mg

100 mg

TEQUIN
(gatifloxacin)
BRISTOL-MYERS SQUIBB

200 mg

400 mg

TESSALON
(benzonatate)
FOREST PHARMACEUTICALS

100 mg

200 mg

TIAZAC
(diltiazem HCl)
FOREST PHARMACEUTICALS

120 mg

180 mg

240 mg

300 mg

360 mg

420 mg

Extended-Release Capsules

TOPAMAX
(topiramate)
ORTHO-MCNEIL

25 mg

100 mg

200 mg

TOPAMAX SPRINKLE
(topiramate)
ORTHO-MCNEIL

15 mg

25 mg

TOPROL-XL
(metoprolol succinate)
ASTRAZENECA

25 mg

50 mg

100 mg

200 mg

Extended-Release Tablets

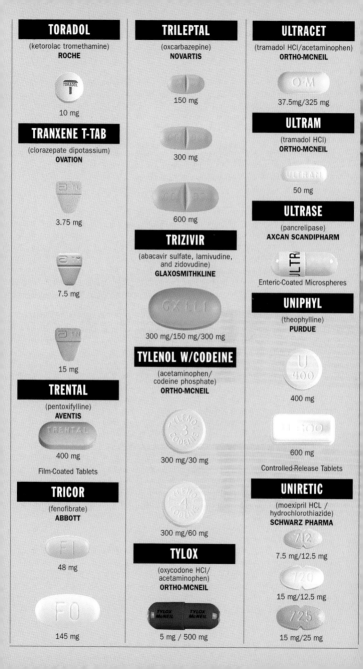

TORADOL
(ketorolac tromethamine)
ROCHE

10 mg

TRANXENE T-TAB
(clorazepate dipotassium)
OVATION

3.75 mg

7.5 mg

15 mg

TRENTAL
(pentoxifylline)
AVENTIS

400 mg

Film-Coated Tablets

TRICOR
(fenofibrate)
ABBOTT

48 mg

145 mg

TRILEPTAL
(oxcarbazepine)
NOVARTIS

150 mg

300 mg

600 mg

TRIZIVIR
(abacavir sulfate, lamivudine,
and zidovudine)
GLAXOSMITHKLINE

300 mg/150 mg/300 mg

TYLENOL W/CODEINE
(acetaminophen/
codeine phosphate)
ORTHO-MCNEIL

300 mg/30 mg

300 mg/60 mg

TYLOX
(oxycodone HCl/
acetaminophen)
ORTHO-MCNEIL

5 mg / 500 mg

ULTRACET
(tramadol HCl/acetaminophen)
ORTHO-MCNEIL

37.5mg/325 mg

ULTRAM
(tramadol HCl)
ORTHO-MCNEIL

50 mg

ULTRASE
(pancrelipase)
AXCAN SCANDIPHARM

Enteric-Coated Microspheres

UNIPHYL
(theophylline)
PURDUE

400 mg

600 mg

Controlled-Release Tablets

UNIRETIC
(moexipril HCL /
hydrochlorothiazide)
SCHWARZ PHARMA

7.5 mg/12.5 mg

15 mg/12.5 mg

15 mg/25 mg

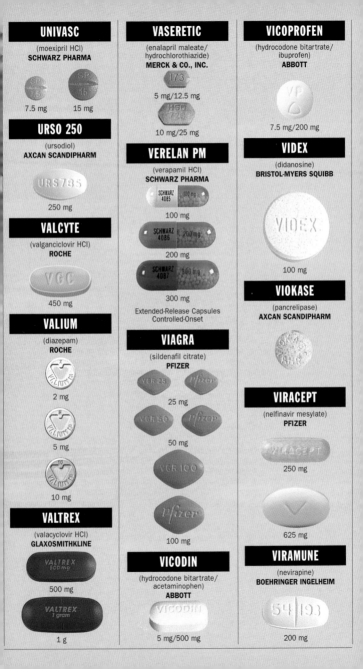

UNIVASC

(moexipril HCl)
SCHWARZ PHARMA

7.5 mg   15 mg

URSO 250

(ursodiol)
AXCAN SCANDIPHARM

URS785

250 mg

VALCYTE

(valganciclovir HCl)
ROCHE

VGC

450 mg

VALIUM

(diazepam)
ROCHE

2 mg

5 mg

10 mg

VALTREX

(valacyclovir HCl)
GLAXOSMITHKLINE

VALTREX
500 mg

500 mg

VALTREX
1 gram

1 g

VASERETIC

(enalapril maleate/
hydrochlorothiazide)
MERCK & CO., INC.

173

5 mg/12.5 mg

MSD
718

10 mg/25 mg

VERELAN PM

(verapamil HCl)
SCHWARZ PHARMA

SCHWARZ 100 mg
4085

100 mg

SCHWARZ 200 mg
4086

200 mg

SCHWARZ 300 mg
4087

300 mg

Extended-Release Capsules
Controlled-Onset

VIAGRA

(sildenafil citrate)
PFIZER

VGR 25   Pfizer

25 mg

VGR 50   Pfizer

50 mg

VGR 100

Pfizer

100 mg

VICODIN

(hydrocodone bitartrate/
acetaminophen)
ABBOTT

VICODIN

5 mg/500 mg

VICOPROFEN

(hydrocodone bitartrate/
ibuprofen)
ABBOTT

VP

7.5 mg/200 mg

VIDEX

(didanosine)
BRISTOL-MYERS SQUIBB

VIDEX

100 mg

VIOKASE

(pancrelipase)
AXCAN SCANDIPHARM

SK&F
AHR

VIRACEPT

(nelfinavir mesylate)
PFIZER

VIRACEPT

250 mg

625 mg

VIRAMUNE

(nevirapine)
BOEHRINGER INGELHEIM

54 193

200 mg

VIREAD
(tenofovir disoproxil fumarate)
GILEAD SCIENCES, INC.
300 mg

VIVACTIL
(protriptyline HCl)
ODYSSEY PHARMACEUTICALS
5 mg
10 mg

VOLTAREN
(diclofenac sodium)
NOVARTIS
25 mg   50 mg
75 mg

VOLTAREN-XR
(diclofenac sodium)
NOVARTIS
100 mg

VYTORIN
(ezetimibe/simvastatin)
MERCK/SCHERING-PLOUGH
10/10 mg   10/20 mg
10/40 mg
10/80 mg

WELCHOL
(colesevelam HCl)
SANKYO PHARMA
625 mg

WELLBUTRIN
(bupropion HCl)
GLAXOSMITHKLINE
75 mg
100 mg

WELLBUTRIN SR
(bupropion HCl)
GLAXOSMITHKLINE
100 mg
150 mg
200 mg
Sustained-Release Tablets

WELLBUTRIN XL
(bupropion HCl)
GLAXOSMITHKLINE
150 mg   300 mg
Extended-Release Tablets

XANAX
(alprazolam)
PHARMACIA & UPJOHN
0.25 mg
0.5 mg
1 mg
2 mg

XANAX XR
(alprazolam)
PHARMACIA & UPJOHN
0.5 mg
1 mg
2 mg
3 mg
Extended-Release Tablets

XENICAL
(orlistat)
ROCHE
120 mg

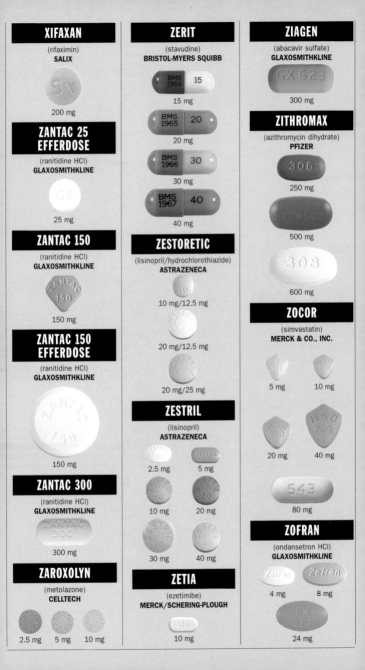

XIFAXAN
(rifaximin)
SALIX

SX

200 mg

ZANTAC 25 EFFERDOSE
(ranitidine HCl)
GLAXOSMITHKLINE

GS

25 mg

ZANTAC 150
(ranitidine HCl)
GLAXOSMITHKLINE

ZANTAC 150

150 mg

ZANTAC 150 EFFERDOSE
(ranitidine HCl)
GLAXOSMITHKLINE

ZANTAC 150

150 mg

ZANTAC 300
(ranitidine HCl)
GLAXOSMITHKLINE

ZANTAC 300

300 mg

ZAROXOLYN
(metolazone)
CELLTECH

2.5 mg   5 mg   10 mg

ZERIT
(stavudine)
BRISTOL-MYERS SQUIBB

BMS 1964 | 15

15 mg

BMS 1965 | 20

20 mg

BMS 1966 | 30

30 mg

BMS 1967 | 40

40 mg

ZESTORETIC
(lisinopril/hydrochlorothiazide)
ASTRAZENECA

141

10 mg/12.5 mg

20 mg/12.5 mg

20 mg/25 mg

ZESTRIL
(lisinopril)
ASTRAZENECA

2.5 mg   5 mg

10 mg   20 mg

30 mg   40 mg

ZETIA
(ezetimibe)
MERCK/SCHERING-PLOUGH

414

10 mg

ZIAGEN
(abacavir sulfate)
GLAXOSMITHKLINE

GX G23

300 mg

ZITHROMAX
(azithromycin dihydrate)
PFIZER

306

250 mg

ZTM 500

500 mg

308

600 mg

ZOCOR
(simvastatin)
MERCK & CO., INC.

5 mg   10 mg

MSD 749

20 mg   40 mg

543

80 mg

ZOFRAN
(ondansetron HCl)
GLAXOSMITHKLINE

Zofran   Zofran

4 mg   8 mg

GX CF7

24 mg

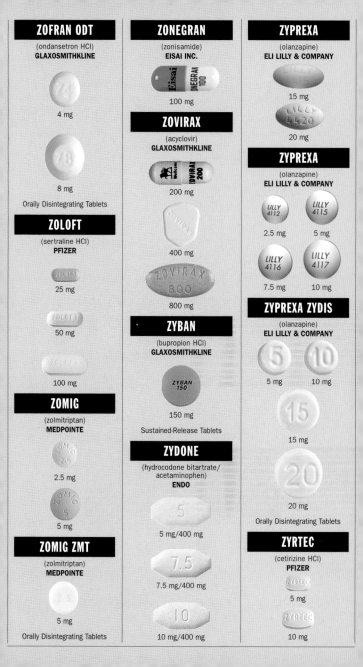

ZOFRAN ODT
(ondansetron HCl)
GLAXOSMITHKLINE

4 mg

8 mg

Orally Disintegrating Tablets

ZOLOFT
(sertraline HCl)
PFIZER

25 mg

50 mg

100 mg

ZOMIG
(zolmitriptan)
MEDPOINTE

2.5 mg

5 mg

ZOMIG ZMT
(zolmitriptan)
MEDPOINTE

5 mg

Orally Disintegrating Tablets

ZONEGRAN
(zonisamide)
EISAI INC.

100 mg

ZOVIRAX
(acyclovir)
GLAXOSMITHKLINE

200 mg

400 mg

800 mg

ZYBAN
(bupropion HCl)
GLAXOSMITHKLINE

150 mg

Sustained-Release Tablets

ZYDONE
(hydrocodone bitartrate/
acetaminophen)
ENDO

5 mg/400 mg

7.5 mg/400 mg

10 mg/400 mg

ZYPREXA
(olanzapine)
ELI LILLY & COMPANY

15 mg

20 mg

ZYPREXA
(olanzapine)
ELI LILLY & COMPANY

2.5 mg

5 mg

7.5 mg

10 mg

ZYPREXA ZYDIS
(olanzapine)
ELI LILLY & COMPANY

5 mg

10 mg

15 mg

20 mg

Orally Disintegrating Tablets

ZYRTEC
(cetirizine HCl)
PFIZER

5 mg

10 mg

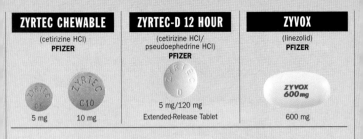

ZYRTEC CHEWABLE	ZYRTEC-D 12 HOUR	ZYVOX
(cetirizine HCl) **PFIZER**	(cetirizine HCl/ pseudoephedrine HCl) **PFIZER**	(linezolid) **PFIZER**
5 mg 10 mg	5 mg/120 mg Extended-Release Tablet	600 mg

Note: While every effort has been made to ensure the faithful reproduction of the product photos in this section, changes in medication size, color, and design are always a possibility. Likewise, all available dosage forms and strengths may not be pictured. When in doubt, it's best to confirm a product's identity with your doctor or pharmacist.

■ *Storage instructions…*
Procardia and Procardia XL can be stored at room temperature. Protect from moisture, light, humidity, and excessive heat.

What side effects may occur?

Side effects cannot be anticipated. If any develop or change in intensity, inform your doctor as soon as possible. Only your doctor can determine whether it is safe for you to continue taking Procardia or Procardia XL.

■ *Side effects may include:*
Constipation, cough, dizziness, fatigue, flushing, giddiness, headache, heartburn, heat sensation, light-headedness, mood changes, muscle cramps, nasal congestion, nausea, sore throat, swelling of arms, legs, hands, and feet, tremors, wheezing

Why should this drug not be prescribed?

Procardia should not be used if you have ever had an allergic reaction to it or are sensitive to it or other calcium channel blockers (Adalat, Calan, others). Make sure your doctor is aware of any drug reactions you have experienced.

Special warnings about this medication

Procardia and Procardia XL may cause your blood pressure to become too low, which may make you feel light-headed or faint. This is more likely to happen when you start taking the medication and when the amount you take is increased. It is also more likely to occur if you are also taking a beta-blocker heart medication such as Tenormin or Inderal. Your doctor should check your blood pressure when you start taking Procardia or Procardia XL and continue monitoring it while your dosage is being adjusted.

Procardia XL can be used for high blood pressure; plain Procardia should be used only for angina—*not* for high blood pressure.

Do not take Procardia for the first week or two following a heart attack, or if you are in danger of a heart attack.

There is a remote possibility of experiencing increased angina when you start taking Procardia or Procardia XL, or when your dosage is increased. If this happens, contact your doctor immediately.

You may have angina pain if you suddenly stop taking beta-blockers when beginning Procardia therapy. Your doctor will taper you off the other drug.

If you have tight aortic stenosis (a narrowing of the aortic valve that obstructs blood flow from the heart to the body) and have been taking a beta-blocker, your doctor will monitor you carefully while you are taking Procardia or Procardia XL.

If you develop swelling of the arms, hands, legs, and feet, your doctor can prescribe a diuretic (water pill) to relieve the problem.

Procardia XL should be used cautiously if you have any stomach or intestinal narrowing.

Notify your doctor or dentist that you are taking Procardia if you have a medical emergency, and before you have surgery or dental treatment.

This drug is not recommended for use in children.

Possible food and drug interactions when taking this medication

If Procardia or Procardia XL is taken with certain other drugs, the effects of either could be increased, decreased, or altered. It is especially important to check with your doctor before combining Procardia or Procardia XL with the following:

Cimetidine (Tagamet)
Digoxin (Lanoxin)
Quinidine (Quinaglute, Quinidex)

Taking Procardia with grapefruit juice can dramatically increase the effect of the drug. Do not combine the two.

Special information if you are pregnant or breastfeeding

The effects of Procardia and Procardia XL during pregnancy have not been adequately studied, although new animal research points to possible birth defects in humans. If you are pregnant or plan to become pregnant, inform your doctor immediately. It is not known whether Procardia or Procardia XL appears in breast milk and can affect a nursing infant. If this medication is essential to your health, your doctor may advise you to discontinue breastfeeding until your treatment is finished.

Recommended dosage

ADULTS

The usual starting dose of Procardia and Adalat is one 10-milligram capsule, 3 times a day. The usual range is 10 to 20 milligrams 3 times a day. Some people may need 20 to 30 milligrams, 3 or 4 times a day. Usually you will not take more than 120 milligrams in a day and should take no more than 180 milligrams.

The starting dose of Procardia XL and Adalat CC is usually a 30- or 60-milligram tablet, taken once daily. Your doctor may increase the dose over 1 to 2 weeks if not satisfied with the way the drug is working. Doses above 120 milligrams per day are not recommended.

Although no serious side effects have been reported when Procardia XL is stopped, your doctor will probably have you lower the dose gradually under close supervision.

Overdosage

Any medication taken in excess can have serious consequences. If you suspect an overdose, seek medical treatment immediately.

■ *Symptoms of Procardia overdose may include:*
Dizziness, drowsiness, nausea, severe drop in blood pressure, slurred speech, weakness

PROCHIEVE
Pronounced: PRO-cheev
Generic name: Progesterone gel

Why is this drug prescribed?
Prochieve is a vaginal gel used to treat progesterone deficiency in women undergoing infertility treatment. It is also prescribed to restore menstruation in women whose menstrual periods have stopped.

Most important fact about this drug
If you are undergoing infertility treatment, it is very important that you strictly adhere to the medication schedule your doctor has planned for you. Administering the dose at the wrong time or forgetting to take a dose can jeopardize your chances of getting pregnant and maintaining a pregnancy.

How should you take this medication?
1. Remove the applicator from the sealed wrapper. Do not remove the twist-off tab yet.
2. Hold the applicator by the thick end. Shake several times like a thermometer to be sure the contents are at the thin end.
3. Hold the applicator by the flat section of the thick end. Twist off and throw away the tab at the other end. Do not squeeze the thick end while twisting the tab. This could force some gel to be released before it is inserted.
4. Gently insert the thin end of the applicator into the vagina. You can do this while in a sitting position or when lying on your back with your knees bent.
5. Squeeze the thick end of the applicator to deposit the gel. Remove the applicator and throw it away. Do not be concerned if a small amount of gel is left in the applicator; you will still be receiving the appropriate dose.

For altitudes above 2,500 feet: Follow step 1 above, then use a lancet to puncture a hole in the flat section of the thick end; this will relieve the difference in air pressure between the inside and outside of the applicator caused by high altitudes. Follow steps 2 through 4 above. For step 5, place your thumb or finger over the hole before squeezing the applicator to dispense the gel.

Note that if your doctor prescribes the 8% gel, you cannot substitute 2 tubes of the 4% gel, as the proper amount of drug will not be absorbed.

■ *If you miss a dose...*
Take it as soon as you remember. If it is almost time for your next dose, skip the one you missed and take the next one as scheduled.

■ *Storage instructions...*
Store at room temperature.

What side effects may occur?

Side effects cannot be anticipated. If any develop or change in intensity, inform your doctor as soon as possible. Only your doctor can determine if it is safe for you to continue taking Prochieve.

■ *Side effects may include:*
Abdominal pain, acne, allergy, back pain, bloating, breast pain, cramps, depression, dizziness, fatigue, flu-like symptoms, frequent urination, gas, gastrointestinal discomfort, genital itching, headache, hot flushes, increased appetite, increased sweating, infections, insomnia, leg pain, migraine, mood swings, muscle pain, nausea, nervousness, pain, painful menstruation, rash, sleep problems, sleepiness, thirst, tremor, upper respiratory tract infection, vaginal discharge, yeast infection

Why should this drug not be prescribed?

You cannot use Prochieve if you are allergic to progesterone or if you have unusual vaginal bleeding that has not been evaluated by a doctor.

You must also avoid the drug if you have liver disease, known or suspected cancer of the breast or genitals, or a history of blood clots, especially in the legs, lungs, or eyes.

If you've had a miscarriage and your doctor suspects some tissue is still in the uterus (sometimes called a *missed miscarriage*), you cannot use Prochieve.

Special warnings about this medication

Before starting progesterone therapy, your doctor will need to do a complete gynecological exam, including a Pap smear, to rule out cancer. Be sure to tell the doctor about any unusual vaginal bleeding before using Prochieve.

Progesterone therapy can cause blood clots in susceptible individuals. Call your doctor immediately if you develop any of the following: pain in the calves or chest, shortness of breath, coughing up blood, severe headache, severe vomiting, dizziness, faintness, changes in vision or speech, and weakness or numbness in an arm or leg.

Be sure to tell the doctor if you develop fluid retention while using Prochieve, especially if you also have a condition that could be aggravated by excess fluid, such as epilepsy, migraine, asthma, and heart or kidney dysfunction.

Use Prochieve with caution if you have a history of depression, since the drug can aggravate this condition.

A small percentage of patients taking a combination of progesterone and estrogen develop blood sugar problems. If you have diabetes, the doctor will monitor your blood sugar levels carefully during treatment with Prochieve.

Possible food and drug interactions when taking this medication

There are no known drug interactions with Prochieve. However, other vaginal medications should not be taken at the same time. Be sure to tell the doctor if you take any other vaginal medications and ask about the best time to administer each one.

Special information if you are pregnant or breastfeeding

Prochieve is used in women who are undergoing infertility treatment. Rare cases of birth defects have been reported in women who used Prochieve during early pregnancy, although a definite cause/effect relationship has not been established.

Because progesterone is excreted in breast milk, be sure to tell the doctor if you're nursing.

Recommended dosage

To Treat Infertility

The usual dose is one application of Prochieve 8% gel once or twice a day. One application of the 8% gel delivers 90 milligrams of progesterone.

To Restore Menstrual Periods

The usual dose is one application of Prochieve 4% gel every other day as directed by your doctor, for a total of 6 doses. One application of the 4% gel delivers 45 milligrams of progesterone. If needed, the doctor may increase your dose by switching you to the 8% gel.

Overdosage

Any medication taken in excess can have serious consequences. If you suspect an overdose, seek medical attention immediately.

PROCHLORPERAZINE
Pronounced: pro-klor-PEAR-ah-zine

Why is this drug prescribed?

Prochlorperazine is used to control severe nausea and vomiting. It is also used to treat symptoms of the mental disorder schizophrenia, and is occasionally prescribed for anxiety.

Most important fact about this drug

Prochlorperazine may cause tardive dyskinesia—involuntary muscle spasms and twitches in the face and body. This condition may be permanent. It appears to be most common among the elderly, especially women. Ask your doctor for information about this possible risk.

How should you take this medication?

Never take more prochlorperazine than prescribed. It can increase the risk of serious side effects.

If you are using the suppository form of prochlorperazine and find it is too soft to insert, you can chill it in the refrigerator for about 30 minutes or run cold water over it before removing the wrapper.

To insert a suppository, first remove the wrapper and moisten the suppository with cold water. Then lie down on your side and use a finger to push the suppository well up into the rectum.

- *If you miss a dose...*
  Take the forgotten dose as soon as you remember. If it is almost time for the next dose, skip the one you missed and go back to your regular schedule. Never try to catch up by doubling the dose.
- *Storage instructions...*
  Store at room temperature. Protect from heat and light.

What side effects may occur?

Side effects cannot be anticipated. If any develop or change in intensity, inform your doctor as soon as possible. Only your doctor can determine if it is safe for you to continue taking Prochlorperazine.

- *Side effects may include:*
  Blurred vision, dizziness, drowsiness, jaundice, low blood pressure, menstrual irregularities, Neuroleptic Malignant Syndrome (see *Special warnings about this medication*), skin reactions

Why should this drug not be prescribed?

Do not take prochlorperazine if you are sensitive to or have ever had an allergic reaction to prochlorperazine or other phenothiazine drugs such as Thorazine, Prolixin, Triavil, Mellaril, or Stelazine.

Prochlorperazine should not be given to children who are undergoing surgery.

Special warnings about this medication

Never take large amounts of alcohol, barbiturates, or narcotics when taking prochlorperazine. Serious problems can result.

Prochlorperazine should be used with caution if you are being treated for a brain tumor, intestinal blockage, heart disease, breast cancer, seizures, glaucoma, or an abnormal bone marrow or blood condition such as leukemia. Also use caution if you're exposed to pesticides or extreme heat.

If you suddenly stop taking prochlorperazine, you may experience a change in appetite, dizziness, nausea, vomiting, and tremors. Therapy should be discontinued only under a doctor's supervision.

Due to its ability to prevent vomiting, prochlorperazine can mask symptoms of an overdose of other drugs. It could also mask symptoms of brain tumor, intestinal blockage, and the neurological condition known as Reye's syndrome.

Prochlorperazine should be used cautiously in children suffering from dehydration or an acute illness such as chickenpox, measles, or other infection. The drug should be avoided altogether in children and adolescents who have symptoms that could indicate Reye's syndrome, including persistent or recurrent vomiting, listlessness, irritability, combativeness, and disorientation.

Prochlorperazine can cause a potentially fatal group of symptoms called Neuroleptic Malignant Syndrome (NMS). Symptoms include extremely high body temperature, rigid muscles, mental changes, irregular pulse or blood pressure, rapid heartbeat, excessive sweating, and changes in heart rhythm. Alert your doctor immediately if these symptoms develop. Prochlorperazine therapy will need to be discontinued.

This drug may impair your ability to drive a car or operate potentially dangerous machinery. Do not participate in any activities that require full alertness if you are unsure about your ability.

While taking prochlorperazine, try to stay out of the sun. Use sunblock and wear protective clothing. Your eyes may become more sensitive to sunlight, too, so keep sunglasses handy.

Prochlorperazine interferes with your ability to shed extra heat. Be cautious in hot weather.

People taking prochlorperazine for a prolonged period should see their doctor for regular evaluations, since side effects can get worse over time.

Prochlorperazine may cause false positive phenylketonuria (PKU) tests.

Possible food and drug interactions when taking this medication

If prochlorperazine is taken with certain other drugs, the effects of either could be increased, decreased, or altered. It is especially important to check with your doctor before combining prochlorperazine with the following:

Anticoagulants such as Coumadin
Antiseizure drugs such as Dilantin and Tegretol
Guanethidine (Ismelin)
Lithium (Lithobid, Eskalith)
Narcotic painkillers such as Demerol and Tylenol with Codeine

Other central nervous system depressants such as Xanax, Valium, Seconal, and Halcion
Propranolol (Inderal)
Thiazide diuretics such as Dyazide

Special information if you are pregnant or breastfeeding

Prochlorperazine is not usually recommended for pregnant women. However, your doctor may prescribe it for severe nausea and vomiting if the potential benefits of the drug outweigh the potential risks. Prochlorperazine appears in breast milk and may affect a nursing infant. If this drug is essential to your health, your doctor may recommend that you stop breastfeeding until your treatment is finished.

Recommended dosage

ADULTS

To Control Severe Nausea and Vomiting
Tablets: The usual dosage is one 5-milligram or 10-milligram tablet 3 or 4 times a day.
  Spansule capsules: The usual starting dose is one 15-milligram capsule on getting out of bed or one 10-milligram capsule every 12 hours.
  The usual rectal dosage (suppository) is 25 milligrams, taken 2 times a day.

Non-psychotic Anxiety
Tablets: The usual dose is 5 milligrams, taken 3 or 4 times a day.
  Spansule capsules: The usual starting dose is one 15-milligram capsule on getting up or one 10-milligram capsule every 12 hours.
  Treatment should not continue for longer than 12 weeks, and daily doses should not exceed 20 milligrams.

Relatively Mild Schizophrenia
The usual dose is 5 or 10 milligrams, taken 3 or 4 times daily.

Moderate to Severe Schizophrenia
Dosages usually start at 10 milligrams, taken 3 or 4 times a day. If needed, dosage may be gradually increased; 50 to 75 milligrams daily has been helpful for some people.

More Severe Schizophrenia
Dosages may range from 100 to 150 milligrams per day.

CHILDREN

Children under 2 years of age or weighing less than 20 pounds should not be given prochlorperazine. If a child becomes restless or excited after taking prochlorperazine, do not give the child another dose.

Severe Nausea and Vomiting
An oral or rectal dose of Prochlorperazine is usually not needed for more than 1 day.

Children 20 to 29 pounds: The usual dose is 2½ milligrams 1 or 2 times daily. Total daily amount should not exceed 7.5 milligrams.

Children 30 to 39 pounds: The usual dose is 2½ milligrams 2 or 3 times daily. Total daily amount should not exceed 10 milligrams.

Children 40 to 85 pounds: The usual dose is 2½ milligrams 3 times daily, or 5 milligrams 2 times daily. Total daily amount should not exceed 15 milligrams.

Schizophrenia
Children 2 to 5 years old: The starting oral or rectal dose is 2½ milligrams 2 or 3 times daily. Do not exceed 10 milligrams the first day and 20 milligrams thereafter.

Children 6 to 12 years old: The starting oral or rectal dose is 2½ milligrams 2 or 3 times daily. Do not exceed 10 milligrams the first day and 25 milligrams thereafter.

OLDER ADULTS

In general, older people take lower dosages of prochlorperazine. Because they may develop low blood pressure while taking the drug, the doctor should monitor them closely. Older people (especially women) may be more susceptible to tardive dyskinesia—a possibly permanent condition. Tardive dyskinesia causes involuntary muscle spasms and twitches in the face and body. Consult your doctor for more information about these potential risks.

Overdosage
An overdose of prochlorperazine can be fatal. If you suspect an overdose, seek medical help immediately.

■ *Symptoms of prochlorperazine overdose may include:*
Agitation, coma, convulsions, dry mouth, extreme sleepiness, fever, intestinal blockage, irregular heart rate, restlessness

Progesterone *See Prometrium, page 1172.*

Progesterone gel *See Prochieve, page 1165.*

Promethazine *See Phenergan, page 1085.*

Promethazine with Codeine *See Phenergan with Codeine, page 1089.*

PROMETRIUM

Pronounced: pro-ME-tree-um
Generic name: Progesterone

Why is this drug prescribed?

Prometrium is prescribed for postmenopausal women who are taking estrogen (hormone replacement therapy); it prevents a buildup of the lining of the uterus and abnormal bleeding. Prometrium also may be prescribed to restore menstruation if your menstrual periods have stopped.

Most important fact about this drug

Prometrium increases the risk of blood clots, which can lead to phlebitis, breathing problems, vision problems, or stroke. If you experience any symptoms that might suggest the onset of a clot-related disorder—pain with swelling, warmth, and redness in a leg vein, coughing or shortness of breath, loss of vision or double vision, migraine, or weakness or numbness in an arm or leg—stop taking Prometrium and see your doctor immediately.

How should you take this medication?

Take Prometrium as directed by your doctor. If Prometrium is prescribed to prevent abnormal buildup of the uterine lining, you will take it once a day for 12 days in a 28-day cycle. If it is prescribed to treat missed menstrual periods, you will take it for 10 days. Prometrium is taken in the evening.

■ *If you miss a dose...*
Take it as soon as you remember. If it is almost time for your next dose, skip the one you missed and go back to your regular schedule. Never take 2 doses at the same time.

■ *Storage instructions...*
Store at room temperature. Protect from light and moisture.

What side effects may occur?

Side effects cannot be anticipated. If any develop or change in intensity, inform your doctor as soon as possible. Only your doctor can determine if it is safe for you to continue taking Prometrium.

■ *Side effects may include:*
Abdominal cramping, back pain, bloating, breast tenderness or pain, chest pain, constipation, coughing, depression, diarrhea, dizziness, emotional instability, fatigue, headache, hot flashes, irritability, joint pain, muscle pain, nausea, night sweats, swelling of hands and feet, upper respiratory infection, urinary problems, vaginal discharge, vaginal dryness, viral infection, vomiting, worry

Why should this drug not be prescribed?

Do not take Prometrium if you have ever had an allergic reaction to it. Prometrium contains peanut oil, so you should also avoid this medication if you are allergic to peanuts.

Do not take Prometrium if you are pregnant or have had an incomplete miscarriage. Avoid it if you have ever had a blood clotting disorder or a stroke. Do not take this drug if you have breast or genital cancer, unexplained vaginal bleeding, or severe liver disease.

Special warnings about this medication

To rule out cancer and other problems before you start taking Prometrium, your doctor will give you a complete physical exam, including examination of your breasts and pelvic organs. You also should have a Pap test (cervical smear). Tell your doctor if you experience any irregular vaginal bleeding while taking this medication.

Remember that Prometrium can cause clot-related disorders. Check with your doctor immediately if you experience any of the warning signs listed in *Most important fact about this drug.*

Prometrium may cause some degree of fluid retention. If you have a medical condition that could be made worse by fluid retention—such as epilepsy, migraine, asthma, or a heart or kidney problem—make sure your doctor knows about it.

Prometrium makes some women depressed. If you've suffered from serious depression in the past, alert your doctor if you think you're having a relapse. You will probably need to stop taking Prometrium.

Prometrium has a slight effect on insulin and blood sugar levels. If you have diabetes, your doctor will want to watch you closely while you are taking this drug.

Prometrium may make you dizzy or drowsy. Do not drive or operate machinery until you know how this medication affects you. If you experience extreme drowsiness or dizziness, the doctor may tell you to take Prometrium at bedtime.

Because progesterone is processed in the liver and kidneys, the doctor will monitor you closely if you have a mild liver or kidney disorder. If you have severe liver disease, the drug should not be used at all.

In rare cases, women taking Prometrium suffer a sudden drop in blood pressure that can cause them to faint.

Possible food and drug interactions when taking this medication

Tell the doctor if you're taking the antifungal medication ketoconazole (Nizoral) or a similar drug. It's possible that it may increase Prometrium's effect.

Special information if you are pregnant or breastfeeding

Because the possibility of harm to a developing infant cannot be ruled out, Prometrium should not be taken during pregnancy.

Prometrium appears in breast milk. The drug is recommended for nursing mothers only if it is clearly necessary.

Recommended dosage

ADULTS

To Prevent Abnormal Buildup of the Uterine Lining
For women taking daily conjugated estrogen tablets, the usual dosage of Prometrium is 200 milligrams taken each evening for 12 days in a 28-day cycle.

To Restore Menstrual Periods
The usual dose is 400 milligrams taken each evening for 10 days.

Overdosage
Although no specific information is available, any medication taken in excess can have serious consequences. If you suspect an overdose of Prometrium, seek medical attention immediately.

Pronestyl *See Procanbid, page 1159.*

Propafenone *See Rythmol, page 1284.*

PROPECIA
Pronounced: pro-PEE-she-ah
Generic name: Finasteride

Why is this drug prescribed?
Propecia is a remedy for baldness in men with mild to moderate hair loss on the top of the head and the front of the mid-scalp area. It increases hair growth, improves hair regrowth, and slows down hair loss. It works only on scalp hair and does not affect hair on other parts of the body.

You may begin to see improvement as early as 3 months after you begin taking Propecia, but for many men it takes longer. The improvement lasts only as long as you take the drug; if you stop, new hair growth will cease and hair loss will resume.

Propecia is a low-dose form of Proscar, a drug prescribed for prostate enlargement.

Most important fact about this drug
Propecia should not be used by women. If taken during pregnancy, it can cause abnormal development of a male baby's genital organs.

How should you take this medication?

For maximum benefit, take Propecia regularly once a day. It can be taken with or without food.

■ *If you miss a dose…*
Take it as soon as you remember. If it is almost time for your next dose, skip the one you missed and go back to your regular schedule. Do not take 2 doses at the same time.

■ *Storage instructions…*
Store at room temperature in a closed container away from moisture.

What side effects may occur?

Propecia's side effects are primarily sexual, and relatively uncommon—they strike one or two men in a hundred. If any side effects develop or change in intensity, inform your doctor as soon as possible. Only your doctor can determine if it is safe for you to continue taking Propecia.

■ *Side effects may include:*
Breast tenderness and enlargement, decreased amount of semen per ejaculation, decreased sex drive, impotence, itching, rash, swelling, testicular pain

Why should this drug not be prescribed?

Due to the drug's effect on male babies, women should avoid Propecia if there is any chance that they may be pregnant.

Do not use Propecia if it gives you an allergic reaction, or if you've ever had an allergic reaction to its chemical twin, Proscar.

Special warnings about this medication

If there's even a possibility that they're pregnant, women should avoid handling a crushed or broken Propecia tablet for fear of absorbing some of the active ingredient through the skin. Whole tablets are safe to handle thanks to a protective outer coating.

Use Propecia with caution if you have liver problems.

Propecia lowers readings of the PSA screening test for prostate cancer. If you're scheduled to have your PSA level checked, make sure the doctor knows you're taking Propecia.

Possible food and drug interactions when taking this medication

No significant drug interactions have been reported.

Special information if you are pregnant or breastfeeding

Avoid even touching the active ingredient in Propecia if there's a chance that you're pregnant.

Recommended dosage

ADULT MEN

The recommended dosage, for men only, is 1 tablet daily.

Overdosage

Although no specific information is available on Propecia overdose, any medication taken in excess can have serious consequences. If you suspect an overdose, seek medical attention immediately.

PROPINE

Pronounced: PROH-peen
Generic name: Dipivefrin hydrochloride

Why is this drug prescribed?

Propine is used to treat chronic open-angle glaucoma, the most common form of the disease. In glaucoma, the fluid inside the eyeball is under abnormally high pressure, a condition which can cause vision problems or even blindness.

Propine belongs to a class of medication called *prodrugs,* drugs that generally are not active by themselves, but are converted in the body to an active form. This makes for better absorption, stability, and comfort and reduces side effects.

Most important fact about this drug

There is no cure for glaucoma. Propine and similar drugs can keep ocular pressure under control, but only as long as you take them. You will probably need to continue treatment for life; and you must be sure to take the medication regularly.

How should you use this medication?

Use this medication exactly as prescribed. If you use too much, or use it too often, Propine may cause side effects.

Wash your hands before and after you use the eyedrops. Once the drops are in your eye, keep your eye closed for 1 to 2 minutes, applying pressure to the inside corner of your eye, so the medicine can be properly absorbed.

To keep the medication free of contamination, do not touch the applicator tip to your eye or any other surface.

A number appears on the cap of the dropper bottle to tell you what dose you are taking. When you are ready to take the first dose, make sure the number 1 appears in the window. After each dose, replace the cap and rotate it to the next number. Turn until you hear a click.

■ *If you miss a dose...*
   Apply it as soon as you remember. If it is almost time for your next dose, skip the one you missed and go back to your regular schedule. Never apply more than 1 dose at a time.
■ *Storage instructions...*
   Keep Propine in the plastic dropper bottle it came in.

What side effects may occur?

Side effects cannot be anticipated. If any develop or change in intensity, inform your doctor as soon as possible. Only your doctor can determine if it is safe for you to continue taking Propine.

■ *Side effects may include:*
   Burning and stinging, red eye

Why should this drug not be prescribed?

If you are sensitive to or have ever had an allergic reaction to Propine or any of its ingredients, you should not use this medication. Make sure your doctor is aware of any drug reactions you have experienced.

Unless you are directed to do so by your doctor, do not use this medication if you have narrow-angle glaucoma.

Special warnings about this medication

Propine may cause vision problems, including blurry vision, for a short time after the eyedrops are applied. If this occurs, make sure you do not drive, use machinery, or participate in any hazardous activity that requires clear vision.

Possible food and drug interactions when taking this medication

No significant interactions have been reported.

Special information if you are pregnant or breastfeeding

The effects of Propine during pregnancy have not been adequately studied. If you are pregnant or plan to become pregnant, inform your doctor immediately. Propine may appear in breast milk and could affect a nursing infant. If this medication is essential to your health, your doctor may advise you to discontinue breastfeeding your baby until your treatment is finished.

Recommended dosage

ADULTS

The usual dose is 1 drop in the eye(s) every 12 hours. It usually takes about 30 minutes for Propine to start working. You should feel the maximum effects of the drug within 1 hour.

CHILDREN

The safety and effectiveness of Propine have not been established in children.

Overdosage

Any medication taken in excess can have serious consequences. If you suspect an overdose of Propine, seek medical attention immediately.

Propoxyphene See Darvocet-N, page 385.

Propranolol See Inderal, page 676.

Propranolol with Hydrochlorothiazide See Inderide, page 680.

PROSCAR

Pronounced: PRAHS-car
Generic name: Finasteride

Why is this drug prescribed?

Proscar is prescribed to help shrink an enlarged prostate.

The prostate, a chestnut-shaped gland present in males, produces a liquid that forms part of the semen. This gland completely encloses the upper part of the urethra, the tube through which urine flows out of the bladder. Many men over age 50 suffer from a benign (noncancerous) enlargement of the prostate. The enlarged gland squeezes the urethra, obstructing the normal flow of urine. Resulting problems may include difficulty in starting urination, weak flow of urine, and the need to urinate urgently or frequently. Sometimes surgical removal of the prostate is necessary.

By shrinking the enlarged prostate, Proscar may alleviate the various associated urinary problems, making surgery unnecessary.

Some doctors are also prescribing Proscar for baldness and as a preventive measure against prostate cancer.

Most important fact about this drug

Different men have different responses to Proscar:

You may experience early relief from your urinary problems.
You may need to take the drug for 6 months or even a year before
   noticing any improvement.
Or you may find that, even after a year of treatment, Proscar simply
   has not helped you.

How should you take this medication?

You may take Proscar either with a meal or between meals.

■ *If you miss a dose...*
Take it as soon as you remember. If it is almost time for your next dose, skip the one you missed and go back to your regular schedule. Never take 2 doses at the same time.

■ *Storage instructions...*
Store at room temperature in a tightly closed container. Protect from light.

What side effects may occur?
Side effects cannot be anticipated. If any develop or change in intensity, inform your doctor as soon as possible. Only your doctor can determine if it is safe for you to continue taking Proscar.

■ *Side effects may include:*
Decreased amount of semen per ejaculation, decreased sex drive, impotence

Why should this drug not be prescribed?
Proscar should never be taken by a woman or a child.

Do not take Proscar if you are sensitive to it or have ever had an allergic reaction to it.

Special warnings about this medication
Benign enlargement of the prostate is not the only condition that can cause male urinary inefficiency and discomfort. Other possibilities include infection, obstruction, cancer of the prostate, and bladder disorders. Before prescribing Proscar, your doctor will want to do various tests to determine the cause of your urinary problems.

Even if Proscar does relieve your urinary symptoms, periodic checkups are necessary to test for possible development of cancer of the prostate. Proscar is not an effective treatment for prostate cancer.

Check the patient information that comes in the Proscar package for new information every time you renew your prescription.

Possible food and drug interactions when taking this medication
No significant drug interactions have been reported.

Special information if you are pregnant or breastfeeding
If accidentally absorbed by a pregnant woman who is carrying a male fetus, Proscar may cause abnormal development of the unborn baby's genital organs. Any woman who is pregnant or who may become pregnant should therefore never even touch a crushed Proscar tablet.

Recommended dosage

ADULTS

The recommended dosage, for men only, is one 5-milligram tablet per day.

Overdosage

Although no specific information is available, any medication taken in excess can have serious consequences. If you suspect an overdose of Proscar, seek medical attention immediately.

PROSOM

Pronounced: PROE-som
Generic name: Estazolam

Why is this drug prescribed?

ProSom, a sleeping pill, is given for the short-term treatment of insomnia. Insomnia may involve difficulty falling asleep, frequent awakenings during the night, or too-early morning awakening.

Most important fact about this drug

A chemical cousin of Valium and similar tranquilizers, ProSom is potentially addictive; thus, you should plan on taking this drug only as a temporary sleeping aid. Even after relatively short-term use of ProSom, you may experience some withdrawal symptoms when you stop taking the medication.

How should you take this medication?

Take ProSom exactly as prescribed by your doctor. A typical schedule is 1 tablet at bedtime. For small, physically run-down, or older people, one-half a tablet may be a safer starting dose.

Avoid drinking alcoholic beverages while taking ProSom.

If you have ever had seizures, do not abruptly stop taking ProSom, even if you are taking antiseizure medication. Instead, taper off from ProSom under your doctor's supervision.

Even if you have never had seizures, it is better to taper off from ProSom than to stop taking the medication abruptly. Experience suggests that tapering off can help prevent drug withdrawal symptoms.

Typically, the only withdrawal symptoms caused by ProSom are mild and temporary insomnia or irritability. Occasionally, however, withdrawal can involve considerable discomfort or even danger, with symptoms such as abdominal and muscle cramps, convulsions, sweating, tremors, and vomiting.

■ *If you miss a dose...*
Take at bedtime only as needed. It is not necessary to make up a missed dose.

■ *Storage instructions...*
Store at room temperature.

What side effects may occur?

Side effects cannot be anticipated. If any develop or change in intensity, inform your doctor as soon as possible. Only your doctor can determine whether it is safe for you to continue taking ProSom.

■ *Side effects may include:*
Abnormal coordination, constipation, decreased movement or activity, dizziness, dry mouth, general feeling of illness, hangover, headache, leg and foot pain, memory problems, nausea, nervousness, sleepiness, weakness

Why should this drug not be prescribed?

Do not take ProSom if you are sensitive or allergic to it, or if you have ever had an adverse reaction to another Valium-type medication.

Do not take ProSom if you are pregnant or planning to become pregnant. Drugs in this class may cause damage to the unborn child.

Special warnings about this medication

Since ProSom may cloud your thinking, impair your judgment, or interfere with your normal physical coordination, do not drive, climb, or perform hazardous tasks until you know your reaction to this medication. It is important to remember that the tablet you took in the evening may continue to affect you well into the following day.

If you are older or physically run-down, or if you have liver or kidney damage or breathing problems, you will be particularly vulnerable to side effects from ProSom, and you should use this medication with special caution.

Possible food and drug interactions when taking this medication

Do not drink alcohol while you are taking ProSom; this combination could make you comatose or dangerously slow your breathing.

For the same reason, do not combine ProSom with any other medication that might calm or slow the functioning of your central nervous system. Among such drugs are:

Antihistamines such as Benadryl and Chlor-Trimeton
Antiseizure drugs such as Dilantin, Tegretol, and Depakene
Barbiturates such as phenobarbital
Major tranquilizers such as Haldol and Mellaril
MAO inhibitors such as the antidepressants Nardil and Parnate
Narcotics such as Percodan and Tylox
Tranquilizers such as Valium and Xanax

If you smoke, you will tend to process and eliminate ProSom fairly quickly compared with a nonsmoker.

Special information if you are pregnant or breastfeeding

If you are pregnant, you must not take ProSom; it could cause birth defects in your child.

When a pregnant woman takes ProSom or a similar medication shortly before giving birth, her baby is likely to have poor muscle tone (flaccidity) and/or experience drug withdrawal symptoms.

Because ProSom is thought to pass into breast milk, you should not take this medication while breastfeeding.

Recommended dosage

ADULTS

The recommended initial dose is 1 milligram at bedtime; however, some people may need a 2-milligram dose.

CHILDREN

There is no information on the safety and effectiveness of ProSom in children under age 18.

OLDER ADULTS

The recommended usual dosage for older adults is 1 milligram. However, some people may require only 0.5 milligram.

Overdosage

Any medication taken in excess can have serious consequences. If you suspect an overdose, seek medical attention immediately.

■ *Symptoms of a ProSom overdose may include:*
  Confusion, depressed breathing, drowsiness and eventually coma, lack of coordination, slurred speech

PROTONIX

Pronounced: PRO-ton-iks
Generic name: Pantoprazole sodium

Why is this drug prescribed?

Protonix blocks the production of stomach acid. It is prescribed to heal a condition called erosive esophagitis (a severe inflammation of the passage to the stomach) brought on by a persistent backflow of stomach acid (gastroesophageal reflux disease). Later, it may be prescribed to maintain healing and prevent a relapse. It is also used in the treatment of conditions marked by constant overproduction of stomach acid, such as Zollinger-Ellison syndrome.

Protonix is a member of the proton pump inhibitor class of acid blockers, which includes AcipHex, Nexium, Prilosec, and Prevacid.

Most important fact about this drug
Protonix is highly effective. In most patients, stomach acid secretion drops 85 to 95 percent after a single week of treatment.

How should you take this medication?
Protonix may be taken with or without food. Do not chew, crush, or split the delayed-release tablets. If you are taking antacids, you may continue to do so.

■ *If you miss a dose...*
Take it as soon as you remember. If it is almost time for your next dose, skip the one you missed and go back to your regular schedule. Never take 2 doses at once.

■ *Storage instructions...*
Store Protonix at room temperature.

What side effects may occur?
Side effects cannot be anticipated. If any develop or change in intensity, tell your doctor as soon as possible. Only your doctor can determine if it is safe for you to continue taking Protonix.

■ *Side effects may include:*
Abdominal pain, burping, diarrhea, gas, headache, insomnia, nausea, rash, vomiting

Why should this drug not be prescribed?
If Protonix gives you an allergic reaction, you'll be unable to use it.

Special warnings about this medication
Protonix has been known to cause several extremely rare—but very serious—side effects, including severe allergic reaction, severe swelling of the face and throat, eye damage, dangerous skin reactions, and inflammation of the pancreas. Seek emergency care immediately if you begin to have difficulty breathing or swallowing, or begin to develop blisters, eruptions, or peeling skin.

If you have a liver condition, make sure the doctor is aware of it. A dosage adjustment may be needed for anyone with serious liver disease.

Protonix has not been tested for safety or effectiveness in children.

Possible food and drug interactions when taking this medication
If Protonix is taken with certain other drugs, the effects of either could be increased, decreased, or altered. It is especially important to check with your doctor before combining Protonix with the following:

Ampicillin (Omnipen)
Iron
Ketoconazole (Nizoral)
Warfarin (Coumadin)

Special information if you are pregnant or breastfeeding

Although no harmful effects during pregnancy are known, there's no definite proof of safety either. Protonix is therefore recommended during pregnancy only if clearly needed. If you are pregnant or plan to become pregnant, inform your doctor immediately.

There is a possibility that Protonix may appear in breast milk, causing serious side effects in the nursing infant. If you have to take the drug, you should not plan on breastfeeding.

Recommended dosage

ADULTS

Erosive Esophagitis

The usual dose is 40 milligrams once a day for up to 8 weeks. If your esophagus hasn't healed in that time, your doctor may prescribe an additional 8-week course of therapy. The same dose is used to maintain healing.

Overproduction of Stomach Acid

The usual starting dose is 40 milligrams twice a day. The doctor may increase the dose if necessary. Doses as high as 240 milligrams per day have been used. Treatment may continue for years.

Overdosage

Any medication taken in excess can have serious consequences. Although little is known about Protonix overdose in humans, in animal studies it interferes with coordination and reduces activity. If you suspect an overdose, seek medical attention immediately.

Protriptyline *See Vivactil, page 1576.*

PROVENTIL

Pronounced: Proh-VEN-till
Generic name: Albuterol sulfate
Other brand names: AccuNeb, Proventil HFA, Ventolin HFA,
   Volmax Extended-Release Tablets, VoSpire Extended-
   Release Tablets

Why is this drug prescribed?

Drugs containing albuterol are prescribed for the prevention and relief of bronchial spasms that narrow the airway. This especially applies to the treatment of asthma. Some brands of this medication are also used for the prevention of bronchial spasm due to exercise.

Most important fact about this drug

Do not take albuterol more frequently than your doctor recommends. Increasing the number of doses can be dangerous and may actually make symptoms of asthma worse.

If the dose your doctor recommends does not provide relief of your symptoms, or if your symptoms become worse, consult your doctor immediately.

How should you take this medication?

If you are taking extended-release tablets, swallow them whole with some liquid—never chew or crush them.

Shake the inhalation aerosol canister well before using and make sure it's firmly seated in the plastic mouthpiece. Before using it for the first time, prime the canister with 4 sprays into the air away from your face. Prime it with 2 sprays whenever it has not been used for at least 4 days. Use only the adapter that comes with the product; do not use this adapter with any other product. Wash the plastic mouthpiece with warm running water at least once a week to prevent medication buildup and blockage.

If you are using an inhalation solution, be sure to protect it from contamination. Keep the tip of the dropper away from the lip of the bottle or any other surface. Do not use the solution if it changes color or becomes cloudy.

■ *If you miss a dose…*
   Take the forgotten dose as soon as you remember; then take any remaining doses for that day at equally spaced intervals. Never take a double dose.

■ *Storage instructions…*
   AccuNeb, Proventil syrup, and Proventil solution for inhalation can be kept in the refrigerator or at room temperature. Proventil aerosol can be stored at temperatures as low as 60 degrees Fahrenheit, but should be at room temperature before use. Protect from excessive heat.

Ventolin nebules must be used within 2 weeks of being removed from the refrigerator.

Store VoSpire tablets at room temperature in a tight, light-resistant container.

Volmax tablets should be kept refrigerated.

What side effects may occur?

Side effects cannot be anticipated. If any develop or change in intensity, inform your doctor as soon as possible. Only your doctor can determine if it is safe for you to continue taking albuterol.

■ *Side effects may include:*

Aggression, agitation, allergic reaction, anxiety, back pain, chest pain or discomfort, chills and fever, coordination problems, cough, decreased appetite, depression, difficulty speaking, diabetes, diarrhea, dizziness, drowsiness, dry mouth and throat, excitement, fluid retention and swelling, flushing, general bodily discomfort, headache, heart palpitations, heartburn, hives, increased appetite, increased blood pressure, increased difficulty breathing, indigestion, irritability, labored breathing, leg cramps, light-headedness, muscle cramps, muscle spasm, nasal inflammation, nausea, nervousness, nightmares, nosebleed, overactivity, rapid heartbeat, rash, respiratory infection or disorder, restlessness, ringing in the ears, shakiness, sleeplessness, slowed movement, stomachache, stuffy nose, sweating, swelling of mouth and throat, taste sensation on inhalation, throat irritation, tooth discoloration, tremors, unusual taste, urinary problems, vomiting, weakness, wheezing

Why should this drug not be prescribed?

If you are sensitive to or have ever had an allergic reaction to albuterol or other bronchodilators, you should not take this medication. Make sure that your doctor is aware of any drug reactions that you have experienced.

Special warnings about this medication

When taking albuterol inhalation aerosol, you should not use other inhaled medications before checking with your doctor.

Make sure the doctor is aware of it if you have a heart condition, seizure disorder, high blood pressure, abnormal heartbeat, overactive thyroid gland, or diabetes. Call your doctor immediately if you notice any change in heartbeat or pulse while taking this medication.

You may have an immediate, serious allergic reaction to the first dose of albuterol, causing symptoms such as hives, rash, and swelling of the mouth, throat, lips, and tongue. The drug has been known to cause life-threatening bronchial spasms, especially with the first dose from a new canister or vial. There have also been rare reports of skin reddening and peeling in children taking albuterol syrup.

Do not exceed your doctor's recommended dose of albuterol. If you need more than usual, check with your doctor. Your asthma may be getting unstable, and you may need another medication. Do not, however, change your medication without first consulting your doctor or pharmacist.

Possible food and drug interactions when taking this medication
Use albuterol inhalation aerosol with other aerosol bronchodilators only if your doctor recommends it.

If albuterol is taken with certain other drugs, the effects of either could be increased, decreased, or altered. It is especially important to check with your doctor before combining albuterol with the following:

  Antidepressants classified as MAO inhibitors, such as Nardil and
    Parnate, and tricyclic antidepressants such as Elavil, Norpramin,
    Pamelor, and Tofranil
  Beta-blockers (heart and blood pressure drugs such as Inderal,
    Tenormin, and Sectral)
  Digoxin (Lanoxin)
  Drugs similar to albuterol, such as Alupent, Brethine, Isuprel, and
    epinephrine
  Drugs that lower potassium levels (water pills such as Lasix and
    HydroDIURIL)

Special information if you are pregnant or breastfeeding
The effects of albuterol during pregnancy have not been adequately studied. If you are pregnant or plan to become pregnant, inform your doctor immediately. It is not known whether albuterol appears in breast milk. If this drug is essential to your health, your doctor may advise you to stop nursing your baby until your treatment is finished.

Recommended dosage

ADULTS

Inhalation Aerosol
If you are being treated for a sudden or severe bronchial spasm or the prevention of asthma symptoms, the usual dosage of albuterol inhalation aerosol is 2 inhalations repeated every 4 to 6 hours. More frequent use is not recommended. In some individuals, 1 inhalation every 4 hours may be sufficient.

To prevent exercise-induced bronchial spasm, the usual dosage is 2 inhalations, 15 minutes prior to exercise.

Tablets
The usual starting dose for adults and children 12 years of age and older is 2 or 4 milligrams 3 to 4 times a day. Dosage should not exceed 32 milligrams per day.

Syrup
The usual starting dose for adults and children over 12 years of age is 1 or 2 teaspoonfuls 3 or 4 times a day. Dosage should not exceed 4 teaspoonfuls 4 times a day.

Proventil Inhalation Solution
The usual dosage for adults and children 12 years of age and older is 2.5 milligrams administered 3 to 4 times daily by nebulization. Do not use more often or in higher doses. To administer 2.5 milligrams, use the entire contents of a unit-dose bottle of the 0.083% solution or dilute 0.5 milliliter of the 0.5 percent solution with 2.5 milliliters of sterile normal saline solution.

Proventil Repetabs, Volmax Extended-Release Tablets,
and VoSpire Extended-Release Tablets
The usual recommended dosage for adults and children 12 years of age and older is 8 milligrams every 12 hours. In some people, 4 milligrams every 12 hours may be sufficient. If the desired effect is not achieved with the standard dosage, your doctor may increase doses to a maximum of 32 milligrams per day, divided into two 16-milligram doses spaced 12 hours apart. Those taking standard tablets or syrup can switch to extended-release tablets. One extended-release tablet every 12 hours is equivalent to one 2-milligram standard tablet every 6 hours.

CHILDREN

Inhalation Aerosol
The usual dose of albuterol inhalation aerosol for children aged 4 and over (12 and over for Proventil) is 2 inhalations every 4 to 6 hours. To prevent exercise-induced bronchial spasm, the dose is 2 inhalations 15 minutes prior to exercise.

Tablets
The usual starting dose for children 6 to 12 years of age is 2 milligrams 3 or 4 times a day. The dose can be increased with caution but should not exceed 24 milligrams per day. Safety and effectiveness in children under 6 have not been established.

Syrup
The usual starting dose for children 6 to 12 years of age is 1 teaspoonful 3 to 4 times a day. The dosage should not exceed 3 teaspoonfuls 4 times a day. For children 2 to 6 years of age, the starting dose is 0.1 milligram per 2.2 pounds of body weight, to a maximum of 4 milligrams 3 times a day.

Proventil Repetabs, Volmax Extended-Release Tablets,
and VoSpire Extended-Release Tablets
The usual starting dosage for children 6 to 12 years of age is 4 milligrams every 12 hours. The dosage can be increased with caution but should not exceed 24 milligrams per day.

AccuNeb Inhalation Solution
The usual starting dose for children 2 to 12 years of age is 0.63 or 1.25 milligrams 3 or 4 times daily by nebulization. To administer, use the entire contents of the prescribed unit-dose vial. The 1.25-milligram dosage may be more helpful for children 6 to 12 with more severe asthma, and for children 11 to 12.

OLDER ADULTS

Oral Dosage
The usual starting dose of tablets or syrup is 2 milligrams 3 or 4 times a day. If needed, the dosage may be increased gradually to as much as 8 milligrams 3 or 4 times a day.

Overdosage

■ *Symptoms of albuterol overdose may include:*
Dizziness, dry mouth, fatigue, general feeling of illness, headache, high or low blood pressure, insomnia, nausea, nervousness, radiating chest pain, rapid or irregular heartbeat, seizures, tremors

Heart attack and even death have been associated with abuse of albuterol inhalation. Exaggerated side effects may also be a sign of an overdose. If you suspect an overdose, seek medical attention immediately.

PROVERA
Pronounced: pro-VAIR-uh
Generic name: Medroxyprogesterone acetate

Why is this drug prescribed?
Provera is derived from the female hormone progesterone. You may be given Provera if your menstrual periods have stopped or a female hormone imbalance is causing your uterus to bleed abnormally. Provera is also prescribed to prevent abnormal growth of the uterine lining in women taking estrogen replacement therapy.

Other forms of medroxyprogesterone, such as Depo-Provera, are used as a contraceptive injection and prescribed in the treatment of endometrial cancer.

Some doctors prescribe Provera to treat endometriosis, menopausal symptoms, premenstrual tension, aggressive sexual behavior in men, and sleep apnea (temporary failure to breathe while sleeping).

Most important fact about this drug
You should never take Provera during the first 4 months of pregnancy. During this formative period, even a few days of treatment with Provera might put your unborn baby at increased risk for birth defects. If you take

Provera and later discover that you were pregnant when you took it, discuss this with your doctor right away.

How should you take this medication?

Provera may be taken with or between meals.

Do not change from one brand to another without consulting your doctor or pharmacist.

- *If you miss a dose...*
  Take it as soon as you remember. If it is almost time for your next dose, skip the one you missed and go back to your regular schedule. Never take 2 doses at the same time.
- *Storage instructions...*
  Store at room temperature.

What side effects may occur?

Side effects cannot be anticipated. If any develop or change in intensity, inform your doctor as soon as possible. Only your doctor can determine if it is safe for you to continue taking Provera.

- *Side effects may include:*
  Acne, anaphylaxis (life-threatening allergic reaction), blood clot in a vein, lungs, or brain, breakthrough bleeding (between menstrual periods), breast tenderness or sudden or excessive flow of milk, cervical erosion or changes in secretions, depression, excessive growth of hair, fever, fluid retention, hair loss, headache, hives, insomnia, itching, lack of menstruation, menstrual flow changes, spotting, nausea, rash, skin discoloration, sleepiness, weight gain or loss, yellowed eyes and skin

Why should this drug not be prescribed?

Provera should never be taken during pregnancy. Avoid it if you even suspect you're pregnant. Doctors once prescribed Provera as a test for pregnancy, but no longer do so for 2 reasons:

- Quicker, safer pregnancy tests are now available.
- If you are in fact pregnant, Provera might injure the baby.

Similarly, Provera used to be given to try to prevent miscarriage. However, doctors now believe that this treatment is not only ineffective but also potentially harmful to the baby.

Do not take Provera if you have:

- Cancer of the breast or genital organs
- Liver disease or a liver condition
- A dead fetus still in the uterus
- Undiagnosed bleeding from the vagina

Do not take Provera if you have, or have ever developed, blood clots. Avoid it, too, if it gives you an allergic reaction.

Special warnings about this medication

Before you start to take Provera, your doctor will give you a complete physical exam, including examination of your breasts and pelvic organs. You should also have a cervical smear (Pap test).

Provera may cause some degree of fluid retention. If you have a medical condition that could be made worse by fluid retention—such as epilepsy, migraine, asthma, or a heart or kidney problem—make sure your doctor knows about it.

Provera may mask the onset of menopause. In other words, while taking Provera you may continue to experience regular menstrual bleeding even if your menopause has started.

Provera may make you depressed, especially if you have suffered from depression in the past. If you become seriously depressed, tell your doctor; you should probably stop taking Provera.

If you are diabetic, Provera could make your diabetes worse; your doctor will want to watch you closely while you are taking this drug.

There is some concern that Provera, like birth control pills, may increase your risk for a blood clot in a vein. If you experience any symptoms that might suggest the onset of such a condition—pain with swelling, warmth, and redness in a leg vein, coughing or shortness of breath, vision problems, migraine, or weakness or numbness in an arm or leg—see your doctor immediately.

Tell your doctor right away if you lose some or all of your vision or you start seeing double. You may have to stop taking the medication.

Possible food and drug interactions when taking this medication

If Provera is taken with certain other drugs, the effects of either may be increased, decreased, or altered. It is especially important to check with your doctor before combining Provera with aminoglutethimide (Cytadren).

Special information if you are pregnant or breastfeeding

You should not take Provera during pregnancy. If you are pregnant or plan to become pregnant, inform your doctor immediately.

Provera appears in breast milk. If you are a new mother, you may need to choose between taking Provera and breastfeeding your baby.

Recommended dosage

ADULTS

To Restore Menstrual Periods

Provera Tablets are taken in dosages of 5 to 10 milligrams daily for 5 to 10 days. Make sure you discuss what effect this will have on your menstrual cycle with your doctor. You should have bleeding 3 to 7 days after you stop taking Provera.

Abnormal Uterine Bleeding Due to Hormonal Imbalance

Beginning on the 16th or 21st day of your menstrual cycle, you will take 5 to 10 milligrams daily for 5 to 10 days. Make sure you discuss what effect this will have on your menstrual cycle with your doctor. You should have bleeding 3 to 7 days after you stop taking Provera.

To Accompany Estrogen Replacement Therapy

The recommended regimen is 5 or 10 milligrams of Provera a day for 12 to 14 days each month, beginning on either Day 1 or Day 16 of the cycle.

Overdosage

Although no specific information is available, any medication taken in excess can have serious consequences. If you suspect an overdose of Provera, seek medical attention immediately.

PROVIGIL

Pronounced: PRO-vi-jil
Generic name: Modafinil

Why is this drug prescribed?

Provigil is a stimulant drug used to treat unusually sleepy people who have been diagnosed with narcolepsy, obstructive sleep apnea/hypopnea syndrome, or shift work sleep disorder. You should be diagnosed with one of these sleep disorders before taking Provigil, since sleepiness can be a symptom of other medical conditions.

Most important fact about this drug

Provigil will not cure any sleep disorder; it merely treats the symptom of sleepiness. This medication should not be used in place of getting enough sleep. You should follow your doctor's advice about maintaining good sleep habits.

Provigil, like other stimulants, has the potential for abuse. It can alter your mood, perception, thinking, and feelings, providing an artificial lift and potentially leading to a certain degree of dependence (although discontinuation of the drug does not produce physical withdrawal symptoms). Make a point of taking only the prescribed dose; never increase the dose or take additional doses.

How should you take this medication?

Food does not reduce the effectiveness of this medication. However, it will delay the onset of action by approximately 1 hour.

■ *If you miss a dose...*
Take it as soon as possible. If you don't remember until the next day, skip the dose you missed and go back to your regular schedule. Do not take a double dose.

■ *Storage instructions…*
Store at room temperature.

What side effects may occur?
Side effects cannot be anticipated. If any develop or change in intensity, tell your doctor as soon as possible. Only your doctor can determine if it is safe for you to continue taking Provigil.

■ *Side effects may include:*
Anxiety, depression, diarrhea, difficulty sleeping, dizziness, dry mouth, headache, infection, loss of appetite, loss of muscle strength, lung problems, nausea, nervousness, prickling or tingling feeling, runny nose, sore throat

Why should this drug not be prescribed?
If Provigil gives you an allergic reaction, you'll need to avoid it.

Special warnings about this medication
If you have high blood pressure, liver or kidney problems, or a history of psychosis or drug abuse, use Provigil with caution. Be sure your doctor knows your medical history before you begin this medication.

Provigil should be avoided by people with certain types of heart disease such as mitral valve prolapse. If you've ever had a heart problem, be sure to check with the doctor before using this drug.

Provigil may impair your judgment, thinking, or motor skills. You should not drive a car or operate hazardous machinery until you know how this medication affects you.

Oral and implantable contraceptives are less effective while you are taking Provigil. You should use an additional method of contraception while you are taking Provigil and for one month after discontinuing this medication.

Possible food and drug interactions when taking this medication
The effect of combining Provigil with alcohol has not been studied. It's considered wise to avoid alcohol while taking the drug.

If Provigil is taken with certain other drugs, the effects of either could be increased, decreased, or altered. It is especially important to check with your doctor before combining Provigil with any of the following:

Antidepressants such as Effexor, Elavil, Pamelor, Paxil, Prozac, and Tofranil
Carbamazepine (Tegretol)
Clomipramine (Anafranil)
Cyclosporine (Sandimmune)
Diazepam (Valium)
Itraconazole (Sporanox)
Ketoconazole (Nizoral)

MAO inhibitors such as the antidepressants Nardil and Parnate
Methylphenidate (Ritalin)
Oral contraceptives and hormonal implants
Phenobarbital
Phenytoin (Dilantin)
Propranolol (Inderal)
Rifampin (Rifater)
Theophylline (Theo-Dur)
Warfarin (Coumadin)

Special information if you are pregnant or breastfeeding

The possibility of harmful effects during pregnancy has not been ruled
out. If you become pregnant or plan to become pregnant, tell your doctor
immediately. Provigil is recommended during pregnancy only if the need
for therapy outweighs the potential risk.

It is not known whether Provigil appears in breast milk. Tell your doctor if you are breastfeeding an infant. Nursing mothers should use
Provigil with caution and only when clearly needed.

Recommended dosage

ADULTS

The usual dose of Provigil is 200 milligrams taken as a single dose in the
morning.

CHILDREN

Not for children under 16.

OLDER ADULTS

People over 65 may need a lower dose if they have liver or kidney disease,
which reduce the body's ability to metabolize this medication.

Overdosage

Any medication taken in excess can cause symptoms of overdose. If you
suspect an overdose, seek medical treatment immediately.

■ *Symptoms of Provigil overdose may include:*
   Aggressiveness, agitation, anxiety, confusion, diarrhea, fluttering
   heartbeat, insomnia, irritability, nausea, nervousness, sleep disturbances, slow blood clotting, tremor

PROZAC

Pronounced: PRO-zak
Generic name: Fluoxetine hydrochloride
Other brand names: Prozac Weekly, Sarafem

Why is this drug prescribed?

Prozac is prescribed for the treatment of depression—that is, a continuing depression that interferes with daily functioning. The symptoms of major depression often include changes in appetite, sleep habits, and mind/body coordination; decreased sex drive; increased fatigue; feelings of guilt or worthlessness; difficulty concentrating; slowed thinking; and suicidal thoughts.

Prozac is also prescribed to treat obsessive-compulsive disorder. An obsession is a thought that won't go away; a compulsion is an action done over and over to relieve anxiety. The drug is also used in the treatment of bulimia (binge eating followed by deliberate vomiting). It has also been used to treat other eating disorders and obesity.

In addition, Prozac is used to treat panic disorder, including panic associated with agoraphobia (a severe fear of being in crowds or public places). People with panic disorder usually suffer from panic attacks—feelings of intense fear that develop suddenly, often for no reason. Various symptoms occur during the attacks, including a rapid or pounding heartbeat, chest pain, sweating, trembling, and shortness of breath.

In children and adolescents, Prozac is used to treat major depression and obsessive-compulsive disorder.

Prozac Weekly is approved for treating major depression.

Under the brand name Sarafem, the active ingredient in Prozac is also prescribed for the treatment of premenstrual dysphoric disorder (PMDD), formerly known as premenstrual syndrome (PMS). Symptoms of PMDD include mood problems such as anxiety, depression, irritability or persistent anger, mood swings, and tension. Physical problems that accompany PMDD include bloating, breast tenderness, headache, and joint and muscle pain. Symptoms typically begin 1 to 2 weeks before a woman's menstrual period and are severe enough to interfere with day-to-day activities and relationships.

Prozac belongs to the class of drugs called selective serotonin re-uptake inhibitors (SSRIs). Serotonin is one of the chemical messengers believed to govern moods. Ordinarily, it is quickly reabsorbed after its release at the junctures between nerves. Re-uptake inhibitors such as Prozac slow this process, thereby boosting the levels of serotonin available in the brain.

Most important fact about this drug

Serious, sometimes fatal, reactions have been known to occur when Prozac is used in combination with other antidepressant drugs known as

MAO inhibitors, including Nardil and Parnate; and when Prozac is discontinued and an MAO inhibitor is started. Never take Prozac with one of these drugs or within at least 14 days of discontinuing therapy with one of them; and allow 5 weeks or more between stopping Prozac and starting an MAO inhibitor. Be especially cautious if you have been taking Prozac in high doses or for a long time.

In addition, Prozac should never be combined with thioridazine (Mellaril) due to the risk of life-threatening drug interactions; and a minimum of 5 weeks should be allowed between stopping Prozac and starting Mellaril.

If you are taking any prescription or nonprescription drugs, notify your doctor before taking Prozac.

How should you take this medication?
Prozac should be taken exactly as prescribed by your doctor.

Prozac usually is taken once or twice a day. To be effective, it should be taken regularly. Make a habit of taking it at the same time you do some other daily activity.

It may be 4 weeks before you feel any relief from your depression, but the drug's effects should last about 9 months after a 3-month treatment regimen. For obsessive-compulsive disorder, the full effect may take 5 weeks to appear.

■ *If you miss a dose...*
Take the forgotten dose as soon as you remember. If several hours have passed, skip the dose. Never try to catch up by doubling the dose.
■ *Storage instructions...*
Store at room temperature.

What side effects may occur?
Side effects cannot be anticipated. If any develop or change in intensity, inform your doctor as soon as possible. Only your doctor can determine if it is safe for you to continue taking Prozac.

■ *Side effects may include:*
Abnormal dreams, abnormal ejaculation, abnormal vision, anxiety, diarrhea, diminished sex drive, dizziness, dry mouth, flu-like symptoms, flushing, gas, headache, impotence, insomnia, itching, loss of appetite, nausea, nervousness, rash, sex-drive changes, sinusitis, sleepiness, sore throat, sweating, tremors, upset stomach, vomiting, weakness, yawning

Why should this drug not be prescribed?
If you are sensitive to or have ever had an allergic reaction to Prozac or similar drugs such as Paxil and Zoloft, you should not take this medication. Make sure that your doctor is aware of any drug reactions that you have experienced.

Do not take this drug while using an MAO inhibitor (see *Most important fact about this drug*). You should also not use Prozac if you are taking Mellaril (thioridazine). Likewise, do not start taking Mellaril within 5 weeks of stopping Prozac.

Special warnings about this medication

In clinical studies, antidepressants increased the risk of suicidal thinking and behavior in children and adolescents with depression and other psychiatric disorders. Anyone considering the use of Prozac or any other antidepressant in a child or adolescent must balance this risk with the clinical need. Prozac is approved for treating major depression in children 8 years and older and for treating obsessive-compulsive disorder in children 7 years and older.

Additionally, the progression of major depression is associated with a worsening of symptoms and/or the emergence of suicidal thinking or behavior in both adults and children, whether or not they are taking antidepressants. Individuals being treated with Prozac and their caregivers should watch for any change in symptoms or any new symptoms that appear suddenly—especially agitation, anxiety, hostility, panic, restlessness, extreme hyperactivity, and suicidal thinking or behavior—and report them to the doctor immediately. Be especially observant at the beginning of treatment or whenever there is a change in dose.

Unless you are directed to do so by your doctor, do not take this medication if you are recovering from a heart attack or if you have liver disease or diabetes.

Prozac may cause you to become drowsy or less alert and may affect your judgment. Therefore, driving or operating dangerous machinery or participating in any hazardous activity that requires full mental alertness is not recommended.

While taking this medication, you may feel dizzy or light-headed or actually faint when getting up from a lying or sitting position. If getting up slowly doesn't help or if this problem continues, notify your doctor.

If you develop a skin rash or hives while taking Prozac, discontinue use of the medication and notify your doctor immediately.

Prozac should be used with caution if you have a history of mania or seizures. You should discuss all of your medical conditions with your doctor before taking this medication.

Prozac can occasionally cause decreased appetite and weight loss, especially in depressed people who are already underweight and in those with bulimia. If you notice changes in your weight or appetite, tell your doctor.

Antidepressants such as Prozac can potentially cause stomach bleeding, especially when combined with nonsteroidal anti-inflammatory drugs (NSAIDs) such as aspirin, ibuprofen (Advil, Motrin), naproxen (Aleve), and ketoprofen (Orudis KT). Consult your doctor before combining Prozac with NSAIDs or blood-thinning medications.

There have been rare reports of prolonged seizures in people who received electroconvulsive therapy (ECT) while taking Prozac. To date, there are no clinical studies establishing the benefit of combined treatment with Prozac and ECT.

Possible food and drug interactions when taking this medication

Never take Prozac with MAO inhibitors or thioridazine (Mellaril) (see *Most important fact about this drug*).

Do not drink alcohol while taking this medication.

If Prozac is taken with certain other drugs, the effects of either could be increased, decreased, or altered. It is especially important to check with your doctor before combining Prozac with the following:

Alprazolam (Xanax)
Any other antidepressants
Carbamazepine (Tegretol)
Clozapine (Clozaril)
Diazepam (Valium)
Digitoxin (Crystodigin)
Drugs that impair brain function, such as sleep aids and narcotic painkillers
Flecainide (Tambocor)
Haloperidol (Haldol)
Lithium (Eskalith)
Nonsteroidal anti-inflammatory drugs (NSAIDs) such as aspirin, ibuprofen (Advil, Motrin), naproxen (Aleve), and ketoprofen (Orudis KT)
Phenytoin (Dilantin)
Pimozide (Orap)
Sumatriptan (Imitrex)
Tryptophan
Vinblastine (Velban)
Warfarin (Coumadin)

Special information if you are pregnant or breastfeeding

The effects of Prozac during pregnancy have not been adequately studied. If you are pregnant or plan to become pregnant, inform your doctor immediately. This medication appears in breast milk, and breastfeeding is not recommended while you are taking Prozac.

Recommended dosage

DEPRESSION

It may take 4 weeks before the full antidepressant effect of Prozac is seen.

Adults

The recommended starting dose is 20 milligrams a day, usually taken in the morning. If needed, your doctor may gradually increase the dose up to a maximum of 80 milligrams a day. The usual daily dose ranges from 20 to 60 milligrams. Daily doses above 20 milligrams should be taken in the morning or in two smaller doses taken in the morning and at noon.

Children 8 Years and Older

The usual starting dose is 10 or 20 milligrams a day. Children starting at 10 milligrams will have their dose increased to 20 milligrams a day after 1 week. Underweight children may need to remain at the 10-milligram dose.

Prozac Weekly

You need to wait at least 7 days after stopping your daily dose of Prozac before switching to the once-weekly formulation. One Prozac Weekly capsule contains 90 milligrams of medication.

OBSESSIVE-COMPULSIVE DISORDER

It may take 5 weeks before the full effects of Prozac are seen.

Adults

The recommended starting dose is 20 milligrams a day, usually taken in the morning. If needed, your doctor may gradually increase the dose up to a maximum of 80 milligrams a day. The usual daily dose ranges from 20 to 60 milligrams. Daily doses above 20 milligrams should be taken in the morning or in two smaller doses taken in the morning and at noon.

Children 7 Years and Older

The recommended starting dose is 10 milligrams a day. After 2 weeks, your doctor will increase the dose to 20 milligrams. If needed, your doctor may further increase the dose up to a maximum of 60 milligrams a day. The recommended dosage range for underweight children is 10 to 30 milligrams a day.

BULIMIA

Adults

The recommended dose is 60 milligrams a day taken in the morning. Your doctor may start you at a lower dose and gradually increase it over a period of several days.

PANIC DISORDER

Adults

The recommended starting dose is 10 milligrams a day. After 1 week, your doctor will increase the dose to 20 milligrams. If no improvement is seen after several weeks, your doctor may increase the dose to a maximum of 60 milligrams a day.

PREMENSTRUAL DYSPHORIC DISORDER

Adults
The usual dose of Sarafem is 20 milligrams a day. Your doctor will instruct you to take the dose either every day of the month or only during the 2 weeks before menstruation begins (the luteal phase of your cycle). If there's no improvement after several weeks, the dose can be increased, usually to 60 milligrams a day. The maximum dose is 80 milligrams daily.

DOSAGE ADJUSTMENT

For all indications, your doctor may need to prescribe a lower dose if you are elderly, have liver disease, or are taking other medications.

Overdosage

Any medication taken in excess can have serious consequences. An overdose of Prozac can be fatal. In addition, combining Prozac with certain other drugs can cause symptoms of overdose. If you suspect an overdose, seek medical attention immediately.

■ *Common symptoms of Prozac overdose include:*
Nausea, rapid heartbeat, seizures, sleepiness, vomiting
■ *Other symptoms of Prozac overdose include:*
Coma, delirium, fainting, high fever, irregular heartbeat, low blood pressure, mania, rigid muscles, sweating, stupor

PSORCON

Pronounced: SORE-kon
Generic name: Diflorasone diacetate

Why is this drug prescribed?

Psorcon is prescribed for the relief of the inflammation and itching of skin disorders that respond to the application of steroids (hormones produced by the body that have potent anti-inflammatory effects).

Psorcon is available in ointment and cream forms, and in emollient ointment and cream.

Most important fact about this drug

When you use Psorcon, you inevitably absorb some of the medication through your skin and into the bloodstream. Too much absorption can lead to unwanted side effects elsewhere in the body. To keep this problem to a minimum, avoid using large amounts of Psorcon over large areas, and do not cover it with airtight dressings such as plastic wrap or adhesive bandages unless specifically told to by your doctor.

How should you use this medication?
Use this medication exactly as prescribed.
Psorcon is for use only on the skin. Be careful to keep it out of your eyes.

■ *If you miss a dose...*
Apply it as soon as you remember. If it is almost time for the next dose, skip the one you missed and go back to your regular schedule.

■ *Storage instructions...*
Store at room temperature.

What side effects may occur?
Side effects cannot be anticipated. If any develop or change in intensity, inform your doctor as soon as possible. Only your doctor can determine if it is safe for you to continue taking Psorcon.

■ *Side effects may include:*
Burning, dryness, eruptions resembling acne, excessive discoloring of the skin, excessive growth of hair, inflammation around the mouth, inflammation of hair follicles, irritation, itching, prickly heat, secondary infection, severe inflammation of the skin, softening of the skin, stretch marks, stretching or thinning of the skin

Why should this drug not be prescribed?
If you are sensitive to or have ever had an allergic reaction to diflorasone diacetate or other drugs of this type (antifungals, steroids), you should not take this medication. Make sure your doctor is aware of any drug reactions you have experienced.

Special warnings about this medication
Remember that absorption of Psorcon through the skin can affect the whole body. Although it's unusual (most common if Psorcon is spread over large areas of the skin), you could develop symptoms of steroid excess such as weight gain, reddening and rounding of the face and neck, growth of excess body and facial hair, high blood pressure, emotional disturbances, loss of energy due to high blood sugar, and increase in frequency of urination.

Do not use this drug for any disorder other than the one for which it was prescribed.

The treated skin area should not be bandaged, covered, or wrapped unless otherwise directed by your doctor. Avoid covering a treated area with waterproof diapers or plastic pants. They can cause unwanted absorption of Psorcon.

If an irritation or allergic reaction develops while you are using Psorcon, notify your doctor.

Possible food and drug interactions when taking this medication
No interactions with food or other drugs have been reported.

Special information if you are pregnant or breastfeeding

If you are pregnant or plan to become pregnant, inform your doctor before using Psorcon. In general, women who are pregnant should not use steroids extensively, in large amounts, or over long periods of time. It is not known whether this medication appears in breast milk. If this drug is essential to your health, your doctor may advise you to discontinue breastfeeding until treatment with this medication is finished.

Recommended dosage

ADULTS

Psorcon ointment should be applied as a thin film over the affected area from 1 to 3 times a day, depending on the severity or resistant nature of the condition. The emollient ointment may be applied up to 4 times daily.

Psorcon cream should be applied twice a day. The emollient cream may be applied up to 3 times a day.

Your doctor may recommend airtight bandages for the management of psoriasis (a chronic skin disorder) or other stubborn skin conditions. If an infection develops, you should stop using airtight dressings.

CHILDREN

Your doctor will limit the use of Psorcon for your child to the smallest amount that is effective. Long-term treatment may interfere with the growth and development of children.

Overdosage

An acute overdosage is unlikely with the use of Psorcon; however, long-term or prolonged use can produce side effects throughout your body. If you suspect an overdose, seek medical attention immediately.

PULMICORT RESPULES

Pronounced: PULL-mi-cort
Generic name: Budesonide

Why is this drug prescribed?

Budesonide, the active ingredient in Pulmicort Respules, is an anti-inflammatory steroid medication. Inhaled on a regular basis, Pulmicort helps prevent asthma attacks.

Pulmicort Respules are prescribed for children 12 months to 8 years of age. They are given by nebulizer (a device that produces a fine spray). Adults and children over 6 can use another form of budesonide, Pulmicort Turbuhaler, that's taken with an inhaler. Both types of Pulmicort are preventive medicines. They will not relieve an acute or life-threatening episode of asthma.

Most important fact about this drug
Because steroids can suppress the immune system, children taking Pulmicort may become more susceptible to infections, and their infections could be more severe. Be careful to protect the child from exposure to infectious diseases such as chickenpox and measles. If the youngster is exposed, contact your doctor immediately.

How should you take this medication?
Use Pulmicort Respules exactly as directed. The effectiveness of this medication depends on its regular use. Your doctor will prescribe the lowest effective dose. Do not use more or less medication than the amount prescribed. When starting therapy, carefully read the instructions that come with the medication. The child's asthma symptoms may begin to improve in 2 to 8 days, although you may not see the maximum benefit for 4 to 6 weeks. If symptoms do not improve or get worse, contact your doctor.

Pulmicort Respules contain a liquid suspension of budesonide for administration with a jet nebulizer connected to a mouthpiece or face mask. Do not use an ultrasonic nebulizer, and do not mix Pulmicort with other medications. Gently shake the Respule in a circular motion before use. Avoid exposing the eyes to the medication. To decrease the risk of developing a fungus infection in the mouth, have the child rinse with water, without swallowing, after each dose. Wash the child's face after using the face mask.

■ *If you miss a dose...*
  Give it as soon as you remember. If it is almost time for the next dose, skip the one you missed and go back to the regular schedule. Do not give 2 doses at once.
■ *Storage instructions...*
  Store Pulmicort Respules upright at room temperature. Do not refrigerate or freeze. When you open the aluminum foil envelope containing the Respules, record the date on the back of the envelope. Keep unused Respules in the envelope protected from light. Use any individually opened Respules promptly. You should discard any unused Respules two weeks after opening the envelope.

What side effects may occur?
Side effects cannot be anticipated. If any develop or change in intensity, inform your doctor as soon as possible. Only your doctor can determine if it is safe for you to continue taking Pulmicort.

■ *Side effects may include:*
  Abdominal pain, conjunctivitis (pinkeye), cough, diarrhea, ear infection or inflammation, fever, fungal infection in mouth, headache, nasal or sinus inflammation, nosebleed, pain, rash, respiratory infection,

stomach or intestinal inflammation, throat inflammation, viral infection, vomiting, wheezing

Why should this drug not be prescribed?

If the child is allergic to budesonide, this drug cannot be used. In addition, Pulmicort cannot be used to treat severe asthma attacks.

Special warnings about this medication

If the youngster is switching to Pulmicort from an oral steroid medication, your doctor will be careful to reduce the oral dosage very gradually. Taking oral steroids suppresses the natural production of steroids by the adrenal gland, and it takes months for production to return to normal after the oral steroids are stopped. In the meantime, the body will be unusually vulnerable to stress.

There have been reports of death during and immediately after transfer from oral steroids to inhaled steroids, so your doctor will monitor the child carefully during this period. People who have been taking high doses of oral steroids for an extended period of time are especially prone to problems, particularly when the oral steroids have been almost completely stopped. At that point, any stress from trauma, surgery, or infection (especially stomach or intestinal inflammation) is more likely to trigger adverse events.

If the child experiences a period of stress or a severe asthma attack during the switch to Pulmicort, begin giving the oral medication again (in large doses) and contact your doctor immediately. The child should carry a medical identification card indicating that he or she may need additional medication during periods of stress or a severe asthma attack.

Transfer from oral steroids to Pulmicort may unmask allergic conditions previously controlled by the oral drugs, such as nasal inflammation, conjunctivitis (pinkeye), and eczema. Transfer from oral steroids may also be accompanied by withdrawal symptoms, including joint or muscle pain, fatigue, and depression, even while Pulmicort is improving the child's asthma symptoms.

Like other inhaled asthma medications, Pulmicort occasionally triggers an asthma attack. If this occurs, immediately administer a fast-acting inhaled bronchodilator, stop using Pulmicort, and contact your doctor. The youngster will need to switch to a different asthma medication. Also alert your doctor immediately if the usual doses of the child's fast-acting bronchodilator no longer work. Oral steroids may be needed for a while.

Steroid medications can stunt growth in children and teenagers. Your doctor will prescribe the lowest effective dose of Pulmicort in order to minimize this problem, and will monitor the child's growth carefully.

While using this medication, some people develop fungal infections in the mouth and throat. If this occurs, your doctor can prescribe antifungal medication while the child continues to use Pulmicort. Individuals with tuberculosis, ocular herpes simplex, or any untreated fungal, bacterial, viral, or parasitic infection should use inhaled steroids with caution. Caution is also in order if the child has liver disease.

In rare instances, inhaled steroids have been known to cause glaucoma (increased pressure in the eye) and cataracts.

Possible food and drug interactions when taking this medication

If Pulmicort is taken with certain other drugs, the effects of either can be increased, decreased, or altered. It is especially important to check with your doctor before combining Pulmicort with ketoconazole (Nizoral).

Special information if you are pregnant or breastfeeding

This medication is not intended for women of childbearing age, but you should know that budesonide is recommended during pregnancy only if clearly needed. In addition, steroids make their way into breast milk and are not recommended for nursing mothers.

Recommended dosage

CHILDREN 12 MONTHS TO 8 YEARS OF AGE

The usual dosage depends on the child's previous treatments for asthma.

If fast-acting bronchodilators alone have been used previously, the usual starting dose is 0.5 milligrams daily. (A dose of 0.25 milligram taken once daily may be prescribed if the child has failed to respond to non-steroidal therapy.) The maximum long-term dosage is 0.5 milligram daily.

If inhaled steroids have been used previously, the usual starting dose is 0.5 milligram. The maximum long-term dosage is 1 milligram daily.

If oral steroids have been used previously, the usual starting dose is 1 milligram. The maximum long-term dosage is also 1 milligram daily.

The daily dosage may be taken in a single dose or divided into 2 doses if once-daily treatment does not adequately control asthma symptoms. Once asthma symptoms are controlled, the dose may be gradually lowered.

Children already taking oral steroids will continue to do so while starting therapy with Pulmicort Respules. After one week, the doctor will lower the dose of the oral steroids, then gradually lower it further at 1- or 2-week intervals.

Overdosage

Excessive doses of steroid medications taken for long periods can stunt growth or cause a condition called Cushing's syndrome. Symptoms of this condition include weight gain, a moon-shaped face, muscle wasting, weakness, and poor wound healing. If you think a problem is developing, check with your doctor immediately.

PULMICORT TURBUHALER

Pronounced: PULL-mi-cort
Generic name: Budesonide

Why is this drug prescribed?

Budesonide, the active ingredient in Pulmicort Turbuhaler, is an anti-inflammatory steroid medication. Inhaled on a regular basis, Pulmicort helps prevent asthma attacks. It is sometimes prescribed in addition to oral steroids, and may reduce or eliminate the need for them.

Pulmicort Turbuhaler is used to treat asthma in adults and children over age 6. Children 12 months to 8 years of age can be treated with another form of budesonide, Pulmicort Respules, which is given by nebulizer. Both types of Pulmicort are preventive medicines. They will not relieve an acute or life-threatening episode of asthma.

Most important fact about this drug

Because steroids can suppress the immune system, people taking Pulmicort may become more susceptible to infections, and their infections could be more severe. If you are taking Pulmicort, avoid exposure to infectious diseases such as chickenpox and measles. If you are exposed, contact your doctor immediately.

How should you take this medication?

Use Pulmicort Turbuhaler exactly as directed. The effectiveness of this medication depends on its regular use. Your doctor will prescribe the lowest effective dose. Do not take more or less medication than the amount prescribed. When starting therapy, carefully read the instructions that come with the inhaler. Your asthma symptoms may begin to improve in 24 hours, although you may not see the maximum benefit for 1 to 2 weeks or longer. If your symptoms do not improve or get worse, contact your doctor.

Pulmicort Turbuhaler delivers a dose of medication in dry powder form. To ensure the correct dose, the inhaler must be held in an upright position, with the mouthpiece on top, during priming and loading.

Before its first use, each new inhaler must be primed. To prime the inhaler, hold it upright and turn the brown grip fully to the right, then fully to the left until it clicks. Repeat this procedure a second time. The unit is now primed.

The inhaler must be loaded with medication immediately prior to each use. As you did when priming the unit, turn the brown grip fully to the right, then fully to the left until it clicks.

During inhalation, the inhaler must be held in an upright (mouthpiece up) or horizontal position. Do not shake the inhaler. Place the mouthpiece between your lips and inhale forcefully and deeply. The Pulmicort powder is then delivered to the lungs. Do not exhale through the inhaler.

You may not taste or sense any medication entering the lungs when inhaling from the Turbuhaler. This lack of sensation is not a cause for concern, and does not mean that you'll fail to receive the medication's benefits.

To decrease the risk of developing a fungus infection in the mouth, rinse it with water, without swallowing, after each dose. Do not use the inhaler with a spacer. Do not bite or chew the mouthpiece.

■ *If you miss a dose…*
Take it as soon as you remember. If it is almost time for your next dose, skip the one you missed and go back to your regular schedule. Do not take 2 doses at once.

■ *Storage instructions…*
Keep the Pulmicort Turbuhaler clean at all times. Replace the cover securely after each opening. Store with the cover tightened in a dry place at room temperature. Discard the unit when a red mark appears in the indicator window.

What side effects may occur?
Side effects cannot be anticipated. If any develop or change in intensity, inform your doctor as soon as possible. Only your doctor can determine if it is safe for you to continue taking Pulmicort.

■ *Side effects may include:*
Aching joints, back pain, cough, fever, flu-like symptoms, fungal infection in mouth, headache, indigestion, nasal and sinus inflammation, pain, respiratory infection, sore throat, weakness

Why should this drug not be prescribed?
If you are allergic to budesonide, you cannot use Pulmicort. In addition, Pulmicort cannot be used to treat severe asthma attacks.

Special warnings about this medication
If you are switching to Pulmicort from an oral steroid medication, your doctor will be careful to reduce your oral dosage very gradually. Taking oral steroids suppresses the natural production of steroids by the adrenal gland, and it takes months for production to return to normal after the oral steroids are stopped. In the meantime, the body will be unusually vulnerable to stress.

There have been reports of death during and immediately after transfer from oral steroids to inhaled steroids, so your doctor will monitor you carefully during this period. People who have been taking high doses of oral steroids for an extended period of time are especially prone to problems, particularly when the oral steroids have been almost completely stopped. At that point, any stress from trauma, surgery, or infection (especially stomach or intestinal inflammation) is more likely to trigger adverse events.

If you experience a period of stress or a severe asthma attack during your switch to Pulmicort, you should begin taking your oral medication again (in large doses) and contact your doctor immediately. You should carry a medical identification card indicating that you may need additional medication during periods of stress or a severe asthma attack.

Transfer from oral steroids to Pulmicort may unmask allergic conditions previously controlled by those steroids, such as nasal inflammation, conjunctivitis (pinkeye), and eczema. Transfer from oral steroids may also be accompanied by withdrawal symptoms, including joint or muscle pain, fatigue, and depression, even while Pulmicort is improving your asthma symptoms.

Like other inhaled asthma medications, Pulmicort occasionally triggers an asthma attack. If this occurs, immediately use a fast-acting inhaled bronchodilator, stop using Pulmicort, and contact your doctor. You'll need to switch to a different asthma medication. Also alert your doctor immediately if the usual doses of your fast-acting bronchodilator no longer work. You may need to take oral steroids for a while.

Steroid medications can stunt growth in children and teenagers. Your doctor will prescribe the lowest effective dose of Pulmicort in order to minimize this problem, and will monitor the child's growth carefully.

While using this medication, some people develop fungal infections in the mouth and throat. If this occurs, the doctor can prescribe antifungal medication while you continue to use Pulmicort. People with tuberculosis, ocular herpes simplex, or any untreated fungal, bacterial, viral, or parasitic infection should use inhaled steroids with caution. Caution is also in order if you have liver disease.

In rare instances, inhaled steroids have been known to cause glaucoma (increased pressure in the eye) and cataracts.

Possible food and drug interactions when taking this medication
If Pulmicort is taken with certain other drugs, the effects of either can be increased, decreased, or altered. It is especially important to check with your doctor before combining Pulmicort with the following:

 Antibiotics such as clarithromycin (Biaxin) and erythromycin
    (E.E.S., Ery-Tab, PCE)
 Antifungal medications such as ketoconazole (Nizoral) and
    itraconazole (Sporanox)

Special Information if you are pregnant or breastfeeding
Pulmicort does not appear to harm the developing infant during pregnancy. Nevertheless, the possibility for harm cannot be ruled out. This medication should be used during pregnancy only if it is clearly needed.

Steroids make their way into breast milk. Because they could affect the nursing infant, you'll need to either discontinue breastfeeding or stop taking this medication.

Recommended dosage

ADULTS

The usual dosage depends on your previous treatments for asthma.

If you have previously been using only fast-acting bronchodilators, the usual starting dose is 200 to 400 milligrams twice a day. The maximum long-term dosage is 400 milligrams twice daily.

If you have previously been using inhaled steroids, the usual starting dose is 200 to 400 milligrams twice a day (or once daily in the morning or evening if your asthma has been well controlled). The maximum long-term dosage is 800 milligrams twice daily.

If you have previously been taking oral steroids, the usual starting dose is 400 to 800 milligrams twice a day. The maximum long-term dosage is 800 milligrams twice daily.

If you are taking oral steroids, you will continue to do so while starting Pulmicort Turbuhaler. After one week, the doctor will lower your dose of oral steroids, then gradually lower it further at 1- or 2-week intervals.

CHILDREN AGE 6 AND OLDER

As with adults, the child's usual dosage depends on previous treatments.

If the child has previously been using only a fast-acting bronchodilator, the usual starting dose is 200 milligrams twice a day. The maximum long-term dosage is 400 milligrams twice daily.

If the child has previously been using inhaled steroids, the usual starting dose is 200 milligrams twice daily. (A once-a-day dose of 200 or 400 milligrams may be prescribed instead.) The maximum long-term dosage is 400 milligrams twice daily.

If the child has previously been taking oral steroids, the highest recommended dose is 400 milligrams taken twice a day. As with adults, the dosage of oral steroids will be gradually reduced while the child continues to take Pulmicort.

Overdosage

Excessive doses of steroid medications taken for long periods can stunt growth or cause a condition called Cushing's syndrome. Symptoms of this condition include weight gain, a moon-shaped face, muscle wasting, weakness, and poor wound healing. If you think a problem is developing, check with your doctor immediately.

PYRIDIUM

Pronounced: pie-RI-di-um
Generic name: Phenazopyridine hydrochloride

Why is this drug prescribed?

Pyridium is a urinary tract analgesic that helps relieve the pain, burning, urgency, frequency, and irritation caused by infection, trauma, catheters, or various surgical procedures in the lower urinary tract. Pyridium is indicated for short-term use and can only relieve symptoms; it is not a treatment for the underlying cause of the symptoms.

Most important fact about this drug

Pyridium produces an orange to red color in urine, and may stain fabric. Staining of contact lenses has also been reported.

How should you take this medication?

Take Pyridium after meals, exactly as prescribed.

■ *If you miss a dose...*
Take it as soon as you remember. If it is almost time for your next dose, skip the one you missed and go back to your regular schedule. Never take 2 doses at the same time.

■ *Storage instructions...*
Store at room temperature.

What side effects may occur?

Side effects cannot be anticipated. If any occur or change in intensity, inform your doctor as soon as possible. Only your doctor can determine if it is safe for you to continue taking Pyridium.

■ *Side effects may include:*
Headache, itching, rash, severe allergic reaction (rash, difficulty breathing, fever, rapid heartbeat, convulsions), upset stomach

Why should this drug not be prescribed?

Pyridium should be avoided if you have kidney disease, or if you are sensitive to or have ever had an allergic reaction to it.

Special warnings about this medication

If your skin or the whites of your eyes develop a yellowish tone, it may indicate that your kidneys are not eliminating the medication as they should. Notify your doctor immediately. If you are older, your doctor will watch you more closely, since the kidneys work less effectively as we age.

Possible food and drug interactions when taking this medication

No interactions have been reported.

Special information if you are pregnant or breastfeeding

The effects of Pyridium during pregnancy have not been adequately studied. If you are pregnant or plan to become pregnant, inform your doctor immediately. To date, there is no information on whether Pyridium appears in breast milk. If this medication is essential to your health, your doctor may advise you to stop breastfeeding until your treatment with Pyridium is finished.

Recommended dosage

ADULTS

The usual dose is two 100-milligram tablets or one 200-milligram tablet 3 times a day after meals.

You should not take Pyridium for more than 2 days if you are also taking an antibiotic for the treatment of a urinary tract infection.

Overdosage

Any medication taken in excess can have serious consequences. If you suspect an overdose, seek emergency medical treatment immediately.

■ *Symptoms of Pyridium overdose may include:*
Blood disorders, bluish skin color, impaired kidney and liver function

Quazepam See Doral, page 472.

QUESTRAN

Pronounced: KWEST-ran
Generic name: Cholestyramine
Other brand name: Questran Light

Why is this drug prescribed?

Questran is used to lower cholesterol levels in the blood of people with primary hypercholesterolemia (too much LDL cholesterol). Hypercholesterolemia is a genetic condition characterized by a lack of the LDL receptors that remove cholesterol from the bloodstream.

This drug can be used to lower cholesterol levels in people who also have hypertriglyceridemia, a condition in which an excess of fat is stored in the body.

This drug may also be prescribed to relieve itching associated with gallbladder obstruction.

It is available in two forms: Questran and Questran Light. The same instructions apply to both.

Most important fact about this drug

It's important to remember that Questran is a supplement to—not a substitute for—diet, exercise, and weight loss. To get the full benefit of the medication, you need to stick to the diet and exercise program prescribed by your doctor. All these efforts to keep your cholesterol levels normal are important because together they may lower your risk of heart disease.

How should you take this medication?

Never take Questran in its dry form. Always mix it with water or other liquids *before* taking it. For Questran, use 2 to 6 ounces of liquid per packet or level scoopful; for Questran Light, use 2 to 3 ounces. Soups or fruits with a high moisture content, such as applesauce or crushed pineapple, can be used in place of beverages.

■ *If you miss a dose...*
Take the forgotten dose as soon as you remember. If it is almost time for the next dose, skip the one you missed and go back to your regular schedule. Never try to catch up by doubling the dose.

■ *Storage instructions...*
Store at room temperature. Protect from moisture and high humidity.

What side effects may occur?

Side effects cannot be anticipated. If any develop or change in intensity, inform your doctor as soon as possible. Only your doctor can determine if it is safe for you to continue taking Questran.

■ *Side effects may include:*
Constipation

Why should this drug not be prescribed?

If you are sensitive to or have ever had an allergic reaction to Questran or similar drugs such as Colestid, you should not take this medication. Make sure that your doctor is aware of any drug reactions that you have experienced.

Unless you are directed to do so by your doctor, do not take this medication if you are being treated for gallbladder obstruction.

Special warnings about this medication

If you have phenylketonuria, a genetic disorder, check with your doctor before taking Questran Light because this product contains phenylalanine.

If you are being treated for any disease that contributes to increased blood cholesterol, such as hypothyroidism (reduced thyroid function), diabetes, nephrotic syndrome (kidney and blood vessel disorder), dysproteinemia, obstructive liver disease, or alcoholism, or if you are taking any drugs that may raise cholesterol levels, consult your doctor before taking this medication. Caution is also in order if your kidney function is poor.

Questran should begin to reduce cholesterol levels during the first month of therapy. If adequate reduction of cholesterol is not obtained, your doctor may increase the dosage or add other cholesterol-lowering drugs. Therefore, it is important that your doctor check your progress regularly.

Questran does not cure the tendency to have high cholesterol levels; it merely helps control it. To maintain healthy levels, you therefore must continue taking the drug as directed.

The use of this medication may produce or worsen constipation and aggravate hemorrhoids. If this happens, inform your doctor. To prevent constipation, the doctor may increase your dosage very slowly, and ask you to drink more fluids, take more fiber, or take a stool softener. If severe constipation develops anyway, the doctor may switch to a different drug.

The prolonged use of Questran may change acidity in the bloodstream, especially in younger and smaller individuals in whom the doses are relatively higher. Again, it is important that you or your child be checked by your doctor on a regular basis.

Sipping Questran or holding it in your mouth for a long period can lead to tooth discoloration, enamel erosion, or decay. Be sure to brush and floss regularly.

Possible food and drug interactions when taking this medication
If Questran is taken with certain other drugs, the effects of either could be increased, decreased, or altered. It is especially important to check with your doctor before taking Questran with the following:

Digitalis (Lanoxin, Crystodigin)
Estrogens and progestins (hormones)
Oral diabetes drugs such as DiaBeta and Diabinese
Penicillin G (Pentids, others)
Phenobarbital
Phenylbutazone (Butazolidin)
Propranolol (Inderal)
Spironolactone (Aldactazide, Aldactone)
Tetracycline (Achromycin V)
Thiazide-type water pills such as Diuril
Thyroid medication such as Synthroid
Warfarin (Coumadin)

Your doctor may recommend that you take other medications at least 1 hour before or 4 to 6 hours after you take Questran.

If you are taking a drug such as digitalis (Lanoxin), stopping Questran could be hazardous, since you might experience exaggerated effects of the other drug. Consult your doctor before discontinuing Questran.

This drug may interfere with normal digestion and absorption of fats, including fat-soluble vitamins such as A, D, E, and K. If supplements of vitamins A, D, E, and K are essential to your health, your doctor may prescribe an alternative form of these vitamins.

There are no special considerations regarding alcohol use with this medication.

Special information if you are pregnant or breastfeeding
The effects of Questran during pregnancy have not been adequately studied. If you are pregnant or plan to become pregnant, inform your doctor
immediately. Because this medication can interfere with vitamin absorption, you may need to increase your vitamin intake before the baby is born
and while nursing an infant.

Recommended dosage

ADULTS

The recommended starting dose is 1 single-dose packet or 1 level scoopful, 1 to 2 times daily. The usual maintenance dosage is a total of 2 to 4
packets or scoopfuls daily divided into 2 doses preferably at mealtime
(usually before meals). The maximum daily dose is 6 packets or scoopfuls. Although the recommended dosing schedule is 2 times daily, your
doctor may ask you to take Questran in up to 6 smaller doses per day.

CHILDREN

Experience with the use of Questran in infants and children is limited. If
this medication is essential to your child's health, follow your doctor's
recommended dosing schedule.

Overdosage
No ill effects from an overdose have been reported. The main potential
harm of an overdose would be obstruction of the stomach and intestines.
If you suspect an overdose, seek medical attention immediately.

Quetiapine See Seroquel, page 1303.

Quibron-T/SR See Theo-Dur, page 1432.

Quinapril See Accupril, page 6.

Quinapril with Hydrochlorothiazide See Accuretic,
   page 9.

QUINIDINE SULFATE
Pronounced: KWIN-ih-dyne

Why is this drug prescribed?
Quinidine is used to correct certain types of irregular heart rhythms and
to slow an abnormally fast heartbeat.

Most important fact about this drug
It is important to take only the prescribed amount of this medication—no
more and no less. Try to keep your doses at regularly spaced intervals,
and be sure not to miss any.

How should you take this medication?

Take quinidine exactly as prescribed.

■ *If you miss a dose...*
Take it as soon as you remember, if it is within 2 hours of your scheduled time. If you do not remember until later, skip the dose you missed and go back to your regular schedule. Do not take 2 doses at once.
■ *Storage instructions...*
Store at room temperature in a tightly closed container, away from light.

What side effects may occur?

Side effects cannot be anticipated. If any develop or change in intensity, inform your doctor as soon as possible. Only your doctor can determine if it is safe for you to continue taking quinidine.

■ *Side effects include:*
Abdominal pain, diarrhea, hepatitis, inflammation of the esophagus (gullet), loss of appetite, nausea, vomiting

Another possible side effect is a sensitivity reaction called cinchonism. Symptoms include blurred or double vision, confusion, delirium, diarrhea, headache, intolerance to light, hearing loss, ringing in the ears, vertigo, and vomiting.

Why should this drug not be prescribed?

Do not take this medication if you have ever had an allergic reaction to quinidine. Also avoid this medication if quinine or quinidine causes you to bruise easily.

Quinidine is prescribed only for certain specific types of heart irregularity, and should be avoided when other irregularities are present. It could also prove harmful if you have myasthenia gravis (abnormal muscle weakness) or a similar condition.

Special warnings about this medication

Quinidine is reserved for certain kinds of dangerously rapid heart irregularities. It works well for some people, providing them with significant symptomatic relief. However, you should know that—on average for all cases—it has not been shown to improve chances of long-term survival, and could actually lower the odds.

Remember, too, that under certain conditions (slow heart rate, low potassium or magnesium levels) quinidine can *cause* certain types of heart irregularity. It can also cause the condition known as heart block, and should be used with caution if you have partial heart block.

Also use quinidine cautiously if you have kidney or liver disease. Your doctor will check your blood count and liver and kidney function periodically during long-term therapy.

There have been rare cases of severe allergic reaction to quinidine, especially during the first few weeks of therapy. Discuss any allergic reactions you have experienced with your doctor.

Do not confuse quinidine with quinine, which, although related, is used to treat malaria.

Possible food and drug interactions when taking this medication

Concentrations of digoxin (Lanoxin) in your blood may increase or even double when this drug is taken with quinidine. Your doctor may need to reduce the amount of digoxin you take.

A decrease in your salt intake can lead to a higher blood level of quinidine. Try to keep the salt in your diet constant. Grapefruit juice may also have an impact on quinidine levels. It's best to avoid it.

If quinidine are taken with certain other drugs, the effects of either could be increased, decreased, or altered. It is especially important to check with your doctor before combining quinidine with the following:

Amiodarone (Cordarone)
Antacids containing magnesium, such as Maalox and Mylanta
Antispasmodic drugs such as Bentyl
Aspirin
Beta-blocking blood pressure medications such as Inderal and
　Tenormin
Blood thinners such as Coumadin
Certain antidepressants such as Elavil and Tofranil
Certain diuretic drugs such as Diamox and Daranide
Cimetidine (Tagamet)
Codeine
Decamethonium
Digitoxin (Crystodigin)
Diltiazem (Cardizem)
Disopyramide (Norpace)
Felodipine (Plendil)
Haloperidol (Haldol)
Hydrocodone (Vicodin)
Ketoconazole (Nizoral)
Major tranquilizers such as Stelazine and Thorazine
Mexiletine (Mexitil)
Nicardipine (Cardene)
Nifedipine (Procardia)
Nimodipine (Nimotop)
Phenobarbital
Phenytoin (Dilantin)
Physostigmine (Antilirium)
Procainamide (Procanbid)
Reserpine (Diupres)
Rifampin (Rifadin)

Sodium bicarbonate
Sucralfate (Carafate)
Thiazide diuretics such as Dyazide and HydroDIURIL
Verapamil (Calan)

Special Information if you are pregnant or breastfeeding

The effects of quinidine during pregnancy have not been adequately studied. If you are pregnant or plan to become pregnant, inform your doctor immediately. Quinidine appears in breast milk and can affect a nursing infant. If this medication is essential to your health, your doctor may advise you to discontinue breastfeeding until your treatment is finished.

Recommended dosage

ADULTS

The usual dosage is 300 milligrams every 8 to 12 hours.

Overdosage

Any medication taken in excess can have serious consequences. If you suspect an overdose, seek medical treatment immediately.

■ *The symptoms of Quinidex Extentabs overdose may include:*
Abnormal heart rhythms, blurred or double vision, confusion, delirium, diarrhea, headache, intolerance to light, loss of hearing, low blood pressure, ringing in the ears, vertigo, vomiting

Qvar Inhalation Aerosol *See Beclomethasone, page 193.*

Rabeprazole *See AcipHex, page 19.*

Raloxifene *See Evista, page 545.*

Ramipril *See Altace, page 77.*

Ranitidine *See Zantac, page 1609.*

RAPTIVA

Pronounced: rap-TEE-vuh
Generic name: Efalizumab

Why is this drug prescribed?

Psoriasis is a skin disease that is caused, in part, by an overactive immune system. Raptiva belongs to a class of drugs called immunosuppressives, which decrease the activity of the immune system. It is prescribed for patients with severe plaque psoriasis who can no longer control their disease with medications applied to the skin.

Most important fact about this drug

Raptiva, like other immunosuppressive agents, has the potential to increase the risk of serious infections and cancer. Call your doctor immediately if you are diagnosed with cancer or your psoriasis worsens. Also contact your doctor if you develop an infection, excessive bleeding, or unusual bruising.

How should you take this medication?

Raptiva is administered once a week, as an injection under the skin (also called a subcutaneous injection). If you will be giving the injection to yourself or another person, the doctor will instruct you on how to prepare and inject the medication. The usual sites for injection are the upper leg, upper arm, abdomen, or buttocks. The injection site should be rotated each week. Do not change the dose or stop taking Raptiva without first talking to your doctor.

Once Raptiva has been mixed, it should be used right away. If you are unable to inject the medication immediately, you may let the mixture sit at room temperature for up to 8 hours before injecting it. However, do not use the mixture once 8 hours has passed; throw it away and mix a new solution instead.

Do not use the solution if it appears discolored or has particles floating in it. Throw it out and mix a new solution instead.

■ *If you miss a dose...*
Call your doctor to find out when to take your next dose and what schedule you should follow after that.

■ *Storage instructions...*
Raptiva should be stored in its original carton in the refrigerator. Do not freeze the medication. Protect the vial from exposure to light.

What side effects may occur?

Side effects cannot be anticipated. If any develop or change in intensity, tell your doctor as soon as possible. Only your doctor can determine if it is safe to continue using Raptiva.

■ *Common side effects may include:*
Acne, backache, chills, fever, flu-like symptoms, headache, infections, muscle aches, nausea, pain

There have been very rare reports of more serious side effects during Raptiva treatment. These include cancer (mainly skin cancer), serious and possibly life-threatening infections, and low blood cell platelets, which can lead to abnormal bleeding.

Why should this drug not be prescribed?

You should not use Raptiva if you have an active infection, cancer, or an impaired immune system. You must also avoid Raptiva if you've ever had an allergic reaction to it.

Special warnings about this medication

Many people experience a reaction the first time they receive a dose of Raptiva. Symptoms include headache, fever, nausea, vomiting, muscle aches, and chills, which usually occur within 2 days following the first two injections. To minimize these side effects, the first dose of Raptiva will be lower than the following doses.

Your psoriasis may worsen or new forms of psoriasis may appear while you're using Raptiva or after treatment has stopped. Tell your doctor right away if your symptoms worsen or if a new rash appears.

Raptiva may affect the ability of your blood to clot. Be sure to inform your doctor immediately if you develop bleeding gums, unusual bruising, or purplish red spots on your skin.

Do not undergo phototherapy while taking Raptiva.

Be sure to throw away all syringes and needles after one use. Do not save them for later.

Possible food and drug interactions when taking this medication

If Raptiva is taken with certain other drugs, the effects of either drug could be increased, decreased, or altered. It is especially important to check with your doctor before taking the following medications:

Immunosuppressive drugs such as cyclosporine (Neoral, Sandimmune) and methotrexate (Rheumatrex, Trexall)
Vaccines

Special information if you are pregnant or breastfeeding

The effects of Raptiva during pregnancy have not been adequately studied. If you are pregnant, planning to become pregnant, or if you become pregnant within 6 weeks of stopping Raptiva, inform your doctor immediately.

It is not known if Raptiva appears in breast milk. If this drug is essential to your health, your doctor may advise you to stop breastfeeding until your treatment is finished.

Recommended dosage

ADULTS

To avoid an allergic reaction the first time you inject Raptiva, the recommended initial dose is 0.7 milligram per 2.2 pounds of body weight. Thereafter, the recommended dose is 1 milligram per 2.2 pounds of body weight, injected once a week. Individual doses should not exceed a total of 200 milligrams. Raptiva should be injected on the same day each week.

Overdosage

There have been very few reports of Raptiva overdose. However, any medication taken in excess can have serious consequences. If you suspect an overdose, seek emergency treatment immediately.

RAZADYNE

Pronounced: RAZ-ah-dine
Generic name: Galantamine

Why is this drug prescribed?

Razadyne can delay or even reverse mental decline in some patients with mild to moderate Alzheimer's disease. It is thought to work by boosting levels of the chemical messenger acetylcholine in the brain. (In Alzheimer's disease, the cells that produce acetylcholine slowly deteriorate.)

Razadyne is a temporary remedy. It doesn't work for everyone, and it doesn't halt the underlying disease.

Most important fact about this drug

Razadyne therapy starts at a low dose and increases over several months. It is important to wait 4 weeks between dosage adjustments. If treatment with Razadyne is interrupted for several days or longer, the patient will need to start over again at the lowest dose, increasing the dose at 4-week intervals until the former dose is achieved.

How should you take this medication?

Razadyne should be taken twice a day, preferably with the morning and evening meals. The drug is available in tablet form and as an oral solution. If you are using the solution, draw the required amount into the measuring pipette that comes with the bottle, then empty the pipette into 3 to 4 ounces of a non-alcoholic beverage. Stir well and administer immediately.

■ *If you miss a dose...*
Give it as soon as you remember. If it is almost time for the next dose, skip the one you missed and go back to the regular schedule. Do not give 2 doses at once.

■ *Storage instructions...*
Both the tablets and the oral solution may be stored at room temperature. Do not freeze the solution.

What side effects may occur?

Side effects cannot be anticipated. If any develop or change in intensity, inform your doctor as soon as possible. Only your doctor can determine if it is safe to continue giving Razadyne.

■ *Side effects may include:*
Abdominal pain, anemia, blood in urine, depression, diarrhea, dizziness, fatigue, headache, inability to sleep, indigestion, loss of appetite, nausea, runny nose, sleepiness, tremor, urinary tract infection, vomiting, weight loss

Why should this drug not be prescribed?

Razadyne cannot be used if it gives the patient an allergic reaction. This drug is not recommended for patients with severe liver disease or kidney disease.

Special warnings about this medication

Use Razadyne with caution if the patient has severe asthma, obstructive lung disease, or a history of stomach ulcers.

Razadyne can slow the heart rate and cause fainting episodes. Be especially cautious if the patient has a heart irregularity.

Before surgery, make sure the doctor knows about the use of Razadyne.

Possible food and drug interactions when taking this medication

If Razadyne is taken with certain other drugs, the effect of either may be increased, decreased, or altered. It is especially important to check with your doctor before combining Razadyne with the following:

Certain Parkinson's drugs such as Artane and Cogentin
Cimetidine (Tagamet)
Erythromycin (E.E.S., Eryc, PCE)
Ketoconazole (Nizoral)
Meclizine (Antivert)
Nonsteroidal anti-inflammatory drugs such as Motrin and Voltaren
Paroxetine (Paxil)
Urinary tract medications such as Urispas and Urecholine.

Special information if you are pregnant or breastfeeding

Razadyne is not usually prescribed for women of childbearing age. It should be used during pregnancy only if the potential benefit justifies the risk to the developing baby. Razadyne should not be used by nursing mothers.

Recommended dosage

ADULTS

The recommended starting dose of Razadyne is 4 milligrams twice a day. Four weeks later, the dose should be increased to 8 milligrams twice a day. After waiting an additional 4 weeks, the doctor may increase the dose to 12 milligrams twice a day if necessary.

For patients with mild to moderate liver problems and kidney problems, dosage should not exceed 16 milligrams per day.

Overdosage

Any medication taken in excess can have serious consequences. A massive overdose of Razadyne could prove fatal. If you suspect an overdose, seek medical attention immediately.

■ *Symptoms of Razadyne overdose may include:*
Convulsions, drooling, fainting, incontinence, low blood pressure, muscle weakness, severe nausea, slow or irregular heartbeat, stomach cramps, sweating, teary eyes, twitching, weak breathing, vomiting

Rebetol *See Ribavirin, page 1258.*

REGLAN

Pronounced: REG-lan
Generic name: Metoclopramide hydrochloride

Why is this drug prescribed?

Reglan increases the contractions of the stomach and small intestine, helping the passage of food. It is given to treat the symptoms of diabetic gastroparesis (stomach paralysis), a condition in which the stomach does not contract. These symptoms include vomiting, nausea, heartburn, feeling of indigestion, persistent fullness after meals, and appetite loss. Reglan is also used, for short periods, to treat heartburn in people with gastroesophageal reflux disorder (backflow of stomach contents into the esophagus). In addition, it is given to prevent nausea and vomiting caused by cancer chemotherapy and surgery.

Most important fact about this drug

Reglan may cause mild to severe depression. If you have suffered from depression in the past, make sure your doctor is aware of it. Reglan may not be the best drug for you.

How should you take this medication?

Reglan is usually taken 30 minutes before a meal. If you suffer from heartburn that occurs only intermittently or only at certain times of day, your doctor may want you to schedule your Reglan therapy around those times.

You will probably take Reglan for only 4 to 12 weeks. Continuous treatment beyond 12 weeks is not recommended.

If you have diabetic stomach paralysis that tends to recur, your doctor may want you to take Reglan at the first sign of a recurrence.

■ *If you miss a dose...*
Take it as soon as you remember. If it is almost time for your next dose, skip the one you missed and go back to your regular schedule. Do not take 2 doses at once.

■ *Storage instructions...*
Store at room temperature.

What side effects may occur?

Side effects cannot be anticipated. If any develop or change in intensity, inform your doctor as soon as possible. Only your doctor can determine if it is safe for you to continue taking Reglan.

■ *Side effects may include:*
Drowsiness, fatigue, restlessness

In addition, Reglan may cause symptoms similar to those of Parkinson's disease, such as slow movements, rigidity, tremor, or a mask-like facial appearance.

Especially in older people, Reglan may produce tardive dyskinesia, a syndrome of jerky or writhing involuntary movements, particularly of the tongue, face, mouth, or jaw. In children and adults under 30, Reglan may cause involuntary movements of the arms and legs, and sometimes loud or labored breathing, usually in the first day or two of treatment.

Reglan may cause intense restlessness with associated symptoms such as anxiety, agitation, foot-tapping, pacing, inability to sit still, jitteriness, and insomnia. These symptoms may disappear as your body gets used to Reglan, or if your dosage is reduced.

Why should this drug not be prescribed?

Do not take Reglan if you are sensitive to it or have ever had an allergic reaction to it.

You should not take Reglan if you have a condition such as obstruction, perforation, or hemorrhage of the stomach or small bowel that might be aggravated by increased stomach and small-bowel movement.

If you have pheochromocytoma (a nonmalignant tumor that causes hypertension), do not take Reglan; it could trigger a dangerous jump in blood pressure.

Do not take Reglan if you have epilepsy; it could increase the frequency and severity of seizures.

If you are taking a drug that is likely to cause side effects such as tremors, jerks, grimaces, or writhing movements, do not take Reglan; it could make such symptoms more severe.

Reglan is not recommended for patients under 18 years of age.

Special warnings about this medication

If you have Parkinson's disease, you should be given Reglan cautiously or not at all, since the drug may make your Parkinson's symptoms worse.

Because Reglan may make you drowsy and impair your coordination, you should not drive, climb, or perform hazardous tasks until you know how the medication affects you.

Use Reglan with caution if you have high blood pressure. Be careful, too, if you have cirrhosis or congestive heart failure. Under these conditions, Reglan may cause fluid retention and heart problems. If this happens during the first few weeks of Reglan therapy, you'll have to stop taking the drug.

Possible food and drug interactions when taking this medication

If Reglan is taken with certain other drugs, the effects of either could be increased, decreased, or altered. It is especially important to check with your doctor before combining Reglan with the following:

Acetaminophen (Tylenol)
Alcoholic beverages
Antispasmodic drugs such as Bentyl and Pro-Banthine
Cimetidine (Tagamet)
Cyclosporine (Sandimmune)
Digoxin (Lanoxin)
Insulin
Levodopa (Sinemet)
MAO inhibitor antidepressants such as Nardil and Parnate
Narcotic painkillers such as Percocet and Demerol
Sleeping pills such as Dalmane, Halcion, and Restoril
Tetracycline (Sumycin, others)
Tranquilizers such as Valium and Xanax

If you take insulin for diabetes, your insulin dosage or dosing schedule may have to be adjusted while you are taking Reglan.

Special information if you are pregnant or breastfeeding

The effects of Reglan during pregnancy have not been adequately studied. If you are pregnant or plan to become pregnant, inform your doctor immediately. Reglan should be used during pregnancy only if it is clearly needed. Reglan appears in breast milk. Your doctor may recommend that you discontinue Reglan while you are breastfeeding your baby.

Recommended dosage

ADULTS

Symptoms of Gastroesophageal Reflux
The usual dose is 10 to 15 milligrams of Reglan, up to 4 times a day, 30 minutes before each meal and at bedtime, depending upon the symptoms being treated and the effectiveness of the dose. Treatment usually lasts no longer than 12 weeks.

If symptoms occur only intermittently or at specific times of the day, your doctor may give you a single dose of up to 20 milligrams as a preventive measure.

Symptoms Associated with Diabetic Gastroparesis or Gastric Stasis
The usual dose is 10 milligrams 30 minutes before each meal and at bedtime for 2 to 8 weeks.

OLDER ADULTS

Relief of Symptomatic Gastroesophageal Reflux
Older adults may need only 5 milligrams per dose.

Overdosage
Any medication taken in excess can have serious consequences. If you suspect an overdose, seek medical attention immediately.

■ *Symptoms of Reglan overdose may include:*
Disorientation, drowsiness, involuntary movements

RELAFEN
Pronounced: *REL-ah-fen*
Generic name: *Nabumetone*

Why is this drug prescribed?
Relafen, a nonsteroidal anti-inflammatory drug, is used to relieve the inflammation, swelling, stiffness, and joint pain associated with rheumatoid arthritis and osteoarthritis (the most common form of arthritis).

Most important fact about this drug
You should have frequent checkups by your doctor if you take Relafen regularly. Ulcers or internal bleeding can occur with or without warning.

How should you take this medication?
Relafen can be taken with or without food. Take it exactly as prescribed.

■ *If you miss a dose...*
Take the forgotten dose as soon as you remember. If it is almost time for your next dose, skip the one you missed and go back to your regular schedule. Never take a double dose.

■ *Storage instructions...*
Keep this medication in the container it came in, tightly closed, and away from moist places and direct light. It can be stored at room temperature.

What side effects may occur?

Side effects cannot be anticipated. If any develop or change in intensity, inform your doctor as soon as possible. Only your doctor can determine whether it is safe for you to continue taking Relafen.

■ *Side effects may include:*
Abdominal pain, constipation, diarrhea, dizziness, fluid retention, gas, headache, indigestion, itching, nausea, rash, ringing in ears

Why should this drug not be prescribed?

Do not take this medication if you are sensitive to or have ever had an allergic reaction to Relafen, or if you have had asthma attacks, hives, or other allergic reactions caused by Relafen, aspirin, or other nonsteroidal anti-inflammatory drugs.

Special warnings about this medication

Stomach and intestinal ulcers can occur without warning. Remember to get regular checkups.

Make sure your doctor knows if you have kidney or liver disease. Relafen should be used with caution.

This drug can cause fluid retention and swelling. It should be used with caution if you have congestive heart failure or high blood pressure.

Relafen can cause increased sensitivity to sunlight.

Possible food and drug interactions when taking this medication

If Relafen is taken with certain other drugs, the effects of either could be increased, decreased, or altered. It is especially important to check with your doctor before combining Relafen with blood-thinning drugs such as Coumadin and aspirin.

Other drugs with which Relafen could possibly interact include:

Diuretics such as HydroDIURIL and Lasix
Lithium (Eskalith)
Methotrexate

Special information if you are pregnant or breastfeeding

The effects of Relafen during pregnancy have not been adequately studied. If you are pregnant or plan to become pregnant, inform your doctor immediately. Relafen may appear in breast milk and could affect a nursing infant. If this medication is essential to your health, your doctor may advise you to discontinue breastfeeding until your treatment with Relafen is finished.

Recommended dosage

ADULTS

The usual starting dose is 1,000 milligrams taken as a single dose. Dosage may be increased up to 2,000 milligrams per day, taken once or twice a day.

CHILDREN

The safety and effectiveness of this drug in children have not been established.

Overdosage

Overdoses of nonsteroidal anti-inflammatory drugs such as Relafen have been known to cause stomach bleeding, elevated blood pressure, kidney failure, impaired breathing, and coma, though these effects are rare.

■ *Warning signs of overdose include:*
   Drowsiness, lack of energy, nausea, vomiting, stomach pain

If you suspect an overdose, seek medical attention immediately.

RELENZA
Pronounced: rell-EN-zuh
Generic name: Zanamivir

Why is this drug prescribed?
Relenza is an antiviral drug that hastens recovery from the flu. Victims who begin taking Relenza within the first 2 days of their illness typically start to feel improvement a day earlier than they would otherwise. The drug is believed to work by interfering with the spread of virus particles inside the respiratory tract.

Most important fact about this drug
There is no evidence that Relenza protects you from catching the flu, and it will not prevent you from spreading the flu virus to others.

How should you take this medication?
Relenza is delivered directly to the lungs by oral inhalation from a Diskhaler device. To benefit from the drug, you must begin taking it within 48 hours of feeling the first symptoms of flu, and must finish the entire 5-day course of treatment.

Be sure to take two doses on the first day, allowing at least 2 hours between them. On the following days, take a dose every 12 hours (morning and evening). Do not puncture a blister containing the drug until you are ready to use it.

Children should use this drug only under the supervision of an adult.

■ *If you miss a dose...*
Take it as soon as you remember. If it is almost time for your next dose, skip the one you missed and go back to your regular schedule. Do not take 2 doses at the same time.

■ *Storage instructions...*
Store at room temperature.

What side effects may occur?

Symptoms experienced during Relenza therapy are virtually the same as those associated with untreated flu. Problems reported during clinical tests are listed below.

■ *Side effects may include:*
Abdominal pain, bronchitis, cough, diarrhea, dizziness, ear infection, headache, fatigue, fever, hives, joint pain, muscle ache, nasal infection, nasal symptoms, nausea, sinus inflammation, throat infection, vomiting

Why should this drug not be prescribed?

If Relenza gives you an allergic reaction, you cannot use this drug.

Special warnings about this medication

Relenza has been known to cause serious and potentially fatal breathing problems, especially in people who have asthma or other chronic pulmonary disorders. If you develop breathing difficulties such as wheezing or shortness of breath, stop taking Relenza and call your doctor immediately.

Relenza is generally not recommended for anyone with a chronic pulmonary disease. If you do use it under these circumstances, be extremely cautious, and make sure that you have a fast-acting inhaled bronchodilator (Proventil Inhaler or Ventolin Inhaler) available and ready to use whenever you take it. If you use an inhaled bronchodilator regularly and have a dose scheduled at the same time as Relenza, use the bronchodilator first.

Relenza can also cause serious allergic reactions. If you experience swelling of the face, tongue, or throat, or develop a skin rash, stop taking this medication and contact your doctor.

Serious bacterial infections may begin with flu-like symptoms or may coexist with the flu. Relenza has no effect on such infections.

Relenza has not been tested in people with medical conditions severe enough for possible hospitalization. Use it with caution if you have any kind of serious health problem in addition to the flu.

Possible food and drug interactions when taking this medication
Interactions are considered unlikely.

Special information if you are pregnant or breastfeeding
The effects of Relenza during pregnancy have not been adequately studied. If you are pregnant or plan to become pregnant, inform your doctor. It is not known whether Relenza appears in breast milk. Caution is recommended if you are breastfeeding.

Recommended dosage
The recommended dose for adults and children 7 years and older is 2 inhalations (one 5-milligram blister per inhalation) twice a day, approximately 12 hours apart, for 5 days. Safety and efficacy have not been established for children under 7.

Overdosage
Substantially increased doses of Relenza have caused no increase in adverse reactions. Nevertheless, if you suspect an overdose of Relenza, it would be wise to check with your doctor.

RELPAX
Pronounced: RELL-packs
Generic name: Eletriptan hydrobromide

Why is this drug prescribed?
Relpax is used to treat migraine headaches with or without the presence of auras (visual disturbances that precede an attack, such as halos or flickering lights). It shortens the duration of the headache but will not prevent attacks.

Most important fact about this drug
Relpax should only be used during a genuine attack of classic migraine. Do not attempt to prevent migraines with this drug, and do not use it for tension headaches, cluster headaches, or unusual types of migraine such as hemiplegic or basilar migraine.

How should you take this medication?
Take 1 dose of Relpax as soon as your symptoms appear. If the first dose does not relieve the headache, check with your doctor before taking a second one.

 If the headache goes away but returns later, a second dose may be taken if 2 hours have elapsed since the first dose. Do not take more than 80 milligrams of Relpax in a 24-hour period.

■ *If you miss a dose…*
Relpax is not intended for regular use and should be taken only to relieve an acute migraine attack.

■ *Storage instructions…*
Store at room temperature.

What side effects may occur?
Side effects cannot be anticipated. If any develop or change in intensity, inform your doctor as soon as possible. Only your doctor can determine if it is safe for you to continue taking Relpax.

■ *Side effects may include:*
Chest tightness or pressure, dizziness, dry mouth, headache, nausea, sleepiness, tingling, weakness

Why should this drug not be prescribed?
You should not use Relpax if you have ever had a heart attack or if you have ever had any of the following vascular problems: angina, cardiovascular disease, coronary artery vasospasm, ischemic bowel disease, ischemic heart disease, peripheral vascular disease, Prinzmetal's angina, stroke, transient ischemic attacks, or uncontrolled high blood pressure.

You cannot take Relpax if you have severe liver impairment.

Relpax should never be taken within 24 hours of other migraine or headache medication (see *Possible food and drug interactions when taking this medication*).

If Relpax causes an allergic reaction, you will not be able to use it.

Special warnings about this medication
In rare cases, medications similar to Relpax have caused heart attack, stroke, and certain types of ischemia (restricted blood flow to an area). Call your doctor immediately if you experience chest pains, shortness of breath, sudden numbness or weakness on one side of the body, trouble speaking or seeing, loss of balance, bloody diarrhea, or stomach pain.

If you are at risk for stroke or heart disease, your doctor may perform cardiovascular tests to be sure it is safe for you to take Relpax. Your doctor may ask you to take the first dose of Relpax in the office, where you can be monitored for cardiac side effects.

Since Relpax can make you drowsy or dizzy, do not participate in activities that require full alertness until you are certain of the drug's effect.

Relpax can cause a slight increase in blood pressure, especially in people with kidney problems and the elderly. Your doctor will monitor you closely to make sure your blood pressure stays at a safe level. If you develop high blood pressure that can't be controlled, you'll have to stop taking Relpax.

Possible food and drug interactions when taking this medication
If Relpax is taken with certain other drugs, the effects of either could be increased, decreased, or altered. Never take Relpax within 24 hours of using another migraine or headache drug, including:

Almotriptan (Axert)
Dihydroergotamine (DHE-45, Migranal)
Ergotamine (Cafergot)
Frovatriptan (Frova)
Methysergide (Sansert)
Naratriptan (Amerge)
Rizatriptan (Maxalt, Maxalt-MLT)
Sumatriptan (Imitrex)
Zolmitriptan (Zomig)

You should also refrain from using Relpax within 72 hours of taking the following:

Clarithromycin (Biaxin)
Itraconazole (Sporanox)
Ketoconazole (Nizoral)
Nefazodone (Serzone)
Nelfinavir (Viracept)
Ritonavir (Norvir)
Troleandomycin (TAO)

Special information if you are pregnant or breastfeeding
The effects of Relpax in pregnancy have not been adequately studied. If you are pregnant or plan to become pregnant, inform your doctor immediately.

Relpax is excreted in breast milk. If you are nursing an infant, discuss your treatment options with your physician.

Recommended dosage

ADULTS

When a headache begins, take one 20-milligram or 40-milligram tablet. If the first dose does not relieve the headache, check with your doctor before taking a second one.

If the headache goes away but returns later, a second dose may be taken if 2 hours have elapsed since the first dose. Do not take more than 80 milligrams of Relpax in a 24-hour period.

Relpax is not recommended for use in children under 18 years old.

Overdosage
Any medication taken in excess can have serious consequences. If you suspect an overdose, seek medical attention immediately.

REMERON

Pronounced: REM-ur-on
Generic name: Mirtazapine
Other brand name: Remeron SolTab

Why is this drug prescribed?

Remeron is prescribed for the treatment of major depression—that is, a continuous depressed mood that interferes with everyday life. The symptoms of major depression often include changes in appetite and weight, difficulty sleeping, loss of interest in pleasurable activities, constant fidgeting or a slowdown in movement, fatigue, feelings of guilt or worthlessness, difficulty concentrating, slowed thinking, and suicidal thoughts.

Remeron is thought to work by adjusting the balance of the brain's natural chemical messengers, especially norepinephrine and serotonin. It belongs to the class of drugs known as tetracyclics and is chemically unrelated to other antidepressants such as serotonin re-uptake inhibitors and MAO inhibitors.

Most important fact about this drug

Remeron makes some people drowsy or less alert, and may affect judgment and thinking. Don't drive or participate in any hazardous activity that requires full mental alertness until you know whether Remeron has this effect on you.

How should you take this medication?

Remeron may be taken with or without food. It is preferable to take it in the evening before you go to sleep. Even though you may begin to feel better in 1 to 4 weeks, continue taking this medication exactly as prescribed. Regular daily doses are needed for the drug to work properly.

If you are using Remeron SolTabs, an orally disintegrating form of the drug, make sure your hands are dry before removing the tablet from the blister pack and immediately place the tablet on your tongue. Do not attempt to split the tablet; it will fall apart rapidly and can be swallowed with saliva.

■ *If you miss a dose…*
Take the forgotten dose if you remember within a few hours. Otherwise, skip the dose. Never try to catch up by doubling the dose.
■ *Storage instructions…*
Store at room temperature in a tight, light-resistant container.

What side effects may occur?

Side effects cannot be anticipated. If any develop or change in intensity, tell your doctor as soon as possible. Only your doctor can determine if it is safe for you to continue taking Remeron.

■ *Side effects may include:*
Abnormal dreams and thinking, constipation, dizziness, dry mouth, flu-like symptoms, increased appetite, sleepiness, weakness, weight gain

Why should this drug not be prescribed?

If you have ever had an allergic reaction to Remeron or similar drugs such as Ludiomil and Desyrel, you should not take this medication. Be sure to tell your doctor about any drug reactions you have experienced.

You should also avoid Remeron if you are taking the antidepressants Nardil or Parnate (see *Special warnings about this medication*).

Special warnings about this medication

In clinical studies, antidepressants increased the risk of suicidal thinking and behavior in children and adolescents with depression and other psychiatric disorders. Anyone considering the use of Remeron or any other antidepressant in a child or adolescent must balance this risk with the clinical need. Remeron has not been studied in children or adolescents and is not approved for treating anyone less than 18 years old.

Additionally, the progression of major depression is associated with a worsening of symptoms and/or the emergence of suicidal thinking or behavior in both adults and children, whether or not they are taking antidepressants. Individuals being treated with Remeron and their caregivers should watch for any change in symptoms or any new symptoms that appear suddenly—especially agitation, anxiety, hostility, panic, restlessness, extreme hyperactivity, and suicidal thinking or behavior—and report them to the doctor immediately. Be especially observant at the beginning of treatment or whenever there is a change in dose.

Serious, sometimes fatal reactions have been known to occur when drugs such as Remeron are taken in combination with other drugs known as MAO inhibitors, including the antidepressants Nardil and Parnate. Never take Remeron with one of these drugs or within 14 days of discontinuing therapy with one of them; and allow at least 14 days between stopping Remeron and starting an MAO inhibitor.

If you develop flu-like symptoms, a sore throat, chills or fever, mouth sores, or any other signs of infection, call your doctor; these symptoms may signal a serious underlying condition.

Remeron tends to raise cholesterol levels in some people. If you have a cholesterol problem, be sure to mention it to your doctor before starting therapy with Remeron.

Remeron should be used with caution if you have active liver or kidney disease, or heart or blood pressure problems. Also be sure to tell your doctor if you have a history of seizures, mania (extremely high spirits), hypomania (mild excitability), drug use, or any other physical or emotional problems.

While first taking this medication, you may feel dizzy or light-headed, especially when getting up from a lying or sitting position. If getting up slowly doesn't help, or if this problem continues, notify your doctor.

If you must avoid phenylalanine, do not use the SolTab form of Remeron, which contains this substance.

Possible food and drug interactions when taking this medication

Never combine Remeron with an MAO inhibitor; and do not drink alcohol while taking this medication. If Remeron is taken with certain other drugs, the effects of either could be increased, decreased, or altered. It is especially important to check with your doctor before combining Remeron with tranquilizers such as Valium, Xanax, and Ativan.

Special information if you are pregnant or breastfeeding

The effects of Remeron during pregnancy have not been adequately studied. If you are pregnant or plan to become pregnant, tell your doctor immediately. It is not known whether Remeron appears in breast milk. However, because many drugs do make their way into breast milk, you should tell your doctor if you are breastfeeding or plan to breastfeed.

Recommended dosage

ADULTS

The usual starting dose is 15 milligrams taken daily before going to sleep. Depending upon your response, your dosage may be increased to as much as 45 milligrams a day.

CHILDREN

The safety and effectiveness of Remeron have not been established in children.

Overdosage

Any medication taken in excess can have serious consequences. If you suspect an overdose, seek medical attention immediately.

■ *Symptoms of Remeron overdose include:*
  Drowsiness, impaired memory, mental confusion, rapid heartbeat

Renova *See Retin-A and Renova, page 1242.*

Repaglinide See Prandin, page 1116.

REQUIP

Pronounced: REE-kwip
Generic name: Ropinirole hydrochloride

Why is this drug prescribed?

Requip helps relieve the signs and symptoms of Parkinson's disease. Caused by a deficit of dopamine (one of the brain's chief chemical messengers), this disorder is marked by progressive muscle stiffness, tremor, and fatigue. Requip works by stimulating dopamine receptors in the brain, thus promoting better, easier movement.

Requip can be taken with or without levodopa (usually prescribed as Sinemet), another drug used to treat the symptoms of Parkinson's disease.

Most important fact about this drug

Requip is not a cure for Parkinson's disease. However, it does alleviate symptoms of the disease, and it can shorten the "off" periods of immobility that patients on long-term levodopa therapy often begin to experience.

How should you take this medication?

Take 3 doses a day, with or without food. If the drug upsets your stomach, combining it with food may relieve the problem. If you are also taking levodopa, its dosage may be gradually decreased when you start therapy with Requip.

■ *If you miss a dose...*
   Take it as soon as you remember. If it is almost time for your next dose, skip the one you missed and go back to your regular schedule. Do not take 2 doses at once.
■ *Storage instructions...*
   Store at room temperature away from light.

What side effects may occur?

Side effects cannot be anticipated. If any develop or change in intensity, inform your doctor as soon as possible. Only your doctor can determine if it is safe for you to continue taking Requip.

■ *Side effects may include:*
   Abdominal pain, abnormal dreaming, abnormal muscle movements, abnormal vision, amnesia, anxiety, arthritis, bronchitis, confusion, constipation, decreased muscle movements, diarrhea, difficulty breathing, dizziness, drowsiness, dry mouth, eye problems, fainting, falling, fatigue, hallucinations, headache, increased sweating, indigestion, joint pain, leg swelling, nausea, nervousness, pain, paralysis, respiratory tract infection, runny nose, sinus inflammation, skin tingling,

sore throat, swelling, tremor, urinary tract infection, viral infections, vomiting, weakness

Why should this drug not be prescribed?

If Requip gives you an allergic reaction, you will not be able to continue using it.

Special warnings about this medication

At the start of Requip therapy and whenever the dose is increased, you face a slightly increased risk of a fainting spell or other symptoms of low blood pressure such as dizziness, nausea, sweating, and light-headedness, particularly when you get up suddenly after sitting or reclining for a prolonged period. To avoid such symptoms, be careful to stand up slowly.

A few patients—especially older ones—also develop hallucinations. Let your doctor know if this occurs. You may have to stop Requip therapy.

Use Requip with caution if you have heart disease. There is also a slight chance of developing respiratory difficulties or problems with your eyesight. If you find it hard to breathe, have any swelling, or develop problems with your vision, alert your doctor at once.

If you are taking Sinemet with Requip, you may experience jerking muscle movements. Tell your doctor. He will need to decrease your dose of Sinemet.

With other Parkinson's medications, a sudden dose reduction has been known to cause high fever, muscle stiffness, and loss of consciousness. Although this has not happened with Requip, be alert for such problems and contact your doctor immediately if they occur.

Requip may cause drowsiness, and some people have reported falling asleep without warning during their daily activities. Do not drive a car or operate machinery until you know how the drug affects you. If you find that Requip makes you sleepy or that you're suddenly falling asleep in the middle of routine activities, tell your doctor; he will probably discontinue the drug.

Requip may also cause darkening of your skin and eye color. Tell your doctor if you notice any change.

Possible food and drug interactions when taking this medication

If Requip is taken with certain other drugs, the effects of either can be increased, decreased, or altered. It is especially important to check with your doctor before combining Requip with the following:

Alcohol
Antidepressants such as Elavil, Pamelor, and Tofranil
Ciprofloxacin (Cipro)
Drugs that contain levodopa such as Dopar, Larodopa, and Sinemet
Estrogen medications such as ethinyl estradiol (Estinyl)

Major tranquilizers such as Haldol, Mellaril, Navane, Prolixin, and Thorazine

Metoclopramide (Reglan)

Tranquilizers such as the benzodiazepines Ativan, Librium, Valium, and Xanax

Special information if you are pregnant or breastfeeding

Although the effects of Requip during pregnancy have not been adequately studied in humans, birth defects have occurred in animals. If you are pregnant or plan to become pregnant, inform your doctor immediately.

Requip may inhibit production of breast milk. There is also a possibility that it will appear in breast milk and affect the nursing infant. If this medication is essential to your health, your doctor may advise you to discontinue breastfeeding.

Recommended dosage

ADULTS

Requip is taken 3 times a day. During the first week of therapy, each dose is 0.25 milligram. During the second week, the amount rises to 0.5 milligram. In the third week, it increases to 0.75 milligram, and in the fourth week reaches 1 milligram (3 milligrams daily). If necessary, your doctor will gradually increase the dosage further, up to a maximum of 24 milligrams per day.

If you need to stop Requip therapy, the doctor will discontinue the drug gradually over a 7-day period, reducing the number of doses from 3 to 2 per day for the first 4 days, then to once a day for the remaining 3 days.

Overdosage

Any medication taken in excess can have serious consequences. If you suspect an overdose, seek medical treatment immediately.

■ *Symptoms of Requip overdose may include:*
Agitation, chest pain, confusion, drowsiness, facial muscle movements, grogginess, increased jerkiness of movement, nausea, symptoms of low blood pressure (dizziness, light-headedness) upon standing, vomiting

RESTASIS

Pronounced: REH-stay-sis
Generic name: Cyclosporine

Why is this drug prescribed?

Restasis is a medicated eyedrop that increases tear production. It is used to relieve the symptoms of dry eye syndrome, including burning, redness, dryness, grittiness, and the sensation of a foreign object stuck in the eye.

Most important fact about this drug

Do not use Restasis to treat eye dryness that is related to an infection.

How should you take this medication?

Use Restasis solution only in the eyes; never swallow it. Turn each individual, single-use vial upside down a few times before using to mix the solution (it should look white with no streaks). After opening the vial, immediately insert the drops into one or both eyes; throw away any remaining medication when you're done.

To prevent contamination of the solution, do not touch the tip of the vial to any surface, to your eyelids, or to the surrounding area of the eye.

If you wear contact lenses, wait at least 15 minutes after using Restasis before inserting your lenses. This will prevent them from absorbing the medication. It's okay to use lubricating eye drops or artificial tears during treatment with Restasis, but you should wait 15 minutes after using one product before using the other one.

■ *If you miss a dose...*
Take it as soon as you remember. If it is almost time for your next dose, skip the one you missed and go back to your regular schedule. Do not take 2 doses at once.

■ *Storage instructions...*
Store at room temperature.

What side effects may occur?

Side effects cannot be anticipated. If any develop or change in intensity, tell your doctor as soon as possible. Only your doctor can determine if it is safe to continue using Restasis.

■ *Side effects may include:*
Burning in the eye

Why should this drug not be prescribed?

Do not use Restasis if you currently have an eye infection. Also avoid the drug if you've ever had an allergic reaction to it.

Special warnings about this medication

Be sure to tell the doctor if you've ever had herpes in either eye. Restasis has not been studied in people who have a history of eye-related herpes infection.

If you wear contact lenses, talk to your doctor before using Restasis. People with reduced tear production generally should not wear contact lenses.

Restasis has not been studied in children less than 16 years old.

Possible food and drug interactions when taking this medication

No interactions with Restasis have been reported.

Special information if you are pregnant or breastfeeding

Restasis has not been adequately studied in pregnant women. Before using the drug, let your doctor know if you are pregnant or plan to become pregnant.

It is not known whether Restasis appears in breast milk. If you plan to breastfeed, discuss your medication options with your doctor.

Recommended dosage

The usual dose is 1 drop in each affected eye twice a day, about 12 hours apart.

Overdosage

There is no information on Restasis overdose. However, any medication taken in excess can have serious consequences. If you suspect an overdose, seek medical attention immediately.

RESTORIL

Pronounced: RES-tah-rill
Generic name: Temazepam

Why is this drug prescribed?

Restoril is used for the relief of insomnia (difficulty in falling asleep, waking up frequently at night, or waking up early in the morning). It belongs to a class of drugs known as benzodiazepines.

Most important fact about this drug

Sleep problems are usually temporary, requiring treatment for only a short time, usually 1 or 2 days and no more than 2 to 3 weeks. Insomnia that lasts longer than this may be a sign of another medical problem. If you find you need this medicine for more than 7 to 10 days, be sure to check with your doctor.

How should you take this medication?
Take this medication exactly as directed; never take more than the prescribed amount.

■ *If you miss a dose...*
Take only as needed.
■ *Storage instructions...*
Keep this medication in the container it came in, tightly closed, and out of the reach of children. Store it at room temperature.

What side effects may occur?
Side effects cannot be anticipated. If any develop or change in intensity, inform your doctor as soon as possible. Only your doctor can determine if it is safe for you to continue taking Restoril.

■ *Side effects may include:*
Dizziness, drowsiness, fatigue, headache, nausea, nervousness, sluggishness
■ *Side effects due to rapid decrease in dose or abrupt withdrawal from Restoril:*
Abdominal and muscle cramps, convulsions, feeling of discomfort, inability to fall asleep or stay asleep, sweating, tremors, vomiting

Why should this drug not be prescribed?
If you are pregnant or plan to become pregnant, you should not take this medication. It poses a potential risk to the developing baby.

Special warnings about this medication
When you take Restoril every night for more than a few weeks, it loses its effectiveness to help you sleep. This is known as tolerance. You can also develop physical dependence on this drug, especially if you take it regularly for more than a few weeks, or take high doses.

When you first start taking Restoril, until you know whether the medication will have any carryover effect the next day, use extreme care while doing anything that requires complete alertness such as driving a car or operating machinery.

If you are severely depressed or have suffered from severe depression, in the past, consult your doctor before taking this medication.

If you have kidney or liver problems or chronic lung disease, make sure your doctor is aware of it.

After you stop taking Restoril, you may have more trouble sleeping than you had before you started taking it. This is called *rebound insomnia* and should clear up after 1 or 2 nights.

Possible food and drug interactions when taking this medication
Restoril may intensify the effects of alcohol. Do not drink alcohol while taking this medication.

If Restoril is taken with certain other drugs, the effects of either could be increased, decreased, or altered. It is especially important to check with your doctor before combining Restoril with the following:

Antidepressant drugs such as Elavil, Nardil, Parnate, and Tofranil
Antihistamines such as Benadryl
Barbiturates such as phenobarbital and Seconal
Major tranquilizers such as Mellaril and Thorazine
Narcotic pain relievers such as Percocet and Demerol
Tranquilizers such as Valium and Xanax

Special information if you are pregnant or breastfeeding

Do not take Restoril if you are pregnant or planning to become pregnant. There is an increased risk of birth defects. This drug may appear in breast milk and could affect a nursing infant. If this medication is essential to your health, your doctor may advise you to discontinue breastfeeding until your treatment with this medication is finished.

Recommended dosage

ADULTS

The usual recommended dose is 15 milligrams at bedtime; however, 7.5 milligrams may be all that is necessary, while some people may need 30 milligrams. Your doctor will tailor your dose to your needs.

CHILDREN

The safety and effectiveness of Restoril have not been established in children under 18 years of age.

OLDER ADULTS

The doctor will prescribe the smallest effective amount in order to avoid side effects such as oversedation, dizziness, confusion, and lack of muscle coordination. The usual starting dose is 7.5 milligrams.

Overdosage

Any medication taken in excess can have serious consequences. If you suspect an overdose, seek medical attention immediately.

■ *The symptoms of Restoril overdose may include:*
Coma, confusion, diminished reflexes, low blood pressure, labored or difficult breathing, sleepiness

RETIN-A AND RENOVA

Pronounced: Ret-in-A, Re-NO-va
Generic name: Tretinoin
Other brand name: Avita

Why is this drug prescribed?

Retin-A, Avita, and Renova contain the skin medication tretinoin. Retin-A and Avita are used in the treatment of acne. Renova is prescribed to reduce fine wrinkles, discoloration, and roughness on facial skin (as part of a comprehensive program of skin care and sun avoidance).

Retin-A is available in liquid, cream, or gel form, and in a stronger gel called Retin-A Micro. Avita comes only as a gel. Renova is available in cream form only.

Most important fact about this drug

While using Retin-A, Avita, or Renova, keep exposure to sunlight, including sunlamps, to a minimum. If you have a sunburn, do not use the medication until you have fully recovered. Use of sunscreen products (at least SPF 15) and protective clothing over treated areas is recommended when exposure to the sun cannot be avoided. Weather extremes, such as wind and cold, may be irritating and should also be avoided while using these products.

How should you use this medication?

Retin-A and Avita should be applied once a day, in the evening, to the skin where acne appears, using enough to lightly cover the affected area. The liquid form may be applied using a fingertip, gauze pad, or cotton swab. If you use gauze or cotton, avoid oversaturation, which might cause the liquid to run into areas where treatment is not intended.

Renova is also applied once daily in the evening. Use only enough to lightly cover the affected area. Before you use Renova, wash your face with a mild soap, pat your skin dry, and wait 20 to 30 minutes. Then apply a dab of Renova cream the size of a pea and spread it lightly over your face, avoiding your eyes, ears, nostrils, mouth, and open wounds.

You may use cosmetics while being treated with these products; however, you should thoroughly cleanse the areas to be treated before applying the medication.

If your skin becomes too dry, you may want to use petroleum jelly or another emollient during the day.

If there is no immediate improvement, or new blemishes appear, don't get discouraged; it takes weeks for the medicine to take effect. Continue applying the prescribed amount. (Do not increase the dosage; it may irritate your skin.)

Do not stop treatment when improvement finally occurs. You must continue therapy to maintain the beneficial effect.

■ *If you miss a dose...*
Resume your regular schedule the next day.
■ *Storage instructions...*
Store at ordinary room temperature. Do not freeze Renova.

What side effects may occur?

If you have sensitive skin, the use of Avita or Retin-A may cause your skin to become excessively red, puffy, blistered, or crusted. If this happens, notify your doctor, who may recommend that you discontinue the medication until your skin returns to normal, or adjust the medication to a level that you can tolerate.

An unusual darkening of the skin or lack of color of the skin may occur temporarily with repeated application of Avita or Retin-A.

Side effects of these medications are generally not severe and may include burning, dry skin, itching, peeling, redness, and stinging.

Why should this drug not be prescribed?

If you are sensitive to or have ever had an allergic reaction to either of these products, avoid using them.

The safety and effectiveness of long-term use of Retin-A in the treatment of disorders other than acne have not been established.

The safety and effectiveness of Renova 0.05% cream have not been established in children under age 18, adults over age 50, and people with heavily pigmented or sun-damaged skin, nor in periods of greater than 48 weeks of daily use.

The safety and effectiveness of Renova 0.02% cream have not been established in children under age 18, adults over age 71, and people with sun-damaged skin, nor in periods of greater than 52 weeks of daily use.

Special warnings about this medication

Be sure to keep these products away from the eyes, mouth, angles of the nose, and mucous membranes.

The medication may cause a brief feeling of warmth or slight stinging when applied. If it causes an abnormal irritation, redness, blistering, or peeling of the skin, notify your doctor. He may suggest that you use the medication less frequently, discontinue use temporarily, or discontinue use altogether. If a severe sensitivity reaction or chemical irritation occurs, you will probably need to stop using the drug.

If you have eczema (skin inflammation consisting of itching and small blisters that ooze and crust over) or other chronic skin conditions, use these products with extreme caution, as they may cause severe irritation.

During the early weeks of acne therapy, a worsening of the condition may occur due to the action of Avita or Retin-A on deep, previously unseen areas of inflammation. This is not a reason to discontinue therapy, but do notify your doctor if it occurs.

Retin-A gel and Avita are flammable and should be kept away from heat and flame.

Renova will not eliminate wrinkles, repair damage done by the sun, or reverse the aging process. After you stop using Renova, it is best to continue using a sunscreen and avoiding the sun.

Possible food and drug interactions when taking this medication

If these medications are used with certain other drugs, the effects of either could be increased, decreased, or altered. It is especially important to check with your doctor before combining Avita or Retin-A with the following:

Preparations containing benzoyl peroxide, such as Benzac AC Wash 5, Benzshave, Desquam-E, PanOxyl

Preparations containing sulfur (ointments and other preparations used to treat skin disorders and infections)

Resorcinol (a drug, used in ointments to treat acne, that causes skin to peel)

Salicylic acid (a drug that kills bacteria and fungi and causes skin to peel)

Resting your skin is recommended between use of the above preparations and treatment with Avita or Retin-A.

Do not use Renova if you are taking other drugs that increase sensitivity to sunlight. These include:

Certain antibiotics, including Cipro, Noroxin, and tetracycline

Major tranquilizers such as Thorazine and Mellaril

Sulfa drugs such as Bactrim and Septra

Thiazide drugs (water pills) such as Diuril and HydroDIURIL

Caution should be exercised when using Avita, Retin-A, or Renova in combination with other topical medications, medicated or abrasive soaps and cleansers, soaps and cosmetics that have a strong drying effect, products with high concentrations of alcohol, astringents, spices, or lime (especially the peel), permanent wave solutions, electrolysis, hair depilatories or waxes, or other preparations that may dry or irritate the skin.

Special information if you are pregnant or breastfeeding

The effects of Retin-A during pregnancy have not been adequately studied. If you are pregnant or plan to become pregnant, inform your doctor immediately.

Do not use Renova or Avita during pregnancy or if there is a good chance that you will become pregnant.

It is not known whether the drug appears in breast milk. Use with caution when breastfeeding.

Recommended dosage

RETIN-A AND AVITA

Apply once a day in the evening.

You should begin to notice results after 2 to 3 weeks of treatment. More than 6 or 7 weeks of treatment are needed before consistent beneficial effects appear.

Once acne has responded satisfactorily, it may be possible to maintain the improvement with less frequent applications or other dosage forms. However, any change in formulation, drug concentration, or dose frequency should be closely monitored by your doctor to determine your tolerance and response.

RENOVA

Apply just enough to lightly cover the affected area once daily at bedtime. Do not apply more than the recommended amount; it will not improve results and may cause increased discomfort. You will see the most improvement during the first 24 weeks of therapy. After that, Renova will simply maintain the improvement. When therapy is stopped, the improvement will gradually diminish.

Overdosage

Applying Avita, Retin-A, or Renova excessively will not produce faster or better results, and marked redness, peeling, or discomfort could occur.

RETROVIR
Pronounced: reh-troh-VEER
Generic name: Zidovudine

Why is this drug prescribed?

Retrovir is prescribed for adults infected with human immunodeficiency virus (HIV). HIV causes the immune system to break down so that it can no longer respond effectively to infection, leading to the fatal disease known as acquired immune deficiency syndrome (AIDS). Retrovir slows down the progress of HIV. Combining Retrovir with other drugs such as Epivir and Crixivan can help slow the progression.

Retrovir is also prescribed for HIV-infected children over 3 months of age who have symptoms of HIV or who have no symptoms but, through testing, have shown evidence of impaired immunity.

Retrovir taken during pregnancy often prevents transmission of HIV from mother to child.

Signs and symptoms of HIV disease are significant weight loss, fever, diarrhea, infections, and problems with the nervous system.

Most important fact about this drug

The long-term effects of treatment with zidovudine are unknown. However, treatment with this drug may lead to blood diseases, including granulocytopenia (a severe blood disorder characterized by a sharp decrease of certain types of white blood cells called granulocytes) and severe anemia requiring blood transfusions. This is especially true in women, individuals who are overweight, people who have been using this medication for a long time, people with more advanced HIV, and those who start treatment later in the course of their infection.

Also, because Retrovir is not a cure for HIV infections or AIDS, those who are infected may continue to develop complications, including opportunistic infections (exotic infections that develop when the immune system falters). Therefore, frequent blood counts by your doctor are strongly advised. Notify your doctor immediately of any changes in your general health.

How should you take this medication?

Take this medication exactly as prescribed by your doctor. Do not share this medication with anyone and do not exceed your recommended dosage. Take it at even intervals every 4 hours around the clock (children every 6 hours).

If you are pregnant, take the drug 5 times a day.

■ *If you miss a dose...*
Take it as soon as you remember. If it is almost time for your next dose, skip the one you missed and go back to your regular schedule. Do not take 2 doses at once.

■ *Storage instructions...*
Tablets, capsules, and syrup should be stored at room temperature; keep capsules away from moisture.

What side effects may occur?

Side effects cannot be anticipated. If any develop or change in intensity, inform your doctor as soon as possible. Only your doctor can determine if it is safe for you to continue taking Retrovir.

The frequency and severity of side effects associated with the use of Retrovir are greater in people whose infection is more advanced when treatment is started. Sometimes it is difficult to distinguish side effects from the underlying signs of HIV disease or the infections caused by HIV.

■ *Side effects may include:*
Cough, diarrhea, difficult or labored breathing, ear pain, discharge or swelling, enlarged liver, enlarged spleen, fever, general feeling of illness, headache, loss of appetite, mouth sores, nausea, nasal discharge or congestion, rash, swollen lymph nodes, vomiting

Why should this drug not be prescribed?

If you have ever had a life-threatening allergic reaction to Retrovir or any of its ingredients, you should not take this drug.

Special warnings about this medication

This drug has been studied for only a limited period of time. Long-term safety and effectiveness are not known, especially for people who are in a less advanced stage of AIDS or AIDS-related complex (the condition that precedes AIDS), and for those using the drug over a prolonged period of time.

Retrovir can cause an enlarged liver and the chemical imbalance known as lactic acidosis. This serious and sometimes fatal side effect is more likely in women, people who are overweight, and those who have been taking drugs such as Retrovir for an extended period. Signs of lactic acidosis include fatigue, nausea, abdominal pain, and a feeling of unwellness. Contact your doctor if you experience any of these symptoms. Treatment with Retrovir may have to be discontinued.

If you develop a blood disease, you may require a blood transfusion, and your doctor may reduce your dose or take you off the drug altogether. Make sure your doctor monitors your blood count on a regular basis.

The use of Retrovir has *not* been shown to reduce the risk of transmission of HIV to others through sexual contact or blood contamination or to nursing infants.

Retrovir should be used with extreme caution by people who have a bone marrow disease.

Some people taking Retrovir develop a sensitization reaction, often signaled by a rash. If you notice a rash developing, notify your doctor.

Contact your doctor immediately if you develop shortness of breath, muscle weakness, abdominal pain, or any unexpected problems while being treated with Retrovir.

Because few data are available concerning the use of this drug in people with impaired kidney or liver function, check with your doctor before using Retrovir if you have either problem.

Like other HIV drugs, Retrovir sometimes causes a redistribution of body fat, resulting in added weight around the waist, a "buffalo hump" of fat on the upper back, breast enlargement, and wasting of the face, arms, and legs. It's not known why this occurs, or what long-term effects it might have.

Possible food and drug interactions when taking this medication

If Retrovir is taken with certain other drugs, the effects of either could be increased, decreased, or altered. It is especially important to check with your doctor before combining Retrovir with the following:

Atovaquone (Mepron)
Doxorubicin (Adriamycin, a cancer drug)

Fluconazole (Diflucan)
Ganciclovir (Cytovene)
Interferon (Intron A, Roferon-A)
Methadone
Nelfinavir (Viracept)
Phenytoin (Dilantin, a seizure medication)
Probenecid (Benemid, an antigout drug)
Ribavirin (Virazole)
Rifampin (Rifadin)
Ritonavir (Norvir)
Stavudine (Zerit)
Valproic acid (Depakene, a seizure medication)

Do not take Retrovir with Combivir or Trizivir, which contain the same active ingredient.

Special information if you are pregnant or breastfeeding

The effects of Retrovir during pregnancy are under study. Use during pregnancy has been shown to protect the developing baby from contracting HIV. If you are pregnant or plan to become pregnant, inform your doctor immediately.

Since HIV can be passed on through breast milk to a nursing infant, do not breastfeed your baby.

Recommended dosage

ADULTS

All dosages of Retrovir must be very closely monitored by your physician. The following dosages are general; your physician will tailor the dose to your specific condition.

Tablets, Capsules, and Syrup

The usual dose of Retrovir, in combination with other HIV drugs, is 600 milligrams a day, divided into smaller doses.

If you are pregnant, the usual dosage is 100 milligrams in capsules, tablets, or syrup 5 times a day, beginning at 14 weeks of pregnancy, until you go into labor. You will then be given the drug intravenously until the baby is born. The baby will get Retrovir every 6 hours until it is 6 weeks old.

CHILDREN

The usual starting dose for children 6 weeks to 12 years of age is determined by body size. While the dose should not exceed 200 milligrams every 8 hours, it must still be individually determined. The drug is given along with other HIV medications.

Overdosage

Any medication taken in excess can have serious consequences. If you suspect an overdose, seek emergency medical treatment immediately.

■ *Symptoms of Retrovir overdose may include:*
Fatigue, headache, nausea, vomiting

REVIA

Pronounced: reh-VEE-uh
Generic name: Naltrexone hydrochloride

Why is this drug prescribed?

ReVia is prescribed to treat alcohol dependence and narcotic addiction. ReVia is not a cure. You must be ready to make a change and be willing to undertake a comprehensive treatment program that includes profes-sional counseling, support groups, and close medical supervision.

Most important fact about this drug

Before taking ReVia for narcotic addiction, you must be drug-free for at least 7 to 10 days. You must also be free of any drug withdrawal symp-toms. If you think you are still in withdrawal, be sure to tell your doctor, since taking ReVia while narcotics are still in your system could cause se-rious physical problems. Your doctor will perform tests to confirm your drug-free condition.

How should you take this medication?

It is important to take ReVia on schedule as directed by your doctor, and to follow through with your counseling and support group therapy.

If you take small doses of heroin or other narcotic drugs while taking ReVia, they will have no effect. Large doses combined with ReVia can be fatal.

■ *If you miss a dose...*
Take the missed dose as soon as possible. If you do not remember until the next day, skip the missed dose and go back to your regular dosing schedule. Do not take 2 doses at once.
■ *Storage instructions...*
No special measures are needed.

What side effects may occur?

Side effects cannot be anticipated. If any side effects develop or change in intensity, tell your doctor immediately. Only your doctor can determine whether it is safe for you to continue taking ReVia.

- *Side effects of treatment for alcoholism may include:*
  Dizziness, fatigue, headache, nausea, nervousness, sleeplessness,
  vomiting
- *Side effects of treatment for narcotic addiction may include:*
  Abdominal pain/cramps, anxiety, difficulty sleeping, headache, joint
  and muscle pain, low energy, nausea and/or vomiting, nervousness

Why should this drug not be prescribed?

If you are sensitive to or have ever had an allergic reaction to ReVia, you
should not take it. If you have acute hepatitis (liver disease) or liver failure, do not start therapy with ReVia. Remember, too, that you must be
narcotic-free before beginning ReVia therapy.

Special warnings about this medication

Since ReVia may cause liver damage when taken at high doses, if you develop symptoms that signal possible liver problems, you should stop taking ReVia immediately and see your doctor as soon as possible. These
symptoms include abdominal pain lasting more than a few days, white
bowel movements, dark urine, or yellowing of your eyes. Your doctor
may periodically test your liver function while you are on ReVia therapy.
Caution is also advisable if you have kidney problems.

If you are narcotic-dependent and accidentally take ReVia, you may experience severe withdrawal symptoms lasting up to 48 hours, including
confusion, sleepiness, hallucinations, vomiting, and diarrhea. If this occurs, seek help immediately.

Do not attempt to use narcotics while taking ReVia. Small doses will
have no effect, and large doses could lead to coma or even death.

Ask your doctor to give you a ReVia medication card to alert medical
personnel that you are taking ReVia in case of an emergency. Carry this
card with you at all times. If you do require medical treatment, be sure to
tell the doctor that you are taking ReVia. You should also tell your dentist
and pharmacist that you are taking ReVia.

The safety of ReVia in children under 18 years of age has not been established.

Possible food and drug interactions when taking this medication

Since studies to evaluate the interaction of ReVia with drugs other than
narcotics have not been performed, do not take any medications, either
over-the-counter or prescription, without first notifying your doctor.

Do not use Antabuse while you are taking ReVia; both drugs can damage your liver.

Do not take Mellaril (a drug used to treat depression and anxiety) while
on ReVia therapy, as the combination may make you feel very sleepy and
sluggish.

While taking ReVia, avoid medicines that contain narcotics, including
cough and cold preparations such as Actifed-C, Ryna-C, and Dimetane-

DC; antidiarrheal medications such as Lomotil; and narcotic painkillers such as Percodan, Tylox, and Tylenol No. 3.

Special information if you are pregnant or breastfeeding

The effects of ReVia during pregnancy have not been adequately studied. If you are pregnant or are planning to become pregnant, tell your doctor immediately. ReVia should be used during pregnancy only if clearly needed. ReVia may appear in breast milk. If this medication is essential to your health, your doctor may tell you to discontinue breastfeeding your baby until your treatment with ReVia is finished.

Recommended dosage

ALCOHOLISM

The usual starting dose is 50 milligrams once a day.

NARCOTIC DEPENDENCE

The usual starting dose is 25 milligrams once a day. If no withdrawal symptoms occur, the doctor may increase the dosage to 50 milligrams a day.

Overdosage

Any medication taken in excess can have serious consequences. If you suspect an overdose of ReVia, seek medical attention immediately.

REYATAZ
Pronounced: RAY-ah-taz
Generic name: Atazanavir sulfate

Why is this drug prescribed?

Reyataz is used with other medications to treat human immunodeficiency virus (HIV) infection. HIV causes the immune system to break down so that it can no longer fight off other infections. This leads to acquired immune deficiency syndrome (AIDS).

HIV thrives by taking over the immune system's vital CD4 cells (white blood cells) and using their inner workings to make additional copies of itself. Reyataz belongs to a class of HIV drugs called protease inhibitors, which work by interfering with an important step in the virus's reproductive cycle.

Reyataz is approved for used only in combination with other anti-HIV medications.

Most important fact about this drug

Reyataz must be taken exactly as your doctor prescribes. Like many anti-HIV drugs, Reyataz can affect the action of other medications. Before you start taking Reyataz, make sure your doctor knows about all the medicines you take, including over-the-counter drugs. Do not start a new medication without talking to your doctor, and also alert him or her when you stop taking any medication.

How should you take this medication?

Take Reyataz exactly as prescribed by your doctor. Do not change your dose or stop taking Reyataz without first talking to your doctor.

The amount of HIV in your blood may increase if you stop taking Reyataz even for a short time. Be careful not to miss any doses of Reyataz or other anti-HIV medications. It's also important to renew the medication promptly when your supply of pills starts to run low.

Always take Reyataz with a meal or snack to increase absorption of the drug. Do not open the capsules; swallow them whole.

If you are taking antacids or Videx, take Reyataz either 2 hours before or 1 hour after those medications.

■ *If you miss a dose...*
Take the forgotten dose as soon as you remember, then take the next scheduled dose at its regular time. If you are scheduled to take your next dose in 6 hours or less, do not take the missed dose. Just wait and take the next dose at its scheduled time. Do not take 2 doses at once.

■ *Storage instructions...*
Store at room temperature and protect from moisture.

What side effects may occur?

Side effects cannot be anticipated. If any develop or change in intensity, tell your doctor as soon as possible. Only your doctor can determine if it is safe for you to continue using Reyataz.

■ *Side effects may include:*
Abdominal pain, burning of hands or feet, depression, diarrhea, difficulty sleeping, dizziness, fever, headache, heartbeat irregularities, muscle numbness, nausea, pain, rash, redistribution of body fat, tingling, vomiting, yellow skin or eyes

Why should this drug not be prescribed?

You cannot take Reyataz if you develop an allergic reaction to the drug. If you take certain other medications you should not use Reyataz (see *Possible food and drug interactions*).

Special warnings about this medication

Reyataz is not a cure for HIV infection or AIDS. It also does not reduce your chance of passing HIV infection to others through sexual contact or through contact with your blood. Therefore, you should still continue to avoid practices that could spread HIV.

You could develop a rash while taking Reyataz. If the rash becomes severe, let your doctor know; you may have to stop taking this drug.

If you have ever had liver problems, use Reyataz with caution. The drug can worsen existing liver disease, especially if you have a history of hepatitis.

Treatment with HIV drugs such as Reyataz sometimes causes a redistribution of body fat, resulting in added weight around the waist, a "buffalo hump" of fat on the upper back, breast enlargement, and wasting of the face, arms, and legs. It's not known why this occurs, or what long-term effects it might have.

You may develop a condition called immune reconstitution syndrome, which is a reaction of your immune system that causes your body to develop an inflammatory response to certain secondary infections. If you suspect that you may have a secondary infection, contact your doctor immediately.

Some people taking HIV drugs such as Reyataz develop diabetes or high blood sugar. Those who already have diabetes may experience a worsening of their symptoms. If you're taking a diabetes medication, your doctor may have to adjust your dosage.

If you have the blood-clotting disorder hemophilia, you may have more bleeding problems when taking Reyataz.

Possible food and drug interactions when taking this medication

If you take the following medications, you should not use Reyataz. The combination may cause reduced effectiveness, resistance to Reyataz or other HIV drugs, serious or life-threatening side effects, or even death.

Cisapride
Ergot-based drugs such as Cafergot and Methergine
Indinavir (Crixivan)
Irinotecan (Camptosar)
Lovastatin (Mevacor)
Midazolam (Versed)
Pimozide (Orap)
Proton pump inhibitors such as esomeprazole (Nexium), omeprazole (Prilosec), and pantoprazole (Protonix)
Rifampin (Rifadin, Rifater, Rifamate, Rimactane)
Simvastatin (Zocor)
St. John's wort
Triazolam (Halcion)

If Reyataz is taken with certain other drugs, the effects of either could be increased, decreased, or altered. It is especially important to check with your doctor before combining Reyataz with the following:

Antiarrhythmic drugs that correct abnormal heart rhythms, such as amiodarone (Cordarone), Bepridil (Vascor), quinidine, and lidocaine
Antidepressants such as amitriptyline (Elavil), desipramine (Norpramin), doxepin (Sinequan), imipramine (Tofranil), protriptyline (Vivactil), and trimipramine (Surmontil)

Antifungal medications such as ketoconazole (Nizoral) and itraconazole (Sporanox)

Anti-ulcer drugs such as nizatidine (Axid), famotidine (Pepcid AC), cimetidine (Tagamet), and ranitidine (Zantac)

Atorvastatin (Lipitor)

Beta-blockers such as atenolol (Tenormin)

Calcium channel blockers such as diltiazem (Cardizem), felodipine (Plendil), nifedipine (Procardia), nicardipine (Cardene), and verapamil (Isoptin SR)

Clarithromycin (Biaxin)

Cyclosporine (Sandimmune, Neoral)

Didanosine (Videx)

Efavirenz (Sustiva)

Erectile dysfunction drugs such as sildenafil (Viagra), tadalafil (Cialis), and vardenafil (Levitra)

HIV drugs known as protease inhibitors, such as fosamprenavir (Lexiva), indinavir (Crixivan), and ritonavir (Norvir)

Nevirapine (Viramune)

Oral contraceptives containing ethinyl estradiol and norethindrone

Rifabutin (Mycobutin)

Saquinavir (Invirase, Fortovase)

Sirolimus (Rapamune)

Tacrolimus (Prograf)

Tenofovir (Viread)

Warfarin (Coumadin)

Voriconazole (VFend) should not be taken if you are using Reyataz and Norvir together.

Reyataz should be taken 2 hours before or 1 hour after antacids (Maalox, Mylanta) or buffered medications (Videx).

Be sure to tell your doctor and pharmacist about all medications you take, both prescription and over-the-counter. Alert them when you stop taking a medication too.

Special information if you are pregnant or breastfeeding

If you are pregnant or plan to become pregnant, inform your doctor immediately. The effects of Reyataz during pregnancy have not been well studied.

You should not breastfeed if you have HIV, since the virus appears in breast milk and can infect a nursing infant.

Recommended dosage

ADULTS

For Adults Who Have Never Taken HIV Medications
The recommended dose of Reyataz is two 200-milligram capsules once a day, for a total of 400 milligrams.

*For Adults Who **Have** Taken HIV Medications*
The recommended once-daily dose of Reyataz is two 150-milligram capsules (for a total of 300 milligrams) plus 100 milligrams of ritonavir (Norvir).

If you take Sustiva or a buffered formulation of Videx, your doctor may tell you to use a different dosage.

Adults with Reduced Liver Function
If you have moderate liver problems, your doctor may reduce your dosage to 300 milligrams once a day.

CHILDREN

Because Reyataz has not been well studied in children under age 16, there isn't enough information to recommend a dose. The drug is not recommended for use in babies under the age of 3 months.

Overdosage
Any medication taken in excess can have serious consequences. If you suspect an overdose, seek emergency treatment immediately. A possible sign of Reyataz overdose may include yellowing of the skin or whites of the eyes.

Rheumatrex *See Methotrexate, page 834.*

RHINOCORT AQUA
Pronounced: RYE-no-kort
Generic name: Budesonide

Why is this drug prescribed?
Rhinocort Aqua is an anti-inflammatory steroid nasal spray. It is prescribed for relief of the symptoms of hay fever and similar allergic nasal inflammations.

Most important fact about this drug
Because steroids can suppress the immune system, people taking Rhinocort Aqua may become more susceptible to infections, and their infections could be more severe. Anyone taking Rhinocort Aqua or other corticosteroids who has not had infections such as chickenpox and measles should avoid exposure to them. If you are taking Rhinocort Aqua and are exposed, tell your doctor immediately.

How should you take this medication?
Before using Rhinocort Aqua Nasal Spray, shake the container gently and prime the pump by spraying it 8 times. If used daily, the pump does not need to be reprimed. If not used for 2 consecutive days, reprime with 1 spray or until a fine mist appears. If not used for more than 14 days, rinse

the applicator and reprime with 2 sprays or until a fine mist appears. Discard the bottle after 120 sprays, since the amount of drug in each spray will decline substantially after that point.

Relief may begin within 10 hours. Most improvement occurs during the first 1 or 2 days, but it may take as long as 2 weeks to achieve the maximum benefits. If symptoms do not improve after 2 weeks, or the condition grows worse, check with your doctor.

Do not use doses that are larger than recommended.

■ *If you miss a dose...*
Take the forgotten dose as soon as you remember. If it is almost time for your next dose, skip the one you missed and go back to your regular schedule. Never take two doses at the same time.

■ *Storage instructions...*
Store at room temperature with the valve up. Do not freeze. Protect from light.

What side effects may occur?
Side effects cannot be anticipated. If any develop or change in intensity, inform your doctor as soon as possible. Only your doctor can determine if it is safe for you to continue taking Rhinocort.

■ *Side effects may include:*
Nosebleeds, sore throat

Why should this drug not be prescribed?
If you develop an infection of your nose and throat, stop using Rhinocort Aqua and call your doctor. If you already have tuberculosis or any other kind of infection, be sure your doctor knows about it.

Do not use Rhinocort Aqua if you have recently had nasal ulcers, nasal surgery or a nasal injury; this drug would slow the healing process. You will also need to avoid Rhinocort if it gives you an allergic reaction.

Special warnings about this medication
If you have been taking a steroid in tablet form, such as prednisone, and are switched to Rhinocort Aqua, you may have symptoms of withdrawal, such as joint or muscle pain, lethargy, and depression. If you have been taking another steroid for a long time for asthma, your asthma may get worse if your medication is cut back too quickly. Using Rhinocort Aqua with another steroid drug can decrease the body's normal ability to make its own steroid chemicals.

Use this drug with caution in children and teenagers. It can affect their rate of growth.

Possible food and drug interactions when taking this medication
Talk to your doctor before using Rhinocort Aqua if you already take prednisone or any other steroid medication.

If Rhinocort Aqua is taken with certain other drugs, its effects could be increased. It is especially important to check with your doctor before combining Rhinocort Aqua with the following:

Cimetidine (Tagamet)
Clarithromycin (Biaxin)
Erythromycin (E.E.S., Ery-Tab, PCE)
Itraconazole (Sporanox)
Ketoconazole (Nizoral)

Special information if you are pregnant or breastfeeding

In large doses, this drug has caused fetal harm in laboratory animals. If you are pregnant or plan to become pregnant, inform your doctor immediately. Rhinocort Aqua should be used during pregnancy only if clearly needed. The effect of this drug on nursing infants is also unknown, although we do know that similar drugs have been found in breast milk. It should be used with caution by women who breastfeed.

Recommended dosage

ADULTS

The recommended starting dose for adults and children over 12 is 64 micrograms per day administered as 1 spray in each nostril once a day. The maximum recommended dose is 256 micrograms per day, administered as 4 sprays per nostril once a day.

CHILDREN

The recommended starting dose for children between 6 and 12 years of age is 64 micrograms per day administered as one spray per nostril once a day. The maximum recommended dose for children in this age group is 128 micrograms per day, administered as 2 sprays per nostril once a day. The safety and effectiveness of Rhinocort Aqua in children under 6 have not been established.

Overdosage

Any medication taken in excess can have serious consequences. If you suspect an overdose, seek medical attention immediately.

Symptoms of long-term overdose with Rhinocort Aqua stem from a condition called hypercorticism, when the body produces an excess of its own steroid chemicals.

■ *Symptoms of overdose may include:*
Diabetes, easy bruising, fat around the waist and on the upper back, high blood pressure, lowered resistance to infection, menstrual problems, moon face, muscle weakness and wasting, poor healing, thin skin

RIBAVIRIN

Pronounced: RY-bah-vy-rin
Brand names: Copegus, Rebetol

Why is this drug prescribed?

In combination with certain interferon drugs, ribavirin is prescribed to treat chronic hepatitis C. Copegus is taken with the interferon drug Pegasys, and Rebetol is taken with the interferon drugs Intron A or PEG-Intron. Ribavirin is always used with one of the other drugs. By itself, it is ineffective against hepatitis C.

Most important fact about this drug

Extreme care should be taken to avoid pregnancy when a woman or her partner is taking ribavirin. The drug poses a significant risk of serious harm to developing infants, even at lower doses, and it can also cause abnormalities in a man's sperm. The doctor will want to see a negative pregnancy report immediately before starting ribavirin therapy; and pregnancy tests should be done every month during therapy and for six months after it stops. Use at least two forms of birth control during treatment and for six months afterwards.

How should you take this medication?

Copegus is available as tablets; Rebetol is available in capsule and oral solution forms. Make sure you drink plenty of water while taking ribavirin, especially when you first begin treatment. Ribavirin may be taken with or without food when used in combination therapy with Intron A, but whichever way you choose, do it consistently. When ribavirin is used in combination therapy with Pegasys or PEG-Intron, you should take the dose with food.

■ *If you miss a dose...*
Take it as soon as you remember. If it is almost time for your next dose, skip the one you missed and go back to your regular schedule. Never take 2 doses at once.

■ *Storage instructions...*
Store at room temperature.

What side effects may occur?

Side effects cannot be anticipated. If any develop or change in intensity, tell your doctor immediately. Only your doctor can determine whether it is safe for you to continue taking ribavirin.

■ *Side effects may include:*
Anemia (possibly severe), anxiety, blood disorders, chills, depression, dizziness, fatigue, fever, hair loss, headache, insomnia, irritability, joint or muscle pain, nausea, shortness of breath, skin problems, vomiting, weight loss

Why should this drug not be prescribed?

Do not take ribavirin if you:

- Are pregnant or planning to become pregnant during treatment or during the 6 months after treatment has ended, or if you're breastfeeding. If you're a man and have a female partner who fits these criteria, you must also avoid ribavirin.
- Have hepatitis caused by your immune system attacking your liver (autoimmune hepatitis)
- Have certain blood disorders, such as thalassemia major or sickle-cell anemia
- Have severe or unstable heart disease or liver disease
- Have severe kidney dysfunction
- Have ever had an allergic reaction to any of the ingredients in Copegus or Rebetol

Special warnings about this medication

Within two weeks of starting treatment with ribavirin, about 1 patient in 10 develops a severe form of anemia. Your doctor will order blood tests periodically to check for this condition. Severe anemia is a serious condition that can lead to a potentially fatal heart attack. Ribavirin should be used with caution if you have a heart condition. Your doctor will perform heart tests such as an ECG before you begin treatment and will monitor your heart closely while you are taking ribavirin. You may have to discontinue therapy if you develop heart-related problems or if your heart condition gets worse.

Treatment with ribavirin and interferon drugs can have other serious side effects, including depression and suicidal thoughts (especially in adolescents), blood disorders, pancreas and lung problems, diabetes, autoimmune disorders, and infections. If you develop symptoms of these conditions, your doctor may have to discontinue treatment with ribavirin.

The risk of side effects is greater for individuals with poor kidney function. If you have this problem, your doctor will monitor you closely and adjust your dosage if necessary. Since many older adults have impaired kidney, liver, and heart function, the dosage of ribavirin is often decreased for these individuals.

The safety and effectiveness of ribavirin treatment have not been established for individuals with organ transplants, uncontrolled liver disease, and hepatitis B or unstable HIV infection. Your doctor will have your liver function tested before you begin taking ribavirin.

Possible food and drug interactions when taking this medication

If you are taking didanosine (Videx), treatment with ribavirin is not recommended. Serious and even fatal reactions have occurred.

If ribavirin is taken with certain other drugs, the effects of either could be increased, decreased, or altered. It is especially important to check with your doctor before combining ribavirin with HIV drugs known as nucleoside analogues, such as Combivir, Epivir, Retrovir, and Zerit.

Special information if you are pregnant or breastfeeding

Ribavirin may cause birth defects or death in the developing infant. Neither a woman nor her partner should take ribavirin while she is pregnant. Use two forms of contraception if either partner is taking ribavirin. Continue using two forms of contraception for 6 months after treatment is finished. If pregnancy occurs during ribavirin therapy or within 6 months afterwards, contact your doctor immediately.

It is not known whether ribavirin appears in breast milk. Because of the potential for serious adverse effects on the nursing infant, you should not breastfeed your baby while taking ribavirin.

Recommended dosage

Your doctor will determine the best dose based on your condition and how your body responds to the drug. Your dosage will be lowered if you develop anemia while taking ribavirin.

TREATMENT WITH COPEGUS AND PEGASYS

Adults 18 Years of Age and Older

The dosage depends on your body weight. The usual dose for individuals weighing less than 165 pounds is 500 milligrams in the morning and 500 milligrams at night. For individuals weighing 165 pounds or more, the usual dose is 600 milligrams in the morning and at night. Certain people, including those infected with HIV, may have to take 400 milligrams in the morning and at night. You should take your dose with food.

The recommended duration of treatment for people who have not taken an interferon drug previously is 24 to 48 weeks.

TREATMENT WITH REBETOL AND INTRON A

Adults

The dosage depends on your body weight. The usual dose for individuals weighing 165 pounds or less is 400 milligrams in the morning and 600 milligrams at night. The usual daily dose for individuals weighing more than 165 pounds is 600 milligrams in the morning and at night.

The recommended duration of treatment for people who have not taken an interferon drug previously is 24 to 48 weeks. If you've taken interferon in the past and have had a relapse, the recommended duration of treatment is 24 weeks.

Children 3 Years of Age and Older

Children who weigh 134 pounds or more will usually take the adult dose listed above. For children who weigh less than 134 pounds, the doctor will adjust the dose accordingly based on the child's weight.

TREATMENT WITH REBETOL AND PEG-INTRON

Adults 18 Years of Age and Older
The usual dose is 400 milligrams in the morning and 400 milligrams at night. You should take your dose with food.

Overdosage
No adverse effects of ribavirin overdose have been reported. Nevertheless, any medication taken in excess may have serious consequences. If you suspect an overdose of ribavirin, seek medical attention immediately.

RIDAURA
Pronounced: ri-DOOR-ah
Generic name: Auranofin

Why is this drug prescribed?
Ridaura, a gold preparation, is given to help treat rheumatoid arthritis. Ridaura is taken by mouth, unlike other gold compounds, which are given by injection. It is recommended only for people who have not been helped sufficiently by nonsteroidal anti-inflammatory drugs (Anaprox, Dolobid, Indocin, Motrin, and others). Ridaura should be part of a comprehensive arthritis treatment program that includes non-drug forms of therapy.

You are most likely to benefit from Ridaura if you have active joint inflammation, especially in the early stages.

Most important fact about this drug
Unlike anti-inflammatory medications, Ridaura does not take effect immediately. In fact, you may have to wait for 3 to 6 months to get any benefit from Ridaura. Ridaura prevents or suppresses joint swelling, but does not cure rheumatoid arthritis.

How should you take this medication?
Read the patient information sheet provided with Ridaura, and take the medication exactly as prescribed.

You should observe good oral hygiene during therapy with Ridaura.

■ *If you miss a dose...*
If you take 1 dose a day, take the missed dose as soon as you remember. If you do not remember until the next day, skip the dose you missed and go back to your regular schedule.

If you take more than 1 dose a day, take the missed dose as soon as you remember. If it is almost time for your next dose, skip the one you missed and go back to your regular schedule.

Do not take 2 doses at once.

■ *Storage instructions...*
Store at room temperature in a tightly closed, light-resistant container.

What side effects may occur?

Side effects cannot be anticipated. If any side effects develop or change in intensity, tell your doctor immediately. Only your doctor can determine whether it is safe for you to continue taking Ridaura. Ridaura causes loose stools or diarrhea in about half of all people who take it; there may also be indigestion, abdominal pain and gas, loss of appetite, vomiting, or nausea.

Why should this drug not be prescribed?

Do not take Ridaura if you have ever had any of the following reactions to a medication containing gold:

Anaphylaxis (life-threatening allergic reaction)
Blood or bone marrow abnormality
Fibrosis (scar tissue formation) in the lungs
Serious bowel inflammation
Skin peeling off in sheets

Special warnings about this medication

You should be monitored especially closely while taking Ridaura if you have any of the following:

History of a bone marrow abnormality
Inflammatory bowel disease
Kidney disease
Liver disease
Skin rash

Your doctor may order periodic blood and urine tests to check for unwanted effects.

Like other medications containing gold, Ridaura may cause serious blood abnormalities. If you start to bruise easily, or develop small red or purplish skin discolorations, see your doctor. He or she will have you stop taking Ridaura and will do some blood tests, including a platelet count.

Ridaura may cause protein or microscopic amounts of blood to spill into your urine. If a urine test shows that this is happening, your doctor will take you off of Ridaura immediately.

Gold compounds may cause your skin to become more sensitive to sunlight, so you may need to limit your exposure to the sun and wear a sunscreen.

Possible food and drug interactions when taking this medication

If Ridaura is taken with certain other drugs, the effects of either could be increased, decreased, or altered. It is especially important to check with your doctor before combining Ridaura with the following:

Penicillamine (Cuprimine)
Phenytoin (Dilantin)

Special information if you are pregnant or breastfeeding

If you are pregnant or plan to become pregnant, inform your doctor immediately. Because Ridaura may cause birth defects, it should not be taken during pregnancy.

Likewise, you should not take Ridaura while breastfeeding; although there are no data on Ridaura, injected gold appears in breast milk. If you are a new mother, you may have to choose between taking Ridaura and breastfeeding your baby.

Recommended dosage

The usual dosage of Ridaura is 6 milligrams daily in a single dose or divided into 2 smaller doses. After 6 months, your doctor may increase the dose to 9 milligrams, divided into 3 doses. Ridaura is prescribed only for adults.

Overdosage

Any medication taken in excess can have serious consequences. If you suspect an overdose of Ridaura, seek medical attention immediately.

Rifampin, Isoniazid, and Pyrazinamide *See Rifater, below.*

RIFATER

Pronounced: RIF-a-tur
Generic ingredients: Rifampin, Isoniazid, Pyrazinamide

Why is this drug prescribed?

Rifater is a combination antibiotic used to treat the initial phase of tuberculosis. After a 2-month period, your doctor may prescribe another combination of antituberculosis drugs (Rifamate), which can be continued for longer periods.

Most important fact about this drug

Isoniazid, one of the components of Rifater, sometimes causes liver damage. Contact your doctor immediately if you develop yellowing of the eyes or skin, fatigue, weakness, loss of appetite, nausea, or vomiting.

How should you take this medication?

Take Rifater exactly as prescribed. Do not stop without consulting your doctor. It is important to take all of the drug prescribed for you, even if you feel better, and not to miss any doses.

Take Rifater on an empty stomach, either 1 hour before or 2 hours after a meal, with a full glass of water. Wait at least 1 hour before taking an antacid, as antacids may interfere with the drug.

If needed, your doctor may suggest taking vitamin B$_6$ while you are on Rifater therapy.

■ *If you miss a dose...*
Take it as soon as you remember. If it is almost time for the next dose, skip the one you missed and go back to your regular schedule. Never take 2 doses at once.

■ *Storage instructions...*
Store at room temperature. Protect from moisture.

What side effects may occur?

Side effects cannot be anticipated. If any develop or change in intensity, tell your doctor as soon as possible. Only your doctor can determine if it is safe for you to continue taking Rifater.

■ *Side effects may include:*
Angina (crushing chest pain), anxiety, bone pain, chest pain, chest tightness, cough, coughing up blood, diabetic coma, diarrhea, difficulty breathing, digestive pain, fast, fluttery heartbeat, headache, hepatitis, hives, itching, joint pain, nausea, numbness or tingling of the legs, rash, reddened skin, skin peeling or flaking, sleeplessness, sweating, swelling of the legs, vomiting, yellowing of skin and eyes

Why should this drug not be prescribed?

Do not take this medication if you have ever had an allergic reaction to or are sensitive to rifampin, isoniazid, or pyrazinamide. If you have serious liver disease or have ever had a severe side effect from isoniazid (such as fever, chills, and arthritis), do not take Rifater. Also, if you have a history of liver disease or have had acute and painful joint swelling (gout), avoid this drug.

Special warnings about this medication

Rifater may cause your urine, sputum, sweat, and tears to turn a red-orange color. This is to be expected and is not harmful. The drug may also permanently discolor contact lenses.

Since Rifater may cause eye problems, you should have a complete eye examination before starting therapy and periodically during Rifater treatment.

Limit the amount of alcohol you drink while on this medicine. Daily users of alcohol may be more prone to liver problems.

Use this medicine with caution if you have diabetes or kidney disease.

When rifampin, one of the drugs in Rifater, is taken at high doses (more than 600 milligrams once or twice a week), it is likely that side effects may increase, including flu-like symptoms such as fever, chills, fatigue, weakness, upset stomach, and shortness of breath.

Possible food and drug interactions when taking this medication
If Rifater is taken with certain other drugs, the effects could be increased, decreased, or altered. Consider another form of birth control if you are taking oral contraceptives, since Rifater lowers their effectiveness. Also check with your doctor before combining Rifater with the following:

Antacids such as Maalox and Tums
Anticonvulsants such as Dilantin, Depakene, Mysoline, and Tegretol
Barbiturates such as phenobarbital and Nembutal
Blood pressure medicines such as Inderal, Tenormin, and Vasotec
Blood thinners such as Coumadin
Chloramphenicol (Chloromycetin)
Ciprofloxacin (Cipro)
Clofibrate (Atromid-S)
Cotrimoxazole (Bactrim, Septra)
Cycloserine (Seromycin)
Cyclosporine (Sandimmune)
Dapsone
Diabetes medications such as Diabinese and Orinase
Disulfiram (Antabuse)
Fluconazole (Diflucan)
Haloperidol (Haldol)
Heart medications such Calan, Cardizem, Lanoxin, Mexitil, Norpace,
    Procardia, Quinidex, and Tonocard
Itraconazole (Sporanox)
Ketoconazole (Nizoral)
Levodopa (Sinemet)
Narcotic analgesics such as Darvon, Demerol, Percocet, and
    Percodan
Nortriptyline (Pamelor)
Probenecid (Benemid)
Progestins such as Megace
Steroid drugs such as Deltasone and Prelone
Sulfasalazine (Azulfidine)
Theophylline (Theolair, Slo-Phyllin, Theo-Dur)
Tranquilizers such as Valium and Xanax

Foods such as cheese, fish, and red wine may cause reactions if you are taking a medicine containing isoniazid. Call your doctor immediately if fast or fluttery heartbeat, flushing, sweating, headache, or lightheadedness occurs while you are taking this medication.

Special information if you are pregnant or breastfeeding

If you are pregnant or plan to become pregnant, tell your doctor immediately. You may need to discontinue the drug. If needed for preventive treatment, Rifater should be started after delivery. An ingredient in Rifater may cause postnatal hemorrhaging in the mother and baby when given during the last few weeks of pregnancy.

Rifater can pass into breast milk and may affect the nursing infant. Your doctor may recommend that you stop breastfeeding until your treatment with Rifater is finished.

Recommended dosage

ADULTS

Take once a day, as follows:

If you weigh 97 pounds or less: 4 tablets
If you weigh 98 to 120 pounds: 5 tablets
If you weigh 121 pounds or more: 6 tablets

CHILDREN

The safety and effectiveness of Rifater in children under the age of 15 have not been established.

Overdosage

Any medication taken in excess can have serious consequences. An untreated overdose of Rifater can be fatal. If you suspect an overdose, seek medical attention immediately.

■ *Symptoms of Rifater overdose may include:*
Blurred vision, coma, dizziness, hallucinations, increasing tiredness or sluggishness, liver enlargement or tenderness, nausea, seizures, shallow or difficult breathing, slurring of speech, stupor, vomiting, yellow eyes and skin

Rifaximin See Xifaxan, page 1600.

Risedronate See Actonel, page 29.

RISPERDAL

Pronounced: RIS-per-dal
Generic name: Risperidone
Other brand name: Risperdal M-Tab

Why is this drug prescribed?

Risperdal is prescribed for the treatment of schizophrenia, a severe mental disorder that can cause delusions (false beliefs) and hallucinations.

It is also used for the short-term treatment of mania associated with bipolar disorder. Risperdal is thought to work by muting the impact of dopamine and serotonin, two of the brain's key chemical messengers.

Most important fact about this drug

Risperdal may cause tardive dyskinesia, a condition that causes involuntary muscle spasms and twitches in the face and body. This condition can become permanent and is most common among older people, especially women. Tell your doctor immediately if you begin to have any involuntary movement. You may need to discontinue Risperdal therapy.

Drugs such as Risperdal may increase the risk of death in elderly people with dementia-related psychosis. Risperdal is not approved for use in such patients.

How should you take this medication?

Do not take more or less of this medication than prescribed. Higher doses are more likely to cause unwanted side effects.

Risperdal may be taken with or without food.

Risperdal oral solution comes with a calibrated pipette to use for measuring. The oral solution can be taken with water, coffee, orange juice, or low-fat milk, but not with cola drinks or tea.

Risperdal orally disintegrating tablets (M-Tabs) come in blister packs and should not be removed from the package until you are ready to take them. When it's time for your dose, use dry fingers to peel back the foil of the blister pack to remove the tablet; do not push the tablet through the foil because this could damage the tablet. Immediately place the tablet on your tongue. The medication dissolves in the mouth quickly and can be swallowed with or without liquid. You should not split or chew the orally disintegrating tablets.

■ *If you miss a dose...*
Take it as soon as you remember. If it is almost time for your next dose, skip the one you missed and go back to your regular schedule. Do not take 2 doses at once.

■ *Storage instructions...*
Store at room temperature. Protect tablets from light and moisture; protect oral solution from light and freezing.

What side effects may occur?

Side effects cannot be anticipated. If any develop or change in intensity, tell your doctor as soon as possible. Only your doctor can determine if it is safe for you to continue taking Risperdal.

■ *Side effects may include:*
Agitation, anxiety, constipation, dizziness, hallucination, headache, indigestion, insomnia, rapid or irregular heartbeat, restlessness, runny nose, sleepiness, vomiting, weight change

Why should this drug not be prescribed?

If you are sensitive to or have ever had an allergic reaction to Risperdal or other major tranquilizers, you should not take this medication.

Risperdal should not be used to treat elderly patients who have dementia because the drug could increase the risk of stroke.

Special warnings about this medication

You should use Risperdal cautiously if you have kidney, liver, or heart disease, seizures, breast cancer, thyroid disorders, or any other diseases that affect the metabolism (conversion of food into energy and tissue). Use caution, too, if you've had a stroke or mini-strokes, suffer from fluid loss or dehydration, or expect to be exposed to extremes of temperature.

Be aware that Risperdal may mask signs and symptoms of drug overdose and of conditions such as intestinal obstruction, brain tumor, and Reye's syndrome (a dangerous neurological condition that may follow viral infections, usually occurring in children). Risperdal can also cause difficulty when swallowing, which in turn can cause a type of pneumonia.

Risperdal may cause Neuroleptic Malignant Syndrome (NMS), a condition marked by muscle stiffness or rigidity, fast heartbeat or irregular pulse, increased sweating, high fever, and high or low blood pressure. Unchecked, this condition can prove fatal. Call your doctor immediately if you notice any of these symptoms. Risperdal therapy should be discontinued.

Certain antipsychotic drugs, including Risperdal, are associated with an increased risk of developing high blood sugar, which on rare occasions has led to coma or death. See your doctor right away if you develop signs of high blood sugar, including dry mouth, unusual thirst, increased urination, and tiredness. If you have diabetes or have a high risk of developing it, see your doctor regularly for blood sugar testing.

People at high risk for suicide attempts will be prescribed the lowest dose possible to reduce the risk of intentional overdose.

This drug may impair your ability to drive a car or operate potentially dangerous machinery. Do not participate in any activities that require full alertness if you are unsure of your ability.

Risperdal is prescribed for the short-term treatment of rapid-onset bipolar mania; it is not approved for preventing future episodes. The effectiveness of the drug for treating mania for more than 3 weeks has not been studied.

Risperdal can cause orthostatic hypotension (low blood pressure when rising to a standing position), with dizziness, rapid heartbeat, and fainting, especially when you first start to take it. If you develop this problem, report it to your doctor. He can adjust your dose to reduce the symptoms.

Be sure to tell your doctor if you have phenylketonuria and must avoid the amino acid phenylalanine, since Risperdal M-Tabs contains this substance.

The safety and effectiveness of Risperdal have not been studied in children.

Possible food and drug interactions when taking this medication

If Risperdal is taken with certain other drugs, the effects of either can be increased, decreased, or altered. It is especially important to check with your doctor before combining Risperdal with the following:

Blood pressure medicines such as Aldomet, Procardia, and Vasotec
Bromocriptine mesylate (Parlodel)
Carbamazepine (Tegretol)
Clozapine (Clozaril)
Fluoxetine (Prozac)
Levodopa (Sinemet, Larodopa)
Paroxetine (Paxil)
Phenobarbital
Phenytoin (Dilantin)
Quinidine
Rifampin (Rifadin, Rimactane)
Valproic acid (Depakene, Depakote)

Risperdal tends to increase the effect of blood pressure medicines.

You may experience drowsiness and other potentially serious effects if Risperdal is combined with alcohol and other drugs that slow the central nervous system such as Valium, Percocet, Demerol, or Haldol.

Check with your doctor before taking any new medications.

Special information if you are pregnant or breastfeeding

The safety and effectiveness of Risperdal during pregnancy have not been adequately studied. If you are pregnant or plan to become pregnant, tell your doctor immediately. Risperdal makes its way into breast milk, so women taking Risperdal must avoid breastfeeding.

Recommended dosage

SCHIZOPHRENIA

Adults

Doses of Risperdal can be taken once a day, or divided in half and taken twice daily. The usual dose on the first day is 2 milligrams or 2 milliliters of oral solution. On the second day, the dose increases to 4 milligrams or milliliters, and on the third day it rises to 6 milligrams or milliliters. Further dosage adjustments can be made at intervals of 1 week. Over the long term, typical daily doses range from 2 to 8 milligrams or milliliters.

BIPOLAR MANIA (SHORT-TERM TREATMENT OF ACUTE EPISODES)

Adults

The recommended starting dose is 2 to 3 milligrams (or milliliters of oral solution) per day, given as a single dose. If needed, the doctor will adjust the dose by 1 milligram at intervals of at least 24 hours. The effective dosage range is 1 to 6 milligrams a day.

DOSAGE ADJUSTMENT

The doctor may prescribe lower doses if you are weak, elderly, have liver or kidney disease, or have a high risk for low blood pressure. The usual starting dose is 0.5 milligram (or 0.5 milliliter of oral solution) twice a day. The doctor may switch you to a once-a-day dosing schedule after the first 2 to 3 days of treatment.

If needed, each dose may be increased by increments of no more than 0.5 milligram. Increases to dosages above 1.5 milligrams twice a day should generally me made at intervals of at least 1 week.

You may also need your Risperdal dose adjusted if you're taking certain medications, including Dilantin, Paxil, phenobarbital, Prozac, Rifadin, and Tegretol.

Overdosage

Any medication taken in excess can have serious consequences. If you suspect an overdose of Risperdal, seek medical attention immediately.

■ *Symptoms of Risperdal overdose may include:*
  Drowsiness, low blood pressure, rapid heartbeat, sedation

Risperidone See Risperdal, page 1266.

RITALIN

Pronounced: RIT-ah-lin
Generic name: Methylphenidate hydrochloride
Other brand names: Concerta, Metadate, Methylin

Why is this drug prescribed?

Ritalin and other brands of methylphenidate are mild central nervous system stimulants used in the treatment of attention deficit hyperactivity disorder in children. With the exceptions of Ritalin LA, Concerta, and Metadate CD, these products are also used in adults to treat narcolepsy (an uncontrollable desire to sleep).

When given for attention deficit disorder, this drug should be an integral part of a total treatment program that includes psychological, educational, and social measures. Symptoms of attention deficit disorder include continual problems with moderate to severe distractibility, short attention span, hyperactivity, emotional changeability, and impulsiveness.

Most important fact about this drug

Excessive doses of this drug over a long period of time can produce addiction. It is also possible to develop tolerance to the drug, so that larger doses are needed to produce the original effect. Because of these dangers, be sure to check with your doctor before making any change in dosage; and withdraw the drug only under your doctor's supervision.

How should you take this medication?

Follow your doctor's directions carefully. It is recommended that methylphenidate be taken 30 to 45 minutes before meals. If the drug interferes with sleep, give the child the last dose before 6 P.M. Ritalin-SR, Ritalin LA, Metadate CD, Methylin ER, and Concerta are long-acting forms of the drug, taken less frequently. They should be swallowed whole, never crushed or chewed. (Ritalin LA and Metadate CD may also be given by sprinkling the contents of the capsule on a tablespoon of cool applesauce and administering immediately, followed by a drink of water.)

■ *If you miss a dose...*
  Give it to the child as soon as you remember. Give the remaining doses for the day at regularly spaced intervals. Do not give 2 doses at once.

■ *Storage instructions...*
  Keep out of reach of children. Store below 86 degrees Fahrenheit in a tightly closed, light-resistant container. Protect Ritalin-SR from moisture.

What side effects may occur?

Side effects cannot be anticipated. If any develop or change in intensity, inform your doctor as soon as possible. Only your doctor can determine if it is safe for you to continue giving this drug.

■ *Side effects may include:*
  Inability to fall or stay asleep, nervousness

These side effects can usually be controlled by reducing the dosage and omitting the drug in the afternoon or evening.

In children, loss of appetite, abdominal pain, weight loss during long-term therapy, inability to fall or stay asleep, and abnormally fast heartbeat are more common side effects.

Why should this drug not be prescribed?

This drug should not be prescribed for anyone experiencing anxiety, tension, and agitation, since the drug may aggravate these symptoms.

Anyone sensitive or allergic to this drug should not take it.

This medication should not be taken by anyone with the eye condition known as glaucoma, anyone who suffers from tics (repeated, involuntary twitches), or someone with a family history of Tourette's syndrome (severe and multiple tics).

This drug is not intended for use in children whose symptoms may be caused by stress or a psychiatric disorder.

This medication should not be used for the prevention or treatment of normal fatigue, nor should it be used for the treatment of severe depression.

This drug should not be taken during treatment with drugs classified as monoamine oxidase inhibitors, such as the antidepressants Nardil and Parnate, nor during the 2 weeks following discontinuation of these drugs.

Special warnings about this medication

Your doctor will do a complete history and evaluation before prescribing this drug. He or she will take into account the severity of the symptoms, as well as your child's age.

This drug should not be given to children under 6 years of age; safety and effectiveness in this age group have not been established.

There is no information regarding the safety and effectiveness of long-term treatment in children. However, suppression of growth has been seen with the long-term use of stimulants, so your doctor will watch your child carefully while he or she is taking this drug.

Blood pressure should be monitored in anyone taking this drug, especially those with high blood pressure.

Some people have had visual disturbances such as blurred vision while being treated with this drug.

The use of this drug by anyone with a seizure disorder is not recommended. Be sure your doctor is aware of any problem in this area. Caution is also advisable for anyone with a history of emotional instability or substance abuse, due to the danger of addiction.

Possible food and drug interactions when taking this medication

If this medication is taken with certain other drugs, the effects of either can be increased, decreased, or altered. It is especially important to check with your doctor before combining this drug with the following:

Antidepressant drugs such as Tofranil, Anafranil, Norpramin, and Effexor
Antiseizure drugs such as phenobarbital, Dilantin, and Mysoline
Blood thinners such as Coumadin
Clonidine (Catapres-TTS)
Drugs that restore blood pressure, such as EpiPen
Guanethidine (Ismelin)
MAO inhibitors (drugs such as the antidepressants Nardil and Parnate)
Phenylbutazone

Special information if you are pregnant or breastfeeding

The effects of this drug during pregnancy have not been adequately studied. If you are pregnant or plan to become pregnant, inform your doctor immediately. It is not known if this drug appears in breast milk. If this medication is essential to your health, your doctor may advise you to discontinue nursing your baby until your treatment with this medication is finished.

Recommended dosage

ADULTS

Ritalin and Methylin Tablets
The average dosage is 20 to 30 milligrams a day, divided into 2 or 3 doses, preferably taken 30 to 45 minutes before meals. Some people may need 40 to 60 milligrams daily, others only 10 to 15 milligrams. Your doctor will determine the best dose.

Ritalin-SR, Methylin ER, and Metadate ER Tablets
These tablets keep working for 8 hours. They may be used in place of Ritalin tablets if they deliver a comparable dose over an 8-hour period.

CHILDREN

This drug should not be given to children under 6 years of age.

Ritalin and Methylin Tablets
The usual starting dose is 5 milligrams taken twice a day, before breakfast and lunch; your doctor will increase the dose by 5 to 10 milligrams a week. Your child should not take more than 60 milligrams in a day. If you do not see any improvement over a period of 1 month, check with your doctor. He or she may wish to discontinue the drug.

Ritalin-SR, Methylin ER, and Metadate ER Tablets
These tablets continue working for 8 hours. Your doctor will decide if they should be used in place of the regular tablets.

Ritalin LA Capsules
The recommended starting dose is 20 milligrams once daily in the morning. At weekly intervals, the doctor may increase the dose by 10 milligrams, up to a maximum of 60 milligrams once a day.

Concerta Tablets
The recommended starting dose is 18 milligrams once daily in the morning. At weekly intervals, your doctor may increase the dose in 18-milligram steps, up to a maximum of 54 milligrams each morning.

Metadate CD Capsules
The recommended starting dose is 20 milligrams once daily before breakfast. If necessary, the doctor may increase the dose in 20-milligram steps to a maximum of 60 milligrams once a day.

Your doctor will periodically discontinue the drug in order to reassess your child's condition. Drug treatment should not, and need not, be indefinite and usually can be discontinued after puberty.

Overdosage

If you suspect an overdose, seek medical attention immediately.

■ *Symptoms of Ritalin overdose may include:*
Agitation, confusion, convulsions (may be followed by coma), delirium, dryness of mucous membranes, enlarging of the pupil of the eye, exaggerated feeling of elation, extremely elevated body temperature, flushing, hallucinations, headache, high blood pressure, irregular or rapid heartbeat, muscle twitching, sweating, tremors, vomiting

Ritonavir See Norvir, page 978.

Rivastigmine See Exelon, page 548.

Rizatriptan See Maxalt, page 812.

ROBAXIN

Pronounced: Ro-BAKS-in
Generic name: Methocarbamol

Why is this drug prescribed?

Robaxin is prescribed, along with rest, physical therapy, and other measures, for the relief of pain due to severe muscular injuries, sprains, and strains.

Most important fact about this drug

Robaxin is not a substitute for the rest or physical therapy needed for proper healing.

Although the drug may temporarily make an injury feel better, do not let that tempt you into pushing your recovery. Lifting or exercising too soon may further damage the muscle.

How should you take this medication?

Take Robaxin exactly as prescribed. Do not take a larger dose or use more often than directed.

■ *If you miss a dose...*
If only an hour or so has passed, take it as soon as you remember. If you do not remember until later, skip the dose and go back to your regular schedule. Do not take 2 doses at once.
■ *Storage instructions...*
Store at room temperature in a tightly closed container.

What side effects may occur?

Side effects cannot be anticipated. If any develop or change in intensity, inform your doctor as soon as possible. Only your doctor can determine if it is safe for you to continue taking Robaxin.

■ *Side effects may include:*

Abnormal taste, allergic reaction, amnesia, blurred vision, confusion, dizziness, double vision, drop in blood pressure and fainting, drowsiness, fever, flushing, headache, hives, indigestion, insomnia, itching, light-headedness, nasal congestion, nausea, pinkeye, poor coordination, rash, seizures, slowed heartbeat, uncontrolled eye movement, vertigo, vomiting, yellow eyes and skin

Why should this drug not be prescribed?

If you are sensitive to or have ever had an allergic reaction to Robaxin or other drugs of this type, you should not take this medication. Make sure your doctor is aware of any drug reactions you have experienced.

Special warnings about this medication

Robaxin can cause drowsiness and dizziness. Do not drive a car or operate potentially dangerous machinery until you know how the drug affects you.

Tell your doctor if you have kidney or liver disease. These conditions may affect Robaxin's effectiveness.

Avoid or be careful using alcoholic beverages.

Robaxin may darken urine to brown, green, or black.

Possible food and drug interactions when taking this medication

If Robaxin is taken with certain other drugs, the effects of either can be increased, decreased, or altered. It is especially important to check with your doctor before combining Robaxin with drugs that slow the nervous system, including:

Alcohol

Drugs for myasthenia gravis, including Mestinon, Prostigmin, and Tensilon

Narcotic pain relievers such as Percocet and Tylenol with Codeine

Sleep aids such as Halcion and Seconal

Tranquilizers such as Valium and Xanax

Special information if you are pregnant or breastfeeding

There have been rare reports of harm to the developing baby following use of Robaxin during pregnancy. Pregnant women should take this drug only if the potential benefits clearly outweigh the possible risks. If you are pregnant or plan to become pregnant, inform your doctor immediately. It is not known if this drug appears in breast milk. If this medication is essential to your health, your doctor may advise you to discontinue breast-feeding your baby until your treatment is finished.

Recommended dosage

ADULTS

Robaxin
The usual starting dose is 3 tablets taken 4 times a day. The usual long-term dose is 2 tablets taken 4 times a day.

Robaxin-750
The usual starting dose is 2 tablets taken 4 times a day. The usual long-term dose is 1 tablet taken every 4 hours or 2 tablets taken 3 times a day.

CHILDREN

The safety and effectiveness of Robaxin have not been established in children.

Overdosage

Any drug taken in excess can have dangerous consequences. If you suspect an overdose of Robaxin, seek emergency medical treatment immediately.

■ *Symptoms of Robaxin overdose may include:*
Blurred vision, coma, drowsiness, low blood pressure, nausea, seizures

ROCALTROL

Pronounced: Ro-CAL-trol
Generic name: Calcitriol

Why is this drug prescribed?

Rocaltrol is a synthetic form of vitamin D used to treat people on dialysis who have hypocalcemia (abnormally low blood calcium levels) and resulting bone damage. Rocaltrol is also prescribed to treat low blood calcium levels in people who have hypoparathyroidism (decreased functioning of the parathyroid glands). When functioning correctly, these glands help control the level of calcium in the blood.

Rocaltrol is also prescribed for *hyper*parathyroidism (*increased* functioning of the parathyroid glands) and resulting bone disorders in people with kidney disease who are not yet on dialysis.

Most important fact about this drug

While you are taking Rocaltrol, your doctor may want you to follow a special diet or take calcium supplements. This is an important part of your therapy. On the other hand, too high a calcium level can be harmful. If you are already taking any medications containing calcium or calcium supplements, make sure you doctor knows about it.

How should you take this medication?
Be sure to get enough fluids and avoid dehydration while taking Rocaltrol.

■ *If you miss a dose...*
If you take 1 dose every other day, and you remember before the next day, take the forgotten dose immediately, then go back to your regular schedule. If you do not remember until the next day, take the dose immediately, skip a day, then go back to your regular schedule.

If you take 1 dose every day, take it as soon as you remember. Then go back to your regular schedule. If you do not remember until the next day, skip the dose you missed and go back to your regular schedule.

If you take Rocaltrol more than once a day, take the forgotten dose as soon as you remember. If it is almost time for your next dose, skip the one you missed and go back to your regular schedule.

Do not take 2 doses at once.

■ *Storage instructions...*
Keep capsules and oral solution away from heat and light.

What side effects may occur?
Side effects cannot be anticipated. If any develop or change in intensity, inform your doctor as soon as possible. Only your doctor can determine if it is safe for you to continue taking Rocaltrol.

■ *Side effects occurring early may include:*
Bone pain, constipation, dry mouth, extreme sleepiness, headache, loss of appetite, metallic taste, muscle pain, nausea, vomiting, weakness

■ *Side effects occurring later may include:*
Abnormal thirst, apathy, arrested growth, decreased sex drive, dehydration, elevated blood cholesterol levels, excessive urination, extremely high body temperature, high blood pressure, inflamed eyes, intolerance to light, irregular heartbeat, itchy skin, kidney problems, loss of appetite, nighttime urination, runny nose, sensory disturbances, urinary tract infections, wasting of muscles or other tissues, weight loss, yellowish skin

Excessive amounts of Vitamin D may cause abnormally high calcium levels in the blood.

Why should this drug not be prescribed?
You should not use Rocaltrol if you have high blood levels of calcium, or if you have vitamin D poisoning. You should also avoid Rocaltrol if it, or any similar drug, has given you an allergic reaction in the past.

Special warnings about this medication

You should not take additional doses of vitamin D while taking Rocaltrol. People who are on dialysis should not take antacids containing magnesium (such as Maalox) while taking Rocaltrol.

Your doctor will monitor your calcium levels while you are taking Rocaltrol because excessive calcium levels can be very dangerous. If this problem develops, your doctor will need to stop Rocaltrol therapy temporarily and prescribe a lower dose when treatment resumes.

While taking Rocaltrol, you should have an adequate daily intake of calcium (at least 600 milligrams a day), either from foods (such as milk and dairy products) or from a calcium supplement. Your doctor will estimate your daily calcium intake before you take this drug to see if you will require more calcium.

Possible food and drug interactions when taking this medication

If Rocaltrol is taken with certain other drugs, the effects of either could be increased, decreased, or altered. It is especially important to check with your doctor before combining Rocaltrol with the following:

Antacids containing magnesium, such as Maalox
Calcium supplements
Cholestyramine (Questran)
Digitalis (Lanoxin)
Ketoconazole (Nizoral)
Phenobarbital
Phenytoin (Dilantin)
Steroid medications such as prednisone
Thiazide water pills such as Dyazide and HydroDIURIL
Vitamin D pills

Special information if you are pregnant or breastfeeding

The effects of Rocaltrol during pregnancy have not been adequately studied. If you are pregnant or plan to become pregnant, inform your doctor immediately. Pregnant women should use Rocaltrol only if the possible benefit outweighs any possible risk to the unborn baby.

Rocaltrol may appear in breast milk. Because it may affect a nursing infant, you should not use Rocaltrol while you are breastfeeding.

Recommended dosage

ADULTS

For People on Dialysis
The suggested beginning dose is 0.25 microgram daily. Your doctor may increase the dose by 0.25 microgram daily at 4- to 8-week intervals if needed. Most people on dialysis require a dose of 0.5 to 1 microgram a day.

People with normal or only slightly low blood calcium levels may find it helpful to take 0.25 microgram every other day.

For Low Calcium Levels Due to Hypoparathyroidism
The suggested beginning dose is 0.25 microgram daily, taken in the morning. Your doctor may increase the dose at 2- to 4-week intervals.

For most adults, regular doses ranging from 0.5 to 2 micrograms daily are effective.

For People Not Yet on Dialysis
The recommended starting dose is 0.25 microgram a day, increased to 0.5 microgram if necessary.

CHILDREN

For Low Calcium Levels Due to Hypoparathyroidism
The starting dose is 0.25 microgram, taken in the morning.

For most children 6 years and older, doses ranging from 0.5 to 2 micrograms per day are effective.

Children from 1 to 5 years old are usually given 0.25 to 0.75 microgram a day. Doses have not been established for hypoparathyroidism in infants under 1 year, or for pseudohypoparathyroidism (a special form of the disorder) in children under 6.

For Children not yet on Dialysis
The recommended starting dose for children 3 years and older is 0.25 microgram a day, increased to 0.5 microgram if necessary.

For children less than 3 years old, the daily starting dose is 10 to 15 nanograms per 2.2 pounds of body weight.

Overdosage
Any medication taken in excess can have serious consequences. Severe overdosage of Rocaltrol may cause serious effects, such as extremely high blood levels of calcium. Warning signs include the symptoms listed under early side effects. If you suspect an overdose, seek medical help immediately.

Rolaids *See Antacids, page 114.*

Ropinirole *See Requip, page 1235.*

Rosiglitazone *See Avandia, page 160.*

Rosiglitazone with Metformin *See Avandamet, page 155.*

Rosuvastatin *See Crestor, page 358.*

ROWASA

Pronounced: ROH-ace-ah
Generic name: Mesalamine
Other brand names: Asacol, Canasa, Pentasa

Why is this drug prescribed?

Rowasa Suspension Enema, Pentasa, and Asacol are used to treat mild to moderate ulcerative colitis (inflammation of the large intestine and rectum). Rowasa Suspension Enema is also prescribed for inflammation of the lower colon, and inflammation of the rectum.

Rowasa Suppositories and Canasa Suppositories are used to treat inflammation of the rectum.

Most important fact about this drug

Mesalamine, the active ingredient in these products, has been known to cause side effects such as:

Bloody diarrhea
Cramping
Fever
Rash
Severe headache
Sudden, severe stomach pain

If you develop any of these symptoms, stop taking this medication and consult your doctor.

How should you use this medication?

To use Rowasa Suspension Enema:
1. Rowasa Suspension Enema comes in boxes of 7 bottles each. After the foil on the box has been unwrapped, all Rowasa Suspension Enemas should be used promptly, following your doctor's instructions. The Suspension Enema is normally off-white to tan in color, but may darken over time once its foil cover is unwrapped. You may still use the enema if it is slightly discolored, but do not use Rowasa Suspension Enema if it is dark brown. If you have any questions about using Rowasa Suspension Enema, contact your doctor.
2. Use Rowasa Suspension Enema at bedtime.
3. Shake the bottle thoroughly.
4. Uncover the applicator tip.
5. You may find it easier to use Rowasa Suspension Enema if you lie down on your left side, extending your left leg and bending your right leg forward for a comfortable balance. An alternative position is on your knees with your hips in the air and your head and shoulders down on the bed.

6. Pointing the applicator tip slightly towards the navel, gently insert the tip into the rectum.
7. Tilt the bottle slightly towards the back, then squeeze it slowly to discharge the contents.
8. Remain in position for at least 30 minutes to allow thorough distribution of the medicine. Retain the enema all night (8 hours) for best results.

To use Rowasa or Canasa Suppositories:
1. Rowasa Suppositories should be used twice a day. Canasa Suppositories can be used 2 or 3 times a day.
2. You should handle the suppositories as little as possible, because they are designed to melt at body temperature.
3. Remove one suppository from the strip of suppositories.
4. While holding the suppository upright, carefully remove the wrapper.
5. Using gentle pressure, insert the suppository (with the pointed end first) completely into the rectum. A small amount of lubricating gel may be used on the tip of the suppository to assist insertion.
6. The suppository should be retained for 1 to 3 hours or longer for best results.

To take Pentasa or Asacol:
Swallow the capsule or tablet whole. Do not break, crush, or chew it before swallowing.

You may notice what looks like small beads in your stool. These are just empty shells that are left after the medication has been absorbed into your body. However, if this continues, check with your doctor.

■ *If you miss a dose...*
Take it as soon as you remember. If it is almost time for your next dose, skip the one you missed and go back to your regular schedule. Never take 2 doses at the same time.

■ *Storage instructions...*
Store these products at room temperature. Keep suppositories away from direct heat, light, and humidity. Do not refrigerate.

What side effects may occur?
Side effects cannot be anticipated. If any side effects develop or change in intensity, tell your doctor immediately. Only your doctor can determine whether it is safe to continue using this medication.

■ *Side effects generally include:*
Diarrhea, dizziness, flu-like symptoms, gas, headache, nausea, stomach pain

■ *Other typical side effects may include:*
Abdominal pain, acne, back pain, belching, bloating, chest pain, chills, constipation, fever, hair loss, hemorrhoids, indigestion, insomnia, itching, joint pain, leg pain, liver disorders, menstrual problems, mus-

cle pain, nasal inflammation, rash, rectal pain or bleeding, sore throat, stomach and intestinal bleeding, sweating, swelling of the arms and legs, tiredness, urinary burning, vomiting, weakness

Why should this drug not be prescribed?

These products should not be used by anyone who is allergic or sensitive to mesalamine or their other ingredients.

Pentasa, Canasa, and Asacol should not be used if you are allergic or sensitive to salicylates (aspirin), foods, preservatives, or dyes.

Special warnings about this medication

Your doctor should check your kidney function while you are taking mesalamine, especially if you have a history of kidney disease or you are using other anti-inflammatory drugs such as Dipentum.

Because older adults tend to have weaker kidneys, mesalamine is more likely to trigger side effects within this age group. The drug also seems more prone to cause blood disorders in older adults. If you are 65 or older, be sure to tell the doctor about any change in your health.

You should use mesalamine cautiously if you are allergic to sulfasalazine (Azulfidine). If you develop a rash or fever, you should stop using the medication and notify your doctor.

Some people using mesalamine have developed flare-ups of their colitis. Inflammation of the pancreas has also been reported.

Rare cases of pericarditis, in which the membrane surrounding the heart becomes inflamed, have been reported with products containing mesalamine. Symptoms may include chest, neck, and shoulder pain, and shortness of breath.

Rowasa Suspension Enema contains a sulfite that may cause allergic reactions in some people. These reactions may include shock and severe, possibly fatal asthma attacks. Most people aren't sensitive to sulfites. However, some people with asthma might be sensitive and should take any medication containing sulfites cautiously.

Rowasa Suspension Enema may stain clothes and fabrics. Canasa Suppositories can also stain surfaces, including marble, granite, plastic, and painted surfaces.

Possible food and drug interactions when taking this medication

If these products are taken with certain other drugs, the effects of either could be increased, decreased, or altered. It is especially important to check with your doctor before combining Rowasa Suspension Enema, Rowasa Suppositories, and Canasa Suppositories with sulfasalazine (Azulfidine).

Special information if you are pregnant or breastfeeding

Pregnant women should use mesalamine only if clearly needed. Mesalamine has been found in breast milk. If this medication is essential to your health, your doctor may advise you to discontinue breastfeeding until your treatment is finished.

Recommended dosage

ADULTS

Rowasa Suspension Enema
The usual dose is 1 rectal enema (60 milliliters) per day, preferably used at bedtime and retained for about 8 hours. Treatment time usually lasts from 3 to 6 weeks, although improvement may be seen within 3 to 21 days.

Suppositories
The usual dose is 1 rectal suppository (500 milligrams) 2 times a day. To get the most benefit from the suppository, it should be retained for 1 to 3 hours or longer. Treatment time usually lasts from 3 to 6 weeks, although improvement may be seen within 3 to 21 days. The dosage of Canasa may be increased to 3 suppositories daily if response is unsatisfactory after 2 weeks of therapy.

Pentasa Capsules
The usual dose is 4 capsules taken 4 times a day for a total of 16 capsules daily.

Asacol Tablets
The recommended dose for the treatment of ulcerative colitis is 2 tablets 3 times a day for 6 weeks.

To prevent a relapse, the usual dosage is 4 tablets a day, taken in 2 or more smaller doses, for 6 months.

CHILDREN

Safety and effectiveness in children have not been established.

Overdosage

There have been no proven reports of serious effects resulting from overdoses of Rowasa or Canasa.

■ *An overdose of Pentasa or Asacol could cause any of the following symptoms:*
Confusion, diarrhea, drowsiness, headache, hyperventilation, ringing in the ears, sweating, vomiting

Any medication taken in excess can have serious consequences. If you suspect an overdose, seek medical attention immediately.

Roxicet *See Percocet, page 1073.*

Rynatan *See Trinalin, page 1502.*

RYTHMOL

Pronounced: RITH-mol
Generic name: Propafenone

Why is this drug prescribed?

Rythmol is used to help correct certain life-threatening heartbeat irregularities (ventricular arrhythmias).

Most important fact about this drug

There is a possibility that Rythmol may cause new heartbeat irregularities or make the existing ones worse. Rythmol is therefore used only for serious problems, and should be accompanied by periodic electrocardiograms (EKGs) prior to and during treatment. Discuss this with your doctor.

How should you take this medication?

Rythmol may be taken with food or on an empty stomach.

Take Rythmol exactly as prescribed. It works best when there is a constant amount of the drug in the blood, so you should take it at evenly spaced intervals.

- *If you miss a dose...*
  Unless otherwise instructed by your doctor, take the forgotten dose as soon as possible. However, if it is almost time for your next dose or more than 4 hours have passed, skip the missed dose and go back to your regular schedule. Never take a double dose.
- *Storage instructions...*
  Keep this medication in the container it came in, tightly closed, away from direct light, at room temperature.

What side effects may occur?

Side effects cannot be anticipated. If any develop or change in intensity, inform your doctor as soon as possible. Only your doctor can determine if it is safe for you to continue taking Rythmol.

The most common side effects affect the digestive, cardiovascular, and nervous systems. The most serious are heartbeat abnormalities.

- *Side effects may include:*
  Constipation, dizziness, heartbeat abnormalities, nausea, unusual taste in the mouth, vomiting

Why should this drug not be prescribed?

Do not take Rythmol if you have ever had an allergic reaction to or are sensitive to it. Your doctor will not prescribe Rythmol if you are suffering from any of the following conditions:

Abnormally slow heartbeat
Certain heartbeat irregularities, such as atrioventricular block or sick
    sinus syndrome, that have not been corrected by a pacemaker
Cardiogenic shock (shock due to a weak heart)
Chronic bronchitis or emphysema
Congestive heart failure that is not well controlled
Mineral (electrolyte) imbalance
Severely low blood pressure

Special warnings about this medication

If you have congestive heart failure, this condition must be brought under
full medical control before you start taking Rythmol.

If you have a pacemaker, the pacemaker's settings must be monitored—
and possibly reprogrammed—while you are taking Rythmol.

There is some risk that Rythmol may interfere with your body's normal
ability to manufacture blood cells. Too few white blood cells may cause
signs and symptoms that mimic infection. If you experience fever, chills,
or sore throat while taking Rythmol—especially during the first 3 months
of treatment—notify your doctor right away.

Rythmol may cause a lupus-like illness characterized by rashes and
arthritic symptoms. If you have been taking Rythmol and testing shows
that your blood contains ANA (antinuclear antibodies), your doctor may
want to discontinue the medication.

Possible food and drug interactions when taking this medication

If Rythmol is taken with certain other drugs, the effects of either could be
increased, decreased, or altered. It is especially important to check with
your doctor before combining Rythmol with the following:

Beta-blockers such as Inderal and Lopressor
Cimetidine (Tagamet)
Cyclosporine (Neoral, Sandimmune)
Digoxin (Lanoxin)
Local anesthetics (such as Novocain used during dental work)
Quinidine (Cardioquin)
Rifampin (Rifadin)
Theophylline (Theo-Dur, Uni-Dur)
Warfarin (blood thinners such as Coumadin)

There may be certain other psychiatric, antidepressant, antifungal, or antibiotic drugs that could possibly cause a reaction if combined with Rythmol. Be sure to tell your doctor if you are taking any of these types of
medications.

Special information if you are pregnant or breastfeeding

If you are pregnant or plan to become pregnant, inform your doctor immediately. Because of a possible risk of birth defects, Rythmol is not rec-

ommended during pregnancy unless the benefit to the mother outweighs the potential risk to the unborn baby.

It is not known whether Rythmol appears in breast milk. You are advised not to take Rythmol if you are breastfeeding a baby. If treatment with Rythmol is essential to your health, your doctor may advise you to stop breastfeeding until your treatment is finished.

Recommended dosage

ADULTS

In most cases, treatment with Rythmol begins in the hospital.

Your doctor will tailor your dosage according to your individual condition and the presence of other disorders.

The usual initial dose of Rythmol is 150 milligrams every 8 hours. Your doctor may increase the dosage depending on how you respond to the initial dosage. The maximum recommended daily dosage of Rythmol is 900 milligrams.

CHILDREN

Safety and effectiveness have not been established in children.

OLDER ADULTS

The doctor will increase the dosage more slowly at the beginning of treatment.

Overdosage

Any medication taken in excess can have serious consequences. If you suspect an overdose of Rythmol, seek medical attention immediately.

■ *Symptoms of Rythmol overdose, which are usually most severe within the first 3 hours of taking the medication, may include:*
Convulsions (rarely), heartbeat irregularities, low blood pressure, sleepiness

Salmeterol *See Serevent, page 1300.*

Salsalate *See Disalcid, page 458.*

SANDIMMUNE

Pronounced: SAN-dim-ewn
Generic name: Cyclosporine
Other brand name: Neoral

Why is this drug prescribed?

Sandimmune is given after organ transplant surgery to help prevent rejection of organs (kidney, heart, or liver) by holding down the body's immune system. It is also used to avoid long-term rejection in people previously treated with other immunosuppressant drugs, such as Imuran.

Neoral is a newer formulation of Sandimmune's active ingredient, cyclosporine. In addition to prevention of organ rejection, it is prescribed for certain severe cases of rheumatoid arthritis and psoriasis.

Some doctors also prescribe Sandimmune to treat alopecia areata (localized areas of hair loss), aplastic anemia (shortage of red and white blood cells and platelets), Crohn's disease (chronic inflammation of the digestive tract), and nephropathy (kidney disease). Sandimmune is sometimes used in the treatment of severe skin disorders, including psoriasis and dermatomyositis (inflammation of the skin and muscles causing weakness and rash). The drug is also used in procedures involving bone marrow, the pancreas, and the lungs.

Sandimmune is always given with prednisone or a similar steroid. It is available in capsules and liquid, or as an injection.

Most important fact about this drug

If you take Sandimmune orally over a period of time, your doctor will monitor your blood levels of cyclosporine to make sure your body is receiving the correct amount of Sandimmune. The reason for this repeated testing is that the absorption of this drug by the body is erratic. Constant monitoring is necessary to prevent toxicity due to overdosing or to prevent possible organ rejection due to underdosing. It is important to note that Sandimmune may need to be taken by mouth for an indefinite period following surgery.

How should you take this medication?

Take the Sandimmune capsule or oral liquid at the same time every day. You may take the medication either with a meal or between meals, but be consistent.

To make Sandimmune oral liquid more palatable, you may mix it with room-temperature milk, chocolate milk, or orange juice. Try to use the same beverage as often as possible. Neoral oral solution may be mixed with room-temperature orange or apple juice. It does not taste good in milk. Use a container made of glass, not plastic. Never let the mixture stand; drink it as soon as you prepare it. To make sure you get your full dose, rinse the glass with a little more liquid and drink that too.

You should maintain good dental hygiene and see your dentist frequently for cleaning to prevent tenderness, bleeding, and gum enlargement.

After you use the dosage syringe to transfer the oral solution to a glass, dry the outside of the syringe with a clean towel and put it away. Do not rinse or wash it. If you do have to clean it, make sure it is thoroughly dry before you use it again.

You may notice an odor when you open the capsule container; this is nothing to worry about and will soon dissipate.

Neoral should start to work on rheumatoid arthritis in 4 to 8 weeks, and on psoriasis in 2 weeks. Psoriasis is usually controlled within 12 to 16 weeks; you should not take the drug for more than a year.

■ *If you miss a dose...*
If fewer than 12 hours have passed, take it as soon as you remember. If it is almost time for the next dose, skip the one you missed and go back to your regular schedule. Do not take 2 doses at once.

■ *Storage instructions...*
Store both the capsules and the oral solution at room temperature. Do not store the liquid in the refrigerator. Keep the liquid from freezing. Sandimmune liquid, once opened, must be used within 2 months.

What side effects may occur?
Side effects cannot be anticipated. If any appear or change in intensity, inform your doctor immediately. Only your doctor can determine if it is safe for you to continue taking Sandimmune. The principal side effects of Sandimmune are high blood pressure, hirsutism (unusual growth of hair), kidney damage, excessive growth of the gums, and tremor.

■ *Other side effects may include:*
Abdominal discomfort, acne, breathing difficulty, convulsions, coughing, cramps, diarrhea, flu-like symptoms, flushing, headache, liver damage, lymph system tumor, muscle, bone, or joint pain, nasal inflammation, nausea, numbness or tingling, sinus inflammation, vomiting, wheezing

Why should this drug not be prescribed?
Do not take these products if you have ever had an allergic reaction to them. Avoid Sandimmune by injection if you have ever had an allergic reaction to an injection of the drug or you are especially sensitive to castor oil.

Avoid taking Neoral for arthritis or psoriasis if you have a kidney condition, high blood pressure, or cancer. While taking the drug, you should avoid most other psoriasis treatment, including ultraviolet light, coal tar, methotrexate, and radiation.

Special warnings about this medication

When your immune system is suppressed by Sandimmune, you are at increased risk of infection and of certain malignancies, including skin cancer and lymph system cancer.

High-dose Sandimmune is toxic to the liver and kidneys and may cause serious kidney damage. Because this toxicity has symptoms similar to those of transplant rejection, you must be monitored closely. If your body is trying hard to reject a transplanted organ, your doctor will probably allow the rejection to occur rather than give you a very high dose of Sandimmune.

This drug can raise blood pressure, especially in older people. If high blood pressure develops while you are taking Neoral for transplant rejection, the doctor will prescribe blood pressure medication. If it develops while you are taking the drug for arthritis or psoriasis, the doctor may lower your dose.

Sandimmune and Neoral are not directly interchangeable. Your doctor may need to adjust the dosage if you switch.

Brain disorders have developed in patients taking this drug, sometimes leading to convulsions, loss of movement, vision problems, impaired consciousness, and psychiatric disturbances. The chance of convulsions is greater if you are taking high doses of steroid drugs, particularly methylprednisolone (Medrol). Brain-related disorders usually clear up once Sandimmune is discontinued.

Use a barrier method of contraception, such as diaphragms or condoms, during Sandimmune therapy. Do not use oral contraceptive pills without your doctor's approval.

Do not try to change dosage forms without consulting your doctor.

If you take Neoral for arthritis or psoriasis, the condition will eventually return when you stop taking the drug, generally within 1 or 2 months. Neoral treatments for psoriasis should be replaced with other types of therapy after 1 year.

Possible food and drug interactions when taking this medication

Avoid getting immunizations while you are taking Sandimmune. The drug may make vaccinations less effective or increase your risk of contracting an illness from a live vaccine.

If taking Neoral for psoriasis, remember to avoid other psoriasis treatments.

Avoid grapefruit and grapefruit juice while taking this drug. Also avoid the antidepressant herb St. John's wort. This over-the-counter herbal remedy reduces the effect of Sandimmune and Neoral, and can lead to organ rejection.

If Sandimmune is taken with certain other drugs, the effects of either could be increased, decreased, or altered. It is especially important to check with your doctor before combining Sandimmune with the following:

Allopurinol (Zyloprim)
Amiodarone (Cordarone)
Amphotericin B (Abelcet, Fungizone)
Atorvastatin (Lipitor)
Bromocriptine (Parlodel)
Calcium-blocking heart and blood pressure medications such as Adalat, Calan, Cardene, Cardizem, and Procardia
Carbamazepine (Tegretol)
Cimetidine (Tagamet)
Clarithromycin (Biaxin)
Colchicine
Danazol (Danocrine)
Diclofenac (Cataflam, Voltaren)
Digoxin (Lanoxicaps, Lanoxin)
Erythromycin (E.E.S., Erythrocin, others)
Fluconazole (Diflucan)
Fluvastatin (Lescol)
Gentamicin (Garamycin)
Indinavir (Crixivan)
Itraconazole (Sporanox)
Ketoconazole (Nizoral)
Lovastatin (Mevacor)
Melphalan (Alkeran)
Methotrexate
Methylprednisolone (Depo-Medrol, Medrol, Solu-Medrol)
Metoclopramide (Reglan)
Nafcillin (Unipen)
Nelfinavir (Viracept)
Nonsteroidal anti-inflammatory drugs such as Clinoril and Naprosyn
Octreotide (Sandostatin)
Orlistat (Xenical)
Phenobarbital
Phenytoin (Dilantin)
Potassium-sparing diuretics (Aldactone, Dyrenium, Midamor)
Pravastatin (Pravachol)
Prednisolone (Delta-Cortef, Prelone)
Quinupristin (Synercid)
Ranitidine (Zantac)
Rifampin (Rifadin, Rifamate, Rimactane)
Ritonavir (Norvir)
Saquinavir (Fortovase)
Simvastatin (Zocor)
Tacrolimus (Prograf)
Ticlopidine (Ticlid)
Tobramycin (Nebcin)

Trimethoprim/sulfamethoxazole (Bactrim, Septra)
Vancomycin (Vancocin)

Special information if you are pregnant or breastfeeding

The effects of Sandimmune in pregnancy have not been adequately studied. If you are pregnant or plan to become pregnant, inform your doctor immediately. Sandimmune should be used during pregnancy only if the benefit justifies the potential risk to the unborn child. Since Sandimmune appears in breast milk, it should not be used during breastfeeding. If you are a new mother, you may need to choose between taking Sandimmune and breastfeeding your baby.

Recommended dosage

ADULTS

Transplant Rejection
Your doctor will tailor your dosage of Sandimmune in accordance with your body's response. Expect a single dose of 15 milligrams per 2.2 pounds of body weight 4 to 12 hours before a transplant and 1 dose daily for 1 to 2 weeks after the operation. After that, the doctor may keep you on a daily dose of 5 to 10 milligrams per 2.2 pounds of body weight.

The dosage of Neoral depends on the type of transplant and the other drugs you are taking. It is always taken twice a day.

Psoriasis or Rheumatoid Arthritis
The starting dosage is 2.5 milligrams of Neoral per 2.2 pounds of body weight divided into 2 doses per day. Your doctor may gradually increase the daily dose to a maximum of 4 milligrams per 2.2 pounds.

CHILDREN

Dosage is generally the same for children as for adults, though somewhat higher doses are sometimes needed. Both drugs have been used to prevent transplant rejection in small children. Neoral has not been tested for arthritis or psoriasis in children under 18.

Overdosage

Although no specific information is available, an overdose of Sandimmune would be expected to cause liver and kidney problems. Any medication taken in excess can have serious consequences. If you suspect an overdose of Sandimmune, seek medical attention immediately.

Saquinavir See Fortovase, page 603.

Sarafem See Prozac, page 1195.

SECTRAL

Pronounced: SEK-tral
Generic name: Acebutolol hydrochloride

Why is this drug prescribed?

Sectral, a type of medication known as a beta-blocker, is used in the treatment of high blood pressure and abnormal heart rhythms. When used to treat high blood pressure, it is effective used alone or in combination with other high blood pressure medications, particularly with a thiazide-type diuretic. Beta-blockers decrease the force and rate of heart contractions, thus reducing pressure within the circulatory system.

Most important fact about this drug

If you have high blood pressure, you must take Sectral regularly for it to be effective. Since blood pressure declines gradually, it may be several weeks before you get the full benefit of Sectral; and you must continue taking it even if you are feeling well. Sectral does not cure high blood pressure; it merely keeps it under control.

How should you take this medication?

Sectral can be taken with or without food. Take it exactly as prescribed, even if your symptoms have disappeared.

Try not to miss any doses. If this medication is not taken regularly, your condition may worsen.

■ *If you miss a dose...*
Take the forgotten dose as soon as you remember. If it's within 4 hours of your next scheduled dose, skip the one you missed and go back to your regular schedule. Never take 2 doses at the same time.

■ *Storage instructions...*
Store at room temperature. Keep the container tightly closed. Protect from light.

What side effects may occur?

Side effects cannot be anticipated. If any develop or change in intensity, inform your doctor as soon as possible. Only your doctor can determine if it is safe for you to continue taking Sectral.

■ *Side effects may include:*
Abnormal vision, chest pain, constipation, cough, decreased sexual ability, depression, diarrhea, dizziness, fatigue, frequent urination, gas, headache, indigestion, joint pain, nasal inflammation, nausea, shortness of breath or difficulty breathing, strange dreams, swelling due to fluid retention, trouble sleeping, weakness

Why should this drug not be prescribed?

If you have heart failure, inadequate blood supply to the circulatory system (cardiogenic shock), heart block (a type of irregular heartbeat), or a severely slow heartbeat, you should not take this medication.

Special warnings about this medication

If you have had severe congestive heart failure in the past, Sectral should be used with caution.

Sectral should not be stopped suddenly. This can cause increased chest pain and heart attack. Dosage should be gradually reduced.

If you suffer from asthma, seasonal allergies, other bronchial conditions, coronary artery disease, or kidney or liver disease, this medication should be used with caution.

Ask your doctor if you should check your pulse while taking Sectral. This medication can cause your heartbeat to become too slow.

This medication may mask the symptoms of low blood sugar or alter blood sugar levels. If you are diabetic, discuss this with your doctor.

Notify your doctor or dentist that you are taking Sectral if you have a medical emergency, or before you have any surgery.

Tell your doctor if you are taking over-the-counter cold medications and nasal drops. They may interact with Sectral.

If you experience difficulty breathing, or develop hives or large areas of swelling, seek medical attention immediately. You may be having a serious allergic reaction to the medicine. Sectral can also make other severe allergies worse.

Possible food and drug interactions when taking this medication

If Sectral is taken with certain other drugs, the effects of either could be increased, decreased, or altered. It is especially important to check with your doctor before combining Sectral with the following:

Albuterol (the airway-opening drug Ventolin)
Certain blood pressure medicines such as reserpine (Diupres)
Certain over-the-counter cold remedies and nasal drops such as
    Afrin, Neo-Synephrine, and Sudafed
Nonsteroidal anti-inflammatory drugs such as Motrin and Voltaren
Oral diabetes drugs such as Micronase

Special information if you are pregnant or breastfeeding

The effects of Sectral during pregnancy have not been adequately studied. If you are pregnant or plan to become pregnant, inform your doctor immediately. Sectral appears in breast milk and could affect a nursing infant. If this medication is essential to your health, your doctor may advise you to discontinue breastfeeding until your treatment with Sectral is finished.

Recommended dosage

ADULTS

Hypertension

The usual initial dose for mild to moderate high blood pressure is 400 milligrams per day. It may be taken in a single daily dose or in 2 doses of 200 milligrams each. The usual daily dosage ranges from 200 to 800 milligrams.

People with severe high blood pressure may take up to 1,200 milligrams per day divided into 2 doses. Sectral may be taken alone or in combination with another high blood pressure medication.

Irregular heartbeat

The usual starting dosage is 400 milligrams per day divided into 2 doses. Your doctor may gradually increase the dose to 600 to 1,200 milligrams per day. If your doctor wants you to stop taking this medication, he or she will have you taper off over a period of 2 weeks.

CHILDREN

The safety and effectiveness of Sectral have not been established in children.

OLDER ADULTS

Your doctor will determine the dosage based on your particular needs. Do not take more than 800 milligrams per day.

Overdosage

Any medication taken in excess can have serious consequences. If you suspect an overdose, seek medical attention immediately.

■ *There is no specific information available on Sectral; however, overdose symptoms seen with other beta-blockers include:*
Difficulty breathing, extremely slow heartbeat, irregular heartbeat, low blood pressure, low blood sugar, seizures, severe congestive heart failure

Selegiline *See Eldepryl, page 502.*

SEMPREX-D

Pronounced: SEM-precks-D
Generic ingredients: Acrivastine, Pseudoephedrine hydrochloride

Why is this drug prescribed?

Semprex-D is an antihistamine and decongestant drug that relieves sneezing, running nose, itching, watery eyes, and stuffy nose caused by seasonal allergies such as hay fever.

Most important fact about this drug

Semprex-D may cause drowsiness. Do not drive or operate dangerous machinery or participate in any hazardous activity that requires full mental alertness until you know how you react to this medication.

How should you take this medication?

Take Semprex-D exactly as prescribed by your doctor. Do not take more of this drug or use it more often than your doctor recommends.

■ *If you miss a dose...*
   Take it as soon as you remember. If it is almost time for your next dose, skip the one you missed and go back to your regular schedule. Never take 2 doses at the same time.
■ *Storage instructions...*
   Store at room temperature in a dry place; protect the drug from light.

What side effects may occur?

Side effects cannot be anticipated. If any develop or change in intensity, inform your doctor as soon as possible. Only your doctor can determine if it is safe for you to continue taking Semprex-D.

■ *Side effects may include:*
   Cough, dizziness, drowsiness, dry mouth, headache, indigestion, menstrual problems, nausea, nervousness, skin eruptions, sleeplessness, sore throat, weakness, wheezing

Severe allergic reactions are rare. There have been isolated reports of swelling of the throat, lips, neck, face, hands, or feet. Pseudoephedrine, one of the ingredients of this drug, has also been known to cause rapid or fluttery heartbeat.

Why should this drug not be prescribed?

You should not take Semprex-D if you are sensitive to or have ever had an allergic reaction to acrivastine, pseudoephedrine, or similar drugs such as Actifed, Dimetane, Trinalin, or Seldane-D. Make sure your doctor is aware of any drug reactions you have experienced.

Avoid using Semprex-D if you have extremely high blood pressure or severe heart problems.

Do not take this drug within 14 days of taking any drug known as an MAO inhibitor, including the antidepressants Nardil and Parnate.

Special warnings about this medication

Use this drug with caution if you have high blood pressure, diabetes, heart problems, peptic ulcer or other stomach problems, or an enlarged prostate gland. Use Semprex-D with care, too, if you have increased eye pressure, an overactive thyroid gland, or kidney disease. Make sure the doctor has taken these conditions into account.

Antihistamines are more likely to cause dizziness, extreme calm (sedation), bladder obstruction, and low blood pressure in the elderly (over age 60). The elderly are also more likely to have more side effects from the decongestant (pseudoephedrine) in Semprex-D.

Possible food and drug interactions when taking this medication

If Semprex-D is taken with certain other drugs, the effects of either could be increased, decreased, or altered. It is especially important to check with your doctor before combining this drug with the following:

Alcoholic beverages
Blood pressure medications such as Inderal and Lopressor
MAO inhibitors, including the antidepressants Nardil and Parnate
Other antihistamines such as Actifed, Seldane-D, and Entex
Other decongestants such as Quibron and Rynatan

Special information if you are pregnant or breastfeeding

The effects of Semprex-D during pregnancy have not been adequately studied. If you are pregnant or plan to become pregnant, tell your doctor immediately.

It is not known whether acrivastine appears in breast milk, but pseudoephedrine does. If the drug is essential to your health, your doctor may tell you to stop nursing until your treatment is finished.

Recommended dosage

ADULTS

The usual dose for adults and children 12 years of age and older is 1 capsule, taken by mouth, every 4 to 6 hours, 4 times a day.

CHILDREN

The safety and effectiveness of Semprex-D in children less than 12 years old have not been established.

Overdosage

Although there have been few reports of overdosage with Semprex-D, overdosage with similar drugs has caused a variety of serious symptoms. If you suspect an overdose of Semprex-D, seek medical attention immediately.

■ *Symptoms of overdose may include:*
Anxiety, convulsions, difficulty breathing, drowsiness, fear, hallucinations, heart failure with low blood pressure, irregular heartbeat, loss of consciousness, painful urination, paleness, restlessness, sleeplessness, tenseness, trembling, weakness

Septra *See Bactrim, page 188.*

Serax *See Omeprazole, page 996.*

SERENTIL

Pronounced: seh-REN-til
Generic name: Mesoridazine besylate

Why is this drug prescribed?

Serentil is prescribed to treat schizophrenia, the crippling psychological disorder that causes its victims to lose touch with reality, often triggering hallucinations, delusions, and disorganized thought. Because of its dangerous side effects, this medication is recommended only after at least two other drugs have failed to provide relief.

Most important fact about this drug

Serentil may cause dangerous and even fatal cardiac irregularities by prolonging a part of the heartbeat known as the QT interval. The likelihood of such irregularities increases when Serentil is combined with other medications known to prolong the QT interval, such as the heart medications Cordarone, Inderal, Quinaglute, Quinidex, and Rythmol. Never combine these drugs with Serentil, and check with your doctor before taking any other new medications.

Symptoms of a possible heart irregularity include palpitations, dizziness, and fainting. Call your doctor immediately if you experience any of these symptoms.

How should you take this medication?

Take Serentil exactly as directed by your doctor. If you are taking Serentil in a liquid concentrate form, you can dilute it with distilled water, orange juice, or grape juice just before swallowing it.

If Serentil is given by injection, you should remain lying down for at least one-half hour after the injection.

■ *If you miss a dose...*
Take it as soon as you remember. If it is almost time for your next dose, skip the one you missed and go back to your regular schedule. Do not take 2 doses at once.

■ *Storage instructions...*
Store at room temperature in a tightly closed container. Protect from light.

What side effects may occur?
Side effects cannot be anticipated. If any develop or change in intensity, inform your doctor as soon as possible. Only your doctor can determine if it is safe to continue taking Serentil. Side effects generally occur when high doses are given early in treatment.

■ *Side effects may include:*
Blurred vision, drowsiness, dry mouth, impotence, incontinence, low blood pressure, muscle rigidity, nausea, rash, slowed heartbeat, tremor, vomiting

Why should this drug not be prescribed?
You should not take Serentil if you have a history of heartbeat irregularities, or you are taking other medications that may cause an irregular heartbeat (see *Most important fact about this drug*). Serentil should not be combined with other substances that slow the nervous system, such as alcohol, barbiturates (sleep aids), and narcotics (painkillers), nor should it be given to anyone in a comatose state. People who have shown a hypersensitivity to Serentil cannot take this drug.

Special warnings about this medication
Before using Serentil, tell your doctor if you have a history of heart problems. The doctor will perform tests to check the health of your heart before prescribing this medication.

Serentil can cause tardive dyskinesia, a condition marked by involuntary muscle spasms and twitches in the face and body, including chewing movements, puckering, puffing the cheeks, and sticking out the tongue. This condition may be permanent and appears to be most common among older adults, especially older women. Ask your doctor for more information about this possible risk.

Drugs such as Serentil can cause a potentially fatal condition called Neuroleptic Malignant Syndrome (NMS). Symptoms include high fever, rigid muscles, irregular pulse or blood pressure, rapid heartbeat, excessive perspiration, and changes in heart rhythm. If you have these symptoms, contact your doctor immediately. Serentil therapy should be discontinued.

This type of drug can cause vision problems. Tell your doctor if you have a change in your vision while taking this medication.

Serentil may impair your ability to drive a car or operate machinery. Do not participate in any activities that require full alertness until you are sure of your reaction to this drug.

Serentil should be used with caution if you have ever had breast cancer. The drug stimulates production of a hormone that promotes the growth of certain types of tumors.

Serentil may cause a condition called agranulocytosis, a dangerous drop in the number of certain kinds of white blood cells. Symptoms include fever, lethargy, sore throat, and weakness.

Possible food and drug interactions when taking this medication

Remember that Serentil must never be combined with alcohol, barbiturates, or narcotics. It's also best to avoid combining it with other drugs prescribed for schizophrenia, depression, or anxiety, or with the spasm-quelling drug atropine (Donnatal). Be careful, too, to avoid exposure to phosphorus insecticides.

Special information if you are pregnant or breastfeeding

The effects of Serentil during pregnancy have not been adequately studied. If you are pregnant or plan to become pregnant, tell your doctor immediately. Pregnant women should use Serentil only if clearly needed.

It is not known whether Serentil appears in breast milk. Check with your doctor before deciding to breastfeed.

Recommended dosage

Your doctor will tailor the dose of Serentil to your needs. Once your symptoms improve, the doctor will gradually reduce the dosage to the lowest effective dose.

ADULTS

Tablets and Oral Solution
The usual starting dose of Serentil tablets or oral solution is 50 milligrams taken 3 times daily. Over the long term, the usual daily dose ranges from 100 to 400 milligrams per day.

CHILDREN

The safety and effectiveness of Serentil in children have not been established.

Overdosage

An overdose of Serentil can be fatal. If you suspect an overdose, seek medical attention immediately.

■ *Symptoms of Serentil overdose include:*
Absence of reflexes, agitation, blurred vision, coma, confusion, convulsions, difficulty breathing, disorientation, drowsiness, dry mouth, enlarged pupils, heartbeat irregularities, heart failure or arrest, high

temperature, nasal congestion, overactive reflexes, rigid muscles, stupor, swollen throat, throat spasms, vomiting

SEREVENT
Pronounced: SER-ah-vent
Generic name: Salmeterol xinafoate
Other brand name: Serevent Diskus

Why is this drug prescribed?
Serevent relaxes the muscles in the walls of the bronchial tubes, allowing the passageways to expand and carry more air. Taken regularly (twice a day), the drug is used in the treatment of asthma and chronic obstructive pulmonary disease (COPD), including emphysema and chronic bronchitis. A relatively long-acting medication, it is recommended only for the type of asthma patient who needs shorter-acting bronchodilators such as Alupent and Ventolin on a frequent, regular basis.

Serevent is available in an aerosol inhaler and as Serevent Diskus inhalation powder. Both forms of Serevent can be used with or without inhaled or oral steroid therapy.

Most important fact about this drug
Serevent is intended only for long-term prevention of symptoms, and should not be used more than twice a day. Do not use it to treat acute asthma attacks, and do not attempt to relieve worsening asthma by increasing the frequency of your doses. (Your doctor will prescribe a short-acting bronchodilator to relieve acute attacks.)

Seriously worsening asthma is a dangerous—even life-threatening—condition that needs immediate medical attention. Alert your doctor if your short-acting bronchodilator is becoming less effective or you need more inhalations than usual. Also consider it a warning sign if you need 4 or more inhalations daily for 2 days or more in a row, or find that you are finishing a 200-dose canister in less than 8 weeks.

How should you take this medication?
Use no more than the prescribed dose and follow package directions closely. Space your 2 daily doses approximately 12 hours apart, in the morning and evening. To be effective, the drug must be used regularly every day.

Serevent aerosol inhaler must be shaken thoroughly before each use. Test-spray the inhaler 4 times before the first use and whenever 4 weeks have passed since the last use. Avoid spraying in the eyes.

Serevent Diskus should never be used with a spacer. Always activate the Diskus device in a level, horizontal position. Never exhale into the Diskus device, and always keep it dry. Do not wash the mouthpiece or any other part of the device. Never attempt to take the Diskus apart.

You may be able to taste or feel the medication delivered by the Diskus. However, whether you can sense the delivery of a dose or not, never take more inhalations than what your doctor prescribes.

■ *If you miss a dose...*
Take it as soon as you remember. If it is almost time for your next dose, skip the one you missed and go back to your regular schedule. Never double your dose.

■ *Storage instructions...*
Store the Serevent aerosol inhaler and Serevent Diskus at room temperature, away from direct sunlight and freezing temperatures. Leave the aerosol inhaler canister with the nozzle end down. Keep the Diskus in a dry place. Throw away the Diskus inhalation device after every blister has been used (when the dose indicator reads "0") or 6 weeks after the blisters have been removed from their foil pouch.

What side effects may occur?

Side effects cannot be anticipated. If any develop or change in intensity, inform your doctor as soon as possible. Only your doctor can determine if it is safe for you to continue using Serevent.

■ *Side effects may include:*
Asthma, back pain, bronchitis, chest congestion, cough, diarrhea, dizziness, headache, nasal inflammation, pallor, respiratory tract infection, sinus headache, sinus infection, sinus problems, sore throat, stomachache, tremor

Why should this drug not be prescribed?

If Serevent gives you an allergic reaction, you cannot continue using it.

Special warnings about this medication

Serevent is not for the treatment of seriously worsening asthma, and should not be started if your asthma is deteriorating.

If you are taking inhaled or oral steroid medications for your asthma, continue using them along with Serevent. This drug does not replace them.

A safety study found that one of the ingredients in Serevent, salmeterol, may be associated with rare cases of serious asthma attacks or asthma-related death. If you're concerned, talk with the doctor about your options. Do not, however, stop using Serevent without first consulting your doctor.

Very rarely, Serevent has triggered allergic reactions in people with severe milk allergy. If you develop an allergic reaction (throat irritation, choking, hives, face and throat swelling, rash, and wheezing) after using Serevent, call your doctor immediately. Likewise, if symptoms of asthma or chronic lung disease get worse after inhaling Serevent, stop using it, take a short-acting bronchodilator, and check with your doctor at once.

Although such effects are rare, Serevent can cause an increase in blood pressure and heart rate. Use this medication carefully if you have high blood pressure, heart disease, or an irregular heartbeat. Caution is also advised if you have a seizure disorder or an overactive thyroid.

Serevent aerosol inhaler can be given to children 12 years of age and older. The Diskus inhalation powder can be given to children 4 and older.

Do not stop Serevent therapy without a doctor's guidance. Your symptoms could worsen without the medication.

Possible food and drug interactions when taking this medication
If Serevent is taken with certain other drugs, the effects of either drug could be increased, decreased, or altered. It is especially important to check with your doctor before combining Serevent with the following:

Airway-opening medications such as Alupent, Proventil, and Ventolin
Blood pressure medications known as beta-blockers, including
    Inderal, Lopressor, and Tenormin
MAO inhibitors such as the antidepressants Marplan, Nardil, and
    Parnate
Tricyclic antidepressants such as Elavil and Tofranil
Water pills (diuretics) such as furosemide (Lasix) and
    hydrochlorothiazide (HydroDIURIL)

Special information if you are pregnant or breastfeeding
Serevent has not been adequately tested in pregnant women and is recommended only if its benefits clearly outweigh potential risks. Check with your doctor immediately if you are pregnant or are planning a pregnancy. Serevent's effects during breastfeeding are also unknown. You and your doctor should decide whether to discontinue nursing or give up Serevent.

Recommended dosage

SEREVENT AEROSOL INHALER

Asthma and Chronic Pulmonary Disease
The usual dose is 2 inhalations (42 micrograms) twice a day (morning and evening) 12 hours apart.

Prevention of Exercise-induced Asthma
Take 2 inhalations at least 30 to 60 minutes before exercise. Do not take another dose for 12 hours. (If you are on a twice-daily dosage schedule, do **not** take additional Serevent before exercise.)

SEREVENT DISKUS INHALATION POWDER

Asthma and Chronic Pulmonary Disease
The usual dose is 1 inhalation (50 micrograms) twice a day (morning and evening).

Prevention of Exercise-induced Asthma
Take 1 inhalation at least 30 minutes before exercise. Do not take another dose for 12 hours. (If you are on a twice-daily dosage schedule, do *not* take additional Serevent before exercise.)

Overdosage
Any medication taken in excess can have serious consequences. If you suspect an overdose, seek medical attention immediately.

■ *Symptoms of Serevent overdose may include:*
Angina (chest pain), dizziness, dry mouth, fatigue, flu-like symptoms, headache, heart irregularities, high blood sugar, high or low blood pressure, insomnia, muscle cramps, nausea, nervousness, rapid heartbeat, seizures, tremor

Serophene *See Clomiphene Citrate, page 307.*

SEROQUEL
Pronounced: SER-oh-kwell
Generic name: Quetiapine fumarate

Why is this drug prescribed?
Seroquel is prescribed for the treatment of schizophrenia, a mental disorder marked by delusions (false beliefs), hallucinations, disrupted thinking, and loss of contact with reality. It is also used for the short-term treatment of mania associated with bipolar disorder.

Seroquel is the first in a new class of antipsychotic medications. Researchers believe that it works by diminishing the action of dopamine and serotonin, two of the brain's chief chemical messengers.

Most important fact about this drug
Seroquel may cause tardive dyskinesia, a condition characterized by uncontrollable muscle spasms and twitches in the face and body. This problem can be permanent, and appears to be most common among older adults, especially women.

How should you take this medication?
Your doctor will increase your dose gradually until the drug takes effect. If you stop Seroquel for more than 1 week, you'll need to build up to your ideal dosage once again.

■ *If you miss a dose...*
Take it as soon as you remember. If it is almost time for the next dose, skip the one you missed and go back to your regular schedule. Do not take 2 doses at once.

■ *Storage instructions...*
Store at room temperature.

What side effects may occur?

Side effects cannot be anticipated. If any develop or change in intensity, inform your doctor as soon as possible. Only your doctor can determine if it is safe for you to continue taking Seroquel.

■ *Side effects may include:*
Abdominal pain, constipation, diminished movement, dizziness, drowsiness, dry mouth, excessive muscle tone, headache, indigestion, low blood pressure (especially upon standing), nasal inflammation, neck rigidity, rapid or irregular heartbeat, rash, sleepiness, tremor, uncontrollable movements, weakness

Why should this drug not be prescribed?

If Seroquel gives you an allergic reaction, you will not be able to use this drug.

Special warnings about this medication

Call your doctor immediately if you develop muscle stiffness, confusion, irregular or rapid heartbeat, excessive sweating, and high fever. These are signs of Neuroleptic Malignant Syndrome (NMS), a serious—and potentially fatal—reaction to the drug. Be especially wary if you have a history of heart attack, heart disease, heart failure, circulation problems, or irregular heartbeat.

Particularly during the first few days of therapy, Seroquel can cause low blood pressure, with accompanying dizziness, fainting, and rapid heartbeat. To minimize these effects, your doctor will increase your dose gradually. If you are prone to low blood pressure, take blood pressure medication, or become dehydrated, use Seroquel with caution.

Seroquel also tends to cause drowsiness, especially at the start of therapy, and can impair your judgment, thinking, and motor skills. Until you are certain of the drug's effect, use caution when operating machinery or driving a car.

Certain antipsychotic drugs, including Seroquel, are associated with an increased risk of developing high blood sugar, which on rare occasions has led to coma or death. See your doctor right away if you develop signs of high blood sugar, including dry mouth, unusual thirst, increased urination, and tiredness. If you have diabetes or have a high risk of developing it, see your doctor regularly for blood sugar testing.

People at high risk of suicide attempts should be prescribed the lowest dose possible to reduce the risk of intentional overdose.

Seroquel should be used cautiously in older people and those with Alzheimer's disease. Antipsychotic drug treatment has been associated with swallowing and breathing problems in these patients.

Animal studies suggest that Seroquel may increase the risk of breast cancer, although human studies have not confirmed such a risk. If you have a history of breast cancer, see your doctor regularly for checkups.

If you are having problems with your vision, tell your doctor. There is a chance that Seroquel may cause cataracts, and you may be asked to see an eye doctor when you start Seroquel therapy, and every 6 months thereafter.

Seroquel poses a very slight risk of seizures, especially if you are over 65, or have epilepsy or Alzheimer's disease. The drug can also suppress an underactive thyroid, and generally causes a minor increase in cholesterol levels. There is also a remote chance that it will trigger a prolonged and painful erection.

Other antipsychotic medications have been known to interfere with the body's temperature-regulating mechanism, causing patients to overheat. Although this problem has not occurred with Seroquel, caution is still advisable. Avoid exposure to extreme heat, strenuous exercise, and dehydration.

Seroquel is prescribed for the short-term treatment of rapid-onset bipolar mania; it is not approved for preventing future episodes. The effectiveness of the drug for treating mania for more than 3 weeks has not been studied.

The safety and effectiveness of Seroquel have not been studied in children.

Possible food and drug interactions when taking this medication

Seroquel increases the effects of alcohol. Avoid alcoholic beverages while on Seroquel therapy.

If Seroquel is taken with certain other drugs, the effects of either could be increased, decreased, or altered. It is especially important to check with your doctor before combining Seroquel with the following:

Barbiturates such as phenobarbital
Carbamazepine (Tegretol)
Cimetidine (Tagamet)
Erythromycin (Eryc, Ery-Tab)
Fluconazole (Diflucan)
Itraconazole (Sporanox)
Ketoconazole (Nizoral)
Levodopa (Laradopa, Sinemet)
Lorazepam (Ativan)
Phenytoin (Dilantin)
Rifampin (Rifadin, Rifamate, Rimactane)
Steroid medications such as hydrocortisone and prednisone
Thioridazine (Mellaril)

Special information if you are pregnant or breastfeeding

The possibility of harm to a developing baby has not been ruled out. You should take Seroquel during pregnancy only if the benefits outweigh this potential risk. Notify your doctor as soon as you become pregnant or decide to become pregnant.

It is not known whether Seroquel appears in breast milk, and breast-feeding is not recommended.

Recommended dosage

SCHIZOPHRENIA

Adults

The usual dosage range is 300 to 400 milligrams a day, divided into 2 or 3 smaller doses. Doses as low as 150 milligrams a day sometimes prove effective, and the dose rarely exceeds 750 milligrams per day. Doses above 800 milligrams per day have not been tested for safety. The dose is gradually increased over 4 days until the most effective dose is reached, using the following schedule: *Day 1:* Take 25 milligrams twice a day. *Days 2, 3, and 4:* The doctor will increase each daily dose by 25 to 50 milligrams, taken either 2 or 3 times a day. *Day 5 and up:* If needed, the doctor may increase each dose by 25 to 50 milligrams every 2 or more days.

BIPOLAR MANIA (SHORT-TERM TREATMENT OF ACUTE EPISODES)

Adults

The usual dosage range is 400 to 800 milligrams a day. Doses above 800 milligrams a day have not been tested for safety. The dosage will be gradually increased over 4 to 6 days until the most effective dose is reached, using the following schedule: *Day 1:* Take 50 milligrams twice a day. *Day 2:* The doctor will increase the dose to 100 milligrams twice a day. *Day 3:* The doctor will increase the dose to 150 milligrams twice a day. *Day 4:* The doctor will increase the dose to 200 milligrams twice a day. *Days 5 and 6:* If needed, the doctor may increase each dose by no more than 200-milligram increments to a total daily dose of 800 milligrams.

DOSAGE ADJUSTMENT

If you have liver problems, you may be started at 25 milligrams a day. The doctor will increase the dose as needed in increments of 25 to 50 milligrams a day based on your body's response.

The dosage may also need to be lowered if you are weak, elderly, or prone to low blood pressure reactions. You may also need your dose adjusted if you're taking certain drugs, including Dilantin, Tegretol, and phenobarbital.

Overdosage

Any medication taken in excess can have serious consequences. If you suspect an overdose, seek medical help immediately.

■ *Symptoms of Seroquel overdose may include:*
Dizziness, drowsiness, fainting, rapid heartbeat

Sertraline *See Zoloft, page 1646.*

Sibutramine *See Meridia, page 824.*

Sildenafil *See Viagra, page 1554.*

SILVADENE CREAM 1%

Pronounced: SIL-vuh-deen
Generic name: Silver sulfadiazine

Why is this drug prescribed?

Silvadene Cream 1% is applied directly to the skin. The cream is used along with other medications to prevent and treat wound infections in people with second- and third-degree burns. It is effective against a variety of bacteria as well as yeast.

Most important fact about this drug

Silvadene is a sulfa derivative. If burn wounds cover extensive areas of the body, Silvadene may be absorbed into the bloodstream, and if you have ever had an allergic reaction to sulfa drugs, such as Bactrim or Septra, this could lead to a similar reaction. Make sure your doctor is aware of any drug reactions you have experienced.

How should you use this medication?

Silvadene cream is for external use only.

Bathe the burned area daily.

You should continue using Silvadene Cream until the area has healed or is ready for skin grafting.

Clean your skin and apply Silvadene with a sterile, gloved hand. Apply a thin layer (about one-sixteenth of an inch) to the affected area.

■ *If you miss a dose…*
Keep the burn areas covered with Silvadene at all times. Reapply the medicine if it is rubbed or washed off.

■ *Storage instructions…*
Silvadene can be stored at room temperature.

What side effects may occur?

Side effects cannot be anticipated. If any side effects develop or change in intensity, tell your doctor immediately. Only your doctor can determine whether it is safe for you to continue using Silvadene.

■ *Side effects may include:*
Areas of dead skin, burning sensation, red and raised rash on the body, skin discoloration

Why should this drug not be prescribed?
You should not use Silvadene if you are allergic to sulfa drugs such as Bactrim or Septra.

Do not use Silvadene at the end of pregnancy, on premature infants, or on newborn infants during the first 2 months of life.

Special warnings about this medication
Make sure your doctor knows about any kidney or liver problems you may have. If either organ becomes impaired, it may be necessary to stop using Silvadene.

There is a small chance of fungal infection when using Silvadene.

Possible food and drug interactions when using this medication
If Silvadene is used with certain other drugs, the effects of either could be increased, decreased, or altered. It is especially important to check with your doctor before combining Silvadene with the following:

Topical enzyme preparations such as Panafil and Santyl, that contain collagenase, papain, or sutilains

Special information if you are pregnant or breastfeeding
If you are pregnant or plan to become pregnant, inform your doctor immediately.

The safety of Silvadene during pregnancy has not been fully studied, but you definitely should not take this drug at the end of your pregnancy, as it can lead to complications for the baby.

Although it is not known whether Silvadene appears in breast milk, other sulfa drugs are excreted in breast milk and can cause harm to a nursing infant. If this medication is essential to your health, your doctor may advise you to stop breastfeeding until your treatment is finished.

Recommended dosage
Apply Silvadene Cream 1% to the affected area once or twice daily to a thickness of one-sixteenth of an inch. Treatment with Silvadene should be continued until your doctor is satisfied that healing has occurred or determines that the burn site is ready for grafting.

Overdosage
Any medication taken in excess can have serious consequences. If you suspect an overdose, seek medical treatment immediately.

Silver sulfadiazine *See Silvadene Cream 1%, page 1307.*

Simvastatin See Zocor, page 1638.

SINEMET CR

Pronounced: SIN-uh-met see-are
Generic ingredients: Carbidopa, Levodopa

Why is this drug prescribed?

Sinemet CR is a controlled-release tablet that may be given to help relieve the muscle stiffness, tremor, and weakness caused by Parkinson's disease. It may also be given to relieve Parkinson's-like symptoms caused by encephalitis (brain fever), carbon monoxide poisoning, or manganese poisoning.

Sinemet CR contains two drugs, carbidopa and levodopa. The drug that actually produces the anti-Parkinson's effect is levodopa. Carbidopa prevents vitamin B_6 from destroying levodopa, thus allowing levodopa to work more efficiently.

Parkinson's drugs such as Sinemet CR relieve the symptoms of the disease, but are not a permanent cure.

Most important fact about this drug

There is also a regular, non-controlled-release form of this medication, which is called Sinemet. Over a period of hours, Sinemet CR, the controlled-release form, gives a smoother release of the drug than regular Sinemet. If you have been taking regular Sinemet, be aware that you may need a somewhat higher dosage of Sinemet CR to get the same degree of relief. Your first morning dose of Sinemet CR may take as much as an hour longer to start working than your first morning dose of regular Sinemet.

How should you take this medication?

Take Sinemet CR after meals, rather than before or between meals. Swallow the tablets whole without chewing or crushing them.

Sinemet CR releases its ingredients slowly over a period of 4 to 6 hours. It is important to follow a careful schedule, taking your doses at the same time every day.

You should not change the prescribed dosage or add another product for Parkinson's disease without first consulting your doctor.

Sinemet CR works best when there is a constant amount in the blood. Try not to miss any doses, and take them at evenly spaced intervals day and night.

■ *If you miss a dose...*
If you forget to take a dose, take it as soon as you remember. If it is almost time for your next dose, skip the one you missed and go back to your regular schedule. Do not take 2 doses at once.

■ *Storage instructions…*
Store at room temperature in a tightly closed container.

What side effects may occur?
Side effects from Sinemet CR cannot be anticipated. If any develop or change in intensity, inform your doctor immediately.

Only your doctor can determine if it is safe for you to continue taking Sinemet CR.

■ *Side effects may include:*
Confusion, hallucinations, nausea, uncontrollable twitching or jerking

Why should this drug not be prescribed?
Do not take Sinemet CR if you are sensitive to or have ever had an allergic reaction to its ingredients.

Sinemet CR should not be prescribed if you have a suspicious, undiagnosed mole or a history of melanoma.

Special warnings about this medication
Make sure your doctor knows if you have any of the following:

Bronchial asthma
Cardiovascular or lung disease (severe)
Endocrine (glandular) disorder
History of active peptic ulcer
History of heart attack or heartbeat irregularity
Kidney disorder
Liver disorder
Wide-angle glaucoma (pressure in the eye)

Your doctor will monitor your liver, blood, kidney, and heart functions during extended therapy with Sinemet CR.

If you have been taking levodopa alone, you should stop taking levodopa for at least 12 hours before starting to take Sinemet CR.

The carbidopa contained in Sinemet CR cannot eliminate side effects caused by levodopa. Since carbidopa helps levodopa reach your brain, Sinemet CR may, in fact, produce some levodopa side effects—particularly twitching, jerking, or writhing—sooner and at a lower dosage than levodopa alone or even regular Sinemet. If such involuntary movements develop while you are taking Sinemet CR, you may need a dosage reduction.

Like levodopa, Sinemet CR may cause depression. Make sure your doctor knows if you have mental or emotional problems.

Muscle rigidity, high temperature, rapid heartbeat or breathing, sweating, blood pressure changes, and mental changes may occur when Sinemet CR is reduced suddenly or discontinued. If you stop taking this medication abruptly, your doctor should monitor your condition carefully.

You may see a red, brown, or black coloration in your saliva, urine, or sweat. This is not harmful, but may stain your clothes. Too much stomach acid can interfere with absorption of the medication.

Possible food and drug interactions when taking this medication

If Sinemet CR is taken with certain other drugs, the effects of either could be increased, decreased, or altered. It is especially important to check with your doctor before combining Sinemet CR with the following:

Antacids such as Di-Gel, Maalox, and Mylanta
Antihypertensives such as Aldomet and Clonidine
Antiseizure drugs such as Dilantin
Antispasmodic drugs such as Artane and Cogentin
High-protein foods
Isoniazid (Nydrazid)
Major tranquilizers such as Haldol, Mellaril, Risperdal, and Thorazine
MAO inhibitors such as the antidepressants Nardil and Parnate and the Parkinson's drug Eldepryl
Methionine drugs such as Pedameth
Metoclopramide (Reglan)
Papaverine (Pavabid)
Pyridoxine (Vitamin B_6)
Tranquilizers such as Dalmane, Valium, and Xanax
Tricyclic antidepressants such as Elavil and Tofranil

If you have been taking an MAO inhibitor such as Nardil or Parnate, you must discontinue it at least 2 weeks before starting to take Sinemet CR.

A high-protein diet may impair the effectiveness of Sinemet CR. Iron supplements can also reduce its effect.

Special information if you are pregnant or breastfeeding

If you are pregnant or plan to become pregnant, inform your doctor immediately. Sinemet CR should be used during pregnancy only if the benefit outweighs the potential risk to the unborn child. It is not known whether Sinemet CR appears in breast milk. If this medication is essential to your health, your doctor may advise you to stop nursing your baby until your treatment with this drug is finished.

Recommended dosage

Your doctor will tailor your individual dosage carefully, depending on your response to previous therapy and symptoms.

ADULTS

For patients with mild to moderate symptoms, the initial recommended dose is 1 tablet of Sinemet CR taken 2 times a day.

Starting doses should be spaced out every 4 to 8 hours and then adjusted to each patient's individual response.

The usual long-term dose is 2 to 8 tablets per day, taken in divided doses every 4 to 8 hours during the waking day.

Higher doses (12 or more tablets per day) and shorter intervals (less than 4 hours) have been used, but are not usually recommended.

When doses of Sinemet CR are given at intervals of less than 4 hours, and/or if the divided doses are not equal, it is recommended that the smaller doses be given at the end of the day.

An interval of at least 3 days between dosage adjustments is recommended.

Dosage adjustment of Sinemet CR may be necessary if your doctor prescribes additional medications.

CHILDREN

Use of Sinemet CR in children under 18 is not recommended.

Overdosage

Too much Sinemet CR may cause muscle twitches, inability to open the eyes, or other symptoms of levodopa overdosage. Like other medications, Sinemet CR taken in excess can have serious consequences. If you suspect symptoms of a Sinemet CR overdose, seek medical attention immediately.

SINEQUAN

Pronounced: SIN-uh-kwan
Generic name: Doxepin hydrochloride

Why is this drug prescribed?

Sinequan is used in the treatment of depression and anxiety. It helps relieve tension, improve sleep, elevate mood, increase energy, and generally ease the feelings of fear, guilt, apprehension, and worry most people experience. It is effective in treating people whose depression and/or anxiety is psychological, associated with alcoholism, or a result of another disease (cancer, for example) or psychotic depressive disorders (severe mental illness). It is in the family of drugs called tricyclic antidepressants.

Most important fact about this drug

Serious, sometimes fatal, reactions have occurred when Sinequan is used in combination with drugs known as MAO inhibitors, including the antidepressants Nardil and Parnate. Any drug of this type should be discontinued at least 2 weeks prior to starting treatment with Sinequan, and you should be carefully monitored by your doctor.

If you are taking any prescription or nonprescription drugs, consult your doctor before taking Sinequan.

How should you take this medication?

Take this medication exactly as prescribed. It may take several weeks for you to feel better.

■ *If you miss a dose...*
If you are taking several doses a day, take the missed dose as soon as you remember, then take any remaining doses for that day at evenly spaced intervals. If it is almost time for your next dose, skip the one you missed and go back to your regular schedule. Never take 2 doses at the same time.

If you are taking a single dose at bedtime and do not remember until the next morning, skip the dose. Do not take a double dose to make up for a missed one.

■ *Storage instructions...*
Store at room temperature.

What side effects may occur?

Side effects cannot be anticipated. If any develop or change in intensity, inform your doctor as soon as possible. Only your doctor can determine if it is safe for you to continue taking Sinequan.

■ *Side effects may include:*
Blurred vision, constipation, dizziness, drowsiness, dry mouth, itchy or scaly skin (pruritus), light sensitivity, low blood pressure, nausea, rapid or irregular heartbeat, rash, trouble urinating, water retention

Why should this drug not be prescribed?

If you are sensitive to or have ever had an allergic reaction to Sinequan or similar antidepressants, you should not take this medication. Make sure that your doctor is aware of any drug reactions that you have experienced.

Unless you are directed to do so by your doctor, do not take this medication if you have the eye condition known as glaucoma or difficulty urinating.

Special warnings about this medication

In clinical studies, antidepressants increased the risk of suicidal thinking and behavior in children and adolescents with depression and other psychiatric disorders. Anyone considering the use of Sinequan or any other antidepressant in a child or adolescent must balance this risk with the clinical need. Sinequan is not approved for treating anyone less than 12 years old.

Additionally, the progression of major depression is associated with a worsening of symptoms and/or the emergence of suicidal thinking or behavior in both adults and children, whether or not they are taking antidepressants. Individuals being treated with Sinequan and their caregivers should watch for any change in symptoms or any new symptoms that appear suddenly—especially agitation, anxiety, hostility, panic, restlessness, extreme hyperactivity, and suicidal thinking or behavior—and report them to the doctor immediately. Be especially observant at the beginning of treatment or whenever there is a change in dose.

Sinequan may cause you to become drowsy or less alert; driving or operating dangerous machinery or participating in any hazardous activity that requires full mental alertness is not recommended.

Notify your doctor or dentist that you are taking Sinequan if you have a medical emergency, and before you have surgery or dental treatment.

Possible food and drug interactions when taking this medication

Alcohol increases the danger of a Sinequan overdose. Do not drink alcohol while taking this medication.

Never combine Sinequan with drugs known as MAO inhibitors. Medications in this category include the antidepressants Nardil and Parnate.

If you are switching from Prozac, wait at least 5 weeks after your last dose of Prozac before starting Sinequan.

If Sinequan is taken with certain other drugs, the effects of either could be increased, decreased, or altered. It is especially important to check with your doctor before combining Sinequan with the following:

Antidepressants that act on serotonin, such as Celexa, Lexapro, Paxil, Prozac, and Zoloft
Carbamazepine (Tegretol)
Cimetidine (Tagamet)
Clonidine (Catapres)
Flecainide (Tambocor)
Guanethidine (Ismelin)
Major tranquilizers such as Compazine, Mellaril, and Thorazine
Other antidepressants such as Elavil and Serzone
Propafenone (Rythmol)
Quinidine (Quinidex)
Tolazamide (Tolinase)

Special information if you are pregnant or breastfeeding

The effects of Sinequan during pregnancy have not been adequately studied. If you are pregnant or planning to become pregnant, inform your doctor immediately. Sinequan may appear in breast milk and could affect a nursing infant. If this medication is essential to your health, your doctor may advise you to discontinue breastfeeding your baby until your treatment is finished.

Recommended dosage

ADULTS

The starting dose for mild to moderate illness is usually 75 milligrams per day. This dose can be increased or decreased by your doctor according to individual need. The usual ideal dose ranges from 75 milligrams per day to 150 milligrams per day, although it can be as low as 25 to 50 milligrams per day. The total daily dose can be given once a day or divided into smaller doses. If you are taking this drug once a day, the recommended dose is 150 milligrams at bedtime.

The 150-milligram capsule strength is intended for long-term therapy only and is not recommended as a starting dose.

For more severe illness, gradually increased doses of up to 300 milligrams may be required as determined by your doctor.

CHILDREN

Safety and effectiveness have not been established for use in children under 12 years of age.

OLDER ADULTS

Due to a greater risk of drowsiness and confusion, older people are usually started on a low dose.

Overdosage

An overdose of this drug can be fatal. If you experience any of these symptoms, seek medical attention immediately.

■ *Symptoms of Sinequan overdose may include:*
   Agitation, coma, confusion, convulsions, dilated pupils, disturbed concentration, drowsiness, hallucinations, high or low body temperature, irregular heartbeat, overactive reflexes, rigid muscles, severely low blood pressure, stupor, vomiting

SINGULAIR

Pronounced: sing-you-LAIR
Generic name: Montelukast sodium

Why is this drug prescribed?

Singulair is used for long-term prevention of asthma. It reduces the swelling and inflammation that tend to close up the airways, and relaxes the walls of the bronchial tubes, expanding the airways and permitting more air to pass through.

Singulair is also used to relieve the stuffy, runny nose and sneezing caused by seasonal allergies.

Most important fact about this drug

Singulair alleviates the ongoing symptoms of asthma, but it won't stop an acute asthma attack. For that you need a fast-acting, orally inhaled airway opener such as Alupent or Proventil.

How should you take this medication?

Take a Singulair tablet once daily, whether or not you have any symptoms. The tablet can be taken with or without food.

If you have asthma, or asthma plus allergies, take Singulair in the evening. If you have only allergies, you can take Singulair at any time.

The oral granules should be given directly in the child's mouth. The granules can also be mixed with a spoonful of one of the following soft foods: applesauce, carrots, rice, or ice cream. The food should be cold or at room temperature.

The granules should not be dissolved in liquids before giving them to your child. However, the child can drink liquids after the granules have been swallowed. Do not open the granules packet until your child is ready to take them. Once the packet is opened, the full dose of medication must be given within 15 minutes. Throw away any unused portion of the granules; do not store them for future use.

■ *If you miss a dose...*
Take it as soon as you remember. If it is almost time for your next dose, skip the one you missed and go back to your regular schedule. Do not take 2 doses at once.

■ *Storage instructions...*
Store at room temperature, away from moisture and light.

What side effects may occur?

Side effects cannot be anticipated. If any develop or change in intensity, inform your doctor as soon as possible. Only your doctor can determine if it is safe for you to continue taking Singulair.

■ *Side effects may include:*
Abdominal pain, abnormal dreams, allergic reaction, bronchitis, bruising, cough, dental pain, diarrhea, difficulty breathing or swallowing, dizziness, drowsiness, ear infection, ear pain, eczema, eye inflammation, fatigue, fever, flu, hallucinations, headache, hives, indigestion and other digestive problems, infection, insomnia, irritability, itching, laryngitis, leg pain, muscle aches and cramps, nasal congestion, nausea, pancreatitis, pneumonia, rash, restlessness, runny nose, seizures, sinus pain, skin inflammation, sneezing, sore throat, swelling due to fluid retention, swelling of the mouth or throat, upper respiratory infection, tendency to bleed easily, thirst, viral infection, vomiting

Why should this drug not be prescribed?

If Singulair gives you an allergic reaction, you cannot continue using the drug.

Special warnings about this medication

After you begin taking Singulair, your doctor may be able to slowly reduce the dosage of other asthma medications such as inhaled steroids. However, Singulair is not a complete replacement for such drugs, so you should not abruptly stop using them unless your doctor recommends it. If your asthma symptoms get worse or you develop a rash, numbness, or heart problems as you reduce your dose of steroids, check with your doctor. Such reactions usually result from a reduction in oral steroid therapy.

If your asthma gets worse after exercise, you'll need to continue using a short-acting inhaled airway opener to prevent the problem and relieve attacks.

If you are allergic to aspirin and other nonsteroidal anti-inflammatory drugs (NSAIDs), you should continue to avoid them. Singulair does not remedy this problem.

If you have difficulty breathing while taking Singulair, or find that you need your orally inhaled bronchodilator more often than usual (or require more puffs than prescribed), notify your doctor.

If you have a child with phenylketonuria—an inability to process phenylalanine that quickly leads to mental retardation—you should be aware that Singulair chewable tablets contain this substance.

Possible food and drug interactions when taking this medication

If Singulair is taken with certain other drugs, the effects of either could be increased, decreased, or altered. It is especially important to check with your doctor before combining Singulair with the following:

Phenobarbital
Rifampin (Rifadin, Rifamate, Rimactane)

Special information if you are pregnant or breastfeeding

Singulair should be used during pregnancy only if clearly needed. If you are pregnant or plan to become pregnant, inform your doctor immediately.

It is not known whether Singulair appears in breast milk. Because many drugs do make their way into breast milk, use Singulair with caution if you are breastfeeding.

Recommended dosage

ADULTS AND CHILDREN 15 AND OVER

Asthma
The usual dose is one 10-milligram tablet once a day in the evening.

Allergies
The usual dose is one 10-milligram tablet once a day taken at any time.

CHILDREN 6 TO 14 YEARS OLD

Asthma
The usual dose is one 5-milligram chewable tablet once a day in the evening.

Allergies
The usual dose is one 5-milligram chewable tablet once a day taken at any time.

CHILDREN 2 TO 5 YEARS OLD

Asthma
The dosage is one 4-milligram chewable tablet or one packet of 4-milligram oral granules per day, taken in the evening.

Allergies
The dosage is one 4-milligram chewable tablet or one packet of 4-milligram oral granules per day, taken at any time.

CHILDREN 12 TO 23 MONTHS OLD

Asthma
The dosage is one packet of 4-milligram oral granules taken once a day in the evening.

The safety and effectiveness of Singulair for treating asthma in children under 12 months have not been studied.

Allergies
Singulair is not approved for treating allergies in children under 2 years old.

Overdosage
Little is known about the effects of Singulair overdose. However, any medication taken in excess can have serious consequences. If you suspect an overdose, seek medical attention immediately.

SKELAXIN
Pronounced: skell-AX-in
Generic name: Metaxalone

Why is this drug prescribed?
Along with rest and physical therapy, Skelaxin is prescribed for the relief of painful musculoskeletal conditions. Researchers aren't sure how the drug works, but suspect that its effectiveness stems from its sedative properties.

Most important fact about this drug
Skelaxin should be avoided by anyone with significant liver or kidney problems.

How should you take this medication?
No special instructions apply. Take exactly as prescribed.

■ *If you miss a dose...*
   Take the forgotten dose as soon as you remember. However, if it is almost time for your next dose, skip the one you missed and return to your regular schedule. Do not take 2 doses at once.

■ *Storage instructions...*
   Store at room temperature.

What side effects may occur?

Side effects cannot be anticipated. If any develop or change in intensity, tell your doctor as soon as possible. Only your doctor can determine if it is safe to continue using Skelaxin.

■ *Side effects may include:*
   Dizziness, drowsiness, headache, irritability, nausea, nervousness, stomach upset, vomiting

Why should this drug not be prescribed?

You'll need to avoid this drug if it causes an allergic reaction. Do not take it if you have a tendency to anemia or a significant liver or kidney condition.

Special warnings about this medication

If you have any problems with your liver, the doctor will monitor your liver function carefully.

Safety and effectiveness in children 12 and under have not been established.

Possible food and drug interactions when using this medication

There is no information on potential interactions.

Special information if you are pregnant or breastfeeding

It's best to avoid using Skelaxin during pregnancy—particularly early pregnancy—unless the potential benefits clearly outweigh the possible risks. If you are pregnant or plan to become pregnant, notify your doctor immediately.

It is not known whether Skelaxin makes its way into breast milk. Breastfeeding while using the drug is not recommended.

Recommended dosage

ADULTS

The usual dose for adults and children over 12 is 800 milligrams (2 tablets) 3 or 4 times a day.

Overdosage

There have been no reports of major Skelaxin overdose. However, any medication taken in excess can have serious consequences. If you suspect an overdose, seek medical attention immediately.

■ *Possible symptoms of Skelaxin overdose may include:*
  Depressed breathing, sedation

Slo-Bid *See Theo-Dur, page 1432.*

Slow-K *See Micro-K, page 851.*

Sodium fluoride *See Luride, page 804.*

SODIUM SULAMYD
Pronounced: SOH-dee-um SOO-lah-mid
Generic name: Sulfacetamide sodium
Other brand name: Bleph-10

Why is this drug prescribed?
Sodium Sulamyd is used in the treatment of eye inflammations, corneal ulcer, and other eye infections. It may be used along with an oral sulfa drug to treat a serious eye infection called trachoma.

Most important fact about this drug
Sodium Sulamyd is similar to oral sulfa drugs such as Bactrim, Gantanol, and Gantrisin. If you are allergic to any of these medications, you may also be allergic to Sodium Sulamyd. In addition, if you have taken one of these medications in the past, you may have developed a hidden allergy to sulfa drugs that might show up when you take Sodium Sulamyd. Be alert for a rash, itching, or other signs of allergy. If any of these symptoms develops, stop taking Sodium Sulamyd immediately and consult your doctor.

How should you use this medication?
Sodium Sulamyd is available in eyedrop and ointment form. Use it exactly as prescribed. Your doctor may tell you to use both the eye drops and the ointment.

To apply Sodium Sulamyd, pull down your lower eyelid to form a pouch, then squeeze in the medication. To avoid contaminating the eyedrops or the ointment, do not touch your eye with the dropper bottle or the tip of the tube. Keep the dropper bottle or tube poised slightly above your eye as you instill the drops or squeeze out the ointment.

■ *If you miss a dose...*
  Apply it as soon as you remember. If it is almost time for your next dose, skip the one you missed and go back to your regular schedule.
■ *Storage instructions...*
  Store at room temperature. Protect the ointment from excessive heat.

What side effects may occur?

Side effects cannot be anticipated. If any develop or change in intensity, inform your doctor as soon as possible. Only your doctor can determine if it is safe for you to continue taking this medication.

Sodium Sulamyd may irritate your eye, causing stinging and burning. The irritation usually lasts only a short time. If it is very painful or lasts for a long time, you may have to stop using the medication.

In rare cases, people using Sodium Sulamyd have developed a severe blistering skin rash. Be alert for skin reactions. If a rash appears, stop using Sodium Sulamyd and call your doctor.

Why should this drug not be prescribed?

Do not use Sodium Sulamyd if you have ever had an allergic reaction to or are sensitive to this medication or any other sulfa drug.

Special warnings about this medication

Stay in close touch with your doctor while using Sodium Sulamyd. In some cases, an eye ointment may actually delay healing of the cornea. If you have a pus-producing eye infection, the pus may inactivate Sodium Sulamyd. Since sulfa drugs do not kill fungi, it is possible to develop a fungus infection in your eye while using Sodium Sulamyd.

Possible food and drug interactions when taking this medication

Sodium Sulamyd should not be used with medications containing silver. Check with your doctor if you are unsure of any medications you are taking.

Special information if you are pregnant or breastfeeding

If you are pregnant or plan to become pregnant, inform your doctor immediately. There is no information about the safety of Sodium Sulamyd during pregnancy.

It is not known whether Sodium Sulamyd appears in breast milk. If Sodium Sulamyd is essential to your health, it may be necessary to stop breastfeeding during treatment.

Recommended dosage

SODIUM SULAMYD OPHTHALMIC SOLUTION 30%

Inflamed Eyes or Corneal Ulcer
Place 1 drop inside the lower eyelid every 2 hours or less frequently; your doctor will determine the schedule according to the severity of the infection.

Trachoma (Contagious Inflammation)
Use 2 drops every 2 hours.

SODIUM SULAMYD OPHTHALMIC SOLUTION 10%

Place 1 or 2 drops inside the lower eyelid every 2 or 3 hours during the day, less often at night.

SODIUM SULAMYD OPHTHALMIC OINTMENT 10%

Apply a small amount of the ointment 4 times daily and at bedtime. The ointment may be used at the same time as either of the solutions.

Overdosage

Although no specific information is available on overdose with Sodium Sulamyd, any medication used in excess can have serious consequences. If you suspect you may have used too much Sodium Sulamyd, seek medical attention immediately.

SOMA

Pronounced: SOE-muh
Generic name: Carisoprodol

Why is this drug prescribed?

Soma is used, along with rest, physical therapy, and other measures, for the relief of acute, painful muscle strains and spasms.

Most important fact about this drug

Soma alone will not heal your muscles. You need to follow the program of physical therapy, rest, or exercise that your doctor prescribes. Do not attempt any more physical activity than your doctor recommends, even though Soma temporarily makes it seem feasible.

How should you take this medication?

Take Soma exactly as prescribed by your doctor.

■ *If you miss a dose...*
Take it as soon as you remember if only an hour or so has passed. If you do not remember until later, skip the dose you missed and go back to your regular schedule. Do not take 2 doses at once.

■ *Storage instructions...*
Store at room temperature in a tightly closed container.

What side effects may occur?

Side effects cannot be anticipated. If any develop or change in intensity, inform your doctor as soon as possible. Only your doctor can determine if it is safe for you to continue taking Soma.

■ *Side effects may include:*
Agitation, depression, dizziness, drowsiness, facial flushing, fainting, headache, hiccups, inability to fall or stay asleep, irritability, light-

headedness upon standing up, loss of coordination, nausea, rapid heart rate, stomach upset, tremors, vertigo, vomiting

Allergic reactions usually seen between the first and fourth doses of Soma in patients who have never taken this drug before include itching, red welts on the skin, and skin rash. A more severe allergic reaction may include symptoms such as asthmatic attacks, dizziness, fever, low blood pressure, shock, stinging of the eyes, swelling due to fluid retention, and weakness.

Why should this drug not be prescribed?
If you are sensitive to or have ever had an allergic reaction to Soma or drugs of this type, such as meprobamate (Miltown), you should not take this medication. Make sure your doctor is aware of any drug reactions you have experienced.

Unless you are directed to do so by your doctor, do not take this medication if you have porphyria (an inherited blood disorder).

Special warnings about this medication
In rare cases, the first dose of Soma may cause unusual symptoms that appear within minutes or hours of taking the medication. Symptoms reported include: agitation, confusion, disorientation, dizziness, double vision, enlargement of pupils, extreme weakness, exaggerated feeling of well-being, lack of coordination, speech problems, temporary loss of vision, and temporary paralysis of arms and legs. These symptoms usually subside within a few hours. If you experience any of them, contact your doctor immediately.

Soma may impair the mental or physical abilities you need to drive a car or operate dangerous machinery. Do not participate in hazardous activities until you know how this drug affects you.

If you have a history of drug dependence, make sure your doctor is aware of it before you start taking this medication.

Withdrawal symptoms, including abdominal cramps, chilliness, headache, insomnia, and nausea, have occurred in people who suddenly stop taking Soma.

Take this drug cautiously if you have any kidney or liver problems.

Possible food and drug interactions when taking this medication
Soma may intensify the effects of alcohol. Be careful drinking alcoholic beverages while you are taking this medication.

If Soma is taken with certain other drugs, the effects of either could be increased, decreased, or altered. It is especially important to check with your doctor before combining Soma with the following:

Antidepressant drugs such as Elavil, Nardil, and Tofranil
Major tranquilizers such as Haldol, Stelazine, and Thorazine
Sedatives such as Halcion and Nembutal
Tranquilizers such as Librium, Valium, and Xanax

Special information if you are pregnant or breastfeeding

The effects of Soma during pregnancy have not been adequately studied. If you are pregnant or plan to become pregnant, inform your doctor immediately. This drug appears in breast milk and could affect a nursing infant. If this medication is essential to your health, your doctor may advise you to discontinue breastfeeding until your treatment is finished.

Recommended dosage

ADULTS

The usual dosage of Soma is one 350-milligram tablet, taken 3 times daily and at bedtime.

CHILDREN

The safety and effectiveness of Soma have not been established in children under 12 years of age.

Overdosage

A severe overdose of Soma can be fatal. If you suspect an overdose, seek medical help immediately.

■ *Symptoms of Soma overdose may include:*
Breathing difficulty, coma, shock, stupor

SONATA
Pronounced: Sah-NAH-ta
Generic name: Zaleplon

Why is this drug prescribed?

Sonata is prescribed for people who have trouble falling asleep at bedtime. Because it has a short duration of action, it doesn't help those who suffer from frequent awakenings during the night or those who wake too early in the morning. It is intended only for short-term use (7 to 10 days).

Most important fact about this drug

Problems with sleep are usually temporary and require only short-term treatment with medication. Call your doctor immediately if it seems the medication is making the problem worse, or if you notice any unusual changes in your thinking or behavior, such as hallucinations, amnesia, agitation, or a lack of inhibition. The emergence of new symptoms could be a sign of an undiagnosed medical or psychiatric condition.

How should you take this medication?

Sonata is very fast-acting and should be taken only at bedtime.

■ *If you miss a dose...*
Take Sonata only when you're ready to sleep. Never double your dose.
■ *Storage instructions...*
Store at room temperature in a light-resistant container.

What side effects may occur?
Side effects cannot be anticipated. If any develop or change in intensity, inform your doctor as soon as possible. Only your doctor can determine if it is safe for you to continue taking Sonata.

■ *Side effects may include:*
Abdominal pain, amnesia, dizziness, drowsiness, eye pain, headache, memory loss, menstrual pain, nausea, sleepiness, tingling, weakness

Why should this drug not be prescribed?
Sonata is not recommended for people with severe liver disease and is best avoided during pregnancy. Do not take it if you are allergic to any of its ingredients. It contains the coloring agent FD&C Yellow No. 5, which causes a reaction in some individuals. This allergic reaction is more likely in people who are sensitive to aspirin.

Special warnings about this medication
Do not take Sonata unless you plan to be in bed for at least four hours after taking it. If you need to be alert and active in less than four hours, your performance could be impaired. Never attempt to drive a car or operate other dangerous machinery right after taking Sonata.

Use Sonata only for temporary relief of insomnia; sleep medicines tend to lose their effect when taken for more than a few weeks. Remember, too, that taking sleeping pills for extended periods or in high doses can lead to physical dependence and the danger of a withdrawal reaction when the drug is abruptly stopped. Be especially wary if you've ever had addiction problems with alcohol or other drugs.

Severe allergic reactions—including life-threatening ones that can cause severe breathing problems—have been reported and may require immediate medical care. Signs of a severe reaction include agitation, difficulty breathing, sudden drop in blood pressure, fainting, tingling sensations, itchy and flushed skin, hives, and swelling. If you are allergic to FD&C Yellow No. 5 (tartrazine), you'll probably want to avoid Sonata, which contains this substance.

The safety and effectiveness of Sonata have not been studied in children.

Possible food and drug interactions when taking this medication
Avoid alcoholic beverages when taking Sonata; the drug increases alcohol's effect. Also forgo high-fat meals immediately before taking Sonata; they tend to slow or reduce the drug's effect.

If Sonata is used with certain other drugs, the effects of either could be increased, decreased, or altered. It is especially important to check with your doctor before combining Sonata with the following:

Carbamazepine (Tegretol)
Cimetidine (Tagamet)
Diphenhydramine (Benadryl)
Imipramine (Tofranil)
Phenobarbital
Rifampin (Rifadin)
Thioridazine (Mellaril)

Special information if you are pregnant or breastfeeding

Sonata can affect a developing baby, especially during the last weeks before delivery, and is therefore not recommended for use during pregnancy. This drug also appears in breast milk and should not be used if you are nursing your baby.

Recommended dosage

ADULTS

The usual dose is 10 milligrams taken once daily at bedtime. Your doctor may adjust the dose to your individual need, especially if you are in a weakened condition or have a low body weight. A dose of 5 milligrams is recommended if you have liver disease or use the drug cimetidine.

OLDER ADULTS

The usual dose for older adults is 5 milligrams, as they may be more sensitive to the effects of Sonata.

Overdosage

An overdose of drugs such as Sonata can be fatal. If you suspect an overdose, seek medical attention immediately.

▨ *Symptoms of Sonata overdose may include:*
Drowsiness, mental confusion, grogginess, lack of coordination, flaccid muscles, labored breathing, coma

Sorbitrate *See Isordil, page 697.*

SORIATANE

Pronounced: *sore-EYE-ah-tane*
Generic name: *Acitretin*

Why is this drug prescribed?

Soriatane is prescribed for several types of severe psoriasis, a chronic skin condition that causes inflamed red patches with silvery scales. In more severe cases, the skin thickens with painful patches that fill with pus and crust over, sometimes on large portions of the body. Psoriasis can appear anywhere, but most commonly erupts on the chest and back, elbows and knees, feet and hands, scalp, and fingernails. Soriatane is used when milder forms of treatment have failed.

It's important to remember that Soriatane does not cure psoriasis; it merely helps keep it under control. Your condition may return if you stop treatment.

Most important fact about this drug

Soriatane must never be taken during pregnancy, as it can cause severe birth defects and physical abnormalities in a developing baby. You must not become pregnant while taking Soriatane, and you must also avoid becoming pregnant for a full 3 years after you stop taking it.

Before starting Soriatane therapy, women of childbearing age must receive birth control counseling and sign a detailed consent form stating they understand the consequences of birth control failure, the risk of birth defects, and the warning not to use alcohol (see *Special warnings about this medication*). You must have two negative pregnancy tests, one when you and your doctor decide on a course of Soriatane therapy and one immediately before starting treatment. You must take monthly pregnancy tests and continue to receive regular birth control counseling while using this drug.

In addition, you must use two forms of reliable birth control for at least 1 month prior to starting treatment, as well as for the entire time you take Soriatane and for a full 3 years after discontinuing therapy. It can take 3 years for this drug to be eliminated from the body.

You cannot choose progestin mini-pill products (such as Micronor, Nor-QD, and Ovrette) as a form of birth control because Soriatane interferes with their effectiveness. It is not yet known whether Soriatane interferes with the reliability of other hormone-based contraceptives (combination estrogen/progestin birth control pills, implants, and injections). A qualified counselor or doctor must clearly explain what kinds of birth control are effective. Women taking Soriatane who have previously taken the drug Tegison (etretinate) must continue to follow the birth control requirements for Tegison.

Your doctor can give you a referral for free birth control counseling and pregnancy testing. If you accidentally become pregnant, miss a menstrual period, or have unprotected sex while taking Soriatane, stop taking the drug and call your doctor immediately.

How should you take this medication?

Take Soriatane with food, exactly as prescribed by your doctor, at about the same time each day. Symptoms sometimes worsen after treatment begins, and it may take several months for your condition to improve.

...ou miss a dose...

Take the forgotten dose as soon as you remember. However, if it is almost time for your next dose, skip the one you missed and return to your regular schedule. Do not take 2 doses at once.

■ *Storage instructions:...*

Store at room temperature, away from light and humidity, in a child-proof container.

What side effects may occur?

Side effects cannot be anticipated. If any develop or change in intensity, tell your doctor as soon as possible. Only your doctor can determine if it is safe to continue using Soriatane.

■ *Side effects may include:*

Abnormal bone growth or pain, abnormal skin changes (itching, peeling, rash, sensitivity, thinning), blood clot, changes in blood sugar or cholesterol and triglyceride (blood fat) levels, depression, eye symptoms (dryness, pain, redness, sensitivity), heart attack, inflammation of the pancreas, joint pain, lip inflammation, liver disorders, muscle weakness, numbness or swelling of the hands or feet, stroke, thoughts of suicide or self-injury, vision problems (blurring, difficulty seeing at night)

Why should this drug not be prescribed?

Do not take Soriatane if it causes an allergic reaction or if you have ever had an allergic reaction to other drugs like it (retinoids such as Accutane and Tegison). You must also avoid this drug if you have kidney or liver disease, or if you have abnormally high cholesterol or triglyceride levels.

You must not take Soriatane if you are pregnant or if you plan to become pregnant within the next 3 years (see *Most important fact about this drug*).

Soriatane must never be taken with the drugs methotrexate (Rheumatrex and Trexall) or tetracycline antibiotics (such as Achromycin V and Sumycin). The combination can cause serious, sometimes life-threatening illness.

Special warnings about this medication

You must not become pregnant while taking Soriatane or within 3 years of taking it (see *Most important fact about this drug*).

Do not drink alcohol or take products containing alcohol while using Soriatane and for at least 2 months after discontinuing treatment. Combining alcohol with this drug causes a chemical change that makes it stay in your system longer. Read the labels on all foods and over-the-counter products to make sure they do not contain alcohol.

Soriatane causes significant changes in the level of sugar and fats in the blood. People with a history of alcoholism, diabetes, heart disease, or high levels of cholesterol or triglycerides, as well as those who are overweight, must be closely monitored when taking Soriatane.

People with degenerative spine or bone conditions must be checked regularly during treatment with Soriatane, since the drug can cause changes in their condition. Drugs like Soriatane are known to cause skeletal and bone growth problems in children. The safety and effectiveness of Soriatane have not been studied in children.

Soriatane may cause mental and behavioral changes. If you start to have symptoms of depression or aggression while taking Soriatane, or if you have thoughts of suicide or self-injury, call the doctor immediately.

Because eye conditions can worsen during Soriatane treatment, you must be carefully monitored by your doctor. The drug can cause decreased night vision and can interfere with the ability to drive or operate a vehicle safely at night. It can also interfere with the ability to wear contact lenses. Be sure to report any vision and eye problems to your doctor right away.

Soriatane increases the effects of sunlight. To prevent burning, do not stay in the sun for long periods; wear protective clothing, sunglasses, and sunscreen; and avoid using sunlamps or tanning beds. If you're being treated with phototherapy—that is, light therapy specifically used for certain skin conditions—your doctor may decrease the dosage of light while you're taking Soriatane.

Both men and women being treated with Soriatane may not give blood for at least 3 years.

Possible food and drug interactions when taking this medication

Do not drink alcohol or take products that contain alcohol while using Soriatane (see *Special warnings about this medication*). Always check labels for alcohol content.

Avoid taking vitamin supplements that contain vitamin A without your doctor's approval. Soriatane is chemically related to vitamin A, and taking too much can cause harmful side effects or a toxic overdose.

If you take the herb St. John's wort, do not use hormonal estrogen/progestin pills, implants, or injections as a form of birth control. Women who take these products together can become pregnant. Make sure your doctor knows about any over-the-counter products you are taking.

If Soriatane is taken with certain other drugs, the effects of either could be increased, decreased, or altered. It is especially important to check with your doctor before combining Soriatane with the following:

Birth control mini-pills containing progestin, such as Micronor, Nor-QD, and Ovrette
Demeclocycline (Declomycin)
Doxycycline (Doryx, Vibramycin)
Etretinate (Tegison)
Methotrexate (Rheumatrex, Trexall)

ycline (Dynacin, Minocin)
Retinoids such as isotretinoin (Accutane) and tretinoin (Vesanoid)
Phenytoin (Dilantin)
Tetracycline (Achromycin V, Sumycin)

Special information if you are pregnant or breastfeeding

If taken during pregnancy, Soriatane can cause severe birth defects and physical abnormalities in a developing baby (see *Most important fact about this drug*). Do not take Soriatane if you are pregnant or plan to become pregnant within 3 years after you stop taking it.

Do not take Soriatane if you're breastfeeding, as it can harm a nursing baby.

Recommended dosage

ADULTS

The recommended dose is 25 to 50 milligrams once a day, taken with your main meal. The pharmacist who fills your prescription will also provide you with a Soriatane medication guide.

Overdosage

Any medication taken in excess can have serious consequences. If you suspect an overdose, seek emergency treatment immediately.

After an overdose of Soriatane, all women of childbearing age must take a pregnancy test. They must also be counseled on the risk of birth defects and the need to use two effective forms of birth control for the next 3 years.

■ *Symptoms of overdose may include:*
Headache, vertigo (dizziness and a feeling that you or the room is spinning or moving)

SPECTAZOLE CREAM

Pronounced: SPEK-tah-zole
Generic name: Econazole nitrate

Why is this drug prescribed?

Spectazole cream is prescribed for fungal skin diseases commonly called ringworm (tinea). It is used to treat athlete's foot (tinea pedis), jock itch (tinea cruris), a fungus infection of the entire body (tinea corporis), and a skin infection that causes yellow- or brown-colored skin eruptions (tinea versicolor). It is also prescribed for yeast infections of the skin caused by candida fungus (cutaneous candidiasis).

Most important fact about this drug

Do not use Spectazole in or near the eyes.

How should you use this medication?

Use Spectazole Cream exactly as prescribed by your doctor.

Continue using the medication for the full time prescribed even if your symptoms have been relieved.

When applied, the cream should completely cover the affected area.

■ *If you miss a dose...*
Apply it as soon as you remember. If it is almost time for your next dose, skip the one you missed and go back to your regular schedule.

■ *Storage instructions...*
Store at room temperature.

What side effects may occur?

Side effects cannot be anticipated. If any develop or change in intensity, inform your doctor as soon as possible. Only your doctor can determine whether it is safe for you to continue using Spectazole.

■ *Side effects may include:*
Burning, itching, skin redness, stinging

Why should this drug not be prescribed?

Spectazole Cream should not be used if you are sensitive to it or have ever had an allergic reaction to any of its ingredients.

Special warnings about this medication

If you develop an irritation or an allergic reaction to Spectazole, stop using the cream and inform your doctor.

Spectazole is only for external use.

Possible food and drug interactions when taking this medication

No interactions have been reported.

Special information if you are pregnant or breastfeeding

Spectazole should be used during the first trimester (3 months) of pregnancy only if it is essential to your health, and during the remainder of your pregnancy only if your doctor feels it is clearly needed. If you are pregnant or plan to become pregnant, inform your doctor immediately. Spectazole may appear in breast milk and could affect a nursing infant. If this medication is essential to your health, your doctor may advise you to stop breastfeeding until your treatment with Spectazole is finished.

Recommended dosage

ATHLETE'S FOOT, JOCK ITCH, TINEA CORPORIS, TINEA VERSICOLOR

Apply sufficient Spectazole Cream to completely cover the affected area once a day. Athlete's foot is treated for 1 month; jock itch and tinea corporis are treated for 2 weeks. Tinea versicolor is usually treated for 2 weeks.

CUTANEOUS CANDIDIASIS

Apply sufficient Spectazole Cream to completely cover the affected area 2 times a day, once in the morning and once in the evening. Cutaneous candidiasis is treated for 2 weeks.

Overdosage

Although no specific information is available on Spectazole Cream overdosage, any medication used in excess can have serious consequences. If you suspect an overdose, seek medical attention immediately.

SPECTRACEF

Pronounced: SPEK-trah-sef
Generic name: Cefditoren

Why is this drug prescribed?

Spectracef cures mild to moderate bacterial infections of the skin, throat, and respiratory tract. Among these infections are pneumonia, strep throat, and tonsillitis. Spectracef is also prescribed for acute flare-ups of chronic bronchitis. Spectracef is a cephalosporin antibiotic.

Most important fact about this drug

If you are allergic to either penicillin or cephalosporin antibiotics (such as Ceftin, Lorabid, or Suprax), consult your doctor *before* taking Spectracef. An allergy to either type of medication may indicate a possible allergy to Spectracef, and if a reaction does occur, it could be extremely severe. Seek medical attention immediately if you develop any signs of an allergic reaction, including rash, hives, breathing problems, or swelling of the face or throat.

How should you take this medication?

Spectracef should be taken with meals to enhance absorption. Do not take it with antacids such as Tums or other medications that reduce stomach acid.

To make certain your infection is completely cleared up, take all of the medication exactly as your doctor prescribes, even if you begin to feel better after the first few days.

Certain antibiotics are known to interfere with oral contraceptives; however, it's okay to take Spectracef if you're using birth control pills.

■ *If you miss a dose...*
Take it as soon as you remember. If it is almost time for your next dose, skip the one you missed and go back to your regular schedule. Do not take 2 doses at once.

■ *Storage instructions...*
Store at room temperature; protect from light and moisture.

What side effects may occur?

Side effects cannot be anticipated. If any develop or change in intensity, tell your doctor as soon as possible. Only your doctor can determine if it is safe to continue using Spectracef.

■ *Side effects may include:*
Diarrhea, headache, nausea, vaginal infection

Why should this drug not be prescribed?

If you are sensitive to or have ever had an allergic reaction to Spectracef or other cephalosporin antibiotics, such as Suprax, do not take this medication.

You cannot use Spectracef if you have a deficiency of the amino acid carnitine, or if you have a problem metabolizing carnitine. You should also avoid the drug if you're allergic to milk protein, since Spectracef contains this substance. However, being lactose intolerant should not prevent you from using Spectracef.

Special warnings about this medication

Notify your doctor if you have had allergic reactions to penicillins or other cephalosporin antibiotics.

If you have a history of gastrointestinal disease, particularly colitis, take Spectracef with caution. If you develop diarrhea while taking Spectracef, check with your doctor. The problem could be a sign of a serious condition.

Be sure to tell your doctor if you have kidney problems. Your dosage may have to be lowered.

Spectracef should be used only for short-term treatment. Taking this medication for too long could lead to a deficiency of the amino acid carnitine. Certain people, especially those with kidney problems or decreased muscle mass, are more likely to develop a carnitine deficiency.

Cephalosporin antibiotics such as Spectracef could interfere with blood clotting. Especially at risk are people who have kidney or liver problems, are undernourished, or have been taking blood thinners or long-term antibiotic treatment.

Repeated use of Spectracef may result in an overgrowth of bacteria that do not respond to the medication and can cause a secondary infection. Therefore, do not save this medication for use at another time. Take this medication only when directed to do so by your doctor.

Possible food and drug interactions when taking this medication

If Spectracef is taken with certain other drugs, the effects of either could be increased, decreased, or altered. It is especially important to check with your doctor before combining Spectracef with the following:

Antacids such as Tums, Rolaids, or Maalox
Blood thinners such as warfarin (Coumadin)
Probenecid (Benemid)
Ulcer drugs known as H₂ blockers such as famotidine (Pepcid)

Special information if you are pregnant or breastfeeding

The effects of Spectracef during pregnancy or labor and delivery have not been adequately studied. If you are pregnant or plan to become pregnant, tell your doctor immediately.

Animal studies show that Spectracef can appear in breast milk. If this medication is essential to your health, your doctor may advise you to stop breastfeeding until your treatment is finished.

Recommended dosage

ADULTS AND CHILDREN 12 YEARS AND OLDER

Acute Flare-ups of Chronic Bronchitis
The usual dose is 400 milligrams twice a day for 10 days.

Pharyngitis, Tonsillitis, and Skin Infections
The usual dose is 200 milligrams twice a day for 10 days.

Community-acquired Pneumonia
The usual dose is 400 milligrams twice a day for 14 days.
If you have kidney disease, the dose may be lower.

CHILDREN LESS THAN 12 YEARS OLD

Spectracef has not been studied in children less than 12 years old and should not be used in this age group.

Overdosage

Although no specific information is available, an overdose of cephalosporin antibiotics has been known to cause nausea, vomiting, stomach problems, and convulsions. Any medication taken in excess can have serious consequences. If you suspect an overdose of Spectracef, seek medical attention immediately.

SPIRIVA HANDIHALER

Pronounced: speer-REE-vah
Generic name: Tiotropium bromide

Why is this drug prescribed?

Spiriva is used for the long-term, once-a-day treatment of bronchial spasms (wheezing) associated with chronic obstructive pulmonary disease, including chronic bronchitis and emphysema. It comes as a capsule containing dry powder, which is inhaled through the mouth using the HandiHaler device. When inhaled, Spiriva opens up narrow air passages, allowing more oxygen to reach the lungs.

Most important fact about this drug
Spiriva is not for initial use in sudden attacks of wheezing when fast action is needed—that is, Spiriva is not for "rescue therapy."

How should you take this medication?
Spiriva capsules are designed to be used only with the HandiHaler inhalation device. The capsules should not be swallowed. You should try to use the inhaler about the same time every day.

Spiriva capsules are packaged as a blister card containing 2 strips. Each strip has 3 capsules. When removing a capsule from the blister card, peel back only the foil that is covering the capsule you are about to use. The capsule's effectiveness may be reduced if it is not used immediately after the foil is opened. If you accidentally remove the foil covering any of the other capsules, you must throw them away.

When you're ready to take the medication, use the HandiHaler device as follows:

1. Open the dust cap, and then open the mouthpiece.
2. Place the capsule in the center chamber. Close the mouthpiece until you hear a click. Leave the dust cap open.
3. Hold the HandiHaler device with the mouthpiece upward and press the piercing button that will make holes in the capsule to allow the powder to come out.
4. Before inhaling the powder, breathe out completely, but not into the mouthpiece.
5. Place the inhaler's mouthpiece in your mouth, make a seal with your lips, keep your head upright, and breathe in slowly and deeply with your mouth. Breathe in quickly enough that you hear the capsule vibrate.
6. Hold your breath for as long as is comfortable; at the same time, remove the HandiHaler from your mouth.
7. When you're done, breathe out completely, seal your lips around the mouthpiece again, and inhale a second time as before.
8. Remove the capsule from the inhaler and discard. You may notice that a tiny amount of powder is still left in the capsule; this is normal.

Avoid getting the Spiriva powder into your eyes. It can cause blurred vision.

■ *If you miss a dose...*
Take it as soon as you remember. If it is almost time for your next dose, skip the one you missed and go back to your regular schedule. Do not take 2 doses at once.

■ *Storage instructions…*
Store at room temperature. Do not store capsules in the HandiHaler. Keep capsules away from moisture and extreme temperatures, such as in the refrigerator or in direct sunlight.

What side effects may occur?
Side effects cannot be anticipated. If any develop or change in intensity, tell your doctor as soon as possible. Only your doctor can determine if it is safe to continue using Spiriva.

■ *Side effects may include:*
Abdominal pain, constipation, dry mouth, chest pain, common cold, indigestion, infection, muscle pain, nosebleeds, rash, runny nose or nasal inflammation, sinus infection, sore throat, urinary tract infection, vomiting, yeast infection

Why should this drug not be prescribed?
You should not take Spiriva if you have an allergic reaction to it, or if you are allergic to atropine or any of its derivatives, including ipratropium (Atrovent).

Special warnings about this medication
An immediate allergic reaction (hives, swelling, or rash) is possible when you first use this drug. Inhaled medications such as Spiriva can also cause wheezing in some people. If you have an allergic reaction or you start wheezing, stop using Spiriva and contact your doctor.

Spiriva could worsen certain medical conditions. Use this drug cautiously if you have narrow-angle glaucoma (high pressure inside the eye), an enlarged prostate, or obstruction in the neck of the bladder. Also tell your doctor if you have kidney problems.

Possible food and drug interactions when taking this medication
The use of Spiriva together with other anticholinergic drugs, such as Atrovent, has not been studied and is not recommended.

Always tell your doctor about any medication you're taking, including over-the-counter products and dietary supplements.

Special information if you are pregnant or breastfeeding
Spiriva has not been studied in pregnant women. This drug should be used during pregnancy only if the benefits outweigh the potential risks. Notify your doctor immediately if you are pregnant or plan to become pregnant.

It is not known whether Spiriva appears in breast milk. If using Spiriva is essential to your health, you doctor may recommend that you discontinue breastfeeding while using this medication.

Recommended dosage

ADULTS

The recommended dose is the contents of one capsule, taken once a day, with the HandiHaler device.

Spiriva has not been studied in children.

Overdosage

Any medication taken in excess can have serious consequences. If you suspect an overdose, seek medical treatment immediately.

■ *Symptoms of overdose may include:*
Abdominal pain, blurred vision, confusion or memory problems, dry mouth, glaucoma, inability to concentrate, increased heart rate, severe constipation, urinary difficulty, urinary retention, trembling

---

Spironolactone See *Aldactone, page 64.*

Spironolactone with Hydrochlorothiazide See *Aldactazide, page 61.*

SPORANOX
Pronounced: SPORE-ah-nocks
Generic name: Itraconazole

Why is this drug prescribed?

Sporanox capsules are used to treat three types of serious fungal infection: blastomycosis, histoplasmosis, and aspergillosis. Blastomycosis can affect the lungs, bones, and skin. Histoplasmosis can affect the lungs, heart, and blood. Aspergillosis can affect the lungs, kidneys, and other organs. The drug is also prescribed for onychomycosis, which infects the toenails and fingernails. Additionally, Sporanox is used against fungal infections in people with weak immune systems, such as AIDS patients.

Sporanox oral solution is used to treat candidiasis (fungal infection) of the mouth, throat, and gullet (esophagus), and for other fungal infections in people with weakened immunity and fever.

Most important fact about this drug

Be sure to take Sporanox for as long as your doctor prescribes. It will take 3 months or more to cure some infections completely. If you stop taking Sporanox too soon, the infection may return.

How should you take this medication?

Take Sporanox exactly as prescribed. To make sure the capsules are properly absorbed, you should take them after a full meal; the oral solution should be taken without food. A cola drink can help some people absorb the capsules better. Continue taking Sporanox until all the medication is gone. Do not take antacids within 1 hour before or 2 hours after taking Sporanox.

Swish the oral solution, 10 milliliters at a time, in your mouth for a few seconds before swallowing it.

Mouth and throat candidiasis should clear up in several days.

The oral solution and capsules cannot be used interchangeably.

■ *If you miss a dose...*
Take the forgotten dose as soon as you remember. If it is almost time for the next dose, skip the one you missed and go back to your regular schedule. Never try to catch up by doubling the dose.

■ *Storage instructions...*
Store at room temperature. Protect the capsules from light and moisture. Do not freeze the oral solution.

What side effects may occur?
Side effects cannot be anticipated. If any develop or change in intensity, inform your doctor as soon as possible. Only your doctor can determine if it is safe for you to continue taking Sporanox.

■ *Side effects may include:*
Anxiety, bursitis, diarrhea, fatigue, fever, gas, headache, high blood pressure, indigestion, injury, muscle pain, nasal and sinus inflammation, nausea, pain, rash, respiratory infection, swelling due to water retention, urinary infection, vomiting

■ *Additional side effects that may be seen with the oral solution are:*
Back pain, blood in the urine, breathing difficulty, chest pain, cough, dehydration, difficulty swallowing, hemorrhoids, hot flushes, impaired speech, inflamed mouth, insomnia, pneumonia, shivering, sweating, vision problems, weight loss

People being treated for onychomycosis may experience stomach and intestinal disorders or rash, or, less commonly, headache, lightheadedness upon standing up, low blood pressure, muscle pain, a sick feeling, or vertigo.

Why should this drug not be prescribed?
If you are sensitive to or have ever had an allergic reaction to Sporanox or similar antifungal drugs such as Nizoral, you should not take this medication. Make sure that your doctor is aware of any drug reactions that you have experienced.

Sporanox can have a negative effect on the heart. It should not be used for fungal nail infections in people with cardiac problems such as congestive heart failure.

Serious heart problems, such as irregular heartbeats and even death, have occurred in people who have taken Sporanox at the same time as cisapride, levacetylmethadol, pimozide, or cholesterol-lowering drugs known as statins, such as Mevacor and Zocor. Never take these drugs with Sporanox, and avoid Halcion, Quinidex, Versed, and Tikosyn as well.

During pregnancy, Sporanox should not be used for treatment of fungal nail infections.

If you have cystic fibrosis or a low white blood cell count, taking Sporanox is not advised.

Special warnings about this medication

In rare cases, Sporanox has been known to cause liver failure and even death, sometimes within the first week of treatment. Sporanox treatment is strongly discouraged if you have liver disease or have experienced liver toxicity from other drugs. If you take Sporanox continuously for more than a month, your doctor should monitor your liver function periodically. If you develop such symptoms of liver disease as unusual fatigue, loss of appetite, nausea, vomiting, jaundice, dark urine, or pale stool, stop taking Sporanox and contact your doctor immediately.

People with cardiac problems such as congestive heart failure should avoid Sporanox unless the benefit clearly outweighs the danger. In fact, anyone who is even at risk of heart failure should use Sporanox with caution. Risk factors include heart and lung disorders and kidney failure. If you experience swelling—especially in the feet and ankles—or difficulty breathing while taking Sporanox, stop taking this medication and contact your doctor immediately.

If you develop any nerve disorders while taking Sporanox, see your doctor. Treatment will probably need to be discontinued.

Possible food and drug interactions when taking this medication

If Sporanox is taken with certain other drugs, the effects of either could be increased, decreased, or altered. It is especially important to check with your doctor before combining Sporanox with any of the following:

Acid-blocking drugs such as Tagamet, Pepcid, and Zantac
Alprazolam (Xanax)
Atorvastatin (Lipitor)
Blood-thinning drugs such as Coumadin
Buspirone (BuSpar)
Busulfan (Myleran)
Caffeine-containing agents such as Cafergot
Calcium channel blockers such as Cardene, Norvasc, and Procardia
Carbamazepine (Tegretol)
Cilostazol (Pletal)
Clarithromycin (Biaxin)
Cyclosporine (Sandimmune, Neoral)
Diazepam (Valium)
Disopyramide (Norpace)
Dofetilide (Tikosyn)

Digoxin (Lanoxin)
Docetaxel (Taxotere)
Eletriptan (Relpax)
Erythromycin (E-Mycin, Ery-Tab, and others)
Indinavir (Crixivan)
Isoniazid
Levacetylmethadol
Lovastatin (Mevacor)
Methylprednisolone (Medrol)
Midazolam (Versed)
Nevirapine (Viramune)
Oral diabetes medications such as DiaBeta, Diabinese, Glucotrol,
    Micronase, Orinase, and Tolinase
Phenobarbital
Phenytoin (Dilantin)
Pimozide (Orap)
Quinidine (Quinidex)
Rifabutin (Mycobutin)
Rifampin (Rifadin, Rimactane)
Ritonavir (Norvir)
Saquinavir (Invirase)
Simvastatin (Zocor)
Sirolimus (Rapamune)
Tacrolimus (Prograf)
Triazolam (Halcion)
Trimetrexate (Neutrexin)
Vinblastine (Velban)

Special information if you are pregnant or breastfeeding

The effects of Sporanox during pregnancy have not been adequately studied. If you are pregnant or plan to become pregnant, inform your doctor immediately. You should not take Sporanox to treat onychomycosis if you are or may become pregnant. In any event, Sporanox should not be used during pregnancy if the problem is a nail infection. In other cases, check with your doctor before you take Sporanox.

Sporanox appears in breast milk and could affect a nursing infant. If this medication is essential to your health, your doctor may advise you to discontinue breastfeeding until your treatment with Sporanox is finished.

Recommended dosage

ADULTS

Blastomycosis and Histoplasmosis
The usual dose is two 100-milligram capsules, taken after a full meal once a day. If you feel no improvement, or if there is evidence that the fungal

disease has spread, your doctor will increase the dose 100 milligrams at a time to a maximum of 400 milligrams a day. Daily dosages above 200 milligrams a day should be divided into 2 smaller doses.

Aspergillosis
The usual dose is 200 to 400 milligrams a day. Treatment usually continues for a minimum of 3 months, until tests indicate that the fungal infection has subsided.

Onychomycosis
The usual dose for a toenail infection, whether or not fingernails are also involved, is 200 milligrams once a day for 12 weeks.

If only fingernails are infected, treatment is given in two 7-day-long sessions during which you take 200 milligrams of Sporanox twice a day, with a 3-week rest period between sessions.

Candidiasis, Mouth and Throat
The usual dose is 20 milliliters of oral solution a day for 1 to 2 weeks. If the infection does not go away, your dose will be changed to 10 milliliters twice a day.

Candidiasis, Esophagus
The usual dose is 10 milliliters of oral solution a day for at least 3 weeks. You should continue the treatment for 2 weeks after your symptoms clear up. If necessary, the doctor may increase the dose to 20 milliliters a day.

Fungal Infections in People with Weakened Immunity and Fever
Recommended treatment starts with 200-milligram injections twice a day for 2 days followed by 200 milligrams injected once a day for up to 14 days. This may be followed by 20 milliliters of oral solution twice a day for up to a total of 28 days of treatment

CHILDREN

The safety and effectiveness of Sporanox in children have not been established.

Overdosage
Any drug taken in excess can have dangerous consequences. If you suspect an overdose, seek emergency medical treatment immediately.

STALEVO

Pronounced: stuh-LEE-voh
Generic ingredients: Carbidopa, Levodopa, Entacapone

Why is this drug prescribed?

Stalevo is used to help relieve symptoms of Parkinson's disease, including tremors, muscle stiffness and rigidity, slowness of movement, and poor balance or coordination.

Stalevo contains a combination of three drugs, carbidopa and levodopa (the active ingredients in Sinemet), and entacapone (the active ingredient in Comtan). The drug that actually relieves the symptoms of Parkinson's is levodopa. Carbidopa and entacapone both keep the body from breaking down levodopa too quickly, thus allowing the drug's effects to last longer. Stalevo can be used instead of Sinemet and Comtan by people who are taking those medicines separately or when the benefits of levodopa aren't lasting as long as they used to.

Keep in mind that Stalevo is not a cure for Parkinson's disease; it merely helps keep the symptoms under control.

Most important fact about this drug

You should never take Stalevo with certain antidepressants known as monoamine oxidase (MAO) inhibitors, such as phenelzine (Nardil) and tranylcypromine (Parnate). Combining Stalevo with these drugs could cause serious—and possibly life-threatening—side effects. This type of antidepressant should be discontinued at least 2 weeks before beginning therapy with Stalevo.

However, Stalevo may be combined with the drug selegiline (Eldepryl), which is a different type of MAO inhibitor that is often prescribed for Parkinson's disease. Always check with your doctor before taking any type of MAO inhibitor.

How should you take this medication?

Stalevo may be taken with or without food. Never chew, crush, or break the tablets. Do not change the prescribed dosing regimen or add any Parkinson's medications without first consulting your doctor.

■ *If you miss a dose...*
If you forget to take a dose, take it as soon as you remember. If it is almost time for your next dose, skip the one you missed and go back to your regular schedule. Do not take 2 doses at once.

■ *Storage instructions...*
Store at room temperature.

What side effects may occur?

Side effects cannot be anticipated. If any develop or change in intensity, tell your doctor as soon as possible. Only your doctor can determine if it is safe to continue using Stalevo.

■ *Side effects may include:*
Abdominal pain, back pain, confusion, constipation, diarrhea, dizziness, fatigue, hallucinations, involuntary movements or tremor, nausea (especially at the start of therapy), slow movements or difficulty making voluntary movements, uncontrollable twitching or jerking, urine discoloration, vomiting

Why should this drug not be prescribed?

You should not use Stalevo if you have ever had an allergic reaction to any of its components: carbidopa, levodopa, entacapone (Comtan), or the carbidopa/levodopa combination found in Sinemet.

Do not take Stalevo if you have glaucoma. You must also avoid the drug if you have any suspicious, undiagnosed skin lesion or mole, or a history of melanoma.

Special warnings about this medication

Stalevo may cause or exacerbate depression, hallucinations, psychosis, or suicidal thoughts. If you develop any of these symptoms, tell your doctor right away. Also make sure the doctor knows if you have a history of mental or emotional problems.

Stalevo can make some medical conditions worse. Be sure your doctor knows if you have any of the following:

Asthma
Endocrine (glandular) disorder
Glaucoma (high pressure in the eye)
Heart or lung disease (severe)
History of heart attack or irregular heartbeat
History of peptic ulcer
Kidney disorder
Liver disorder
Undiagnosed skin lesions

Muscle rigidity, high temperature, rapid heartbeat or breathing, sweating, blood pressure changes, involuntary twitching or jerking movements, and mental changes may occur when Stalevo is reduced suddenly or discontinued. If you stop taking this medicine abruptly, your doctor should monitor your condition carefully.

Stalevo may lower blood pressure, causing symptoms such as dizziness, nausea, fainting, and sweating. Be careful about standing up too quickly, especially after lying down or sitting for a long time. Give yourself ample time to understand how the medication affects you before you attempt to drive a car or operate machinery.

Possible food and drug interactions when taking this medication

Stalevo should never be combined with certain MAO inhibitors such as the antidepressants Nardil and Parnate (see *Most important fact about this drug*).

If Stalevo is taken with certain other drugs, the effects of either could be increased, decreased, or altered. It is especially important to consult your doctor before combining Stalevo with the following:

Ampicillin (Principen)
Apomorphine (Uprima)
Asthma medications
Blood pressure medication
Chloramphenicol (Chloromycetin)
Cholestyramine (Questran)
Dobutamine
Dopamine
Epinephrine or norepinephrine (such as Epi-Pen)
Erythromycin (E-Mycin, Erythrocin, and others)
Isoniazid (Laniazid, Nydrazid, Rifater)
Major tranquilizers such as chlorpromazine, Haldol, Mellaril, and
    Risperdal
Methyldopa (Aldomet)
Metoclopramide (Reglan)
Papaverine (Cerespan, Pavabid, and others)
Phenytoin (Dilantin)
Probenecid (Benemid)
Pyridoxine (vitamin B6)
Rifampin or rifampicin (Rifadin, Rifater, Rimactane)
Tricyclic antidepressants such as Elavil and Tofranil

Iron supplements or a high-protein diet may reduce the effectiveness of Stalevo.

Special information if you are pregnant or breastfeeding

The effects of Stalevo during pregnancy have not been studied. Notify your doctor if you are pregnant or plan to become pregnant. Stalevo should be used only if the potential benefits outweigh the potential risks.

It is not known whether Stalevo appears in breast milk. Your doctor may recommend that you discontinue breastfeeding while you are taking Stalevo.

Recommended dosage

ADULTS

Your doctor will tailor your individual dosage carefully, depending on your response to previous therapy and symptoms. If you are already taking carbidopa/levodopa and entacapone as two separate medications, you will start a Stalevo regimen that matches what you were previously taking.

Stalevo may be taken up to 8 times a day. It is available in 3 different strengths:

- 12.5 milligrams carbidopa/50 milligrams levodopa/200 milligrams entacapone
- 25 milligrams carbidopa/100 milligrams levodopa/ 200 milligrams entacapone
- 37.5 milligrams carbidopa/150 milligrams levodopa/200 milligrams entacapone

Overdosage

An overdose of Stalevo can have potentially serious effects and may require hospitalization. If you suspect an overdose, seek medical treatment immediately.

- *Symptoms of overdose may include:*
  Abdominal pain, loose stools, low blood pressure, mental disturbances (depression, psychosis, hallucinations, suicidal thoughts), rapid heartbeat

STARLIX
Pronounced: STAR-licks
Generic name: Nateglinide

Why is this drug prescribed?

Starlix combats high blood sugar levels in people with type 2 diabetes (the kind that does not require insulin shots). Insulin speeds the transfer of sugar from the bloodstream to the body's cells, where it's burned to produce energy. In diabetes, the body either fails to make enough insulin, or is unable to properly use what's available. Starlix attacks the problem from the production angle, stimulating the pancreas to secrete more insulin.

Starlix can be used alone or combined with another diabetes drug, such as Actos, Avandia, or Glucophage, that tackles the other part of the problem, working to improve the body's response to whatever insulin it makes. Starlix is prescribed only when diet and exercise—or the other drug alone—has failed to control blood sugar levels.

Most important fact about this drug

Always remember that Starlix is an aid to, not a substitute for, good diet and exercise. Failure to follow a sound diet and exercise plan can lead to serious complications, such as dangerously high or low blood sugar levels. Remember, too, that Starlix is not an oral form of insulin, and cannot be used in place of insulin shots.

How should you take this medication?

Starlix should be taken before each meal, anywhere from 30 minutes to the moment before you begin to eat. If you skip a meal, skip your Starlix dose as well; wait until your next meal before taking the medication.

■ *If you miss a dose...*
   Wait until your next meal, then take your regular dose. Never take 2 doses at the same time.
■ *Storage instructions...*
   Store at room temperature in a tightly closed container.

What side effects may occur?

Side effects cannot be anticipated. If any develop or change in intensity, inform your doctor as soon as possible. Only your doctor can determine if it is safe for you to continue taking Starlix.

■ *Side effects may include:*
   Back pain, diarrhea, dizziness, flu-like symptoms, joint infection, upper respiratory infection

Starlix, like all oral diabetes drugs, can cause hypoglycemia (low blood sugar). This risk is increased by missed meals, alcohol, other diabetes medications, and excessive exercise. Hypoglycemia is more likely in older or malnourished people and those with poorly functioning adrenal or pituitary glands. To avoid low blood sugar, take Starlix only at meals and closely follow the dietary and exercise regimen suggested by your doctor.

■ *Symptoms of mild low blood sugar may include:*
   Blurred vision, cold sweats, dizziness, fast heartbeat, fatigue, headache, hunger, light-headedness, nausea, nervousness
■ *Symptoms of more severe low blood sugar may include:*
   Coma, disorientation, pale skin, seizures, shallow breathing

Mild hypoglycemia can usually be corrected by eating sugar or a sugar-based product. If symptoms of severe low blood sugar develop, contact your doctor immediately. Severe hypoglycemia should be considered a medical emergency, and prompt medical attention is essential.

Why should this drug not be prescribed?

If you have type 1 (insulin-dependent) diabetes, you cannot use Starlix. The drug also cannot be used for diabetic ketoacidosis (a life-threatening medical emergency caused by insufficient insulin and marked by excessive thirst, nausea, fatigue, pain below the breastbone, and fruity-smelling breath).

If you are already taking a drug that promotes insulin secretion, such as Micronase, you should not switch to Starlix or add it to your current drug. In addition, Starlix is not for you if you have been taking other antidiabetic drugs for a long time, or if Starlix gives you an allergic reaction.

Special warnings about this medication

You should periodically test your blood or urine for abnormal sugar (glucose) levels. Even people with well-controlled diabetes may find that injury, infection, surgery, or fever results in a temporary loss of blood sugar control. At such times, the doctor may recommend that you take insulin instead of Starlix.

The effectiveness of any antidiabetic drug, including Starlix, may decrease with time. This may occur because of either a diminished responsiveness to the medication or a worsening of the diabetes.

If you have liver disease, use Starlix with caution. Also, be aware that dialysis treatments may reduce the effectiveness of the drug.

The safety and effectiveness of Starlix in children have not been established.

Possible food and drug interactions when taking this medication

If Starlix is taken with certain other drugs, the effects of either could be increased, decreased, or altered. It is especially important to check with your doctor before combining Starlix with the following:

> Airway-opening drugs such as Alupent and Proventil
> Aspirin
> Beta-blockers such as the blood pressure medications Inderal and Tenormin
> Corticosteroids such as prednisone (Deltasone)
> Decongestants such as Sudafed
> MAO inhibitors such as the antidepressants Nardil and Parnate
> Nonsteroidal anti-inflammatory drugs such as Advil, Motrin, and Naprosyn
> Salicylates such as the arthritis drugs Disalcid and Trilisate
> Thiazide diuretics such as the water pills Esidrix and HydroDIURIL
> Thyroid medications such as Synthroid

Be careful about drinking alcohol, since excessive alcohol consumption can cause low blood sugar. Also be careful when having a liquid meal; it could reduce the effectiveness of the drug.

Special information if you are pregnant or breastfeeding

Because the effects of Starlix on the unborn child have not been adequately studied, this drug should not be used during pregnancy. Since studies suggest the importance of maintaining normal blood sugar levels during pregnancy, you may need to take insulin instead.

It is not known whether Starlix appears in breast milk. Because of potential harm to the baby, you'll need to choose between breastfeeding and continuing treatment with Starlix.

Recommended dosage

ADULTS

Take Starlix shortly before meals. The usual dose of Starlix, whether taken alone or combined with Actos, Avandia, or Glucophage, is 120 milligrams three times a day. If your doctor finds that your glycosylated hemoglobin (HbA1C) levels are near normal before you start taking the drug, you may use the lower dose of 60 milligrams three times a day.

Overdosage

An overdose of Starlix can cause low blood sugar. (For symptoms, see *What side effects may occur?*) Mild hypoglycemia can usually be corrected by eating sugar or a sugar-based product. If your symptoms persist or worsen, seek medical attention immediately.

Stavudine *See Zerit, page 1618.*

Stimate *See DDAVP, page 390.*

STRATTERA
Pronounced: stra-TER-uh
Generic name: Atomoxetine hydrochloride

Why is this drug prescribed?
Strattera is used in the treatment of Attention Deficit Hyperactivity Disorder (ADHD), a condition marked by either constant activity, a persistent inability to stay focused, or both. Medications such as Strattera should always be part of a comprehensive treatment program that includes psychological, educational, and social measures designed to remedy the problem.

Strattera is the first ADHD medication to avoid classification as a controlled substance (a drug with potential for abuse). It is thought to work by boosting levels of norepinephrine, one of the brain chemicals responsible for regulating activity. It is prescribed for children and adults.

Most important fact about this drug
During clinical trials, researchers found that Strattera slowed children's average rate of growth. It's not known whether final adult height and weight are affected, but the manufacturer recommends interrupting use of the drug if a child is not growing or gaining weight at the expected rate.

How should you take this medication?
Take Strattera exactly as prescribed; higher than recommended doses provide no additional benefit. Strattera may be taken with or without food.

- *If you miss a dose...*
  Take the forgotten dose as soon as you remember, but take no more than the prescribed daily total during any 24-hour period.
- *Storage instructions...*
  Store at room temperature.

What side effects may occur?
Side effects cannot be anticipated. If any develop or change in intensity, tell your doctor as soon as possible. Only your doctor can determine if it is safe to continue using Strattera.

- *Side effects in children may include:*
  Appetite loss, constipation, cough, crying, diarrhea, dizziness, drowsiness, dry mouth, ear infection, fatigue, headache, indigestion, influenza, irritability, mood swings, nausea, runny nose, skin inflammation, stomach pain, vomiting, weight loss
- *Side effects in adults may include:*
  Abnormal dreams, abnormal orgasms, appetite loss, chills, constipation, diminished sex drive, dizziness, dry mouth, ejaculation disorders, erection problems, fatigue or sluggishness, fever, headache, hot flushes, impotence, indigestion, insomnia, gas, menstrual problems, muscle pain, nausea, palpitations, prostate inflammation, sinusitis, skin inflammation, sleep disorder, sweating, tingling, urinary problems, weight loss

Why should this drug not be prescribed?
Do not take Strattera within 2 weeks of taking any drug classified as an MAO inhibitor, such as the antidepressants Nardil and Parnate. The combination can cause severe—even fatal—reactions, including symptoms such as high fever, rigid muscles, rapid changes in heart rate, delirium, and coma.

You should also avoid Strattera if you have narrow-angle glaucoma (high pressure in the eye), or if the drug causes an allergic reaction.

Special warnings about this medication
Strattera can speed up the heart and boost blood pressure. Use it with caution if you have high blood pressure, a rapid heart rate, heart disease, or any other circulation problem.

On the other hand, Strattera can also cause an attack of low blood pressure when you first stand up. Use it with caution if you have a condition, such as severe dehydration, that can cause low blood pressure.

Because Strattera sometimes causes sluggishness, be careful when operating machinery or driving until you know how the drug affects you.

Possible food and drug interactions when taking this medication

Remember that Strattera must never be combined with MAO inhibitors (see *Why should this drug not be prescribed?*). Also, your doctor will probably prescribe a lower dose of Strattera if you are taking one of the following:

    Fluoxetine (Prozac)
    Paroxetine (Paxil)
    Quinidine (Quinidex)

Due to the possibility of boosted effects, you should check with your doctor before combining Strattera with the following:

    Proventil and similar asthma medications
    Drugs that raise blood pressure, such as the phenylephrine in some
      over-the-counter cold medications.

If you are unsure about a particular medication—whether prescription or over-the-counter—make a point of asking your doctor.

Special information if you are pregnant or breastfeeding

Strattera has not been studied in pregnant women. If you are pregnant or plan to become pregnant, notify your doctor immediately. Strattera should not be taken during pregnancy unless its benefits justify the potential risk to the baby.

It is not known whether Strattera makes its way into breast milk. Caution is warranted if you plan to nurse.

Recommended dosage

The daily dose of Strattera can be taken as a single dose in the morning, or divided into 2 equal doses taken in the morning and late afternoon or early evening.

CHILDREN

For children and teenagers weighing up to 154 pounds, the usual starting dosage is 0.5 milligram per 2.2 pounds of body weight per day. After at least 3 days, the doctor may increase the daily total to a recommended level of 1.2 milligrams per 2.2 pounds. Daily doses should never exceed 1.4 milligrams per 2.2 pounds or a total of 100 milligrams, whichever is less.

Strattera has not been tested in children under 6.

ADULTS

For adults and teenagers weighing over 154 pounds, the usual starting dosage is 40 milligrams per day. After at least 3 days, the doctor may increase the daily total to a recommended level of 80 milligrams. After another 2 to 4 weeks, dosage may be increased to a maximum of 100 milligrams daily

If you have liver problems, your dosage will be reduced.

Overdosage
There is limited information on Strattera overdose. However, any medication taken in excess can have serious consequences. If you suspect an overdose, seek medical treatment immediately.

■ *Signs of a Strattera overdose may include:*
Abnormal behavior, agitation, dilated pupils, dry mouth, hyperactivity, rapid heartbeat, sleepiness, stomach problems

STRIANT
Pronounced: STRIE-ant
Generic name: Testosterone buccal system

Why is this drug prescribed?
Striant is a hormone replacement product for men who have hypogonadism, a low level of the male hormone testosterone. The condition is marked by symptoms such as impotence and decreased interest in sex, lowered mood, fatigue, and decreases in bone density and lean body mass. Testosterone replacement therapy helps correct these problems.

The term "buccal" refers to the cheek. When the Striant buccal system is applied to the gum, medication is absorbed through the cheek.

Most important fact about this drug
To keep testosterone levels consistent, the buccal system should be replaced every 12 hours.

How should you take this medication?
Apply the buccal system to alternate sides of the mouth with each application. Remember that Striant is designed to stick to the gum or inner cheek; do **not** chew or swallow it.

Striant buccal system looks like a white to off-white tablet that is curved on one side and flat on the other. Open the Striant packet and apply the curved side against your gum above the right or left incisor tooth (the tooth just to the right or left of your two front teeth). The flat side should be facing the inside of your upper lip. Hold it in place by putting a finger over your lip and against the buccal system for 30 seconds to be sure it sticks.

If the system does not stick to the gum properly—or if it falls off within the first 8 hours—it should be removed and a new Striant system applied. This new system counts as your first dose and needs to be replaced at your next scheduled dose, even if 12 hours have not passed.

If the system falls off after the first 8 hours but before 12 hours, replace it with a new Striant system and skip your next scheduled dose until the following day.

Brushing your teeth, rinsing with mouthwash, chewing gum, and drinking alcohol do not appear to significantly alter the effectiveness of Striant. Check to see that the buccal system is in place following these activities, and if it becomes dislodged, follow the instructions above.

■ *If you miss a dose...*
Take it as soon as you remember. If the buccal system is replaced within 4 hours of your next scheduled dose, skip that dose and wait until the next day to replace the buccal system.

■ *Storage instructions...*
Store at room temperature and protect from heat and moisture. Do not use damaged blister packs.

What side effects may occur?
Side effects cannot be anticipated. If any develop or change in intensity, inform your doctor as soon as possible. Only your doctor can determine if it is safe for you to continue using Striant.

■ *Side effects may include:*
Bitter taste, gum or mouth irritation, gum pain, gum tenderness, headache

Why should this drug not be prescribed?
You cannot use Striant if you have had breast cancer or prostate cancer, or if you are allergic to testosterone. Striant is not intended for use by women.

Special warnings about this medication
Before using Striant, you should be aware that prolonged, high-dose therapy with male hormones is associated with liver disease and in some cases, liver cancer. Breast enlargement is also a common problem.

Remember too that older men who take male hormones are at higher risk for developing prostate disease or prostate cancer. Your doctor should examine you carefully before prescribing Striant if you have a medical profile that increases your risk for prostate cancer.

Inform your doctor if you experience breathing disturbances, especially during sleep. Testosterone replacement therapy tends to worsen sleep apnea, a condition that causes breathing to stop temporarily during sleep. Obese men and those with chronic lung disease are especially at risk.

You should periodically inspect the gum area where Striant is applied and report any irritations or changes in appearance to your physician.

If you have a history of heart, kidney, or liver disease and develop swelling in the hands, feet, or ankles, stop using Striant and alert your doctor immediately. Also contact your doctor if you develop too frequent or persistent erections, nausea, vomiting, or changes in breathing or skin color.

This drug has not been tested in males under 18 years of age.

Possible food and drug interactions when taking this medication

If Striant is taken with certain other drugs, the effects of either could be increased, decreased, or altered. It is especially important to check with your doctor before combining Striant with the following:

Insulin
Oxyphenbutazone
Steroids such as prednisone (Deltasone)

Special information if you are pregnant or breastfeeding

Striant is not indicated for use in women and must not be used by pregnant women or nursing mothers.

Recommended dosage

The recommended dose is one buccal system applied to the gum twice a day, in the morning and evening, about 12 hours apart. Each delivery system contains 30 milligrams of testosterone.

Overdosage

Any medication taken in excess can have serious consequences. If you suspect an overdose, seek medical attention immediately.

Sucralfate See Carafate, page 243.

SULAR

Pronounced: SOO-lar
Generic name: Nisoldipine

Why is this drug prescribed?

Sular controls high blood pressure. A long-acting tablet, Sular may be used alone or in combination with other blood pressure medications.

Sular is a type of medication called a calcium channel blocker. It inhibits the flow of calcium through the smooth muscles of the heart, delaying the passage of nerve impulses, slowing down the heart, and expanding the blood vessels. This eases the heart's workload and reduces your blood pressure.

Most important fact about this drug

You must take Sular regularly for it to be effective. Since blood pressure declines gradually, it may be several weeks before you get the full benefit of Sular, and you must continue taking it even if you are feeling well. Sular does not cure high blood pressure; it merely keeps it under control.

How should you take this medication?

Take Sular exactly as prescribed. Swallow the tablets whole. They should not be crushed, chewed, or divided. Avoid eating high-fat meals with

Sular, as the medication will not work properly. Do not consume grape-fruit products before or after taking Sular.

■ *If you miss a dose...*
Take it as soon as you remember. If it is almost time for your next dose, skip the one you missed and go back to your regular schedule. Never take 2 doses at the same time.

■ *Storage instructions...*
Store at room temperature in a tight, light-resistant container. Protect from moisture.

What side effects may occur?
Side effects cannot be anticipated. If any develop or change in intensity, tell your doctor as soon as possible. Only your doctor can determine if it is safe for you to continue taking Sular.

■ *Side effects may include:*
Dizziness, flushing, headache, heart palpitations, sinus inflammation, sore throat, swelling of the hands and feet

Why should this drug not be prescribed?
Avoid Sular if you have ever had an allergic reaction to it, or to similar cal-cium channel blockers such as Plendil and Procardia.

Special warnings about this medication
If you have a heart condition or liver disease, be sure the doctor is aware of it. Sular should be used with caution.

Sular may cause an excessive drop in blood pressure, especially when you are first taking the medication or when the dosage is increased. Low blood pressure can also become a problem if you are taking other blood pressure medications. If you develop symptoms of low blood pressure such as dizziness or light-headedness, call your doctor.

If you have angina (chest pain) or clogged coronary arteries, there is a remote possibility that Sular will make the condition worse—or even trigger a heart attack—when you first start taking the drug or its dosage is increased. Your doctor should be especially cautious if you have angina, heart failure, or other heart problems, particularly if you are also taking a medication known as a beta-blocker, such as Tenormin.

Possible food and drug interactions when taking this medication
If Sular is taken with certain other drugs, the effects of either could be in-creased, decreased, or altered. It is especially important to check with your doctor before combining Sular with the following:

Atenolol (Tenormin)
Cimetidine (Tagamet)
Phenytoin (Dilantin)
Quinidine (Quinidex)

Special information if you are pregnant or breastfeeding

The effects of Sular during pregnancy have not been adequately studied. If you are pregnant or plan to become pregnant, tell your doctor immediately. It is not known whether Sular makes its way into breast milk. Your doctor will advise you whether to stop taking Sular or forgo breastfeeding.

Recommended dosage

ADULTS

Your doctor will adjust the dosage to your individual needs. The usual starting dose is 20 milligrams once a day. At weekly intervals, the doctor may make 10-milligram increases in the dosage, depending on how your blood pressure responds. For the long term, the usual dosage ranges from 20 to 40 milligrams once daily. Doses above 60 milligrams are not recommended.

OLDER ADULTS

The usual starting dose is 10 milligrams. Dosage is adjusted upward according to your needs.

CHILDREN

Safety and effectiveness have not been established.

Overdosage

Any medication taken in excess can have serious consequences. Although no specific information is available, extremely low blood pressure is the most likely symptom of a Sular overdose. If you suspect an overdose, seek medical attention immediately.

Sulfacetamide See Sodium Sulamyd, page 1320.

Sulfacetamide and Sulfur See Avar, page 165.

Sulfasalazine See Azulfidine, page 185.

Sulfisoxazole See Gantrisin, page 612.

Sulindac See Clinoril, page 305.

Sumatriptan See Imitrex, page 670.

Sumycin See Tetracycline, page 1422.

SUPRAX

Pronounced: SUE-praks
Generic name: Cefixime

Why is this drug prescribed?

Suprax, a cephalosporin antibiotic, is prescribed for bacterial infections of the chest, ears, urinary tract, and throat and for uncomplicated gonorrhea.

Most important fact about this drug

If you are allergic to either penicillin or cephalosporin antibiotics in any form, consult your doctor *before* taking Suprax. An allergy to either type of medication may signal an allergy to Suprax, and if a reaction occurs, it could be extremely severe. If you take the drug and feel signs of a reaction, seek medical attention immediately.

How should you take this medication?

Suprax can be taken with or without food. If the medication causes stomach upset, take it with meals. Food, however, will slow down the rate at which medication is absorbed into your bloodstream.

If you are taking a liquid form of Suprax, use the specially marked measuring spoon to measure each dose accurately. Shake well before using.

It is important that you finish taking all of this medication even if you are feeling better, in order to obtain the medicine's maximum benefit.

■ *If you miss a dose...*
If you are taking this medication once a day and you forget to take a dose, take it as soon as you remember. Wait at least 10 to 12 hours before taking your next dose. Then return to your regular schedule.

If you are taking this medication 2 times a day and you forget to take a dose, take it as soon as you remember and take your next dose 5 to 6 hours later. Then go back to your regular schedule.

If you are taking this medication 3 times a day and you forget to take a dose, take it as soon as you remember and take your next dose 2 to 4 hours later. Then return to your regular schedule.

■ *Storage instructions...*
Suprax liquid may be kept for 14 days, either at room temperature or in the refrigerator. Keep the bottle tightly closed. Do not store in damp places. Keep out of reach of children and away from direct light and heat. Discard any unused portion after 14 days.

What side effects may occur?

Side effects cannot be anticipated. If any develop or change in intensity, inform your doctor as soon as possible. Only your doctor can determine if it is safe for you to continue taking Suprax.

■ *Side effects may include:*
Abdominal pain, gas, indigestion, loose stools, mild diarrhea, nausea, vomiting

Why should this drug not be prescribed?

If you are sensitive to or have ever had an allergic reaction to Suprax, other cephalosporin antibiotics, or any form of penicillin, you should not take this medication. Make sure that your doctor is aware of any drug reactions that you have experienced.

Special warnings about this medication

Notify your doctor if you have had allergic reactions to penicillins or other cephalosporin antibiotics.

If you have a history of stomach or intestinal disease such as colitis, check with your doctor before taking Suprax.

If your symptoms of infection do not improve within a few days, or if they get worse, notify your doctor immediately.

If you suffer nausea, vomiting, or severe diarrhea while taking Suprax, check with your doctor before taking a diarrhea medication. Some of these medications, such as Lomotil and Paregoric, may make your diarrhea worse or cause it to last longer.

If you are a diabetic, it is important to note that Suprax may cause false urine-sugar test results. Notify your doctor that you are taking this medication before being tested for sugar in the urine. Do not change diet or dosage of diabetes medication without first consulting with your doctor.

When prescribing Suprax, your doctor may perform laboratory tests to make certain it is effective against the bacteria causing the infection. Some bacteria do not respond to Suprax, so do not give it to other people or use it for other infections.

If you have a kidney disorder, check with your doctor before taking Suprax. You may need a reduced dose of this medication because of your medical condition.

Repeated use of Suprax may result in an overgrowth of bacteria that do not respond to the medication and can cause a secondary infection. Therefore, do not save this medication for use at another time. Take this medication only when directed to do so by your doctor.

Possible food and drug interactions when taking this medication

When Suprax and the seizure medication Tegretol are used together, the amount of Tegretol in the bloodstream may show an increase. Suprax may also increase the effect of anticlotting drugs such as Coumadin.

Special information if you are pregnant or breastfeeding

The effects of Suprax during pregnancy have not been adequately studied. If you are pregnant or plan to become pregnant, inform your doctor immediately. Suprax may appear in breast milk and could affect a nursing infant. If this medication is essential to your health, your doctor may advise you to discontinue breastfeeding your baby until your treatment with this medication is finished.

Recommended dosage

ADULTS

Infections Other than Gonorrhea
The usual adult dose is 400 milligrams daily. This may be taken as a single 400-milligram tablet once a day or as a 200-milligram tablet every 12 hours. If you have kidney disease, the dose may be lower.

Uncomplicated Gonorrhea
A single 400-milligram oral dose is usually prescribed.

CHILDREN

The safety and effectiveness of Suprax in children less than 6 months old have not been established. The usual child's dose is 8 milligrams of liquid per 2.2 pounds of body weight per day. This may be given as a single dose or in 2 half doses every 12 hours. Children weighing more than 110 pounds or older than 12 years of age should be treated with an adult dose.

If your child has a middle ear infection (otitis media), your doctor will probably prescribe Suprax suspension. The tablet form is less effective against this type of infection.

OLDER ADULTS

Your doctor may start you on a low dosage because this drug is eliminated from your body by the kidneys and kidney function tends to decrease with age.

Overdosage

Any medication taken in excess can cause symptoms of overdose. If you suspect an overdose, seek medical attention immediately.

■ *Symptoms of Suprax overdose may include:*
Blood in the urine, diarrhea, nausea, upper abdominal pain, vomiting

Surfak Liqui-Gels *See Colace, page 317.*

SURMONTIL

Pronounced: SIR-mon-til
Generic name: Trimipramine maleate

Why is this drug prescribed?

Surmontil is used to treat depression. It is a member of the family of drugs known as tricyclic antidepressants.

Most important fact about this drug

Serious, sometimes fatal, reactions have been known to occur when drugs such as Surmontil are taken with another type of antidepressant called an MAO inhibitor. Drugs in this category include Nardil and Parnate. Do not take Surmontil within 2 weeks of taking one of these drugs. Make sure your doctor and pharmacist know of all the medications you are taking.

How should you take this medication?

Surmontil may be taken in 1 dose at bedtime. Alternatively, the total daily dosage may be divided into smaller amounts taken during the day. If you are on long-term therapy with Surmontil, the single bedtime dose is preferred.

It is important to take Surmontil exactly as prescribed, even if the drug seems to have no effect. It may take up to 4 weeks for its benefits to appear.

Surmontil can make your mouth dry. Sucking hard candy or chewing gum can help this problem.

■ *If you miss a dose...*
Take it as soon as you remember. If it is almost time for the next dose, skip the one you missed and go back to your regular schedule. Do not take 2 doses at once. If you take Surmontil once a day at bedtime and you miss a dose, do not take it in the morning. It could cause disturbing side effects during the day.

■ *Storage instructions...*
Store at room temperature in a tightly closed container. Capsules in blister strips should be protected from moisture.

What side effects may occur?

Side effects cannot be anticipated. If any develop or change in intensity, inform your doctor as soon as possible. Only your doctor can determine if it is safe for you to continue taking Surmontil.

■ *Side effects may include:*
Allergic reactions, blood disorders, blurred vision, breast development in men, confusion, dry mouth, heartbeat irregularities, high blood pressure, insomnia, lack of coordination, low blood pressure, stomach and intestinal problems, urination problems

Why should this drug not be prescribed?

Surmontil should not be used if you are recovering from a recent heart attack.

You should not take Surmontil if you are sensitive to it or have ever had an allergic reaction to it or to similar drugs such as Tofranil.

Special warnings about this medication

In clinical studies, antidepressants increased the risk of suicidal thinking and behavior in children and adolescents with depression and other psychiatric disorders. Anyone considering the use of Surmontil or any other antidepressant in a child or adolescent must balance this risk with the clinical need. Surmontil has not been studied in children.

Additionally, the progression of major depression is associated with a worsening of symptoms and/or the emergence of suicidal thinking or behavior in both adults and children, whether or not they are taking antidepressants. Individuals being treated with Surmontil and their caregivers should watch for any change in symptoms or any new symptoms that appear suddenly—especially agitation, anxiety, hostility, panic, restlessness, extreme hyperactivity, and suicidal thinking or behavior—and report them to the doctor immediately. Be especially observant at the beginning of treatment or whenever there is a change in dose.

Use Surmontil cautiously if you have a seizure disorder, the eye condition known as glaucoma, heart disease, or a liver disorder. Also use caution if you have thyroid disease or are taking thyroid medication. People who have had problems urinating should also be careful about taking Surmontil.

Nausea, headache, and a general feeling of illness may result if you suddenly stop taking Surmontil. This does not mean you are addicted, but you should follow your doctor's instructions closely when discontinuing the drug.

This drug may impair your ability to drive a car or operate potentially dangerous machinery. Do not participate in any activities that require full alertness if you are unsure of the drug's effect on you.

Possible food and drug interactions when taking this medication

People who are taking antidepressants known as MAO inhibitors (Parnate and Nardil) should not take Surmontil. Wait 2 weeks after stopping an MAO inhibitor before you begin taking Surmontil.

If Surmontil is taken with certain other drugs, the effects of either could be increased, decreased, or altered. It is especially important to check with your doctor before combining Surmontil with the following:

Antidepressants such as Desyrel and Wellbutrin
Antidepressants that act on serotonin, such as Paxil, Prozac, and Zoloft
Antispasmodic drugs such as Donnatal and Cogentin

Cimetidine (Tagamet)
Drugs for heart irregularities, such as Rythmol and Tambocor
Guanethidine (Ismelin)
Local anesthetics containing epinephrine
Local decongestants such as Dristan Nasal Spray
Major tranquilizers such as Thorazine and Mellaril
Quinidine
Stimulants such as EpiPen, Proventil, and Sudafed
Thyroid medications such as Synthroid

Extreme drowsiness and other potentially serious effects may result if you drink alcoholic beverages while you are taking Surmontil.

Special information if you are pregnant or breastfeeding

The effects of Surmontil in pregnancy have not been adequately studied. Pregnant women should use Surmontil only when the potential benefits clearly outweigh the potential risks.

There is no information on whether Surmontil appears in breast milk. The doctor may have you stop breastfeeding until your treatment is finished.

Recommended dosage

ADULTS

The usual starting dose is 75 milligrams per day, divided into equal smaller doses. Your doctor may gradually increase your dose to 150 milligrams per day, divided into smaller doses. Doses over 200 milligrams a day are not recommended. Doses in long-term therapy may range from 50 to 150 milligrams daily. You can take this total daily dosage at bedtime or spread it throughout the day.

CHILDREN

Safety and effectiveness of Surmontil in children have not been established.

OLDER ADULTS AND ADOLESCENTS

Dosages usually start at 50 milligrams per day. Your doctor may increase the dose to 100 milligrams a day, if needed.

Overdosage

Any medication taken in excess can have serious consequences. An overdose of Surmontil can be fatal. If you suspect an overdose, seek medical help immediately.

■ *Symptoms of Surmontil overdose may include:*
Agitation, coma, confusion, convulsions, dilated pupils, disturbed concentration, drowsiness, hallucinations, high fever, irregular heart

rate, low body temperature, muscle rigidity, overactive reflexes, severely low blood pressure, stupor, vomiting

You may also have any of the symptoms listed under *What side effects may occur?*

SUSTIVA
Pronounced: suss-TEE-vah
Generic name: Efavirenz

Why is this drug prescribed?
Sustiva is one of the growing number of drugs used to fight HIV infection. HIV, the human immunodeficiency virus, weakens the immune system until it can no longer fight off infections, leading to the fatal disease known as AIDS (acquired immune deficiency syndrome).

Like other drugs for HIV, Sustiva works by impairing the virus's ability to multiply. However, when taken alone it may prompt the virus to become resistant. Sustiva is therefore always taken with at least one other HIV medication, such as Retrovir or Crixivan. Even when used properly, it may remain effective for only a limited time.

Most important fact about this drug
Though Sustiva can slow the progress of HIV, it is not a cure. HIV-related infections remain a danger, so frequent checkups and tests are still advisable.

How should you take this medication?
Be sure to take Sustiva every day, exactly as prescribed. Take the drug on an empty stomach, preferably at bedtime. Taking it at bedtime reduces the likelihood of side effects such as dizziness, impaired concentration, weakness, abnormal dreams, or drowsiness.

■ *If you miss a dose...*
Take it as soon as you remember. If it is almost time for the next dose, skip the one you missed and go back to your regular schedule. Do not double the dose.

■ *Storage instructions...*
Store at room temperature.

What side effects may occur?
Side effects cannot be anticipated. If any develop or change in intensity, inform your doctor as soon as possible. Only your doctor can determine if it is safe for you to continue taking Sustiva.

■ *Side effects may include:*
Abnormal dreaming, abnormal thinking, agitation, amnesia, confusion, cough, diarrhea, dizziness, drowsiness, fatigue, feelings of well-being,

fever, hallucinations, headache, impaired concentration, insomnia, loss of identity, nausea, skin rash, vomiting

Why should this drug not be prescribed?

Do not take Sustiva with the following medications. The combination could cause serious—even life-threatening—effects such as heart irregularities or disrupted breathing.

Ergot-based migraine medications such as D.H.E. 45, Ergostat, and Sansert
Midazolam (Versed)
Triazolam (Halcion)

If Sustiva gives you an allergic reaction, you cannot continue using it.

Special warnings about this medication

If you develop delusions, inappropriate behavior, severe depression, or suicidal thoughts, call your doctor immediately. Sustiva could be the cause, and may have to be discontinued. If you've suffered mental illness, substance abuse, or depression in the past, make sure the doctor is aware of this before therapy begins.

Roughly half the people taking Sustiva develop symptoms such as dizziness, lack of concentration, or drowsiness. Avoid driving or operating machinery while these symptoms occur. They are likely to improve with continued therapy, generally within 2 to 4 weeks.

One of the most common side effects of Sustiva is skin rash. Most rashes usually clear up on their own. However, for roughly 1 patient in 100, the drug causes a severe rash associated with blistering, skin peeling, and fever. If you develop this type of rash, call your doctor. You may have to stop taking Sustiva.

Because Sustiva has occasionally caused convulsions, use the drug with caution if you have a history of seizures. Your doctor will monitor you closely during treatment with Sustiva if you're also taking antiseizure drugs such as phenytoin (Dilantin), carbamazepine (Tegretol), or phenobarbital.

Another side effect seen in some people receiving drugs for HIV is a redistribution of body fat, leading to extra fat around the middle, a "buffalo hump" on the back, and wasting in the arms, legs, and face. Researchers don't know whether this represents a long-term health problem or not.

In a few patients, Sustiva has toxic effects on the liver. If you've had hepatitis or must take other medications that could damage the liver, your doctor will probably check your liver function regularly.

Sustiva also has a tendency to raise cholesterol levels in some patients. If you have a cholesterol problem, your doctor may test for this as well.

Remember that Sustiva does not completely eliminate HIV from the body. The virus can still be passed to others during sex or through blood contamination.

Possible food and drug interactions when taking this medication

Be sure to avoid combining Sustiva with Versed, Halcion, or any of the migraine medications listed under *Why should this drug not be prescribed?*

If Sustiva is taken with certain other drugs, the effects of either could be increased, decreased, or altered. It is especially important to check with your doctor before combining Sustiva with the following:

Alcohol
Amprenavir (Agenerase)
Carbamazepine (Tegretol)
Clarithromycin (Biaxin)
Indinavir (Crixivan)
Itraconazole (Sporanox)
Ketoconazole (Nizoral)
Methadone (Dolophine)
Nelfinavir (Viracept)
Oral contraceptives containing ethinyl estradiol, such as Estinyl, Ovcon, and Ovral
Phenobarbital
Phenytoin (Dilantin)
Rifabutin (Mycobutin)
Rifampin (Rifadin and Rimactane)
Ritonavir (Norvir)
Saquinavir (Fortovase and Invirase)
St. John's wort
Warfarin (Coumadin)

Special information if you are pregnant or breastfeeding

Sustiva may be capable of harming a developing baby and should not be taken during pregnancy. Before you begin Sustiva therapy, your doctor will test to make sure that you're not pregnant. While taking the drug, you should use both a barrier type of contraceptive and a second method such as contraceptive pills.

Avoid breastfeeding. HIV infection can be passed to a nursing infant through breast milk.

Recommended dosage

ADULTS

The recommended dose is 600 milligrams once a day, in combination with other HIV medications.

CHILDREN

For children 3 years of age and older, weighing between 22 and 88 pounds, the recommended dose is based upon weight. Children weighing more than 88 pounds receive the 600-milligram adult dose.

Overdosage

Any medication taken in excess can have serious consequences. If you suspect an overdose, seek medical attention immediately.

■ *Symptoms of Sustiva overdose may include:*
Increased nervous system symptoms (such as dizziness, weakness, confusion, impaired concentration, and hallucinations); involuntary muscle contractions

SYMBYAX

Pronounced: SIM-bee-ax
Generic ingredients: Olanzapine, Fluoxetine hydrochloride

Why is this drug prescribed?

Symbyax is used to treat depressive episodes associated with bipolar disorder. Bipolar disorder, sometimes called manic-depressive illness, is a condition in which a person's mood swings from depression to excessive excitement.

Symbyax is a combination of the active ingredients in Prozac (fluoxetine, used to treat depression and other conditions) and Zyprexa (olanzapine, used to treat the manic phase of bipolar disorder as well as other conditions).

Most important fact about this drug

If you have bipolar disorder, you may think about, or try to commit, suicide. You also may think about harming others. If you have any of these thoughts, tell your doctor immediately or go to an emergency center. If your doctor feels that you are at risk for these symptoms, he or she will monitor you closely while you are taking Symbyax.

Drugs such as Symbyax may increase the risk of death in elderly people with dementia-related psychosis. Symbyax is not approved for use in such patients.

Serious, sometimes fatal reactions have been known to occur when fluoxetine, one of the ingredients in Symbyax, is taken with other antidepressant drugs called MAO inhibitors, including Nardil and Parnate. Such reactions have also occurred when fluoxetine is discontinued and an MAO inhibitor is started. Never take Symbyax with an MAO inhibitor, or within 14 days of discontinuing therapy with an MAO inhibitor. Allow 5 weeks or more between stopping Symbyax and starting an MAO inhibitor. Be especially careful if you have been taking Symbyax in high doses or for a long time.

If you are taking any prescription or nonprescription medications, notify your doctor before taking Symbyax (see *Possible food and drug interactions when taking this medication*).

How should you take this medication?

Symbyax can be taken with or without food. It is best to take it in the evening. Take Symbyax exactly as prescribed. Keep taking the medication even if your mood improves. Never change your dosage or stop taking Symbyax without consulting your doctor.

■ *If you miss a dose...*
Take the forgotten dose as soon as you remember. However, if it is almost time for your next dose, skip the one you missed and return to your regular schedule. Do not take 2 doses at once.

■ *Storage instructions...*
Store at room temperature. Keep the container tightly closed and protect the drug from moisture.

What side effects may occur?

Side effects cannot be anticipated. If any develop or change in intensity, tell your doctor as soon as possible. Only your doctor can determine if it is safe to continue using Symbyax.

■ *Side effects may include:*
Abnormal thinking, increased appetite, lack of coordination, sleepiness, sore throat, tremor, water retention (especially in the arms and legs), weakness, weight gain

Why should this drug not be prescribed?

Symbyax is a combination of the ingredients in Prozac and Zyprexa. You cannot use Symbyax if you have experienced an allergic reaction to any of its ingredients, or to Prozac or Zyprexa. Make sure that your doctor is aware of any drug reaction that you have experienced.

Do not take Symbyax with an MAO inhibitor (see *Most important fact about this drug*) or with thioridazine (Mellaril) (see *Possible food and drug interactions while taking this medication*).

Special warnings about this medication

In clinical studies, antidepressants increased the risk of suicidal thinking and behavior in children and adolescents with depression and other psychiatric disorders. Anyone considering the use of Symbyax or any other antidepressant in a child or adolescent must balance this risk with the clinical need. Symbyax is not approved for use in children.

Additionally, the progression of major depression is associated with a worsening of symptoms and/or the emergence of suicidal thinking or behavior in both adults and children, whether or not they are taking antidepressants. Individuals being treated with Symbyax and their caregivers should watch for any change in symptoms or any new symptoms that appear suddenly—especially agitation, anxiety, hostility, panic, restlessness, extreme hyperactivity, and suicidal thinking or behavior—and report them to the doctor immediately. Be especially observant at the beginning of treatment or whenever there is a change in dose.

Certain antipsychotic drugs—including olanzapine, one of the ingredients in Symbyax—are associated with an increased risk of developing high blood sugar, which on rare occasions has led to coma or death. See your doctor right away if you develop signs of high blood sugar, including dry mouth, unusual thirst, increased urination, and tiredness. If you have diabetes or have a high risk of developing it, see your doctor regularly for blood sugar testing.

Use Symbyax with caution if you have a history of heart disease, heart rhythm problems, stroke, seizures, or liver problems. Also be cautious if you're at risk of developing low blood pressure (for example, when you're dehydrated).

Symbyax has not been studied in people with certain diseases. However, the individual ingredients in this drug have been known to cause problems in people with specific illnesses. Be sure to tell the doctor if you've ever had any of the following: heart attack, heart disease, an enlarged prostate, high or low blood pressure, abnormal bleeding, narrow-angle glaucoma, paralysis of the intestines, trouble swallowing, Alzheimer's disease, or dementia (if you're older than 65).

Symbyax can cause dizziness and even fainting when getting up from sitting or lying down. If you experience this, notify your doctor.

The ingredients in this drug could cause an allergic reaction. Tell your doctor immediately if you develop a skin rash or hives.

Olanzapine and other antipsychotic drugs can cause a condition called Neuroleptic Malignant Syndrome (NMS). Symptoms include high fever, muscle rigidity, irregular pulse or blood pressure, rapid or irregular heartbeat, and excessive sweating. If these symptoms appear, contact your doctor immediately.

Symbyax could increase the risk of developing tardive dyskinesia, a condition marked by slow, rhythmic, involuntary movements. This problem is more likely to surface in older adults, especially women. If it does, your doctor may have you stop taking Symbyax.

Symbyax could trigger a manic episode. Your doctor will watch you closely for symptoms of mania.

Medications such as Symbyax can interfere with the regulation of body temperature. Do not get overheated or become dehydrated while taking Symbyax. Avoid extreme heat and drink plenty of fluids.

Symbyax sometimes causes drowsiness. It can impair your judgment, thinking, and motor skills. Use caution while driving, and don't operate dangerous machinery until you know how the drug affects you.

Serotonin-boosting antidepressants such as fluoxetine, one of the ingredients in Symbyax, could potentially cause stomach bleeding. This is especially likely when serotonin boosters are combined with nonsteroidal anti-inflammatory drugs (NSAIDs) such as aspirin, ibuprofen (Advil, Motrin), naproxen (Aleve), and ketoprofen (Orudis KT). Consult your doctor before combining Symbyax with NSAIDs or blood-thinning medications.

Animal studies suggest that olanzapine, one of the ingredients in Symbyax, may increase the risk of breast cancer, although human studies have not confirmed such a risk. If you have a history of breast cancer, see your doctor regularly for checkups.

Prolonged seizures have occurred in people receiving electroconvulsive therapy (ECT) while taking fluoxetine, one of the ingredients in Symbyax. To date, there are no clinical studies establishing the benefit of combined treatment with fluoxetine and ECT.

Possible food and drug interactions when taking this medication

Avoid alcohol while taking Symbyax. The combination can cause a sudden drop in blood pressure.

Never combine Symbyax with MAO inhibitors (see *Most important fact about this drug*).

Do not take Symbyax with thioridazine (Mellaril). Wait at least 5 weeks between stopping Symbyax and starting thioridazine.

Be careful using Symbyax with Zyprexa, Zyprexa Zydis, Prozac, Prozac Weekly, or Sarafem. Symbyax contains the same active ingredients as these medications.

Be careful about combining Symbyax with aspirin or nonsteroidal anti-inflammatory drugs (NSAIDs) such as ibuprofen, or with other drugs that affect blood clotting. The combination may increase the risk of bleeding.

If Symbyax is taken with certain other drugs, the effects of either can be increased, decreased, or altered. Ask your doctor before taking any other prescription or over-the-counter medication. It is especially important to check before combining Symbyax with the following:

Antidepressants known as tricyclics, such as Elavil
Blood pressure medications
Carbamazepine (Tegretol)
Clozapine (Clozaril)
Diazepam (Valium)
Drugs that boost the effect of dopamine, such as the Parkinson's
  medications Mirapex, Parlodel, Permax, and Requip
Fluvoxamine
Haloperidol (Haldol)
Levodopa (Larodopa)
Lithium (Eskalith)
Phenytoin (Dilantin)
Pimozide (Orap)
Sumatriptan (Imitrex)
Tryptophan
Warfarin (Coumadin)

Let the doctor know if you smoke cigarettes, since this could affect how your body processes Symbyax.

Special information if you are pregnant or breastfeeding

If you are pregnant or plan to become pregnant, notify your doctor immediately. Symbyax should be used during pregnancy only if absolutely necessary.

You should not breastfeed while taking Symbyax. The drug may pass into breast milk and harm your baby.

Recommended dosage

ADULTS

The usual starting dose is one capsule containing 6 milligrams of olanzapine and 25 milligrams of fluoxetine, taken once a day in the evening. If needed, the doctor may gradually increase the dose. The usual dosage range is 6 to 12 milligrams of olanzapine and 25 to 50 milligrams of fluoxetine.

The doctor may adjust your dosage if you have liver problems, a high risk of low blood pressure, or a combination of factors that may slow your body's processing of Symbyax (female, older age, nonsmoker).

CHILDREN

The safety and effectiveness of Symbyax have not been studied in children.

Overdosage

Overdose with fluoxetine, one of the ingredients in Symbyax, can be fatal. There have been reports of patients dying after overdosing on fluoxetine and olanzapine taken as separate drugs at the same time. If you suspect an overdose, seek emergency treatment immediately.

■ *Symptoms of overdose may include:*
Aggressive behavior, agitation, coma, confusion, convulsions, heart problems, irregular or fast heartbeat, loss of consciousness, problems with muscle coordination, problems with speech, sleepiness, sluggishness

SYNALGOS-DC

Pronounced: SIN-al-gose dee-cee
Generic ingredients: Dihydrocodeine bitartrate,
  Aspirin, Caffeine

Why is this drug prescribed?

Synalgos-DC is a narcotic analgesic prescribed for the relief of moderate to moderately severe pain.

Most important fact about this drug

Narcotics such as Synalgos-DC can be habit-forming or addicting if they are taken over long periods of time.

How should you take this medication?

Take Synalgos-DC exactly as prescribed. Do not increase the amount you take without your doctor's approval.

Avoid or reduce use of alcohol while taking Synalgos-DC.

■ *If you miss a dose...*
If you take this drug on a regular schedule, take the forgotten dose as soon as you remember. If it is almost time for your next dose, skip the one you missed and go back to your regular schedule. Do not take 2 doses at once.

■ *Storage instructions...*
Store at room temperature in a tightly closed container.

What side effects may occur?

Side effects cannot be anticipated. If any develop or change in intensity, inform your doctor as soon as possible. Only your doctor can determine if it is safe for you to continue taking Synalgos-DC.

■ *Side effects may include:*
Constipation, dizziness, drowsiness, itching, light-headedness, nausea, sedation, skin reactions, vomiting

Why should this drug not be prescribed?

If you are sensitive to or have ever had an allergic reaction to Synalgos-DC, other narcotic pain relievers, or aspirin, you should not take this medication.

Make sure your doctor is aware of any drug reactions you have experienced.

Special warnings about this medication

Synalgos-DC may cause you to become drowsy or less alert; therefore, you should not drive or operate dangerous machinery or participate in any hazardous activity that requires full mental alertness until you know how this drug affects you.

If you have ever been dependent on or addicted to drugs, consult your doctor before taking Synalgos-DC.

If you are being treated for a stomach ulcer or blood clotting disorder, consult your doctor before taking this medication.

Possible food and drug interactions when taking this medication

Synalgos-DC slows brain activity and intensifies the effects of alcohol. Therefore, you should reduce your intake of alcoholic beverages or avoid them altogether.

If Synalgos-DC is taken with certain other drugs, the effects of either could be increased, decreased, or altered. It is especially important to check with your doctor before combining Synalgos-DC with the following:

Narcotic pain relievers such as Demerol and Percocet
Sedatives such as Halcion and Seconal
Tranquilizers such as Valium and Xanax

Taking blood thinners such as Coumadin in combination with Synalgos-DC may cause internal bleeding.

The use of Synalgos-DC in combination with antigout medications such as Benemid may alter its effects.

Special information if you are pregnant or breastfeeding

The effects of Synalgos-DC during pregnancy have not been adequately studied. If you are pregnant or plan to become pregnant, inform your doctor immediately. This drug may appear in breast milk and could affect a nursing infant. If this medication is essential to your health, your doctor may advise you to discontinue breastfeeding until your treatment is finished.

Recommended dosage

ADULTS

Your doctor will prescribe a dosage based on the severity of your pain and how you respond to this medication. The usual dose of Synalgos-DC is 2 capsules taken every 4 hours as needed.

CHILDREN

The safety and effectiveness of this medication have not been established in children 12 years of age and under.

OLDER ADULTS

Synalgos-DC should be taken with caution by older adults or anyone in a weakened or run-down condition. Therefore, your doctor will adjust the dosage accordingly.

Overdosage

Although no specific information is available, any medication taken in excess can have serious consequences. If you suspect an overdose of Synalgos-DC, seek medical attention immediately.

SYNAREL

Pronounced: SIN-er-el
Generic name: Nafarelin acetate

Why is this drug prescribed?

Synarel is used to relieve the symptoms of endometriosis, including menstrual cramps or low back pain during menstruation, painful inter-course, painful bowel movements, and abnormal and heavy menstrual bleeding. Endometriosis is a condition in which fragments of the tissue that lines the uterus are found in the other parts of the pelvic cavity. Synarel is also used to treat unusually early puberty in children of both sexes.

Some doctors prescribe Synarel as a contraceptive for both men and women.

Most important fact about this drug

Although Synarel usually stops ovulation and menstruation, there is still a possibility of becoming pregnant while taking the medication. Since Synarel could harm a fetus, be sure to use a non-hormonal, barrier form of birth control such as condoms and diaphragms. If you should become pregnant, stop the drug and tell your doctor immediately.

How should you take this medication?

Take this medication exactly as prescribed.

Synarel is sprayed into one nostril in the morning and the other nostril in the evening. If your doctor increases the dose, you will spray Synarel into both nostrils morning and evening.

Try not to sneeze during or immediately after spraying Synarel into your nostrils.

Wait 2 hours after taking Synarel before using a decongestant spray or drops.

You should not use Synarel for more than 6 months. If your symptoms recur after you have finished taking the medication, your doctor will usu-ally not prescribe it again.

Before you use each new bottle of Synarel for the first time, you have to prime the spray pump. Remove the plastic wrap from the spray bottle and hold it in an upright position pointed away from you. Applying pres-sure evenly to the shoulders, push down quickly and firmly 7 to 10 times. Usually the spray will appear after about 7 pumps. Priming need only be done once.

To use the Synarel Nasal Spray Unit, follow these steps:
1. Gently blow your nose to clear both nostrils.
2. Remove the safety clip and clear plastic dust cover from the spray bottle.

3. Bend your head forward a little and put the spray tip into one nostril. Close the other nostril with your finger.
4. Applying pressure evenly to the shoulders, quickly and firmly pump the sprayer one time while gently sniffing in.
5. Remove the sprayer from your nose and tilt your head backwards for a few seconds. Do not take additional sprays unless your doctor has specifically instructed you to do so.
6. Wipe tip of the pump with a soft cloth or tissue after each use.

■ *If you miss a dose...*
Take it as soon as you remember. If it is almost time for your next dose, skip the one you missed and go back to your regular schedule. Never try to catch up by doubling the dose.

Try not to miss any doses. If you miss successive doses, bleeding and ovulation can start again, and you could become pregnant.

■ *Storage instructions...*
Store the Synarel bottle upright at room temperature. Protect from excessive heat and freezing. Keep away from light.

What side effects may occur?
Side effects cannot be anticipated. If any develop or change in intensity, inform your doctor as soon as possible. Only your doctor can determine whether it is safe for you to continue taking Synarel.

■ *Side effects may include:*
Acne, decrease in breast size, decreased sex drive, depression, dry skin, hair growth, headaches, hot flashes, insomnia, muscle pain, nasal inflammation, nasal irritation, oily skin, rapidly shifting or changing emotions, swelling due to fluid retention, vaginal dryness, weight gain

When Synarel is used in the treatment of early puberty, it causes body odor and a transient increase in the amount of pubic hair.

Why should this drug not be prescribed?
Do not take Synarel is you are sensitive to it or have ever had an allergic reaction to it or to any of its ingredients.

Your doctor should not prescribe Synarel if you have undiagnosed vaginal bleeding between menstrual periods.

You should not take Synarel if you are pregnant or breastfeeding.

Special warnings about this medication
Because Synarel works by temporarily reducing the body's production of estrogen, you may experience some of the same changes that normally occur at the time of menopause, when the body's production of estrogen decreases naturally. For the first 2 months after you start using Synarel, you may have some irregular vaginal bleeding. This will stop by itself.

Your menstrual periods should stop completely during Synarel therapy. If you continue to bleed regularly, or if you spot or bleed between periods, inform your physician immediately. Vaginal bleeding can occur if you are not following your doctor's instructions carefully or if you need a higher dosage of the medication.

Synarel can cause vaginal dryness. If this is a problem, especially during sexual intercourse, you may want to use a vaginal lubricant. Ask your doctor or pharmacist for a recommendation.

Synarel may cause a small amount of bone loss over the course of your treatment. If you consume large amounts of alcohol, smoke, have a strong family history of osteoporosis, or use drugs that can reduce bone mass such as anticonvulsants or steroids, discuss your condition with your doctor before using Synarel. It may be wiser for you to take another medication.

If your nasal passages become inflamed, your doctor may prescribe a medication to relieve your congestion while you are taking Synarel.

Possible food and drug interactions when taking this medication
No interactions have been reported.

Special information if you are pregnant or breastfeeding
Although the effects of Synarel during pregnancy have not been adequately studied, it is known that the medication could cause harm to a developing baby. If you are pregnant, inform your doctor immediately. Use a barrier method of birth control to prevent pregnancy while you are taking this medication.

It is not known whether Synarel appears in breast milk. If this drug is essential to your health, your doctor will advise you to discontinue breastfeeding until your treatment with the medication is finished.

Recommended dosage
The recommended dosage of Synarel is 400 micrograms daily, divided into 2 doses—1 spray (200 micrograms) into one nostril in the morning and 1 spray into the other nostril in the evening. Start your treatment between days 2 and 4 of your menstrual cycle.

If the above dosage does not stop your menstrual period after 2 months of treatment, your doctor may increase your dosage to 800 micrograms daily—1 spray into each nostril in the morning and a second spray into each nostril in the evening.

Treatment should last no more than 6 months.

Overdosage
Although there is no information on Synarel overdose, any medication taken in excess can have serious consequences. If you suspect an overdose, seek medical attention immediately.

SYNTHROID

Pronounced: SIN-throid
Generic name: Levothyroxine
Other brand names: Levothroid, Levoxyl, Unithroid

Why is this drug prescribed?

Synthroid, a synthetic thyroid hormone may be given in any of the following cases:

If your own thyroid gland is not making enough hormone

If you have an enlarged thyroid (a goiter) or are at risk for developing a goiter

If you have certain cancers of the thyroid

If your thyroid production is low due to surgery, radiation, certain drugs, or disease of the pituitary gland or hypothalamus in the brain

Most important fact about this drug

If you are taking Synthroid to make up for a lack of natural hormone, it is important to take it regularly at the same time every day. You will probably need to take it for the rest of your life.

How should you take this medication?

Take Synthroid as a single dose, preferably on an empty stomach, one-half to one hour before breakfast. The drug is absorbed better on an empty stomach.

If an infant or child cannot swallow whole tablets, you may crush a Synthroid tablet and mix it into 1 or 2 teaspoonfuls of water.

While taking Synthroid, your doctor will perform periodic blood tests to determine whether you are getting the right amount.

■ *If you miss a dose...*
Take it as soon as you remember. If it is almost time for your next dose, skip the one you missed and go back to your regular schedule. Never take 2 doses at the same time. If you miss 2 or more doses in a row, consult your doctor.

■ *Storage instructions...*
Keep this medication in a tightly closed container. Store it at room temperature, away from light and moisture.

What side effects may occur?

Side effects from Synthroid, other than overdose symptoms, are rare. People who are treated with Synthroid may initially lose some hair, but this effect is usually temporary. You may have an allergic reaction such as a rash or hives. Children may have an increase in pressure within the skull. Excessive dosage or a too rapid increase in dosage may lead to overstimulation of the thyroid gland. Notify your doctor immediately if you develop any if the following symptoms.

■ *Symptoms of overstimulation:*
   Abdominal cramps, anxiety, changes in appetite, change in menstrual periods, chest pain, diarrhea, emotional instability, fatigue, fever, flushing, hair loss, headache, heart attack or failure, heat intolerance, hyperactivity, increased heart rate, irregular heartbeat, irritability, muscle weakness, nausea, nervousness, palpitations, shortness of breath, sleeplessness, sweating, tremors, vomiting, weight loss

Why should this drug not be prescribed?
You should not be treated with Synthroid if you are hypersensitive to thyroid hormone; your thyroid gland is making too much thyroid hormone; you have had a recent heart attack; or your adrenal glands are not making enough corticosteroid hormone. If you are sensitive to dyes, you can take the Synthroid 50-microgram tablet, which is made without color additives.

Although Synthroid will speed up your metabolism, it is not effective as a weight loss drug and should not be used as such. An overdose may cause life-threatening side effects, especially if you take Synthroid with an appetite suppressant medication.

Special warnings about this medication
Synthroid has profound effects on the body. Make sure your doctor is aware of all your medical problems, especially heart disease, clotting disorders, diabetes, and disorders of the adrenal or pituitary glands. The doctor will also need to know about any allergies you may have to food or medicine, and will ask for the names of any medications you take, whether prescription or over-the-counter.

You should receive low doses of Synthroid, under very close supervision, if you are an older person, or if you suffer from high blood pressure, angina (chest pain caused by a heart condition), or other types of heart disease. If you develop chest pain or additional circulatory problems, your dosage may have to be reduced.

If you have diabetes, or if your body makes insufficient adrenal corticosteroid hormone, Synthroid will tend to make your symptoms worse. If you take medication for any of these disorders, the dosage will probably have to be adjusted once you begin taking Synthroid. If diabetes is the problem, you should immediately report to your doctor any change in your glucose readings.

Postmenopausal women on long-term Synthroid therapy may suffer a loss of bone density, increasing the danger of osteoporosis (brittle bones). To minimize the loss, the doctor will prescribe the lowest dosage needed to control symptoms of thyroid deficiency.

Synthroid may cause seizures at the beginning of treatment, although this is rare. You may also notice some hair loss at first, but this is temporary.

It may take a few weeks for Synthroid to begin working, and you may not see any change in your symptoms until then.

Tell your doctor or dentist you are taking Synthroid before you have surgery of any kind.

Tell your doctor if you become pregnant while you are taking Synthroid. Your dose may need to be increased.

Do not switch to another brand of levothyroxine without consulting your doctor.

Excessive doses of Synthroid in infants may cause the top of the skull to close too early. In children, overtreatment can stunt growth.

Possible food and drug interactions when taking this medication
Synthroid can interact with a wide variety of medications. It's advisable to check with your doctor before taking *any* other drug, but you should be especially wary of the following:

Amiodarone (Cordarone)
Androgens (male hormones)
Antacids and antigas medications
Antidepressants such as Elavil, Ludiomil, and Zoloft
Blood pressure drugs such as beta-blockers, nitroprusside, and thiazide diuretics
Blood-thinning drugs such as Coumadin and heparin
Chloral hydrate (a sedative)
Diabetes drugs such as insulin and Micronase
Digitalis-type drugs such as Lanoxin
Estrogen products and oral contraceptives
Furosemide (Lasix)
Growth hormones
Hormone inhibitors such as Cytadren and Tapazole
Iodide
Iron supplements
Kayexalate
Ketamine (Ketalar)
Lithium (Eskalith, Lithobid)
Methadone and heroin
Metoclopramide (Reglan)
Nonsteroidal anti-inflammatory drugs such as phenylbutazone and aspirin
Parkinson's drugs such as Sinemet
Propylthiouracil (a thyroid inhibitor)
Seizure medications such as Dilantin, phenobarbital, and Tegretol
Steroids such as dexamethasone and hydrocortisone
Stimulants such as epinephrine (EpiPen)

Sucralfate (Carafate)

The cancer drugs 5-fluorouracil, 6-mercaptopurine, mitotane, and tamoxifen

The cholesterol-lowering drugs Colestid, Mevacor, and Questran

The immune system drugs interferon and interleukin

The tranquilizers Trilafon and Valium

The tuberculosis drugs aminosalicylate, rifampin, and ethionamide

Theophylline (Theo-Dur)

A high-fiber diet, soy-containing supplements, and walnuts can also interfere with Synthroid's effects.

Special information if you are pregnant or breastfeeding

If you need to take Synthroid because of a thyroid hormone deficiency, you can continue to take the medication during pregnancy. In fact, your doctor will test you regularly and may increase your dose. Once your baby is born, you may breastfeed while continuing to take carefully regulated doses of Synthroid.

Recommended dosage

Your doctor will tailor the dosage to meet your individual requirements, taking into consideration the status of your thyroid gland and other medical conditions you may have. Older adults often require somewhat smaller doses. To make sure the dosage is right for you, the doctor will monitor your thyroid hormone level with periodic blood tests.

Overdosage

An overdose of Synthroid can produce the same symptoms of overstimulation listed under *What side effects may occur?* Confusion and disorientation are also possible, and there have been reports of stroke, shock, coma, and death. If you suspect a massive overdose, seek emergency medical attention immediately.

Tacrine See Cognex, page 314.

Tadalafil See Cialis, page 284.

TAGAMET

Pronounced: TAG-ah-met
Generic name: Cimetidine
Other brand name: Tagamet HB

Why is this drug prescribed?

Tagamet is prescribed for the treatment of certain kinds of stomach and intestinal ulcers and related conditions. These include: active duodenal (upper intestinal) ulcers; active benign stomach ulcers; erosive gastro-esophageal reflux disease (backflow of acid stomach contents); prevention of upper abdominal bleeding in those who are critically ill; and excess acid conditions such as Zollinger-Ellison syndrome (a form of peptic ulcer with too much acid). It is also used for maintenance therapy of duodenal ulcer following the healing of active ulcers. Tagamet is known as a histamine blocker.

Some doctors also use Tagamet to treat acne and to prevent stress-induced ulcers. It may also be used to treat chronic hives, herpesvirus infections (including shingles), abnormal hair growth in women, and overactivity of the parathyroid gland.

Tagamet HB is an over-the-counter version of the drug used to relieve heartburn, acid indigestion, and sour stomach.

Most important fact about this drug
Short-term treatment with Tagamet can result in complete healing of a duodenal ulcer. However, there can be a recurrence of the ulcer after Tagamet has been discontinued. The rate of ulcer recurrence may be slightly higher in people healed with Tagamet rather than other forms of therapy. However, Tagamet is usually prescribed for more severe cases.

How should you take this medication?
You can take Tagamet with or between meals. Do not take antacids within 1 to 2 hours of a dose of Tagamet. Avoid excessive amounts of caffeine while taking this drug.

It may take several days for Tagamet to begin relieving stomach pain. Be sure to continue taking the drug exactly as prescribed even if it seems to have no effect.

Do not take the maximum daily dose of Tagamet HB for more than 2 weeks continuously without consulting your doctor.

■ *If you miss a dose...*
Take it as soon as you remember. If it is almost time for your next dose, skip the one you missed and go back to your regular schedule. Do not take 2 doses at once.

■ *Storage instructions...*
Store at room temperature in a tightly closed container, away from light.

What side effects may occur?
Side effects cannot be anticipated. If any develop or change in intensity, inform your doctor as soon as possible. Only your doctor can determine if it is safe for you to continue taking Tagamet.

■ *Side effects may include:*
Breast development in men, headache

Less common side effects—agitation, anxiety, confusion, depression, disorientation, and hallucinations—may appear in severely ill individuals who have been treated for 1 month or longer. However, these reactions are not permanent and have cleared up within 3 to 4 days of discontinuation of the drug.

Why should this drug not be prescribed?

If you have ever had an allergic reaction to Tagamet, do not take this medication.

Special warnings about this medication

Ulcers may be more difficult to heal if you smoke cigarettes.

If you are being treated for a liver or kidney disorder, make sure the doctor is aware if it.

If you are over 50 years old, have liver or kidney disease, or are severely ill, you may experience temporary mental confusion while taking Tagamet. Notify your doctor.

If you have trouble swallowing or persistent abdominal pain, do not take Tagamet HB; instead, check with your doctor. You may have a serious condition that requires different treatment.

Possible food and drug interactions when taking this medication

If Tagamet is taken with certain other drugs, the effects of either can be increased, decreased, or altered. It is especially important that you check with your doctor before combining Tagamet with the following:

Antidiabetic drugs such as Glucotrol and Micronase
Antifungal drugs such as Diflucan and Nizoral
Aspirin
Augmentin
Benzodiazepine tranquilizers such as Librium and Valium
Beta-blocking blood pressure drugs such as Inderal and Lopressor
Calcium-blocking blood pressure drugs such as Calan, Cardizem, and Procardia
Chlorpromazine (Thorazine)
Cisapride (Propulsid)
Cyclosporine (Sandimmune)
Digoxin (Lanoxin)
Medications for irregular heartbeat, such as Cordarone, Procan, Tonocard, and Quinidex
Metoclopramide (Reglan)
Metronidazole (Flagyl)
Narcotic pain relievers such as Demerol and Morphine
Nicotine (Nicoderm, Nicorette)
Paroxetine (Paxil)
Pentoxifylline (Trental)
Phenytoin (Dilantin)
Quinine

Sucralfate (Carafate)
Theophylline (Theo-Dur, others)
Warfarin (Coumadin)

Avoid alcoholic beverages while taking Tagamet. This medication increases the effects of alcohol.

Antacids can reduce the effect of Tagamet when taken at the same time. If you take an antacid to relieve the pain of an ulcer, the doses should be separated by 1 to 2 hours.

If you need to take an antifungal drug such as Nizoral, you should take it at least 2 hours before you take Tagamet.

Special information if you are pregnant or breastfeeding

The effects of Tagamet during pregnancy have not been adequately studied. If you are pregnant or plan to become pregnant, notify your doctor immediately. Tagamet appears in breast milk and could affect a nursing infant. If this medication is essential to your health, your doctor may advise you to discontinue breastfeeding until treatment with this drug is finished.

Recommended dosage

TAGAMET (ADULTS)

Active Duodenal Ulcer
The usual dose is 800 milligrams once daily at bedtime. However, other doses shown to be effective are:

   300 milligrams 4 times a day with meals and at bedtime
   400 milligrams twice a day, in the morning and at bedtime
   Most people heal in 4 weeks.

If you require maintenance therapy, the usual dose is 400 milligrams at bedtime.

Active Benign Gastric Ulcer
The usual dose is 800 milligrams once a day at bedtime or 300 milligrams taken 4 times a day with meals and at bedtime.

Erosive Gastroesophageal Reflux Disease
The usual dosage is a total of 1,600 milligrams daily divided into doses of 800 milligrams twice a day or 400 milligrams 4 times a day for 12 weeks. The beneficial use of Tagamet beyond 12 weeks has not been firmly established.

Pathological Hypersecretory Condition
The usual dosage is 300 milligrams 4 times a day with meals and at bedtime. Your doctor may adjust your dosage based on your needs, but you should take no more than 2,400 milligrams per day.

TAGAMET (CHILDREN)

Safety and effectiveness have not been established in children under 16 years old. However, your doctor may decide that the potential benefits of Tagamet use outweigh the potential risks. Doses of 20 to 40 milligrams per 2.2 pounds of body weight have been used.

TAGAMET HB

Heartburn, Acid Indigestion, Sour Stomach
The usual dosage is 2 tablets, taken with water, once or up to twice a day. Do not take more than 4 tablets in 24 hours.

Do not give Tagamet HB to children under 12 years unless your doctor tells you to.

Overdosage

Information concerning overdosage is limited. However, respiratory failure, an increased heartbeat, exaggerated side effect symptoms or reactions such as unresponsiveness may be signs of Tagamet overdose. If you experience any of these symptoms, notify your doctor immediately.

TAMBOCOR

Pronounced: TAM-ba-kore
Generic name: Flecainide acetate

Why is this drug prescribed?

Tambocor is prescribed to treat certain heart rhythm disturbances, including paroxysmal atrial fibrillation (a sudden attack or worsening of irregular heartbeat in which the upper chamber of the heart beats irregularly and very rapidly) and paroxysmal supraventricular tachycardia (a sudden attack or worsening of an abnormally fast but regular heart rate that occurs in intermittent episodes).

Most important fact about this drug

Tambocor may sometimes cause or worsen heartbeat irregularities and certain heart conditions, such as heart failure (the inability of the heart to sustain its workload of pumping blood). Before prescribing Tambocor, your doctor will weigh the drug's risks and benefits. Your condition will be monitored throughout your treatment.

How should you take this medication?

In almost every case, your doctor will initiate Tambocor therapy in the hospital.

Take Tambocor exactly as prescribed by your doctor. Serious heartbeat disturbances may result if you do not follow your doctor's instructions, if you miss any regular doses, or if you increase or decrease the dosage without consulting your doctor.

Your doctor may order regular blood tests to monitor your therapy.

■ *If you miss a dose...*
Take it as soon as you remember if it is within 6 hours of your scheduled time. If you do not remember until later, skip the dose you missed and go back to your regular schedule. Do not take 2 doses at once.

■ *Storage instructions...*
Store at room temperature in a tightly closed container, away from light.

What side effects may occur?

Tambocor has a wide variety of possible effects on the heart, including new or worsened heartbeat abnormalities, heart attack, congestive heart failure, and heart block—an interference with the heart's contraction. If any develop, inform your doctor immediately. Only your doctor can determine whether it is safe for you to continue taking Tambocor.

Why should this drug not be prescribed?

Your doctor should not prescribe Tambocor if you have ever had an allergic reaction to it or you are sensitive to it, if you have heart block (without a pacemaker), or if your heart cannot supply enough blood to the body.

Special warnings about this medication

If you have a pacemaker, you should be monitored very closely while taking Tambocor—your pacemaker may need to be adjusted.

If you have liver disease, Tambocor could build up in your system. Your doctor will prescribe the drug only if the benefits outweigh the risks. In addition, you should have frequent blood tests to make sure your dosage is not too high.

If you have a history of congestive heart failure or a weak heart, you may be at increased risk for dangerous cardiac side effects from Tambocor.

If you have very alkaline urine, perhaps caused by a kidney condition or by a strict vegetarian diet, your body will tend to process and eliminate Tambocor rather slowly and you may need a lower than average dosage.

If the potassium levels in your blood are too high or too low, your doctor will want to correct the condition before allowing you to take Tambocor.

If you have kidney failure, your doctor will want to watch you closely.

Possible food and drug interactions when taking this medication

If Tambocor is taken with certain other drugs, the effects of either could be increased, decreased, or altered. It is especially important to check with your doctor before combining Tambocor with the following:

Amiodarone (Cordarone)
Beta-blockers (blood pressure drugs such as Inderal, Sectral, and Tenormin)
Carbamazepine (Tegretol)
Cimetidine (Tagamet)
Diltiazem (Cardizem)
Disopyramide (Norpace)
Nifedipine (Procardia)
Phenobarbital
Phenytoin (Dilantin)
Quinidine (Quinidex)
Verapamil (Calan, Isoptin)

Special information if you are pregnant or breastfeeding

The effects of Tambocor during pregnancy have not been adequately studied. If you are pregnant or plan to become pregnant, inform your doctor immediately. Tambocor should be used during pregnancy only if the benefit justifies the potential risk to the unborn child. Tambocor appears in breast milk. Check with your doctor before breastfeeding your baby.

Recommended dosage

ADULTS

Treatment with Tambocor almost always begins in the hospital.

The usual starting dose is 50 to 100 milligrams every 12 hours, depending on the condition under treatment. Every 4 days, your doctor may increase your dose by 50 milligrams every 12 hours until your condition is under control.

CHILDREN

Children's dosage is based on body surface area and is always supervised by a cardiac physician.

Overdosage

An overdose of Tambocor is likely to cause slowed or rapid heartbeat, other cardiac problems, fainting, low blood pressure, nausea, vomiting, convulsions, and heart failure. Taken even in moderate excess, Tambocor may have serious consequences and can be fatal. If you suspect an overdose, seek medical attention immediately.

TAMIFLU

Pronounced: TAM-ih-floo
Generic name: Oseltamivir phosphate

Why is this drug prescribed?

Tamiflu speeds recovery from the flu. When started during the first 2 days of the illness, it hastens improvement by at least a day. It also can prevent the flu if treatment is started within 2 days after exposure to a flu victim. Tamiflu is one of a new class of antiviral drugs called neuraminidase inhibitors.

As the flu virus takes hold in the body, it forms new copies of itself and spreads from cell to cell. Neuraminidase inhibitors fight the virus by preventing the release of new copies from infected cells. The other drug in this class, Relenza, is taken by inhalation. Tamiflu is taken in liquid or capsule form.

Most important fact about this drug

Tamiflu can prevent the flu as long as you continue taking this medication, but getting a yearly flu shot is still the best way of avoiding the disease entirely. For older adults, those in high-risk situations such as healthcare work, and people with an immune deficiency or respiratory disease, vaccination remains a must.

How should you take this medication?

To provide any benefit, Tamiflu must be started within 2 days of the onset of symptoms or exposure to the flu. If you have the flu, continue taking it twice daily for 5 days, even if you start to feel better. To prevent the flu, take it once a day for at least 7 days. Protection lasts as long as you take the drug.

If Tamiflu upsets your stomach, try taking it with food. Shake the liquid suspension before each use.

■ *If you miss a dose...*
Take it as soon as possible. If it is within 2 hours of your next dose, skip the missed dose and go back to your regular schedule.

■ *Storage instructions...*
Store at room temperature. Keep the blister package dry. Use the liquid suspension within 10 days. It should be refrigerated, but do not freeze.

What side effects may occur?

Most problems noted during tests of Tamiflu were indistinguishable from the symptoms of flu. Here are the reactions that showed up more frequently in patients taking the drug.

■ *Side effects may include:*
Abdominal pain, asthma, bronchitis, cough, diarrhea, ear infection, fatigue, headache, insomnia, nausea, nosebleed, vertigo, vomiting

Why should this drug not be prescribed?
If Tamiflu gives you an allergic reaction, avoid it in the future.

Special warnings about this medication
If you have kidney disease, the doctor may have to cut your daily dose of Tamiflu in half.

The effectiveness of Tamiflu has not been established for people with weakened immune systems. The drug has not been studied in people with liver disease.

Tamiflu works only on the flu virus. It won't stop bacterial infections that may have flu-like symptoms or bacterial infections that may develop while you have the flu. If your symptoms persist, check with your doctor.

Possible food and drug interactions when taking this medication
No interactions have been reported.

Special information if you are pregnant or breastfeeding
It is not known whether Tamiflu is completely safe during pregnancy. If you are pregnant or plan to become pregnant, inform your doctor before taking this medication. Tamiflu may appear in breast milk and could affect a nursing infant. Taking it while breastfeeding is usually not recommended.

Recommended dosage

ADULTS AND CHILDREN 13 AND OLDER

Treatment of Influenza
The usual dosage is 75 milligrams taken twice daily (morning and evening) for 5 days. If you have kidney disease, take a 75-milligram dose once a day.

Prevention of Influenza
The usual dosage is 75 milligrams taken once a day for at least 7 days. If there is a general outbreak of the flu in your community, your doctor may recommend that you continue taking this medication for up to 6 weeks. If you have kidney disease, take a 75-milligram capsule every other day, or 30 milligrams of liquid once a day.

CHILDREN 1 TO 12

Treatment of Influenza
Doses should be given twice daily for 5 days using the dispenser that comes with the liquid suspension. Each dose is determined by the child's weight:

Under 33 pounds: 30 milligrams
33 to 55 pounds: 45 milligrams
51 to 88 pounds: 60 milligrams
Over 88 pounds: 75 milligrams

Tamiflu should not be used to treat the flu in children under 1 year old.

Prevention of Influenza
Tamiflu's ability to prevent the flu in children under age 13 has not been established.

Overdosage
High doses of Tamiflu can cause nausea and vomiting. As with any medication, if you suspect an overdose, seek emergency medical treatment immediately.

Tamoxifen See Nolvadex, page 959.

Tamsulosin See Flomax, page 579.

TARKA

Pronounced: *TAR-kah*
Generic ingredients: *Trandolapril, Verapamil hydrochloride*

Why is this drug prescribed?
Tarka is used to treat high blood pressure. It combines two blood pressure drugs: an ACE inhibitor and a calcium channel blocker. The ACE inhibitor (trandolapril) lowers blood pressure by preventing a chemical in your blood called angiotensin I from converting to a more potent form that narrows the blood vessels and increases salt and water retention. The calcium channel blocker (verapamil hydrochloride) also works to keep the blood vessels open, and eases the heart's workload by reducing the force and rate of your heartbeat.

Most important fact about this drug
Doctors usually prescribe Tarka for patients who have been taking one of its components—trandolapril (Mavik) or sustained-release verapamil (Calan SR, Isoptin SR)—without showing improvement. Like other blood pressure medications, Tarka must be taken regularly for it to be effective. Since blood pressure declines gradually, it may take a few weeks before you get the full benefit of Tarka; and you must continue taking it even if you are feeling well. Tarka does not cure high blood pressure; it merely keeps it under control.

How should you take this medication?
Take each dose with food, exactly as prescribed.

- *If you miss a dose...*
  Take it as soon as you remember. If it is almost time for your next dose, skip the one you missed and go back to your regular schedule. Never take 2 doses at the same time.
- *Storage instructions...*
  Keep the container tightly closed. Store at room temperature.

What side effects may occur?

Side effects cannot be anticipated. If any develop or change in intensity, inform your doctor as soon as possible. Only your doctor can determine if it is safe for you to continue taking Tarka.

- *Side effects may include:*
  Constipation, cough, dizziness, headache, heartbeat irregularities, upper respiratory tract infection

Why should this drug not be prescribed?

Avoid Tarka if you have ever had an allergic reaction to it, or to verapamil or any of the ACE inhibitors, including Capoten, Vasotec, and Zestril.

You should also avoid Tarka if you have low blood pressure or certain types of heart disease or irregular heartbeat. Make sure your doctor is aware of any cardiac problems you may have.

In addition, Tarka is not for you if you have ever developed a swollen throat and difficulty swallowing (angioedema) while taking an ACE inhibitor. Make sure your doctor is aware of the incident.

Special warnings about this medication

Call your doctor immediately if you begin to suffer angioedema while taking Tarka. Warning signs include swelling of the face, lips, tongue, or throat; swelling of the arms and legs; and difficulty swallowing or breathing.

Bee or wasp venom given to prevent an allergic reaction to stings may cause a severe allergic reaction to Tarka. Kidney dialysis can also prompt an allergic reaction to the drug.

Tarka sometimes causes a severe drop in blood pressure. The danger is especially great if you have been taking water pills (diuretics), or if you have heart disease, kidney disease, or a potassium or salt imbalance. Excessive sweating, severe diarrhea, and vomiting are also a threat. They can rob the body of water, causing a dangerous drop in blood pressure. If you feel light-headed or faint, you should lie down and contact your doctor immediately.

Because another of the ACE inhibitors, Capoten, has been known to cause serious blood disorders, your doctor will check your blood regularly while you are taking Tarka. If you develop signs of infection such as a sore throat or a fever, you should contact your doctor at once—an infection could be a signal of blood abnormalities.

Tarka may also affect the liver, so your doctor will perform liver function tests periodically. Report these symptoms of liver problems to your doctor immediately: a generally run-down feeling, fever, pain in the upper right abdomen, or yellowing of the skin or the whites of your eyes.

If you have a heart condition, heart failure, cardiac irregularities, kidney disease, liver disease, diabetes, or Duchenne's dystrophy (the most common type of muscular dystrophy), make certain that your doctor knows about it. Tarka should be used with caution under these circumstances.

Possible food and drug interactions when taking this medication

If Tarka is taken with certain other drugs, the effects of either could be increased, decreased, or altered. It is especially important to check with your doctor before combining Tarka with the following:

Carbamazepine (Tegretol)
Cimetidine (Tagamet)
Cyclosporine (Sandimmune, Neoral)
Digoxin (Lanoxin)
Disopyramide (Norpace)
Diuretics such as Lasix and HydroDIURIL
Drugs classified as beta-blockers, such as Inderal, Lopressor, and
    Tenormin
Flecainide (Tambocor)
Lithium (Lithonate, Lithobid)
Phenobarbital
Potassium-sparing diuretics such as Aldactone, Dyrenium, and
    Midamor
Potassium supplements such as K-Lyte, K-Tabs, and Slow-K
Quinidine (Quinidex)
Rifampin (Rifadin)
Theophylline (Theo-Dur)

Because Tarka can increase the potassium level in your blood, you should avoid salt substitutes that contain potassium unless your doctor approves.

Special information if you are pregnant or breastfeeding

Because of its ACE-inhibitor component (trandolapril), Tarka should not be used during pregnancy. When taken during the last 6 months of pregnancy, ACE inhibitors can cause birth defects, premature birth, and death of the developing or newborn baby. If you become pregnant, inform your doctor immediately.

The verapamil component of Tarka does appear in breast milk and could affect a nursing infant. Do not breastfeed while taking Tarka.

Recommended dosage

ADULTS

Tarka comes in four strengths of trandolapril and sustained-release vera-pamil. Your doctor will prescribe a dose of Tarka that is comparable to the doses you were taking separately. Doses range from 1 to 4 milligrams of trandolapril and 180 to 240 milligrams of verapamil. Tarka is taken once a day with food.

If you have impaired liver or kidney function, your doctor will adjust your dosage accordingly.

CHILDREN

The safety and effectiveness of Tarka in children under 18 have not been established.

OLDER ADULTS

If you are over 65 years old, you may be more sensitive to Tarka. Your doctor will monitor your blood pressure more closely and adjust your medication dose accordingly.

Overdosage

An overdose of Tarka can cause dangerously low blood pressure and life-threatening heart problems. If you suspect an overdose, seek medical treatment immediately.

TASMAR

Pronounced: TAZ-mahr
Generic name: Tolcapone

Why is this drug prescribed?

Tasmar helps to relieve the muscle stiffness, tremor, and weakness caused by Parkinson's disease. When taken with Sinemet (levodopa/carbidopa), it sustains the blood levels of dopamine needed for normal muscle function. Because Tasmar has been known to cause liver failure, it is prescribed only when other Parkinson's drugs fail to control the symptoms.

Like all Parkinson's medications, Tasmar can provide long-term relief of symptoms, but won't cure the underlying disease. If your symptoms do not improve after 3 weeks of Tasmar therapy, your doctor will discontinue the drug.

Most important fact about this drug

During the first few weeks of Tasmar treatment, be prepared for certain side effects that appear most frequently at the start of therapy. Among the possibilities: attacks of dizziness or fainting when you first stand up, hallucinations, nausea, and increased stiffness. These problems tend to diminish with the passage of time or a reduction in your Sinemet dosage. However, they have forced a few people to discontinue Tasmar therapy.

How should you take this medication?
Tasmar works by boosting the efficacy of Sinemet, and will not work without it. It can be taken with either the immediate-release or controlled-release form of the drug (Sinemet or Sinemet CR). You may take it with or without food.

This drug is taken 3 times a day. Always take the first dose of Tasmar with your first dose of Sinemet. Take your second and third doses of Tasmar 6 and 12 hours later. (Your doctor will probably decrease your dose of Sinemet when you start taking Tasmar.)

■ *If you miss a dose...*
Take it as soon as you remember. If it is almost time for your next dose, skip the one you missed and go back to your regular schedule. Do not take 2 doses at once.

■ *Storage instructions...*
Store at room temperature in a tightly sealed container.

What side effects may occur?
Side effects cannot be anticipated. If any develop or change in intensity, inform your doctor as soon as possible. Only your doctor can determine if it is safe for you to continue taking Tasmar.

■ *Side effects may include:*
Abdominal pain, abnormal muscle movements, acid indigestion, breathing difficulty, chest pain, confusion, constipation, decreased muscle movement, diarrhea, dizziness, drowsiness, dry mouth, excessive dreaming, fainting, falling, fatigue, flu, gas, hallucinations, headache, increased muscle movement, loss of appetite, loss of balance, muscle cramps, muscle stiffness, nausea, skin tingling, sleep disturbances, sweating, tiredness, upper respiratory tract infection, urinary tract infection, urine discoloration, vomiting

Why should this drug not be prescribed?
You must not take Tasmar if you have liver disease or have developed liver problems while using this drug. You should also avoid Tasmar if it causes an allergic reaction, or gives you a high temperature, stiff muscles, or a feeling of confusion.

Special warnings about this medication
Because of Tasmar's possible effects on the liver, your doctor should do a blood test to check your liver function before you start Tasmar therapy,

then every 2 weeks for the first year, every 4 weeks for the next 6 months, and every 8 weeks thereafter. In addition, be alert for any sign of developing liver damage, such as clay-colored stools, yellowing of your skin and eyes, fatigue, itching, loss of appetite, nausea, dark urine, and pain in the upper right abdomen. Report any such problems to your doctor immediately.

Especially at the start of therapy, Tasmar can cause severely low blood pressure, marked by nausea, sweating, dizziness, or fainting. To avoid these symptoms, get up very slowly from a seated or reclining position.

Hallucinations are most likely to occur within the first 2 weeks of therapy. If this problem surfaces, report it to your doctor immediately.

Diarrhea, occasionally severe, is also a possibility, typically after 6 to 12 weeks of therapy. If this becomes a problem, let your doctor know. Also be quick to inform your doctor if you develop a high fever, muscle rigidity, or altered consciousness.

Because Tasmar has been known to cause drowsiness and affect mental and motor skills, you should avoid operating machinery or driving until you know how the drug affects you.

Tasmar can cause nausea, especially at the start of therapy, and sometimes increases muscle stiffness. Your Parkinson's symptoms may also increase, along with fever and confusion, when the drug is discontinued. Your doctor will adjust your other medications carefully if Tasmar needs to be stopped.

Possible food and drug interactions when taking this medication

If Tasmar is taken with certain other drugs, the effects of either could be increased, decreased, or altered. It is especially important to check with your doctor before combining Tasmar with the following:

Apomorphine
Desipramine (Norpramin)
Isoproterenol (Isuprel)
MAO inhibitors such as the antidepressants Marplan, Nardil, and Parnate
Methyldopa (Aldomet)
Nervous system depressants such as alcohol and the sedatives phenobarbital and Seconal
Warfarin (Coumadin)

Special information if you are pregnant or breastfeeding

The safety of Tasmar during pregnancy has not been confirmed. If you are pregnant or plan to become pregnant, inform your doctor immediately. You should continue taking the drug only if the benefits clearly outweigh the risk.

It is not known whether Tasmar appears in breast milk. Notify your doctor if you plan to breastfeed.

Recommended dosage

ADULTS

The usual dose is 100 milligrams 3 times daily (every 6 hours). Take no more than a total of 300 milligrams a day unless prescribed by your doctor.

Overdosage

Any medication taken in excess can have serious consequences. If you suspect an overdose, seek medical attention immediately.

■ *Symptoms of Tasmar overdose may include:*
Dizziness, nausea, vomiting

Tazarotene *See Tazorac, below.*

TAZORAC

Pronounced: TAZZ-o-rack
Generic name: Tazarotene

Why is this drug prescribed?

Tazorac gel comes in two strengths, 0.05% and 0.1%. Both strengths are used to treat the type of psoriasis that causes large plaques on the skin. The 0.1% strength is also used to treat mild to moderate facial acne. The drug is chemically related to vitamin A.

Most important fact about this drug

Tazorac may cause severe birth defects. If you are a woman in your child-bearing years, do not use Tazorac if there is any chance that you are pregnant. Your doctor should give you a pregnancy test within 2 weeks of starting Tazorac therapy, and you should take reliable birth control measures as long as you use the drug. If you accidentally become pregnant, stop using Tazorac and call your doctor immediately.

How should you take this medication?

For psoriasis, apply a thin film of Tazorac to the affected areas each evening. Make sure your skin is dry before you begin. Keep the gel away from normal skin.

To treat acne, first wash your face and dry it thoroughly. Then apply a thin film of Tazorac to the acne eruptions. Repeat each evening.

■ *If you miss a dose...*
Apply it as soon as you remember. If it is almost time for the next dose, skip the one you missed and go back to your regular schedule.
■ *Storage instructions...*
Store at room temperature.

What side effects may occur?

Side effects cannot be anticipated. If any develop or change in intensity, inform your doctor as soon as possible. Only your doctor can determine if it is safe for you to continue using Tazorac.

■ *Side effects may include:*
Burning, dry skin, irritation, itching, skin pain, skin peeling, skin reddening, stinging, worsening of psoriasis

Why should this drug not be prescribed?

If Tazorac gives you an allergic reaction, you cannot continue using it.

Special warnings about this medication

Use Tazorac only on affected areas of the skin. Be careful to avoid your eyes and mouth. Tazorac is for external use only.

Avoid prolonged exposure to the sun or sunlamps while using Tazorac. Apply sunscreen (at least SPF 15) and wear protective clothing when you go into the sunlight. If you are normally sensitive to sunlight, be especially cautious. If you have a sunburn, wait until it heals before using Tazorac.

Tazorac may cause a temporary feeling of burning or stinging. If this irritation is excessive, or you develop extreme itching, burning, peeling, or reddening, stop using Tazorac and call your doctor. Do not restart therapy until your skin returns to normal. Never use Tazorac while your skin is inflamed.

While on Tazorac therapy, remember that extreme wind or cold may cause skin irritation.

The safety and effectiveness of this drug have not been tested in children under 12.

Possible food and drug interactions when taking this medication Check with your doctor before combining Tazorac with other skin medications and cosmetics. Skin products that have a drying effect should not be used with Tazorac. If you've been using such products, wait for their effects to disappear before using Tazorac.

Possible food and drug interactions when taking this medication

Certain drugs can increase your sensitivity to sunlight. Check with your doctor before taking any other medication while using Tazorac, and be especially cautious when using the following:

Major tranquilizers such as Compazine, Stelazine, and Thorazine
Quinolone antibiotics such as Cipro, Floxin, and Noroxin
Sulfa drugs such as Bactrim and Septra
Tetracycline antibiotics such as Achromycin V, Minocin, and Vibramycin
Thiazide-type water pills such as Dyazide and HydroDIURIL

Special information if you are pregnant or breastfeeding

Remember that Tazorac may cause birth defects and must never be used during pregnancy. Tazorac may appear in breast milk; use it with caution, if at all, while breastfeeding.

Recommended dosage

ADULTS

Apply the prescribed gel to affected areas once a day in the evening.

Overdosage

Excessive external use of Tazorac can cause redness, peeling, and skin discomfort. An oral overdose produces the same symptoms as an overdose of Vitamin A.

■ *Symptoms of ORAL Tazorac include:*
Abdominal pain, dizziness, dry or cracked lips, facial flushing, headache, lack of coordination and clumsiness, vomiting

TEGRETOL

Pronounced: TEG-re-tawl
Generic name: Carbamazepine
Other brand names: Carbatrol, Epitol, Tegretol-XR

Why is this drug prescribed?

Tegretol is used in the treatment of seizure disorders, including certain types of epilepsy. It is also prescribed for trigeminal neuralgia (severe pain in the jaws) and pain in the tongue and throat.

In addition, some doctors use Tegretol to treat alcohol withdrawal, cocaine addiction, and emotional disorders such as depression and abnormally aggressive behavior. The drug is also used to treat migraine headache and "restless legs" syndrome.

Most important fact about this drug

There are potentially dangerous side effects associated with the use of Tegretol. If you experience symptoms such as fever, sore throat, rash, ulcers in the mouth, easy bruising, or reddish or purplish spots on the skin, you should notify your doctor immediately. These symptoms could be signs of a blood disorder brought on by the drug.

How should you take this medication?

This medication should only be taken with meals, never on an empty stomach.

Shake the suspension well before using.

Tegretol-XR (extended-release) tablets must be swallowed whole; do not crush or chew them and do not take tablets that have been damaged.

■ *If you miss a dose...*
Take it as soon as you remember. If it is almost time for your next dose, skip the one you missed and go back to your regular schedule. Do not take 2 doses at once. If you miss more than 1 dose in a day, check with your doctor.

■ *Storage instructions...*
Store Tegretol at room temperature. Keep the container tightly closed. Protect the tablets from light and moisture. Keep the liquid suspension away from light.

What side effects may occur?

Side effects cannot be anticipated. If any develop or change in intensity, inform your doctor as soon as possible. Only your doctor can determine if it is safe for you to continue taking Tegretol.

■ *Side effects especially at the start of treatment may include:*
Dizziness, drowsiness, nausea, unsteadiness, vomiting

■ *Other side effects may include:*
Allergic reactions, blood pressure changes, bone marrow suppression, hives, rash, sensitivity to light, swelling

Why should this drug not be prescribed?

You should not use Tegretol if you have a history of bone marrow depression (reduced function), a sensitivity to Tegretol, or a sensitivity to tricyclic antidepressant drugs such as amitriptyline (Elavil). You should also not take Tegretol if you are on an MAO inhibitor antidepressant such as Nardil or Parnate, or if you have taken such a drug within the past 14 days.

Tegretol is not a simple pain reliever and should not be used for the relief of minor aches and pains.

Special warnings about this medication

If you have a history of heart, liver, or kidney damage, an adverse blood reaction to any drug, glaucoma, or serious reactions to other drugs, you should discuss this history thoroughly with your doctor before taking this medication.

Anticonvulsant drugs such as Tegretol should not be stopped abruptly , if you are taking the medication to prevent major seizures. There exists the strong possibility of continuous epileptic attacks without return to consciousness, leading to possible severe brain damage and death. Only your doctor should determine if and when you should stop taking this medication.

Since dizziness and drowsiness may occur while taking Tegretol, you should refrain from operating machinery or driving an automobile or participating in any high-risk activity that requires full mental alertness until you know how this drug affects you.

Older adults, especially, can become confused or agitated when taking Tegretol.

Tegretol has been known to cause serious blood, liver, and skin reactions, both early in treatment and after extended use. Alert your doctor immediately if you develop such warning signs as fever, sore throat, rash, ulcers in the mouth, easy bruising or spots in the skin, swollen lymph glands, loss of appetite, nausea or vomiting, or yellowing of the skin and eyes.

The coating of the Tegretol-XR tablet is not absorbed and passes through your body intact. If you notice it in your stool, it is not a cause for alarm.

Possible food and drug interactions when taking this medication

The use of the antiseizure medications phenobarbital, phenytoin (Dilantin), or primidone (Mysoline) may reduce the effectiveness of Tegretol. Take other anticonvulsants along with Tegretol only if your doctor advises it. The use of Tegretol with other anticonvulsants may change thyroid gland function.

All of the following drugs may raise the amount of Tegretol in the blood to harmful levels:

Azithromycin (Zithromax)
Calcium channel blockers such as Calan, Plendil, Procardia, and Sular
Cimetidine (Tagamet)
Clarithromycin (Biaxin)
Danazol (Danocrine)
Diltiazem (Cardizem)
Erythromycin (E-Mycin)
Fluoxetine (Prozac)
Isoniazid (Nydrazid)
Itraconazole (Sporanox)
Ketoconazole (Nizoral)
Loratadine (Claritin)
Niacinamide
Nicotinamide
Propoxyphene (Darvon)
Troleandomycin (Tao)
Valproate (Depakene, Depakote)

The following drugs may also reduce the effectiveness of Tegretol:

Cisplatin (Platinol)
Doxorubicin HCl (Adriamycin)
Felbamate (Felbatol)

Rifampin (Rifadin, Rimactane)
Theophylline (Theo-24, Uniphyl)

When taken with Tegretol, the effectiveness of the following drugs may be reduced: acetaminophen, alprazolam, calcium channel blockers (such as Plendil and Sular), clonazepam, clozapine, corticosteroids such as Pediapred and Decadron, cyclosporine, dicumarol, doxycycline, ethosuximide, haloperidol, itraconazole, lamotrigine, levothyroxine, methadone, methsuximide, midazolam, olanzapine, oral contraceptives, oxcarbazepine, phensuximide, phenytoin, praziquantel, protease inhibitors (such as Crixivan, Norvir, and Viracept), risperidone, theophylline, tiagabine, topiramate, tramadol, tricyclic antidepressants (such as Elavil, Pamelor, and Tofranil), valproic acid, warfarin, ziprasidone, and zonisamide.

Tegretol may increase the effectiveness of clomipramine HCl (Anafranil), phenytoin, or primidone if the drugs are taken together.

Lithium (Eskalith) used with Tegretol may cause harmful nervous system side effects.

If you are taking an oral contraceptive and Tegretol, you may experience blood spotting and your contraceptive may not be completely reliable.

Do not combine Tegretol suspension with other liquid medications such as Thorazine solution or Mellaril liquid. The mixture may congeal internally.

Special information if you are pregnant or breastfeeding

There are no adequate safety studies regarding the use of Tegretol in pregnant women. However, there have been reports of birth defects in infants. Therefore, this medication should be used during pregnancy only if the potential benefits justify the potential risk to the fetus. If you are pregnant or plan on becoming pregnant, you should discuss this with your doctor.

Tegretol appears in breast milk. If you are breastfeeding, your doctor may advise you to discontinue doing so if taking Tegretol is essential to your health.

Recommended dosage

ADULTS

Seizures

The usual dose for adults and children over 12 years of age is 200 milligrams (1 tablet or 2 chewable or extended-release tablets) taken twice daily or 1 teaspoon 4 times a day. Your doctor may increase the dose at weekly intervals by adding 200-milligram doses twice a day for Tegretol-XR or 3 or 4 times per day for the other forms. Dosage should generally not exceed 1,000 milligrams daily in children 12 to 15 years old and 1,200 milligrams daily for adults and children over 15. The usual daily maintenance dosage range is 800 to 1,200 milligrams.

Trigeminal Neuralgia

The usual dose is 100 milligrams (1 chewable or extended-release tablet) twice or one-half teaspoon 4 times on the first day. Your doctor may increase this dose using increments of 100 milligrams every 12 hours or one-half teaspoonful 4 times daily only as needed to achieve freedom from pain. Doses should not exceed 1,200 milligrams daily and are usually in the range of 400 to 800 milligrams a day for maintenance.

CHILDREN

Seizures

The usual dose for children 6 to 12 years old is 100 milligrams twice daily or one-half teaspoon 4 times a day. Your doctor may increase the dose at weekly intervals by adding 100 milligrams twice a day for Tegretol-XR, 3 or 4 times a day for the other forms. Total daily dosage should generally not exceed 1,000 milligrams. The usual daily dosage range for maintenance is 400 to 800 milligrams.

The usual daily starting dose for children under 6 years of age is 10 to 20 milligrams per 2.2 pounds of body weight. The total daily dose is divided into smaller doses taken 2 or 3 times a day for tablets or 4 times a day for suspension. Daily dosage should not exceed 35 milligrams per 2.2 pounds.

OLDER ADULTS

To help determine the ideal dosage, your doctor may decide to periodically check the level of Tegretol in your blood.

Overdosage

Any medication taken in excess can have serious consequences. If you suspect an overdose, seek medical attention immediately. The first signs and symptoms of an overdose of Tegretol appear after 1 to 3 hours.

■ *The most prominent signs of a Tegretol overdose include:*
Absence or low production of urine, coma, convulsions, dizziness, drowsiness, inability to urinate, involuntary rapid eye movements, irregular or reduced breathing, lack of coordination, low or high blood pressure, muscular twitching, nausea, pupil dilation, rapid heartbeat, restlessness, severe muscle spasm, shock, tremors, unconsciousness, vomiting, writhing movements

Telithromycin *See Ketek, page 708.*

Telmisartan *See Micardis, page 847.*

Telmisartan with Hydrochlorothiazide *See Micardis HCT, page 848.*

Temazepam *See Restoril, page 1239.*

TEMOVATE
Pronounced: TIM-oh-vate
Generic name: Clobetasol propionate
Other brand name: Cormax

Why is this drug prescribed?
Temovate and Cormax relieve the itching and inflammation of moderate to severe skin conditions. The scalp application is used for short-term treatment of scalp conditions; the cream, ointment, emollient cream, and gel are used for short-term treatment of skin conditions on the body. The products contain a steroid medication for external use only.

Most important fact about this drug
When you use Temovate, you inevitably absorb some of the medication through your skin and into the bloodstream. Too much absorption can lead to unwanted side effects elsewhere in the body. To keep this problem to a minimum, avoid using large amounts of Temovate over large areas, and do not cover it with airtight dressings such as plastic wrap or adhesive bandages unless specifically told to by your doctor.

How should you use this medication?
Use Temovate exactly as directed. Do not use it more often or for a longer time than ordered. Remember to avoid covering or bandaging the affected area.

Temovate is for use only on the skin. Be careful to keep it out of your eyes. If the scalp application gets into your eyes, flush your eyes with a lot of water.

A thin layer of cream, ointment, or gel should be gently rubbed into the affected area.

Do not use the scalp application near an open flame.

■ *If you miss a dose...*
Apply it as soon as you remember. If it is almost time for the next dose, skip the one you missed and go back to your regular schedule.

■ *Storage instructions...*
Store at room temperature. Do not refrigerate the creams, gel, or scalp application.

What side effects may occur?
Side effects cannot be anticipated. If any develop or change in intensity, inform your doctor as soon as possible. Only your doctor can determine

if it is safe for you to continue using Temovate. This medication is generally well tolerated when used for 2 weeks. However, some side effects have been reported at the affected area.

CREAMS, OINTMENT, GEL

■ *Side effects are infrequent but may include:*
Burning, cracking/fissuring, irritation, itching, numbness of fingers, patches, reddened skin, shrinking of the skin, stinging

SCALP APPLICATION

■ *Side effects may include:*
Burning, stinging

These additional side effects have been known to result from use of topical steroids and may be particularly apt to occur with airtight dressings or higher-strength steroids: acne, allergic skin inflammation, dryness, excessive hair growth, infection, inflammation around the mouth, loss of skin color, prickly heat, skin softening, streaking.

Why should this drug not be prescribed?
All forms of Temovate should be avoided if you are sensitive to or have ever had an allergic reaction to clobetasol propionate, other corticosteroids such as Valisone and Topicort, or any of their ingredients. Do not use the scalp application if you have a scalp infection.

Special warnings about this medication
Temovate is a strong corticosteroid that can be absorbed into the bloodstream. It has caused Cushing's syndrome (a disorder characterized by a moon-shaped face, emotional disturbances, high blood pressure, weight gain, and, in women, abnormal growth of facial and body hair) and changes in blood sugar.

This medication should not be used for any condition other than the one for which it was prescribed.

If your skin becomes irritated, stop using the medication and call your doctor.

Temovate should not be used by children under 12 years of age.

Treatment should not last for more than 2 weeks.

Possible food and drug interactions when using this medication
No interactions have been reported.

Special information if you are pregnant or breastfeeding
Although Temovate is applied to the skin, there is no way of knowing how much medication is absorbed into the bloodstream. Strong corticosteroids have caused birth defects in animals. Temovate, a strong corticosteroid, should be used only if the potential benefits outweigh the potential risks to the unborn baby; limit use to small amounts, on a lim-

ited area, for a short period of time. It is not known whether topical steroids are absorbed in sufficient amounts to appear in breast milk. If Temovate is essential to your health, your doctor may advise you to stop breastfeeding until your treatment with the medication is finished.

Recommended dosage

ADULTS AND CHILDREN 12 YEARS AND OLDER

Apply the medication to the affected area 2 times a day, once in the morning and once at night. Treatment should not last for more than 2 consecutive weeks, and the affected area should not be covered with a bandage. No more than 50 grams or 50 milliliters (approximately one large tube or bottle) should be used per week.

Overdosage

When absorbed into the bloodstream over a prolonged period, Temovate can cause disorders such as Cushing's syndrome. If you suspect an overdose of Temovate, seek medical attention immediately.

Tenofovir disoproxil *See Viread, page 1573.*

TENORETIC

Pronounced: Ten-or-ET-ic
Generic ingredients: Atenolol, Chlorthalidone

Why is this drug prescribed?

Tenoretic is used in the treatment of high blood pressure. It combines a beta-blocker drug and a diuretic. Tenoretic can be used alone or in combination with other high blood pressure medications. Atenolol, the beta-blocker, decreases the force and rate of heart contractions. Chlorthalidone, the diuretic, helps your body produce and eliminate more urine, which helps in lowering blood pressure.

Most important fact about this drug

You must take Tenoretic regularly for it to be effective. Since blood pressure declines gradually, it may be several weeks before you get the full benefit of Tenoretic; and you must continue taking it even if you are feeling well. Tenoretic does not cure high blood pressure; it merely keeps it under control.

How should you take this medication?

Tenoretic can be taken with or without food.

Take this medication exactly as prescribed by your doctor, even if your symptoms have disappeared.

Try not to miss any doses. If this medication is not taken regularly, your condition may worsen.

■ *If you miss a dose...*
Take the forgotten dose as soon as you remember. If it's within 8 hours of your next scheduled dose, skip the one you missed and go back to your regular schedule. Never take 2 doses at the same time.

■ *Storage instructions...*
Store Tenoretic at room temperature in a tightly closed container. Protect from light.

What side effects may occur?

Side effects cannot be anticipated. If any develop or change in intensity, inform your doctor as soon as possible. Only your doctor can determine if it is safe for you to continue taking Tenoretic.

■ *Side effects may include:*
Dizziness, fatigue, nausea, slow heartbeat

Why should this drug not be prescribed?

If you have a slow heartbeat; a history of serious heart block (conduction disorder); inadequate blood supply to the circulatory system (cardiogenic shock); heart failure; or inability to urinate; or if you are sensitive to or have ever had an allergic reaction to Tenoretic, its ingredients or similar drugs, or to other sulfonamide-derived drugs, you should not take this medication. It should also be avoided if you have an untreated adrenal tumor.

Special warnings about this medication

If you have a history of congestive heart failure or certain other heart problems, Tenoretic should be used with caution.

Tenoretic should not be stopped suddenly. It can cause increased chest pain and heart attack. When stopping the drug, your physician will gradually reduce your dosage.

When taking Tenoretic, if you suffer from asthma, seasonal allergies or other bronchial conditions, or liver or kidney disease, your doctor should monitor you more carefully.

Ask your doctor if you should check your pulse while taking Tenoretic. This medication can cause your heartbeat to become too slow or make heartbeat irregularities worse.

This medication may mask the symptoms of low blood sugar or alter blood sugar levels. If you are diabetic, discuss this with your doctor.

Tenoretic can cause you to become drowsy or less alert; therefore, activity that requires full mental alertness is not recommended until you know how you respond to the drug.

Make sure the doctor knows that you are taking Tenoretic if you have a medical emergency, or plan to have surgery.

Possible food and drug interactions when taking this medication

If Tenoretic is taken with certain other drugs, the effects of either could be increased, decreased, or altered. It is especially important to check with your doctor before combining Tenoretic with the following:

Blood pressure medicines containing reserpine
Clonidine (Catapres)
Diltiazem (Cardizem)
Epinephrine (EpiPen)
Insulin
Lithium (Eskalith)
Nasal decongestants
Nonsteroidal anti-inflammatory drugs such as Indocin and Motrin
Other blood pressure drugs
Verapamil (Calan)

Special information if you are pregnant or breastfeeding

When taken during pregnancy, Tenoretic may cause harm to the developing baby. If you are pregnant, or plan to become pregnant, inform your doctor immediately. Tenoretic appears in breast milk and could affect a nursing infant. If this medication is essential to your health, your doctor may advise you to discontinue breastfeeding until your treatment with this medication is finished.

Recommended dosage

ADULTS

Dosage is always individualized.

The usual starting dosage is 1 Tenoretic 50 tablet taken once a day. Your doctor may increase the dosage to 1 Tenoretic 100 tablet taken once a day. Your doctor may gradually add other high blood pressure medications.

Your doctor will adjust your dosage if your kidney function is impaired.

CHILDREN

The safety and effectiveness of Tenoretic have not been established in children.

Overdosage

Any medication taken in excess can have serious consequences. If you suspect an overdose, seek medical attention immediately.

■ *No specific information on Tenoretic is available,*
but common symptoms of overdose with the drug's
atenolol component are:
Congestive heart failure, constricted airways, low blood pressure, low blood sugar, slow heartbeat, sluggishness, wheezing

- *Symptoms of overdose with the chlorthalidone component include:*
  Dizziness, nausea, weakness

TENORMIN

Pronounced: Ten-OR-min
Generic name: Atenolol

Why is this drug prescribed?

Tenormin, a type of medication known as a beta-blocker, is used in the treatment of high blood pressure, angina pectoris (chest pain, usually caused by lack of oxygen in the heart muscle due to clogged arteries), and heart attack. When used for high blood pressure, it is effective alone or combined with other high blood pressure medications, particularly with a thiazide-type water pill (diuretic). Beta-blockers decrease the force and rate of heart contractions.

Occasionally doctors prescribe Tenormin for treatment of alcohol withdrawal, prevention of migraine headache, and bouts of anxiety.

Most important fact about this drug

If you have high blood pressure, you must take Tenormin regularly for it to be effective. Since blood pressure declines gradually, it may be several weeks before you get the full benefit of Tenormin; and you must continue taking it even if you are feeling well. Tenormin does not cure high blood pressure; it merely keeps it under control.

How should you take this medication?

Tenormin can be taken with or without food. Take it exactly as prescribed, even if your symptoms have disappeared.

Try not to miss any doses, especially if you are taking Tenormin once a day. If this medication is not taken regularly, your condition may worsen.

- *If you miss a dose...*
  Take the forgotten dose as soon as you remember. If it's within 8 hours of your next scheduled dose, skip the one you missed and go back to your regular schedule. Never take 2 doses at the same time.
- *Storage instructions...*
  Store Tenormin at room temperature; protect from light.

What side effects may occur?

Side effects cannot be anticipated. If any develop or change in intensity, inform your doctor as soon as possible. Only your doctor can determine if it is safe for you to continue taking Tenormin.

- *Side effects may include:*
  Dizziness, fatigue, nausea, slow heartbeat

Why should this drug not be prescribed?

If you have heart failure, inadequate blood supply to the circulatory system (cardiogenic shock), heart block (conduction disorder), or a severely slow heartbeat, you should not take this medication. You'll also need to avoid it if it gives you an allergic reaction.

Special warnings about this medication

If you have a history of severe congestive heart failure, Tenormin should be used with caution.

Tenormin should not be stopped suddenly. It can cause increased chest pain and heart attack. Dosage should be gradually reduced.

If you suffer from asthma, seasonal allergies or other bronchial conditions, coronary artery disease, or kidney disease, this medication should be used with caution.

Ask your doctor if you should check your pulse while taking Tenormin. This medication can cause your heartbeat to become too slow.

This medication may mask the symptoms of low blood sugar or alter blood sugar levels. If you are diabetic, discuss this with your doctor.

Notify your doctor or dentist that you are taking Tenormin if you have a medical emergency, and before you have surgery or dental surgery.

Tenormin may cause harm to a developing baby when taken during pregnancy. If you are pregnant or become pregnant while taking this medication, inform your doctor immediately.

Possible food and drug interactions when taking this medication

If Tenormin is taken with certain other drugs, the effects of either could be increased, decreased, or altered. It is especially important to check with your doctor before combining Tenormin with the following:

Ampicillin (Omnipen, others)
Calcium-blocking blood pressure drugs such as Calan and Cardizem
Calcium-containing antacids such as Tums
Certain other blood pressure drugs such as reserpine (Diupres)
Clonidine (Catapres)
Epinephrine (EpiPen)
Indomethacin (Indocin)
Insulin
Oral diabetes drugs such as Micronase
Quinidine (Quinidex)

Special information if you are pregnant or breastfeeding

The use of Tenormin during pregnancy may cause harm to a developing baby. If you are pregnant, become pregnant, or plan to become pregnant, inform your doctor immediately. Tenormin appears in breast milk and could affect a nursing infant. If this medication is essential to your health, your doctor may advise you to discontinue breastfeeding until your treatment is finished.

Recommended dosage

ADULTS

Hypertension
The usual starting dose is 50 milligrams a day in 1 dose, alone or with a diuretic. Full effects should be seen in 1 to 2 weeks. Dosage may be increased to a maximum of 100 milligrams per day in 1 dose. Your doctor can and may use this medication with other high blood pressure medications.

Angina Pectoris
The usual starting dose is 50 milligrams in 1 dose a day. Full effects should be seen in 1 week. Dosage may be increased to a maximum of 100 milligrams per day. In some cases, a single dose of 200 milligrams per day may be given. Dosage will be individualized by your doctor.

Heart Attack
This medication may be used in the acute treatment of heart attack. Your doctor will determine the proper dosage.

If you have kidney problems, the doctor will start you with the lowest effective dose, usually 25 milligrams once a day up to a maximum of 50 milligrams daily.

CHILDREN

The safety and effectiveness of Tenormin have not been established in children.

OLDER ADULTS

The doctor will determine the dosage for an older individual, according to his or her needs, especially in the case of reduced kidney function. The usual dosage range is 25 to 50 milligrams a day.

Overdosage

Any medication taken in excess can have serious consequences. If you suspect an overdose, seek medical attention immediately.

■ *Symptoms of Tenormin overdose may include:*
Congestive heart failure, constricted airways, low blood pressure, low blood sugar, slow heartbeat, sluggishness, wheezing

TENUATE

Pronounced: TEN-you-ate
Generic name: Diethylpropion hydrochloride

Why is this drug prescribed?

Tenuate, an appetite suppressant, is prescribed for short-term use (a few weeks) as part of an overall diet plan for weight reduction. It is available in two forms: immediate-release tablets (Tenuate) and controlled-release tablets (Tenuate Dospan). Tenuate should be used with a behavior modification program.

Most important fact about this drug

Tenuate will lose its effectiveness within a few weeks. When this begins to happen, you should discontinue the medicine rather than increase the dosage.

How should you take this medication?

Take this medication exactly as prescribed. Tenuate may be habit-forming and can be addicting.

If you are taking Tenuate Dospan (the controlled-release formulation), do not crush or chew the tablets. Swallow the medication whole.

■ *If you miss a dose...*
If you are taking the immediate-release form of Tenuate, go back to your regular schedule at the next meal.

If you are taking Tenuate Dospan, take the missed dose as soon as you remember. If you do not remember until the next day, skip the dose. Never take 2 doses at once.

■ *Storage instructions...*
Store at room temperature in a tightly closed container. Protect from excessive heat.

What side effects may occur?

Side effects cannot be anticipated. If any develop or change in intensity, inform your doctor as soon as possible. Only your doctor can determine if it is safe for you to continue using Tenuate.

■ *Side effects may include:*
Abdominal discomfort, abnormal redness of the skin, anxiety, blood pressure elevation, blurred vision, breast development in males, bruising, changes in sex drive, chest pain, constipation, depression, diarrhea, difficulty with voluntary movements, dizziness, drowsiness, dryness of the mouth, feelings of discomfort, feelings of elation, feeling of illness, hair loss, headache, hives, impotence, inability to fall or stay asleep, increased heart rate, increased seizures in epileptics, increased sweating, increased volume of diluted urine, irregular heart-

beat, jitteriness, menstrual upset, muscle pain, nausea, nervousness, overstimulation, painful urination, palpitations, pupil dilation, rash, restlessness, shortness of breath or labored breathing, stomach and intestinal disturbances, tremors, unpleasant taste, vomiting

Why should this drug not be prescribed?

If you are sensitive to or have ever had an allergic reaction to Tenuate or other appetite suppressants, you should not take this medication. Make sure your doctor is aware of any drug reactions you have experienced.

Do not take this drug if you have severe hardening of the arteries, an overactive thyroid, glaucoma, or severe high blood pressure, or if you are agitated, have a history of drug abuse, or are taking an MAO inhibitor (antidepressant drug such as Nardil) or have taken one within the last 14 days.

Special warnings about this medication

Tenuate or Tenuate Dospan may impair your ability to engage in potentially hazardous activities. Therefore, make sure you know how you react to this medication before you drive, operate dangerous machinery, or do anything else that requires alertness or concentration.

If you have heart disease or high blood pressure, use caution when taking this medication.

This drug may increase convulsions in some epileptics. Your doctor should monitor you carefully if you have epilepsy.

Psychological dependence has occurred while taking this drug. Talk with your doctor if you find you are relying on this drug to maintain a state of well-being.

The abrupt withdrawal of this medication following prolonged use at high doses may result in extreme fatigue, mental depression, and sleep disturbances.

Possible food and drug interactions when taking this medication

Tenuate or Tenuate Dospan may interact unfavorably with alcohol. Do not drink alcohol while taking this medication.

If Tenuate or Tenuate Dospan is taken with certain other drugs, the effects of either could be increased, decreased, or altered. It is especially important that you consult your doctor before combining Tenuate with the following:

Blood pressure medications such as Ismelin
Insulin
Phenothiazine drugs such as the major tranquilizer Thorazine

Special information if you are pregnant or breastfeeding

The effects of Tenuate or Tenuate Dospan during pregnancy have not been adequately studied. If you are pregnant or plan to become pregnant, inform your doctor immediately. This drug appears in breast milk. If the medication is essential to your health, your doctor may advise you to discontinue breastfeeding until your treatment is finished.

Recommended dosage

ADULTS

Tenuate Immediate-Release
The usual dosage is one 25-milligram tablet taken 3 times a day, 1 hour before meals; you may take 1 tablet in the middle of the evening, if you want, to overcome night hunger.

Tenuate Dospan Controlled-Release
The usual dosage is one 75-milligram tablet taken once daily, swallowed whole, in midmorning.

CHILDREN

Safety and effectiveness have not been established in children below 12 years of age.

Overdosage

Any medication taken in excess can have serious consequences. If you suspect an overdose, seek emergency medical treatment immediately.

■ *Symptoms of Tenuate overdose may include:*
Abdominal cramps, assaultiveness, confusion, depression, diarrhea, elevated blood pressure, fatigue, hallucinations, irregular heartbeat, lowered blood pressure, nausea, overreactive reflexes, panic state, rapid breathing, restlessness, tremors, vomiting

TEQUIN
Pronounced: TEK-win
Generic name: Gatifloxacin

Why is this drug prescribed?

Tequin is a member of the quinolone family of antibiotics. It is used to treat acute sinus infections, skin infections, pneumonia, complications of chronic bronchitis, kidney and urinary tract infections, and gonorrhea.

Most important fact about this drug

Quinolone antibiotics can cause serious and sometimes fatal allergic reactions, sometimes after a single dose. Stop taking this drug and call your doctor immediately if you develop swelling in the tongue, throat, or face; difficulty breathing or swallowing; itching, tingling; rash; hives; rapid or irregular heartbeat; seizures; or any other sign of an allergic reaction.

How should you take this medication?

Tequin should be taken once a day. Swallow the tablet whole. Try to take it at the same time each day.

You may take Tequin with or without food, milk, or calcium supplements. However, you should not take it within 4 hours of taking antacids, dietary supplements, or multivitamins containing iron, magnesium, or zinc. Also leave 4 hours between a dose of Tequin and a dose of Videx (didanosine).

Your doctor will prescribe Tequin only to treat a bacterial infection; it will not cure a viral infection, such as the common cold. It's important to take the full dosage schedule of Tequin, even if you're feeling better in a few days. Not completing the full dosage schedule may decrease the drug's effectiveness and increase the chances that the bacteria may become resistant to Tequin and similar antibiotics.

■ *If you miss a dose...*
Take it as soon as you remember. If it is almost time for your next dose, skip the one you missed and go back to your regular schedule. Never take 2 doses at once.

■ *Storage instructions...*
Store Tequin at room temperature in a tightly sealed container.

What side effects may occur?

Side effects cannot be anticipated. If any develop or change in intensity, tell your doctor as soon as possible. Only your doctor can determine if it is safe for you to continue taking Tequin.

■ *Side effects may include:*
Diarrhea, dizziness, headache, heart palpitations, high blood pressure, labored breathing, nausea, stomach pain, vaginal inflammation, vomiting

Why should this drug not be prescribed?

Do not take this medication if you are allergic to any member of the quinolone family of drugs, including Cipro, Floxin, Levaquin, Maxaquin, Noroxin, Penetrex, and Raxar.

Special warnings about this medication

Tequin can alter the heartbeat. It's best to avoid it if you have an irregular or slow heartbeat, suffer from low potassium levels, or are taking medication to treat an irregular heartbeat. If you or anyone in your family has a history of heart problems, make sure the doctor is aware of it. Contact your doctor if you have palpitations or fainting spells while on Tequin.

Rare cases of peripheral neuropathy (changes or disturbances of the nervous system) have been reported with this type of antibiotic. Contact your doctor if you experience muscle weakness, paralysis, pain or numbness, a burning sensation, or a pins and needles sensation.

Tequin has been known to cause a rupture in the muscle tendons of the hand, shoulder, or heel. Your risk for this type of rupture is greater if you are taking a steroid medication along with Tequin. If you notice any pain and inflammation in a tendon, stop taking this medication and avoid exercise until you have seen your doctor.

Tequin may cause convulsions, increased pressure in the head, psychosis, tremors, restlessness, nervousness, anxiety, light-headedness, confusion, depression, nightmares, insomnia, unfounded suspicions, and hallucinations. If you experience any of these symptoms, stop taking the drug and contact your doctor immediately. Before taking Tequin, let your doctor know if you are prone to seizures.

Tequin may cause dizziness and light-headedness. Do not drive, operate machinery, or participate in activities that require mental alertness or coordination until you know how this medication affects you.

Tequin can disturb blood sugar levels. If you are a diabetic on oral diabetes medications and your blood sugar drops, eat some sugar, stop taking Tequin, and call your doctor. Monitor your blood sugar levels carefully during your entire course of Tequin therapy.

An increase in blood sugar is also possible, especially among older adults, people with poor kidneys, and those taking medications that tend to increase blood sugar. Check with your doctor immediately if you develop warning signs such as frequent urination, thirst, loss of appetite, nausea, vomiting, and drowsiness.

Tequin, used in high doses for short periods of time, may hide or delay the symptoms of syphilis. If you are taking Tequin for gonorrhea, your doctor will test you for syphilis.

You'll also need to be closely monitored if you have kidney disease; your dosage may have to be reduced.

Some of the other drugs in the quinolone family tend to increase sensitivity to the sun. To be on the safe side, avoid excessive exposure to sunlight while taking Tequin.

Like all antibiotics, Tequin occasionally causes a severe and even dangerous form of diarrhea. Alert your doctor if you develop this problem.

Tequin is not recommended for children under 18 years of age.

Possible food and drug interactions when taking this medication

If Tequin is taken with certain other drugs, the effects of either could be increased, decreased, or altered. It is especially important to check with your doctor before combining Tequin with the following:

Antacids containing aluminum or magnesium
Digoxin (Lanoxin)
Insulin
Iron
Nonsteroidal anti-inflammatory drugs such as Motrin and Naprosyn
Oral diabetes drugs such as Diabinese and Micronase

Probenecid
Vitamins containing iron, magnesium, or zinc

Special information if you are pregnant or breastfeeding
Although it's not known for sure, Tequin may be capable of causing harm during pregnancy. It is not recommended for pregnant or breastfeeding women. If you are pregnant, make sure the doctor is aware of it.

Recommended dosage

ADULTS

Acute Sinus Infections
The usual dose is 400 milligrams taken once a day for 10 days.

Bacterial Complications of Chronic Bronchitis
The usual dose is 400 milligrams once a day for 5 days.

Complicated Urinary Tract Infections, Kidney Inflammation, or Skin Infections
The usual dose is 400 milligrams taken once a day for 7 to 10 days.

Uncomplicated Urinary Tract Infections
You may be prescribed 200 milligrams once a day for 3 days. Alternatively, you may be given a single dose of 400 milligrams.

Gonorrhea
The usual treatment is a single dose of 400 milligrams.

Pneumonia
The usual dose is 400 milligrams taken once a day for 7 to 14 days.

Patients with poor kidney function may need smaller doses.

Overdosage
Little is known about Tequin overdose, but any medication taken in excess can have serious consequences. If you suspect an overdose, seek medical attention immediately.

TERAZOL
Pronounced: TER-uh-zawl
Generic name: Terconazole

Why is this drug prescribed?
Terazol is prescribed to treat candidiasis (a yeast-like fungal infection) of the vulva and vagina.

Most important fact about this drug
Keep using Terazol for the full time of treatment, even if the infection seems to have disappeared. If you stop too soon, the infection could re-

turn. You should continue using this medicine during your menstrual period.

How should you use this medication?

Follow these steps to apply Terazol:
1. Load the applicator to the fill line with cream, or unwrap a suppository, wet it with warm water, and place it in the applicator as shown in the instructions you received with the product.
2. Lie on your back with knees drawn up.
3. Gently insert the applicator high into the vagina and push the plunger.
4. Withdraw the applicator and wash it with soap and water.

To protect your clothing, wear a sanitary napkin. Do not use tampons because they will absorb the medicine. Wear cotton underwear—avoid synthetic fabrics such as rayon or nylon. Do not douche unless your doctor tells you to do so.

Dry the genital area thoroughly after a shower, bath, or swim. Change out of a wet bathing suit or damp workout clothes as soon as possible. Moisture encourages the growth of yeast.

Try not to scratch. It can cause more irritation and can spread the infection.

■ *If you miss a dose...*
Apply it as soon as you remember. If it is almost time for your next dose, skip the one you missed and go back to your regular schedule.
■ *Storage instructions...*
Store at room temperature.

What side effects may occur?
Side effects cannot be anticipated. If any develop or change in intensity, inform your doctor as soon as possible. Only your doctor can determine if it is safe for you to continue using Terazol.

■ *Side effects may include:*
Abdominal pain, body pain, burning, genital pain or irritation, headache, menstrual pain

Why should this drug not be prescribed?
If you have ever had an allergic reaction to or are sensitive to terconazole or any other ingredients of Terazol, you should not use this medication. Make sure your doctor is aware of any drug reactions you have experienced.

Special warnings about this medication
If irritation, an allergic reaction, fever, chills, or flu-like symptoms develop while using this medication, notify your doctor.

To avoid re-infection while using Terazol, either avoid sexual intercourse or make sure your partner uses a non-latex condom.

Terazol 3 suppositories can interact with latex products such as diaphragms and certain type of condoms. Use some other method of birth control while you are using Terazol.

Possible food and drug interactions when taking this medication
No interactions have been reported.

Special information if you are pregnant or breastfeeding
Since Terazol is absorbed from the vagina, it should not be used during the first trimester (first 3 months) of pregnancy unless your doctor considers it essential to your health. It is not known whether this drug appears in breast milk. Your doctor may advise you to discontinue breastfeeding your baby while using this medication.

Recommended dosage

ADULTS

Terazol 3 and Terazol 7 Vaginal Cream
The recommended dose is 1 full applicator (5 grams) of cream inserted into the vagina once daily at bedtime. Apply Terazol 3 for 3 consecutive days; apply Terazol 7 for 7.

Terazol 3 Vaginal Suppositories
The recommended dose is 1 suppository inserted into the vagina once daily at bedtime for 3 consecutive days.

CHILDREN

The safety and effectiveness of Terazol have not been established in children.

Overdosage
There has been no reported overdose of this medication. Any medication used in excess, however, can have serious consequences. If you suspect an overdose of Terazol, seek medical attention immediately.

Terazosin *See Hytrin, page 662.*

Terbinafine *See Lamisil, page 722.*

Terbutaline *See Brethine, page 216.*

Terconazole *See Terazol, page 1413.*

TESSALON

Pronounced: TESS-ah-lon
Generic name: Benzonatate

Why is this drug prescribed?

Tessalon is taken for relief of a cough.

Most important fact about this drug

Tessalon should be swallowed whole, not chewed.

How should you take this medication?

Tessalon perles (soft capsules) should be swallowed whole. If chewed, they can produce a temporary numbness of the mouth and throat that could cause choking or a severe allergic reaction.

■ *If you miss a dose...*
Take the forgotten dose as soon as you remember. If it is almost time for your next dose, skip the one you missed and go back to your regular schedule. Never double the dose.
■ *Storage instructions...*
Store Tessalon at room temperature.

What side effects may occur?

Side effects cannot be anticipated. If any occur or change in intensity, inform your doctor as soon as possible. Only your doctor can determine if it is safe to continue taking Tessalon.

■ *Side effects may include:*
Allergic reactions, burning sensation in the eyes, constipation, dizziness, extreme calm (sedation), headache, itching, mental confusion, nausea, numbness in chest, skin eruptions, stuffy nose, upset stomach, vague chilly feeling, visual hallucinations

Why should this drug not be prescribed?

Tessalon should not be used if you are sensitive to or have ever had an allergic reaction to benzonatate or similar drugs (such as local anesthetics).

Special warnings about this medication

Remember to swallow Tessalon perles whole.

Possible food and drug interactions when taking this medication

There have been rare occurrences of bizarre behavior, including confusion and visual hallucinations, when Tessalon is taken with other prescribed drugs. Check with your doctor before taking Tessalon with other medications.

Special information if you are pregnant or breastfeeding

The effects of Tessalon during pregnancy have not been studied adequately. Tessalon should be used during pregnancy only if clearly needed. If you are pregnant or plan to become pregnant, notify your doctor immediately. It is unknown if Tessalon appears in breast milk and could affect a nursing infant. If this medication is essential to your health, your doctor may advise you to stop breastfeeding until your treatment with Tessalon ends.

Recommended dosage

CHILDREN OVER AGE 10 AND ADULTS

The usual dose is a 100-milligram perle 3 times per day, as needed. The maximum dose is 600 milligrams, or 6 perles, a day.

Overdosage

If capsules are chewed or allowed to dissolve in the mouth, numbness of the mouth and throat will develop rapidly. Symptoms of restlessness and tremors may be followed by convulsions.

If you suspect a Tessalon overdose, seek medical attention immediately.

Testim *See AndroGel, page 109.*

Testoderm *See Testosterone Patches, page 1420.*

TESTOPEL

Pronounced: TEST-o-pell
Generic name: Testosterone pellets

Why is this drug prescribed?

Testopel pellets contain testosterone, the sex hormone that is responsible for growth and maintenance of male physical characteristics. Testosterone is a member of the androgen family of steroids responsible for the growth spurt that happens during adolescence. Testopel is used to treat low testosterone levels brought on by age, tumors, injury, radiation, or a condition present from birth. It also is used to stimulate puberty in boys who have a family history of delayed puberty.

In addition, testosterone is sometimes used to treat certain types of breast cancer.

Most important fact about this drug

Testosterone and other androgens can have serious, long-lasting side effects. They should be used only as prescribed by your doctor.

How should you take this medication?

Testopel pellets are implanted under the skin by your doctor. Their effects last for three to four months and sometimes for as long as six months. Your doctor will perform periodic blood tests to make sure that this medication is working correctly and is not having adverse effects.

What side effects may occur?

Side effects cannot be anticipated. If any develop or change in intensity, inform your doctor as soon as possible. Only your doctor can determine if it is safe for you to continue using Testopel.

■ *Side effects may include:*
Abnormal hair growth, acne, anxiety, blood clotting disorders, decreased sperm count, depression, enlarged breasts in men, fluid retention and swelling, frequent and prolonged erections, headache, increased cholesterol levels, increased or decreased sex drive, inflammation and pain at the pellet site, liver disorders, male pattern baldness, nausea, prickling or tingling sensation, yellowing of skin and eyes

Why should this drug not be prescribed?

Men with a history of breast or prostate cancer should not take Testopel. Androgens such as testosterone should never be used by pregnant women.

Special warnings about this medication

In rare instances, Testopel pellets may be expelled due to improper insertion or infection. Contact your doctor if you notice any of the pellets coming out, or if you have an infection with redness, swelling, or pus.

Testopel can cause a buildup of fluids in the body. People with a history of heart, kidney, or liver problems should use Testopel with caution. Contact your doctor if you experience too frequent or persistent erections, nausea, vomiting, changes in skin color, or ankle swelling.

Testopel should be used very cautiously in children. The hormone may cause bones to mature and stop lengthening before they should. If Testopel has been prescribed to treat delayed puberty, the doctor will take x-rays every 6 months to make sure the bones are growing properly.

When given for breast cancer, androgens can leach calcium from the bones and cause a buildup of calcium in the blood. If this happens, androgen therapy must be discontinued.

In people with diabetes, Testopel may reduce blood sugar levels. If you are diabetic, your doctor will want to watch you closely.

You should be aware that men treated with androgens have an increased risk of prostate and liver problems, including prostate and liver cancer.

The safety and effectiveness of Testopel for improving athletic performance have not been established. Due to its potentially serious side effects, it should never be used for that purpose.

Possible food and drug interactions when taking this medication

If Testopel is taken with certain other drugs, the effects of either could be increased, decreased, or altered. It is especially important to check with your doctor before combining Testopel with the following:

Blood-thinning drugs, such as Coumadin
Insulin
Oxyphenbutazone (Oxalid, Tandearil)

Special information if you are pregnant or breastfeeding

Androgens such as Testopel can cause masculinization of the genitals in a developing female baby, and should never be used during pregnancy.

It is not known whether androgens make their way into breast milk. If this drug is essential to your health, your doctor may advise you to discontinue breastfeeding until your treatment is finished.

Recommended dosage

The dosage of Testopel depends on the age of the patient and the condition being treated. The dosage is adjusted according to the medication's effectiveness and any adverse reactions it may trigger.

Testosterone Replacement Therapy in Men

The usual starting dose is 150 to 450 milligrams (2 to 6 pellets) implanted by your doctor every 3 to 6 months. If you are currently getting injections of 75 milligrams of testosterone each week, the doctor will implant 6 pellets; if you are getting 50 milligrams each week, the doctor will use 4 pellets.

Delayed Puberty in Adolescent Boys

The dosage level for delayed puberty is generally lower than the dosage for testosterone replacement therapy. The doctor may begin with a low dosage and gradually increase it as puberty progresses, or begin with a higher dose to induce puberty and then lower the dosage. The doctor will take into account the boy's age and stage in development when determining the dosage. The Testopel pellets usually are implanted for only a limited period, such as 4 to 6 months.

Overdosage

There have been no reports of massive androgen overdose. However, any medication taken in excess can have serious consequences. If you suspect an overdose of Testopel, check with your doctor immediately.

Testosterone buccal system, oral See Striant, page 1351.

Testosterone gel See AndroGel, page 109.

TESTOSTERONE PATCHES

Brand names: Androderm, Testoderm

Why is this drug prescribed?

These patches are prescribed for men with low levels of the male hormone, testosterone. Lack of testosterone can lead to declining interest in sex, impotence, fatigue, depression, and loss of masculine characteristics.

Most important fact about this drug

If you have prostate problems, make sure your doctor is aware of them. Supplementary testosterone may increase the risk of prostate cancer.

How should you use this medication?

The patches deliver steady doses of testosterone through the skin.

TESTODERM

Testoderm patches are applied daily to the skin of the scrotum. They should not be applied elsewhere. Scrotal skin is much thinner than other skin, so you will not get the full dosage if you apply the patch to another part of the body.

For best results, the scrotal skin should be shaved, clean, and dry. Dry-shave the skin; avoid wet shaving or chemical hair removal products. The patch should be worn for 22 to 24 hours per day, every day, for up to 8 weeks.

ANDRODERM

Androderm patches are applied to the skin of the back, abdomen, upper arms, or thigh, but *not* to the scrotum. It's also best to avoid bony areas such as the shoulders and hips as well as areas that get the greatest pressure while you are sleeping or sitting. You should change sites each day of the week, waiting 7 days before re-using a site.

Apply the prescribed number of patches every night. Press each patch firmly in place immediately after opening its pouch. Leave the patches in place for a full 24 hours. The application sites should be clean, dry, and free of irritation.

■ *If you miss a dose...*
Apply it as soon as you remember. If it is almost time for the next application, skip the one you missed and go back to your regular schedule. Do not apply 2 doses at the same time.

■ *Storage instructions...*
Store at room temperature.

What side effects may occur?

Side effects cannot be anticipated. If any develop or change in intensity, inform your doctor as soon as possible. Only your doctor can determine if it is safe for you to continue using the patch.

Among younger men being treated for delayed sexual development, supplementary testosterone can cause breast enlargement; among older men, it increases the odds of prostate cancer. Among men with heart, kidney, or liver disease, it can lead to fluid retention and congestive heart failure. The Testoderm patch sometimes causes itching, discomfort, or irritation. The Androderm patch occasionally causes itching, blisters, burning, or hardening or reddening of the skin.

Why should this drug not be prescribed?

Do not use these patches if you have prostate cancer (or breast cancer). Avoid them if they give you an allergic reaction. The patches are not for use by women.

Special warnings about this medication

Some testosterone may be left on the skin after a patch is removed. Particularly with Testoderm, there is a possibility that your partner could absorb some of the hormone during sex and suffer unwanted changes. If she experiences increased hair growth or an aggravation of acne, inform your doctor.

Also check with your doctor if you have frequent or persistent erections, nausea, vomiting, changes in skin color, or ankle swelling.

Testosterone patches have not been tested in boys under 15 years of age.

Possible food and drug interactions when using this medication

Extra testosterone can decrease the need for blood-thinning drugs and insulin. While using the patch, you should also check with your doctor before taking the anti-inflammatory drug oxyphenbutazone.

Special information if you are pregnant or breastfeeding

Testosterone is intended for use only by males and must not be used by women. If used during pregnancy, it can cause serious harm to the developing baby.

Recommended dosage

TESTODERM

The usual dose is 1 patch per day. The larger patch delivers 6 milligrams of testosterone. The smaller patch delivers 4 milligrams.

ANDRODERM

The usual starting dose is one 5-milligram patch or two 2.5-milligram patches per day. Depending on results, your doctor may increase the dosage to 1 large and 1 small patch (or 3 small patches) daily, or reduce it to 1 small patch per day of testosterone.

Overdosage

Testosterone overdose is very rare, but has been implicated in one case of stroke. Any medication taken in excess can have serious consequences. If you suspect an overdose, seek medical attention immediately.

Testosterone pellets *See Testopel, page 1417.*

TETRACYCLINE

Pronounced: TET-ra-SY-clin
Brand names: Achromycin V, Sumycin

Why is this drug prescribed?

Tetracycline, a broad-spectrum antibiotic, is used to treat bacterial infections such as Rocky Mountain spotted fever, typhus fever, and tick fevers; upper respiratory infections; pneumonia; gonorrhea; amoebic infections; and urinary tract infections. It is also used to help treat severe acne and to treat trachoma (a chronic eye infection) and conjunctivitis (pinkeye). Tetracycline is often an alternative drug for people who are allergic to penicillin.

Most important fact about this drug

Tetracycline should not be used during the last half of pregnancy or in children under the age of 8. It may damage developing teeth and cause permanent discoloration.

How should you take this medication?

Tetracycline should be taken exactly as prescribed by your doctor. Be sure to use the entire prescription. If you are taking a liquid form of the drug, shake well before using.

Do not use outdated tetracycline. Outdated tetracycline is highly toxic to the kidneys.

Do not take antacids containing aluminum, calcium, or magnesium (e.g., Mylanta, Maalox) while taking this medication. They will affect the absorption of the drug.

Take tetracycline 1 hour before or 2 hours after meals. Foods, milk, and some other dairy products affect absorption of the drug.

Tetracycline should be continued for at least 24 to 48 hours after your symptoms have subsided.

■ *If you miss a dose...*
Take it as soon as you remember. If it is almost time for your next dose and you take tetracycline once a day (e.g., for acne), take the dose you

missed, and then take the next one 10 to 12 hours later; if you take it twice a day, take the dose you missed, and then take the next one 5 to 6 hours later; if you take 3 or more doses a day, take the one you missed, and then take the next one 2 to 4 hours later. Then go back to your regular schedule.

■ *Storage instructions...*
Store capsules at room temperature. Keep the liquid form of tetracycline in the refrigerator, but do not allow it to freeze.

What side effects may occur?
Side effects cannot be anticipated. If any occur or change in intensity, inform your doctor as soon as possible. Only your doctor can determine if it is safe for you to continue taking tetracycline.

■ *Side effects may include:*
Anemia, blood disorders, blurred vision and headache (in adults), bulging soft spot on the head (in infants), diarrhea, difficult or painful swallowing, dizziness, extreme allergic reactions, genital or anal sores or rash, hives, inflammation of the large bowel, inflammation of the tongue, inflammation of the upper digestive tract, increased sensitivity to light, loss of appetite, nausea, rash, ringing in the ears, swelling due to fluid accumulation, vision disturbance, vomiting

Why should this drug not be prescribed?
Do not take this medication if you are sensitive to or have ever had an allergic reaction to any tetracycline medication.

Special warnings about this medication
If you have kidney disease, make sure the doctor knows about it. A lower than usual dose of tetracycline may be needed.

Tetracycline drugs can make you more prone to sunburn when you are in sunlight or ultraviolet light. Take appropriate precautions.

Some adults may develop a headache and blurred vision while taking tetracycline, and infants may develop a bulging soft spot on the head. Contact your doctor if you experience or notice these symptoms. They usually disappear soon after the medication is stopped.

As with other antibiotics, use of this medication may cause other infections to develop. Contact your doctor if this occurs.

If you are taking tetracycline over an extended period of time, your doctor will perform blood, kidney, and liver tests periodically.

Possible food and drug interactions when taking this medication
If tetracycline is taken with certain other drugs, the effects of either could be increased, decreased, or altered. It is especially important to check with your doctor before combining tetracycline with the following:

Antacids containing aluminum, calcium, or magnesium, such as Mylanta and Maalox

Blood thinners such as Coumadin

Oral contraceptives

Penicillin (Amoxil, Pen-Vee K, others)

Special information if you are pregnant or breastfeeding

Tetracycline is not recommended for use during pregnancy. It can affect the development of the unborn child's bones and teeth. If you are pregnant or plan to become pregnant, inform your doctor immediately. Tetracycline appears in breast milk and may affect a nursing infant. If this medication is essential to your health, your doctor may recommend that you stop breastfeeding until your treatment is finished.

Recommended dosage

Your doctor will adjust your dose on the basis of the condition to be treated, your age, and risk factors such as kidney problems.

You should use this drug for at least 24 to 48 hours after symptoms and fever have subsided. For a streptococcal infection, doses should be taken for at least 10 days.

ADULTS

For most infections, the usual daily dose is 1 to 2 grams, divided into 2 or 4 equal doses, depending on severity.

Brucellosis

The usual dose is 500 milligrams 4 times daily for 3 weeks; the drug should be accompanied by streptomycin.

Syphilis

You should take a total of 30 to 40 grams, divided into equal doses over a period of 10 to 15 days.

Gonorrhea patients sensitive to penicillin can take tetracycline, starting with 1.5 grams, followed by 0.5 gram every 6 hours for 4 days, to a total dosage of 9 grams.

Urethral, Endocervical, or Rectal Infections in Adults Caused by Chlamydia trachomatis

The usual dose is 500 milligrams 4 times a day for at least 7 days.

CHILDREN 8 YEARS OF AGE AND ABOVE

The usual daily dose is 10 to 20 milligrams per pound of body weight, divided into 2 or 4 equal doses.

Overdosage

Any medication taken in excess can have serious consequences. Seek medical attention immediately if you suspect an overdose of tetracycline.

TEVETEN

Pronounced: TEH-veh-ten
Generic name: Eprosartan mesylate

Why is this drug prescribed?

Teveten is used to treat high blood pressure. It is a member of the family of drugs called angiotensin II receptor blockers. The hormone angiotensin II makes the blood vessels constrict, causing blood pressure to rise. Teveten works by blocking the receptors that respond to angiotensin II. The drug may be prescribed alone or in combination with other medications that help lower blood pressure, such as water pills (diuretics) or calcium channel blockers.

Most important fact about this drug

You must take Teveten regularly for it to be effective. Since blood pressure declines gradually, it may be several weeks before you get the full benefit of Teveten, and you must continue taking it even if you are feeling well. Teveten does not cure high blood pressure; it merely keeps it under control.

How should you take this medication?

Teveten can be taken with or without food. Try to establish a regular routine by taking it at the same time each day, for example in the morning with breakfast. This reduces the chances that you'll forget a dose.

■ *If you miss a dose...*
Take it as soon as possible. If it is almost time for your next dose, skip the one you missed and go back to your regular schedule.

■ *Storage instructions...*
Store at room temperature.

What side effects may occur?

Side effects cannot be anticipated. If any develop or change in intensity, inform your doctor as soon as possible. Only your doctor can determine if it is safe for you to continue taking Teveten.

■ *Side effects may include:*
Cold, cough, runny nose, sore throat

Why should this drug not be prescribed?

Do not take Teveten if you are pregnant, or if you have ever had an allergic reaction to it.

Special warnings about this medication

When Teveten is combined with diuretics, it can cause excessively low blood pressure, especially when you first start taking it. If you develop warning signs such as light-headedness or faintness, call your doctor right away. You may need to have your dosage adjusted or discontinue the medication.

If you have kidney disease, Teveten should be used with caution. Be sure your doctor knows your medical history before you begin this medication so you can be carefully monitored.

Possible food and drug interactions when taking this medication
No interactions have been reported.

Special information if you are pregnant or breastfeeding
Drugs such as Teveten can cause injury or even death to an unborn child when used in the second or third trimester of pregnancy. Stop taking Teveten as soon as you know you are pregnant, and be sure to tell your doctor if you are pregnant or plan to become pregnant. Teveten may appear in breast milk and could affect the nursing infant. If this medication is essential to your health, your doctor may advise you to stop breastfeeding while you are taking Teveten.

Recommended dosage

ADULTS

The usual starting dose of Teveten is 600 milligrams taken once daily. Teveten may also be taken once or twice daily with total doses ranging from 400 to 800 milligrams. If your blood pressure does not go down as expected, your doctor may combine your dose with a diuretic or calcium channel blocker.

CHILDREN

The safety and effectiveness of Teveten have not been established in children.

Overdosage
Although there is limited information available on Teveten overdosage, remember that any medication taken in excess can have serious consequences. Extremely low blood pressure and abnormally slow or rapid heartbeat are possible signs of an overdose with this class of drugs. If you suspect an overdose, seek emergency medical treatment immediately.

TEVETEN HCT

Pronounced: TEH-veh-ten
Generic ingredients: Eprosartan mesylate,
  Hydrochlorothiazide

Why is this drug prescribed?

Teveten HCT is a combination medication used in the treatment of high
blood pressure. One component, eprosartan, belongs to a class of blood
pressure medications that work by preventing the hormone angiotensin
II from constricting the blood vessels, thus allowing blood to flow more
freely and keeping blood pressure down. The other component, hydrochlorothiazide, is a diuretic that increases the output of urine, removing
excess fluid from the body and thus lowering blood pressure.

Most important fact about this drug

You must take Teveten HCT regularly for it to be effective. Since blood
pressure declines gradually, it may be several weeks before you get the
full benefit of this medication, and you must continue to take it even if you
are feeling well. Teveten HCT does not cure high blood pressure; it merely
keeps it under control.

How should you take this medication?

Take Teveten HCT regularly, once a day every day. Schedule it for the
same time each day so that it's easier to remember.

■ *If you miss a dose...*
  Take the forgotten dose as soon as you remember. However, if it is al-
  most time for your next dose, skip the one you missed and return to
  your regular schedule. Do not take 2 doses at once.
■ *Storage instructions...*
  Store at room temperature.

What side effects may occur?

Side effects cannot be anticipated. If any develop or change in intensity,
tell your doctor as soon as possible. Only your doctor can determine if it
is safe to continue using Teveten HCT.

■ *Side effects may include:*
  Back pain, dizziness, fatigue, headache

Many other rare side effects have been reported by people taking the individual components of Teveten HCT. Be sure to tell your doctor about any
new or unusual symptoms you suffer.

Why should this drug not be prescribed?

If you have ever had an allergic reaction to eprosartan, hydrochlorothiazide, or sulfa drugs, you should not take this medication. Also avoid
Teveten HCT if you are unable to urinate.

Special warnings about this medication

Teveten HCT can cause an excessive drop in blood pressure, especially when you first begin taking it. If you feel light-headed or faint, let your doctor know about it. If you actually pass out, stop taking Teveten HCT and see your doctor immediately. The problem is more likely if you suffer from a lack of fluid, due either to inadequate intake or to excessive sweating, diarrhea, or vomiting.

Excessive fluid loss can also lead to a chemical imbalance in the body. Warning signs include dry mouth, thirst, diminished urination, weakness, lack of energy, drowsiness, restlessness, confusion, seizures, muscle pain, muscle fatigue, nausea, vomiting, and rapid heartbeat. Alert your doctor if you develop any of these symptoms.

If you have liver or kidney disease, diabetes, gout, or lupus erythematosus, Teveten HCT should be used with caution. This drug may bring out hidden diabetes. If you are already taking insulin or oral diabetes drugs, your dosage may have to be adjusted. If you have asthma or a history of allergies, you may be at greater risk of an allergic reaction to this medication.

This drug is not approved for children.

Possible food and drug interactions when taking this medication

Unless your doctor approves, avoid potassium supplements and potassium-containing salt substitutes while taking Teveten HCT.

If Teveten HCT is taken with certain other drugs, the effects of either could be increased, decreased, or altered. It is especially important to check with your doctor before combining Teveten HCT with the following:

Alcohol
Barbiturates such as phenobarbital and Seconal
Cholestyramine (Questran)
Colestipol (Colestid)
Diuretics that leave potassium in the body, including amiloride,
    spironolactone, and triamterene
Insulin
Lithium (Eskalith, Lithobid)
Narcotic painkillers such as Demerol, OxyContin, and Percodan
Nonsteroidal anti-inflammatory drugs such as Aleve, Anaprox,
    and Motrin
Other blood pressure medications such as Procardia XL and
    Tenormin
Oral diabetes drugs such as DiaBeta, Diabinese, and Glucotrol
Steroid medications such as prednisone

Special information if you are pregnant or breastfeeding

When used in the second or third trimester of pregnancy, Teveten HCT can cause injury or even death to the unborn child. Alert your doctor as soon as you learn you are pregnant. Teveten HCT should be discontinued as soon as possible.

This drug is not recommended if you plan to breastfeed.

Recommended dosage

ADULTS

Teveten HCT comes in two strengths: 600/12.5 and 600/25 (600 milligrams of eprosartan and either 12.5 milligrams or 25 milligrams of hydrochlorothiazide). The usual starting dose is one 600/12.5 tablet per day. If your blood pressure remains too high, the doctor may increase the dose to one 600/25 tablet per day.

Overdosage

Little is known about overdosage with Teveten HCT. The most likely symptoms would be those of chemical imbalance triggered when the hydrochlorothiazide in the product flushes too much water from the system. These symptoms include thirst, diminished urination, weakness, drowsiness, restlessness, confusion, seizures, muscle pain, nausea, vomiting, and rapid heartbeat. If you suspect an overdose, seek medical attention immediately.

THALITONE
Pronounced: THAL-i-tone
Generic name: Chlorthalidone

Why is this drug prescribed?

Thalitone is a diuretic (water pill) used to treat high blood pressure and fluid retention associated with congestive heart failure, cirrhosis of the liver (a disease of the liver caused by damage to its cells), corticosteroid and estrogen therapy, and kidney disease. When used for high blood pressure, Thalitone may be used alone or in combination with other high blood pressure medications. Diuretics help your body produce and eliminate more urine, which helps lower blood pressure.

Most important fact about this drug

If you have high blood pressure, you must take Thalitone regularly for it to be effective. Since blood pressure declines gradually, it may be several weeks before you get the full benefit of Thalitone; and you must continue taking it even if you are feeling well. Thalitone does not cure high blood pressure; it merely keeps it under control.

How should you take this medication?

Diuretics such as Thalitone increase urination; therefore Thalitone should be taken in the morning.

Do not interchange generic chlorthalidone with Thalitone without consulting your doctor or pharmacist.

Thalitone may be taken with food. Take it exactly as prescribed.

■ *If you miss a dose...*
Take it as soon as you remember. If it is almost time for the next dose, skip the one you missed and go back to your regular schedule. Do not take 2 doses at the same time.

■ *Storage instructions...*
Store at room temperature.

What side effects may occur?

Side effects cannot be anticipated. If any side effects develop or change in intensity, tell your doctor immediately. Only your doctor can determine whether it is safe to continue taking Thalitone.

■ *Side effects may include:*
Allergic reaction, anemia, changes in blood sugar, change in potassium levels (causing such symptoms as dry mouth, excessive thirst, weak or irregular heartbeat, and muscle pain or cramps), constipation, cramping, diarrhea, dizziness, dizziness upon standing up, flaky skin, headache, hives, impotence, inflammation of a lymph or blood vessel, inflammation of the pancreas, itching, loss of appetite, low blood pressure, muscle spasms, nausea, rash, restlessness, sensitivity to light, stomach irritation, tingling or pins and needles, vision changes, vomiting, weakness, yellow eyes and skin

Why should this drug not be prescribed?

If you are unable to urinate or if you have ever had an allergic reaction to or are sensitive to chlorthalidone or other sulfa drugs, do not take Thalitone.

Special warnings about this medication

Diuretics can cause your body to lose too much potassium. Signs of an excessively low potassium level include muscle weakness and rapid or irregular heartbeat. To boost your potassium level, your doctor may recommend eating potassium-rich foods or taking a potassium supplement.

Tell your doctor if you have ever had an allergic reaction to other diuretics or if you have asthma, kidney or liver disease, gout, or lupus.

If you have a history of bronchial asthma, you are more likely to have an allergic reaction to Thalitone.

Be careful in hot weather not to become dehydrated. Contact your doctor if you experience excessive thirst, tiredness, restlessness, drowsiness, muscle pains or cramps, nausea, vomiting, or increased heart rate or pulse.

This medication may aggravate lupus erythematosus, a disease of the connective tissue.

Avoid prolonged exposure to sunlight.

Possible food and drug interactions when taking this medication
Drinking alcohol may increase the chance of dizziness. Do not drink alcohol while taking this medication.

If Thalitone is taken with certain other drugs, the effects of either could be increased, decreased, or altered. It is especially important to check with your doctor before combining Thalitone with the following:

Insulin
Lithium (Eskalith, Lithobid)
Oral diabetes drugs such as Micronase
Other high blood pressure medications such as Aldomet and
  Catapres

Special information if you are pregnant or breastfeeding
Information is not available about the safety of Thalitone during pregnancy. If you are pregnant or plan to become pregnant, inform your doctor immediately. Thalitone may appear in breast milk and could affect a nursing infant. If Thalitone is essential to your health, your doctor may advise you to stop breastfeeding until your treatment is finished.

Recommended dosage
Your doctor will tailor your individual dose to the lowest possible amount that delivers a satisfactory response.

Once desired control of blood pressure or fluid retention has been achieved, your doctor may adjust your dose downward.

HIGH BLOOD PRESSURE

The usual initial dose is a single dose of 15 milligrams. Your doctor may increase the dose to 30 milligrams and then to 45 to 50 milligrams once daily.

FLUID RETENTION

The usual initial dose is 30 to 60 milligrams daily or 60 milligrams on alternate days. Some people may require up to 90 to 120 milligrams at these intervals. Your doctor may be able to lower the dose as treatment continues.

Overdosage
Any medication taken in excess can have serious consequences. If you suspect an overdose, seek medical treatment immediately.

■ *Symptoms of Thalitone overdose may include:*
Confusion, dizziness, nausea, weakness

Theo-24 *See Theo-Dur, page 1432.*

Theochron *See Theo-Dur, page 1432.*

THEO-DUR

Pronounced: THEE-a-door
Generic name: Theophylline
Other brand names: Quibron-T/SR, Slo-bid, T-Phyl, Theo-24,
Theochron, Uni-Dur, Uniphyl

Why is this drug prescribed?

Theo-Dur, an oral bronchodilator medication, is given to treat symptoms of asthma, chronic bronchitis, and emphysema. The active ingredient of Theo-Dur, theophylline, is a chemical cousin of caffeine. It opens the airways by relaxing the smooth muscle that circles the tubes and blood vessels in the lungs.

Most important fact about this drug

Theo-Dur is a controlled-release medication. For an acute attack you should take an immediate-release medication instead of more Theo-Dur. If you develop status asthmaticus (a severe breathing difficulty that does not clear up with your usual medications), do not take extra Theo-Dur; instead, seek medical treatment immediately. Since even a little extra Theo-Dur may constitute an overdose, you should be treated in a place where close monitoring is possible.

Individual doses are determined by a person's response (a decrease in symptoms of asthma). In order to avoid overdosing or underdosing, your doctor will perform regular tests to determine the amount of Theo-Dur in your bloodstream.

You should not change from Theo-Dur to another brand without first consulting your doctor or pharmacist. Products manufactured by different companies may not be equally effective.

How should you take this medication?

Take Theo-Dur exactly as prescribed. Do not change the dose, the time you take it, or how often you take it without consulting your doctor.

This drug is available in two forms. The extended-release tablets should be swallowed whole, not crushed or chewed. The tablets of some brands, including Theo-Dur, are scored; if the doctor prescribes a partial dosage, these tablets should be broken only at the score. You may take the tablets with or without food. If you are taking them on a once-a-day basis, do not take the dose at night.

The other form, Theo-Dur Sprinkle sustained-action capsules, must be taken either 1 hour before or 2 hours after a meal. You may take the capsule whole or open it and empty the contents onto a spoonful of food that is soft but not hot. Without chewing, immediately swallow the spoonful of food and follow it with a glass of cool water or juice. Always take the complete contents of the capsule.

When taking Theo-Dur, you should avoid large amounts of caffeine-containing beverages, such as tea and coffee.

■ *If you miss a dose...*
Take the next dose at the regular time. Do not try to make up the dose you missed.

■ *Storage instructions...*
Store at room temperature. Keep the container tightly closed. Protect from excessive heat, light, and moisture. Make sure this medicine is kept out of reach of children.

What side effects may occur?
Side effects from Theo-Dur cannot be anticipated. Nausea and restlessness may occur when you first start to take Theo-Dur, but will probably disappear as your body becomes used to the drug. If side effects persist, see your doctor; the dosage may be too high.

■ *Other side effects may include:*
Convulsions, diarrhea, disturbances of heart rhythm, excitability, frequent urination, hair loss, headache, heart palpitations, insomnia, irritability, muscle twitching, rash, severe seizures, tremors, vomiting

Why should this drug not be prescribed?
Do not take Theo-Dur if you have ever had an allergic reaction to it or similar drugs.

Do not take Theo-Dur if you have an active peptic ulcer or a seizure disorder such as epilepsy.

Special warnings about this medication
If you are a smoker, your body will tend to process and get rid of Theo-Dur rather quickly; thus, you may need to take more frequent doses than a nonsmoker. Tell your doctor if you start or stop smoking. Even if you quit, the quick-clearance effect may linger for 6 months to 2 years.

You should take Theo-Dur cautiously and under close medical supervision if you are over age 60.

You should also take Theo-Dur cautiously and under close supervision if you have had a sustained high fever, or if you have heart disease, liver disease, heartbeat irregularities, fluid in the lungs, an underactive thyroid gland, the flu or another viral illness, or the symptoms of shock.

Call your doctor immediately if you develop nausea, vomiting, a lasting headache, insomnia, restlessness, or a too rapid heartbeat; if you develop a new illness, especially with a fever; or if an illness you already have gets worse.

Possible food and drug interactions when taking this medication
Theo-Dur interacts with a wide variety of drugs. Consult your doctor before combining any other medication with Theo-Dur. Let your doctor

know whenever another doctor starts you on a new medication or stops an old one. Let every doctor you deal with know you are taking Theo-Dur.

Special information if you are pregnant or breastfeeding

If you are pregnant or plan to become pregnant, inform your doctor immediately. Theo-Dur should not be taken during pregnancy unless it is clearly needed, and unless the benefits to the mother outweigh the potential risk to the developing child.

Theo-Dur does find its way into breast milk; it may make a nursing baby irritable or harm the baby in other ways. If you are a new mother, you will probably need to choose between breastfeeding and taking Theo-Dur.

Recommended dosage

ADULTS

Theo-Dur Extended Release Tablets
The usual initial dose is 1 Theo-Dur 150-milligram tablet every 12 hours. If this is not effective, your doctor will gradually increase the dose until you respond, up to a maximum of 600 milligrams per day. Once you have adjusted to the medication, your doctor may be able to put you on a once-a-day dose schedule.

Theo-Dur Sprinkle
The usual initial dose is no more than 200 milligrams every 12 hours. If this is not effective, your doctor will gradually increase the dose until you respond, up to a maximum of 900 milligrams per day. If a dose every 12 hours is inconvenient, your doctor may divide the daily total into 3 small doses taken every 8 hours.

CHILDREN AGED 6 TO 16

Theo-Dur Extended Release Tablets
Maximum regular daily dosages are calculated by body weight as follows.

Less than 99 pounds: 20 milligrams per 2.2 pounds up to a
   maximum of 600 milligrams
99 pounds or more: 600 milligrams

Theo-Dur Sprinkle
For children under 55 pounds, a liquid preparation is recommended to establish proper dosage before switching to Theo-Dur Sprinkle. Maximum regular daily dosages are calculated by body weight as follows:

Children 6 through 8: 24 milligrams per 2.2 pounds
Children 9 through 11: 20 milligrams per 2.2 pounds
Children 12 through 15: 18 milligrams per 2.2 pounds

OLDER ADULTS

Older adults are more likely than younger people to be seriously affected by Theo-Dur. Anyone over age 60 should not take more than 400 milligrams a day except in special circumstances.

Overdosage

Most of the symptoms listed in the side effects section are actually caused by slight overdosage.

Be aware that a flu shot, influenza itself, or another viral infection may make your usual dose of Theo-Dur act like an overdose. Consult your doctor if you anticipate getting a flu shot, or if you think you have the flu; you may need a temporary dosage reduction.

A mild overdose of Theo-Dur may cause nausea and restlessness. Taking too much over a long period of time may cause serious heartbeat irregularities, convulsions, or even death. If at any time you suspect symptoms of an overdose of Theo-Dur, seek medical attention immediately.

Theophylline *See Theo-Dur, page 1432.*

Theragran *See Multivitamins, page 901.*

Thioridazine *See Mellaril, page 821.*

Thiothixene *See Navane, page 924.*

Thyroid Hormones *See Armour Thyroid, page 127.*

Tiazac *See Cardizem, page 249.*

TIGAN

Pronounced: TIE-gan
Generic name: Trimethobenzamide hydrochloride

Why is this drug prescribed?

Tigan is prescribed to control nausea and vomiting.

Most important fact about this drug

Antiemetics (drugs that prevent or lessen nausea and vomiting) are not recommended for the treatment of simple vomiting in children. Use of Tigan in children should be limited to prolonged vomiting caused by a known disease. Tigan is thought to have an aggravating effect on Reye's syndrome (a potentially fatal childhood disease of the brain that sometimes strikes after a viral infection such as chickenpox). In addition, some of Tigan's side effects can actually be confused with the symptoms of Reye's syndrome.

How should you take this medication?

Take this medication exactly as prescribed.

If you are using the suppository form of Tigan and find it is too soft to insert, you can firm it up by chilling it in the refrigerator for about 30 minutes or running cold water over it before removing the wrapper.

To insert a suppository, first remove the wrapper and moisten the suppository with cold water. Then lie down on your side and use a finger to push the suppository well up into the rectum.

■ *If you miss a dose...*
Take it as soon as you remember. If it is almost time for your next dose, skip the one you missed and go back to your regular schedule. Do not take 2 doses at once.

■ *Storage instructions...*
Store away from heat, light, and moisture.

What side effects may occur?

Side effects cannot be anticipated. If any develop or change in intensity, inform your doctor as soon as possible. Only your doctor can determine if it is safe for you to continue taking Tigan.

■ *Side effects may include:*
Allergic-type skin reactions, blood disorders, blurred vision, coma, convulsions, depression, disorientation, dizziness, drowsiness, headache, muscle cramps, severe muscle spasm, tremors, yellowed eyes and skin

Why should this drug not be prescribed?

If you are sensitive to or have ever had an allergic reaction to Tigan, do not take this medication. Do not use the suppositories if you are allergic to benzocaine or other local anesthetics. Make sure your doctor is aware of any drug reactions you have experienced.

Do not use suppositories in premature or newborn infants.

Special warnings about this medication

Tigan may cause you to become drowsy or less alert. Do not drive or operate dangerous machinery or participate in any hazardous activity that requires full mental alertness until you know how you respond to this drug.

During illnesses such as high fever, inflammation of the brain, inflammation of the digestive tract, or dehydration, Tigan should be used with caution, especially in children, older adults, and anyone in a run-down condition. Under these circumstances, the drug is more likely to cause severe reactions such as convulsions and coma.

Severe vomiting should not be treated with Tigan alone. Your doctor should emphasize restoration of body fluids, the relief of fever, and the relief of the disease causing the vomiting. However, the overconsumption of fluids may result in cerebral edema (excessive accumulation of fluid in the brain).

The antinausea effects of Tigan may make it difficult to diagnose such conditions as appendicitis and may mask signs of drug poisoning due to overdosage of other drugs.

Possible food and drug interactions when taking this medication

The use of alcohol in combination with this drug may produce an unfavorable reaction.

Caution should be exercised when taking Tigan in combination with central nervous system drugs such as phenothiazines (tranquilizers and antiemetics), barbiturates such as phenobarbital, and drugs derived from belladonna, such as Donnatal, if you are dehydrated or have a severe disease with fever, inflammation of the stomach, intestines, or brain.

Special information if you are pregnant or breastfeeding

The effects of Tigan during pregnancy or breastfeeding have not been adequately studied. If you are pregnant or plan to become pregnant, inform your doctor immediately. If you are breastfeeding your baby, consult your doctor before taking this medication.

Recommended dosage

Dosage will be adjusted by your doctor according to your illness, the severity of your symptoms, and how well you do on the drug.

ADULTS

Capsules
The usual dosage is one 300-milligram capsule taken 3 or 4 times per day, as determined by your doctor.

Suppositories
The recommended dosage is 1 suppository (200 milligrams) inserted into the rectum 3 or 4 times per day, as determined by your doctor.

CHILDREN

Capsules
The usual dosage for children weighing 30 to 90 pounds is one or two 100-milligram capsules taken 3 or 4 times per day, as determined by the doctor.

Suppositories
The usual dosage for children weighing under 30 pounds is half a suppository (100 milligrams), inserted into the rectum 3 or 4 times a day, as determined by the doctor.

The usual dosage for children weighing 30 to 90 pounds is one-half to one 200-milligram suppository rectally 3 or 4 times a day, as determined by the doctor.

Pediatric Suppositories
The usual dosage for children weighing under 30 pounds is 1 suppository (100 milligrams) rectally 3 or 4 times a day, as determined by the doctor.

The usual dosage for children weighing 30 to 90 pounds is 1 to 2 suppositories (100 milligrams to 200 milligrams) rectally 3 or 4 times a day, as determined by the doctor.

Overdosage
Although no specific information is available, any medication taken in excess can have serious consequences. If you suspect a Tigan overdose, seek medical attention immediately.

TILADE
Pronounced: TILE-aid
Generic name: Nedocromil sodium

Why is this drug prescribed?
Tilade is an anti-inflammatory medication prescribed for use on a regular basis to control symptoms in people with mild to moderate asthma.

Most important fact about this drug
Tilade must be used regularly to be effective, even if you have no symptoms. It improves your condition, but won't help during an acute attack.

How should you take this medication?
Proper inhalation of Tilade is essential for it to be effective. Make sure you understand how to use the medication correctly, and take exactly the amount prescribed. It may be a week or more before you feel the full effect.

Tilade Inhaler should not be used with other mouthpieces.

Avoid spraying the medication in your eyes.

■ *If you miss a dose...*
To work properly, Tilade must be inhaled every day at regular intervals. If you miss a dose, take it as soon as you remember. If it is almost time for your next dose, skip the one you missed and go back to your regular schedule. Do not take double doses.

■ *Storage instructions...*
Store Tilade Inhaler at room temperature. Because the contents are under pressure, do not puncture, incinerate, or place near heat.

What side effects may occur?
Side effects cannot be anticipated. If any develop or change in intensity, inform your doctor as soon as possible. Only your doctor can determine if it is safe for you to continue using Tilade.

■ *Side effects may include:*
Chest pain, coughing, fever, headache, inflamed nose and sinuses, nausea, sore throat, unpleasant taste, upper respiratory tract infection, wheezing

Why should this drug not be prescribed?

Tilade Inhaler should not be used if you are sensitive to or have ever had an allergic reaction to nedocromil sodium or any of Tilade's other ingredients. Make sure your doctor is aware of any drug reactions you have experienced.

Special warnings about this medication

This medication will not stop an asthma attack. However, you should continue to take it during an attack, along with a bronchodilator (a medication that increases air flow to your lungs) to relieve the acute symptoms.

If your symptoms do not improve or get worse, call your doctor right away; don't try increasing the dose to make the medication work.

Medications that are inhaled can cause coughing and wheezing in some people. If you experience these symptoms, stop taking Tilade and notify your doctor immediately.

Possible food and drug interactions when taking this medication

No interactions have been reported.

Special information if you are pregnant or breastfeeding

The effects of Tilade during pregnancy have not been adequately studied. If you are pregnant or plan to become pregnant, notify your doctor immediately. Tilade may appear in breast milk and could affect a nursing infant. If this medication is essential to your health, your doctor may advise you to discontinue breastfeeding until your treatment is finished.

Recommended dosage

ADULTS AND CHILDREN 6 YEARS OF AGE AND OVER

The recommended dose is 2 inhalations 4 times a day at regular intervals. If you are doing well on that dosage, your doctor may try reducing the dose after a time.

CHILDREN

The safety and effectiveness of Tilade Inhaler have not been established in children under 6 years of age.

Overdosage

A dangerous reaction is unlikely. However, any medication taken in excess can have serious consequences. If you suspect an overdose, seek medical attention immediately.

Timolol *See Timoptic, below.*

TIMOPTIC
Pronounced: Tim-OP-tic
Generic name: Timolol
Other brand names: Betimol, Timoptic-XE

Why is this drug prescribed?
Timoptic is a topical medication (applied directly in the eye) that effectively reduces internal pressure in the eye. Timoptic is used in the treatment of glaucoma to lower elevated eye pressure that could damage vision and, with other glaucoma medications, to further reduce pressure in the eye.

Most important fact about this drug
Although Timoptic eyedrops are applied only to the eye, the medication is absorbed and may have effects in other parts of the body. If you have diabetes, asthma, or other respiratory disease, or decreased heart function, make sure your doctor is aware of the problem.

How should you use this medication?
Timoptic should be used exactly as prescribed by your doctor.

If you are using Timoptic in Ocudose, use the medication as soon as you open the individual unit and throw out any leftover solution.

If you are using Timoptic-XE, invert the closed container and shake it once—and only once—before each use.

If you need to use other eye medications along with Timoptic, use them at least 10 minutes before you instill Timoptic. Allow 5 minutes with Betimol.

If you wear contact lenses, remove them before using Timoptic and wait 15 minutes before reinserting them.

Handle the Timoptic solution carefully to avoid contamination. Do not let the tip of the dispenser actually touch the eye. Do not enlarge the hole in the dispenser tip; it is designed to provide just 1 drop. Do not wash the dispenser tip with water, soap, or any other cleaner.

To administer Timoptic, follow these steps:
1. Wash your hands thoroughly.
2. Tilt your head back and gently pull your lower eyelid down to form a pocket.
3. Turn the bottle upside down, holding it with your thumb or index finger over the Finger Push Area.
4. Press the bottle lightly until a single drop falls into the eye.
5. Repeat steps 3 and 4 with the other eye if necessary.
6. Replace the cap firmly.

- *If you miss a dose...*
  If you use Timoptic once a day, apply it as soon as you remember. If you do not remember until the next day, skip the dose you missed and go back to your regular schedule. Do not take 2 doses at once. If you use it more than once a day, apply it as soon as you remember. If it is almost time for your next dose, skip the one you missed and go back to your regular schedule. Do not take 2 doses at once.
- *Storage instructions...*
  Store at room temperature, protected from light. Keep from freezing.

What side effects may occur?
Side effects cannot be anticipated. If any side effects develop or change in intensity, tell your doctor immediately. Only your doctor can determine whether it is safe to continue using this medication. If Timoptic is absorbed into the bloodstream, it can cause additional side effects.

- *Side effects may include:*
  Burning and stinging on instillation of the drug

Why should this drug not be prescribed?
Do not use Timoptic if you have bronchial asthma, a history of bronchial asthma, or other serious breathing disorders such as emphysema, slow heartbeat, heart block (conduction disorder), active heart failure, or inadequate blood supply to the circulatory system (cardiogenic shock), or if you have ever had an allergic reaction or are sensitive to Timoptic or any of its ingredients.

Special warnings about this medication
Use Timoptic cautiously if you have a history of heart failure or poor circulation to the brain.

Tell your doctor if you have any type of allergy. The frequency and severity of allergic reactions may increase while you are using Timoptic.

Timoptic may mask the symptoms of low blood sugar. If you are diabetic, discuss this possibility with your doctor.

Tell your doctor or dentist that you are using Timoptic if you have a medical emergency or before you have surgery or dental treatment.

Timoptic may mask symptoms of an overactive thyroid. If your doctor suspects you have excessive thyroid function, he or she will manage your case carefully to avoid such symptoms as rapid heartbeat, which can occur when the drug is withdrawn too abruptly.

Timoptic's antiglaucoma effects may decrease if you use the medication for a long time.

Some older individuals may be more sensitive to this product than younger people. If you develop an eye infection, suffer an eye injury, or have eye surgery, check with your doctor. You may need to stop using Timoptic.

Possible food and drug interactions when using this medication

If Timoptic is used with certain other drugs, the effects of either could be increased, decreased, or altered. It is especially important to check with your doctor before combining Timoptic with the following:

Calcium antagonists such as Cardizem and Isoptin
Catecholamine-depleting drugs, such as blood pressure drugs that contain reserpine (Serpasil)
Clonidine (Catapres, Clorpres, Combipres)
Digitalis (Lanoxin)
Epinephrine (EpiPen)
Quinidine (Quinaglute, Quinidex)

Timoptic should not be used with other topical beta-blockers and should be used with caution if you are taking oral beta-blockers such as Inderal and Tenormin.

Special information if you are pregnant or breastfeeding

If you are pregnant or plan to become pregnant, inform your doctor immediately. No information is available about the safety of using Timoptic during pregnancy.

Timolol appears in breast milk and may harm a nursing infant. If using Timoptic is essential to your health, your doctor may advise you to stop breastfeeding until your treatment is finished.

Recommended dosage

ADULTS

Your doctor will tailor an individual Timoptic dosage depending on your medical condition and how you responded to any previous glaucoma treatment.

The usual recommended initial dose is to place 1 drop of 0.25 percent Timoptic in the affected eye(s) twice a day. If you do not respond satisfactorily to this dosage, your doctor may tell you to place 1 drop of 0.5 percent Timoptic in the affected eye(s) twice a day.

The usual dose of Timoptic-XE is 1 drop of either 0.25 percent or 0.5 percent in the affected eye(s) once a day. Invert the closed container and shake it once before you use it.

The usual dose of Betimol is 1 drop of either 0.25 percent or 0.5 percent in the affected eye(s) twice a day.

Overdosage

Seek medical treatment immediately if you think you might have used too much Timoptic. Call your local poison control center or your doctor for assistance.

■ *Symptoms of Timoptic overdose may include:*
Dizziness, headache, heart failure, shortness of breath, slow heartbeat, wheezing

TINDAMAX

Pronounced: TIN-dah-macks
Generic name: Tinidazole

Why is this drug prescribed?

Tindamax is prescribed to treat infections caused by a variety of parasites, including:

1. Trichomoniasis, a common sexually transmitted disease that affects men and women. It can contribute to reduced fertility in both sexes and may enhance the acquisition and transmission of HIV. Trichomoniasis has also been linked to cervical cancer, preterm birth, and postoperative infection. Symptoms in women include yellow or green vaginal discharge (often with a foul odor) and vaginal burning, itching, soreness, or redness. Urination and intercourse may also be painful. Men who are infected with trichomoniasis frequently do not have symptoms and often unknowingly transmit the infection to their partner. When symptoms are present in men, they may include urethral discharge and irritation.

2. Giardiasis, an intestinal infection caused by drinking untreated water. Symptoms include abdominal pain, nausea, vomiting, diarrhea, cramping, bloating, and weight loss.

3. Intestinal amebiasis (commonly known as dysentery), an infection caused by consuming contaminated water or food. Symptoms may include loose stools, stomach pain, and cramping. In more severe cases, symptoms can include severe stomach pain, weight loss, bloody stools, and fever.

4. Amebic liver abscess, a severe and potentially life-threatening infection caused by the same parasite that causes intestinal amebiasis. Symptoms may not be detectable. When symptoms do appear, they can include fever, jaundice, loss of appetite, diarrhea, and intense stomach pain, especially in the upper right-hand side near the liver.

Most important fact about this drug

Do not drink alcohol while taking Tindamax or for 3 days after you stop taking the drug. Combining alcohol with Tindamax can cause stomach cramps, nausea, vomiting, headaches, and flushing. When Tindamax is combined with alcohol and the drug disulfiram (Antabuse), a severe mental disorder can occur. Always check the labels on foods and over-the-counter products to make sure they do not contain alcohol.

How should you take this medication?

Take Tindamax with food at about the same time each day. The drug works best when there's a constant amount in the bloodstream.

For people who cannot swallow tablets, a pharmacist can make Tindamax into a syrup.

■ *If you miss a dose...*
Take the forgotten dose as soon as you remember. However, if it is almost time for your next dose, skip the one you missed and return to your regular schedule. Do not take 2 doses at once.

■ *Storage instructions...*
Store at room temperature.

What side effects may occur?

Side effects cannot be anticipated. If any develop or change in intensity, tell your doctor as soon as possible. Only your doctor can determine if it is safe to continue using Tindamax.

■ *Side effects may include:*
Abdominal pain, appetite loss, bitter or metallic taste, confusion, depression, difficulty breathing, drowsiness, fatigue, headache, loss of consciousness, nausea, skipped heartbeat, vaginal discharge, vomiting, weakness

Although rare, Tindamax has caused seizures and numbness or tingling in the arms, hands, legs, and feet (see *Special warnings about this medication*).

Why should this drug not be prescribed?

Do not use Tindamax if you have ever had an allergic reaction to other drugs in the same class such as metronidazole (Flagyl).

You should not take Tindamax within 2 weeks of the drug disulfiram (Antabuse).

Tindamax should not be used during the first 3 months of pregnancy.

Special warnings about this medication

Use Tindamax cautiously if you have any disease of the central nervous system. In rare cases, the drug has caused seizures or peripheral neuropathy (a painful nerve disorder marked by numbness or tingling in the arms, hands, legs, and feet). If you experience these symptoms, stop taking Tindamax and call your doctor immediately.

Tindamax can make some medical conditions worse. If you have a blood disorder, liver disease, or yeast infection, your doctor will monitor you closely during treatment with Tindamax.

If you're taking Tindamax to treat the sexually transmitted disease trichomoniasis, your partner should be treated at the same time to prevent you from getting infected again.

Possible food and drug interactions when taking this medication
Do not combine Tindamax with alcohol or any product containing alcohol (see *Most important fact about this drug*).

If Tindamax is taken with certain other drugs, the effects of either could be increased, decreased, or altered. It is especially important to check with your doctor before combining Tindamax with the following:

Blood thinners such as warfarin (Coumadin)
Cholestyramine (Questran, Questran Light)
Cimetidine (Tagamet)
Cyclosporine (Neoral, Sandimmune)
Disulfiram (Antabuse)
Fluorouracil (Adrucil)
Fosphenytoin (Cerebyx)
Ketoconazole (Nizoral)
Lithium (Eskalith, Lithobid)
Oxytetracycline (Terramycin)
Phenobarbital
Phenytoin (Dilantin)
Rifampin (Rifadin, Rimactane)
Tacrolimus (Prograf)

Special information if you are pregnant or breastfeeding
If you are pregnant or plan to become pregnant, inform your doctor immediately. Tindamax has not been studied in pregnant women. However, because lab and animal studies indicate that Tindamax does cross the placenta, it should not be used during the first 3 months of pregnancy. Tindamax should only be used in the last 6 months of pregnancy if your doctor decides the benefits outweigh the risks.

Because Tindamax appears in breast milk, you should not take it while breastfeeding. If your doctor decides to treat you with Tindamax, you'll have to avoid breastfeeding while you're taking the drug and for 3 days after the last dose.

Recommended dosage

ADULTS

Trichomoniasis
The treatment consists of a single 2-gram dose. Your sexual partner should be treated at the same time.

Giardiasis
The treatment consists of a single 2-gram dose.

Intestinal Amebiasis
The recommended dose is 2 grams a day for 3 days.

Amebic Liver Abscess
The recommended dose is 2 grams a day for 3 to 5 days.

CHILDREN 3 YEARS OF AGE AND OLDER

Giardiasis
The treatment consists of a single dose based on the child's weight (50 milligrams per 2.2 pounds), up to a maximum of 2 grams.

Intestinal Amebiasis
The daily dose is based on the child's weight (50 milligrams per 2.2 pounds), up to a maximum of 2 grams, taken for 3 days.

Amebic Liver Abscess
The daily dose is based on the child's weight (50 milligrams per 2.2 pounds), up to a maximum of 2 grams, taken for 3 to 5 days. Children who take Tindamax for more than 3 days must be closely monitored.

Overdosage
There are no reported overdoses with Tindamax. However, any medication taken in excess can have serious consequences. If you suspect an overdose, seek emergency treatment immediately.

Tinidazole *See Tindamax, page 1443.*

Tiotropium *See Spiriva HandiHaler, page 1334.*

Tizanidine *See Zanaflex, page 1607.*

Tobramycin *See Tobrex, below.*

TOBREX
Pronounced: TOE-breks
Generic name: Tobramycin
Other brand name: Aktob

Why is this drug prescribed?
Tobrex is an antibiotic applied to the eye to treat bacterial infections.

Most important fact about this drug
In order to clear up your infection completely, keep using Tobrex for the full time of treatment, even if your symptoms have disappeared.

How should you use this medication?

To apply Tobrex eyedrops:
1. Wash your hands thoroughly.
2. Gently pull your lower eyelid down to form a pocket between your eye and eyelid.

3. Brace the bottle on the bridge of your nose or your forehead.
4. Do not let the applicator tip touch your eye or any other surface.
5. Tilt your head back and squeeze the medication into the eye.
6. Close your eyes gently.
7. Keep your eyes closed for 1 to 2 minutes.
8. Do not rinse the dropper.
9. If you are using another eye drop wait 5 to 10 minutes before applying it.

To apply the ointment form of this medication:
1. Tilt your head back.
2. Place a finger on your cheek just under your eye and gently pull down until a V pocket is formed between your eyeball and your lower lid.
3. Place about half an inch of Tobrex in the V pocket. Do not let the tip of the tube touch the eye.
4. Look downward before closing your eye.

■ *If you miss a dose…*
Apply it as soon as you remember. If it is almost time for your next dose, skip the one you missed and go back to your regular schedule.

■ *Storage instructions…*
Store Tobrex at room temperature, away from heat, or in the refrigerator. Do not allow to freeze.

What side effects may occur?
Side effects cannot be anticipated. If any develop or change in intensity, inform your doctor as soon as possible. Only your doctor can determine if it is safe for you to continue to take Tobrex.

■ *Side effects may include:*
Abnormal redness of eye tissue, allergic reactions, lid itching, lid swelling

Why should this drug not be prescribed?
If you are sensitive to or have ever had an allergic reaction to Tobrex or any of its ingredients, you should not use this medication. Make sure your doctor is aware of any drug reactions you have experienced.

Special warnings about this medication
If you experience an allergic reaction to this medication, discontinue use and inform your doctor.
    Continued or prolonged use of Tobrex may result in a growth of bacteria that do not respond to this medication and can cause a secondary infection.

Possible food and drug interactions when taking this medication
If you are taking any other prescription antibiotics for your eyes, check with your doctor before using Tobrex. Using this medication with certain other antibiotics in your system may cause an overdose.

Special information if you are pregnant or breastfeeding

The effects of Tobrex during pregnancy have not been adequately studied. If you are pregnant or plan to become pregnant, inform your doctor immediately. Tobrex may appear in breast milk. Your doctor may advise you to discontinue breastfeeding until your treatment with this medication is finished.

Recommended dosage

ADULTS

Solution

If the infection is mild to moderate, place 1 or 2 drops into the affected eye(s) every 4 hours. In severe infections, place 2 drops into the eye(s) every hour until there is improvement. Then you will be instructed to use less medication before you stop using it altogether.

Ointment

If the infection is mild to moderate, apply a half-inch ribbon into the affected eye(s) 2 or 3 times per day. In severe infections, apply a half-inch ribbon into the affected eye(s) every 3 or 4 hours until there is improvement. Then use less medication before stopping altogether.

CHILDREN

Your doctor will tailor a dose for the child.

Overdosage

Any medication used in excess can have serious consequences. If you suspect an overdose, seek medical assistance immediately.

■ *Symptoms of Tobrex overdose may be similar to side effects. They include:*
Corneal redness and inflammation, excessive eye tearing, lid itching and swelling

Tocainide *See Tonocard, page 1458.*

TOFRANIL

Pronounced: TOE-fra-nil
Generic name: Imipramine hydrochloride
Other brand name: Tofranil-PM

Why is this drug prescribed?

Tofranil is used to treat depression. It is a member of the family of drugs called tricyclic antidepressants.

Tofranil is also used on a short-term basis, along with behavioral therapies, to treat bedwetting in children aged 6 and older. Its effectiveness may decrease with longer use.

Some doctors also prescribe Tofranil to treat bulimia, attention deficit disorder in children, obsessive-compulsive disorder, and panic disorder.

Tofranil-PM, which is usually taken once daily at bedtime, is approved to treat major depression.

Most important fact about this drug

Serious, sometimes fatal, reactions have been known to occur when drugs such as Tofranil are taken with another type of antidepressant called an MAO inhibitor. Drugs in this category include Nardil and Parnate. Do not take Tofranil within 2 weeks of taking one of these drugs. Make sure your doctor and pharmacist know of all the medications you are taking.

How should you take this medication?

Tofranil may be taken with or without food.

You should not take Tofranil with alcohol.

Do not stop taking Tofranil if you feel no immediate effect. It can take from 1 to 3 weeks for improvement to begin.

Tofranil can cause dry mouth. Sucking hard candy or chewing gum can help this problem.

■ *If you miss a dose...*
If you take 1 dose a day at bedtime, contact your doctor. Do not take the dose in the morning because of possible side effects.

If you take 2 or more doses a day, take the forgotten dose as soon as you remember. If it is almost time for your next dose, skip the one you missed and go back to your regular schedule. Do not take 2 doses at once.

■ *Storage instructions...*
Store at room temperature in a tightly closed container.

What side effects may occur?

Side effects cannot be anticipated. If any develop or change in intensity, inform your doctor as soon as possible. Only your doctor can determine if it is safe for you to continue taking Tofranil.

■ *Side effects may include:*
Breast development in males, breast enlargement in females, breast milk production, confusion, diarrhea, dry mouth, hallucinations, hives, high blood pressure, low blood pressure upon standing, nausea, numbness, tremors, vomiting

■ *The most common side effects in children being treated for bedwetting are:*
Nervousness, sleep disorders, stomach and intestinal problems, tiredness

■ *Other side effects in children are:*
Anxiety, collapse, constipation, convulsions, emotional instability, fainting

Why should this drug not be prescribed?

Tofranil should not be used if you are recovering from a recent heart attack.

People who take drugs known as MAO inhibitors, such as the antidepressants Nardil and Parnate, should not take Tofranil. You should not take Tofranil if you are sensitive or allergic to it.

Special warnings about this medication

In clinical studies, antidepressants increased the risk of suicidal thinking and behavior in children and adolescents with depression and other psychiatric disorders. Anyone considering the use of Tofranil or any other antidepressant in a child or adolescent must balance this risk with the clinical need. Tofranil has not been studied in children less than 6 years old. Tofranil-PM is not approved for use in children.

Additionally, the progression of major depression is associated with a worsening of symptoms and/or the emergence of suicidal thinking or behavior in both adults and children, whether or not they are taking antidepressants. Individuals being treated with Tofranil and their caregivers should watch for any change in symptoms or any new symptoms that appear suddenly—especially agitation, anxiety, hostility, panic, restlessness, extreme hyperactivity, and suicidal thinking or behavior—and report them to the doctor immediately. Be especially observant at the beginning of treatment or whenever there is a change in dose.

You should use Tofranil cautiously if you have or have ever had: narrow-angle glaucoma (increased pressure in the eye); difficulty in urinating; heart, liver, kidney, or thyroid disease; or seizures. Also be cautious if you are taking thyroid medication.

General feelings of illness, headache, and nausea can result if you suddenly stop taking Tofranil. Follow your doctor's instructions closely when discontinuing Tofranil.

Tell your doctor if you develop a sore throat or fever while taking Tofranil.

This drug may impair your ability to drive a car or operate potentially dangerous machinery. Do not participate in any activities that require full alertness if you are unsure about your ability.

This drug can make you sensitive to light. Try to stay out of the sun as much as possible while you are taking it.

If you are going to have elective surgery, your doctor will take you off Tofranil.

Both increased and decreased blood sugar levels have been reported during Tofranil therapy. If you have diabetes or low blood sugar (hypoglycemia), your doctor will monitor you closely.

Be sure your doctor knows if you have a history of mental disorders. Tofranil could cause a manic episode in people with bipolar disorder or a psychotic episode in those with schizophrenia.

Unless it's absolutely essential, Tofranil is not recommended for people undergoing electroconvulsive therapy (ECT).

Possible food and drug interactions when taking this medication

Never combine Tofranil with an MAO inhibitor (see *Most important fact about this drug*). If Tofranil is taken with certain other drugs, the effects of either could be increased, decreased, or altered. It is especially important to check with your doctor before combining Tofranil with the following:

Albuterol (Proventil, Ventolin)
Antidepressants that act on serotonin, including Paxil, Prozac
    and Zoloft
Antipsychotic drugs such as chlorpromazine and Mellaril
Barbiturates such as Nembutal and Seconal
Blood pressure medications such as Catapres
Carbamazepine (Tegretol)
Cimetidine (Tagamet)
Decongestants such as Sudafed
Drugs that control spasms, such as Cogentin
Epinephrine (EpiPen)
Flecainide (Tambocor)
Guanethidine
Methylphenidate (Ritalin)
Norepinephrine
Other antidepressants such as Elavil and Pamelor
Phenytoin (Dilantin)
Propafenone (Rythmol)
Quinidine
Thyroid medications such as Synthroid
Tranquilizers and sleep aids such as Halcion, Valium, and Xanax

Extreme drowsiness and other potentially serious effects can result if Tofranil is combined with alcohol or other mental depressants, such as narcotic painkillers (Percocet), sleeping medications (Halcion), or tranquilizers (Valium).

If you are switching from Prozac, wait at least 5 weeks after your last dose of Prozac before starting Tofranil.

Special information if you are pregnant or breastfeeding

The effects of Tofranil during pregnancy have not been adequately studied. Pregnant women should use Tofranil only when the potential benefits clearly outweigh the potential risks. If you are pregnant or plan to become pregnant, inform your doctor immediately. Tofranil may appear in breast milk and could affect a nursing infant. If this medication is essential to your health, your doctor may advise you to stop breastfeeding until your treatment is finished.

Recommended dosage

ADULTS

The usual starting dose is 75 milligrams a day. The doctor may increase this to 150 milligrams a day. The maximum daily dose is 200 milligrams. People who need to take 75 milligrams or more a day may use Tofranil-PM capsules instead of the regular tablets.

CHILDREN

Tofranil is not to be used in children to treat any condition but bedwetting, and its use will be limited to short-term therapy. Safety and effectiveness in children under the age of 6 have not been established. Tofranil-PM should not be used in children for any reason.

Total daily dosages for children should not exceed 2.5 milligrams for each 2.2 pounds of the child's weight.

Doses usually begin at 25 milligrams per day. This amount should be taken an hour before bedtime. If needed, this dose may be increased after 1 week to 50 milligrams (ages 6 through 11) or 75 milligrams (ages 12 and up), taken in one dose at bedtime or divided into 2 doses, 1 taken at mid-afternoon and 1 at bedtime.

OLDER ADULTS AND ADOLESCENTS

People in these two age groups should start with 25 to 50 milligrams per day of Tofranil tablets, since Tofranil-PM capsules are not available in these dosage strengths. The dose may be increased as necessary, but effective dosages usually do not exceed 100 milligrams a day.

Overdosage

Any medication taken in excess can have serious consequences. An overdose of Tofranil can cause death. It has been reported that children are more sensitive than adults to overdoses of Tofranil. If you suspect an overdose, seek medical help immediately.

- *Symptoms of Tofranil overdose may include:*
  Agitation, bluish skin, coma, convulsions, difficulty breathing, dilated pupils, drowsiness, heart failure, high fever, involuntary writhing or jerky movements, irregular or rapid heartbeat, lack of coordination, low blood pressure, overactive reflexes, restlessness, rigid muscles, shock, stupor, sweating, vomiting

Tolazamide See Tolinase, page 1455.

Tolbutamide See Orinase, page 1006.

Tolcapone See Tasmar, page 1390.

TOLECTIN

Pronounced: toe-LEK-tin
Generic name: Tolmetin sodium

Why is this drug prescribed?

Tolectin is a nonsteroidal anti-inflammatory drug used to relieve the inflammation, swelling, stiffness, and joint pain associated with rheumatoid arthritis and osteoarthritis (the most common form of arthritis). It is used for both acute episodes and long-term treatment. It is also used to treat juvenile rheumatoid arthritis.

Most important fact about this drug

You should have frequent checkups with your doctor if you take Tolectin regularly. Ulcers or internal bleeding can occur without warning.

How should you take this medication?

If Tolectin upsets your stomach, it may be taken with food or an antacid, and with a full glass of water. It may also help to prevent upset if you avoid lying down for 20 to 30 minutes after taking the drug.

Take this medication exactly as prescribed by your doctor.

- *If you miss a dose...*
  Take it as soon as you remember. If it is almost time for your next dose, skip the one you missed and go back to your regular schedule. Never take 2 doses at the same time.
- *Storage instructions...*
  Store at room temperature in a tightly closed container, away from light.

What side effects may occur?

Side effects cannot be anticipated. If any develop or change in intensity, inform your doctor as soon as possible. Only your doctor can determine if it is safe for you to continue taking Tolectin.

- *Side effects may include:*
  Abdominal pain, change in weight, diarrhea, dizziness, gas, headache, heartburn, high blood pressure, indigestion, nausea, stomach and intestinal upset, swelling due to fluid retention, vomiting, weakness

Why should this drug not be prescribed?

If you are sensitive to or have ever had an allergic reaction to Tolectin, aspirin, or other nonsteroidal anti-inflammatory drugs, or if you have had asthma, hives, or nasal inflammation caused by aspirin or other nonsteroidal anti-inflammatory drugs, you should not take this medication. Make sure your doctor is aware of any drug reactions you have experienced.

Special warnings about this medication

Tolectin can cause kidney problems, especially if you are elderly, suffer from heart failure or liver disease, or take diuretics.

This drug can also affect the liver. If you develop symptoms such as yellow skin and eyes, notify your doctor. You should be taken off Tolectin.

Do not take aspirin or any other anti-inflammatory medications while taking Tolectin unless your doctor tells you to do so.

Tolectin can cause visual disturbances. If you experience a change in your vision, inform your doctor.

Tolectin prolongs bleeding time. If you are taking blood-thinning medication, this drug should be taken with caution.

This drug can increase water retention. Use with caution if you have heart disease or high blood pressure.

Tolectin causes some people to become drowsy or less alert. If it has this effect on you, driving or operating dangerous machinery or participating in any hazardous activity that requires full mental alertness is not recommended.

Possible food and drug interactions when taking this medication

If Tolectin is taken with certain other drugs, the effects of either could be increased, decreased, or altered. It is especially important to check with your doctor before combining Tolectin with the following:

Aspirin
Blood thinners such as Coumadin
Carteolol (Cartrol)
Diuretics such as Lasix
Glyburide (Micronase)
Lithium (Lithonate)
Methotrexate

Special information if you are pregnant or breastfeeding

The effects of Tolectin during pregnancy have not been adequately studied. If you are pregnant or plan to become pregnant, inform your doctor immediately. Tolectin appears in breast milk and could affect a nursing infant. If this medication is essential to your health, your doctor may advise you to discontinue breastfeeding until your treatment is finished.

Recommended dosage

ADULTS

Rheumatoid Arthritis or Osteoarthritis
The starting dosage is usually 1,200 milligrams a day, divided into 3 doses of 400 milligrams each. Take 1 dose when you wake up, 1 at bedtime, and 1 sometime in between. Your doctor may adjust the dosage

after 1 to 2 weeks. Most people will take a total daily dosage of 600 to 1,800 milligrams usually divided into 3 doses.

You should see the benefits of Tolectin in a few days to a week.

CHILDREN

The starting dose for children 2 years and older is usually a total of 20 milligrams per 2.2 pounds of body weight per day, divided into 3 or 4 smaller doses. Your doctor will advise you on use in children. The usual dose ranges from 15 to 30 milligrams per 2.2 pounds per day.

The safety and effectiveness of Tolectin have not been established in children under 2 years of age.

Overdosage

Although no specific information is available, any medication taken in excess can have serious consequences. If you suspect an overdose of Tolectin, seek medical attention immediately.

TOLINASE

Pronounced: TAHL-in-ace
Generic name: Tolazamide

Why is this drug prescribed?

Tolinase is an oral antidiabetic drug available in tablet form. It lowers the blood sugar level by stimulating the pancreas to release insulin. Tolinase may be given as a supplement to diet therapy to help control type 2 (non-insulin-dependent) diabetes.

There are two type of diabetes: type 1 (insulin-dependent) and type 2 (non-insulin-dependent). Type 1 diabetes usually requires insulin injection for life; type 2 can usually be controlled by dietary changes, exercise, and oral diabetes medications. Occasionally—during stressful periods or times of illness, or if oral medications fail to work—a type 2 diabetic may need insulin injections.

Most important fact about this drug

Always remember that Tolinase is an aid to, not a substitute for, good diet and exercise. Failure to follow a sound diet and exercise plan can lead to serious complications, such as dangerously low blood sugar levels. Remember, too, that Tolinase is not an oral form of insulin, and cannot be used in place of insulin.

How should you take this medication?

Remember that if you are diligent about diet and exercise, you may need Tolinase for only a short period of time. Take it exactly as prescribed.

While you are taking Tolinase, your blood and urine glucose levels should be monitored regularly. Your doctor may also want you to have a periodic glycosylated hemoglobin blood test, which will show how well you have kept your blood sugar down during the weeks preceding the test.

■ *If you miss a dose...*
Take it as soon as you remember. If it is almost time for the next dose, skip the one you missed and go back to your regular schedule. Do not take 2 doses at the same time.

■ *Storage instructions...*
Store at room temperature.

What side effects may occur?

Side effects cannot be anticipated. If any appear or change in intensity, inform your doctor as soon as possible. Only your doctor can determine if it is safe for you to continue taking Tolinase. The most frequently encountered side effects from Tolinase—nausea, a full, bloated feeling, and heartburn—may disappear if the dosage is reduced.

Hives, itching, and rash may appear initially and then disappear as you continue to take the drug. If a skin reaction persists, you should stop taking Tolinase.

Why should this drug not be prescribed?

Do not take Tolinase if you are sensitive to it or have ever had an allergic reaction to it; if you are suffering from diabetic ketoacidosis (a chemical imbalance leading to nausea, vomiting, confusion, and coma); or if you have type 1 (insulin-dependent) diabetes and are not taking insulin.

Special warnings about this medication

It's possible that drugs such as Tolinase may lead to more heart problems than diet treatment alone, or diet plus insulin. If you have a heart condition, you may want to discuss this with your doctor.

Like other oral antidiabetic drugs, Tolinase may produce severe low blood sugar (hypoglycemia) if the dosing is wrong. While taking Tolinase, you are particularly susceptible to episodes of low blood sugar if:

You suffer from a kidney or liver problem;
You have a lack of adrenal or pituitary hormones; or
You are older, run-down, or malnourished.

You are at increased risk for a low blood sugar episode if you are hungry, exercising heavily, drinking alcohol, or using more than one glucose-lowering drug.

Note that an episode of low blood sugar may be difficult to recognize if you are an older person or if you are taking a beta-blocker drug (Inderal, Lopressor, Tenormin, and others).

If switching to Tolinase from chlorpropamide (Diabinese), you should take special care to avoid an episode of low blood sugar.

Stress such as fever, trauma, infection, or surgery may increase blood sugar to the point that you require insulin injections.

Possible food and drug interactions when taking this medication

If Tolinase is taken with certain other drugs, the effects of either could be increased, decreased, or altered. It is especially important to check with your doctor before combining Tolinase with the following:

Airway-opening drugs such as Sudafed and Ventolin
Alcohol
Aspirin or related drugs
Beta-blocking blood pressure medications such as Inderal and Lopressor
Blood-thinning drugs such as Coumadin
Calcium channel blockers such as Calan and Isoptin
Chloramphenicol (Chloromycetin)
Corticosteroids such as Cortef, Decadron, and Medrol
Diuretics such as Esidrix and Diuril
Estrogens such as Premarin and Estraderm
Isoniazid (Nydrazid)
MAO inhibitors (antidepressants such as Nardil and Parnate)
Miconazole (Monistat)
Nicotinic acid
Nonsteroidal anti-inflammatory drugs such as Motrin and Naprosyn
Oral contraceptives
Phenothiazines (antipsychotic drugs such as Mellaril)
Phenytoin (Dilantin)
Probenecid
Rifampin (Rifadin)
Sulfa drugs such as Bactrim and Gantrisin
Thyroid drugs such as Synthroid

Special information if you are pregnant or breastfeeding

If you are pregnant or plan to become pregnant, inform your doctor immediately. Tolinase is not recommended for use during pregnancy, and should not be prescribed if you might become pregnant while taking it.

Control of diabetes during pregnancy is very important, but in most cases it should be accomplished with insulin injections rather than oral antidiabetic drugs.

Tolinase should not be used during breastfeeding because of possible harmful effects on the baby. If you are a new mother, you may need to choose between taking Tolinase and breastfeeding your baby.

Recommended dosage

Your doctor will determine the dosage level based on your needs.

ADULTS

The usual starting dose of Tolinase tablets for the mild to moderately severe type 2 diabetic is 100 to 150 milligrams daily taken with breakfast or the first main meal.

OLDER ADULTS

If you are malnourished, underweight, an older person, or not eating properly, the initial dose is usually 100 milligrams once a day. Failure to follow an appropriate dosage regimen may precipitate hypoglycemia (low blood sugar). If you do not stick to your prescribed dietary regimen, you are more likely to have an unsatisfactory response to this medication.

Overdosage

An overdose of Tolinase can cause an episode of low blood sugar. Mildly low blood sugar without loss of consciousness should be treated with oral glucose, an adjusted meal pattern, and possibly a reduction in the Tolinase dosage. Severely low blood sugar, which may cause coma or seizures, is a medical emergency and must be treated in a hospital. If you suspect an overdose of Tolinase, seek medical attention immediately.

Tolmetin See Tolectin, page 1453.

Tolterodine See Detrol, page 425.

TONOCARD

Pronounced: TAH-nuh-card
Generic name: Tocainide hydrochloride

Why is this drug prescribed?

Tonocard is used to treat severe irregular heartbeat (arrhythmias). Arrhythmias are generally divided into two main types: heartbeats that are faster than normal (tachycardia) and heartbeats that are slower than normal (bradycardia). Irregular heartbeats are often caused by drugs or disease but can occur in otherwise healthy people with no history of heart disease or other illness. Tonocard works differently from other antiarrhythmic drugs, such as quinidine (Quinidex), procainamide (Procan SR), and disopyramide (Norpace). It is similar to lidocaine (Xylocaine) and is effective in treating severe ventricular arrhythmias (irregular heartbeats that occur in the main chambers of the heart).

Most important fact about this drug

Tonocard can cause serious blood and lung disorders in some patients, especially in the first 3 months of treatment. Be sure to notify your doctor if any of the following occurs: painful or difficult breathing, wheezing, cough, easy bruising or bleeding, tremors, palpitations, rash, soreness or ulcers in the mouth, sore throat, fever, and chills.

How should you take this medication?

It is important to take Tonocard on a regular schedule, exactly as prescribed by your doctor. Try not to miss any doses. If this medication is not taken regularly, your condition can worsen.

■ *If you miss a dose…*
If less than 2 hours have passed, take the forgotten dose as soon as you remember. If you are more than 2 hours late, skip the dose. Never try to catch up by taking a double dose.

■ *Storage instructions…*
Keep the container tightly closed, and store it at room temperature. Protect from extreme heat.

What side effects may occur?

Side effects cannot be anticipated. If any develop or change in intensity, inform your doctor as soon as possible. Only your doctor can determine if it is safe for you to continue taking Tonocard.

■ *Side effects may include:*
Confusion/disorientation, diarrhea/loose stools, dizziness/vertigo, excessive sweating, hallucinations, increased irregular heartbeat, lack of coordination, loss of appetite, nausea, nervousness, rash/skin eruptions, tingling or pins and needles, tremor, vision disturbances, vomiting

Why should this drug not be prescribed?

If you have heart block (conduction disorder) and do not have a pacemaker, or if you are sensitive to or have ever had an allergic reaction to Tonocard or certain local anesthetics such as Xylocaine, do not take this medication.

Special warnings about this medication

Be alert for signs of the blood and lung disorders that can occur early in your treatment (see *Most important fact about this drug*).

If you have congestive heart failure, make sure the doctor is aware of it. Tonocard could worsen this condition.

Also make certain that the doctor is aware of any kidney or liver problems that you have. You will need to be monitored more carefully.

Before any kind of surgery, including dental surgery and emergency treatment, make sure the surgeon knows that you are taking Tonocard.

Possible food and drug interactions when taking this medication

If Tonocard is taken with certain other drugs, the effects of either could be increased, decreased, or altered. It is especially important to check with your doctor before combining Tonocard with any of the following:

The anesthetic Lidocaine (Xylocaine)
The blood pressure medicine Metoprolol (Lopressor)
Other antiarrhythmics such as Mexitil, Quinidex, and Procan

Special information if you are pregnant or breastfeeding

The effects of Tonocard during pregnancy have not been adequately studied. However, animal studies have shown an increase in stillbirths and spontaneous abortions. If you are pregnant or plan to become pregnant, inform your doctor immediately. Tonocard may appear in breast milk and could affect a nursing infant. If this medication is essential to your health, your doctor may advise you to discontinue breastfeeding until your treatment is finished.

Recommended dosage

ADULTS

Dosages of Tonocard must be adjusted according to its effects on each individual. Your doctor should monitor you carefully to determine if the dosage you are taking is working properly. He may divide your doses further or make other changes, such as shortening the time between doses, if side effects occur.

The usual starting dose is 400 milligrams every 8 hours.

The usual dose range is between 1,200 and 1,800 milligrams total per day, divided into 3 doses. This medication can be taken in 2 doses a day with careful monitoring by your doctor.

Doses beyond 2,400 milligrams per day are rarely used.

Some people, particularly those with reduced kidney or liver function, may be treated successfully with less than 1,200 milligrams per day.

CHILDREN

The safety and effectiveness of Tonocard in children have not been established.

Overdosage

Any medication taken in excess can have serious consequences. If you suspect an overdose, seek medical attention immediately.

There are no specific reports of Tonocard overdose. However, the first and most important signs of overdose would be expected to appear in the central nervous system. Disorders of the stomach and intestines might follow. Convulsions and heart and lung slowing or stopping might occur.

TOPAMAX

Pronounced: TOW-pah-macks
Generic name: Topiramate

Why is this drug prescribed?

Topamax is an antiepileptic drug, prescribed to control both the mild attacks known as partial seizures and the severe tonic-clonic convulsions known as grand mal seizures. It is typically added to the treatment regimen when other drugs fail to fully control a patient's attacks.

Topamax is also prescribed for the prevention of migraine headaches (also known as prophylactic treatment). However, due to a lack of studies, it's not known whether the drug can treat acute migraine attacks.

Most important fact about this drug

Do not abruptly stop taking Topamax. If the drug isn't withdrawn gradually, the frequency of your seizures could increase.

How should you take this medication?

It is important to take this medication exactly as prescribed. It can be taken with or without food. Avoid breaking the tablets; the medication has a bitter taste.

Topamax capsules may be swallowed whole, or the capsule may be opened and its contents sprinkled on a teaspoonful of soft food. To open the capsule, hold it so you can read the word "top" and carefully twist off the clear portion of the capsule. The drug and food mixture should be swallowed whole and not chewed. Do not store the mixture for future use.

Topamax increases your risk of developing kidney stones. To prevent this problem, be sure to take this medication with plenty of fluids.

- ■ *If you miss a dose…*
  Take it as soon as you remember. If it is almost time for your next dose, skip the one you missed and go back to your regular schedule. Never take 2 doses at once.
- ■ *Storage instructions…*
  Store Topamax at room temperature in a tightly closed container. Protect the tablets from moisture.

What side effects may occur?

Some side effects, such as fatigue, are more likely to surface with high doses of Topamax. Others occur regardless of dosage. While many tend to disappear after the first 8 weeks of therapy, it's still important to report them to your doctor. Only your doctor can determine if it is safe for you to continue taking Topamax.

■ *Side effects may include:*
Abdominal pain, abnormal coordination, abnormal vision, agitation, anxiety, appetite loss, back pain, breast pain, chest pain, confusion, constipation, depression, difficulty with concentration, difficulty with memory, dizziness, double vision, drowsiness, fatigue, flu-like symptoms, indigestion, language problems, leg pain, loss of coordination, menstrual problems, mood problems, nausea, nervousness, nose inflammation, rash, sinusitis, slowing of movements, sore throat, speech problems, tingling or burning sensations, tremors, weakness, weight loss

In children, the more common side effects are abnormal gait, aggressiveness, behavior problems, confusion, constipation, difficulty concentrating, difficulty with memory, difficulty sleeping, dizziness, drowsiness, fatigue, increased muscle movement, increased saliva, injury, loss of appetite, loss of coordination, nausea, nervousness, nosebleed, pneumonia, rash, speech problems, urinary incontinence, viral infection, and weight loss.

Other, less common side effects in children include allergic reaction, digestive inflammation, increased thirst, skin disorders, slowing of movement, vaginal discharge, vision disorders, and weakened reflexes.

Topamax has also been known to cause a number of very rare side effects in adults and children (typically striking less than 1 person in 100). If you develop any unfamiliar problems while taking Topamax, report them to your doctor.

Why should this drug not be prescribed?
If Topamax gives you an allergic reaction, you'll be unable to use the drug.

Special warnings about this medication
Because Topamax sometimes causes confusion, dizziness, fatigue, and problems with coordination and concentration, you should not drive, operate machinery, or participate in any hazardous activity that requires full mental alertness until you are certain how the drug affects you.

Topamax has been known to cause a potentially serious condition known as metabolic acidosis (an increase of acid in the blood). In children, chronic metabolic acidosis may affect growth or cause rickets (a softening or weakness of the bones that can lead to bone deformities). Contact your doctor immediately if you experience symptoms of metabolic acidosis such as rapid breathing, an irregular heartbeat, confusion, lethargy, fatigue, or loss of appetite. Your doctor will decide if you should discontinue taking Topamax. Do not abruptly stop taking this drug on your own; your doctor will gradually taper the dosage to avoid an increase in seizures.

Topamax has been known to trigger severe nearsightedness along with increased pressure inside the eye. The problem usually occurs within 1 month of starting treatment. If you develop blurred vision or eye pain, call your doctor immediately. Discontinuation of the drug may be necessary to prevent permanent vision loss.

In children with chronic diarrhea or untreated kidney disorders, use of Topamax may lead to rickets and reduced growth rates.

Tell your doctor if you have kidney problems or if you are on hemodialysis; your dosage of Topamax may need adjustment. Elderly patients in particular may experience reduced kidney function when taking Topamax. Also make sure the doctor is aware of any liver disorder you may have. Topamax must be used cautiously by individuals with impaired liver function.

Anyone using Topamax, particularly children, should be carefully monitored by their doctor for signs of increased body temperature or decreased sweating, especially during hot weather.

In rare instances, suicide attempts have been reported in people taking Topamax.

Possible food and drug interactions when taking this medication

If Topamax is taken with certain other drugs, the effects of either could be increased, decreased, or altered. It is especially important to check with your doctor before combining Topamax with:

Acetazolamide (Diamox)
Carbamazepine (Tegretol)
Dichlorphenamide (Daranide)
Digoxin (Lanoxin)
Metformin (Glucophage)
Phenytoin (Dilantin)
Oral contraceptives
Valproic acid (Depakene)

Topamax can depress the central nervous system. Be extremely cautious about combining it with alcohol, sedatives, tranquilizers, and other central nervous system depressants.

Special information if you are pregnant or breastfeeding

In animal studies, Topamax has caused harm to the developing fetus, and its safety has not been verified in pregnant humans. It is recommended for use during pregnancy only if the doctor feels that its potential benefit outweighs the potential risk to the infant.

This medication may appear in breast milk, and its possible effect on the nursing infant remains unknown. Check with your doctor if you plan to breastfeed your baby.

Recommended dosage

ADULTS

Seizures

Topamax therapy usually begins with a dose of 50 milligrams once daily during the first week. The daily dosage is then increased each week until, by the eighth week, the patient is taking 200 milligrams twice a day.

If you are also taking Dilantin or Tegretol, the dosage of Topamax may need adjustment.

Prevention of Migraine Headaches

The recommended total daily dose is 100 milligrams a day, taken in 2 divided doses. Your doctor will increase the dose slowly over 4 weeks. The usual regimen is as follows: Week 1: No morning dose; take 25 milligrams at night. Week 2: Take 25 milligrams in the morning and again at night. Week 3: Take 25 milligrams in the morning and 50 milligrams at night. Week 4: Take 50 milligrams in the morning and again at night.

CHILDREN

The usual daily dose for children 2 to 16 years of age is 5 to 9 milligrams for every 2.2 pounds of body weight, divided into 2 doses. Topamax therapy usually begins with a dose of 25 milligrams (or less) once daily during the first week. The daily dosage is then increased each week until the doctor is satisfied with the patient's response. It may take 8 weeks to reach the ideal dose.

DOSAGE ADJUSTMENT

For people with poor kidney function, the dosage is usually cut in half. On the other hand, those undergoing hemodialysis may need a supplemental dose. Likewise, the doctor may adjust your dosage if you have liver problems.

Overdosage

Any medication taken in excess can have serious consequences. If you suspect an overdose of Topamax, seek medical attention immediately.

■ *Symptoms of Topamax overdose may include:*
Abdominal pain, agitation, blurred vision, convulsions, depression, dizziness, double vision, drowsiness, impaired coordination, impaired mental activity, low blood pressure, reduced consciousness, severe diarrhea, sluggishness, speech problems

A Topamax overdose may result in metabolic acidosis (see *Special warnings about this medication*).

TOPICORT

Pronounced: TOP-i-court
Generic name: Desoximetasone

Why is this drug prescribed?

Topicort is a synthetic steroid medication in cream, gel, or ointment form that relieves the inflammation and itching caused by a variety of skin conditions.

Most important fact about this drug

When you use Topicort, you may absorb some of the medication through your skin and into the bloodstream. Too much absorption can lead to unwanted side effects elsewhere in the body. To keep this problem to a minimum, avoid using large amounts of Topicort over large areas, do not use it for extended periods of time, and do not cover it with airtight dressings such as plastic wrap or adhesive bandages unless specifically told to by your doctor.

Children may absorb more medication than adults do.

How should you use this medication?

Topicort is for use only on the skin. Be careful to keep it out of your eyes.

Apply a thin coating of Topicort to the affected area. Rub in gently.

The treated area should not be covered unless your doctor has told you to do so.

If Topicort is being used for an infant or toddler with a genital rash, make sure the diapers or plastic pants are not too tight, so that air can circulate.

■ *If you miss a dose...*
Use Topicort only as needed, in the smallest amount required for relief.
■ *Storage instructions...*
Store Topicort at room temperature.

What side effects may occur?

Side effects cannot be anticipated. If any develop or change in intensity, inform your doctor as soon as possible. Only your doctor can determine if it is safe for you to continue using Topicort. The side effects listed below occur infrequently, but may occur more often if the treated area is covered with a bandage.

■ *Side effects may include:*
Acne-like pimples, blistering, burning of the skin, dryness, excessive growth of hair, infection, inflammation of the hair follicles, irritation, itching, loss of skin pigmentation, prickly heat, skin inflammation around the mouth, rash, redness, softening of the skin, stretch marks on the skin, thinning of the skin

Why should this drug not be prescribed?
Do not use Topicort if you are sensitive to it or have ever had an allergic reaction to any of its ingredients.

Special warnings about this medication
Remember to avoid getting Topicort into your eyes. Do not use Topicort to treat any condition other than the one for which it was prescribed.

Long-term use of steroids such as Topicort may interfere with the growth and development of children. They may also develop headaches or bulging at the top of the head. This drug is not recommended for children under 10.

Avoid covering a treated area with tight waterproof diapers or plastic pants. They can increase unwanted absorption of Topicort.

If your skin becomes irritated or infected, stop using Topicort and call your doctor.

Possible food and drug interactions when using this medication
No interactions have been reported.

Special information if you are pregnant or breastfeeding
Topicort should not be used over large areas, in large amounts, or for long periods of time during pregnancy unless the benefit outweighs any potential risk to the unborn child. If you are pregnant or plan to become pregnant, inform your doctor immediately.

It is not known whether topical steroids are absorbed in sufficient amounts to appear in breast milk. If your doctor considers Topicort essential to your health, he or she may advise you to stop breastfeeding until your treatment with the medication is finished.

Recommended dosage

ADULTS
Apply a thin film of Topicort cream, gel, or ointment to the affected area 2 times a day. Rub in gently.

CHILDREN
Use the smallest amount of Topicort necessary to relieve symptoms. Ask your doctor for specific instructions.

Overdosage
Large doses of steroids such as Topicort applied over a large area or for a long time, especially when the treated area is covered, can cause increases in blood sugar and Cushing's syndrome, a condition characterized by a moon-shaped face, emotional disturbances, high blood pressure, weight gain, and, in women, baldness or growth of body and facial hair. Cushing's syndrome may also trigger the development of diabetes.

If left uncorrected, Cushing's syndrome may become serious. If you suspect your use of Topicort has led to this problem, seek medical attention immediately.

Topiramate *See Topamax, page 1461.*

Toprol-XL *See Lopressor, page 775.*

TORADOL

Pronounced: TOH-rah-dol
Generic name: Ketorolac tromethamine

Why is this drug prescribed?

Toradol, a nonsteroidal anti-inflammatory drug, is used to relieve moderately severe, acute pain. It is prescribed for a limited amount of time (no more than 5 days for adults and as a single dose for children), not for long-term therapy.

Most important fact about this drug

Toradol can cause serious side effects, including ulcers and internal bleeding. Never take it for more than 5 days.

How should you take this medication?

Toradol works fastest when taken on an empty stomach, but an antacid can be taken if it causes upset. Take this medication exactly as prescribed.

Take Toradol with a full glass of water. Also, do not lie down for about 20 minutes after taking it. This will help to prevent irritation of your upper digestive tract.

■ *If you miss a dose...*
If you take Toradol on a regular schedule, take it as soon as you remember. If it is almost time for your next dose, skip the one you missed and go back to your regular schedule. Never take 2 doses at the same time.

■ *Storage instructions...*
Store at room temperature, away from light.

What side effects may occur?

Side effects cannot be anticipated. If any develop or change in intensity, inform your doctor as soon as possible. Only your doctor can determine if it is safe for you to continue using Toradol.

■ *Side effects may include:*
Diarrhea, dizziness, drowsiness, headache, indigestion, nausea, stomach and intestinal pain, swelling due to fluid retention

Why should this drug not be prescribed?

Do not take Toradol if it has ever given you an allergic reaction. Also avoid this medication if you have ever had an allergic reaction—such as nasal polyps (tumors), swelling of the face, limbs, and throat, hives, wheezing, light-headedness—to aspirin or other nonsteroidal anti-inflammatory drugs (NSAIDs) such as Motrin.

Do not take Toradol if you have ever had a peptic ulcer or stomach or intestinal bleeding. Avoid it if you have severe kidney disease or bleeding problems.

Never combine this drug with aspirin, NSAIDs, or probenecid. Make sure your doctor is aware of any drug reactions you have experienced.

Special warnings about this medication

Remember that Toradol has been known to cause peptic ulcers and bleeding. Contact your doctor immediately if you suspect a problem.

This drug should be used with caution if you have kidney or liver disease. It may cause liver inflammation or kidney problems in some people.

Toradol is not recommended for long-term use, since side effects increase over time. This medication should be taken for no more than 5 days.

If you are an older adult, use this drug cautiously.

Toradol can increase water retention. If you have heart disease or high blood pressure, use this drug with care.

This medication can prolong bleeding time. If you are taking blood-thinning medication, take Toradol with caution.

Possible food and drug interactions when using this medication

If Toradol is taken with certain other drugs, the effects of either could be increased, decreased, or altered. It is especially important to check with your doctor before combining Toradol with the following:

ACE inhibitor drugs such as the blood pressure medications Capoten and Vasotec
Antidepressants such as Prozac
Antiepileptic drugs (Dilantin, Tegretol)
Aspirin and other nonsteroidal anti-inflammatory drugs such as Motrin
Blood thinners such as Coumadin
Lithium (Eskalith, Lithobid)
Major tranquilizers such as Navane
Methotrexate (Rheumatrex)
Probenecid
Tranquilizers such as Xanax
Water pills such as Lasix and Dyazide

Special information if you are pregnant or breastfeeding

Toradol should not be taken late in pregnancy; during this period, it can harm the developing baby. If you are pregnant or plan to become pregnant, inform your doctor immediately. Toradol appears in breast milk and could affect a nursing infant. This medication should not be used while you are breastfeeding.

Recommended dosage

ADULTS

Your doctor will give you Toradol intravenously or intramuscularly to start, then have you switch to the tablets. Most patients take 2 tablets for the first dose (20 milligrams) and then 1 tablet (10 milligrams) every 4 to 6 hours. You should not take more than 40 milligrams per day and should not take Toradol for more than 5 days in all.

CHILDREN

For children under 16, the doctor may prescribe a single dose of Toradol, by intravenous or intramuscular injection, after an operation. Toradol is not recommended for children under 2.

OLDER ADULTS

Doses are usually lower for people over 65, those with kidney problems, and those who weigh less than 110 pounds. Your doctor will tailor the best dosage for you.

Overdosage

Any medication taken in excess can have serious consequences. If you suspect an overdose, seek medical attention immediately.

■ *Symptoms of Toradol overdose may include:*
  Drowsiness, nausea, stomach pain, vomiting

In rare cases, the victim may develop stomach bleeding, high blood pressure, kidney failure, impaired breathing, or coma. Severe allergic reactions are also possible.

Torsemide See Demadex, page 400.

T-Phyl See Theo-Dur, page 1432.

Tramadol See Ultram, page 1521.

Tramadol and Acetaminophen See Ultracet, page 1519.

Trandate See Normodyne, page 964.

Trandolapril See Mavik, page 809.

Trandolapril with Verapamil *See Tarka, page 1387.*

Transderm-Nitro *See Nitroglycerin, page 952.*

TRANXENE
Pronounced: TRAN-zeen
Generic name: Clorazepate dipotassium
Other brand names: Tranxene-SD, Tranxene-SD Half Strength

Why is this drug prescribed?
Tranxene belongs to a class of drugs known as benzodiazepines. It is used in the treatment of anxiety disorders and for short-term relief of the symptoms of anxiety.

It is also used to relieve the symptoms of acute alcohol withdrawal and to help in treating certain convulsive disorders such as epilepsy.

Most important fact about this drug
Tranxene can be habit-forming if taken regularly over a long period. You may experience withdrawal symptoms if you stop using this drug abruptly. Consult your doctor before discontinuing Tranxene or making any change in your dose.

How should you take this medication?
Tranxene should be taken exactly as prescribed by your doctor.

■ *If you miss a dose...*
  Take it as soon as you remember if it is within an hour or so of your scheduled time. If you do not remember until later, skip the dose you missed and go back to your regular schedule. Do not take 2 doses at once.
■ *Storage instructions...*
  Store at room temperature. Protect from excessive heat.

What side effects may occur?
Side effects cannot be anticipated. If any develop or change in intensity, inform your doctor as soon as possible. Only your doctor can determine if it is safe for you to continue taking Tranxene.

■ *Side effects may include:*
  Blurred vision, depression, difficulty sleeping or falling asleep, dizziness, drowsiness, dry mouth, double vision, fatigue, genital and urinary tract disorders, headache, irritability, lack of muscle coordination, mental confusion, nervousness, skin rashes, slurred speech, stomach and intestinal disorders, tremors

■ *Side effects due to a rapid decrease in dose or abrupt*
  withdrawal from Tranxene may include:
Abdominal cramps, convulsions, diarrhea, difficulty sleeping or falling
asleep, hallucinations, impaired memory, irritability, muscle aches,
nervousness, tremors, vomiting

Why should this drug not be prescribed?

If you are sensitive to or have ever had an allergic reaction to Tranxene,
you should not take this medication. Make sure your doctor is aware of
any drug reactions you have experienced.

Do not take this medication if you have the eye condition known as
acute narrow-angle glaucoma.

Anxiety or tension related to everyday stress usually does not require
treatment with such a strong drug. Discuss your symptoms thoroughly
with your doctor.

Tranxene is not recommended for use in more serious conditions such
as depression or severe psychological disorders.

Special warnings about this medication

Tranxene may cause you to become drowsy or less alert; therefore, you
should not drive or operate dangerous machinery or participate in any
hazardous activity that requires full mental alertness until you know how
this drug affects you.

If you are being treated for anxiety associated with depression, your
doctor will prescribe the lowest dose possible to avoid the risk of overdose. Do not increase your dose without consulting the doctor.

The elderly and people in a weakened condition are more apt to become unsteady or oversedated when taking Tranxene.

If you have to take Tranxene for a long period of time, the doctor will
need to monitor your blood counts and liver function.

Possible food and drug interactions when taking this medication

Tranxene slows down the central nervous system and may intensify the
effects of alcohol. Do not drink alcohol while taking this medication.

If Tranxene is taken with certain other drugs, the effects of either could
be increased, decreased, or altered. It is especially important to check
with your doctor before combining Tranxene with the following:

Antidepressant drugs known as MAO inhibitors (Nardil, Parnate) and
     other antidepressants such as Elavil and Prozac
Antipsychotic drugs such as Mellaril and chlorpromazine
Barbiturates such as Nembutal and Seconal
Narcotic pain relievers such as Demerol and Percodan
Any other drugs that slow down the central nervous system

Special information if you are pregnant or breastfeeding

The effects of Tranxene during pregnancy have not been adequately studied. However, because there is an increased risk of birth defects associated with this class of drug, its use during pregnancy should be avoided. Tranxene may appear in breast milk and could affect a nursing infant. If this medication is essential to your health, your doctor may advise you to discontinue breastfeeding until your treatment with this medication is finished.

Recommended dosage

ANXIETY

Adults

The usual daily dosage is 30 milligrams divided into several smaller doses. A normal daily dose can be as little as 15 milligrams. Your doctor may increase the dosage gradually to as much as 60 milligrams, according to your individual needs.

Tranxene can also be taken in a single bedtime dose. The initial dose is 15 milligrams, but your doctor will adjust the dosage to suit your individual needs.

Tranxene-SD, a 22.5-milligram tablet, and Tranxene-SD Half Strength, an 11.25-milligram tablet, can be taken once every 24 hours. Your doctor may switch you to this form of the drug after you have been taking Tranxene for several weeks.

Older Adults

The usual starting dose is 7.5 to 15 milligrams per day.

ACUTE ALCOHOL WITHDRAWAL

Tranxene can be used in a multi-day program for relief of the symptoms of acute alcohol withdrawal.

Dosages are usually increased in the first 2 days from 30 to 90 milligrams and then reduced over the next 2 days to lower levels. After that, your doctor will gradually lower the dose still further, and will take you off the drug when you are ready.

WHEN USED WITH ANTIEPILEPTIC DRUGS

Tranxene can be used in conjunction with antiepileptic drugs. Follow the recommended dosages carefully to avoid drowsiness.

Adults and Children over 12 Years Old

The starting dose is 7.5 milligrams 3 times a day. Your doctor may increase the dosage by 7.5 milligrams per week to a maximum of 90 milligrams a day.

Children 9 to 12 Years Old
The starting dose is 7.5 milligrams twice a day. Your doctor may increase the dosage by 7.5 milligrams a week to a maximum of 60 milligrams a day.

The safety and effectiveness of Tranxene in children under 9 years of age have not been established.

Overdosage
Any medication taken in excess can have serious consequences. If you suspect an overdose, seek medical treatment immediately.

■ *Symptoms of Tranxene overdose may include:*
Coma, low blood pressure, sedation

Tranylcypromine *See Parnate, page 1037.*

TRAVATAN
Pronounced: TRAV-a-tan
Generic name: Travoprost

Why is this drug prescribed?
Travatan is an eyedrop that reduces excessive pressure in the eye (often a result of the condition called open-angle glaucoma). Travatan works by promoting drainage of the fluid that fills the eye. It is usually prescribed when you cannot use other remedies or the other drugs have not been effective.

Most important fact about this drug
Over a period of months or years, Travatan may permanently darken the color of your iris and eyelid. It also may increase the darkness, length, and thickness of your eyelashes. If you need Travatan in only one eye, this may cause a noticeable difference.

How should you take this medication?
To apply Travatan, gently pull your lower eyelid down to form a pocket then place a drop of the medication in the pouch.

Do not place Travatan in the eyes while wearing contact lenses. Remove the lenses before administering Travatan and wait 15 minutes before reinserting them.

Handle the Travatan solution carefully. Do not allow the tip of the bottle to come in contact with your eye or any surface. This could contaminate the solution and lead to an infection that seriously damages the eye.

If you need to use another eye medication along with Travatan, the drugs should be applied at least 5 minutes apart.

■ *If you miss a dose...*
Take it as soon as you remember. If it is almost time for your next dose, skip the one you missed and go back to your regular schedule. Do not take 2 doses at once.

■ *Storage instructions...*
Store at room temperature. Throw away any unused medication after 6 weeks.

What side effects may occur?

Side effects cannot be anticipated. If any develop or change in intensity, inform your doctor as soon as possible. Only your doctor can determine if it is safe for you to continue taking Travatan.

■ *Side effects may include:*
Decreased visual sharpness, eye discomfort, eye pain or itching, redness in the eye (affects 35 to 50 percent of patients), sensation of a foreign body in the eye

Why should this drug not be prescribed?

You should avoid this medication if you are allergic to travoprost, benzalkonium chloride, or any of Travatan's other ingredients.

Special warnings about this medication

Infections from contaminated eye products can lead to serious damage or even loss of vision. If you have an eye injury or infection, or if you have eye surgery, ask your doctor if you should continue to use the Travatan container.

Contact your doctor immediately if you develop any adverse eye reactions while using Travatan, especially conjunctivitis (pinkeye) and eyelid reactions.

Use Travatan with caution if you have an inflammation of the iris or swelling of the macular part of the eye.

The safety and effectiveness of Travatan in children have not been established.

Possible food and drug interactions when taking this medication

No interactions have been reported.

Special information if you are pregnant or breastfeeding

Travatan has been found to cause miscarriages in animal studies. Since there are no adequate and well-controlled studies in pregnant women, Travatan should not be used if you're pregnant or planning to become pregnant unless the benefit outweighs the potential risk to the baby.

It is not known whether Travatan appears in breast milk, but caution is advised.

Recommended dosage

ADULTS

Place one drop in the affected eye(s) once a day in the evening. Do not apply more often; this will decrease the effectiveness of the medication.

Overdosage

There is no information on overdosage. However, any medication taken in excess can have serious consequences. If you suspect a Travatan overdose, seek medical help immediately.

Travoprost See *Travatan, page 1473.*

Trazodone See *Desyrel, page 422.*

TRENTAL

Pronounced: TREN-tall
Generic name: Pentoxifylline

Why is this drug prescribed?

Trental is a medication that reduces the viscosity or stickiness of your blood, allowing it to flow more freely. It helps relieve the painful leg cramps caused by intermittent claudication, a condition that results when hardening of the arteries reduces the leg muscles' blood supply.

Some doctors also prescribe Trental for dementia, strokes, circulatory and nerve problems caused by diabetes, and Raynaud's syndrome (a disorder of the blood vessels in which exposure to cold causes the fingers and toes to turn white). The drug is also used to treat impotence and to increase sperm motility in infertile men.

Most important fact about this drug

Trental can ease the pain in your legs and make walking easier but should not replace other treatments such as physical therapy or surgery.

How should you take this medication?

Trental comes in controlled-release tablets. Do not break, crush, or chew the tablets; swallow them whole. Take Trental exactly as prescribed.

■ *If you miss a dose...*
  Take it as soon as you remember. If it is almost time for your next dose, skip the one you missed and go back to your regular schedule. Never take 2 doses at the same time.
■ *Storage instructions...*
  Keep this medication in the container it came in, tightly closed and away from light. Store it at room temperature.

What side effects may occur?

Side effects cannot be anticipated. If any develop or change in intensity, inform your doctor as soon as possible. Only your doctor can determine if it is safe for you to continue taking Trental.

Trental's side effects are fairly uncommon.

■ *Side effects may include:*

Allergic reaction (symptoms include: swelling of face, lips, tongue, throat, arms, or legs, sore throat, fever and chills, difficulty swallowing, chest pain), anxiety, bad taste in the mouth, blind spot in vision, blurred vision, brittle fingernails, chest pain (sometimes crushing), confusion, conjunctivitis (pinkeye), constipation, depression, difficult or labored breathing, dizziness, dry mouth/thirst, earache, excessive salivation, flu-like symptoms, fluid retention, general body discomfort, headache, hives, indigestion, inflammation of the gallbladder, itching, laryngitis, loss of appetite, low blood pressure, nosebleeds, rash, seizures, sore throat/swollen neck glands, stuffy nose, tremor, vomiting, weight change

Why should this drug not be prescribed?

Do not take Trental if you have recently had a stroke or bleeding in the retina of your eye.

If you are sensitive to or have ever had an allergic reaction to Trental, caffeine, theophylline (medication for asthma or other breathing disorders), or theobromine, do not take this medication. Make sure that your doctor is aware of any drug reactions that you have experienced.

Special warnings about this medication

If you are taking a blood thinner, or have recently had surgery, peptic ulcers, or other disorders that involve bleeding, the doctor should test your blood periodically.

Most people tolerate Trental well, but there have been occasional cases of crushing chest pain, low blood pressure, and irregular heartbeat in people with heart disease and brain disorders.

Possible food and drug interactions when taking this medication

If Trental is taken with certain other drugs, the effects of either could be increased, decreased, or altered. It is especially important to check with your doctor before combining Trental with the following:

Blood pressure medications such as Vasotec and Cardizem SR
Blood-thinning drugs such as Coumadin
Clot inhibitors such as Persantine
Theophylline (Theo-Dur)
Ulcer medicines such as Tagamet

Special information if you are pregnant or breastfeeding

The effects of Trental during pregnancy have not been adequately studied. If you are pregnant or plan to become pregnant, inform your doctor immediately. Trental appears in breast milk and could affect a nursing infant. If this medication is essential to your health, your doctor may advise you to discontinue breastfeeding until your treatment with this medication is finished.

Recommended dosage

ADULTS

The usual dosage of Trental in controlled-release tablets is one 400-milligram tablet 3 times a day with meals.

While the effect of Trental may be seen within 2 to 4 weeks, it is recommended that treatment be continued for at least 8 weeks.

Any stomach or central nervous system (affecting the brain and spinal cord) side effects are related to the dose. If any of these side effects occurs, the dosage should be lowered to 1 tablet 2 times a day, for a total of 800 milligrams a day. If side effects persist at this lower dosage, your doctor may consider stopping this drug.

CHILDREN

The safety and effectiveness of this drug in children have not been established.

Overdosage

Any medication taken in excess can have serious consequences. If you suspect symptoms of a Trental overdose, seek medical attention immediately. Symptoms appear within 4 to 5 hours and may last for 12 hours.

■ *Symptoms of Trental overdose may include:*
Agitation, convulsions, fever, flushing, loss of consciousness, low blood pressure, sleepiness

Tretinoin See Retin-A and Renova, page 1242.

Trexall See Methotrexate, page 834.

Triamcinolone See Azmacort, page 180.

TRIAVIL

Pronounced: TRY-uh-vill
Generic ingredients: Amitriptyline hydrochloride,
Perphenazine

Why is this drug prescribed?

Triavil is used to treat anxiety, agitation, and depression. Triavil is a combination of a tricyclic antidepressant (amitriptyline) and a tranquilizer (perphenazine).

Triavil can also help people with schizophrenia (distorted sense of reality) who are depressed and people with insomnia, fatigue, loss of interest, loss of appetite, or a slowing of physical and mental reactions.

Most important fact about this drug

Triavil may cause tardive dyskinesia—a condition marked by involuntary muscle spasms and twitches in the face and body. This condition may be permanent and appears to be most common among the elderly, especially women. Ask your doctor for information about this possible risk.

How should you take this medication?

Triavil may be taken with or without food. You should not take it with alcohol. In addition, Triavil should not be taken within 2 hours of antacids or diarrhea medication.

■ *If you miss a dose...*
Take it as soon as you remember. If it is within 2 hours of your next dose, skip the one you missed and go back to your regular schedule. Do not take 2 doses at once.

■ *Storage instructions...*
Store at room temperature in a tightly closed container. Protect Triavil 2-10 tablets from light.

What side effects may occur?

Side effects cannot be anticipated. If any develop or change in intensity, inform your doctor as soon as possible. Only your doctor can determine if it is safe for you to continue taking Triavil.

■ *Side effects may include:*
Disorientation, dry mouth, high or low blood pressure, nervous system disorders, sedation

Why should this drug not be prescribed?

You should not be using Triavil if you are taking drugs that slow down the central nervous system, including alcohol, barbiturates, analgesics, antihistamines, or narcotics.

Triavil should not be used if you are recovering from a recent heart attack, or if you have an abnormal bone marrow condition. Avoid Triavil if you have ever had an allergic reaction to phenothiazines or amitriptyline.

People who are taking antidepressant drugs known as MAO inhibitors (including Nardil and Parnate) should not take Triavil.

Special warnings about this medication

In clinical studies, antidepressants increased the risk of suicidal thinking and behavior in children and adolescents with depression and other psychiatric disorders. Anyone considering the use of Triavil or any other antidepressant in a child or adolescent must balance this risk with the clinical need. Triavil is not approved for use in children.

Additionally, the progression of major depression is associated with a worsening of symptoms and/or the emergence of suicidal thinking or behavior in both adults and children, whether or not they are taking antidepressants. Individuals being treated with Triavil and their caregivers should watch for any change in symptoms or any new symptoms that appear suddenly—especially agitation, anxiety, hostility, panic, restlessness, extreme hyperactivity, and suicidal thinking or behavior—and report them to the doctor immediately. Be especially observant at the beginning of treatment or whenever there is a change in dose.

Before using Triavil, tell your doctor if you have ever had the following: glaucoma (high pressure in the eye); difficulty urinating; breast cancer; breathing problems; seizures; heart, liver, kidney, or thyroid disease; or if you are exposed to extreme heat or pesticides. Be aware that Triavil may mask signs of brain tumor, intestinal blockage, and overdose of other drugs.

Nausea, headache, and a general ill feeling can result if you suddenly stop taking Triavil. Follow your doctor's instructions closely when discontinuing Triavil. If your dose is gradually reduced, you may experience irritability, restlessness, and dream and sleep disturbances, but these effects will not last.

This drug may impair your ability to drive a car or operate potentially dangerous machinery. Do not participate in any activities that require full alertness if you are unsure about your ability.

If you develop a fever that has no other cause, stop taking Triavil and call your doctor.

Drugs such as Triavil are known to trigger a potentially fatal condition known as Neuroleptic Malignant Syndrome (NMS). Symptoms include high fever, muscle rigidity, unstable blood pressure, rapid or irregular heartbeat, and excessive sweating. If any of these symptoms develop, contact your doctor immediately.

Triavil could make you more sensitive to sunlight. Be careful to stay out of the sun, wear protective clothing, and use sunblock.

Triavil could also trigger a manic episode in people with bipolar disorder, although the drug's tranquilizing effects seem to reduce this risk.

While taking this medication, you may feel dizzy or light-headed or actually faint when getting up from a lying or sitting position. If getting up more slowly doesn't help or if the problem continues, contact your doctor.

Tell the doctor or dentist you're taking Triavil before having any surgery, dental work, or diagnostic procedure. Triavil could interact with anesthetics, muscle relaxants, and other drugs used during surgical procedures.

Possible food and drug interactions when taking this medication

Triavil contains the same active ingredients as Elavil and Trilafon and should not be used with these drugs.

If Triavil is taken with certain other drugs, the effects of either could be increased, decreased, or altered. It is especially important to check with your doctor before combining Triavil with the following:

Airway-opening drugs such as Proventil
Antidepressants classified as MAO inhibitors, including Nardil and Parnate
Antidepressants that boost serotonin, including fluvoxamine, Paxil, Prozac, and Zoloft
Antihistamines such as Benadryl
Antiseizure drugs such as Dilantin
Antispasmodic drugs such as Bentyl
Atropine (Donnatal)
Barbiturates such as phenobarbital
Blood pressure medications
Blood-thinning drugs such as Coumadin
Cimetidine (Tagamet)
Disulfiram (Antabuse)
Epinephrine (EpiPen)
Ethchlorvynol (Placidyl)
Flecainide (Tambocor)
Fluoxetine (Prozac)
Fluphenazine (Prolixin)
Furazolidone (Furoxone)
Guanethidine
Major tranquilizers such as Haldol
Narcotic analgesics such as Percocet
Phosphorus insecticides
Propafenone (Rythmol)
Quinidine
Thioridazine (Mellaril)
Thyroid medications such as Synthroid

Extreme drowsiness and other potentially serious effects can result if Triavil is combined with alcohol or other central nervous system depressants such as narcotics, painkillers, and sleep medications.

Special information if you are pregnant or breastfeeding
Triavil may cause false positive results on pregnancy tests. Triavil should not be used by pregnant women or mothers who are breastfeeding.

Recommended dosage
Your doctor will individualize your dose.

You should not take more than 4 tablets of Triavil 4-50 or 8 tablets of any other strength in one day. It may be a few days to a few weeks before you notice any improvement.

ADULTS

Non-Psychotic Anxiety and Depression
The usual dose is 1 tablet of Triavil 2-25 or 4-25 taken 3 or 4 times a day, or 1 tablet of Triavil 4-50 taken twice a day.

Anxiety in People with Schizophrenia
The usual dose is 2 tablets of Triavil 4-25 taken 3 times a day. Your doctor may tell you to take another tablet of Triavil 4-25 at bedtime, if needed.

If you need to keep taking Triavil, your doctor will probably have you take 1 tablet of Triavil 2-25 or 4-25 from 2 to 4 times a day or 1 tablet of Triavil 4-50 twice a day.

CHILDREN

Children should not use Triavil.

OLDER ADULTS AND ADOLESCENTS

Anxiety
The usual dose is 1 tablet of Triavil 4-10, taken 3 or 4 times a day. People in these age groups usually take Triavil at lower doses.

Overdosage
Any medication taken in excess can have serious consequences. An overdose of Triavil can be fatal. If you suspect an overdose, seek medical help immediately.

■ *Symptoms of Triavil overdose may include:*
Abnormalities of posture and movements, agitation, coma, convulsions, dilated pupils, drowsiness, extreme low body temperature, eye movement problems, heart failure, high fever, overactive reflexes, rapid or irregular heartbeat, rigid muscles, stupor, very low blood pressure, vomiting

Triaz *See Desquam-E, page 421.*

Triazolam *See Halcion, page 643.*

TRICOR

Pronounced: TRY-core
Generic name: Fenofibrate
Other brand name: Lofibra

Why is this drug prescribed?

Tricor is used, along with a special diet, to treat people with very high levels of triglycerides (a fatty substance in the blood). Tricor also improves cholesterol levels by lowering total cholesterol—including "bad" LDL cholesterol—and raising "good" HDL cholesterol. It works by promoting the dissolution and elimination of fat particles in the blood.

Tricor is usually added to a treatment regimen only when other measures have failed to produce adequate results. Often, diet and exercise are enough to bring blood fats under control. Likewise, it's sometimes sufficient to simply treat an underlying problem such as diabetes, underactive thyroid, kidney disease, liver dysfunction, or alcoholism. And in some cases, just discontinuing a medication is enough to do the job. For instance, certain water pills and beta-blocker heart medications are capable of causing a massive increase in triglyceride levels. Estrogen replacement therapy is another potential culprit.

Whatever your other treatment measures may be, it's important to remember that Tricor is intended to supplement them, rather than replace them outright. To get the full benefit of the medication, you need to stick to the diet, exercise program, and other treatments your doctor prescribes. All these efforts to keep your cholesterol and triglyceride levels normal are important because together they may lower your risk of heart disease. If you're judged to be at high risk of heart disease, current guidelines call for considering drug therapy when LDL levels reach 130. For people at lower risk, the cutoff is 160. For those at little or no risk, it's 190.

Most important fact about this drug

Drugs such as Tricor have caused rare cases of a muscle-wasting disease called rhabdomyolysis. The chances of this problem rise dramatically when Tricor is combined with another type of cholesterol-lowering drug called statins. Among these drugs are Altocor, Lescol, Lipitor, Mevacor, Pravachol, and Zocor. Avoid combining Tricor with any of them unless your doctor feels it's absolutely necessary. Inform the doctor immediately if you develop muscle pain or weakness, especially if these symptoms are accompanied by fatigue or fever: You'll probably have to stop taking Tricor.

How should you take this medication?

Tricor should be taken with meals. If you've also been prescribed a cholesterol-lowering drug such as Questran or Colestid, take Tricor at least 1 hour before or 4 to 6 hours after the other drug to make sure Tricor is properly absorbed.

■ *If you miss a dose...*
Take it as soon as you remember. If it is almost time for your next dose, skip the one you missed and go back to your regular schedule. Never take 2 doses at the same time.

■ *Storage instructions...*
Store at room temperature and protect from moisture.

What side effects may occur?
Side effects cannot be anticipated. If any develop or change in intensity, inform your doctor as soon as possible. Only your doctor can determine if it is safe for you to continue taking Tricor.

■ *Side effects may include:*
Abdominal pain, back pain, headache, respiratory disorders

Why should this drug not be prescribed?
You should not take Tricor if you have liver or gallbladder disease, or severe kidney problems. You'll also have to avoid Tricor if it gives you an allergic reaction.

Special warnings about this medication
Tricor has the potential to cause gallstones. Your doctor will discontinue the drug if gallstones develop.

Tricor may also affect liver function. Your doctor should perform periodic blood tests to monitor the health of your liver.

Tricor has not been tested in children.

Possible food and drug interactions when taking this medication
If Tricor is taken with certain other drugs, the effects of either could be increased, decreased, or altered. It is especially important to check with your doctor before combining Tricor with the following:

Blood thinners such as warfarin (Coumadin)
Cholesterol-lowering drugs Colestid and Questran
Cyclosporine (Sandimmune, Neoral)
Statins (the cholesterol-lowering drugs Altocor, Lescol, Lipitor, Mevacor, Pravachol, and Zocor)

Special information if you are pregnant or breastfeeding
Pregnancy tests have not been conducted in humans, but high doses of Tricor have proven harmful in animal studies. If you are pregnant or plan to become pregnant, inform your doctor immediately.

Tricor should not be used by breastfeeding mothers. If this drug is essential to your health, your doctor will advise you to stop breastfeeding your baby.

Recommended dosage

ADULTS

High Cholesterol Levels or a Combination of High Cholesterol and High Triglycerides
The initial dose of Tricor is 160 milligrams per day.

High Triglyceride Levels
The starting dose of Tricor ranges from 54 to 160 milligrams per day. The usual starting dose of Lofibra is 67 milligrams a day. Your doctor may increase the dose every 4 to 8 weeks if your triglycerides do not improve. The maximum dose of Tricor is 160 milligrams a day. For Lofibra, the maximum dose is about 200 milligrams a day.

OLDER ADULTS

The starting dose of Tricor for older adults and those with poor kidney function is 54 milligrams per day. For Lofibra, the starting dose is 67 milligrams a day.

Overdosage

There is no information on the effects of a Tricor overdose. However, any medication taken in excess can have serious consequences. If you suspect an overdose, seek medical attention immediately.

TRIDESILON

Pronounced: tri-DESS-ill-on
Generic name: Desonide
Other brand name: DesOwen

Why is this drug prescribed?

Tridesilon is a steroid preparation that relieves the itching and inflammation of a variety of skin problems. It is applied directly to the skin.

Most important fact about this drug

When you use Tridesilon, you inevitably absorb some of the medication through your skin and into the bloodstream. Too much absorption can lead to unwanted side effects elsewhere in the body. To keep this problem to a minimum, avoid using large amounts of Tridesilon over large areas, and do not cover it with airtight dressings such as plastic wrap or adhesive bandages unless specifically told to by your doctor.

How should you use this medication?

Use Tridesilon exactly as directed by your doctor. Shake lotion well before using.

Tridesilon is for use only on the skin. Be careful to keep it out of your eyes.

Remember to avoid wrapping the treated area with bandages or other coverings unless your doctor has told you to do so.

■ *If you miss a dose...*
Apply it as soon as you remember. If it is almost time for the next dose, skip the one you missed and go back to your regular schedule.

■ *Storage instructions...*
Store at room temperature.

What side effects may occur?

Side effects cannot be anticipated. If any develop or change in intensity, notify your doctor as soon as possible. Only your doctor can determine if it is safe for you to continue using Tridesilon. Many of the side effects listed below are rare, but may occur more often if the affected area is covered with a bandage or treated for a long time.

■ *Side effects may include:*
Acne, additional infections, allergic reactions of the skin, burning and stinging, dryness, excessive hair growth, irritation, itching, loss of skin color, prickly heat, rash, scaly skin, skin inflammation around the mouth, skin loss, skin peeling or redness, skin softening, stretch marks, worsening of the condition

■ *Side effects that may occur in children include:*
Delayed weight gain, headaches, slowed growth

Why should this drug not be prescribed?

You should not take this medication if you are sensitive or allergic to any of its ingredients.

Because steroid medications may interfere with their growth and development, children should be given the lowest strength that provides effective therapy. The safety and effectiveness of DesOwen in children have not been established.

Special warnings about this medication

If an irritation develops, or if your skin condition does not heal within 2 weeks, inform your doctor.

Avoid covering a treated area with waterproof diapers or plastic pants. They can increase unwanted absorption of Tridesilon.

Large doses of steroids applied over a large area, and long-term use of these preparations, especially when the treated areas are covered, can cause increases in blood sugar or sugar in the urine, Cushing's syndrome (a condition characterized by a moon-shaped face, emotional disturbances, high blood pressure, weight gain, and, in women, growth of body hair), and effects on the adrenal gland, pituitary, and hypothalamus.

Possible food and drug interactions when using this medication
No interactions have been reported.

Special information if you are pregnant or breastfeeding
Although Tridesilon is applied to the skin, there is no way of knowing how much medication is absorbed into the bloodstream. The more powerful steroids have caused birth defects in animals. In general, these preparations should not be used extensively, in large amounts, or for prolonged periods of time by pregnant women. They should be used only if the potential benefits outweigh the potential risks to the unborn baby. If you are pregnant or plan to become pregnant, inform your doctor immediately. It is not known whether steroid creams and ointments are absorbed in sufficient amounts to appear in breast milk. If your doctor considers Tridesilon essential to your health, he or she may advise you to stop breastfeeding until your treatment with the medication is finished.

Recommended dosage

ADULTS AND CHILDREN
Tridesilon should be applied to the affected area as a thin film, from 2 to 4 times a day, depending on the severity of the condition. Apply DesOwen 2 or 3 times daily.

A bandage or other covering may be prescribed by your doctor to apply over the affected area for psoriasis or conditions that are not responding as well as expected.

Overdosage
Any medication taken in excess can have serious consequences. With overuse or misuse of Tridesilon, too much medicine can enter the body, causing increases in blood sugar and Cushing's syndrome, with symptoms such as a moon-shaped face, emotional disturbances, high blood pressure, weight gain, and, in women, growth of body and facial hair.

TRIFLUOPERAZINE HYDROCHLORIDE
Pronounced: TRY-flue-oh-pear-ah-zine

Why is this drug prescribed?
Trifluoperazine is used for the treatment of schizophrenia (severe disruptions in thought and perception). It is also prescribed for anxiety that does not respond to ordinary tranquilizers.

Most important fact about this drug
Trifluoperazine may cause tardive dyskinesia—a condition marked by involuntary muscle spasms and twitches in the face and body. This condition may be permanent and appears to be most common among the

elderly, especially women. Ask your doctor for information about this possible risk.

How should you take this medication?

If taking trifluoperazine in a liquid concentrate form, you will need to dilute it with a liquid such as a carbonated beverage, coffee, fruit juice, milk, tea, tomato juice, or water. You can also use puddings, soups, and other semi-solid foods. Trifluoperazine should be diluted just before you take it.

You should not take trifluoperazine with alcohol.

■ *If you miss a dose...*
If you take 1 dose a day, take the dose you missed as soon as you remember. Then go back to your regular schedule. If you do not remember until the next day, skip the missed dose and go back to your regular schedule.

If you take more than 1 dose a day, take the dose you missed if it is within an hour or so of the scheduled time. If you do not remember until later, skip the missed dose and go back to your regular schedule. Do not take 2 doses at once.

■ *Storage instructions...*
Store at room temperature. Protect the concentrate from light.

What side effects may occur?

Side effects cannot be anticipated. If any develop or change in intensity, inform your doctor as soon as possible. Only your doctor can determine if it is safe for you to continue taking trifluoperazine.

■ *Side effects may include:*
Blood disorders, convulsions, dry mouth, headache, muscle stiffness or rigidity, nausea, restlessness, Parkinson's-like movements, tardive dyskinesia (see *Most important fact about this drug*).

Why should this drug not be prescribed?

You should not be using trifluoperazine if you have liver damage, or if you are taking central nervous system depressants such as alcohol, barbiturates, or narcotic pain relievers. Trifluoperazine should not be used if you have an abnormal bone marrow or blood condition.

Special warnings about this medication

You should use trifluoperazine cautiously if you have ever had a brain tumor, breast cancer, intestinal blockage, the eye condition called glaucoma, heart or liver disease, or seizures. Be cautious, too, if you are exposed to certain pesticides or extreme heat. Be aware that trifluoperazine may hide the signs of overdose of other drugs and may make it more difficult for your doctor to diagnose intestinal obstruction, brain tumor, and the dangerous neurological condition called Reye's syndrome.

Tell your doctor if you have ever had an allergic reaction to any major tranquilizer similar to trifluoperazine.

Dizziness, nausea, vomiting, and tremors can result if you suddenly stop taking trifluoperazine. Follow your doctor's instructions when discontinuing this drug.

Tell your doctor immediately if you experience symptoms such as a fever or sore throat, mouth, or gums. These signs of infection may signal the need to stop trifluoperazine treatment. Notify your doctor, too, if you develop flu-like symptoms with fever.

Trifluoperazine can cause Neuroleptic Malignant Syndrome (NMS), a dangerous—and possibly life-threatening—condition marked by high body temperature, rigid muscles, irregular pulse or blood pressure, rapid or abnormal heartbeat, excessive sweating, and high fever. Seek medical attention immediately if you develop any of these symptoms.

This drug may impair your ability to drive a car or operate potentially dangerous machinery, especially during the first few days of treatment. Do not participate in any activities that require full alertness if you are unsure about your ability.

If you have any trouble with your vision, tell your doctor. Trifluoperazine has been known to cause vision problems.

Trifluoperazine concentrate contains a sulfite that may cause allergic reactions in some people, especially in those with asthma.

Possible food and drug interactions when taking this medication

Extreme drowsiness and other potentially serious effects can result if trifluoperazine is combined with alcohol, tranquilizers such as Valium, narcotic painkillers such as Percocet, antihistamines such as Benadryl, and barbiturates such as phenobarbital.

If trifluoperazine is taken with certain other drugs, the effects of either could be increased, decreased, or altered. It is especially important to check with your doctor before combining trifluoperazine with the following:

Antiseizure drugs such as Dilantin
Atropine (Donnatal)
Blood thinners such as Coumadin
Guanethidine
Lithium (Lithobid, Eskalith)
Propranolol (Inderal)
Thiazide diuretics such as Dyazide

Special information if you are pregnant or breastfeeding

Pregnant women should use trifluoperazine only if clearly needed. The effects of trifluoperazine during pregnancy have not been adequately studied. If you are pregnant or plan to become pregnant, inform your doctor immediately. Trifluoperazine appears in breast milk and may affect a nursing infant. If this medication is essential to your health, your doctor may have you discontinue breastfeeding while you are taking it.

Recommended dosage

ADULTS

Nonpsychotic Anxiety
Doses usually range from 2 to 4 milligrams daily. This amount should be divided into 2 equal doses and taken twice a day. Do not take more than 6 milligrams a day or take the medication for more than 12 weeks.

Schizophrenia
The usual starting dose is 4 to 10 milligrams a day, divided into 2 equal doses; doses range from 15 to 40 milligrams daily.

CHILDREN

Doses are based on the child's weight and the severity of his or her symptoms.

Schizophrenia in Children 6 to 12 Years Old
Who Are Closely Monitored or Hospitalized
The starting dose is 1 milligram a day, taken all at once or divided into 2 doses. Your doctor will increase the dosage gradually, up to 15 milligrams a day.

OLDER ADULTS

Older people usually take trifluoperazine at lower doses. Because you may develop low blood pressure while taking this drug, your doctor will watch you closely. Older people (especially older women) may be more susceptible to tardive dyskinesia—a possibly permanent condition characterized by involuntary muscle spasms and twitches in the face and body. Consult your doctor for information about these potential risks.

Overdosage

Any medication taken in excess can have serious consequences. If you suspect an overdose of trifluoperazine, seek medical help immediately.

■ *Symptoms of trifluoperazine overdose may include:*
Agitation, coma, convulsions, difficulty breathing, difficulty swallowing, dry mouth, extreme sleepiness, fever, intestinal blockage, irregular heart rate, low blood pressure, restlessness

TRIHEXYPHENIDYL HYDROCHLORIDE
Pronounced: try-HEX-ih-FEN-ih-dil

Why is this drug prescribed?

Trihexyphenidyl is used, in conjunction with other drugs, for the relief of certain symptoms of Parkinson's disease, a brain disorder that causes muscle tremor, stiffness, and weakness. It is also used to control certain side effects induced by antipsychotic drugs such as Thorazine and Haldol. Trihexyphenidyl works by correcting the chemical imbalance that causes Parkinson's disease.

Most important fact about this drug

Trihexyphenidyl is not a cure for Parkinson's disease; it merely minimizes and reduces the frequency of symptoms such as tremors.

How should you take this medication?

You may take trihexyphenidyl either before meals or after meals, whichever you find more convenient. Your doctor will probably start you on a small amount and increase the dosage gradually. Take trihexyphenidyl exactly as prescribed.

If the medication makes your mouth feel dry, try chewing gum, sucking mints, or simply sipping water.

Trihexyphenidyl comes in tablet and liquid form. With either, you will probably need to take 3 or 4 doses a day.

Once you have reached the dosage that is best for you, your doctor may switch you to sustained-release capsules (sequels), which are to be taken only once or twice a day. Do not open or crush the sequels. Always swallow them whole.

■ *If you miss a dose...*
Take it as soon as you remember. If it is within 2 hours or your next dose, skip the one you missed and go back to your regular schedule. Do not take 2 doses at the same time.

■ *Storage instructions...*
Store at room temperature. Do not allow the liquid to freeze.

What side effects may occur?

Side effects cannot be anticipated. If any develop or change in intensity, inform your doctor as soon as possible. Only your doctor can determine if it is safe for you to continue taking trihexyphenidyl.

■ *Side effects may include:*
Blurred vision, dry mouth, nausea, nervousness

These side effects, which appear in 30 to 50 percent of all people who take trihexyphenidyl, tend to be mild. They may disappear as your body gets used to the drug; if they persist, your doctor may want to lower your dosage slightly.

Why should this drug not be prescribed?

Do not take trihexyphenidyl if you are known to be sensitive to it or if you have ever had an allergic reaction to it or to other anti-Parkinson's medications of this type.

Special warnings about this medication

The elderly are highly sensitive to drugs such as trihexyphenidyl and should use it with caution.

Trihexyphenidyl can reduce the body's ability to perspire, one of the key ways your body prevents overheating. Avoid excess sun or exercise that can cause you to become overheated.

If you have any of the following conditions, make sure your doctor knows about them, since trihexyphenidyl could make them worse:

Enlarged prostate
Glaucoma
Stomach/intestinal obstructive disease
Urinary tract obstructive disease

It is important to stick to the prescribed dosage; taking larger amounts could lead to an overdose.

Your doctor should watch you carefully if you have heart, liver, or kidney disease or high blood pressure, and should check your eyes frequently. You should also be watched for the development of any allergic reactions.

Possible food and drug interactions when taking this medication

If you take trihexyphenidyl along with any of the drugs listed below, your doctor may need to adjust the dosage of trihexyphenidyl, the other medication, or possibly both.

Amantadine (Symmetrel)
Amitriptyline (Elavil)
Chlorpromazine (Thorazine)
Doxepin (Sinequan)
Haloperidol (Haldol)

Special information if you are pregnant or breastfeeding

No specific information is available concerning the use of trihexyphenidyl during pregnancy or breastfeeding. If you are pregnant or plan to become pregnant while taking trihexyphenidyl, inform your doctor immediately.

Recommended dosage

Your doctor will individualize the dose to your needs, starting with a low dose and then increasing it gradually, especially if you are over 60 years of age.

ADULTS

Parkinson's Disease
The usual starting dose, in tablet or liquid form, is 1 milligram on the first day.

After the first day, your doctor may increase the dose by 2 milligrams at intervals of 3 to 5 days, until you are taking a total of 6 to 10 milligrams a day.

Your total daily dose will depend upon what is found to be the most effective level. For many people, 6 to 10 milligrams is most effective. Some, however, may require a total daily dose of 12 to 15 milligrams.

Drug-induced Parkinsonism

Your doctor will have to determine by trial and error the size and frequency of the dose of trihexyphenidyl needed to control the tremors and muscle rigidity that sometimes result from commonly used tranquilizers.

The total daily dosage usually ranges between 5 and 15 milligrams, although, in some cases, symptoms have been satisfactorily controlled on as little as 1 milligram daily.

Your doctor may start you on 1 milligram of trihexyphenidyl a day. If your symptoms are not controlled in a few hours, he or she may slowly increase the dose until satisfactory control is achieved.

Use of Trihexyphenidyl with Levodopa

When trihexyphenidyl is used at the same time as Levodopa, the usual dose of each may need to be reduced. Your doctor will adjust the dosages carefully, depending on the side effects and the degree of symptom control. Trihexyphenidyl dosage of 3 to 6 milligrams daily, divided into equal doses, is usually adequate.

Trihexyphenidyl Tablets and Liquid

You will be able to handle the total daily intake of trihexyphenidyl tablets or liquid best if the medication is divided into 3 doses and taken at mealtimes. If you are taking high doses (more than 10 milligrams daily), your doctor may divide them into 4 parts, so that you take 3 doses at mealtimes and the fourth at bedtime.

Overdosage

Overdosage with trihexyphenidyl may cause agitation, delirium, disorientation, hallucinations, or psychotic episodes.

■ *Other symptoms may include:*
Clumsiness or unsteadiness, fast heartbeat, flushing of skin, seizures, severe drowsiness, shortness of breath or troubled breathing, trouble sleeping, unusual warmth

If you suspect an overdose of trihexyphenidyl, seek medical attention immediately.

TRILAFON

Pronounced: TRILL-ah-fon
Generic name: Perphenazine

Why is this drug prescribed?

Trilafon is used to treat schizophrenia and to control severe nausea and vomiting in adults. It is a member of the phenothiazine family of antipsychotic medications, which includes such drugs as Mellaril, Stelazine, and Thorazine.

Most important fact about this drug

Trilafon can cause tardive dyskinesia, a condition marked by involuntary muscle spasms and twitches in the face and body, including chewing movements, puckering, puffing the cheeks, and sticking out the tongue. This condition may be permanent and appears to be most common among older adults, especially older women. Ask your doctor for more information about this possible risk.

How should you take this medication?

Trilafon should be taken exactly according to physician instructions and for no longer than necessary.

- *If you miss a dose...*
  If it is within an hour or so after the scheduled time, take the forgotten dose as soon as you remember. If you do not remember until later, skip the dose and go back to your regular schedule. Never take 2 doses at once.
- *Storage instructions...*
  Trilafon should be stored at room temperature.

What side effects may occur?

Side effects cannot be anticipated. If any develop or change in intensity, inform your doctor as soon as possible. Only your doctor can determine if it is safe to continue taking Trilafon.

- *Side effects may include:*
  Aching or numbness of the limbs, brain swelling, breast milk production, diarrhea, drowsiness, dry mouth, low blood pressure upon standing, nausea, rapid or irregular heartbeat, restlessness, salivation, seizures, vomiting

Why should this drug not be prescribed?

People who are comatose or who are at reduced levels of consciousness or alertness should not take Trilafon. Nor should those who are taking large amounts of any substance that slows brain function, including barbiturates, alcohol, narcotics, painkillers, and antihistamines.

Trilafon should also be avoided by people who have blood disorders, liver problems, or brain damage. It cannot be taken by anyone who is hypersensitive to its ingredients or to related drugs.

Special warnings about this medication

Use Trilafon with caution if you have any of the following: glaucoma (high pressure in the eye); difficulty urinating; breast cancer; breathing problems; or heart, liver, kidney, or thyroid disease. Caution is also advised if you are exposed to extreme heat or pesticides. Be aware that Trilafon may mask signs of brain tumor, intestinal blockage, and overdose of other drugs.

Drugs such as Trilafon can trigger a potentially fatal condition known as Neuroleptic Malignant Syndrome (NMS). Symptoms include high fever, muscle rigidity, unstable blood pressure, rapid or irregular heartbeat, and excessive sweating. If any of these symptoms develop, see your doctor immediately.

Trilafon should be used cautiously in people who are severely depressed and may be at risk for suicide. These patients should be watched closely for signs of suicidal thoughts and behavior. The doctor will prescribe the lowest amount of drug possible to avoid the risk of overdose.

While taking this medication, you may feel dizzy or light-headed or actually faint when getting up from a lying or sitting position. If getting up more slowly doesn't help or if the problem continues, contact your doctor.

Also report any significant increase in body temperature to the doctor. It could be an early warning that you cannot tolerate the drug.

Alert your physician before taking Trilafon if you are going through alcohol withdrawal, suffer from convulsions or seizures, or have a depressive disorder. You'll have to use the drug with caution.

Trilafon could make you more sensitive to sunlight. Be sure to stay out of the sun, wear protective clothing, and use sunblock.

Tell the doctor or dentist you're taking Trilafon before having any surgery, dental work, or diagnostic procedure. Trilafon could interact with anesthetics, muscle relaxants, and other drugs used during surgical procedures.

Be aware that Trilafon may impair the mental or physical abilities needed to drive a car or operate heavy machinery. Avoid activities that require full alertness until you know how the drug affects you.

Stomach inflammation, dizziness, nausea, vomiting, and tremors may result if Trilafon is stopped suddenly. Therapy should be discontinued only under a doctor's supervision.

Trilafon is not recommended for children under the age of 12 years.

Possible food and drug interactions when taking this medication

If Trilafon is taken with certain other drugs, the effects of either could be increased, decreased, or altered. It is especially important to check with your doctor before combining Trilafon with the following:

Antidepressants such as Elavil, Nardil, Prozac, and Triavil
Antihistamines such as Benadryl and Tavist
Antipsychotic medications such as chlorpromazine and Mellaril
Antiseizure drugs such as Dilantin
Atropine (Donnatal)
Barbiturates such as Nembutal and Seconal
Blood pressure medications
Drugs that quell spasms, such as Levsin
Narcotic painkillers such as Percodan and Vicodin
Phosphorus insecticides
Tranquilizers and sleep aids such as Halcion, Valium, and Xanax

Extreme drowsiness and other potentially serious effects can result if Trilafon is combined with alcohol or other central nervous system depressants such as narcotics, painkillers, and sleep medications.

Special information if you are pregnant or breastfeeding

Trilafon may cause false positive results on pregnancy tests. If you are pregnant or plan to become pregnant, tell your doctor immediately. The safe use of Trilafon during pregnancy has not been established. The benefits of using this medication must be weighed against the possible hazards to the mother and child.

Drugs similar to Trilafon appear in breast milk. If this medication is essential to your health, the doctor may advise you to avoid breastfeeding until your treatment is finished.

Recommended dosage

The dosage of Trilafon is adjusted according to the severity of the condition and the drug's effect. Doctors aim for the lowest effective dose.

SCHIZOPHRENIA

The usual initial dosage of Trilafon tablets is 4 to 8 milligrams 3 times daily, up to a maximum daily dose of 24 milligrams. Hospitalized patients are usually given 8 to 16 milligrams 2 to 4 times daily, up to a maximum daily dose of 64 milligrams.

SEVERE NAUSEA AND VOMITING IN ADULTS

For this problem, the usual dosage of Trilafon tablets is 8 to 16 milligrams daily, divided into smaller doses. Up to 24 milligrams daily is occasionally necessary.

Overdosage

Anyone suspected of overdosing on Trilafon should be hospitalized immediately for emergency treatment.

■ *Symptoms of Trilafon overdose may include:*
Coma, convulsions (in children), stupor

Victims may also exhibit symptoms such as rigid muscles, twitches and involuntary movements, hair-trigger reflexes, loss of coordination, rolling eyeballs, and slurred speech.

TRILEPTAL

Pronounced: tri-LEP-tal
Generic name: Oxcarbazepine

Why is this drug prescribed?

Trileptal helps reduce the frequency of partial epileptic seizures, a form of epilepsy in which neural disturbances are limited to a specific region of the brain and the victim remains conscious throughout the attack. Trileptal may be prescribed by itself to treat the problem in adults. It can also be used in combination with other seizure medications in adults and in children as young as 4 years old.

Most important fact about this drug

Trileptal can cause drowsiness, dizziness, and loss of coordination, which could impair your ability to drive a vehicle or operate dangerous machinery. Do not attempt hazardous activities until you know how the drug affects you.

How should you take this medication?

Take Trileptal exactly as prescribed by your doctor. Stopping Trileptal suddenly could cause an increase in the frequency of your seizures. Trileptal may be taken with or without food.

Trileptal is available in tablets and an oral suspension, which can be used interchangeably.

To administer a dose of the oral suspension:

1. Shake the bottle well and remove the cap.
2. Push the plunger all the way down in the dosing syringe provided with the bottle.
3. With the bottle upright, push the syringe firmly into the plastic adapter on the neck of the bottle.
4. With the syringe in place, turn the bottle upside down.
5. Slowly pull the plunger out until a small amount of medicine enters the syringe. Push the plunger back in far enough to force out any large air bubbles trapped in the syringe.
6. Slowly pull the plunger out until the top edge of the black ring is level with the marker for the prescribed dose.
7. Turn the bottle upright and twist the syringe free from the plastic adapter.
8. Push the plunger to empty the syringe. The medicine can be dropped directly into the mouth or into a small glass of water. If using water, stir the medicine, then drink the entire glass.

9. Rinse the syringe with warm water and allow it to dry. Replace the cap on the bottle.

■ *If you miss a dose…*
Take it as soon as you remember. If it is almost time for your next dose, skip the one you missed and go back to your regular schedule. Do not take 2 doses at once. If you miss more than 1 dose in a day, check with your doctor.

■ *Storage instructions…*
Store in a tightly closed container at room temperature.

What side effects may occur?
Side effects cannot be anticipated. If any develop or change in intensity, inform your doctor as soon as possible. Only your doctor can determine if it is safe for you to continue taking Trileptal.

■ *Side effects may include:*
Abnormal gait, dizziness, double vision, headache, involuntary movement of the eyeballs, nausea, sleepiness, tremor, uncoordinated muscle movement, visual disturbances, vomiting, weakness

Why should this drug not be prescribed?
If Trileptal gives you an allergic reaction, you won't be able to use it.

Special warnings about this medication
A significant number (25 to 30 percent) of people who are sensitive to carbamazepine (Tegretol) also experience sensitivity to Trileptal. If you've had a problem with Tegretol, make sure the doctor is aware of it. Trileptal is prescribed under such circumstances only if there's no better alternative.

Trileptal can lead to a loss of sodium from the blood, resulting in a serious medical condition which, left untreated, could lead to convulsions, coma, and death. Your doctor should carefully monitor your blood sodium levels during treatment with Trileptal. Alert the doctor immediately if you develop warning signs such as nausea, headache, sluggishness, confusion, loss of feeling, or an increase in the frequency or severity of seizures.

If you have kidney disease, your doctor will prescribe a lower dosage of Trileptal. Be sure your doctor knows your medical history before you start therapy.

Possible food and drug interactions when taking this medication
Alcohol can intensify the sedative effects of Trileptal. Avoid alcohol while taking this drug.

If Trileptal is taken with certain other drugs, the effects of either could be increased, decreased, or altered. It is especially important to check with your doctor before combining Trileptal with the following:

Calcium channel blockers such as verapamil (Calan) or felodipine
(Plendil)
Carbamazepine (Tegretol)
Phenobarbital
Phenytoin (Dilantin)
Oral contraceptives
Valproic acid (Depakene)

Special Information if you are pregnant or breastfeeding

Although it's not known for sure, there is good reason to believe that
Trileptal can cause birth defects. If you are pregnant or are planning to become pregnant, tell your doctor immediately. Trileptal should be used
during pregnancy only if the potential benefits justify the risk.

Trileptal appears in breast milk and could cause serious side effects in
a nursing infant. Check with your doctor. You'll probably need to make a
choice between breast feeding and continuing your Trileptal therapy.

Recommended dosage

ADULTS

Trileptal Taken Alone
The usual starting dose is 300 milligrams twice daily. Your doctor may
gradually increase the dose to 600 milligrams twice daily. In people with
kidney disorders, the starting dose is 150 milligrams twice daily.

Changing from Another Antiepileptic Medication to Trileptal
The usual starting dose is 300 milligrams twice daily. Your doctor will
gradually increase the dose over a period of 2 to 4 weeks, while reducing
the other medication over a period of 3 to 6 weeks. The final dosage of
Trileptal is typically 1,200 milligrams twice daily.

Trileptal Combined with Another Antiepileptic Medication
The usual starting dose is 300 milligrams twice daily. Your doctor may increase the dose to 600 milligrams twice daily.

CHILDREN 4 TO 16 YEARS OLD

For children the dosage of Trileptal is based on body weight.

Trileptal Taken Alone
Your child's doctor will gradually increase the dose every 3 days until the
most effective dose is reached. The usual dose ranges from 300 to 1,050
milligrams taken twice daily.

Changing from Another Antiepileptic Medication to Trileptal
Your child's doctor will gradually increase the dose of Trileptal while reducing the other medication over a period of 3 to 6 weeks. The doctor will increase the dose of Trileptal weekly until the most effective dose is reached.
The usual dose ranges from 300 to 1,050 milligrams taken twice daily.

Trileptal Combined with Another Antiepileptic Medication
After a 2-week buildup, the dosage typically ranges from 450 to 900 milligrams taken twice daily.

Overdosage

There is little information on Trileptal overdose. However, any medication taken in excess can have serious consequences. If you suspect an overdose, seek medical treatment immediately.

Tri-Levlen *See Oral Contraceptives, page 1000.*

TRILISATE

Pronounced: TRILL-ih-sate
Generic name: Choline magnesium trisalicylate

Why is this drug prescribed?

Trilisate, a nonsteroidal, anti-inflammatory medication, is prescribed for the relief of the signs and symptoms of rheumatoid arthritis (chronic joint inflammation disease), osteoarthritis (degenerative joint disease), and other forms of arthritis. This drug is used in the long-term management of these diseases and especially for flare-ups of severe rheumatoid arthritis.

Trilisate may also be prescribed for the treatment of acute painful shoulder, for mild to moderate pain in general, and for fever.

In children, this medication is prescribed for severe conditions—such as juvenile rheumatoid arthritis—that require relief of pain and inflammation.

Most important fact about this drug

Because there is a possible association between the development of the rare but serious nerve disorder known as Reye's syndrome and the use of medicines containing salicylates or aspirin during bouts of chickenpox or flu, Trilisate should not be used by children or teenagers during these illnesses unless otherwise advised by their doctor.

How should you take this medication?

Trilisate is available in tablet or liquid form. Take Trilisate exactly as prescribed by your doctor.

■ *If you miss a dose...*
If you take Trilisate on a regular schedule, take the forgotten dose as soon as you remember. If it is almost time for your next dose, skip the one you missed and go back to your regular schedule. Do not take 2 doses at once.

■ *Storage instructions...*
Store at room temperature.

What side effects may occur?

Side effects cannot be anticipated. If any develop or change in intensity, inform your doctor as soon as possible. Only your doctor can determine if it is safe for you to continue taking Trilisate.

■ *Side effects may include:*
Constipation, diarrhea, heartburn, indigestion, nausea, ringing in the ears, stomach pain and upset, vomiting

Why should this drug not be prescribed?

If you are sensitive to or have ever had an allergic reaction to Trilisate or drugs of this type, such as aspirin, you should not take this medication. Make sure your doctor is aware of any drug reactions you have experienced.

Special warnings about this medication

Use Trilisate with caution if you have severe or recurring kidney or liver disorder, gastritis (inflammation of the stomach lining), or a stomach or intestinal ulcer. Be cautious, too, if you routinely have 3 or more alcoholic drinks per day. This increases the risk of stomach problems.

If you are an asthmatic allergic to aspirin, tell your doctor before taking Trilisate.

It may be 2 to 3 weeks before you feel the effect of this medication.

If you are an older adult, you are more likely to suffer side effects from Trilisate.

Possible food and drug interactions when taking this medication

If Trilisate is taken with certain other drugs, the effects of either could be increased, decreased, or altered. It is especially important to check with your doctor before combining Trilisate with the following:

Antacids such as Gaviscon and Maalox
Antigout medications
Blood thinners such as Coumadin
Carbonic anhydrase inhibitors such as acetazolamide (Diamox) used to treat heart failure, the eye condition called glaucoma, and certain convulsive disorders
Diabetes medications such as insulin, Micronase, and Tolinase
Methotrexate, an anticancer drug
Other salicylates used to reduce fever, inflammation, and pain, such as aspirin
Phenytoin (the seizure medication Dilantin)
Steroids such as prednisone
Valproic acid (the seizure medication Depakene)

Special information if you are pregnant or breastfeeding

The effects of Trilisate during pregnancy have not been adequately studied. If you are pregnant or plan to become pregnant, inform your doctor immediately. This drug does appear in breast milk and could affect a nursing infant. If this medication is essential to your health, your doctor may advise you not to breastfeed until your treatment is finished.

Recommended dosage

ADULTS

In rheumatoid arthritis, osteoarthritis, more severe arthritis, and acute painful shoulder, the recommended starting dose is 1,500 milligrams taken 2 times a day or 3,000 milligrams taken once a day. Your doctor will adjust the dosage based on your response to this medication.

If you have a kidney disorder, your doctor will monitor you and adjust your dose accordingly.

For mild to moderate pain or to reduce a high fever, the usual dosage is 2,000 to 3,000 milligrams per day, divided into 2 equal doses, as recommended by your doctor.

CHILDREN

For reduction of inflammation or pain, the recommended dose for children is determined by weight. The usual dose for children who weigh 81 pounds or less is 50 milligrams per 2.2 pounds of body weight, taken twice a day. For heavier children, the usual dose is 2,250 milligrams per day, divided into 2 doses.

Trilisate liquid can be taken by younger children and by adults who are unable to swallow a tablet.

OLDER ADULTS

The usual dosage is 2,250 milligrams divided into 3 doses of 750 milligrams each.

Overdosage

Any medication taken in excess can have serious consequences. If you suspect an overdose, seek medical treatment immediately. An overdose of Trilisate can be fatal.

◼ *Symptoms of Trilisate overdose may include:*
Confusion, diarrhea, dizziness, drowsiness, headache, hearing impairment, rapid breathing, ringing in the ears, sweating, vomiting

Trimethobenzamide *See Tigan, page 1435.*

Trimethoprim with Sulfamethoxazole *See Bactrim, page 188.*

Trimipramine *See Surmontil, page 1359.*

Trimox *See Amoxil, page 95.*

TRINALIN

Pronounced: TRIN-uh-lin
Generic ingredients: Azatadine maleate,
Pseudoephedrine sulfate
Other brand name: Rynatan

Why is this drug prescribed?

Trinalin and Rynatan are long-acting antihistamine/decongestants that relieve nasal stuffiness and middle ear congestion caused by hay fever and ongoing nasal inflammation. They can be used alone or with antibiotics and analgesics such as aspirin or acetaminophen. Azatadine, the antihistamine in these products, reduces itching and swelling and dries up secretions from the nose, eyes, and throat. Pseudoephedrine, the decongestant, reduces nasal congestion and makes breathing easier.

Most important fact about this drug

This medication may cause drowsiness. You should not drive or operate dangerous machinery or participate in any hazardous activity that requires full mental alertness until you know how you react to this medication.

How should you take this medication?

Take this medication as indicated; do not take more than your doctor has prescribed.

■ *If you miss a dose...*
If you take Trinalin on a regular schedule, take the forgotten dose as soon as you remember. If it is almost time for your next dose, skip the one you missed and go back to your regular schedule. Do not take 2 doses at once.

■ *Storage instructions...*
Store at room temperature.

What side effects may occur?

Side effects cannot be anticipated. If any develop or change in intensity, inform your doctor as soon as possible. Only your doctor can determine if it is safe for you to continue taking this medication.

■ *Side effects may include:*
Abdominal cramps, acute inflammation of the inner ear, anemia, anxiety, blood disorders, blurred vision, chest pain, chills, confusion, constipation, convulsions, diarrhea, difficulty breathing, dilated pupils, disturbed coordination, dizziness, dry mouth, nose, and throat, early menstruation, exaggerated feeling of well-being, excessive perspiration, excitement, extreme calm (sedation), fatigue, fear, fluttery heart-

beat, frequent urination, hallucinations, headache, high blood pressure, hives, hysteria, increased chest congestion, increased sensitivity to light, insomnia, irregular heartbeat, irritability, loss of appetite, low blood pressure, nausea, nervousness, painful or difficult urination, pale skin, rapid heartbeat, rash, restlessness, ringing in the ears, severe allergic reaction, sleepiness, stuffy nose, tension, tightness in chest, tingling or pins and needles, tremor, upset stomach, urinary retention, vertigo, vomiting, weakness, wheezing

Why should this drug not be prescribed?

These products should be avoided if you have narrow-angle glaucoma or difficulty urinating, if you are taking one of the antidepressant drugs known as MAO inhibitors or have taken one within the past 2 weeks, if you have severe high blood pressure, severe heart disease, or an overactive thyroid, or if you are sensitive to or have ever had an allergic reaction to any of its ingredients.

This drug should not be used to treat asthma and other lower respiratory tract diseases.

Special warnings about this medication

These products should be used with care if you have a peptic ulcer or other upper intestinal obstruction, bladder obstruction due to an enlarged prostate or other bladder problems, a history of bronchial asthma, heart disease, high blood pressure, increased eye pressure, or diabetes.

Pseudoephedrine can be habit-forming at high doses. Remember that this medication can make you feel drowsy. Be careful driving, operating machinery, or using appliances.

The products may cause dizziness, extreme calm (sedation), and low blood pressure in people aged 60 and over. It is also more likely to cause such side effects as confusion, convulsions, hallucinations, and death in this age group.

Possible food and drug interactions when taking this medication

Alcohol may increase the effects of this medication. Do not drink alcohol while taking this medication.

If this medication is taken with certain other drugs, the effects of either could be increased, decreased, or altered. It is especially important to check with your doctor before combining Trinalin with the following:

Alcohol
Antacids such as Maalox
Barbiturates such as phenobarbital
Beta-blocking blood pressure drugs such as Tenormin and Inderal
Blood thinners such as Coumadin
Digitalis (Lanoxin)
Drugs for depression such as Prozac and Elavil

High blood pressure drugs such as Aldomet, Diupres, Hydropres, and Inversine

Kaolin (Kaopectate)

MAO inhibitor drugs such as the antidepressants Nardil and Parnate

Sedatives such as Nembutal and Seconal

Tranquilizers such as Xanax and Valium

Special information if you are pregnant or breastfeeding

Although the effects of these products during pregnancy have not been adequately studied, antihistamines have caused severe reactions in premature and newborn babies when used in the last 3 months of pregnancy. If you are pregnant or plan to become pregnant, notify your doctor immediately. The drugs may appear in breast milk and could affect a nursing infant. If this medication is essential to your health, your doctor may advise you to discontinue breastfeeding until your treatment is finished.

Recommended dosage

ADULTS AND CHILDREN 12 AND OVER

The usual dosage is 1 tablet twice a day.

Children under age 12 should not take these products.

Overdosage

Any medication taken in excess can have serious consequences. An overdose of these products can be fatal. If you suspect an overdose, seek medical attention immediately.

■ *Symptoms of overdose may include:*
Anxiety, bluish color caused by lack of oxygen, blurred vision, chest pain, coma, convulsions, decreased mental alertness, delusions, difficulty sleeping, difficulty urinating, dizziness, excitement, extreme calm (sedation), exaggerated sense of well-being, fluttery heartbeat, giddiness, hallucinations, headache, high blood pressure/low blood pressure, irregular heartbeat, lack of muscle coordination, muscle tenseness, muscle weakness, nausea, perspiration, rapid heartbeat, restlessness, ringing in the ears, temporary interruption of breathing, thirst, tremors, vomiting

■ *Overdose symptoms more common in children may include:*
Dry mouth, fixed, dilated pupils, flushing, overstimulation, stomach and intestinal problems, very high body temperature

Tri-Norinyl *See Oral Contraceptives, page 1000.*

Triphasil *See Oral Contraceptives, page 1000.*

Trivora *See Oral Contraceptives, page 1000.*

TRIZIVIR

Pronounced: TRY-zuh-vir
Generic ingredients: Abacavir, Lamivudine, Zidovudine

Why is this drug prescribed?

Trizivir combines three drugs used to fight HIV, the deadly virus that undermines the immune system, leaving the body ever more vulnerable to infection, and eventually leading to AIDS. The components of Trizivir are all members of the category of HIV drugs known as nucleoside analogs:

Abacavir (also called Ziagen)
Lamivudine (also called Epivir or 3TC)
Zidovudine (also called Retrovir, AZT, or ZDV)

Trizivir may be prescribed alone or in combination with other HIV drugs. It reduces the amount of HIV in the bloodstream, but does not completely cure the disease. You may still develop the rare infections and other complications that accompany HIV. Remember, too, that Trizivir does not reduce the risk of transmitting the virus to others.

Most important fact about this drug

The abacavir (Ziagen) component of this medication can cause a serious, possibly fatal allergic reaction. You should stop taking Trizivir and seek immediate medical attention if you develop any of the following symptoms: abdominal pain, body aches, cough, diarrhea, extreme fatigue, fever, general ill feeling, nausea, severely peeling skin, shortness of breath, skin rash, sore throat, vomiting. These symptoms usually appear during the first 6 weeks of therapy, but may occur any time during treatment. If they do occur, do not take another dose of Trizivir until you've seen your doctor.

If you have to stop taking Trizivir because of this allergic reaction, you must never take Trizivir or Ziagen again. Once you've had such a reaction, taking either drug could lead to death within hours.

When your prescription for Trizivir is filled, the pharmacist will give you a warning card that lists the symptoms of an allergic reaction. Be sure to read it and to carry it with you.

How should you take this medication?

Trizivir is usually taken twice a day, with or without food. It is important to take the medication exactly as prescribed and not to miss any doses. Be sure to refill your prescription before your supply runs out. If HIV drugs are stopped for even a short time, the virus can increase rapidly and may become harder to treat.

■ *If you miss a dose…*
    Take it as soon as you remember. If it is almost time for your next dose, skip the one you missed and go back to your regular schedule.

■ *Storage instructions...*
Store Trizivir tablets at room temperature.

What side effects may occur?

Side effects cannot be anticipated. If any develop or change in intensity, inform your doctor as soon as possible. Only your doctor can determine if it is safe for you to continue taking Trizivir.

■ *Side effects may include:*
Abdominal cramps, abdominal pain, allergic reaction, blisters in the mouth or eyes, blood and lymph disorders, breast enlargement in males, chills, cough, depression, diarrhea, dizziness, enlarged spleen, fatigue, fever, hair loss, headache, heart problems, high blood sugar, hives, ill feeling, indigestion, inflamed blood vessels, insomnia and other sleep problems, joint pain, liver problems, loss of appetite, mouth inflammation, muscle pain or weakness, nasal symptoms, nausea, pain or tingling in the hands or feet, pancreatitis, redistribution of body fat, seizures, severely peeling skin, skin rash, vomiting, weakness, wheezing

Why should this drug not be prescribed?

Do not take Trizivir if you have ever had an allergic reaction to its abacavir component (either in Trizivir itself or as the drug Ziagen).

You also cannot take Trizivir if you weigh less than 90 pounds or have severe kidney disease.

Special warnings about this medication

Trizivir has been known to cause liver problems and a serious medical condition called lactic acidosis. This condition is more likely to develop in women, people who are overweight, those at risk of liver disease, and patients who have been taking nucleoside analogs for a long time. Your doctor will perform blood tests to monitor for lactic acidosis. In addition, be alert for warning signs of the problem, such as persistent nausea and fatigue, and notify your doctor if they occur. Be sure to let your doctor know if you've had liver problems in the past. Trizivir is not recommended under these circumstances.

Treatment with Trizivir can cause serious blood disorders including anemia (low red blood cell count) and neutropenia (low white cell count). You will need to have frequent blood tests performed while you are taking Trizivir.

Prolonged treatment with Trizivir has the potential to cause diseases of the muscles. Be sure to tell your doctor about any muscle pain or weakness you experience.

If you also have the liver infection hepatitis B, there is a chance that it will get worse if treatment with Trizivir is discontinued.

Treatment with HIV drugs, including Trizivir, sometimes causes a redistribution of body fat, resulting in added weight around the waist, a "buffalo hump" of fat on the upper back, breast enlargement, and wasting of the face, arms, and legs. It's not known why this occurs, or what long-term effects it might have.

Possible food and drug interactions when taking this medication

Do not combine Trizivir with Epivir, Combivir, Retrovir, or Ziagen, since these drugs contain ingredients included in Trizivir. Also avoid Zerit while taking Trizivir.

In addition, if Trizivir is taken with certain other drugs, the effects of either may be increased, decreased, or altered. It is especially important to check with your doctor before combining Trizivir with the following:

Alcohol
Atovaquone (Mepron)
Doxorubicin (Adriamycin, Doxil, Rubex)
Drugs used for bone marrow suppression and cancer therapy
Fluconazole (Diflucan)
Ganciclovir (Cytovene)
Interferon-alfa (Intron, Roferon)
Methadone
Nelfinavir (Viracept)
Probenecid (Benemid)
Ribavirin (Virazole)
Ritonavir (Norvir, Kaletra)
Trimethoprim/sulfamethoxazole (Bactrim, Septra)
Valproic acid (Depakene)
Zalcitabine (Hivid)

Special information if you are pregnant or breastfeeding

Trizivir has not been studied in pregnant women and should be used only if the benefit to the mother outweighs the potential risk to the developing baby.

Because the virus can be passed to a baby through breast milk, breastfeeding is not recommended for mothers with HIV.

Recommended dosage

ADULTS

The recommended dose of Trizivir is 1 tablet twice daily with or without food.

CHILDREN

Trizivir is not intended for children and adolescents who weigh less than 90 pounds. Teenagers who weigh more than 90 pounds receive the adult dose.

Overdosage

Any medication taken in excess can have serious consequences. If you suspect an overdose, seek medical attention immediately.

■ *Symptoms of Trizivir overdose may include:*
Confusion, dizziness, drowsiness, headache, lack of energy, nausea, vomiting

T-Stat *See Erythromycin, Topical, page 524.*

Tums *See Antacids, page 114.*

TUSSIONEX

Pronounced: TUSS-ee-uh-nex
Generic ingredients: Hydrocodone polistirex,
Chlorpheniramine polistirex

Why is this drug prescribed?

Tussionex Extended-Release Suspension is a cough suppressant/antihistamine combination used to relieve coughs and the upper respiratory symptoms of colds and allergies. Hydrocodone, a mild narcotic similar to codeine, is believed to work directly on the cough center. Chlorpheniramine, an antihistamine, reduces itching and swelling and dries up secretions from the eyes, nose, and throat.

Most important fact about this drug

This medication can cause considerable drowsiness and make you less alert. You should not drive or operate machinery or participate in any activity that requires full mental alertness until you know how you react to Tussionex.

How should you take this medication?

Tussionex should be taken exactly as prescribed.

It should not be diluted with other liquids or mixed with other drugs. Shake well before using.

■ *If you miss a dose...*
If you take Tussionex on a regular schedule, take the forgotten dose as soon as you remember. If it is almost time for your next dose, skip the one you missed and go back to your regular schedule. Do not take 2 doses at once.

■ *Storage instructions...*
Store at room temperature in a tightly closed container.

What side effects may occur?
Side effects cannot be anticipated. If any develop or change in intensity, inform your doctor as soon as possible. Only your doctor can determine if it is safe for you to continue taking Tussionex.

■ *Side effects may include:*
Anxiety, constipation, decreased mental and physical performance, difficulty breathing, difficulty urinating, dizziness, drowsiness, dry throat, emotional dependence, exaggerated feeling of depression, exaggerated sense of well-being, extreme calm (sedation), fear, itching, mental clouding, mood changes, nausea, rash, restlessness, sluggishness, tightness in chest, vomiting

Why should this drug not be prescribed?
Do not take Tussionex if you are sensitive to or have ever had an allergic reaction to hydrocodone or chlorpheniramine. Make sure your doctor is aware of any drug reactions you have experienced.

Special warnings about this medication
Tussionex contains a mild narcotic that can cause dependence and tolerance when the drug is used for several weeks. However, it is unlikely that dependence will develop when Tussionex is used for the short-term treatment of a cough.

Like all narcotics, Tussionex may produce slowed or irregular breathing. If you have lung disease or a breathing disorder, use this medication cautiously.

Use Tussionex with care if you have the eye condition known as narrow-angle glaucoma, asthma, an enlarged prostate gland, urinary difficulties, an intestinal disorder, liver or kidney disease, an underactive thyroid gland, or Addison's disease (a disorder of the adrenal glands), or if you have recently suffered a head injury.

Extra caution should be used when giving Tussionex to the elderly and those in a weakened condition.

Remember that Tussionex can cause drowsiness.

Narcotics can cause intestinal blockage or mask a severe abdominal condition.

Possible food and drug interactions when taking this medication
Tussionex may increase the effects of alcohol. Do not drink alcohol while taking this medication.

If Tussionex is taken with certain other drugs, the effects of either could be increased, decreased, or altered. It is especially important to check with your doctor before combining Tussionex with the following:

Antispasmodic medications such as Bentyl and Cogentin
Major tranquilizers such as Compazine and Thorazine

MAO inhibitor drugs (antidepressant drugs such as Nardil and Parnate)

Medications for anxiety such as Valium and Xanax

Medications for depression such as Elavil and Prozac

Other antihistamines such as Benadryl

Other narcotics such as Demerol and Percocet

Special information if you are pregnant or breastfeeding

The safety of Tussionex during pregnancy has not been adequately studied. However, babies born to mothers who have been taking narcotics regularly before delivery will be born addicted. If you are pregnant or plan to become pregnant, inform your doctor immediately. Tussionex may appear in breast milk and could affect a nursing infant. If this medication is essential to your health, your doctor may recommend that you stop breastfeeding until your treatment with Tussionex is finished.

Recommended dosage

ADULTS

The usual dose is 1 teaspoonful (5 milliliters) every 12 hours. Do not take more than 2 teaspoonfuls in 24 hours.

CHILDREN AGED 6 TO 12

The usual dose is one-half teaspoonful every 12 hours. Do not take more than 1 teaspoonful in 24 hours.

Tussionex is not recommended for children under 6 years old.

Overdosage

Any medication taken in excess can have serious consequences. A narcotic overdose can be fatal. If you suspect an overdose, seek medical treatment immediately.

■ *Symptoms of Tussionex overdose may include:*
Blue skin color due to lack of oxygen, cardiac arrest, cold and clammy skin, decreased or difficult breathing, extreme sleepiness leading to stupor or coma, low blood pressure, muscle flabbiness, slow heartbeat, temporary cessation of breathing

TUSSI-ORGANIDIN NR

Pronounced: TUSS-ee or-GAN-i-din
Generic ingredients: Guaifenesin, Codeine phosphate
Other brand name: Brontex

Why is this drug prescribed?

Tussi-Organidin NR is used to relieve coughs and chest congestion in adults and children. It contains guaifenesin, which helps thin and loosen mucus in the lungs, making it easier to cough up. It also contains a cough suppressant, the narcotic codeine.

Most important fact about this drug

Tussi-Organidin NR may cause you to become drowsy or less alert. Alcohol will intensify this effect. Driving, operating dangerous machinery, or participating in any hazardous activity that requires your full mental alertness is not recommended until you know how you react to this medication.

How should you take this medication?

Take Tussi-Organidin NR exactly as described. When giving the liquid to a child, use a calibrated dropper to measure the dose.

■ *If you miss a dose...*
Take the missed dose as soon as you remember. If it is almost time for your next dose, skip the one you missed and go back to your regular schedule. Never take 2 doses at once.
■ *Storage instructions...*
Store at room temperature in a tightly closed container, away from light.

What side effects may occur?

Side effects cannot be anticipated. If any side effects develop or change in intensity, tell your doctor as soon as possible. Only your doctor can determine whether it is safe to continue taking Tussi-Organidin NR.

■ *Side effects may include:*
Constipation, nausea, pinpoint pupils of the eye, vomiting

At higher doses, this medication may also cause light-headedness, drowsiness, slowed breathing, and an exaggerated sense of well-being.

Why should this drug not be prescribed?

Do not take Tussi-Organidin NR if you are allergic to codeine or guaifenesin.

Special warnings about this medication

Because it contains codeine, Tussi-Organidin NR may cause drug dependence and tolerance with continued use.

Do not use this product in children under 2 years of age. Be cautious if the child has an allergy.

Do not take Tussi-Organidin NR for the constant cough brought on by smoking, asthma, chronic bronchitis, or emphysema unless your doctor recommends it. If your cough lasts for more than 1 week, tends to come back, or is accompanied by fever, rash, or persistent headache, check with your doctor

Be sure to tell the doctor if you have any breathing problems, a severe abdominal condition, kidney or liver problems, an underactive thyroid gland, or an enlarged prostate. Also alert the doctor if you suffer from seizures, have had a head injury, or have recently had stomach, intestinal, or urinary tract surgery.

Possible food and drug interactions when taking this medication

If Tussi-Organidin NR is taken with certain other drugs, the effects of either could be increased, decreased, or altered. It is especially important to check with your doctor before combining Tussi-Organidin NR with the following:

Alcohol
Antihistamines such as Actifed and Benadryl
Drugs used to treat anxiety or depression, such as Librium and Prozac
Sedatives such as Dalmane

Special information if you are pregnant or breastfeeding

If you are pregnant or plan to become pregnant, inform your doctor immediately. The safety of Tussi-Organidin NR during pregnancy has not been established. Tussi-Organidin NR should not be taken if you are breastfeeding.

Recommended dosage

ADULTS AND CHILDREN 12 YEARS AND OLDER

Tussi-Organidin NR
The usual dosage is 2 teaspoonfuls every 4 hours, not to exceed 12 teaspoonfuls in 24 hours.

Brontex
The usual dosage is 1 tablet or 4 teaspoonfuls every 4 hours. Do not take more than 6 tablets in a 24-hour period.

CHILDREN 6 TO 12 YEARS OF AGE

Tussi-Organidin NR
The usual dosage is 1 teaspoonful every 4 hours, not to exceed 6 teaspoonfuls in 24 hours.

Brontex
The usual dosage is 2 teaspoonfuls every 4 hours. Do not give tablets.

CHILDREN 2 TO 6 YEARS OF AGE

Tussi-Organidin NR
Your doctor will determine the dosage according to weight. The recommended total daily dosage is 1 milligram per 2.2 pounds of body weight, divided into 4 small doses.

Overdosage
Any medication taken in excess can have serious consequences. If you suspect an overdose, seek medical treatment immediately.

■ *Symptoms of Tussi-Organidin NR overdose may include:*
Alternate periods of not breathing and rapid, deep breathing, bluish skin coloration, cold and clammy skin, constriction of the pupils of the eyes, delirium, delusions, double vision, excitement, extreme sleepiness progressing to stupor or coma, flaccid muscles, hallucinations, low blood pressure, restlessness, slow heartbeat, slow, shallow, or labored breathing, speech disturbances, vertigo

TYLENOL
Pronounced: TIE-len-all
Generic name: Acetaminophen
Other brand name: Aspirin Free Anacin

Why is this drug prescribed?
Tylenol is a fever- and pain-reducing medication that is widely used to relieve simple headaches and muscle aches; the minor aches and pains associated with the common cold; backache; toothache; minor pain of arthritis; and menstrual cramps.

Most important fact about this drug
Do not use Tylenol to relieve pain for more than 10 days, or to reduce fever for more than 3 days unless your doctor has specifically told you to do so.

How should you take this medication?
Follow the dosing instructions on the label. Do not take more Tylenol than is recommended.

■ *If you miss a dose…*
Take this medication only as needed.
■ *Storage instructions…*
Store at room temperature. Protect extra strength gelcaps and geltabs from high humidity and excessive heat. Keep the extended relief caplets away from high heat.

What side effects may occur?
Tylenol is relatively free of side effects. Rarely, an allergic reaction may occur. If you develop any allergic symptoms such as rash, hives, swelling, or difficulty breathing, stop taking Tylenol immediately and notify your doctor.

Special warnings about this medication

Stop taking Tylenol and check with your doctor if you develop new symptoms, if redness or swelling are present, if pain gets worse or lasts more than 10 days, or if fever gets worse or lasts more than 3 days. Children's and Junior Strength Tylenol should not be used for more than 5 days for pain, or 3 days for fever.

If you generally drink 3 or more alcoholic beverages per day, check with your doctor about using Tylenol and other acetaminophen-containing products, and never take more than the recommended dosage. There is a possibility of damage to the liver when large amounts of alcohol and acetaminophen are combined.

Possible food and drug interactions when taking this medication

If Tylenol is taken with certain other drugs the effects of either could be increased, decreased, or altered. It is especially important to check with your doctor before combining Tylenol with the following:

Alcohol
Cholestyramine (Questran)
Isoniazid (Nydrazid)
Nonsteroidal anti-inflammatory drugs such as Dolobid and Motrin
Oral contraceptives
Phenytoin (Dilantin)
Warfarin (Coumadin)
Zidovudine (Retrovir)

Tylenol should not be used with other products containing acetaminophen.

Special information if you are pregnant or breastfeeding

As with all medications, ask your doctor or healthcare professional whether it is safe for you to use Tylenol while you are pregnant or breastfeeding.

Recommended dosage

ADULTS AND CHILDREN 12 YEARS AND OLDER

Tylenol Regular Strength
The usual dose is 2 tablets every 4 to 6 hours. Do not take more than 12 caplets or tablets in 24 hours.

Tylenol Extra Strength
The usual dose is 2 pills or tablespoonfuls every 4 to 6 hours. Do not take more than 8 pills or tablespoonfuls in 24 hours.

Tylenol Extended Relief
The usual dose is 2 caplets every 8 hours, not to exceed 6 caplets in any 24 hour period. Swallow each caplet whole. Do not crush, chew, or dissolve the caplets.

CHILDREN 6 TO 12 YEARS OLD

Tylenol Regular Strength
One-half to 1 tablet every 4 to 6 hours. Children in this age group should not be given more than 5 doses in 24 hours.

Junior Strength Tylenol
All doses of Junior Strength Tylenol chewable tablets may be repeated every 4 hours, up to 5 times a day. The usual dose for children 6 to 8 years of age is 2 tablets; 9 to 10 years, 2½ tablets; 11 years, 3 tablets; 12 years, 4 tablets

Children's Tylenol
All doses of Children's Tylenol may be repeated every 4 hours, but not more than 5 times daily. Chewable tablets: The usual dose for children 6 to 8 years of age is 4 tablets; 9 to 10 years, 5 tablets; 11 to 12 years, 6 tablets. Suspension liquid (a special cup for measuring dosage is provided): The usual dose for children 6 to 8 years of age is 2 teaspoons; 9 to 10 years, 2½ teaspoons; 11 to 12 years, 3 teaspoons.

CHILDREN UNDER 6 YEARS OLD

Children's Tylenol
All doses of Children's Tylenol may be repeated every 4 hours, but not more than 5 times daily. Children under 2 years old should be given Children's Tylenol only on the advice of a physician. Chewable tablets: The usual dose for children 2 to 3 years of age is 2 tablets; 4 to 5 years, 3 tablets. Suspension liquid (a special cup for measuring dosage is provided): The usual dose for children 4 to 11 months of age is ½ teaspoon; 12 to 23 months, ¾ teaspoon; 2 to 3 years, 1 teaspoon; 4 to 5 years, 1½ teaspoons.

Infants' Tylenol Concentrated Drops
The usual dose for children 0 to 3 months of age is 0.4 milliliter; 4 to 11 months, 0.8 milliliter; 12 to 23 months, 1.2 milliliters; 2 to 3 years, 1.6 milliliters.

Overdosage
Any medication taken in excess can have serious consequences. If you suspect an overdose, seek medical attention immediately. Massive doses of Tylenol may cause liver damage.

■ *Symptoms of Tylenol overdose may include:*
Excessive perspiration, exhaustion, general discomfort, nausea, vomiting

TYLENOL WITH CODEINE

Pronounced: TIE-len-awl with CO-deen
Generic ingredients: Acetaminophen, Codeine phosphate
Other brand name: Phenaphen with Codeine

Why is this drug prescribed?

Tylenol with Codeine, a narcotic analgesic, is used to treat mild to moderately severe pain. It contains two drugs—acetaminophen and codeine. Acetaminophen, an antipyretic (fever-reducing) analgesic, is used to reduce pain and fever. Codeine, a narcotic analgesic, is used to treat pain that is moderate to severe.

People who are allergic to aspirin can take Tylenol with Codeine.

Most important fact about this drug

Tylenol with Codeine contains a narcotic (codeine) and, even if taken in prescribed amounts, can cause physical and psychological addiction if taken for a long enough time.

Addiction may be more of a risk for a person who has been addicted to alcohol or drugs. Be sure to follow your doctor's instructions carefully when taking Tylenol with Codeine (or any other drugs that contain a narcotic).

How should you take this medication?

Tylenol with Codeine may be taken with meals or with milk (but not with alcohol).

■ *If you miss a dose...*
If you take this medication on a regular schedule, take the forgotten dose as soon as you remember. If it is almost time for your next dose, skip the one you missed and go back to your regular schedule. Do not take 2 doses at once.

■ *Storage instructions...*
Store away from heat, light, and moisture. Keep the liquid from freezing.

What side effects may occur?

Side effects cannot be anticipated. If any develop or change in intensity, inform your doctor as soon as possible. Only your doctor can determine if it is safe for you to continue taking Tylenol with Codeine.

■ *Side effects may include:*
Dizziness, light-headedness, nausea, sedation, shortness of breath, vomiting

Why should this drug not be prescribed?
You should not use Tylenol with Codeine if you are sensitive to either acetaminophen (Tylenol) or codeine.

Special warnings about this medication
You should take Tylenol with Codeine cautiously and only according to your doctor's instructions, as you would take any medication containing a narcotic. Make sure your doctor is aware of any problems you have had with drug or alcohol addiction.

Tylenol with Codeine tablets contain a sulfite that may cause allergic reactions in some people. These reactions may include shock and severe, possibly life-threatening, asthma attacks. People with asthma are more likely to be sensitive to sulfites.

If you have experienced a head injury, consult your doctor before taking Tylenol with Codeine.

If you have stomach problems, such as an ulcer, check with your doctor before taking Tylenol with Codeine. Tylenol with Codeine may obscure the symptoms of stomach problems, making them difficult to diagnose and treat.

If you have ever had liver, kidney, thyroid, or adrenal disease, difficulty urinating, or an enlarged prostate, consult your doctor before taking Tylenol with Codeine.

If you generally drink 3 or more alcoholic beverages per day, check with your doctor before using Tylenol with Codeine and other acetaminophen-containing products, and never take more than the recommended dosage. There is a possibility of damage to the liver when large amounts of alcohol and acetaminophen are combined.

This drug may cause drowsiness and impair your ability to drive a car or operate potentially dangerous machinery. Do not participate in any activities that require full attention when using this drug until you are sure of its effect on you.

Possible food and drug interactions when taking this medication
Alcohol may increase the sedative effects of Tylenol with Codeine. Therefore, do not drink alcohol while you are taking this medication.

If Tylenol with Codeine is taken with certain other drugs, the effects of either could be increased, decreased, or altered. It is especially important to check with your doctor before combining Tylenol with Codeine with the following:

Antidepressants such as Elavil, Nardil, Parnate, and Tofranil
Drugs that control spasms, such as Cogentin
Major tranquilizers such as Clozaril and Thorazine
Other narcotic painkillers such as Darvon
Tranquilizers such as Valium and Xanax

Special information if you are pregnant or breastfeeding

It is not known if Tylenol with Codeine could injure a baby, or if it could affect a woman's reproductive capacity. Using any medication that contains a narcotic during pregnancy may cause babies to be born with a physical addiction to the narcotic. If you are pregnant or plan to become pregnant, you should not take Tylenol with Codeine unless the potential benefits clearly outweigh the possible dangers. As with other narcotic painkillers, taking Tylenol with Codeine shortly before delivery (especially at higher dosages) may cause some degree of breathing difficulty in the mother and newborn.

Some studies (but not all) have reported that codeine appears in breast milk and may affect a nursing infant. Therefore, nursing mothers should use Tylenol with Codeine only if the potential gains are greater than the potential hazards.

Recommended dosage

ADULTS

Dosage will depend on how severe your pain is and how you respond to the drug.

To Relieve Pain

A single dose may contain from 15 to 60 milligrams of codeine phosphate and from 300 to 1,000 milligrams of acetaminophen. The maximum dose in a 24-hour period should be 360 milligrams of codeine phosphate and 4,000 milligrams of acetaminophen. Your doctor will determine the amounts of codeine phosphate and acetaminophen taken in each dose. Doses may be repeated up to every 4 hours.

Single doses above 60 milligrams of codeine do not give enough pain relief to balance the increased number of side effects.

Adults may also take Tylenol with Codeine elixir (liquid). Tylenol with Codeine elixir contains 120 milligrams of acetaminophen and 12 milligrams of codeine phosphate per teaspoonful.

The usual adult dose is 1 tablespoonful every 4 hours as needed.

CHILDREN

The safety of Tylenol with Codeine elixir has not been established in children under 3 years old.

Children 3 to 6 years old may take 1 teaspoonful 3 or 4 times daily.

Children 7 to 12 years old may take 2 teaspoonsful 3 or 4 times daily.

OLDER ADULTS

Older people and anyone in a weakened or run-down condition should use Tylenol with Codeine cautiously.

Overdosage

Any medication taken in excess can cause symptoms of overdose. Severe overdosage of Tylenol with Codeine can cause death. If you suspect an overdose, seek medical attention immediately.

■ *Symptoms of Tylenol with Codeine overdose may include:*
Bluish skin, cold and clammy skin, coma due to low blood sugar, decreased, irregular, or stopped breathing, extreme sleepiness progressing to stupor or coma, general bodily discomfort, heart attack, kidney failure, liver failure, low blood pressure, muscle weakness, nausea, slow heartbeat, sweating, vomiting

Tylox *See Percocet, page 1073.*

ULTRACET
Pronounced: UL-tra-set.
Generic ingredients: Tramadol hydrochloride, Acetaminophen

Why is this drug prescribed?
Ultracet is used to treat moderate to severe pain for a period of 5 days or less. It contains two pain-relieving agents. Tramadol, known technically as an opioid analgesic, is a narcotic pain reliever. Acetaminophen is the active ingredient in the over-the-counter pain remedy Tylenol.

Most important fact about this drug
Take only the amount and number of doses prescribed. Exceeding the recommended dosage can lead to reduced breathing, liver damage, seizures, and death.

How should you take this medication?
Follow dosage recommendations strictly, and stop taking the drug as soon as possible.

■ *If you miss a dose...*
Take this drug only as needed. Never take 2 doses at once.
■ *Storage instructions...*
Store Ultracet in a tight container at room temperature.

What side effects may occur?
■ *Side effects may include:*
Constipation, increased sweating, sleepiness

Why should this drug not be prescribed?
Avoid Ultracet if you have had an allergic reaction to either of its active ingredients, or to any other narcotic pain reliever. Do not take this drug if you have been drinking, or have taken any other narcotic drug, sleep aid,

tranquilizer, or antidepressant; your consciousness or breathing could be compromised. Avoid this drug if you've ever been dependent on other narcotic pain relievers.

Special warnings about this medication

Ultracet has caused serious and even fatal allergic reactions in some people, typically after the first dose. Seek medical help immediately if you begin to have trouble breathing or break out in hives or blisters.

Ultracet may cause seizures, particularly in those with epilepsy, a history of seizures, or at special risk for seizures, such as people with head trauma, metabolic disorders, or central nervous system infections, and those going through alcohol or drug withdrawal.

Inform your doctor if you have had a head injury, as Ultracet can increase pressure around the brain. Also let the doctor know if you have liver disease, since Ultracet can affect the liver.

Do not take this drug if you will be driving a car or operating dangerous machinery. Ultracet may impair the mental and physical abilities needed for driving

Ultracet poses a danger of mental and physical addiction. Never exceed the prescribed dosage. If you experience withdrawal symptoms—which can occur if you stop taking the drug abruptly—consult your doctor for a tapering regimen. Withdrawal symptoms include anxiety, chills, diarrhea, hallucinations, insomnia, nausea, pain, erection of hair, sweating, tremors, and upper respiratory symptoms.

The safety and effectiveness of Ultracet have not been established in children under the age of 16 years.

Possible food and drug interactions when taking this medication

If Ultracet is taken with certain other drugs, the effects of either may be increased, decreased, or altered. It is especially important to check with your doctor before combining Ultracet with the following:

Acetaminophen-containing products such as Tylenol
Antidepressant drugs classified as MAO inhibitors, including Nardil and Parnate
Antipsychotic drugs such as Haldol and Thorazine
Carbamazepine (Tegretol)
Cyclobenzaprine (Flexeril)
Digoxin (Lanoxin)
Other narcotic pain relievers such as Percodan and Vicodin
Promethazine (Phenergan)
Serotonin-boosting antidepressants such as Paxil and Prozac
Sleep aids such as Halcion and Restoril
Tranquilizers such as Valium and Xanax
Tricyclic antidepressants such as Elavil and Tofranil
Warfarin (Coumadin)

Special information if you are pregnant or breastfeeding

Taken during pregnancy, Ultracet can be fatal to the developing baby, or lead to seizures and withdrawal symptoms in the newborn. If you are pregnant, inform your doctor immediately.

Ultracet appears in breast milk and is not recommended for nursing mothers.

Recommended dosage

ADULTS

The usual dose of Ultracet is two tablets every 4 to 6 hours as needed for pain relief up to a maximum of 8 tablets per day for no more than 5 days.

If you have kidney problems, the doctor may reduce the dose to 2 tablets every 12 hours. Older adults may also receive a low dose.

Overdosage

An Ultracet overdose can be fatal. If you suspect an overdose, seek emergency treatment immediately.

■ *Symptoms of Ultracet overdose may include:*
Cardiac arrest, coma, depressed breathing, generally ill feeling, lethargy, loss of appetite, nausea, pallor, profuse perspiration, seizures, vomiting

ULTRAM

Pronounced: UL-tram
Generic name: Tramadol hydrochloride

Why is this drug prescribed?

Ultram is prescribed to relieve moderate to moderately severe pain.

Most important fact about this drug

You should not drive a car, operate machinery, or perform any other potentially hazardous activities until you know how this drug affects you.

How should you take this medication?

It's important to take Ultram exactly as prescribed. Do not increase the dosage or length of time you take this drug without your doctor's approval.

■ *If you miss a dose...*
Take it as soon as you remember. However, if it is almost time for your next dose, skip the one you missed and go back to your regular schedule. Never take 2 doses at once.

■ *Storage instructions...*
Store in a tightly closed container at room temperature.

What side effects may occur?

Side effects cannot be anticipated. If any develop or change in intensity, tell your doctor as soon as possible. Only your doctor can determine if it is safe for you to continue taking Ultram.

■ *Side effects may include:*

Agitation, anxiety, bloating and gas, constipation, convulsive movements, diarrhea, dizziness, drowsiness, dry mouth, feeling of elation, hallucinations, headache, indigestion, itching, nausea, nervousness, sweating, tremor, vomiting, weakness

Why should this drug not be prescribed?

Avoid Ultram if it has ever given you an allergic reaction. Also avoid Ultram after taking large doses of sleeping pills such as Halcion, Dalmane, and Restoril; narcotic pain relievers such as Demerol, morphine, Darvon, and Percocet; or psychotherapeutic drugs such as antidepressants and tranquilizers. And do not take Ultram after drinking excessive amounts of alcohol.

Special warnings about this medication

If you have stomach problems such as an ulcer, make sure your doctor is aware of them. Ultram may hide the symptoms, making them difficult to diagnose and treat.

Ultram can cause mental and physical addiction. If you've ever had a problem with narcotic painkillers such as Percocet, Demerol, or morphine, you should avoid this drug. Withdrawal symptoms may occur if you stop taking Ultram abruptly. Such symptoms include anxiety, sweating, insomnia, pain, nausea, tremor; diarrhea, and respiratory problems. A gradual decrease in dosage will help prevent these symptoms.

Do not take more than the recommended dose of Ultram, since larger doses have been known to cause seizures, especially if you have epilepsy or are taking medications that also increase the risk of seizures. Among such medications are almost all antidepressant drugs, plus narcotics and major tranquilizers such as Loxitane and Stelazine.

If you have liver or kidney disease, be sure your doctor knows about it. Your dosage may have to be reduced.

Before you have any kind of surgery, make sure the doctor knows you are taking Ultram.

If you have any kind of breathing problem, use Ultram with caution or take a different kind of painkiller. Ultram can impair respiration, especially if taken with alcohol.

If you have experienced a head injury, consult your doctor before taking Ultram. The medication's effects may be stronger and could hide warning signs of serious trouble.

Possible food and drug interactions when taking this medication
Ultram may increase the drowsiness caused by alcohol. Do not drink alcohol while taking this medication.

Avoid Ultram, too, if you are taking the seizure medication Tegretol.

If Ultram is taken with certain other drugs, the effects of either could be increased, decreased, or altered. It is especially important to check with your doctor before combining Ultram with the following:

Cyclobenzaprine (Flexeril)
Drugs known as MAO inhibitors, including the antidepressants
    Nardil and Parnate
Tricyclic antidepressants such as Elavil, Norpramin, and Tofranil
Major tranquilizers such as Stelazine and Thorazine
Narcotic pain relievers (Darvon, Demerol, morphine, Percocet)
Promethazine (Mepergan, Phenergan)
Quinidine (Quinidex)
Serotonin-boosting antidepressants such as Paxil, Prozac, and Zoloft
Sleeping pills (Dalmane, Halcion, Restoril)
Tranquilizers (Valium, Xanax)

Special information if you are pregnant or breastfeeding
There have been reports of serious harm to developing babies when Ultram was used during pregnancy. If you are pregnant or plan to become pregnant, tell your doctor immediately.

Ultram appears in breast milk and may affect a nursing infant. If this medication is essential to your health, your doctor may advise you to discontinue breastfeeding until your treatment is finished.

Recommended dosage

ADULTS

The usual starting dose for chronic pain is 25 milligrams once a day in the morning. The daily dosage is then increased every 3 days until it reaches 200 milligrams taken in four doses of 50 milligrams each. After the phase-in period, Ultram may be taken in doses of 50 to 100 milligrams every 4 to 6 hours, depending on the severity of pain. If rapid pain relief is needed, the phase-in steps can be skipped, though side effects will be more likely. The maximum dosage under any circumstances is 400 milligrams a day (300 milligrams for those over age 75).

For people with kidney problems, the usual starting dose is 50 to 100 milligrams every 12 hours; and the maximum per day is 200 milligrams. For those with cirrhosis, the usual dose is 50 milligrams every 12 hours.

CHILDREN

The safety and effectiveness of Ultram in children under 16 years of age have not been established.

Overdosage

An overdose of Ultram can be fatal. If you suspect an overdose, seek emergency medical treatment immediately.

■ *Symptoms of Ultram overdose include:*
Cardiac arrest, coma, dfficult or slowed breathing, drowsiness, seizures

Ultrase *See Pancrease, page 1030.*

ULTRAVATE

Pronounced: ULL-trah-vate
Generic name: Halobetasol propionate

Why is this drug prescribed?

Ultravate is a high-potency steroid medication that relieves the itching and inflammation caused by a wide variety of skin disorders. It is available in cream and ointment formulations.

Most important fact about this drug

Some of the medication in Ultravate is inevitably absorbed through the skin and into the bloodstream. If applied over a large area, or under an airtight dressing, the drug can cause a number of unwanted side effects, including increased sugar in your blood and urine and a set of symptoms called Cushing's syndrome, characterized by a moon-shaped face, emotional disturbances, high blood pressure, weight gain, and growth of body hair in women. Use no more of this medication than your doctor directs, and do not bandage or wrap the affected area unless the doctor specifically recommends it.

How should you take this medication?

Use Ultravate only on the skin. Do not apply it to the face, groin, or armpits, and be careful to keep it out of your eyes.

When treating an infant's diaper area, do not use tight diapers or plastic pants, which can increase absorption of the drug.

■ *If you miss a dose...*
Apply the forgotten dose as soon as you remember. However, if it is almost time for your next dose, skip the one you missed and return to your regular schedule.
■ *Storage instructions...*
Store at room temperature.

What side effects may occur?

Side effects cannot be anticipated. If any develop or change in intensity, tell your doctor as soon as possible. Only your doctor can determine if it is safe to continue using Ultravate.

■ *Side effects may include:*
Burning, itching, stinging

Why should this drug not be prescribed?
Do not use Ultravate to treat red eruptions around the mouth (perioral dermatitis) or the red facial patches caused by rosacea. Avoid Ultravate if it causes an allergic reaction.

Special warnings about this medication
Use of steroid medications can lead to a slowdown in the body's production of natural steroids and result in a shortage when the medication is stopped. To reduce the likelihood of this problem, use Ultravate for no more than 2 weeks at a time, and apply it only to small areas.

When used on children, steroid creams and ointments have been known to stunt growth and raise pressure inside the skull, resulting in headaches, bulges on the head, and loss of vision. Ultravate is not recommended for children under 12.

Possible food and drug interactions when using this medication
No interactions have been reported.

Special information if you are pregnant or breastfeeding
In studies with animals, steroid medications have caused harm during pregnancy. Use Ultravate while pregnant only if the possible benefits outweigh the possible risks to the baby.

Steroids do make their way into breast milk, and can cause harm to a nursing infant. Use Ultravate with caution while breastfeeding.

Recommended dosage
Once or twice a day, gently and completely rub into the affected skin a thin layer of Ultravate. Do not use more than 50 grams per week, and do not continue treatment for more than 2 weeks.

Overdosage
Applied in excessive quantities, Ultravate can produce the problems discussed under *Most important fact about this drug.* If you suspect an overdose, check with your doctor immediately.

Uni-Dur *See Theo-Dur, page 1432.*

Uniphyl *See Theo-Dur, page 1432.*

UNIRETIC

Pronounced: you-nih-RET-ick
Generic ingredients: Moexipril hydrochloride,
  Hydrochlorothiazide

Why is this drug prescribed?

Uniretic combines two types of blood pressure medication. The first, moexipril hydrochloride, is an ACE (angiotensin-converting enzyme) inhibitor. It works by preventing a chemical in your blood called angiotensin I from converting into a more potent form (angiotensin II) that increases salt and water retention in the body and causes the blood vessels to constrict—two actions that tend to increase blood pressure.

To aid in clearing excess water from the body, Uniretic also contains hydrochlorothiazide, a diuretic that promotes production of urine. Diuretics often wash too much potassium out of the body along with the water. However, the ACE inhibitor part of Uniretic tends to keep potassium in the body, thereby canceling this unwanted effect.

Uniretic is not used for the initial treatment of high blood pressure. It is saved for later use, when a single blood pressure medication is not sufficient for the job.

Most important fact about this drug

You must take Uniretic regularly for it to be effective, and you must continue taking it even if you are feeling well. Like other blood pressure medications, Uniretic does not cure high blood pressure; it merely keeps it under control.

How should you take this medication?

Take Uniretic once a day, 1 hour before a meal. Try not to miss any doses. Stopping Uniretic suddenly could cause a rise in blood pressure.

■ *If you miss a dose...*
   Take it as soon as you remember. If it is almost time for your next dose, skip the one you missed and go back to your regular schedule. Never take 2 doses at the same time.
■ *Storage instructions...*
   Store at room temperature, away from moisture, in a tightly closed container.

What side effects may occur?

Side effects cannot be anticipated. If any develop or change in intensity, inform your doctor as soon as possible. Only your doctor can determine if it is safe for you to continue taking Uniretic.

■ *Side effects may include:*
   Abdominal pain, back pain, bronchitis, chest pain, cough, diarrhea, dizziness, fatigue, fever, flu-like symptoms, headache, impotence, in-

creased blood sugar, indigestion, infection, inflammation of the nasal passages, pain, rash, sinus inflammation, sore throat, swelling, tension, upper respiratory tract infection, urinary tract infection, vertigo

Why should this drug not be prescribed?

Do not take Uniretic if you've had a severe reaction called angioedema (swelling of the face, arms, legs, and throat) to any other ACE inhibitor (for example, Capoten, Prinivil, or Zestril). Avoid this drug, too, if you've had an allergic reaction to either of its ingredients, or to any sulfa drug. (Allergic reactions to Uniretic are more likely if you have a history of allergy or bronchial asthma.)

If you have problems with urination, do not take this drug.

Special warnings about this medication

Contact your doctor immediately if you develop swelling around your lips, tongue, or throat, or in your arms and legs, or if you begin to have difficulty breathing or swallowing. You may need emergency room treatment.

If you have poor kidneys, use Uniretic with caution. For people with severe kidney disease, Uniretic is not recommended at all. Your doctor should test your kidney function at the start of treatment, and continue to monitor it as long as you take the drug.

Uniretic can cause light-headedness, especially during the first few days of treatment. If you faint, stop taking the medication and call your doctor immediately.

Uniretic can cause a severe drop in blood pressure if you lose too much liquid through excessive sweating, severe diarrhea, or vomiting. Contact your doctor immediately if you develop one of these problems.

Low blood pressure is especially dangerous if you have congestive heart failure or other heart conditions. Your doctor should monitor your pressure with extra care if that's the case.

This drug should be used with caution if you are on dialysis. There have been reports of extreme allergic reactions during dialysis in people taking ACE inhibitors such as the one in Uniretic. A severe reaction is also more likely if you've ever had desensitization treatments with bee or wasp venom.

If you have liver disease or a disease of connective tissue called lupus erythematosus, Uniretic should be used with caution. Tell your doctor immediately if you notice a yellowish color to your skin or the whites of your eyes.

While taking Uniretic, do not use potassium supplements, salt substitutes that contain potassium, or diuretics that leave potassium levels high (such as Dyrenium and Moduretic) unless your doctor recommends it.

Diuretics such as the one in Uniretic sometimes leave the body with too little sodium, chloride, or potassium, leading to symptoms such as dry mouth, thirst, weakness, sluggishness, drowsiness, restlessness, muscle pain or cramps, muscular fatigue, low urine output, rapid heartbeat, nausea, and vomiting. If you develop any of these symptoms, alert your doctor.

Uniretic can aggravate diabetes or high cholesterol. If you have one of these conditions, your doctor should closely monitor your blood sugar or cholesterol levels.

If you develop unusual or increased coughing, tell your doctor. Contact your doctor immediately if you develop a sore throat or fever; they could be signs of a more serious illness.

If you are having a surgical procedure that requires anesthesia, make sure the doctor knows that you are taking Uniretic.

Possible food and drug interactions when taking this medication

If Uniretic is taken with certain other drugs, the effects of either could be increased, decreased, or altered. It is especially important to check with your doctor before combining Uniretic with the following:

ACTH
Alcohol
Barbiturates such as phenobarbital and Seconal
Cholestyramine (Questran)
Colestipol (Colestid)
Diabetes medications such as glyburide and insulin
Guanabenz (Wytensin)
Lithium (Lithobid, Lithonate)
Narcotics such as Percocet
Nonsteroidal anti-inflammatory painkillers such as Motrin
    and Naprosyn
Potassium-sparing diuretics such as Dyrenium and Moduretic
Potassium supplements such as Slow-K
Propantheline (Pro-Banthine)
Salt substitutes containing potassium
Steroid medications such as prednisone (Deltasone)

Special information if you are pregnant or breastfeeding

ACE inhibitors such as Uniretic have been shown to cause injury and even death of the developing baby when used during the second and third trimesters of pregnancy. If you are pregnant, contact your doctor immediately for instructions on how to safely discontinue Uniretic. If you plan to become pregnant, discuss the situation with your doctor as soon as possible.

Researchers do not know whether Uniretic appears in breast milk. If Uniretic is essential to your health, your doctor may advise you to stop breastfeeding while you are taking the drug.

Recommended dosage

ADULTS

Dosages of this drug are always tailored to the individual's response. The doctor will probably start with a relatively low dosage, then after 2 or 3 weeks adjust it upward if necessary. In general, the daily dose of moexipril should not exceed 30 milligrams. For hydrochlorothiazide, the maximum is 50 milligrams a day.

Your doctor may prescribe other blood pressure medications along with Uniretic.

CHILDREN

The safety and effectiveness of Uniretic have not been established in children.

Overdosage

Any medication taken in excess can have serious consequences. If you suspect an overdose, seek medical attention immediately.

■ *Symptoms of Uniretic overdose include:*
Dehydration (loss of body fluids), low blood pressure, low levels of sodium, potassium, and chloride

Unithroid *See Synthroid, page 1375.*

UNIVASC
Pronounced: YOO-ni-vask
Generic name: Moexipril hydrochloride

Why is this drug prescribed?
Univasc is used in the treatment of high blood pressure. It is effective when used alone or with thiazide diuretics that help rid the body of excess water. Univasc belongs to a family of drugs called angiotensin-converting enzyme (ACE) inhibitors. It works by preventing the transformation of a hormone in your blood called angiotensin I into a more potent substance that increases salt and water retention in your body. Univasc also enhances blood flow throughout your blood vessels.

Most important fact about this drug
You must take Univasc regularly for it to be effective. Since blood pressure declines gradually, it may be several weeks before you get the full benefit of Univasc; and you must continue taking it even if you are feeling well. Univasc does not cure high blood pressure; it merely keeps it under control.

How should you take this medication?

Univasc should be taken 1 hour before a meal. Try to get into the habit of taking your medication at the same time each day, such as 1 hour before breakfast, so that it is easier to remember. Always take Univasc exactly as prescribed.

■ *If you miss a dose...*
  Take the forgotten dose as soon as you remember. If it is almost time for the next dose, skip the one you missed and go back to your regular schedule. Never try to catch up by doubling the dose.

■ *Storage instructions...*
  Store at room temperature in a tightly closed container, away from moisture.

What side effects may occur?

Side effects cannot be anticipated. If any develop or change in intensity, tell your doctor as soon as possible. Only your doctor can determine if it is safe for you to continue taking Univasc.

■ *Side effects may include:*
  Cough, diarrhea, dizziness, flu-like symptoms

If you develop swelling of your face, around the lips, tongue, or throat; swelling of arms and legs; sore throat; or difficulty breathing or swallowing, stop taking the drug and contact your doctor immediately. You may need emergency treatment.

Why should this drug not be prescribed?

If you have ever had an allergic reaction to Univasc or other ACE inhibitors such as Capoten, Vasotec, and Zestril, you should not take this medication.

Special warnings about this medication

Your doctor will check your kidney function when you start taking Univasc and watch it carefully for the first few weeks.

Univasc can cause low blood pressure, especially if you are taking high doses of diuretics. You may feel light-headed or faint, especially during the first few days of therapy. If these symptoms occur, contact your doctor. Your dosage may need to be adjusted or discontinued. If you actually faint, stop taking the drug and contact your doctor immediately.

If you have congestive heart failure or other heart or circulatory disorders, use this drug with caution. Be cautious, too, if you have kidney disease, diabetes, or a collagen-vascular disease such as lupus erythematosus or scleroderma.

Excessive sweating, severe diarrhea, or vomiting could make you lose too much water, causing your blood pressure to become too low. Call your doctor if you have any of those conditions.

If you notice a yellow coloring to your skin or the whites of your eyes, stop taking the drug and notify your doctor immediately. You could be developing liver problems.

If you are using bee or wasp venom to prevent severe reactions to stings, you may have an allergic reaction to Univasc.

Some people on dialysis have had an allergic reaction to this type of drug (ACE inhibitor).

If you develop a persistent, dry cough, tell your doctor. It may be due to the medication and, if so, will disappear if you stop taking Univasc. If you develop a sore throat or fever, you should contact your doctor immediately. It could indicate a more serious illness.

Do not take potassium supplements or salt substitutes containing potassium without talking to your doctor first. In a medical emergency and before you have surgery, notify your doctor or dentist that you are taking Univasc.

Possible food and drug interactions when taking this medication

If Univasc is taken with certain other drugs, the effects of either could be increased, decreased, or altered. It is especially important to check with your doctor before combining Univasc with the following:

Diuretics (Diuril, HydroDIURIL, Lasix)
Lithium (Eskalith, Lithobid)
Potassium-sparing diuretics (Aldactone, Maxzide, Moduretic)
Potassium supplements (Slow-K)

Special information if you are pregnant or breastfeeding

Univasc can cause injury or death to developing and newborn babies if taken during the second and third trimesters of pregnancy. If you are pregnant and are taking Univasc, contact your doctor immediately. It is not known whether Univasc appears in human breast milk. Therefore, Univasc should be used with caution if you are breastfeeding.

Recommended dosage

ADULTS

For people not taking a diuretic drug, the usual starting dose is 7.5 milligrams taken once a day, an hour before a meal. The dosage after that can range from 7.5 to 30 milligrams per day, either taken in a single dose or divided into 2 equal doses daily. The maximum dose is 60 milligrams per day. Your doctor will closely monitor the effect of this drug and adjust it according to your individual needs.

People already taking a diuretic should stop taking it, if possible, 2 to 3 days before starting Univasc. This reduces the possibility of fainting or light-headedness. If the diuretic cannot be discontinued, the starting dosage of Univasc should be 3.75 milligrams. If Univasc alone does not control your blood pressure, your doctor will have you start taking a diuretic again.

For people with kidney problems, the usual starting dose is 3.75 milligrams a day; your doctor may gradually raise the dose to a maximum of 15 milligrams a day.

CHILDREN

The safety and effectiveness of Univasc have not been established in children.

Overdosage

Although there is no specific information available, a sudden drop in blood pressure would be the most likely symptom of Univasc overdose.

If you suspect an overdose, seek medical attention immediately.

URISED

Pronounced: YOUR-i-said
Generic ingredients: Methenamine, Methylene blue, Phenyl
salicylate, Benzoic acid, Atropine sulfate, Hyoscyamine

Why is this drug prescribed?

Urised relieves lower urinary tract discomfort caused by inflammation or diagnostic procedures. It is used to treat urinary tract infections including cystitis (inflammation of the bladder and ureters), urethritis (inflammation of the urethra), and trigonitis (inflammation of the mucous membrane of the bladder). Methenamine, the major component of this drug, acts as a mild antiseptic by changing into formaldehyde in the urinary tract when it comes in contact with acidic urine.

Most important fact about this drug

Urised may give a blue to blue-green color to urine and discolor stools as well.

How should you take this medication?

To avoid stains on your skin, mouth, or teeth, make sure your hands are dry before handling the tablets, swallow them quickly, and wash them down with plenty of liquid.

If your mouth gets dry during Urised therapy, hard candy or gum, saliva substitute, or crushed ice may provide temporary relief.

Take this medication exactly as prescribed; do not take more than the recommended dose.

Drinking plenty of fluids will help the medication work better and relieve discomfort.

■ *If you miss a dose...*
Take it as soon as you remember. If it is almost time for your next dose, skip the one you missed and go back to your regular schedule. Never take 2 doses at the same time.

■ *Storage instructions...*
Store Urised at room temperature, in a dry place.

What side effects may occur?
Side effects cannot be anticipated. If any develop or change in intensity, inform your doctor as soon as possible. Only your doctor can determine if it is safe for you to continue taking Urised.

■ *Side effects with long-term use may include:*
Acute urinary retention (in men with an enlarged prostate), blurry vision, difficulty urinating, dizziness, dry mouth, flushing, rapid pulse, skin rash

Why should this drug not be prescribed?
Urised should be avoided if you have glaucoma, a bladder blockage, cardiospasm, or a disorder that obstructs the passage of food through the stomach. Also avoid Urised if you are sensitive to or have ever had an allergic reaction to any of its ingredients.

Special warnings about this medication
Urised should be used cautiously if you have heart disease or have ever had a reaction to medications that are chemically similar to atropine.

Your doctor may ask you to check your urine with phenaphthazine paper to see if it is acidic. Urine acidifiers, such as vitamin C, may be recommended if the urine is not acidic enough.

Possible food and drug interactions when taking this medication
If Urised is taken with certain other drugs, the effects of either could be increased, decreased, or altered. It is especially important to check with your doctor before combining Urised with the following:

Acetazolamide (Diamox)
Potassium supplements such as Slow-K
Sodium bicarbonate antacids such as Alka-Seltzer
Sulfa drugs such as Bactrim, Gantanol, Gantrisin, and Septra

Drugs and foods that produce alkaline urine (such as sodium bicarbonate, antacids, and orange juice) should be limited.

Special information if you are pregnant or breastfeeding
The effects of Urised during pregnancy have not been adequately studied. If you are pregnant or plan to become pregnant, inform your doctor immediately. Urised may appear in breast milk and could affect a nursing in-

fant. If this medication is essential to your health, your doctor may advise you to stop breastfeeding until your treatment with Urised ends.

Recommended dosage

ADULTS

The usual dose is 2 tablets 4 times a day.

CHILDREN 6 YEARS AND OLDER

The dosage must be determined by your doctor.

CHILDREN UNDER 6 YEARS

Use is not recommended in children under 6 years old.

Overdosage

Any medication taken in excess can have serious consequences. If you suspect an overdose, seek medical treatment immediately.

■ *Symptoms of Urised overdose may include:*
Abdominal pain, bladder and abdominal irritation, bloody diarrhea, bloody urine, burning pain in throat and mouth, circulatory collapse, coma, dilated pupils (large pupils), dizziness, dry nose, mouth, and throat, elevated blood pressure, extremely high body temperature, headache, hot, dry, flushed skin, painful and frequent urination, pallor (paleness), pounding heartbeat (pounding sensation against the chest), rapid heartbeat (increased pulse rate), respiratory failure, ringing in ears, sweating, vomiting, weakness, white sores in mouth

URISPAS

Pronounced: YOUR-eh-spaz
Generic name: Flavoxate hydrochloride

Why is this drug prescribed?

Urispas prevents spasms in the urinary tract and relieves the painful or difficult urination, urinary urgency, excessive nighttime urination, pubic area pain, frequency of urination, and inability to hold urine caused by urinary tract infections. Urispas is taken in combination with antibiotics to treat the infection.

Most important fact about this drug

Urispas can cause blurred vision and drowsiness. Be careful driving, operating machinery, or performing any activity that requires complete mental alertness until you know how you will react to this medication.

How should you take this medication?

Take this medication exactly as prescribed. Urispas may make your mouth dry. Sucking on a hard candy, chewing gum, or melting bits of ice in your mouth can provide relief.

■ *If you miss a dose...*
Take it as soon as you remember. If it is almost time for your next dose, skip the one you missed and go back to your regular schedule. Do not take 2 doses at once.

■ *Storage instructions...*
Store away from heat, light, and moisture.

What side effects may occur?

Side effects cannot be anticipated. If any develop or change in intensity, notify your doctor as soon as possible. Only your doctor can determine whether it is safe for you to continue taking Urispas.

■ *Side effects may include:*
Allergic skin reactions, including hives, blurred vision and vision changes, drowsiness, dry mouth, fluttery heartbeat, headache, high body temperature, mental confusion (especially in the elderly), nausea, nervousness, painful or difficult urination, rapid heartbeat, vertigo, vomiting

Why should this drug not be prescribed?

You should not take Urispas if you have stomach or intestinal blockage, muscle relaxation problems (especially the sphincter muscle), abdominal bleeding, or urinary tract blockage.

Special warnings about this medication

Use Urispas cautiously if you have the eye condition known as glaucoma.

Possible food and drug interactions when taking this medication

No interactions involving Urispas have been noted.

Special information if you are pregnant or breastfeeding

The effects of Urispas during pregnancy have not been adequately studied. If you are pregnant or plan to become pregnant, inform your doctor immediately. Urispas may appear in breast milk and could affect a nursing infant. If this medication is essential to your health, your doctor may advise you to stop breastfeeding until your treatment is finished.

Recommended dosage

ADULTS AND CHILDREN OVER AGE 12

The usual dose of Urispas is one or two 100-milligram tablets 3 or 4 times a day.

When your symptoms have improved, your doctor may reduce the dosage.

CHILDREN

The safety and effectiveness of Urispas in children under 12 years of age have not been established.

Overdosage

Any medication taken in excess can have serious consequences. If you suspect an overdose of Urispas, seek medical attention immediately.

■ *Symptoms of Urispas overdose may include:*
Convulsions, decreased ability to sweat (warm, red skin, dry mouth, and increased body temperature), hallucinations, increased heart rate and blood pressure, mental confusion

UROXATRAL

Pronounced: yur-OX-ah-trall
Generic name: Alfuzosin hydrochloride

Why is this drug prescribed?

Uroxatral is used to treat the symptoms of an enlarged prostate—a condition technically known as benign prostatic hyperplasia or BPH. The walnut-sized prostate gland surrounds the urethra (the duct that drains the bladder). If the gland becomes enlarged, it can squeeze the urethra, interfering with the flow of urine. This can cause difficulty in starting urination, a weak flow of urine, and the need to urinate urgently or more frequently. Uroxatral doesn't shrink the prostate. Instead, it relaxes the muscle around it, freeing the flow of urine and decreasing urinary symptoms.

Most important fact about this drug

Uroxatral can cause dizziness and even fainting, especially in the first few hours after taking it. Be very careful about driving, operating machinery, or performing dangerous tasks during this period.

How should you take this medication?

Uroxatral should be taken with the same meal each day. Do not crush or chew the tablets.

■ *If you miss a dose...*
Take the forgotten dose as soon as you remember. However, if it is almost time for your next dose, skip the one you missed and return to your regular schedule. Do not take 2 doses at once.
■ *Storage instructions...*
Store at room temperature. Protect the medicine from heat, light, and moisture.

What side effects may occur?

Side effects cannot be anticipated. If any develop or change in intensity, tell your doctor as soon as possible. Only your doctor can determine if it is safe to continue using Uroxatral.

■ *Side effects may include:*
Dizziness, fatigue, headache, upper respiratory tract infection

This side effects list is not complete. If you have any questions about side effects you should consult your doctor. Report any new or continuing symptoms to your doctor right away.

Why should this drug not be prescribed?

If you have moderate or severe liver problems, you should not use Uroxatral. You should also avoid the drug if you have ever had an allergic reaction to it. Make sure your doctor is aware of any drug reactions you might have experienced.

Special warnings about this medication

Benign enlargement of the prostate is not the only condition that can cause male urinary inefficiency and discomfort. Other possibilities include infection, obstruction, cancer of the prostate, and bladder disorders. Before prescribing Uroxatral, your doctor will want to do various tests to determine the cause of your urinary problems.

Stop taking Uroxatral immediately and call your doctor if symptoms of angina pectoris (chest pain due to a heart condition) start or get worse.

Be sure to tell your doctor about any history of electrical problems with your heart (QT prolongation) before you start taking Uroxatral. Also let the doctor know if you have any problems with your kidneys or liver.

Possible food and drug interactions when taking this medication

If Uroxatral is taken with certain other drugs, the effects of either could be increased, decreased, or altered. It is especially important to check with your doctor before combining Uroxatral with the following:

Alpha-blockers (used to treat high blood pressure or BPH) such as carvedilol (Coreg), doxazosin (Cardura), prazosin (Minipress), tamsulosin (Flomax)
Atenolol (Tenormin)
Cimetidine (Tagamet)
Diltiazem (Cardizem)
Itraconazole (Sporanox)
Ketoconazole (Nizoral)
Ritonavir (Norvir)

Special information about pregnancy and breastfeeding

Uroxatral should not be used by women.

Recommended dosage

ADULT MALES

The recommended dosage is one 10-milligram tablet daily, taken immediately after the same meal each day.

Overdosage

Any medication taken in excess can have serious consequences. If you suspect an overdose of Uroxatral, seek emergency treatment immediately. Symptoms of an overdose may include low blood pressure.

Urso 250 *See Actigall, page 24.*

Ursodiol *See Actigall, page 24.*

VAGIFEM
Pronounced: vaj-I-fem
Generic name: Estradiol vaginal tablets

Why is this drug prescribed?

As estrogen levels decline during menopause, vaginal tissues tend to shrink and lose their elasticity—sometimes producing a condition known as atrophic vaginitis. Inserted in the vagina on a regular basis, Vagifem tablets provide a local source of estrogen replacement without passing through the rest of the system. This helps relieve such symptoms of atrophic vaginitis as vaginal dryness, soreness, and itching.

Most important fact about this drug

Because estrogen replacement therapy is not advisable if you are in any danger of developing cancer, your doctor should take a complete medical and family history—and do a complete physical exam—before prescribing Vagifem. As a general rule, you should have an examination at least once a year while using this product.

How should you take this medication?

Each Vagifem tablet comes in its own disposable applicator. Insert the applicator as far into the vagina as you find comfortable, stopping when the applicator is half inside. Gently press the plunger in the applicator until you hear a click and the plunger is fully depressed. This will release the Vagifem tablet. Conclude by gently removing the applicator and discarding it as you would a tampon applicator.

The Vagifem tablet can be inserted at any time of day, but it's advisable to do each insertion around the same time.

■ *If you miss a dose...*
Apply it as soon as you remember. If it is almost time for your next dose, skip the one you missed and return to your regular schedule. Never try to catch up by doubling the dose.

■ *Storage instructions...*
Store at room temperature.

What side effects may occur?

Side effects cannot be anticipated. If any develop or change in intensity, tell your doctor as soon as possible. Only your doctor can determine if it is safe to continue using Vagifem.

■ *Side effects may include:*
Abdominal pain, allergic reactions, back pain, genital itching, headache, skin rash, upper respiratory infection, vaginal spotting or discharge, yeast infection

Why should this drug not be prescribed?

Do not use Vagifem if there is any chance that you have breast cancer or any other cancer stimulated by estrogen. Avoid Vagifem if there is a possibility that you are pregnant. Do not use Vagifem if estrogen products have given you clotting problems in the past, or if you currently have phlebitis or other clotting disorders. Also avoid Vagifem if you have unexplained genital bleeding or the metabolic disorder known as porphyria, and do not use this product if it causes an allergic reaction.

Special warnings about this medication

Estrogen replacement therapy is associated with a slight increase in the chances of heart disease, high blood pressure, blood clots, gallbladder disease, excessive calcium levels, and cancer of the uterus. There is also mounting evidence that it may increase the risk of breast cancer.

Because of these possibilities, get in touch with your doctor right away if you develop any of the following:

Abdominal pain, tenderness, or swelling
Abnormal bleeding from the vagina
Breast lumps
Coughing up blood
Difficulty with speech
Dizziness or fainting
Pain in your chest or calves
Severe headache or vomiting
Sudden shortness of breath
Vision changes
Weakness or numbness of an arm or leg
Yellowing of the skin or eyes

Because estrogen can affect the ability to handle blood sugar, diabetic women should use this product with caution. Be alert, too, for signs of fluid retention, which can be especially harmful for people with asthma, epilepsy, migraine, a heart condition, or a kidney disorder. Estrogen has also been known to trigger huge spikes in triglyceride levels, leading to problems in the pancreas.

If you have a liver condition, use Vagifem with caution and make sure your doctor is aware of the situation. Women with liver problems have difficulty processing estrogen.

Any vaginal infection you may have should be cleared up before you begin using Vagifem.

Possible food and drug interactions when using this medication
There is no information on interactions with Vagifem.

Special information if you are pregnant or breastfeeding
Vagifem must not be used during pregnancy, and is not intended for nursing mothers.

Recommended dosage
The usual dosage is 1 tablet a day for the first 2 weeks, then 1 tablet twice weekly. Every 3 to 6 months, the doctor will see if the dosage can be reduced or discontinued.

Overdosage
An overdose from a vaginal tablet is unlikely. An oral overdose of estrogen could be expected to cause the symptoms listed below.

■ *Symptoms of estrogen overdose may include:*
Nausea, vaginal bleeding, vomiting

Valacyclovir See Valtrex, page 1546.

VALCYTE
Pronounced: VAL-site
Generic name: Valganciclovir

Why is this drug prescribed?
Valcyte tablets are used in the treatment of an eye disease called cytomegalovirus (CMV) retinitis, one of the many infections that take hold when the immune system is undermined by AIDS.

Valcyte is also used to prevent CMV disease in people who've had a kidney, heart, or kidney-pancreas transplant. Valcyte is not approved for use in liver transplant patients.

Valcyte is very similar to the CMV medication Cytovene (ganciclovir).

Most important fact about this drug

To avoid an overdose, it is essential to take only the prescribed number of Valcyte tablets each day. These tablets are more potent than Cytovene capsules, and cannot be substituted on a one-for-one basis.

How should you take this medication?

Valcyte is usually taken twice a day for the first 3 weeks, then once a day. It should be taken with food.

Be careful to avoid breaking Valcyte tablets. If a tablet does break, keep the pieces out of direct contact with skin, eyes, and mouth. If contact is unavoidable, wash thoroughly with soap and water and rinse the eyes with plain water.

■ *If you miss a dose...*
 Take it as soon as you remember. If it is almost time for your next dose, skip the one you missed and go back to your regular schedule.
■ *Storage instructions...*
 Store at room temperature.

What side effects may occur?

Side effects cannot be anticipated. If any develop or change in intensity, inform your doctor as soon as possible. Only your doctor can determine if it is safe for you to continue taking Valcyte.

■ *Side effects may include:*
 Abdominal pain, anemia and other blood abnormalities, burning or prickling feeling, diarrhea, fever, graft rejection, headache, high blood pressure, insomnia, mental changes, nausea, retinal detachment, tremors, vision problems, vomiting

Why should this drug not be prescribed?

If Valcyte gives you an allergic reaction, or you've had an allergic reaction to Cytovene, you will not be able to use this medication.

You will not be able to use Valcyte if you are receiving hemodialysis.

Special warnings about this medication

Valcyte may cause low blood counts. You will need to have frequent blood tests to monitor for abnormalities. Your doctor will be especially cautious if you have pre-existing blood problems or if you are taking other medications that can reduce blood counts.

Valcyte can also affect the kidneys, so your doctor will check them frequently. You should be aware that Valcyte is also considered a potential cancer-causing agent, although this possible effect has not been studied.

Valcyte can diminish fertility in both men and women. It may also prove harmful to a developing baby. Women should use birth control while taking Valcyte, and men should use condoms during treatment and for 90 days thereafter.

Convulsions, sedation, dizziness, weakness, and confusion have been reported with the use of Valcyte tablets. If any of these symptoms occur, do not drive, operate machinery, or perform any other task that requires you to be alert.

Valcyte is not a cure for CMV retinitis, and your disease may worsen during or following treatment. You should have an eye exam at least every 4 to 6 weeks while being treated with Valcyte tablets.

Possible food and drug interactions when taking this medication

If Valcyte is taken with certain other drugs, the effects of either could be increased, decreased, or altered. It is especially important to check with your doctor before combining Valcyte with the following:

Didanosine (Videx)
Mycophenolate mofetil (CellCept)
Probenecid
Zidovudine (Retrovir)

Special information if you are pregnant or breastfeeding

Valcyte may cause birth defects and should not be used during pregnancy. It's not certain whether Valcyte appears in breast milk, but it would cause serious side effects if it did. Breastfeeding is not recommended for women taking Valcyte—or for any woman with AIDS, since the disease can be passed to the infant through breast milk.

Recommended dosage

ADULTS

For the Treatment of CMV Retinitis

For active CMV retinitis, the recommended starting dosage is 900 milligrams (two 450-milligram tablets) twice a day for 21 days. The dose can then be decreased to 900 milligrams (two 450-milligram tablets) once a day. Take each dose with food.

Patients who have inactive CMV retinitis can start out at 900 milligrams once daily with food.

For the Prevention of CMV Disease in Heart, Kidney, and Kidney-Pancreas Transplants

The recommended starting dosage is 900 milligrams (two 450-milligram tablets) once a day with food starting within 10 days of transplantation until 100 days posttransplantation.

If you have poor kidney function, your dose will be decreased. If you need hemodialysis, Valcyte cannot be used at all.

Overdosage

Any medication taken in excess can have serious consequences. An overdose of Valcyte can cause blood abnormalities, kidney failure, and liver disorders. If you suspect an overdose, seek medical attention immediately.

■ *Symptoms of Valcyte overdose may include:*
Abdominal pain, convulsions, diarrhea, vomiting, tremors

Valganciclovir See Valcyte, page 1540.

VALIUM

Pronounced: VAL-ee-um
Generic name: Diazepam

Why is this drug prescribed?

Valium is used in the treatment of anxiety disorders and for short-term relief of the symptoms of anxiety. It belongs to a class of drugs known as benzodiazepines.

It is also used to relieve the symptoms of acute alcohol withdrawal, to relax muscles, to relieve the uncontrolled muscle movements caused by cerebral palsy and paralysis of the lower body and limbs, to control involuntary movement of the hands (athetosis), to relax tight, aching muscles, and, along with other medications, to treat convulsive disorders such as epilepsy.

Most important fact about this drug

Valium can be habit-forming or addictive. You may experience withdrawal symptoms if you stop using this drug abruptly. Discontinue or change your dose only on your doctor's advice.

How should you take this medication?

Take this medication exactly as prescribed. If you are taking Valium for epilepsy, make sure you take it every day at the same time.

■ *If you miss a dose...*
Take it as soon as you remember if it is within an hour or so of the scheduled time. If you do not remember until later, skip the dose you missed and go back to your regular schedule. Never take 2 doses at the same time.

■ *Storage instructions...*
Store away from heat, light, and moisture.

What side effects may occur?

Side effects cannot be anticipated. If any develop or change in intensity, inform your doctor as soon as possible. Only your doctor can determine if it is safe for you to continue taking Valium.

■ *Side effects may include:*
Anxiety, drowsiness, fatigue, light-headedness, loss of muscle coordination

■ *Side effects due to a rapid decrease in dose or abrupt withdrawal from Valium:*
Abdominal and muscle cramps, convulsions, sweating, tremors, vomiting

Why should this drug not be prescribed?

If you are sensitive to or have ever had an allergic reaction to Valium, you should not take this medication.

Do not take this medication if you have the eye condition known as acute narrow-angle glaucoma.

Anxiety or tension related to everyday stress usually does not require treatment with such a powerful drug as Valium. Discuss your symptoms thoroughly with your doctor.

Valium should not be prescribed if you are being treated for mental disorders more serious than anxiety.

Special warnings about this medication

Valium may cause you to become drowsy or less alert; therefore, you should not drive or operate dangerous machinery or participate in any hazardous activity that requires full mental alertness until you know how this drug affects you.

If you have liver or kidney problems, use this medication cautiously.

Possible food and drug interactions when taking this medication

Valium slows down the central nervous system and may intensify the effects of alcohol. Do not drink alcohol while taking this medication.

If Valium is taken with certain other drugs, the effects of either could be increased, decreased, or altered. It is especially important to check with your doctor before combining Valium with any of the following:

Antidepressant drugs such as Elavil and Prozac
Antipsychotic drugs such as chlorpromazine and Mellaril
Antiseizure drugs such as Dilantin
Barbiturates such as phenobarbital
Cimetidine (Tagamet)
Digoxin (Lanoxin)
Disulfiram (Antabuse)
Fluoxetine (Prozac)
Isoniazid (Rifamate)
Levodopa (Larodopa, Sinemet)
MAO inhibitors (antidepressant drugs such as Nardil)
Narcotics such as Percocet
Omeprazole (Prilosec)

Oral contraceptives
Propoxyphene (Darvon)
Ranitidine (Zantac)
Rifampin (Rifadin)

Special information if you are pregnant or breastfeeding

Do not take Valium if you are pregnant or planning to become pregnant. There is an increased risk of birth defects.

If this medication is essential to your health, your doctor may advise you to discontinue breastfeeding until your treatment is finished.

Recommended dosage

ADULTS

Treatment of Anxiety Disorders and Short-Term Relief of the Symptoms of Anxiety
The usual dose, depending upon severity of symptoms, is 2 milligrams to 10 milligrams 2 to 4 times daily.

Acute Alcohol Withdrawal
The usual dose is 10 milligrams 3 or 4 times during the first 24 hours, then 5 milligrams 3 or 4 times daily as needed.

Relief of Muscle Spasm
The usual dose is 2 milligrams to 10 milligrams 3 or 4 times daily.

Convulsive Disorders
The usual dose is 2 milligrams to 10 milligrams 2 to 4 times daily.

CHILDREN

Valium should not be given to children under 6 months of age.

The usual starting dose for children over 6 months is 1 to 2.5 milligrams 3 or 4 times a day. Your doctor may increase the dosage gradually if needed.

OLDER ADULTS

The usual dosage is 2 to 2.5 milligrams once or twice a day, which your doctor will increase as needed. Your doctor will limit the dosage to the smallest effective amount because older people are more apt to become oversedated or uncoordinated.

Overdosage

Any medication taken in excess can have serious consequences. If you suspect an overdose, seek medical attention immediately.

■ *Symptoms of Valium overdose may include:*
Coma, confusion, diminished reflexes, sleepiness

Valproic acid *See Depakene, page 407.*

Valsartan *See Diovan, page 451.*

VALTREX

Pronounced: VAL-trex
Generic name: Valacyclovir hydrochloride

Why is this drug prescribed?

Valtrex is used to treat certain herpes infections, including herpes zoster (the painful rash known as shingles), genital herpes, and herpes cold sores on the face and lips.

Most important fact about this drug

Valtrex should not be used by anyone with a weak immune system, such as those with HIV infection or those who have undergone a bone marrow or kidney transplant. Valtrex can cause serious side effects, including death, in such people.

How should you use this medication?

If you are taking Valtrex for shingles, you should start using it as soon as possible after your doctor has made a diagnosis. It's best to see a doctor and start the drug within 48 hours of first noticing the rash. If you wait more than 72 hours after you first get a herpes zoster rash, the medication may not be effective.

If you are using Valtrex for genital herpes, begin taking it at the first sign of an attack. The medication may not be effective if you wait longer than 72 hours after the first attack or 24 hours after a later attack.

If you are taking Valtrex for cold sores, you should start using it at the earliest signs of infection, such as tingling, itching, or burning. If you wait until the cold sore develops, the medication might not work.

You may take Valtrex with or without food.

■ *If you miss a dose...*
Take it as soon as you remember. If it is almost time for your next dose, skip the one you missed and go back to your regular schedule. Do not take 2 doses at the same time.

■ *Storage instructions...*
Store at room temperature.

What side effects may occur?

Side effects cannot be anticipated. If any develop or change in intensity, inform your doctor as soon as possible. Only your doctor can determine if it is safe for you to continue using Valtrex.

■ *Side effects may include:*
Abdominal pain, aggressive behavior, agitation, allergic reactions, coma, confusion, decreased consciousness, depression, diarrhea, dizziness, facial swelling, hallucinations, headache, hepatitis, high blood pressure, joint pain, mania, menstrual problems, nausea, rapid heartbeat, rash, visual abnormalities, vomiting

Why should this drug not be prescribed?

Avoid Valtrex if you are sensitive to it or the similar drug acyclovir (Zovirax).

Special warnings about this medication

High doses of Valtrex have proved dangerous in people whose immune system is compromised because of HIV infection, bone marrow transplant, or kidney transplant.

If your kidneys are not functioning properly, or you are taking drugs that may damage the kidneys such as Neomycin or Streptomycin, Valtrex can make your condition worse or affect your central nervous system (brain and spinal cord).

Effects on the central nervous system are more common in older adults, leading to such symptoms as agitation, confusion, and hallucinations. Their kidneys are also more likely to be affected; and those with kidney problems need a smaller dose. In addition, older adults tend to suffer the pain of shingles for a longer time after healing has begun.

Valtrex relieves the symptoms of genital herpes, but it is not a cure. There's also no evidence that it will prevent transmission of the disease. To avoid spreading the infection, don't have sexual intercourse during a flare-up.

Valtrex is not intended for use in children.

Possible food and drug interactions when taking this medication

If you are taking Valtrex with certain other drugs, the effect of either drug could be increased, decreased, or altered. Check with your doctor before combining Valtrex with cimetidine (Tagamet) and/or probenecid (Benemid).

Special information if you are pregnant or breastfeeding

The effects of Valtrex during pregnancy and breastfeeding have not been adequately studied. If you are pregnant or plan to become pregnant, notify your doctor immediately. If you are nursing and need to use Valtrex, your doctor may advise you to discontinue breastfeeding while using the medication.

Recommended dosage

SHINGLES

The usual dose is 1 gram 3 times a day for 7 days.

GENITAL HERPES

The usual dose for the first attack is 1 gram twice a day for 10 days. For later attacks, the dose is 500 milligrams twice a day for 3 days. To keep the condition from returning, the dose is 1 gram once a day. If you've had less than 10 infections per year, your doctor may prescribe 500 milligrams once a day. The safety and effectiveness of Valtrex treatment beyond 1 year have not been studied.

Patients with kidney problems or HIV infection may need a reduced dosage.

COLD SORES

The recommended dosage is 2 grams twice a day for 1 day, taken about 12 hours apart. Valtrex should not be taken for more than 1 day. The elderly and people with kidney problems may need a reduced dosage.

Overdosage

When taken by people with kidney disorders, excessive doses of Valtrex have been known to cause psychological problems and kidney failure. If you suspect an overdose, check with your doctor immediately.

Vancenase *See Beclomethasone, page 193.*

Vanceril *See Beclomethasone, page 193.*

Vardenafil *See Levitra, page 738.*

VASERETIC

Pronounced: *Vaz-err-ET-ik*
Generic ingredients: *Enalapril maleate, Hydrochlorothiazide*

Why is this drug prescribed?

Vaseretic is used in the treatment of high blood pressure. It combines an ACE inhibitor with a thiazide diuretic. Enalapril, the ACE inhibitor, works by preventing a chemical in your blood called angiotensin I from converting into a more potent form that increases salt and water retention in your body. Enalapril also enhances blood flow throughout your blood vessels. Hydrochlorothiazide, a diuretic, prompts your body to produce and eliminate more urine, which helps in lowering blood pressure.

Most important fact about this drug

You must take Vaseretic regularly for it to be effective. Since blood pressure declines gradually, it may be several weeks before you get the full benefit of Vaseretic; and you must continue taking it even if you are feeling well. Vaseretic does not cure high blood pressure; it merely keeps it under control.

How should you take this medication?

Take this medication exactly as prescribed by your doctor.

■ *If you miss a dose...*
Take it as soon as you remember. If it is almost time for your next dose, skip the one you missed and go back to your regular schedule. Never take 2 doses at the same time.

■ *Storage instructions...*
Keep container tightly closed. Store at room temperature and protect from moisture. Keep out of reach of children.

What side effects may occur?

Side effects cannot be anticipated. If any develop or change in intensity, inform your doctor as soon as possible. Only your doctor can determine if it is safe for you to continue taking Vaseretic.

■ *Side effects may include:*
Cough, diarrhea, dizziness, drop in blood pressure upon standing up, fatigue, headache, impotence, low potassium levels (leading to symptoms such as dry mouth, excessive thirst, weak or irregular heartbeat, muscle pain or cramps), muscle cramps, nausea, rash, tingling or pins and needles, weakness

Why should this drug not be prescribed?

If you are sensitive to or have ever had an allergic reaction to enalapril, hydrochlorothiazide, or similar drugs, or if you are sensitive to other sulfa drugs, you should not take this medication.

If you have a history of angioedema (swelling of face, extremities, and throat) or inability to urinate, you should not take this medication. Tell your doctor of all allergic reactions you have experienced.

Special warnings about this medication

If you develop swelling of your face, eyes, lips, tongue, or throat; swelling of your arms and legs; or difficulty swallowing, you should contact your doctor immediately. You may need emergency treatment.

If you are taking bee or wasp venom to prevent an allergic reaction to stings, you may have a severe allergic reaction to Vaseretic.

If you develop chest pain, a sore throat, or fever, you should contact your doctor immediately. It could indicate a more serious illness.

If you are taking Vaseretic, a complete assessment of your kidney function should be done. Kidney function should continue to be monitored. Some people on dialysis have had a severe allergic reaction to Vaseretic.

If you have liver disease or lupus erythematosus (a form of rheumatism), Vaseretic should be used with caution.

If your skin or the whites of your eyes turn yellow, stop taking Vaseretic and notify your doctor at once.

If you have severe congestive heart failure, you should be carefully watched for low blood pressure.

Excessive sweating, dehydration, severe diarrhea, or vomiting could cause you to lose too much water and cause your blood pressure to become too low. Be careful when exercising and in hot weather.

Vaseretic can cause some people to become drowsy or less alert. If it has this effect on you, driving or operating dangerous machinery or participating in any hazardous activity that requires full mental alertness is not recommended.

If you are diabetic, your blood sugar levels should be monitored.

Vaseretic may increase your sensitivity to sunlight. Be careful to avoid overexposure.

Possible food and drug interactions when taking this medication

Vaseretic may intensify the effects of alcohol. Do not drink alcohol while taking this medication.

If Vaseretic is taken with certain other drugs, the effects of either could be increased, decreased, or altered. It is especially important to check with your doctor before combining Vaseretic with the following:

Alcohol
Barbiturates such as phenobarbital
Certain other antihypertensives
Corticosteroids such as prednisone
Digitalis (Lanoxin)
Insulin
Lithium (Eskalith, Lithonate)
Narcotics (Percocet)
Nonsteroidal anti-inflammatory drugs such as Advil, Motrin, and Naprosyn
Norepinephrine
Oral antidiabetic drugs such as Micronase
Potassium-containing salt substitutes
Potassium-sparing diuretics such as Midamor
Potassium supplements (K-Lyte, K-Tab, others)

Special information if you are pregnant or breastfeeding

Vaseretic can cause birth defects, prematurity, and death to the newborn baby. If you are pregnant or plan to become pregnant and are taking

Vaseretic, contact your doctor immediately to discuss the potential hazard to your unborn child. Vaseretic appears in breast milk and could affect a nursing infant. If this medication is essential to your health, your doctor may advise you to discontinue breastfeeding until your treatment is finished.

Recommended dosage

ADULTS

The doctor will adjust your dosage until your blood pressure is in the desired range. If you are taking the 5 milligrams enalapril/12.5 milligrams hydrochlorothiazide combination, the maximum daily dosage is 4 tablets. For the 10/25 combination, the maximum is 2 tablets.

CHILDREN

The safety and effectiveness of Vaseretic in children have not been established.

OLDER ADULTS

Your doctor will prescribe Vaseretic cautiously, starting with small doses.

Overdosage

Any medication taken in excess can cause symptoms of overdose. If you suspect an overdose, seek medical attention immediately.

- *Symptoms of a Vaseretic overdose may include:*
  Dehydration, low blood pressure

VASOTEC

Pronounced: *VAZ-oh-tek*
Generic name: *Enalapril maleate*

Why is this drug prescribed?

Vasotec is a high blood pressure medication known as an ACE inhibitor. It works by preventing a chemical in your blood called angiotensin I from converting into a more potent form that increases salt and water retention in your body. It is effective when used alone or in combination with other medications, especially thiazide-type diuretics. It is also used in the treatment of congestive heart failure, usually in combination with diuretics and digitalis, and is prescribed as a preventive measure in certain conditions that could lead to heart failure.

Most important fact about this drug

If you have high blood pressure, you must take Vasotec regularly for it to be effective. Since blood pressure declines gradually, it may be several weeks before you get the full benefit of Vasotec; and you must continue taking it even if you are feeling well. Vasotec does not cure high blood pressure; it merely keeps it under control.

How should you take this medication?

Vasotec can be taken with or without food.

Do not use salt substitutes containing potassium without first consulting your doctor.

Take this medication exactly as prescribed by your doctor.

■ *If you miss a dose...*
Take it as soon as you remember. If it is almost time for your next dose, skip the one you missed and go back to your regular schedule. Never take 2 doses at the same time.

■ *Storage instructions...*
Keep container tightly closed. Store at room temperature and protect from moisture.

What side effects may occur?

Side effects cannot be anticipated. If any develop or change in intensity, inform your doctor as soon as possible. Only your doctor can determine if it is safe for you to continue taking Vasotec.

■ *Side effects may include:*
Cough, dizziness, dizziness upon standing, fatigue, headache, low blood pressure, nausea, rash, vomiting, weakness

Why should this drug not be prescribed?

If you are sensitive or have ever had an allergic reaction to Vasotec or similar drugs, or if you have a history of angioedema (swollen throat and difficulty swallowing) related to previous treatment with ACE inhibitors, you should not take this medication. Make sure that your doctor is aware of any drug reactions that you have experienced.

Special warnings about this medication

Vasotec has been known to cause a serious allergic reaction called angioedema. The symptoms are swelling of the face, lips, tongue, or throat; swelling of arms and legs; and difficulty swallowing or breathing. If you notice any of these symptoms, call your doctor immediately.

If you are taking bee or wasp venom to prevent an allergic reaction to stings, you may have a severe allergic reaction to Vasotec.

If you are taking high doses of diuretics and Vasotec, you may develop excessively low blood pressure. You are at special risk if you have heart disease, kidney disease, or a potassium or salt imbalance. Some people on kidney dialysis have had a severe allergic reaction to Vasotec.

There have been cases of serious blood disorders reported with the use of captopril, another ACE inhibitor drug. Your doctor should check your blood regularly while you are taking Vasotec.

ACE inhibitors can cause fetal abnormalities and fetal and newborn deaths when used in pregnancy during the second and third trimesters.

When pregnancy is detected, Vasotec should be discontinued as soon as possible.

If you develop a sore throat or fever, you should contact your doctor immediately. It could indicate a more serious illness. Also, if your skin and the whites of your eyes turn yellow, contact your doctor at once.

Excessive sweating, dehydration, severe diarrhea, or vomiting could prompt you to lose too much water, causing your blood pressure to drop dangerously. Be careful when exercising or when exposed to excessive heat.

Possible food and drug interactions when taking this medication

If Vasotec is taken with certain other drugs, the effects of either could be increased, decreased, or altered. It is especially important to check with your doctor before combining Vasotec with the following:

Diuretics such as Lasix and HydroDIURIL
Lithium (Eskalith, Lithobid)
Nonsteroidal anti-inflammatory drugs such as Advil, Motrin, and Naprosyn
Potassium-containing salt substitutes
Potassium-sparing diuretics such as Dyrenium and Midamor
Potassium supplements such as K-Lyte and K-Tab

Special information if you are pregnant or breastfeeding

Vasotec can cause birth defects, prematurity, and death to the developing or newborn baby. If you are pregnant or plan to become pregnant, inform your doctor immediately. Vasotec appears in breast milk and could affect a nursing infant. If this medication is essential to your health, your doctor may advise you to stop breastfeeding until your treatment with Vasotec is finished.

Recommended dosage

ADULTS

High Blood Pressure

The usual starting dose for people not using diuretics is 5 milligrams taken once a day. The usual dose is 10 to 40 milligrams per day taken as a single dose or divided into 2 smaller doses.

If you are taking a diuretic, your physician may ask you to stop for 2 to 3 days before using Vasotec. Otherwise, he or she may give you an initial dose of 2.5 milligrams of Vasotec under medical supervision before any further medication is prescribed.

If you have a kidney disorder, your dosage will be adjusted according to its severity.

To Treat Heart Failure

This medication can be used in conjunction with digitalis and diuretics in people with heart disease. The usual starting dose is 2.5 milligrams twice a day.

The usual regular dose is 2.5 to 20 milligrams each day, taken in 2 separate doses. The maximum daily dose is 40 milligrams, in 2 separate doses.

To Prevent Heart Failure

The usual starting dose is 2.5 milligrams twice a day, to be gradually increased to 20 milligrams a day divided into smaller doses.

CHILDREN

Vasotec can be prescribed for high blood pressure in children 1 month to 16 years old. Dosage is determined by weight. The usual starting dose is 0.08 milligram per 2.2 pounds of body weight (up to 5 milligrams) once a day. Doses above 40 milligrams have not been tested in children.

Overdosage

Any medication taken in excess can have serious consequences. If you suspect symptoms of a Vasotec overdose, seek medical attention immediately.

A sudden drop in blood pressure is the primary effect of a Vasotec overdose.

Veetids *See Penicillin V Potassium, page 1065.*

Venlafaxine *See Effexor, page 493.*

Ventolin HFA *See Proventil, page 1185.*

Verapamil *See Calan, page 229.*

Verelan *See Calan, page 229.*

VIAGRA

Pronounced: vye-AG-ruh
Generic name: Sildenafil citrate

Why is this drug prescribed?

Viagra is an oral drug for male impotence, also known as erectile dysfunction (ED). It works by dilating blood vessels in the penis, allowing the inflow of blood needed for an erection.

Most important fact about this drug

Viagra causes erections only during sexual excitement. It does not work in the absence of arousal.

How should you take this medication?

Taking Viagra approximately 1 hour before sexual activity works best for most men. Depending on how and when the drug works for you, an interval of one-half hour to as much as 4 hours may prove ideal.

■ *If you miss a dose...*
Viagra is *not* for regular use. Take it only before sexual activity.

■ *Storage instructions...*
Store at room temperature.

What side effects may occur?

Side effects cannot be anticipated. If any develop or change in intensity, inform your doctor as soon as possible. Only your doctor can determine if it is safe for you to continue taking Viagra.

■ *Side effects may include:*
Abnormal vision (color tinge, blurring, sensitivity to light), acid indigestion, diarrhea, flushing, headache, nasal congestion, urinary tract infection

Heart attack, stroke, heart irregularities, dangerous surges in blood pressure, and sudden death have all been reported after use of Viagra, usually in men with existing cardiac risk factors, and typically during or shortly after sex.

Why should this drug not be prescribed?

Do not take Viagra if you are taking any nitrate-based drug, including nitroglycerin patches (Nitro-Dur, Transderm-Nitro), nitroglycerin ointment (Nitro-Bid, Nitrol), nitroglycerin pills (Nitro-Bid, Nitrostat), and isosorbide pills (Dilatrate-SR, Isordil, Sorbitrate). Combining Viagra with these drugs can cause a severe drop in blood pressure.

If Viagra gives you an allergic reaction, do not use it again.

Special warnings about this medication

If you have heart problems severe enough to make sexual activity a danger, you should avoid using Viagra. Use it cautiously—if at all—if you've had a heart attack, stroke, or life-threatening heart irregularities within the past 6 months. Be equally cautious if you have severely high or low blood pressure, heart failure, or unstable angina (crushing heart pain that occurs at any time).

If you take Viagra and develop cardiac symptoms (for example, dizziness, nausea, and chest pain) during sexual activity, do not continue. Alert your doctor to the problem as soon as possible.

If you have a condition that might result in long-lasting erections, such as sickle-cell anemia, multiple myeloma (a disease of the bone marrow), or leukemia, use Viagra with caution. Also use cautiously if you have a genital problem or deformity such as Peyronie's disease. If an erection lasts more than 4 hours, seek treatment immediately. Permanent damage and impotence could result.

If you have a bleeding disorder, a stomach ulcer, or the inherited eye condition known as retinitis pigmentosa, use this medication with caution. Its safety under these circumstances has not yet been studied.

To avoid low blood pressure, do not take the 50-milligram or 100-milligram dose of Viagra within 4 hours of taking an alpha-blocking drug such as Cardura.

Remember that Viagra offers no protection from transmission of sexually transmitted diseases, such as HIV, the virus that causes AIDS.

Possible food and drug interactions when using this medication

If Viagra is taken with certain other drugs, the effects of either could be increased, decreased, or altered. It is especially important to check with your doctor before combining Viagra with the following:

Other impotence remedies, including Caverject and Muse
Alpha-blockers such as doxazosin (Cardura)
Amlodipine (Norvasc)
Cimetidine (Tagamet)
Erythromycin (E-Mycin, Ery-Tab, PCE)
Itraconazole (Sporanox)
Ketoconazole (Nizoral)
Nitrates such as Isordil, Nitro-Bid, and Nitro-Dur
Rifampin (Rifadin, Rimactane)
Ritonavir (Norvir)
Saquinavir (Fortovase, Invirase)

Special information about pregnancy and breastfeeding

Viagra should not be used by women. Its effects during pregnancy and breastfeeding have not been studied.

Recommended dosage

Doses range from 25 to 100 milligrams, depending on the drug's effect. The usual dose is 50 milligrams. If you are over 65, have liver or kidney problems, or are taking erythromycin, ketoconazole, itraconazole, ritonavir, or saquinavir, a dose of 25 milligrams may be sufficient. Your doctor will adjust the dosage if the drug is not working properly for you.

Take Viagra only before sexual activity. The manufacturer recommends a maximum of 1 dose per day (1 dose every 2 days for those taking ritonavir).

To avoid low blood pressure, do not take the 50-milligram or 100-milligram dose of Viagra within 4 hours of taking an alpha-blocking drug such as Cardura.

Overdosage

No overdose of Viagra has been reported. However, any medication taken in excess can have serious consequences. If you suspect an overdose, seek medical attention immediately.

Vibramycin *See Doryx, page 474.*

Vibra-Tabs *See Doryx, page 474.*

VICODIN

Pronounced: VY-koe-din
Generic ingredients: Hydrocodone bitartrate, Acetaminophen
Other brand names: Anexsia, Co-Gesic, Hydrocet, Lorcet,
    Lortab, Maxidone, Norco, Zydone

Why is this drug prescribed?

Vicodin combines a narcotic analgesic (painkiller) and cough reliever with a non-narcotic analgesic for the relief of moderate to moderately severe pain.

Most important fact about this drug

Vicodin can be habit-forming. If you take this drug over a long period of time, you can become mentally and physically dependent on it, and you may find the drug no longer works for you at the prescribed dosage.

How should you take this medication?

Take Vicodin exactly as prescribed. Do not increase the amount you take or the frequency without your doctor's approval. Do not take this drug for any reason other than the one prescribed.

Do not give this drug to others who may have similar symptoms.

■ *If you miss a dose...*
   If you take Vicodin regularly, take the forgotten dose as soon as you remember. If it is almost time for your next dose, skip the one you missed and go back to your regular schedule. Do not take 2 doses at once.

■ *Storage instructions...*
   Store at room temperature in a tightly closed container, away from light.

What side effects may occur?

Side effects cannot be anticipated. If any develop or change in intensity, inform your doctor as soon as possible. Only your doctor can determine if it is safe for you to continue taking Vicodin.

■ *Side effects may include:*

Dizziness, light-headedness, nausea, sedation, vomiting

If these side effects occur, it may help if you lie down after taking the medication.

Why should this drug not be prescribed?

If you are sensitive to or have ever had an allergic reaction to hydrocodone, similar narcotic painkillers, or acetaminophen (Tylenol), you should not take this medication. Make sure your doctor is aware of any drug reactions you have experienced.

Special warnings about this medication

Vicodin may make you drowsy, less alert, or unable to function well physically. Do not drive a car, operate machinery, or perform any other potentially dangerous activities until you know how this drug affects you.

Use caution in taking Vicodin if you have a head injury. Narcotics tend to increase the pressure of the fluid within the skull, and this effect may be exaggerated by head injuries. Side effects of narcotics can interfere in the treatment of people with head injuries.

Use Vicodin with caution if you have a severe liver or kidney disorder, an underactive thyroid gland, Addison's disease (a disease of the adrenal glands), an enlarged prostate, or urethral stricture (narrowing of the tube carrying urine from the bladder).

Older adults and those in a weakened condition should be careful using this drug, since it contains a narcotic.

Narcotics such as Vicodin may interfere with the diagnosis and treatment of people with abdominal conditions.

Hydrocodone suppresses the cough reflex; therefore, be careful using Vicodin after an operation or if you have a lung disease.

High doses of hydrocodone may produce slowed breathing; if you are sensitive to this drug, you are more likely to experience this effect.

Possible food and drug interactions when taking this medication

Hydrocodone slows the nervous system. Alcohol can intensify this effect.

If hydrocodone is taken with certain other drugs, the effects of either may be increased, decreased, or altered. It is especially important to check with your doctor before combining Vicodin with the following:

Antianxiety drugs such as Librium and Valium
Antidepressant medications classified as tricyclics, such as Elavil and Tofranil
Antihistamines such as Tavist

Drugs classified as MAO inhibitors, including the antidepressants
Nardil and Parnate
Major tranquilizers such as Haldol and Thorazine
Other central nervous system depressants such as Halcion and
Restoril
Other narcotic analgesics such as Demerol

Special information if you are pregnant or breastfeeding

The effects of Vicodin in pregnancy have not been adequately studied. Do
not take this drug if you are pregnant or plan to become pregnant unless
you are directed to do so by your doctor. Drug dependence occurs in
newborns when the mother has taken this drug regularly prior to delivery.
If you take it shortly before delivery, the baby's breathing may be slowed.
Acetaminophen does, and hydrocodone may, appear in breast milk and
could affect a nursing infant. If this medication is essential to your health,
your doctor may advise you to discontinue breastfeeding your baby until
your treatment is finished.

Recommended dosage

ADULTS

Your doctor will adjust the dosage according to the severity of the pain
and the way the medication affects you.

The dosages given below are for Vicodin products only. If your doctor
prescribes other brands, your daily dose may vary.

All forms of Vicodin are taken every 4 to 6 hours as needed for pain.
The usual dose of Vicodin is 1 or 2 tablets, up to a maximum of 8 tablets
per day. The usual dose of Vicodin HP is 1 tablet, up to a maximum of 6
tablets per day. For Vicodin ES, the usual dose is 1 tablet, up to a maximum of 5 tablets per day.

CHILDREN

The safety and effectiveness of Vicodin have not been established in children.

Overdosage

Any medication taken in excess can have serious consequences. A severe
overdose of Vicodin can be fatal. If you suspect an overdose, seek emergency medical treatment immediately.

■ *Symptoms of a Vicodin overdose include:*
Blood disorders, bluish tinge to skin, cold and clammy skin, extreme
sleepiness progressing to a state of unresponsiveness or coma, general feeling of bodily discomfort, hearing impairment, heart problems,
heavy perspiration, kidney problems, limp muscles, liver failure, low
blood pressure, nausea, slow heartbeat, troubled or slowed breathing,
vomiting

VICOPROFEN

Pronounced: VY-koe-pro-fen
Generic ingredients: Hydrocodone bitartrate, Ibuprofen

Why is this drug prescribed?

Vicoprofen is a chemical cousin of the well-known painkiller Vicodin. Both products contain the prescription pain medication hydrocodone. However, while Vicodin also includes acetaminophen (the active ingredient in Tylenol), Vicoprofen replaces it with ibuprofen (the active ingredient in Advil).

Vicoprofen relieves acute pain. It is generally prescribed for less than 10 days, and cannot be used in the long-term treatment of osteoarthritis or rheumatoid arthritis.

Most important fact about this drug

Vicoprofen can be habit-forming. If you take this drug over a long period of time, you can become both mentally and physically dependent on it, and you may find that it no longer works for you at the prescribed dose.

How should you take this medication?

Take Vicoprofen exactly as prescribed. Do not increase the amount you take or the number of doses per day without your doctor's approval. Vicoprofen should be used only for pain—and only as needed.

- *If you miss a dose...*
  Take it as soon as you remember. If it is almost time for your next dose, skip the one you missed and go back to your regular schedule. Never take 2 doses at the same time.
- *Storage instructions...*
  Store at room temperature in a tightly sealed, light-resistant container.

What side effects may occur?

Side effects cannot be anticipated. If any develop or change in intensity, inform your doctor as soon as possible. Only your doctor can determine if it is safe for you to continue taking Vicoprofen.

- *Side effects may include:*
  Abdominal pain, anxiety, constipation, diarrhea, dizziness, drowsiness, dry mouth, gas, headache, indigestion, infection, insomnia, itching, loss of strength, nausea, nervousness, sweating, swelling, vomiting

Why should this drug not be prescribed?

If ibuprofen, aspirin, or brands such as Advil, Aleve, and Naprosyn have ever given you asthma, hives, or any other type of allergic attack, do not take this medication. You should also avoid Vicoprofen if you've ever had an allergic reaction to hydrocodone or other narcotic painkillers.

Special warnings about this medication

Vicoprofen can make you drowsy and slow. Do not drive a car, operate machinery, or perform any other potentially dangerous activities until you know how this drug affects you. Alcohol, sedatives, tranquilizers, and other narcotic painkillers can increase drowsiness. Do not combine them with Vicoprofen.

High doses of hydrocodone may produce troubled, irregular, or slowed breathing; if you are sensitive to this drug, or have a head injury, such problems are more likely. Narcotics tend to increase the pressure of the fluid inside the skull, and this effect can be exaggerated by a head injury. Avoid Vicoprofen if possible.

Use Vicoprofen with caution if you have a severe liver or kidney disorder, heart failure, lupus, underactive thyroid or adrenal glands, an enlarged prostate, or any narrowing of the duct that drains the bladder. Caution is also called for in those who are weak, elderly, or dehydrated.

Hydrocodone suppresses the cough reflex; use it cautiously if you have a lung condition or have just had surgery.

The ibuprofen in Vicoprofen has been known to cause ulcers, and stomach bleeding can start without warning. If you've had such problems in the past, make sure the doctor is aware of it. Smoking, drinking, old age, and poor health make stomach problems more likely.

Vicoprofen can prolong bleeding time and cause a decrease in blood cell count. If you are taking a blood-thinning medication, use Vicoprofen with caution. This drug can also cause water retention. Be cautious if you have high blood pressure or poor heart function.

Contact your doctor if you notice any signs of stomach or intestinal bleeding, suffer blurred vision or other eye problems, get a skin rash, or notice any weight gain or swelling. If you have a severe allergic reaction, stop taking the drug and seek medical help immediately.

Possible food and drug interactions when taking this medication

If Vicoprofen is taken with certain other drugs, the effects of either can be increased, decreased, or altered. It is especially important to check with your doctor before combining Vicoprofen with the following:

ACE-inhibitor-type blood pressure and heart drugs such as Capoten and Vasotec
Alcohol
Antidepressants such as Elavil, Norpramin, and Pamelor
Antihistamines such as Benadryl, chlorpheniramine, and Tavist
Aspirin
Blood-thinning drugs such as Coumadin
Drugs that control muscle spasms such as Artane and Cogentin
Lithium (Lithobid, Lithonate)
Major tranquilizers such as Haldol and Thorazine
Methotrexate (Rheumatrex)

Other narcotic painkillers such as Demerol, morphine, and Percocet
Sleeping pills such as Halcion and Restoril
Tranquilizers such as Ativan, Valium, and Xanax
Water pills (diuretics) such as Lasix and HydroDIURIL

Special information if you are pregnant or breastfeeding

Do not take this drug during pregnancy unless directed by your doctor.
Drug dependence occurs in newborns when mothers take narcotics regularly prior to delivery.

Vicoprofen may appear in breast milk and could affect a nursing infant.
If this medication is essential to your health, your doctor may advise you
to discontinue breastfeeding until your treatment is finished.

Recommended dosage

ADULTS

Your doctor will adjust the dosage according to the severity of the pain
and the way the medication affects you. The usual dose is 1 tablet every
4 to 6 hours as needed. Do not take more than 5 tablets a day.

CHILDREN

The safety and effectiveness of Vicoprofen have not been established in
children below 16 years of age.

OLDER ADULTS

A reduced dosage is recommended.

Overdosage

A massive overdose of Vicoprofen can be fatal. If you suspect an overdose, seek medical attention immediately.

■ *Symptoms of Vicoprofen overdose may include:*
Blurred vision, cold and clammy skin, coma, confusion, difficulty
breathing, dizziness, extreme drowsiness, eye problems, headache,
heart attack, inflammation of the skin in the mouth, low blood pressure, muscle weakness, ringing in the ears, skin rash, slowed breathing, slowed heart rate, stomach and intestinal irritation, swelling

Vi-Daylin *See Multivitamins, page 901.*

VIDEX

Pronounced: VIE-decks
Generic name: Didanosine

Why is this drug prescribed?

Videx is one of the drugs used to fight the human immunodeficiency virus (HIV)—the deadly cause of AIDS. Over a period of years, HIV slowly destroys the immune system, leaving the body defenseless against infection. Videx disrupts reproduction of HIV, thereby staving off the immune system's collapse.

Signs and symptoms of advanced HIV infection include diarrhea, fever, headache, infections, problems with the nervous system, rash, sore throat, and significant weight loss.

Most important fact about this drug

Although Videx can slow the progress of HIV, it is not a cure. You may continue to develop complications, including frequent infections. Even if you feel better, regular physical exams and blood counts by your doctor are highly advisable. And notify your doctor immediately if you experience any changes in your general health.

How should you take this medication?

Videx tablets and oral solution should be taken every 12 hours, exactly as prescribed. It is important to keep levels of the drug in your body as constant as possible, so be sure to take every scheduled dose. Videx should be taken on an empty stomach, at least 30 minutes before or 2 hours after a meal. Never take more than the prescribed dose; nerve disorders could result.

Videx Tablets

There should be at least 2 tablets in each dose, but to avoid stomach upset, do not take more than 4 tablets per dose. Do *not* swallow the tablets whole. Instead, take them in one of these three ways:

1. Chew the tablets thoroughly before swallowing.
2. Crush the tablets before you take them.
3. Dissolve the tablets in at least 1 ounce of water, stirring until the particles are evenly dispersed. Swallow the mixture immediately.

If desired, you can add 1 ounce of apple juice to the water/Videx mixture. This combination should be taken within 1 hour of preparation. Be sure to stir it immediately before drinking.

Buffered Powder for Oral Solution

Open the packet and pour the contents into 4 ounces of water. Stir for 2 to 3 minutes, until the powder is completely dissolved. Drink the entire solution immediately. Do not mix with fruit juice.

Videx Pediatric Oral Solution
The pediatric version of Videx comes premixed from the pharmacy. Shake well before using.

Videx EC Delayed Release Capsules
This form is prescribed only when twice-daily dosing is impractical. Take 1 capsule daily on an empty stomach. Do not open the capsule. Swallow it whole.

■ *If you miss a dose...*
Take it as soon as you remember. If it is almost time for your next dose, skip the one you missed and go back to your regular schedule. Do not take 2 doses at once.

■ *Storage instructions...*
Videx tablets and powder can be stored at room temperature. The pediatric oral solution should be stored in a refrigerator and used within 30 days.

What side effects may occur?
The higher your dosage, the greater your chance of side effects. However, it's often hard to tell a side effect from a symptom of the disease. If you think the drug is causing problems, keep taking it until you've checked with your doctor. Only your doctor can determine whether the drug is at fault and adjust your dosage accordingly.

■ *Side effects may include:*
Abdominal pain, chills, diarrhea, fever, headache, itching, nausea, pain, rash, tingling, burning, numbness, or pain in the feet and hands, vomiting, weakness

Why should this drug not be prescribed?
If Videx gives you an allergic reaction, you should not take the drug.

Special warnings about this medication
It's important to remember that Videx will not prevent the spread of HIV through sexual relations or contact with infected blood.

Videx can cause several serious side effects. Severe and even fatal pancreatitis (inflammation of the pancreas) is one possibility, especially if you've had the problem in the past, suffer from kidney disease, or drink alcoholic beverages. Combining Videx with Zerit increases the risk. Check with your doctor immediately if you develop such signs of pancreatitis as stomach pain, nausea, or vomiting; you may have to stop treatment with Videx. If you have any of the risk factors for pancreatitis, make sure the doctor is aware of it.

Videx has also been known to cause serious and even fatal liver damage. Signs of a liver problem include weakness, fatigue, stomach discomfort, dizziness, a cold feeling, and a sudden change in heartbeat. If you develop these symptoms, stop taking Videx and call your doctor immediately. Also be sure to tell the doctor if you've ever had a liver problem or tend to abuse alcohol; the doctor will watch you especially closely.

Videx can also effect the nervous system, causing changes in your eyesight or a feeling of tingling, numbness, or pain in your hands or feet (known as peripheral neuropathy). Alert your doctor immediately if you develop any of these problems. The doctor may need to change the dosage or stop the drug.

Some people receiving drugs for HIV experience a redistribution of body fat, leading to extra fat around the middle, a "buffalo hump" on the back, and wasting in the arms, legs, and face. Researchers don't know whether this represents a long-term health problem or not.

If you are on a sodium-restricted diet, you should be aware that Videx powder contains 1,380 milligrams of sodium per packet. Those with the hereditary disease phenylketonuria should remember that Videx tablets contain phenylalanine.

Possible food and drug interactions when taking this medication

Alcohol increases your risk of developing serious side effects such as pancreatitis.

Severe or even fatal reactions may occur if Videx is combined with tenofovir (Viread) or ribavirin (Rebetol, Virazol). If you need to take Videx while you're using either of these medications, your doctor will monitor you closely. If any of the symptoms of pancreatitis, lactic acidosis, or peripheral neuropathy occur (see *Special warnings about this medication*), contact the doctor immediately.

If Videx is taken with certain other medications, the effect of either may be increased, decreased, or altered. It is especially important to check with your doctor before taking any of the following:

Antacids containing magnesium or aluminum, including Maalox
    and Mylanta
Ganciclovir (Cytovene)
IV pentamidine (Pentam)
Methadone (Dolophine)
Stavudine (Zerit)
Tetracycline

It's best to avoid combining Videx with the gout medication Zyloprim. If you are taking Nizoral or Sporanox, you should allow at least 2 hours to pass before taking Videx. If you've been prescribed the HIV drugs Crixivan or Rescriptor, allow 1 hour to pass before taking Videx. When taking antibiotics known as quinolones, including Cipro, Floxin, and Noroxin, you should take Videx at least 6 hours before the antibiotic, or wait for 2 hours after it. If you've been prescribed the HIV drug Viracept, take it with a light meal 1 hour after Videx.

Special information if you are pregnant or breastfeeding

The effects of Videx during pregnancy have not been adequately studied. If you are pregnant or plan to become pregnant, inform your doctor immediately.

Combining Videx with the HIV drug Zerit seems to increase the danger of serious and even fatal liver reactions during pregnancy. Use this combination with special caution if you're pregnant.

HIV can be passed to a baby through breast milk, so you should not plan on breastfeeding.

Recommended dosage

If you have a kidney or liver problem, your dosage may be reduced.

ADULTS

Tablets

For adults weighing 132 pounds or more, the recommended dose is 200 milligrams every 12 hours. Those weighing less than 132 pounds usually take 125 milligrams every 12 hours.

Buffered Powder for Oral Solution

For adults weighing 132 pounds or more, the recommended dose is 250 milligrams every 12 hours. Those weighing less than 132 pounds usually take 167 milligrams every 12 hours.

Videx EC Delayed-Release Capsules

For adults weighing 132 pounds or more, the recommended dose is 400 milligrams once a day. If you weigh less than 132 pounds, the usual dose is 250 milligrams once a day.

CHILDREN

The recommended dose for pediatric patients 2 weeks of age and older varies according to the child's weight. Videx EC capsules are not prescribed for children.

Overdosage

■ *Symptoms of Videx overdose may include:*
   Abdominal pain, diarrhea, pain, numbness, burning, and tingling in the hands and feet

If you suspect an overdose, seek medical attention immediately.

Viokase *See Pancrease, page 1030.*

VIRACEPT
Pronounced: VYE-ruh-sept
Generic name: Nelfinavir mesylate

Why is this drug prescribed?
Viracept is one of the drugs prescribed to fight HIV, the human immun-odeficiency virus that causes AIDS (acquired immune deficiency syndrome). Once inside the body, HIV spreads through certain key cells in the immune system, weakening the body's ability to fight off other infections. Viracept works by interfering with an important step in the virus's reproductive cycle. This slows the spread of the virus and prolongs the strength of the immune system.

Viracept belongs to the new class of drugs that has successfully reversed the course of HIV infection in many people. Called protease inhibitors, these drugs work better when used in combination with other HIV medications called nucleoside analogues (Retrovir, Hivid, and others) which act against the virus in other ways.

Most important fact about this drug
Although Viracept can keep HIV at bay, it is not a complete cure. If you stop taking the drug, the infection will re-emerge and progress to AIDS, leaving you vulnerable to a host of opportunistic infections (rare infections that develop only when the immune system falters, such as certain types of pneumonia, tuberculosis, and fungal infections). It's imperative, therefore, that you continue to see your doctor regularly and keep all your follow-up appointments.

How should you take this medication?
Take Viracept every day, exactly as prescribed. Do not stop taking it or change the dose without first consulting your doctor.

To achieve higher blood levels of the drug, always take Viracept with a meal or light snack.

If your child is taking Viracept oral powder, mix it with a small amount of water, milk, formula, soy formula, soy milk, or a liquid nutritional product such as Ensure, Sustacal, or Advera, then use within 6 hours. Make sure the child drinks the entire dose. Do not mix the powder with apple juice, applesauce, or orange juice; these combinations will taste bitter.

■ *If you miss a dose...*
Take it as soon as possible. If it is almost time for the next dose, skip the one you missed and go back to your regular schedule. Never double the dose.

■ *Storage instructions...*
Both tablets and powder may be stored at room temperature. Doses of the powder mixed with liquid may be kept for up to 6 hours under refrigeration. Keep container tightly closed.

What side effects may occur?
Side effects cannot be anticipated. If any develop or change in intensity, tell your doctor as soon as possible. Only your doctor can determine if it is safe for you to continue taking Viracept.

The most frequent side effect associated with Viracept is diarrhea. If it develops, it can be controlled with over-the-counter medications such as Imodium A-D.

■ *Side effects may include:*
Abdominal pain, gas, loss of strength, nausea, skin rash

Why should this drug not be prescribed?
If you have ever had an allergic reaction to Viracept or any of its ingredients, do not take this drug.

Special warnings about this medication
Although Viracept reduces the amount of HIV in the blood, its long-term effect on survival is still unknown. We do know, however, that the drug does *not* reduce the risk of passing HIV to others through sexual contact or blood contamination. You will need to continue avoiding practices that spread the virus.

If you have been using oral contraceptives, you'll need to take other measures. Viracept dramatically reduces the effectiveness of the Pill.

Viracept may trigger diabetes or make existing diabetes worse. If this occurs, you may have to start taking insulin or oral diabetes medication, or have your present dosage adjusted.

People with hemophilia type A and B may experience increased bleeding. If this happens, alert your doctor immediately. Make sure, too, that your doctor is aware of any liver problems you may have.

Viracept oral powder contains phenylalanine. If your child has the hereditary disease known as phenylketonuria, do not give the powder form.

Possible food and drug interactions when taking this medication
Do not take Viracept with any of the following medications. The combination could cause serious or even life-threatening problems.

Amiodarone (Cordarone)
Ergot derivatives such as Cafergot, D.H.E., Methergine, and Migranal
Lovastatin (Mevacor)
Midazolam (Versed)
Pimozide (Orap)
Quinidine (Quinaglute, Quinidex)
Rifampin (Rifadin, Rimactane)
Simvastatin (Zocor)
St. John's wort
Triazolam (Halcion)

Viracept may also interact with certain other drugs, and the effects of either could be increased, decreased, or altered. It is especially important to check with your doctor before combining Viracept with the following:

Atorvastatin (Lipitor)
Azithromycin (Zithromax)
Carbamazepine (Tegretol)
Cyclosporine (Neoral, Sandimmune)
Delavirdine (Rescriptor)
Indinavir (Crixivan)
Methadone
Nevirapine (Viramune)
Oral contraceptives
Phenobarbital
Phenytoin (Dilantin)
Rifabutin (Mycobutin)
Ritonavir (Norvir)
Saquinavir (Invirase)
Sildenafil (Viagra)
Sirolimus (Rapamune)
Tacrolimus (Prograf)

If you're also taking the HIV drug didanosine (Videx), be aware that it should be taken on an empty stomach. Since Viracept should be taken with food, you should take your didanosine dose 1 hour before or 2 hours after your Viracept dose.

Special information if you are pregnant or breastfeeding

The effects of Viracept during pregnancy have not been adequately studied. If you are pregnant or plan to become pregnant, tell your doctor immediately.

Do not breastfeed your baby. HIV appears in breast milk and can infect a nursing infant.

Recommended dosage

ADULTS

The recommended dose is 1,250 milligrams (five 250-milligram or two 625-milligram tablets) twice a day or 750 milligrams (three 250-milligram tablets) 3 times a day. Take with a meal or snack.

CHILDREN

Viracept oral powder is available for children who are unable to take tablets. The recommended dose for children 2 to 13 years of age is 20 to 30 milligrams per 2.2 pounds of body weight, 3 times a day with a meal or snack. The oral powder can be measured out with the provided scooper or a teaspoon—your doctor will tell you how much—and mixed with a small amount of water or any other fluid listed under *How should you take this medication?*

The safety and effectiveness of Viracept in children below age 2 have not been established.

Overdosage
Information on acute overdose with Viracept is limited. However, any medication taken in excess can have serious consequences. If you suspect an overdose, seek emergency medical treatment immediately.

VIRAMUNE
Pronounced: VIE-ruh-mewn
Generic name: Nevirapine

Why is this drug prescribed?
Viramune is prescribed for advanced cases of HIV. HIV—the human immunodeficiency virus that causes AIDS—undermines the immune system over a period of years, eventually leaving the body defenseless against infection. Viramune is generally prescribed only after the immune system has declined and infections have begun to appear. It is always taken with at least one other HIV medication such as Retrovir or Videx. If taken alone, it can cause the virus to become resistant. Even if used properly, it may be effective for only a limited time.

Like other drugs for HIV, Viramune works by impairing the virus's ability to multiply.

Most important fact about this drug
The most important side effect of Viramune is a rash which occasionally becomes so serious as to be life-threatening. The rash strikes approximately one in four patients, and becomes severe in about 2 percent. It usually appears during the first 6 weeks of therapy and strikes women more often than men. If you notice any signs of a rash, inform your doctor immediately. If it becomes severe or is accompanied by fever, blisters, mouth sores, red eyes, swelling, muscle or joint aches, or general fatigue, stop taking the drug and call your doctor.

How should you take this medication?
Be sure to take this medication every day, exactly as prescribed. Increase the dosage only when directed. To avoid development of resistance, be careful to take your other HIV drugs as well.

If you are using the oral suspension, shake it gently before each dose. Give it to the child with an oral dosing syringe or dosing cup. After each dose, rinse the cup with water and give the rinse to the child as well.

■ *If you miss a dose...*
Take it as soon as you remember. If it is almost time for the next dose, skip the one you missed and go back to your regular schedule. Do not double the dose.

■ *Storage instructions...*
Store tablets and oral suspension at room temperature in a tightly closed bottle.

What side effects may occur?

Side effects cannot be anticipated. If any develop or change in intensity, inform your doctor as soon as possible. Only your doctor can determine if it is safe for you to continue using Viramune.

■ *Side effects may include:*
Abdominal pain, allergic reactions (including hives, blisters, mouth sores, or swollen mouth and throat), anemia, diarrhea, drowsiness, drug withdrawal, fat redistribution, fatigue, fever, headache, joint pain, liver damage, muscle aches, nausea, rash, tingling, vomiting

Why should this drug not be prescribed?

If Viramune gives you an allergic reaction, you cannot use this drug.
You should also avoid Viramune if you have severe liver impairment.

Special warnings about this medication

Viramune has been known to cause serious—even fatal—liver damage, especially during the first 18 weeks of therapy. People with hepatitis B or C and women with a CD4+ cell count above 250 are more likely to develop this problem. Overall, women are at greater risk than men. If you already have moderate liver impairment, use Viramune with caution, if at all. Warning signs of liver damage include fatigue, a vaguely ill feeling, poor appetite, nausea, yellowish skin or eyes, pale stools, dark urine, and tenderness in the midriff. Check with your doctor immediately if you develop these symptoms. If liver damage has occurred, you'll have to permanently discontinue Viramune therapy.

You should know that HIV medications also cause a redistribution of fat in some people, increasing the amount of fat found around the middle and on the upper back, and reducing the amount of fat in the arms, legs, and face.

Remember that Viramune does not completely eliminate HIV from the body. The virus can still be passed to others during sex or through blood contamination.

Though Viramune can slow the progress of HIV, it is not a cure. HIV-related infections remain a danger, so frequent checkups and tests are still advisable.

Possible food and drug interactions when taking this medication
If Viramune is taken with certain other drugs, the effects of either could
be increased, decreased, or altered. It is especially important to check
with your doctor before combining Viramune with the following:

    Clarithromycin (Biaxin)
    Efavirenz (Sustiva)
    Fluconazole (Diflucan)
    Indinavir (Crixivan)
    Ketoconazole (Nizoral)
    Lopinavir/Ritonavir (Kaletra)
    Methadone (Dolophine)
    Nelfinavir (Viracept)
    Rifabutin (Mycobutin)
    Rifampin (Rifadin, Rimactane)
    Saquinavir (Fortovase)
    St. John's wort
    Zidovudine (Retrovir)

Viramune may interfere with birth control pills and other hormonal
contraceptives. Do not use this form of contraception during Viramune
therapy.
    Also, it's important to talk to your doctor before combining Viramune
with any of the following:

    Antiarrhythmic heart medications such as disopyramide (Norpace)
    Anticonvulsant (seizure) medications such as carbamazepine
        (Tegretol) and clonazepam (Klonopin)
    Antifungal medications such as itraconazole (Sporanox)
    Blood-thinning medications such as warfarin (Coumadin)
    Calcium channel blocker (angina) medications such as diltiazem
        (Cardizem), nifedipine (Procardia), and verapamil (Calan)
    Cancer chemotherapy medications such as cyclophosphamide
        (Cytoxan)
    Immunosuppressant medications such as cyclosporine
        (Sandimmune, Neoral)
    Migraine medications such as ergotamine (Cafergot)
    Opiate agonists (narcotic) pain medications such as fentanyl
        (Duragesic)

Special information if you are pregnant or breastfeeding
If you are pregnant you may be at a higher risk of developing serious—
even fatal—liver damage while taking Viramune. If you are pregnant or
plan to become pregnant, notify your doctor immediately.
    Avoid breastfeeding. HIV can be passed to a nursing infant through
breast milk.

Recommended dosage

ADULTS

For the first 14 days, the dose is 1 tablet a day. If no serious rash appears, the dose is then increased to 1 tablet twice a day. If you miss your doses for more than 7 days, the doctor will have to restart you at the lower initial dose.

CHILDREN

2 Months to 8 Years of Age

For the first 14 days, the dose of oral suspension is 4 milligrams per 2.2 pounds of body weight once a day. If no serious rash appears, the dose is then increased to 7 milligrams per 2.2 pounds twice a day.

8 Years and Older

For the first 14 days, the dose of oral suspension is 4 milligrams per 2.2 pounds of body weight once a day. If no serious rash appears, the dose is then increased to 4 milligrams per 2.2 pounds twice a day.

For both adults and children, total daily dosage should never exceed 400 milligrams (2 tablets).

In certain cases your Viramune dosage may need to be adjusted. Be sure to tell the doctor if you develop a rash within the first 14 days of using Viramune or if you stop taking the drug for more than 7 days. Also tell the doctor if you're undergoing kidney dialysis.

If you develop hepatitis during Viramune treatment, you will have to stop taking the drug.

Overdosage

Any medication taken in excess can have serious consequences. If you suspect an overdose, seek medical attention immediately.

■ *Symptoms of Viramune overdose may include:*
Dizziness, fatigue, fever, headache, insomnia, nausea, rash, reddened bumps on the skin, respiratory problems, swelling, vomiting, weight loss

VIREAD

Pronounced: VEER-ee-ad
Generic name: Tenofovir disoproxil fumarate

Why is this drug prescribed?

Viread is one of the drugs prescribed to fight HIV, the human immunodeficiency virus that causes AIDS (acquired immune deficiency syndrome). HIV attacks the immune system, slowly destroying the body's ability to fight off infection. Viread staves off the attack by interfering with HIV reverse transcriptase, an enzyme the virus needs to reproduce.

Viread lowers the amount of HIV in the blood and may help increase the number of T cells, important agents of the immune system that kill microscopic foreign invaders. It is used in combination with other anti-HIV drugs when these drugs are not effective by themselves.

Most important fact about this drug
Viread does not completely eliminate HIV or totally restore the immune system. There is still a danger of serious infections, so you should be sure to see your doctor regularly for monitoring and tests. Notify your doctor immediately of any changes in your general health.

How should you take this medication?
Be sure to take Viread once a day, every day. Set up a regular schedule so you won't forget, and always get a new supply when the drug runs low. If you don't keep the drug in your system, the virus may develop resistance. Take Viread with meals. Food increases the amount of Viread that reaches the bloodstream.

■ *If you miss a dose...*
Take it as soon as you remember. If it is almost time for your next dose, skip the one you missed and go back to your regular schedule. Do not take 2 doses at once.

■ *Storage instructions...*
Store at room temperature. Throw away any medication that is out of date.

What side effects may occur?
Side effects cannot be anticipated. If any develop or change in intensity, inform your doctor as soon as possible. Only your doctor can determine if it is safe for you to continue taking Viread.

■ *Side effects may include:*
Abdominal pain, diarrhea, gas, headache, loss of appetite, nausea, vomiting, weakness

Why should this drug not be prescribed?
If Viread gives you an allergic reaction, you'll be unable to use it.

Special warnings about this medication
Remember that Viread does not eliminate HIV from the body. The infection can still be passed to others through sexual contact or blood contamination.

Viread should be used with caution if you have liver disease. The drug has been known to cause liver damage and a buildup of lactic acid in the blood—a dangerous and potentially fatal condition. If you are a woman, are overweight, have liver disease, or have used Viread for a long time, you are more likely to develop this condition. Notify your doctor immediately if you develop any signs of lactic acid buildup, including shortness of breath, nausea, vomiting, and stomach/intestinal pain.

If you have a kidney condition, make sure your doctor knows. People with severe kidney problems shouldn't take Viread.

You should know that some people taking HIV medications experience a change in fat distribution, with increased fat in the upper back and neck and loss of fat from the arms, legs, and face.

Viread has not been approved for children.

Possible food and drug interactions when taking this medication

If Viread is taken with certain other drugs, the effects of either could be increased, decreased, or altered. It is especially important to check with your doctor before combining Viread with the following:

Acyclovir (Zovirax)
Cidofovir (Vistide)
Didanosine (Videx)
Ganciclovir (Cytovene)
Valacyclovir (Valtrex)
Valganciclovir (Valcyte)

Special information if you are pregnant or breastfeeding

Although there's no evidence that Viread can harm a developing baby, the drug has not been adequately studied during pregnancy. If you are pregnant or plan to become pregnant, tell your doctor immediately.

Do not breastfeed. HIV appears in breast milk and can infect the nursing infant.

Recommended dosage

ADULTS

The dose is 300 milligrams (1 tablet) taken once a day with a meal.

Overdosage

No information on overdose of Viread is available. However any medication taken in excess can have serious consequences. If you suspect an overdose, seek medical help immediately.

Vistaril *See Atarax, page 142.*

Vitamins with Fluoride *See Poly-Vi-Flor, page 1113.*

VIVACTIL

Pronounced: vi-VAC-til
Generic name: Protriptyline hydrochloride

Why is this drug prescribed?

Vivactil is used to treat the symptoms of mental depression in people who are under close medical supervision. It is particularly suitable for those who are inactive and withdrawn.

Vivactil is a member of the family of drugs called tricyclic antidepressants. Researchers don't know exactly how it works. Unlike the class of antidepressants known as monoamine oxidase (MAO) inhibitors, it does not act primarily through stimulation of the central nervous system. It tends to work more rapidly than some other tricyclic antidepressants. Improvement sometimes begins within a week.

Most important fact about this drug

If you are prone to anxiety or agitation, Vivactil can make the problem worse. It can also exaggerate the symptoms of manic-depression and schizophrenia. If this seems to be happening, let your doctor know immediately. The doctor may have to reduce the dose of Vivactil or add another drug to your regimen.

How should you take this medication?

Take Vivactil exactly as prescribed. Do not take it with alcohol.

■ *If you miss a dose...*
Take it as soon as you remember. If it is almost time for your next dose, skip the one you missed and go back to your regular schedule. Do not take 2 doses at once.

■ *Storage instructions...*
Store at room temperature in a tightly closed container.

What side effects may occur?

Side effects cannot be anticipated. If any develop or change in intensity, inform your doctor as soon as possible. Only your doctor can determine if it is safe for you to continue taking Vivactil.

■ *Side effects may include:*
Anxiety, blood disorders, confusion, decreased libido, dizziness, flushing, headache, impotence, insomnia, low blood pressure, nightmares, rapid or irregular heartbeat, rash, seizures, sensitivity to sunlight, stomach and intestinal problems

Why should this drug not be prescribed?

Due to the possibility of life-threatening side effects, Vivactil must never be taken with drugs classified as monoamine oxidase (MAO) inhibitors, such as the antidepressants Nardil and Parnate. Allow at least 14 days between the last dose of one of these drugs and the first dose of Vivactil.

Vivactil should not be used during recovery from a heart attack. It also cannot be used by anyone who has had an allergic reaction to it.

Special warnings about this medication

In clinical studies, antidepressants increased the risk of suicidal thinking and behavior in children and adolescents with depression and other psychiatric disorders. Anyone considering the use of Vivactil or any other antidepressant in a child or adolescent must balance this risk with the clinical need. Vivactil is not approved for use in children.

Additionally, the progression of major depression is associated with a worsening of symptoms and/or the emergence of suicidal thinking or behavior in both adults and children, whether or not they are taking antidepressants. Individuals being treated with Vivactil and their caregivers should watch for any change in symptoms or any new symptoms that appear suddenly—especially agitation, anxiety, hostility, panic, restlessness, extreme hyperactivity, and suicidal thinking or behavior—and report them to the doctor immediately. Be especially observant at the beginning of treatment or whenever there is a change in dose.

Drugs such as Vivactil sometimes cause heartbeat irregularities. Vivactil should be used with caution by people who have heart problems or a thyroid disorder. Caution is also advisable if you have a history of seizures, difficulty urinating, or glaucoma (high pressure in the eyes); or use alcohol excessively.

This drug is not recommended during electroconvulsive therapy (ECT).

Vivactil should be discontinued several days before any surgery.

Vivactil may impair the physical and/or mental abilities required to drive a car or operate heavy machinery.

Possible food and drug interactions when taking this medication

Remember that Vivactil must never be combined with monoamine inhibitors such as Nardil and Parnate.

If Vivactil is taken with certain other drugs, the effects of either could be increased, decreased, or altered. It is especially important to check with your doctor before combining Vivactil with the following:

Antidepressants that boost serotonin, including Paxil, Prozac, and Zoloft
Antipsychotic medications such as chlorpromazine and Mellaril
Barbiturates such as Nembutal and Seconal
Certain blood pressure medications such as guanethidine
Cimetidine (Tagamet)
Decongestants such as Sudafed
Drugs that quell spasms, such as Donnatal and Levsin
Epinephrine (EpiPen)

Flecainide (Tambocor)
Narcotic painkillers such as Percodan and Vicodin
Norepinephrine
Other antidepressants such as Elavil and Tofranil
Propafenone (Rythmol)
Quinidine
Tramadol (Ultram)
Tranquilizers and sleep aids such as Halcion, Valium, and Xanax

Special information if you are pregnant or breastfeeding

The effects of Vivactil during pregnancy have not been adequately studied. It should be used during pregnancy only if its benefits outweigh the potential risk. If you are pregnant or planning to become pregnant, inform your doctor immediately.

It is not known whether Vivactil makes its way into breast milk. Consult with your doctor before deciding to breastfeed.

Recommended dosage

The doctor will start with a low dose and increase it gradually, watching for side effects and a positive response

ADULTS

The usual adult dosage is 15 to 40 milligrams in 3 or 4 doses per day. The maximum dosage is 60 milligrams daily. Increases are made in the morning dose.

CHILDREN

The safety and effectiveness of Vivactil have not been studied in children.

OLDER ADULTS AND ADOLESCENTS

Lower dosages are recommended for adolescents and older adults. Five milligrams 3 times a day may be given initially, followed by a gradual increase if necessary. Heart function must be monitored in older adults who are taking 20 or more milligrams per day.

Overdosage

An overdose of Vivactil can be fatal. If you suspect an overdose, seek medical help immediately.

- *Critical signs of Vivactil overdose may include:*
  Convulsions, irregular heartbeat, severely low blood pressure, reduced level of consciousness or even coma.
- *Other signs of Vivactil overdose may include:*
  Agitation, confusion, dilated pupils, disturbed concentration, drowsiness, fever, hyperactive reflexes, low body temperature, muscle rigidity, sporadic hallucinations, stupor, vomiting, or any of the other symptoms listed under *What side effects may occur?*

Vivelle *See Estrogen Patches, page 538.*

Volmax *See Proventil, page 1185.*

VOLTAREN

Pronounced: vol-TAR-en
Generic name: Diclofenac sodium
Other brand name: Cataflam (diclofenac potassium)

Why is this drug prescribed?

Voltaren and Cataflam are nonsteroidal anti-inflammatory drugs used to relieve the inflammation, swelling, stiffness, and joint pain associated with rheumatoid arthritis, osteoarthritis (the most common form of arthritis), and ankylosing spondylitis (arthritis and stiffness of the spine). Voltaren-XR, the extended-release form of Voltaren, is used only for long-term treatment. Cataflam is also prescribed for immediate relief of pain and menstrual discomfort.

Most important fact about this drug

You should have frequent checkups by your doctor if you take Voltaren regularly. Ulcers or internal bleeding can occur without warning.

How should you take this medication?

To minimize stomach upset and related side effects, your doctor may recommend taking this medicine with food, milk, or an antacid. However, this may delay onset of relief.

Take this drug with a full glass of water. Also, do not lie down for about 20 minutes after taking it. This will help to prevent irritation in your upper digestive tract.

Take this medication exactly as prescribed.

■ *If you miss a dose...*
If you take this medicine on a regular schedule, take it as soon as you remember. If it is almost time for your next dose, skip the one you missed and go back to your regular schedule. Do not take 2 doses at once.

■ *Storage instructions...*
Store at room temperature. Keep the container tightly closed and protect from moisture.

What side effects may occur?

Side effects cannot be anticipated. If any develop or change in intensity, inform your doctor as soon as possible. Only your doctor can determine if it is safe for you to continue taking Voltaren.

■ *Side effects may include:*
Abdominal bleeding, abdominal pain or cramps, abdominal swelling, anemia, blood clotting problems, constipation, diarrhea, dizziness, fluid retention, gas, headache, heartburn, indigestion, itching, nausea, peptic ulcers, rash, ringing in the ears, vomiting

Why should this drug not be prescribed?
If you have an allergic reaction to Voltaren or Cataflam, or if you have had asthma attacks, hives, or other allergic reactions caused by aspirin or other nonsteroidal anti-inflammatory drugs, you should not take this medication. Make sure your doctor is aware of any drug reactions you have experienced.

Special warnings about this medication
Remember that this medication has been known to cause peptic ulcers and bleeding. Contact your doctor immediately if you suspect a problem.

Use this drug cautiously if you have kidney problems, heart disease, or high blood pressure. It can cause fluid retention.

This medication can also cause liver problems. If you develop signs of liver disease such as nausea, fatigue, lethargy, itching, yellowish eyes and skin, tenderness in the upper right area of your abdomen, or flu-like symptoms, notify your doctor at once.

Rare cases of meningitis (inflammation of the membrane enclosing the brain) have been linked to this medication. If symptoms such as fever and coma develop, alert the doctor immediately.

In rare instances, this drug may also affect your vision. If you notice any problems, stop taking the drug and check with your doctor.

Possible food and drug interactions when taking this medication
If Voltaren or Cataflam is taken with certain other drugs, the effects of either could be increased, decreased, or altered. It is especially important to check with your doctor before combining Voltaren with the following:

Aspirin
Blood thinners such as Coumadin
Cyclosporine (Sandimmune)
Digitalis drugs such as Lanoxin
Diuretics such as Dyazide, Lasix, and Midamor
Insulin or oral antidiabetes medications such as Micronase
Lithium (Eskalith, Lithobid)
Methotrexate
Phenobarbital

Special information if you are pregnant or breastfeeding

Do not take this drug late in your pregnancy; it could harm the baby. Check with your doctor before taking the drug early in pregnancy; it should be used only if necessary. The drug does appear in breast milk and could affect a nursing infant. If this medication is essential to your health, your doctor may advise you to discontinue breastfeeding until your treatment with Voltaren is finished.

Recommended dosage

ADULTS

Osteoarthritis
The usual dose is 100 to 150 milligrams a day, divided into smaller doses of 50 milligrams 2 or 3 times a day (for Voltaren or Cataflam) or 75 milligrams twice a day (for Voltaren). The usual dose of Voltaren-XR (extended-release) is 100 milligrams taken once a day.

Rheumatoid Arthritis
The usual dose is 100 to 200 milligrams a day, divided into smaller doses of 50 milligrams 3 to 4 times a day (for Voltaren or Cataflam), 75 milligrams twice a day (for Voltaren), or 100 milligrams once or twice a day (for Voltaren-XR).

People with rheumatoid arthritis should not take more than 225 milligrams a day.

Ankylosing Spondylitis
The usual dose is 100 to 125 milligrams of Voltaren a day, divided into smaller doses of 25 milligrams 4 times a day, with another 25 milligrams at bedtime if necessary.

Pain and Menstrual Discomfort
The usual starting dose of Cataflam is 50 milligrams every 8 hours as needed, although to provide better relief on the first day doctors sometimes prescribe a starting dose of 100 milligrams followed by two 50-milligram doses. After the first day, you should not take more than 150 milligrams in a day.

CHILDREN

The safety and effectiveness of Voltaren have not been established in children.

Overdosage

Any medication taken in excess can have serious consequences. If you suspect an overdose, seek medical attention immediately.

■ *Symptoms of Voltaren overdose may include:*
Acute kidney failure, drowsiness, loss of consciousness, lung inflammation, nausea, vomiting

VoSpire *See Proventil, page 1185.*

VYTORIN
Pronounced: VIE-tor-in
Generic ingredients: Ezetimibe, Simvastatin

Why is this drug prescribed?
Vytorin is a cholesterol-lowering drug. It is used along with a special diet to lower the amount of fatty material in the blood—triglycerides and LDL (or "bad") cholesterol—that can build up on artery walls and block blood flow. At the same time, Vytorin raises HDL (or "good") cholesterol, which helps prevent fats from building up and clogging the arteries.

Your body needs fat to function properly, but when it accumulates as fatty deposits in the arteries, it increases your risk for heart attack, stroke, and blood vessel disease. Your doctor may prescribe Vytorin if you are at high risk for heart disease and your cholesterol level is above 130, or if you are at low risk for heart disease and your cholesterol level is above 190.

Vytorin is a combination of two drugs, simvastatin (Zocor) and ezetimibe (Zetia). Each works in a different way to lower levels of fat in the blood. Normally, the liver produces most of the cholesterol needed to maintain a healthy balance. Simvastatin works by interrupting the process of cholesterol production, mainly in the liver. Ezetimibe reduces the amount of cholesterol absorbed in the intestines.

Most important fact about this drug
Vytorin is usually prescribed only if diet, exercise, and weight loss fail to bring your cholesterol levels under control. It's important to remember that Vytorin is a supplement—not a substitute—for those other measures. To get the full benefit of the medication, you need to stick to the diet and exercise program prescribed by your doctor. All these efforts to keep your cholesterol levels normal are important because they may lower your risk of heart disease.

How should you take this medication?
Take Vytorin once a day in the evening with or without food.

If you are also using the cholesterol-lowering drugs Colestid, Questran, or WelChol, take Vytorin at least 2 hours before or 4 hours after taking the other medication.

■ *If you miss a dose...*
Take the forgotten dose as soon as you remember. However, if it is almost time for your next dose, skip the one you missed and return to your regular schedule. Do not take 2 doses at once.
■ *Storage instructions...*
Store at room temperature.

What side effects may occur?

Side effects cannot be anticipated. If any develop or change in intensity, tell your doctor as soon as possible. Only your doctor can determine if it is safe to continue using Vytorin.

■ *Side effects may include:*
Allergic reaction including swelling of the face, lips, throat, or tongue, difficulty breathing or swallowing, or rash; flu; gallstones; headache; inflammation of the gallbladder; inflammation of the liver; inflammation of the pancreas; muscle pain, tenderness, or weakness; nausea; numbness or pain in the hands or feet; upper respiratory infection

Why should this drug not be prescribed?

Do not take Vytorin if you are allergic to either ezetimibe (Zetia) or simvastatin (Zocor). You should also not take Vytorin if you have liver disease or if blood tests suggest a liver problem.

If you are pregnant, plan to become pregnant, or have missed a period, do not take Vytorin. In addition, women who are breastfeeding should not use this drug.

Special warnings about this medication

Vytorin can cause the breakdown of muscle tissue, which can lead to serious kidney damage and, in rare cases, death from kidney failure. It is very important to stop taking Vytorin and call your doctor immediately if you have muscle pain, tenderness, or weakness that comes on while taking Vytorin, especially if you also have a fever and feel sick.

Vytorin can make certain medical conditions worse. If you have diabetes, kidney disease, or any kind of muscle disorder, or if you have ever had liver problems, you must be carefully monitored while taking Vytorin.

Because Vytorin can cause liver problems, your doctor will order a blood test to check your liver enzymes before your first dose and again at regular intervals during treatment. You may have to stop taking Vytorin if your liver enzymes become too high.

Because of possible effects on the liver, it is important to limit your alcohol consumption while taking this drug.

Simvastatin and similar drugs have caused cataracts and other serious eye problems in animal studies. Be sure to alert your doctor if you have cataracts or any eye condition that gets worse.

Alert the doctor if you're scheduled to have surgery. You'll probably need to stop taking Vytorin several days beforehand.

Possible food and drug interactions when taking this medication

If Vytorin is taken with certain other drugs, the effects of either could be increased, decreased, or altered. Combining it with the following increases the chance of muscle damage:

Amiodarone (Cordarone)
Antifungal medicines such as itraconazole (Sporanox) and
   ketoconazole (Nizoral)
Benzafibrate
Clarithromycin (Biaxin)
Clofibrate (Atromid-S)
Cyclosporine (Neoral, Sandimmune)
Erythromycin (E-Mycin, Ery-Tab, Erythrocin, and others)
Fenofibrate (Tricor)
Gemfibrozil (Lopid)
Grapefruit juice (large quantities)
HIV medicines called protease inhibitors, such as indinavir
   (Crixivan), nelfinavir (Viracept), ritonavir (Norvir), and saquinavir
   (Fortovase)
Nefazodone
Niacin and nicotinic acid (Niacor, Niaspan)
Verapamil (Calan, Isoptin, Verelan)

Other drugs that may interact with Vytorin include:

Blood-thinning drugs such as warfarin (Coumadin)
Digoxin (Lanoxin)
Propranolol (Inderal, Inderide)

You should also avoid drinking large amounts of alcohol while taking
Vytorin.

Special information if you are pregnant or breastfeeding

Cholesterol is needed for a baby to develop properly. Therefore, you
should not take Vytorin if you are pregnant or if you plan to become pregnant. If you find out you're pregnant during Vytorin treatment, stop taking it and call your doctor. In addition, women who are breastfeeding
should not take Vytorin.

Recommended dosage

ADULTS

The usual starting dose is one 10/20 tablet containing 10 milligrams of
ezetimibe and 20 milligrams of simvastatin taken once a day in the
evening. The doctor may prescribe a lower starting dose (10/10) if you require less aggressive treatment and a higher one (10/40) if you need a
large reduction (more than 55 percent) in LDL cholesterol. Depending on
your body's response, the doctor may increase your dose at 2-week intervals up to a maximum of 10/80 milligrams a day.

If you're taking cyclosporine, the dose of Vytorin should not exceed
10/10 milligrams a day. If you're taking amiodarone or verapamil, the
dose should not exceed 10/20 milligrams a day.

If you have severe kidney disease, the doctor may prescribe a lower dose or have you stop taking Vytorin altogether.

CHILDREN 10 YEARS OF AGE OR OLDER

Vytorin has not been studied in children or adolescents. However, one of the ingredients, simvastatin, is approved for use in children 10 years and older. The recommended starting dose is 10 milligrams once a day in the evening. The dosage may be increased every 4 weeks, as determined by the doctor, up to a maximum of 40 milligrams a day. Girls must have been menstruating for at least 1 year before starting therapy with simvastatin. The drug has not been studied in children less than 10 years old or in doses greater than 40 milligrams a day.

There is limited experience with the use of ezetimibe in children. The drug appears to be metabolized the same as in adults. Ezetimibe is not recommended for children less than 10 years old.

Because of the individual recommendations for simvastatin and ezetimibe, Vytorin is also not recommended for children less than 10 years old.

Overdosage

Although there is no specific information about Vytorin overdose, any medication taken in excess can have serious consequences. If you suspect an overdose, seek emergency treatment immediately.

Warfarin See Coumadin, page 350.

WELCHOL
Pronounced: WELL-call
Generic name: Colesevelam

Why is this drug prescribed?

WelChol is used to lower blood cholesterol levels when diet and exercise prove insufficient. It works by binding with cholesterol-based bile acids to take them out of circulation. This prompts the liver to produce a replacement supply of bile acids, drawing the extra cholesterol it needs out of the bloodstream.

WelChol is sometimes prescribed along with one of the popular statin drugs that fight cholesterol in a different way. Among these drugs are Lescol, Lipitor, Mevacor, Pravachol, and Zocor.

Most important fact about this drug

WelChol is usually added to a treatment regimen only when other measures have failed to produce adequate results. Often, diet and exercise are enough to bring cholesterol levels under control. Likewise, it's sometimes sufficient to simply treat an underlying problem such as diabetes, underactive thyroid, kidney disease, a liver disorder, or alcoholism.

Whatever your other treatment measures may be, it's important to remember that WelChol is intended to supplement them, rather than replace them outright. To get the full benefit of the medication, you need to stick to the diet, exercise program, and other treatments your doctor prescribes. All these efforts to keep your cholesterol levels normal are important because together they may lower your risk of heart disease.

How should you take this medication?
WelChol should be taken at mealtime with a liquid.

■ *If you miss a dose...*
Take it as soon as you remember. If it is almost time for your next dose, skip the one you missed and go back to your regular schedule. Never take 2 doses at the same time.
■ *Storage instructions...*
Store at room temperature and protect from moisture.

What side effects may occur?
WelChol is not absorbed by the body, so it is relatively free of side effects. If any develop or change in intensity, inform your doctor as soon as possible. Only your doctor can determine if it is safe for you to continue taking WelChol.

■ *Side effects may include:*
Constipation, indigestion, muscle aches, sore throat, weakness

Why should this drug not be prescribed?
You should not take WelChol if you have a bowel obstruction or the product gives you an allergic reaction.

Special warnings about this medication
If you have difficulty swallowing or suffer from severe digestive problems, use WelChol with caution; it hasn't been tested under these conditions. The drug has also not been studied in children.

Possible food and drug interactions when taking this medication
No significant interactions are known.

Special information if you are pregnant or breastfeeding
There is no evidence that this drug causes harm during pregnancy. Nevertheless, be sure to let the doctor know if you are pregnant, plan to become pregnant, or are breastfeeding. There is a possibility that WelChol could interfere with the absorption of needed vitamins.

Recommended dosage

ADULTS

The usual dosage is 6 tablets a day, taken as a single dose or divided into 2 doses. If you're taking WelChol with one of the statin drugs, the maximum recommended daily dosage is 6 tablets. If you're taking WelChol alone, the maximum is 7.

Overdosage

Since WelChol is not absorbed by the body, the chances of serious toxicity are low. Still, if you suspect an overdose, call your doctor immediately.

WELLBUTRIN

Pronounced: *Well-BEW-trin*
Generic name: *Bupropion hydrochloride*
Other brand names: *Wellbutrin SR*, *Wellbutrin XL*

Why is this drug prescribed?

Wellbutrin is prescribed to help relieve major depression. Symptoms include a severely depressed mood (for 2 weeks or more) and loss of interest or pleasure in usual activities accompanied by sleep and appetite disturbances, agitation or lack of energy, feelings of guilt or worthlessness, decreased sex drive, inability to concentrate, and sometimes suicidal thoughts or behavior.

Wellbutrin is thought to work by altering levels of the brain chemicals norepinephrine and dopamine. It is not chemically related to other antidepressants such as tricyclics (Elavil), MAO inhibitors (Nardil, Parnate), or serotonin re-uptake inhibitors (Paxil and Prozac).

Most important fact about this drug

Wellbutrin is associated with an increased risk of seizures. This risk is greater at higher doses (approximately 4 in 1,000 patients at dosages of 300 to 450 milligrams a day). Certain factors increase the risk of seizure, including:

A history of eating disorders, including anorexia and bulimia
A history of head trauma or previous seizure
Central nervous system tumor
Excessive use of alcohol, or abrupt withdrawal from alcohol or
    sedatives
Severe liver disease such as cirrhosis
Taking medications that lower the seizure threshold (see *Possible
    food and drug interactions when taking this medication*)

To minimize the risk of seizures, dose increases should be done gradually, and the total daily dose of Wellbutrin should not exceed 450 milligrams. Additionally, the doctor should be aware of all your medical conditions, and you should not take any other medications (both prescription and over-the-counter) unless the doctor approves.

How should you take this medication?
Take Wellbutrin exactly as prescribed by your doctor. The usual dosing regimen is 3 equal doses spaced evenly throughout the day. Allow at least 6 hours between doses. Your doctor will probably start you at a low dosage and gradually increase it; this helps minimize side effects.

You should take Wellbutrin SR, the sustained-release form, in 2 doses, at least 8 hours apart. Wellbutrin XL extended-release tablets should be taken once a day in the morning. Swallow Wellbutrin SR and Wellbutrin XL tablets whole; do not chew, divide, or crush them.

If Wellbutrin works for you, your doctor will probably have you continue taking it for at least several months.

■ *If you miss a dose...*
Take it as soon as you remember. If it is within 4 hours of your next dose, skip the one you missed and go back to your regular schedule. Never take 2 doses at the same time.
■ *Storage instructions...*
Store at room temperature. Protect from light and moisture.

What side effects may occur?
Side effects cannot be anticipated. If any develop or change in intensity, inform your doctor as soon as possible. Only your doctor can determine if it is safe for you to continue taking Wellbutrin.

■ *Side effects of Wellbutrin may include:*
Agitation, constipation, dizziness, dry mouth, excessive sweating, headache, nausea, vomiting, skin rash, sleep disturbances, tremor
■ *Side effects of Wellbutrin SR may include:*
Agitation, constipation, dizziness, dry mouth, insomnia, nausea, rash, sweating, weight loss
■ *Side effects of Wellbutrin XL may include:*
Abdominal pain, agitation, anxiety, constipation, diarrhea, dizziness, dry mouth, heart palpitations, increased urination, insomnia, muscle soreness, nausea, rash, ringing in the ears, sore throat, sweating

Why should this drug not be prescribed?
Do not take Wellbutrin if you are sensitive to or have ever had an allergic reaction to it.

Since Wellbutrin causes seizures in some people, do not take it if you have any type of seizure disorder or if you are taking another medication containing bupropion, such as Zyban, which is used to help quit smoking. If you have a seizure while taking Wellbutrin, stop taking the drug and never take it again.

Do not take Wellbutrin while abruptly giving up alcohol or sedatives, including tranquilizers such as Librium, Valium, and Xanax. Rapid withdrawal increases the risk of seizures.

If you have had any kind of heart trouble or liver or kidney disease, be sure your doctor knows about it before you start taking this drug. It must be used with extreme caution if you have severe cirrhosis of the liver. A reduced dosage may be needed if you have any sort of liver or kidney problem.

You should not take Wellbutrin if you currently have, or formerly had, an eating disorder. For some reason, people with a history of anorexia nervosa or bulimia seem to be more likely to experience Wellbutrin-related seizures. Do not take Wellbutrin if, within the past 14 days, you have taken a monoamine oxidase inhibitor (MAO inhibitor) drug, such as the antidepressants Marplan, Nardil or Parnate. This particular drug combination could cause you to experience a sudden, dangerous rise in blood pressure.

Special warnings about this medication

In clinical studies, antidepressants increased the risk of suicidal thinking and behavior in children and adolescents with depression and other psychiatric disorders. Anyone considering the use of Wellbutrin or any other antidepressant in a child or adolescent must balance this risk with the clinical need. Wellbutrin has not been studied in children or adolescents and is not approved for treating anyone less than 18 years old.

Additionally, the progression of major depression is associated with a worsening of symptoms and/or the emergence of suicidal thinking or behavior in both adults and children, whether or not they are taking antidepressants. Individuals being treated with Wellbutrin and their caregivers should watch for any change in symptoms or any new symptoms that appear suddenly—especially agitation, anxiety, hostility, panic, restlessness, extreme hyperactivity, and suicidal thinking or behavior—and report them to the doctor immediately. Be especially observant at the beginning of treatment or whenever there is a change in dose.

Be sure to let your doctor know if you have heart trouble, liver problems, or kidney disease before you start taking Wellbutrin. Use this drug with extreme caution if you have cirrhosis of the liver.

Stop taking Wellbutrin and call your doctor immediately if you have difficulty breathing or swallowing; notice swelling in your face, lips, tongue, or throat; develop swollen arms and legs; or break out with itchy eruptions. These are warning signs of a potential severe allergic reaction.

Wellbutrin may affect your coordination or judgment and impair your ability to drive or operate dangerous machinery. Avoid activities that require full alertness until you know how the drug affects you.

Like all antidepressants, Wellbutrin could trigger a manic episode in people with bipolar disorder.

Although Wellbutrin occasionally causes weight gain, a more common effect is weight loss: Some 28 percent of people who take this medication lose 5 pounds or more. If depression has already caused you to lose weight, and if further weight loss would be detrimental to your health, Wellbutrin may not be the best antidepressant for you.

Possible food and drug interactions when taking this medication

Do not drink alcohol while you are taking Wellbutrin; an interaction between alcohol and Wellbutrin could increase the possibility of a seizure.

Wellbutrin should not be combined with drugs that lower the seizure threshold, including:

Antidepressants classified as MAO inhibitors, such as Nardil and Parnate
Other antidepressants such as Elavil, Norpramin, Pamelor, Paxil, Prozac, Tofranil, and Zoloft
Antipsychotic drugs such as chlorpromazine, Haldol, Mellaril, and Risperdal
Cocaine
Diabetes medications such as Glucotrol and Prandin
Insulin
Opiates such as heroin and morphine
Sedatives, including benzodiazepines such as Valium and Xanax
Steroid medications such as prednisone
Stimulants, including over-the-counter diet drugs
Theophylline (Theo-24, Uniphyl)

If Wellbutrin is taken with certain other drugs, the effects of either could be increased, decreased, or altered. It is especially important to check with your doctor before combining Wellbutrin with the following:

Beta-blockers (used for high blood pressure and heart conditions) such as Inderal, Lopressor, and Tenormin
Carbamazepine (Tegretol)
Cimetidine (Tagamet)
Cyclophosphamide (Cytoxan)
Heart-stabilizing drugs such as Rythmol and Tambocor
Levodopa (Larodopa)
Nicotine patches such as Habitrol, NicoDerm CQ, and Nicotrol patch
Orphenadrine (Norgesic)
Phenobarbital
Phenytoin (Dilantin)

Special information if you are pregnant or breastfeeding

If you are pregnant or plan to become pregnant, notify your doctor immediately. Wellbutrin should be taken during pregnancy only if clearly needed.

Wellbutrin does pass into breast milk and may cause serious reactions in a nursing baby; therefore, if you are a new mother, you may need to discontinue breastfeeding while you are taking this medication.

Recommended dosage

ADULTS

Wellbutrin
At the beginning, your dose will probably be 200 milligrams per day, taken as 100 milligrams 2 times a day. After at least 3 days at this dose, your doctor may increase the dosage to 300 milligrams per day, taken as 100 milligrams 3 times a day, with at least 6 hours between doses. This is the usual adult dose. The maximum recommended dosage is 450 milligrams per day taken in doses of no more than 150 milligrams each.

Wellbutrin SR
The usual starting dose is 150 milligrams in the morning. After 3 days, if you do well, your doctor will have you take another 150 milligrams at least 8 hours after the first dose. It may be 4 weeks before you feel the benefit and you will take the drug for several months. The maximum recommended dose is 400 milligrams a day, taken in doses of 200 milligrams each.

If you have severe cirrhosis of the liver, your dosage should be no more than 75 milligrams once a day. With less serious liver and kidney problems, the dosage will be reduced as needed.

Wellbutrin XL
The usual starting dose is 150 milligrams taken once a day in the morning. If this dose is well tolerated after a minimum of 3 days, the doctor may increase the dose to 300 milligrams, also taken once a day in the morning. If no improvement is seen after several weeks of treatment, the doctor may increase the dose to a maximum of 450 milligrams once a day.

If you have severe liver damage, use this drug with extreme caution. Your dose should not exceed 150 milligrams every other day. People with mild to moderate liver damage or kidney impairment will be prescribed a lower dose as well.

CHILDREN

The safety and effectiveness in children under 18 years old have not been established.

Overdosage

There have been rare reports of death after an overdose of Wellbutrin. If you suspect an overdose, seek medical attention immediately.

■ *Symptoms of Wellbutrin overdose may include:*
Hallucinations, heart failure, loss of consciousness, rapid heartbeat, seizures

■ *Symptoms of Wellbutrin SR overdose may include:*
Blurred vision, confusion, jitteriness, lethargy, light-headedness, nausea, seizures, vomiting

■ *An overdose that involves other drugs in combination with Wellbutrin may also cause these symptoms:*
Breathing difficulties, coma, fever, rigid muscles, stupor

XALATAN
Pronounced: ZAL-a-tan
Generic name: Latanoprost

Why is this drug prescribed?
Xalatan is used to relieve high pressure within the eye (a hallmark of the condition known as open-angle glaucoma). It can be prescribed alone or with other glaucoma medications.

Most important fact about this drug
Be careful not to let the tip of the Xalatan bottle touch your eye or anything else. Otherwise, the contents could become contaminated. A contaminated solution can cause an eye infection and lead to serious damage, including loss of vision.

How should you use this medication?
Use Xalatan exactly as prescribed. It should be applied only once a day; more frequent administration may reduce its effectiveness. Apply 1 drop to the eye in the evening. If you are using other eye drops to lower pressure, allow at least 5 minutes between applications of the two medications. Contact lenses should be removed before the drug is applied. Wait 15 minutes before reinserting them.

■ *If you miss a dose...*
Apply it as soon as possible. If you don't remember until the next day, skip the dose and go back to your regular schedule. Never double the dose.

■ *Storage instructions...*
Store unopened bottles in the refrigerator. Once opened, the bottles may be stored at room temperature for up to 6 weeks. Protect from light.

What side effects may occur?
Side effects cannot be anticipated. If any develop or change in intensity, inform your doctor as soon as possible. Be especially quick to report pinkeye or any effects on the eyelids. Only your doctor can determine if it is safe for you to continue using Xalatan.

■ *Side effects may include...*
Bloodshot eyes, blurred vision, burning, foreign body sensation, increased pigmentation of the iris, inflammatory disease of the cornea, itching, stinging, upper respiratory infection

Why should this drug not be prescribed?
Do not use Xalatan if you are sensitive or allergic to any of its ingredients.

Special warnings about this medication
Xalatan may gradually turn the eye's iris brown. This change may not be noticed for months or years. Its long-term effects are unknown, but it may be permanent. Ask your doctor about the possibility of mismatched eye color if you will be treating only one eye with Xalatan.

Xalatan may make the eyelids darker. It can gradually change the eyelashes and fine body hair, increasing the length, thickness, color, and number of lashes or hairs. The eyelashes may also start growing in the wrong direction, possibly resulting in irritation to the eye.

If your eye sustains an injury or becomes infected, or you have eye surgery, you may need to start a new bottle of Xalatan. Be sure to check with your doctor.

Xalatan may cause blurred vision. Make certain it does not have this effect on you before you attempt to drive.

Possible food and drug interactions when using this medication
Mixing Xalatan with eyedrops containing thiomersal can cause the formation of solid substances in the eye. To avoid this problem, administer the drops at least 5 minutes apart.

Special information if you are pregnant or breastfeeding
The effects of Xalatan during pregnancy and breastfeeding have not been adequately studied. If you are pregnant or plan to become pregnant, notify your doctor immediately. It is not known whether Xalatan makes it way into breast milk. If you are nursing and need to use Xalatan, your doctor may advise you to discontinue breastfeeding while using the medication.

Recommended dosage
The usual dose is 1 drop in the affected eye once every evening.

Overdosage
Any medication taken in excess can have serious consequences. If you suspect an overdose, seek medical attention immediately.

■ *Symptoms of Xalatan overdose may include:*
Bloodshot eyes, eye irritation

XANAX

Pronounced: ZAN-ax
Generic name: Alprazolam
Other brand name: Xanax XR

Why is this drug prescribed?

Xanax is a tranquilizer used in the short-term relief of symptoms of anxiety or the treatment of anxiety disorders. Anxiety disorder is marked by unrealistic worry or excessive fears and concerns. Anxiety associated with depression is also responsive to Xanax.

Xanax and the extended-release formulation, Xanax XR, are also used in the treatment of panic disorder, which appears as unexpected panic attacks and may be accompanied by a fear of open or public places called agoraphobia. Only your doctor can diagnose panic disorder and best advise you about treatment.

Some doctors prescribe Xanax to treat alcohol withdrawal, fear of open spaces and strangers, depression, irritable bowel syndrome, and premenstrual syndrome.

Most important fact about this drug

Tolerance and dependence can occur with the use of Xanax. You may experience withdrawal symptoms if you suddenly stop using the drug or reduce the dosage too quickly. Withdrawal symptoms are listed under *What side effects may occur?* The drug dosage should be gradually reduced and only your doctor should advise you on how to discontinue or change your dose.

How should you take this medication?

Xanax may be taken with or without food. Take it exactly as prescribed. Do not chew, crush, or break the Xanax XR tablets.

- *If you miss a dose...*
  If you are less than 1 hour late, take it as soon as you remember. Otherwise skip the dose and go back to your regular schedule. Never take 2 doses at the same time.
- *Storage instructions...*
  Store Xanax at room temperature.

What side effects may occur?

Side effects cannot be anticipated. If any develop or change in intensity, inform your doctor as soon as possible. Only your doctor can determine if it is safe for you to continue taking Xanax. Your doctor should periodically reassess the need for this drug.

Side effects of Xanax are usually seen at the beginning of treatment and disappear with continued medication. However, if dosage is increased, side effects will be more likely.

■ *Side effects of Xanax may include:*
Decreased libido, drowsiness, fatigue, impaired coordination, memory impairment, speech difficulties, weight changes

■ *Side effects of Xanax XR may include:*
Constipation, decreased libido, depression, drowsiness, fatigue, impaired coordination, memory problems, mental impairment, nausea, sedation, sleepiness, speech difficulties, weight changes

■ *Side effects due to a rapid decrease in dose or abrupt withdrawal from Xanax or Xanax XR:*
Anxiety, blurred vision, decreased concentration, decreased mental clarity, depression, diarrhea, headache, heightened awareness of noise or bright lights, hot flushes, impaired sense of smell, insomnia, loss of appetite, loss of reality, muscle cramps, nervousness, rapid breathing, seizures, tingling sensation, tremor, twitching, weight loss

Why should this drug not be prescribed?

If you are sensitive to or have ever had an allergic reaction to Xanax or other tranquilizers, you should not take this medication. Also avoid Xanax while taking the antifungal drugs Sporanox or Nizoral. Make sure that your doctor is aware of any drug reactions that you have experienced.

Do not take this medication if you have been diagnosed with the eye condition called narrow-angle glaucoma.

Anxiety or tension related to everyday stress usually does not require treatment with Xanax. Discuss your symptoms thoroughly with your doctor.

Special warnings about this medication

Xanax may cause you to become drowsy or less alert; therefore, driving or operating dangerous machinery or participating in any hazardous activity that requires full mental alertness is not recommended.

If you are being treated for panic disorder, you may need to take a higher dose of Xanax than for anxiety alone. High doses—more than 4 milligrams a day—of this medication taken for long intervals may cause emotional and physical dependence. It is important that your doctor supervise you carefully when you are using this medication.

As with all antianxiety medication, there is a small chance that Xanax could encourage suicidal thoughts or episodes of euphoria known as mania. If you notice any new or unusual symptoms after starting Xanax, call your doctor immediately.

Xanax should be used with caution in elderly or weak patients, and in those with lung disease, alcoholic liver disease, or any disorder that could hinder the elimination of the drug.

Possible food and drug interactions when taking this medication

Xanax may intensify the effect of alcohol. Do not drink alcohol while taking this medication.

Never combine Xanax with Sporanox or Nizoral. These drugs cause a buildup of Xanax in the body.

If Xanax is taken with certain other drugs, the effects of either could be increased, decreased, or altered. It is important to check with your doctor before combining Xanax with the following:

Amiodarone (Cordarone)
Antihistamines such as Benadryl and Tavist
Carbamazepine (Tegretol)
Certain antibiotics such as Biaxin and erythromycin
Certain antidepressant drugs, including Elavil, Norpramin, and Tofranil
Cimetidine (Tagamet)
Cyclosporine (Neoral, Sandimmune)
Digoxin (Lanoxin)
Diltiazem (Cardizem)
Disulfiram (Antabuse)
Ergotamine
Fluoxetine (Prozac)
Fluvoxamine
Grapefruit juice
Isoniazid (Rifamate)
Major tranquilizers such as chlorpromazine and Mellaril
Nefazodone
Nicardipine (Cardene)
Nifedipine (Adalat, Procardia)
Oral contraceptives
Other central nervous system depressants such as Demerol and Valium
Paroxetine (Paxil)
Propoxyphene (Darvon)
Sertraline (Zoloft)

Special information if you are pregnant or breastfeeding

Do not take this medication if you are pregnant or planning to become pregnant. There is an increased risk of respiratory problems and muscular weakness in your baby. Infants may also experience withdrawal symptoms. Xanax may appear in breast milk and could affect a nursing infant. If this medication is essential to your health, your doctor may advise you to stop breastfeeding until your treatment with this medication is finished.

Recommended dosage

ADULTS

Anxiety Disorder
The usual starting dose of Xanax is 0.25 to 0.5 milligram taken 3 times a day. The dose may be increased every 3 to 4 days to a maximum daily dose of 4 milligrams, divided into smaller doses.

Panic Disorder
The usual starting dose of regular Xanax is 0.5 milligram 3 times a day. This dose can be increased by 1 milligram a day every 3 or 4 days. You may be given a dose from 1 up to a total of 10 milligrams, according to your needs. The typical dose is 5 to 6 milligrams a day.

If you're taking Xanax XR, the usual starting dose is 0.5 to 1 milligram once a day taken in the morning. Depending on your response, the dose may be gradually increased by no more than 1 milligram every 3 or 4 days. The usual effective dose is 3 to 6 milligrams a day. Some people may need a larger dose to relieve their symptoms. Others, including older adults and those with liver disease or other serious illnesses, may need to use lower doses.

CHILDREN

The safety and effectiveness of Xanax have not been established in children under 18 years of age.

OLDER ADULTS

The usual starting dose for an anxiety disorder is 0.25 milligram 2 or 3 times daily. The starting dose of Xanax XR is 0.5 milligram once a day. This dose may be gradually increased if needed and tolerated.

PATIENTS SWITCHING FROM XANAX TO XANAX XR

If you're taking divided doses of Xanax, the doctor will switch you to a once-daily dose of Xanax XR that equals the current amount you're taking. If your symptoms return after switching, the dose can be increased as needed.

Overdosage

An overdose of Xanax, alone or after combining it with alcohol, can be fatal. If you suspect an overdose, seek medical attention immediately.

■ *Symptoms of Xanax overdose may include:*
Confusion, coma, impaired coordination, sleepiness, slowed reaction time

XENICAL

Pronounced: ZEN-eh-kal
Generic name: Orlistat

Why is this drug prescribed?

Xenical blocks absorption of dietary fat into the bloodstream, thereby reducing the number of calories you get from a meal. At the usual dosage level, it cuts fat absorption by almost one-third. Combined with a low-calorie diet, it is used to promote weight loss and discourage the return of unwanted pounds.

The drug is prescribed for obese individuals and for overweight people who have other health problems such as high blood pressure, diabetes, or high cholesterol levels. Your weight status is determined by your body mass index (BMI), a comparison of height to weight.

Most important fact about this drug

Along with dietary fat, Xenical decreases the absorption of some fat-soluble vitamins and beta-carotene. To compensate, it is strongly recommended that you take a multivitamin containing vitamins A, E, D, K, and beta-carotene once a day, at least 2 hours before or 2 hours after taking Xenical.

How should you take this medication?

Take a capsule of Xenical during, or up to 1 hour after, each main meal. You should follow a nutritionally balanced, low-calorie diet that provides no more than 30 percent of its calories from fat. If you miss a meal, or the meal contains no fat, you can skip the accompanying dose of Xenical.

■ *If you miss a dose...*
  Resume taking Xenical at the next meal. Don't try to make up the loss with a double dose. The extra drug won't help.
■ *Storage instructions...*
  Store at room temperature, in a tightly sealed container.

What side effects may occur?

Side effects of Xenical are more common during the first year of treatment. If any develop or change in intensity, inform your doctor as soon as possible. Only your doctor can determine if it is safe for you to continue taking Xenical.

■ *Side effects may include:*
  Abdominal discomfort or pain, anxiety, arthritis, back pain, diarrhea, dizziness, earache, fatigue, fatty or oily stools, fecal urgency or incontinence, flu, gas with fecal discharge, gum problems, headache, increased defecation, menstrual problems, muscle pain, nausea, oily

discharge, rectal discomfort or pain, respiratory tract infections, skin rash, sleep problems, tooth problems, urinary tract infections, vaginal inflammation, vomiting

Side effects that usually occur *after* the first year of treatment with Xenical include depression, leg pain, swollen feet, and tendonitis.

Why should this drug not be prescribed?

Do not take Xenical if you suffer from chronic malabsorption syndrome—a condition that prevents nutrients from passing from your stomach into your bloodstream—or from cholestasis, a blockage in the supply of bile needed for digestion. You'll also need to avoid Xenical if it gives you an allergic reaction.

Special warnings about this medication

Weight loss begins within 2 weeks and continues for 6 to 12 months. The effect of using Xenical for more than 2 years is still unknown.

Side effects such as diarrhea and abdominal pain may be worse if you continue eating a high-fat diet or even take a high-fat meal. Limit your fat intake.

Your doctor will test your thyroid function before starting you on Xenical to make sure that your weight problem is not due to an underactive thyroid gland (hypothyroidism). Xenical is not an appropriate remedy for this problem.

Xenical increases the likelihood of kidney stones. Use it with caution if you have a history of this problem.

If you have diabetes, weight loss is likely to reduce your blood sugar levels. If you're taking an oral diabetes medication or insulin, your dose may have to be reduced.

Note that the safety and efficacy of this drug in children younger than 12 years old have not been established.

Possible food and drug interactions when taking this medication

If Xenical is taken with certain other drugs, the effects of either could be increased, decreased, or altered. It is especially important to check with your doctor before combining Xenical with the following:

Cyclosporine (Neoral, Sandimmune)
Warfarin (Coumadin)

Special information if you are pregnant or breastfeeding

The effects of Xenical during pregnancy have not been adequately studied, and the drug is not recommended for pregnant women. If you are pregnant or plan to become pregnant, inform your doctor immediately.

It is not known whether Xenical appears in breast milk. Do not take it while breastfeeding.

Recommended dosage

ADULTS AND CHILDREN 12 YEARS AND OLDER

The recommended dose is one 120-milligram capsule 3 times daily with each main meal containing fat.

Overdosage

The results of a massive overdose of Xenical are unknown, although the drug seems relatively harmless. However, any medication taken in excess can have serious consequences. If you suspect an overdose, seek medical attention.

XIFAXAN
Pronounced: zuh-FAX-in
Generic name: Rifaximin

Why is this drug prescribed?

Xifaxan is an antibiotic prescribed to treat traveler's diarrhea, a bacterial infection in the intestines caused by *Escherichia coli* (also called *E. coli*). Traveler's diarrhea is the result of eating contaminated food or drinking untreated water, usually in foreign countries. Xifaxan is not prescribed for diarrhea that occurs with a fever or bloody stools, or when the diarrhea is not due to *E. coli*.

Most important fact about this drug

Like all antibiotics, Xifaxan could cause a severe inflammation of the colon (known as pseudomembranous colitis). It results from bacterial overgrowth in the colon and ranges in severity from mild to life-threatening. Contact your doctor right away if you develop any of the following:

    Abdominal cramps
    Bloody stools
    Frequent bowel movements
    Low-grade fever
    Watery diarrhea

How should you take this medication?

Xifaxan can be taken with food or on an empty stomach. It is best to take it at evenly spaced intervals throughout the day to keep a constant supply in the bloodstream.

■ *If you miss a dose...*
    Take the forgotten dose as soon as you remember. However, if it is almost time for your next dose, skip the one you missed and return to your regular schedule. Do not take 2 doses at once.

■ *Storage instructions…*
Store at room temperature.

What side effects may occur?
Side effects cannot be anticipated. If any develop or change in intensity, tell your doctor as soon as possible. Only your doctor can determine if it is safe to continue using Xifaxan.

■ *Side effects may include:*
Abdominal pain, constipation, fever or high body temperature, gas, headache, nausea, painful or urgent bowel movements, vomiting

Why should this drug not be prescribed?
Do not take Xifaxan if you are allergic to it or if you have ever had an allergic reaction to other rifamycin antibiotics, such as rifabutin (Mycobutin), rifampin (Rifadin, Rimactane), and rifapentine (Priftin).

Special warnings about this medication
Xifaxan is useful only in cases of diarrhea that are caused by *E. coli*. If your symptoms get worse, if you develop new symptoms such as a fever or bloody diarrhea, or if you do not get better within 1 to 2 days, call your doctor right away. You will probably need to stop taking Xifaxan and start a different treatment.

Possible food and drug interactions when taking this medication
At this time, there are no documented drug interactions with Xifaxan. However, you should always tell the doctor about any medicines you take, including over-the-counter drugs, vitamins, and herbal supplements.

Special information if you are pregnant or breastfeeding
Xifaxan has not been studied in pregnant women and should only be used if the benefits outweigh the potential risks.

It is not known whether Xifaxan appears in human breast milk. If this drug is essential to your health, the doctor may advise you to stop nursing until your treatment is finished.

Recommended dosage

ADULTS AND CHILDREN 12 YEARS AND OLDER

The usual recommended dose is one 200-milligram tablet taken 3 times a day for 3 days.

Xifaxan has not been studied in children less than 12 years old.

Overdosage
While there is no specific overdose information about Xifaxan, any medication taken in excess can have serious consequences. If you suspect an overdose, seek medical attention immediately.

XOPENEX

Pronounced: ZOH-pen-ecks
Generic name: Levalbuterol hydrochloride

Why is this drug prescribed?

Xopenex is a bronchodilator. It works by relaxing the muscles in the walls of the lungs' many tiny airways (bronchioles), allowing them to expand so you can get more air. It is prescribed for asthma.

Most important fact about this drug

If your prescribed dosage of Xopenex does not provide relief, or your symptoms become worse, consult your doctor immediately.

How should you take this medication?

Do not use more Xopenex than prescribed. Increasing the number of doses can be dangerous and may actually make your asthma worse.

Xopenex should be taken only with an inhalation device called a nebulizer. Do not add any other drugs to the nebulizer without first asking your doctor.

■ *If you miss a dose...*
Take the forgotten dose as soon as you remember; then take any remaining doses for that day at equally spaced intervals. Never take a double dose.

■ *Storage instructions...*
Store unopened vials of Xopenex inhalation solution in their protective foil pouch at room temperature, away from light and excessive heat. Once the foil pouch has been opened, the vials should be used within 1 to 2 weeks. Once a vial has been opened, the contents should be used immediately or discarded. The solution should be colorless. If not, throw the vial out.

What side effects may occur?

Side effects cannot be anticipated. If any develop or change in intensity, inform your doctor as soon as possible. Only your doctor can determine if it is safe for you to continue taking Xopenex.

■ *Side effects may include:*
Cough, flu symptoms, nervousness, runny nose, sinus inflammation, tremors, viral infection

■ *Side effects in children may include:*
Diarrhea, fever, headache, hives, increased asthma symptoms, muscle pain, rash, runny nose, sore throat, swollen glands, viral infection, weakness

Why should this drug not be prescribed?

If Xopenex gives you an allergic reaction, you will not be able to use it.

Special warnings about this medication

There is a slight chance of developing an immediate, serious allergic reaction to Xopenex, with symptoms such as hives, rash, mouth and throat swelling, and bronchospasm (constricted airways and difficulty breathing). If this happens, or you experience bronchospasm alone, stop using Xopenex and call your doctor immediately.

If your asthma symptoms get worse despite Xopenex, call your doctor. He may need to add an anti-inflammatory steroid drug such as prednisone or beclomethasone to your treatment regimen.

.Use Xopenex with caution if you have a heart condition, an irregular heartbeat, or high blood pressure. Call your doctor immediately if you notice any change in heartbeat, pulse, or blood pressure. Caution is also advised if you suffer from seizures, an overactive thyroid gland, or diabetes.

Possible food and drug interactions when taking this medication

Xopenex should be used cautiously, if at all, with other bronchodilators such as Proventil, Ventolin, or Primatene Mist.

If Xopenex is taken with certain other drugs, the effects of either could be increased, decreased, or altered. It is especially important to check with your doctor before combining Xopenex with the following:

Antidepressant drugs classified as MAO inhibitors (Marplan, Nardil, Parnate) or tricyclics (Elavil, Tofranil)
Beta-blockers (heart and blood pressure drugs) such as Inderal, Lopressor, and Tenormin
Digoxin (Lanoxin)
Diuretics (water pills) that lower your potassium levels such as Lasix and HydroDIURIL

Special information if you are pregnant or breastfeeding

The effects of Xopenex during pregnancy have not been adequately studied. If you are pregnant or plan to become pregnant, inform your doctor immediately. It is not known whether Xopenex appears in breast milk, but it's considered wise to either give up breastfeeding or discontinue the drug.

Recommended dosage

ADULTS

For adults and children 12 and older, the usual starting dose is 0.63 milligram 3 times a day by nebulizer, every 6 to 8 hours. Your doctor will increase the dose to 1.25 milligrams 3 times a day if you have severe asthma or the lower dose fails to provide relief.

CHILDREN

For children 6 through 11 years old, the usual dosage is 0.31 milligram 3 times a day by nebulizer. A dosage of more than 0.63 milligram 3 times daily is not recommended.

Overdosage

Any medication taken in excess can have serious consequences. If you suspect an overdose of Xopenex, seek medical attention immediately.

■ *Symptoms of Xopenex overdose may include:*
   Chest pain, dizziness, dry mouth, fatigue, flu symptoms, headache, high blood pressure, irregular heartbeat, insomnia, low blood pressure, nausea, nervousness, rapid heartbeat, tremors, seizures

Yasmin *See Oral Contraceptives, page 1000.*

YOCON

Pronounced: YOE-kon
Generic name: Yohimbine hydrochloride
Other brand name: Yohimex

Why is this drug prescribed?

Yocon is used in the treatment of male impotence. The drug is thought to work by stimulating the release of norepinephrine, one of the body's natural chemical regulators. This results in increased blood flow to the penis.

Most important fact about this drug

Yocon does not work for all men. Your doctor will determine if Yocon can be prescribed for you.

How should you take this medication?

Take this medication exactly as prescribed.

■ *If you miss a dose...*
   Take it as soon as you remember. If it is almost time for your next dose, skip the one you missed and go back to your regular schedule. Never take 2 doses at the same time.
■ *Storage instructions...*
   Keep this medication in the container it came in, tightly closed, and out of the reach of children. Store it at room temperature, away from moist places and direct light.

What side effects may occur?

Side effects cannot be anticipated. If any develop or change in intensity, inform your doctor as soon as possible. Only your doctor can determine if it is safe for you to continue taking Yocon.

■ *Side effects may include:*
Decreased urination, dizziness, flushing, headache, increase in blood pressure, increased heart rate, increased motor activity, irritability, nausea, nervousness, tremor

Why should this drug not be prescribed?

Yocon should not be used if you have kidney disease, or if you are sensitive to or have ever had an allergic reaction to yohimbine. Make sure your doctor is aware of any drug reactions you have experienced.

Special warnings about this medication

Yocon is generally not recommended for use by children, the elderly, or men with heart and kidney disease who also have a history of stomach or duodenal ulcer. The drug is also not recommended for men being treated for a psychiatric disorder.

Possible food and drug interactions when taking this medication

It is important that you consult with your doctor before taking Yocon with drugs for depression such as Elavil or other drugs that change mood.

Special information if you are pregnant or breastfeeding

Yocon is not recommended for use in women generally and certainly must not be used during pregnancy.

Recommended dosage

ADULTS

Dosages of this drug are based on experimental research in the treatment of male impotence.

This dosage is one 5.4-milligram tablet, 3 times a day.

If you experience nausea, dizziness, or nervousness, your doctor will reduce the dose to one-half tablet 3 times a day, and then increase it gradually back up to 1 tablet 3 times a day.

CHILDREN

This drug is not for use in children.

OLDER ADULTS

This drug should not be used by older men.

Overdosage

Any medication taken in excess can cause symptoms of overdose. If you suspect an overdose, seek medical attention immediately. No specific symptoms of Yocon overdose have been reported.

Yohimbine See *Yocon,* page 1604.

Yohimex *See Yocon, page 1604.*

ZADITOR
Pronounced: ZA-di-tor
Generic name: Ketotifen fumarate

Why is this drug prescribed?
Zaditor combats the release of chemicals that trigger allergic reactions. Available in eyedrop form, it works within minutes to relieve the itchy eyes brought on by allergies.

Most important fact about this drug
Zaditor is for use in the eyes only. Do not inject or swallow this drug.

How should you take this medication?
To prevent contamination, do not touch the eyelids, eye, or surrounding areas with the dropper tip of the bottle.

■ *If you miss a dose...*
Apply it as soon as you remember. If it is almost time for your next dose, skip the one you missed and go back to your regular schedule. Never apply more than 1 drop at a time.

■ *Storage instructions...*
Keep the bottle tightly closed when it is not in use. Store between 39 and 77 degrees Fahrenheit.

What side effects may occur?
■ *Side effects may include:*
Headache, increased blood flow in the eyelid, runny nose

Why should this drug not be prescribed?
If you are allergic to any of the ingredients in Zaditor, you'll be unable to use it.

Special warnings about this medication
Do not wear contact lenses if your eyes are red or irritated, and do not use Zaditor to treat irritation from contact lenses. If you wear soft contact lenses, wait at least 10 minutes after applying Zaditor before inserting them.

The safety and effectiveness of Zaditor in children below the age of 3 years have not been established.

Possible food and drug interactions when taking this medication
Since Zaditor is not ingested, interactions are unlikely.

Special information if you are pregnant or breastfeeding

The possibility that Zaditor could harm a developing baby has not been ruled out. Inform your doctor immediately if you are pregnant or plan to become pregnant during treatment with the drug.

Researchers do not know whether Zaditor can make its way into breast milk, but caution is advised if you're nursing.

Recommended dosage

The recommended dose is 1 drop in the affected eye(s) twice daily, every 8 to 12 hours.

Overdosage

Overdosage is highly unlikely since swallowing even a whole bottle of Zaditor would give you only a fraction of the amount considered toxic. Nevertheless, if you suspect an overdose, check with your doctor immediately.

Zafirlukast See Accolate, page 4.

Zalcitabine See Hivid, page 652.

Zaleplon See Sonata, page 1324.

ZANAFLEX
Pronounced: ZAN-uh-flecks
Generic name: Tizanidine

Why is this drug prescribed?

Zanaflex relaxes the tense, rigid muscles caused by spasticity. It is prescribed for people with multiple sclerosis, spinal cord injuries, and other disorders that produce protracted muscle spasms. The effect of the drug peaks 1 to 2 hours after each dose and is gone within 3 to 6 hours, so it's best to schedule doses for shortly before the daily activities when relief of spasticity is most important.

Most important fact about this drug

Zanaflex causes drowsiness in almost half the people who use it. It also tends to reduce blood pressure in many people, frequently leading to dizziness and light-headedness. The likelihood of significant drowsiness increases when Zanaflex is combined with other spasticity drugs, such as Lioresal, Klonopin, and Valium. When taking Zanaflex, always be cautious about driving or operating dangerous machinery.

How should you take this medication?

Take Zanaflex exactly as directed. The danger of side effects increases with the size of the dose.

■ *If you miss a dose...*
Doses should be taken only as needed. Allow 6 to 8 hours between doses. Take no more than 3 a day. Never double the dose.

■ *Storage instructions...*
Store at room temperature.

What side effects may occur?
Side effects cannot be anticipated. If any develop or change in intensity, tell your doctor as soon as possible. Only your doctor can determine if it is safe to continue using Zanaflex.

■ *Side effects may include:*
Abnormal movements, blurred vision, constipation, dizziness, drowsiness, dry mouth, flu-like symptoms, frequent urination, low blood pressure, nervousness, runny nose, slow heartbeat, sore throat, speech disorders, urinary and other infections, vomiting, weakness or fatigue

Why should this drug not be prescribed?
You'll need to avoid Zanaflex if it gives you an allergic reaction.

Special warnings about this medication
Researchers have little information on the long-term consequences of using Zanaflex in single doses of more than 8 milligrams, or in total amounts of more than 24 milligrams a day. If you require a higher dosage, previously unrecognized side effects could possibly appear.

Remember that Zanaflex can cause low blood pressure and should be used with caution if you are taking blood pressure medication. Be cautious, too, when first standing up. Dizziness and light-headedness are especially likely at that time.

Zanaflex has been known to cause liver injury in a few patients. If you have a liver condition, make sure the doctor knows about it. Alert your doctor immediately if you develop warning signs of a liver problem such as loss of appetite, nausea, vomiting, or yellow skin or eyes.

You'll need a reduced dose of Zanaflex if you have a kidney problem. Be sure to inform the doctor about your condition, and be quick to report side effects such as dry mouth, drowsiness, dizziness, and weakness. They could be signs that your dose is too high.

Use Zanaflex with caution if spasticity helps you maintain your posture and balance while walking, or helps to increase other functions.

Although there are no reports of eye damage from Zanaflex, it has occurred in animal tests. Be sure to report any vision problems to your doctor.

Zanaflex has not been tested in children.

Possible food and drug interactions when taking this medication
Oral contraceptives tend to boost the amount of Zanaflex in the system. If you are using an oral contraceptive, you'll probably need a smaller dose of this drug.

Alcohol, or any drug that slows the nervous system (including other drugs taken for spasticity), increases the likelihood of drowsiness when taken with Zanaflex.

Special information if you are pregnant or breastfeeding
The effects of Zanaflex during pregnancy have not been adequately studied. It should be used during pregnancy only if clearly needed.

It's likely that Zanaflex makes its way into breast milk, although this has not been confirmed. Check with your doctor before using Zanaflex while nursing.

Recommended dosage

ADULTS

To minimize side effects, the doctor is likely to begin with a dosage of 4 milligrams, then increase the dose gradually. Doses of 8 milligrams provide relief for most people. No more than 3 doses should be taken each 24 hours. The maximum dose per day is 36 milligrams.

Overdosage
An overdose of Zanaflex can impair breathing and lead to coma. If you suspect an overdose, seek emergency treatment immediately.

Zanamivir See Relenza, page 1227.

ZANTAC
Pronounced: ZAN-tac
Generic name: Ranitidine hydrochloride

Why is this drug prescribed?
Zantac is prescribed for the short-term treatment (4 to 8 weeks) of active duodenal ulcer and active benign gastric ulcer, and as maintenance therapy for gastric or duodenal ulcer, at a reduced dosage, after the ulcer has healed. It is also used for the treatment of conditions in which the stomach produces too much acid, such as Zollinger-Ellison syndrome and systemic mastocytosis, for gastroesophageal reflux disease (backflow of acid stomach contents) and for healing—and maintaining healing of—erosive esophagitis (severe inflammation of the esophagus).

Some doctors prescribe Zantac to prevent damage to the stomach and duodenum from long-term use of nonsteroidal anti-inflammatory drugs such as Indocin and Motrin, and to treat bleeding of the stomach and intestine. Zantac is also sometimes prescribed for stress-induced ulcers.

Most important fact about this drug
Zantac helps to prevent the recurrence of gastric or duodenal ulcers and aids the healing of ulcers that do occur.

How should you take this medication?
Take this medication exactly as prescribed by your doctor. Make sure you follow the diet your doctor recommends.

Dissolve Efferdose tablets and granules in 6 to 8 ounces of water before taking them.

You can take an antacid for pain while you are taking Zantac.

- *If you miss a dose...*
  Take it as soon as you remember. If it is almost time for your next dose, skip the one you missed and go back to your regular schedule. Never take 2 doses at the same time.
- *Storage instructions...*
  Store this medication at room temperature in the container it came in, tightly closed and away from moist places and direct light. Keep Zantac Syrup from freezing.

What side effects may occur?
Side effects cannot be anticipated. If any develop or change in intensity, inform your doctor as soon as possible. Only your doctor can determine if it is safe for you to continue taking Zantac.

- *Side effects may include:*
  Headache, sometimes severe

Why should this drug not be prescribed?
If you are sensitive to or have ever had an allergic reaction to Zantac or similar drugs such as Tagamet, you should not take this medication. Make sure that your doctor is aware of any drug reactions that you have experienced.

Special warnings about this medication
A stomach malignancy could be present, even if your symptoms have been relieved by Zantac.

If you have kidney or liver disease, this drug should be used with caution.

If you have phenylketonuria, you should be aware that the Efferdose tablets and granules contain phenylalanine.

Possible food and drug interactions when taking this medication

If Zantac is taken with certain other drugs, the effects of either could be increased, decreased, or altered. It is especially important to check with your doctor before combining Zantac with the following:

Alcohol
Blood-thinning drugs such as Coumadin
Diazepam (Valium)
Diltiazem (Cardizem)
Enoxacin (Penetrex)
Glipizide (Glucotrol)
Glyburide (DiaBeta, Micronase)
Itraconazole (Sporanox)
Ketoconazole (Nizoral)
Metformin (Glucophage)
Nifedipine (Procardia)
Phenytoin (Dilantin)
Procainamide (Procan SR)
Sucralfate (Carafate)
Theophylline (Theo-Dur)
Triazolam (Halcion)

Special information if you are pregnant or breastfeeding

The effects of Zantac in pregnancy have not been adequately studied. If you are pregnant or plan to become pregnant, inform your doctor immediately. Zantac appears in breast milk and could affect a nursing infant. If this medication is essential to your health, your doctor may advise you to discontinue breastfeeding until your treatment with this medication is finished.

Recommended dosage

ADULTS

Active Duodenal Ulcer

The usual starting dose is 150 milligrams 2 times a day or 10 milliliters (2 teaspoonfuls) 2 times a day. Your doctor also might prescribe 300 milligrams or 20 milliliters (4 teaspoonfuls) once a day, after the evening meal or at bedtime, if necessary for your convenience. The dose should be the lowest effective dose. Long-term use should be reduced to a daily total of 150 milligrams or 10 milliliters (2 teaspoonfuls), taken at bedtime.

Other Excess Acid Conditions
(Such as Zollinger-Ellison Syndrome)

The usual dose is 150 milligrams or 10 milliliters (2 teaspoonfuls) 2 times a day. This dose can be adjusted upwards by your doctor.

Benign Gastric Ulcer and Gastroesophageal Reflux Disease (GERD)

The usual dose is 150 milligrams or 10 milliliters (2 teaspoonfuls) 2 times a day. Once an ulcer has cleared up, a single bedtime dose is prescribed to maintain healing. Symptoms of GERD generally improve within 24 hours after the start of therapy.

Erosive Esophagitis

The usual dose is 150 milligrams or 10 milliliters (2 teaspoonfuls) 4 times a day. Maintenance dosage is 150 milligrams or 10 milliliters (2 teaspoonfuls) twice a day.

CHILDREN

Duodenal and Gastric Ulcers

For children 1 month to 16 years of age, the recommended dosage for initial treatment is 2 to 4 milligrams per 2.2 pounds of body weight per day twice daily up to a maximum of 300 milligrams per day. For long-term maintenance of healing, the recommendation is 2 to 4 milligrams per 2.2 pounds of body weight once daily up to a maximum of 150 milligrams per day.

Gastroesophageal Reflux Disease (GERD) and Erosive Esophagitis

For children 1 month to 16 years of age, the usual daily dosage is 5 to 10 milligrams per 2.2 pounds of body weight, divided into two doses.

OLDER ADULTS

People with kidney problems, such as some older adults, typically are given a lower dose. During the therapy with Zantac, the doctor is also more likely to monitor your kidney function if you're over 65.

Overdosage

Any medication taken in excess can have serious consequences. If you suspect an overdose, seek medical attention immediately.

Information concerning Zantac overdosage is limited. However, an abnormal manner of walking, low blood pressure, and exaggerated side effect symptoms may be signs of an overdose.

If you experience any of these symptoms, notify your doctor immediately.

ZAROXOLYN

Pronounced: Zar-OX-uh-lin
Generic name: Metolazone
Other brand name: Mykrox

Why is this drug prescribed?

Zaroxolyn is a diuretic used in the treatment of high blood pressure and other conditions that require the elimination of excess fluid from the body. These conditions include congestive heart failure and kidney disease. When used for high blood pressure, Zaroxolyn can be used alone or with other high blood pressure medications. Diuretics prompt your body to produce and eliminate more urine, which helps lower blood pressure.

Zaroxolyn is also occasionally prescribed for kidney stones.

Most important fact about this drug

If you have high blood pressure, you must take Zaroxolyn regularly for it to be effective. Since blood pressure declines gradually, it may be several weeks before you get the full benefit of Zaroxolyn; and you must continue taking it even if you are feeling well. Zaroxolyn does not cure high blood pressure; it merely keeps it under control.

How should you take this medication?

Take Zaroxolyn exactly as prescribed. Stopping Zaroxolyn suddenly could cause your condition to worsen.

■ *If you miss a dose...*
Take it as soon as you remember. If it is almost time for the next dose, skip the one you missed and go back to your regular schedule. Do not take 2 doses at the same time.

■ *Storage instructions...*
Store at room temperature in a tightly closed, light-resistant container.

What side effects may occur?

Side effects cannot be anticipated. If any develop or change in intensity, inform your doctor as soon as possible. Only your doctor can determine if it is safe for you to continue taking Zaroxolyn.

■ *Side effects may include:*
Artery damage, blood abnormalities, chest pain/discomfort, fainting, inflammation of the pancreas, joint pain, weakness, yellow eyes and skin

Why should this drug not be prescribed?

If you are unable to urinate or have severe liver disease, you should not take this medication.

If you are sensitive to or have ever had an allergic reaction to Zaroxolyn or other diuretics such as HydroDIURIL, you should not take this medication.

Special warnings about this medication

Diuretics can cause your body to lose too much potassium. Signs of an excessively low potassium level include muscle weakness and rapid or irregular heartbeat. To boost your potassium level, your doctor may recommend eating potassium-rich foods or taking a potassium supplement.

If you are taking Zaroxolyn, your doctor will do a complete assessment of your kidney function and continue to monitor it.

Do not interchange Zaroxolyn and other formulations of metolazone such as Mykrox. The brands vary in potency of action.

If you have liver disease, diabetes, gout, or lupus erythematosus (a disease of the immune system), Zaroxolyn should be used with caution.

If you have had an allergic reaction to sulfa drugs, thiazides, or quinethazone, you may be at greater risk for an allergic reaction to this medication. You can have an allergic reaction to Zaroxolyn even if you have never had allergies or asthma.

Dehydration, excessive sweating, severe diarrhea, or vomiting could deplete your fluids and cause your blood pressure to become too low. Be careful when exercising and in hot weather.

Notify your doctor or dentist that you are taking Zaroxolyn if you have a medical emergency and before you have surgery or dental treatment.

Possible food and drug interactions when taking this medication

Zaroxolyn may intensify the effects of alcohol. Avoid drinking alcohol while taking this medication.

If Zaroxolyn is taken with certain other drugs, the effects of either could be increased, decreased, or altered. It is especially important to check with your doctor before combining Zaroxolyn with the following:

ACTH
Antidiabetic drugs such as Micronase
Barbiturates such as phenobarbital
Corticosteroids such as prednisone (Deltasone)
Digitalis glycosides such as Lanoxin
Insulin
Lithium (Lithonate)
Loop diuretics such as furosemide (Lasix)
Methenamine (Mandelamine)
Narcotics such as Percocet
Nonsteroidal anti-inflammatory agents such as Advil, Motrin,
    and Naprosyn
Norepinephrine (Levophed)
Other high blood pressure medications such as Aldomet
Tubocurarine

Special information if you are pregnant or breastfeeding

The effects of Zaroxolyn during pregnancy have not been adequately studied. If you are pregnant or plan to become pregnant, inform your doctor immediately. Zaroxolyn appears in breast milk and could affect a nursing infant. If this medication is essential to your health, your doctor may advise you to discontinue breastfeeding until your treatment is finished.

Recommended dosage

ADULTS

Your doctor will adjust the dosage of this medication to your individual needs and will use the lowest possible dose with the maximum effect. The time it takes for this medication to become effective varies from person to person, depending on the diagnosis.

Most starting doses of this medication will be given once a day.

Edema Due to Heart or Kidney Disorders
The usual dosage is 5 to 20 milligrams once a day.

Mild to Moderate High Blood Pressure
The usual dosage is 2.5 to 5 milligrams once a day.

CHILDREN

The safety and effectiveness of Zaroxolyn in children have not been established.

Overdosage

Any medication taken in excess can have serious consequences. If you suspect an overdose, seek medical attention immediately.

■ *Symptoms of Zaroxolyn overdose may include:*
Difficulty breathing, dizziness, dizziness on standing up, drowsiness, fainting, irritation of the stomach and intestines, lethargy leading to coma

ZEBETA

Pronounced: Zee-BEE-tah
Generic name: Bisoprolol fumarate

Why is this drug prescribed?

Zebeta, a type of medication known as a beta-blocker, is used to treat high blood pressure. Beta-blockers lower blood pressure by decreasing the force and rate of heart contractions, which reduces the heart's demand for oxygen. Zebeta can be used alone or in combination with other high blood pressure medications.

Most important fact about this drug

Zebeta does not cure high blood pressure; it merely keeps it under control. Therefore, you must continue taking it even if you are feeling well. Do not stop taking Zebeta unless instructed to do so by your doctor. This is especially important if you have coronary artery disease. Abruptly stopping Zebeta could cause chest pain, heart rhythm problems, and even heart attack.

How should you take this medication?

Take Zebeta exactly as prescribed, even if your symptoms have disappeared. Try not to miss any doses. If this medication is not taken regularly, your condition may worsen.

■ *If you miss a dose...*
Take the missed dose as soon as possible. However, if it is almost time for your next dose, skip the one you missed and go back to your regular schedule. Never take 2 doses at once.

■ *Storage instructions...*
Store at room temperature in a tightly closed container and protect from moisture.

What side effects may occur?

Side effects cannot be anticipated. If any develop or change in intensity, inform your doctor as soon as possible. Only your doctor can determine whether it is safe for you to continue taking Zebeta.

■ *Side effects may include:*
Diarrhea, dizziness, fatigue, headache, runny nose, swelling, upper respiratory infection

Why should this drug not be prescribed?

Do not take Zebeta if you have inadequate blood supply to the circulatory system (cardiogenic shock), certain types of irregular heartbeat, a slow heartbeat, or severe congestive heart failure

Special warnings about this medication

Do not suddenly stop taking Zebeta (see *Most important fact about this drug*). Use this drug cautiously if you have a history of congestive heart failure, and call your doctor immediately if you develop breathing problems or an extremely slow heartbeat while taking Zebeta.

If you suffer from asthma or other bronchial conditions, coronary artery disease, peripheral vascular disease, or kidney or liver disease, this medication should be used with caution.

Notify your doctor or dentist that you are taking Zebeta if you have a medical emergency, and before you have surgery or dental treatment.

Zebeta causes some people to become drowsy or less alert. You should not drive or operate dangerous machinery or participate in any hazardous activity until you know how the drug affects you.

This medication may mask the symptoms of low blood sugar or alter blood sugar levels. In addition, diabetics who experience a severe drop in blood sugar after taking insulin may suffer a spike in blood pressure if they are also taking Zebeta.

Zebeta could mask symptoms of an overactive thyroid. Abruptly stopping the drug could make the condition worse.

If you have a history of severe allergic reactions that have required epinephrine, you should be aware that Zebeta may make your system unresponsive to the usual effective dose of epinephrine.

Possible food and drug interactions when taking this medication

If Zebeta is taken with certain other drugs, the effects of either could be increased, decreased, or altered. It is especially important to check with your doctor when combining Zebeta with the following:

Calcium-blocking blood pressure drugs such as Calan and Cardizem
Clonidine (Catapres)
Disopyramide (Norpace) and similar drugs used to treat irregular
    heartbeat
Epinephrine (EpiPen)
Guanethidine (Ismelin)
Other beta-blocking blood pressure drugs such as Inderal,
    Lopressor, and Tenormin
Reserpine
Rifampin (Rifadin)

Special information if you are pregnant or breastfeeding

The effects of Zebeta during pregnancy have not been adequately studied. If you are pregnant or plan to become pregnant, inform your doctor immediately. Zebeta should be used only if the benefit outweighs the potential risk.

In animal studies, Zebeta has appeared in breast milk. It is not known if the drug appears in human milk. If this medication is essential to your health, your doctor may advise you to discontinue breastfeeding until your treatment with this medication is finished.

Recommended dosage

ADULTS

Dosage is tailored to each individual's needs. The usual starting dose is 5 milligrams once a day. If this dose is ineffective, the dose may be increased to 10 or 20 milligrams once a day.

If you have asthma, bronchial problems, or kidney or liver disease, the recommended starting dose is 2.5 milligrams a day. Extreme caution should be used if the dose has to be increased.

Zebeta has not been adequately studied in children.

Overdosage

Any medication taken in excess can have serious consequences. If you suspect an overdose of Zebeta, seek medical attention immediately.

■ *Symptoms of Zebeta overdose may include:*
Congestive heart failure (marked by sudden weight gain, swelling of the legs, feet, and ankles, fatigue, and shortness of breath), difficult or labored breathing, low blood pressure, low blood sugar, slow heartbeat

ZERIT

Pronounced: ZAIR-it
Generic name: Stavudine

Why is this drug prescribed?

Zerit is one of the drugs used to fight the human immunodeficiency virus (HIV)—the deadly cause of AIDS. It is usually prescribed for people who have already been taking the HIV drug Retrovir for an extended period. HIV attacks the immune system, slowly destroying the body's ability to fight off infection. Zerit helps stave off the attack by disrupting the virus's ability to reproduce.

Signs and symptoms of HIV infection include diarrhea, fever, headache, infections, problems with the nervous system, rash, sore throat, and significant weight loss.

Most important fact about this drug

Although Zerit can slow the progress of HIV infection, it is not a cure. Because of the continuing danger of complications and infections, you should get frequent physical exams and blood counts. Be sure, too, to notify your doctor immediately if you experience any changes in your general health.

How should you take this medication?

Take Zerit every 12 hours, exactly as prescribed. It's important to keep a constant level of the drug in the body, so be sure to take each dose on schedule. Do not take more than the prescribed amount; nerve disorders could result.

Shake the oral solution vigorously before measuring the dose.
You can take Zerit with or without food.

■ *If you miss a dose…*
Take it as soon as you remember. If it is almost time for your next dose, skip the one you missed and go back to your regular schedule. Do not take 2 doses at once.

■ *Storage instructions…*
Keep the Zerit container tightly closed. Store the capsules at room temperature. Store Zerit oral solution in the refrigerator; throw out any unused medication after 30 days.

What side effects may occur?

Side effects are more likely if you combine Zerit with other drugs that cause similar reactions. Also, the higher your dosage of Zerit, the greater the chance of a problem. However, it's often hard to tell a side effect from a symptom of the disease. If you think the drug is causing problems, keep taking it until you've checked with your doctor. Only your doctor can determine whether the drug is at fault, and adjust your dosage accordingly.

■ *Side effects may include:*
Abdominal pain, allergic reaction, chills, diarrhea, fever, headache, liver damage, loss of appetite, muscle pain, nausea and vomiting, nervous system abnormalities, pain or numbness and tingling in the hands and feet, pancreatitis, rash, sleeplessness

Why should this drug not be prescribed?

If Zerit gives you an allergic reaction, you should not take the drug.

Special warnings about this medication

Remember that Zerit does not prevent the spread of HIV through sexual contact or contact with infected blood.

Zerit has been known to cause severe and even fatal liver damage, especially in women, overweight individuals, and people who have been taking Zerit or similar medications for a long time. The risk increases if you're being treated with a combination of Zerit, Videx, and hydroxyurea. Signs of a liver problem include weakness, fatigue, abdominal pain, nausea, vomiting, and shortness of breath. If you develop these symptoms, call your doctor immediately; treatment with Zerit may have to be stopped. Also be sure to tell the doctor if you've ever had a liver problem or tend to abuse alcohol; the doctor will watch especially closely for any sign of a liver problem.

Zerit can also cause serious and even fatal pancreatitis, especially if you've had the problem in the past, suffer from gallstones, or drink alcoholic beverages. Combining Zerit with Videx increases the risk. Check with your doctor immediately if you develop such signs of pancreatitis as stomach pain, nausea, or vomiting; you may have to stop treatment with Zerit. If you have any of the risk factors for pancreatitis, make sure the doctor is aware of it.

One of the more common and dangerous side effects of Zerit is a problem called peripheral neuropathy, a serious condition in which certain nerves are damaged. If you notice numbness, tingling, or pain in your hands or feet, notify your physician immediately. Treatment with Zerit may have to be stopped.

Another side effect seen in some people receiving drugs for HIV is a redistribution of body fat, leading to extra fat around the middle, a "buffalo hump" on the back, and wasting in the arms, legs, and face. Researchers don't know whether this represents a long-term health problem or not.

The benefit you get from Zerit may not last long. If your symptoms begin to get worse, tell your doctor immediately.

Possible food and drug interactions when taking this medication
Combining Zerit with any of the following drugs may make peripheral neuropathy worse.

Chloramphenicol (Chloromycetin)
Cisplatin (Platinol)
Dapsone
Didanosine (Videx)
Ethambutol (Myambutol)
Hydralazine (Apresoline)
Lithium (Eskalith, Lithobid)
Metronidazole (Flagyl)
Nitrofurantoin (Macrodantin)
Phenytoin (Dilantin)
Vincristine (Oncovin)
Zalcitabine (Hivid)
Zidovudine (Retrovir)

Remember, too, that combination therapy with Zerit, Videx, and hydroxyurea increases the possibility of serious liver problems. Combining Zerit and Videx also increases the risk of pancreatitis.

Special information if you are pregnant or breastfeeding
The possibility that Zerit may harm a developing baby has not been ruled out. The drug should be used during pregnancy only if its benefits seem to outweigh the possible risk. The combination of Zerit and Videx should be used with particular caution during pregnancy due to the danger of liver damage.

Do not breastfeed; HIV can be passed to a newborn infant through breast milk.

Recommended dosage

ADULTS

For adults weighing 132 pounds or more, the usual dose is 40 milligrams every 12 hours. For those under 132 pounds, the dose is 30 milligrams every 12 hours.

CHILDREN

The usual starting dose for children weighing less than 66 pounds is 1 milligram per 2.2 pounds of body weight every 12 hours. Children weighing 66 pounds or more should take the adult dose.

Dosage is often reduced for people with kidney problems.

Overdosage

Numbness, pain, and tingling of the hands and feet can be signs of an overdose. If you suspect an overdose, seek medical attention immediately.

ZESTORETIC

Pronounced: zest-or-ET-ik
Generic ingredients: Lisinopril, Hydrochlorothiazide
Other brand name: Prinzide

Why is this drug prescribed?

Zestoretic is used in the treatment of high blood pressure. It combines an ACE inhibitor drug with a diuretic. Lisinopril, the ACE inhibitor, works by limiting production of a substance that promotes salt and water retention in your body. Hydrochlorothiazide, a diuretic, prompts your body to produce and eliminate more urine, which helps in lowering blood pressure. Combination products such as Zestoretic are usually not prescribed until therapy is already under way.

Most important fact about this drug

You must take Zestoretic regularly for it to be effective. Since blood pressure declines gradually, it may be several weeks before you get the full benefit of Zestoretic; and you must continue taking it even if you are feeling well. Zestoretic does not cure high blood pressure; it merely keeps it under control.

How should you take this medication?

Zestoretic can be taken with or without food once a day. Take it exactly as prescribed.

■ *If you miss a dose...*
   Take the forgotten dose as soon as you remember. If it is almost time for your next dose, skip the one you missed and go back to your regular schedule. Never take a double dose.

■ *Storage instructions...*
   Zestoretic should be stored at room temperature. Keep the container tightly closed.

What side effects may occur?

Side effects cannot be anticipated. If any develop or change in intensity, inform your doctor as soon as possible. Only your doctor can determine if it is safe for you to continue taking Zestoretic.

■ *Side effects may include:*
   Cough, dizziness, dizziness when standing up, fatigue, headache

Why should this drug not be prescribed?

If you are sensitive to or have ever had an allergic reaction to lisinopril or hydrochlorothiazide or if you are sensitive to other ACE inhibitor drugs such as Capoten or sulfa drugs such as Gantrisin, you should not take this medication. You should also avoid this drug if you suffered from angioedema (swelling of face, lips, tongue, throat, arms, or legs) during previous treatment with an ACE inhibitor, or tend to develop the condition for any other reason. You should also avoid Zestoretic if you are unable to urinate. Tell your doctor of all allergic reactions you have experienced.

Special warnings about this medication

If you develop swelling of your face, lips, tongue, or throat, or of your arms and legs, or have difficulty swallowing or breathing, you should stop taking the drug and contact your doctor immediately. You may need emergency treatment.

Zestoretic may cause your blood pressure to become too low. If you feel light-headed, especially during the first few days of treatment, inform your doctor. If you actually faint, stop taking Zestoretic until you have consulted your doctor.

Do not use salt substitutes containing potassium without first consulting your doctor.

Excessive sweating, dehydration, severe diarrhea, or vomiting could cause you to lose too much water and cause your blood pressure to drop dangerously.

If you develop chest pain, a sore throat, or fever and chills, contact your doctor immediately. It could indicate a more serious illness.

Make sure the doctor knows if you have congestive heart failure or other heart problems, diabetes, liver disease, a history of allergy or bronchial asthma, or lupus erythematosus (an arthritis-like disease sometimes accompanied by rashes). Zestoretic should be used cautiously. If you have kidney disease, your doctor should monitor your kidney function regularly.

If you are undergoing desensitization to bee or wasp venom, Zestoretic may cause a severe allergic reaction.

This medication is not recommended for people on dialysis; severe allergic reactions have occurred.

If you notice a yellowish cast to your skin or eyes, stop taking Zestoretic and contact your doctor immediately.

If you are diabetic, your doctor will want to keep an eye on your blood sugar levels.

Before any surgery, make sure your doctor or dentist knows you are taking Zestoretic.

Possible food and drug interactions when taking this medication

Zestoretic may intensify the effects of alcohol. Do not drink alcohol while taking this medication.

If Zestoretic is taken with certain other drugs, the effects of either could be increased, decreased, or altered. It is especially important to check with your doctor before combining Zestoretic with the following:

Barbiturates such as Nembutal and Seconal
Cholestyramine (Questran)
Colestipol (Colestid)
Corticosteroids such as prednisone
High blood pressure drugs such as Aldomet and Procardia XL
Indomethacin (Indocin)
Insulin
Lithium (Lithonate)
Narcotics such as Darvon and Dilaudid
Nonsteroidal anti-inflammatory drugs such as Naprosyn
Oral antidiabetic drugs such as Micronase
Potassium-containing salt substitutes
Potassium-sparing diuretics such as Midamor
Potassium supplements such as K-Dur and Slow-K

Special information if you are pregnant or breastfeeding

During the second and third trimesters, lisinopril can cause birth defects, prematurity, and death in the fetus and newborn. If you are pregnant or plan to become pregnant, contact your doctor immediately to discuss the potential hazard to your unborn child. Zestoretic may appear in breast milk and could affect a nursing infant. If this medication is essential to your health, your doctor may advise you to discontinue breastfeeding until your treatment with this medication is finished.

Recommended dosage

ADULTS

Zestoretic is designed to replace higher doses of either component. Dosages of the lisinopril component range from 10 to 80 milligrams a day; dosages of hydrochlorothiazide typically fall between 6.25 and 50 milligrams daily. If either component, when prescribed alone, fails to control your blood pressure, your doctor may try the Zestoretic combination, starting with either 10 or 20 milligrams of lisinopril and 12.5 milligrams of hydrochlorothiazide, and gradually increasing the dosage as needed.

If you are age 65 or older, or have kidney problems, your doctor will adjust your dosage with caution. This drug is not prescribed for people with severe kidney damage.

CHILDREN

The safety and effectiveness of Zestoretic in children have not been established.

Overdosage

Any medication taken in excess can have serious consequences. If you suspect an overdose, seek medical treatment immediately.

■ *Symptoms of Zestoretic overdose may include:*
Dehydration, low blood pressure

ZESTRIL

Pronounced: ZEST-rill
Generic name: Lisinopril
Other brand name: Prinivil

Why is this drug prescribed?

Zestril is used in the treatment of high blood pressure. It is effective when used alone or when combined with other high blood pressure medications. It may also be used with other medications in the treatment of heart failure, and may be given within 24 hours of a heart attack to improve chances of survival.

Zestril is a type of drug called an ACE inhibitor. It works by reducing production of a substance that increases salt and water retention in your body.

Most important fact about this drug

If you have high blood pressure, you must take Zestril regularly for it to be effective. Since blood pressure declines gradually, it may be several weeks before you get the full benefit of Zestril; and you must continue taking it even if you are feeling well. Zestril does not cure high blood pressure; it merely keeps it under control.

How should you take this medication?

Zestril can be taken with or without food. Take it exactly as prescribed. Stopping Zestril suddenly could cause your blood pressure to rise.

■ *If you miss a dose...*
Take the forgotten dose as soon as you remember. If it is almost time for your next dose, skip the one you missed and go back to your regular schedule. Never take 2 doses at the same time.

■ *Storage instructions...*
Store at room temperature, with the container sealed and dry. Avoid excessive heat or freezing cold.

What side effects may occur?

Side effects cannot be anticipated. If any develop or change in intensity, inform your doctor as soon as possible. Only your doctor can determine if it is safe for you to continue taking Zestril.

■ *Side effects may include:*
Chest pain, cough, diarrhea, dizziness, headache, low blood pressure

Why should this drug not be prescribed?

If you are sensitive to or have ever had an allergic reaction to Zestril or other ACE inhibitors such as Capoten, you should not take this medication. You should also avoid this drug if you suffered from angioedema (swelling of the face, lips, tongue, throat, arms, or legs) during previous treatment with an ACE inhibitor, or have a tendency to develop the condition for any other reason. Make sure your doctor is aware of any drug reactions you have experienced.

Special warnings about this medication

If you develop a sore throat, fever, or swelling of your face, lips, tongue, throat, arms, or legs, or have difficulty swallowing or breathing, you should contact your doctor immediately. You may have a serious side effect of the drug and need emergency treatment.

If you develop abdominal pain with or without nausea and vomiting, contact your doctor. ACE inhibitors such as Zestril have been known to cause intestinal swelling.

If you are being given bee or wasp venom to guard against future reactions, you may have a severe reaction to Zestril.

If you have congestive heart failure or other heart problems, a kidney disorder, or a connective tissue disease such as lupus, you should use this drug with caution. Your doctor may perform periodic blood tests while you are taking this medication.

If you are taking Zestril, a complete assessment of your kidney function should be done and kidney function should continue to be monitored. Zestril is used with great caution after a heart attack if the patient also has kidney problems.

This drug also should be used with caution if you are on dialysis. There have been reports of extreme allergic reactions during dialysis in people taking ACE inhibitor medications such as Zestril.

If you are taking high doses of a diuretic (water pill) and Zestril, you may develop excessively low blood pressure. This problem is also more likely if you are being treated for heart failure.

Zestril may cause some people to become dizzy, light-headed, or faint, especially if they have heart failure or are taking a water pill at the same time. Do not drive, operate dangerous machinery, or participate in any hazardous activity that requires full mental alertness until you are certain Zestril does not have this effect on you.

If you develop chest pain, sore throat, fever, and chills, contact your doctor for medical attention. It could indicate a more serious condition.

If your skin and the whites of your eyes turn yellow, stop taking the medication and contact your doctor.

Avoid salt substitutes that contain potassium. Limit your consumption of potassium-rich foods such as bananas, prunes, raisins, orange juice, and whole and skim milk. Ask your doctor for advice on how much of these foods to consume.

Excessive sweating, dehydration, severe diarrhea, or vomiting could cause you to lose too much water and cause your blood pressure to drop dangerously.

Possible food and drug interactions when taking this medication

If Zestril is taken with certain other drugs, the effects of either could be increased, decreased, or altered. It is especially important to check with your doctor before combining Zestril with any of the following:

Lithium (Lithonate, Eskalith)
Nonsteroidal anti-inflammatory drugs such as indomethacin (Indocin)
Potassium preparations such as K-Phos and Micro-K
Water pills such as HydroDIURIL and Lasix, and others that leave potassium in the body, such as Aldactone and Midamor

Special information if you are pregnant or breastfeeding

If it is taken during the final 6 months of pregnancy, Zestril can cause birth defects, prematurity, and death in the fetus and newborn. If you are pregnant or plan to become pregnant and are taking Zestril, contact your doctor immediately to discuss the potential hazard to your unborn child. Zestril may appear in breast milk and could affect a nursing infant. If this medication is essential to your health, your doctor may advise you to discontinue breastfeeding until your treatment with this medication is finished.

Recommended dosage

ADULTS

High Blood Pressure

For people not on water pills (diuretics), the initial starting dose is usually 10 milligrams taken once a day. Your doctor will increase the dosage until your blood pressure is under control. The long-term dosage usually ranges from 20 to 40 milligrams a day, taken in a single dose.

Diuretic use should, if possible, be stopped before using Zestril. If not, your physician may give an initial dose of 5 milligrams under supervision before any further medication is prescribed.

People with kidney disorders must be carefully monitored, and dosages will be adjusted to the individual's needs, depending on kidney function.

Heart Failure

For this condition, Zestril is usually prescribed along with diuretics and digitalis. The recommended starting dose is 5 milligrams once a day, with the first dose taken under your doctor's supervision. The doctor may increase the dose by up to 10 milligrams at intervals of no less than 2 weeks. Typical long-term dosages range from 5 to 40 milligrams taken once a day.

Heart Attack

The usual dose is 5 milligrams within the first 24 hours after a heart attack, then 5 milligrams 24 hours later, 10 milligrams 48 hours later, and, finally, 10 milligrams once a day for 6 weeks. If low blood pressure is a problem, the doctor may recommend a lower dosage.

CHILDREN 6 YEARS OR OLDER

High Blood Pressure

The usual starting dose is 0.07 milligram per day up to a total of 5 milligrams per day.

Zestril is not recommended in children younger than 6 years old or in children with poor kidney function.

OLDER ADULTS

The physician will adjust the dosage carefully, according to the individual's needs.

Overdosage

Any medication taken in excess can cause symptoms of overdose. If you suspect an overdose, seek medical attention immediately.

A severe drop in blood pressure is the primary sign of a Zestril overdose.

ZETIA

Pronounced: ZEH-tee-uh
Generic name: Ezetimibe

Why is this drug prescribed?

Zetia is a new kind of cholesterol-lowering drug. The older cholesterol-lowering drugs called statins reduce cholesterol by interfering with its production in the body. Zetia acts by diminishing the absorption of dietary cholesterol through the intestines.

Zetia may be taken alone or with a statin drug. Because the two drugs fight cholesterol in different ways, the Zetia/statin combination has a greater impact than either drug alone.

Cholesterol—especially "bad" LDL cholesterol—promotes clogged arteries, increasing the risk of heart attack and stroke. "Good" HDL cholesterol helps to prevent clogged arteries. Zetia lowers the bad cholesterol and raises the good. It also lowers total cholesterol readings and reduces levels of triglycerides (fats in the blood).

Cholesterol-lowering drugs are typically prescribed for people who either have heart disease or are in danger of developing it. For people at high risk of heart disease, current guidelines call for considering drug therapy when LDL levels reach 130. For people at lower risk, the cutoff is 160. For those at little or no risk, it's 190.

Most important fact about this drug

Doctors usually prescribe cholesterol-lowering drugs only after changes in lifestyle have failed to bring cholesterol down to a healthy level. These changes include following a diet low in fat and cholesterol and high in fiber, shedding excess weight, and getting more exercise. It's important to remember that drug therapy is a supplement to—not a substitute for—these other measures. To get the full benefit of the medication, you need to stick to the diet and exercise program recommended by your doctor.

How should you take this medication?

You can take Zetia with or without food. If the doctor has also prescribed a statin drug, you can take Zetia at the same time. If you are also taking Colestid, Questran, or WelChol, take Zetia at least 2 hours before or 4 hours after taking the other medication.

■ *If you miss a dose…*
Take the forgotten dose as soon as you remember. However, if it is almost time for your next dose, skip the one you missed and return to your regular schedule. Do not take 2 doses at once.
■ *Storage instructions…*
Store at room temperature. Protect from moisture.

What side effects may occur?

Side effects cannot be anticipated. If any develop or change in intensity, tell your doctor as soon as possible. Only your doctor can determine if it is safe to continue using Zetia.

■ *Side effects may include:*
Abdominal pain, back pain, diarrhea, joint pain, sinusitis

Other side effects that occur when Zetia is taken with a statin drug include chest pain, dizziness, headache, muscle pain, and upper respiratory infection.

Certain allergic reactions such as hives have also occurred.

Why should this drug not be prescribed?

If Zetia causes an allergic reaction, you'll be unable to use it. Combined therapy with Zetia and a statin drug should be avoided if you have a liver condition or are pregnant or nursing.

Special warnings about this medication

Zetia is not recommended for people with moderate to severe liver disease, or for children under 10.

Possible food and drug interactions when taking this medication

Do not combine Zetia with the cholesterol-lowering drugs called fibrates, including Lopid and Tricor. Check with your doctor before combining Zetia with cyclosporine (Neoral, Sandimmune).

Special information if you are pregnant or breastfeeding

Zetia should be taken during pregnancy only if its benefits outweigh the potential risk to the baby. If you are pregnant or planning to become pregnant, check with your doctor immediately.

Statin drugs pose a definite risk to the baby, so you should never add a statin drug to Zetia therapy during pregnancy.

It's not known whether Zetia makes its way into breast milk. The drug is recommended only if its benefits are thought to outweigh the potential risk.

Recommended dosage

The recommended dose is 10 milligrams once a day.

Overdosage

There is no experience with Zetia overdose. However, any medication taken in excess can have serious consequences. If you suspect an overdose, seek medical attention immediately.

ZIAC

Pronounced: ZIGH-ack
Generic ingredients: Bisoprolol fumarate, Hydrochlorothiazide

Why is this drug prescribed?

Ziac is used to treat high blood pressure. It combines a beta-blocker (bisoprolol, which is the ingredient in the drug Zebeta) with a thiazide diuretic (hydrochlorothiazide). Beta-blockers decrease the force and rate of heart contractions, thus lowering blood pressure. Diuretics help your body produce and eliminate more urine, which also helps lower blood pressure.

Most important fact about this drug

Ziac does not cure high blood pressure; it merely keeps it under control. Therefore, you must continue taking it even if you are feeling well. Do not stop taking Ziac unless instructed to do so by your doctor. This is especially important if you have coronary artery disease. Abruptly stopping Ziac could cause chest pain, heart rhythm problems, and even heart attack.

How should you take this medication?

Take Ziac exactly as prescribed, even if your symptoms have disappeared. Try not to miss any doses. If this medication is not taken regularly, your condition may worsen.

■ *If you miss a dose...*
Take the missed dose as soon as possible. However, if it is almost time for your next dose, skip the one you missed and go back to your regular schedule. Never take 2 doses at once.

■ *Storage instructions...*
Store at room temperature in a tightly closed container.

What side effects may occur?

Side effects cannot be anticipated. If any develop or change in intensity, inform your doctor as soon as possible. Only your doctor can determine whether it is safe for you to continue taking Ziac.

■ *More common side effects may include:*
Dizziness, fatigue

Additional side effects have been reported with Ziac, although it's unknown if the drug was the cause. Be sure to tell your doctor about any unusual or severe symptoms.

Why should this drug not be prescribed?

Do not take Ziac if you have inadequate blood supply to the circulatory system (cardiogenic shock), certain types of irregular heartbeat, a slow heartbeat, bronchial asthma, or severe congestive heart failure. Also avoid the drug if you have trouble urinating.

Do not use Ziac if you have an allergic reaction to the drug or if you're allergic to antibiotics known as sulfonamides (such as Bactrim, Cotrim, and Septra).

Special warnings about this medication

Use Ziac cautiously if you have a history of congestive heart failure.

Do not suddenly stop taking Ziac (see *Most important fact about this drug*). If you have to stop taking the drug, the doctor will gradually lower your dose of Ziac over a period of 2 weeks.

Call your doctor immediately if you develop breathing problems or an extremely slow heartbeat while taking Ziac.

If you suffer from asthma or other bronchial conditions, coronary artery disease, peripheral vascular disease, or kidney or liver disease, this medication should be used with caution.

Notify your doctor or dentist that you are taking Ziac if you have a medical emergency, and before you have surgery or dental treatment.

Ziac causes some people to become drowsy or less alert. You should not drive or operate dangerous machinery or participate in any hazardous activity until you know how the drug affects you.

This medication may mask the symptoms of low blood sugar or alter blood sugar levels. In addition, diabetics who experience a severe drop in blood sugar after taking insulin may suffer a spike in blood pressure if they are also taking Ziac.

If you have a history of severe allergic reactions that have required epinephrine, you should be aware that Ziac may make your system unresponsive to the usual effective dose of epinephrine.

If you have systemic lupus erythematosus, you should be aware that Ziac could make the symptoms worse.

Ziac could mask symptoms of an overactive thyroid. Abruptly stopping the drug could make the condition worse.

In a small number of people, Ziac has interfered with the functioning of the parathyroid, causing blood levels of calcium and phosphate to rise. In rare cases, the drug has also caused gout.

There is a slight chance that Ziac could cause a drop in blood levels of electrolytes such as potassium and magnesium. Call your doctor if you develop any of the following: drowsiness, dry mouth, excessive thirst, low blood pressure, muscle pains or cramps, rapid heartbeat, restlessness, gastrointestinal problems such as nausea and vomiting, weakness or muscle fatigue, or an unusual decrease in urination.

Be aware that Ziac could make you more sensitive to sunlight.

Possible food and drug interactions when taking this medication

If Ziac is taken with certain other drugs, the effects of either could be increased, decreased, or altered. It is especially important to check with your doctor when combining Ziac with the following:

Any other blood pressure drugs, including the calcium-blockers
    diltiazem (Cardizem), disopyramide (Norpace), and verapamil
    (Calan)
Alcohol
Barbiturate sedatives such as Seconal and Nembutal
Cholesterol-lowering drugs such as Colestid and Questran
Clonidine (Catapres)
Diabetes drugs (oral)
Disopyramide (Norpace) and similar drugs used to treat irregular
    heartbeat
Epinephrine (EpiPen)
Guanethidine (Ismelin)
Insulin
Lithium (Eskalith, Lithobid)
Muscle relaxants such as tubocurarine
Nonsteroidal anti-inflammatory drugs such as aspirin, Motrin,
    and Tylenol
Norepinephrine
Painkillers such as codeine and morphine

Reserpine
Rifampin (Rifadin)
Steroids such as prednisone

Special information if you are pregnant or breastfeeding

The effects of Ziac during pregnancy have not been adequately studied. If you are pregnant or plan to become pregnant, inform your doctor immediately. Ziac should be used only if the benefit outweighs the potential risk.

It is not known if Ziac appears in breast milk. If this medication is essential to your health, your doctor may advise you to discontinue breastfeeding until your treatment with this medication is finished.

Recommended dosage

ADULTS

Dosage is tailored to each individual's needs. The usual starting dose is 2.5 milligrams of bisoprolol with 6.25 milligrams of hydrochlorothiazide once a day. If this dose is ineffective, the dose may be increased every 14 days up to a maximum of 20 milligrams bisoprolol/12.5 milligrams hydrochlorothiazide once a day.

If you have asthma, bronchial problems, or kidney or liver disease, the doctor may have you take a very low starting dose. Extreme caution should be used if the dose has to be increased.

Ziac has not been adequately studied in children.

Overdosage

Any medication taken in excess can have serious consequences. If you suspect an overdose of Ziac, seek medical attention immediately.

■ *Symptoms of Ziac overdose may include:*
Abnormal skin sensations, congestive heart failure (marked by sudden weight gain, swelling of the legs, feet, and ankles, fatigue, and shortness of breath), confusion, cramps in the calf muscle, decreased or increased urination, difficult or labored breathing, dizziness, drowsiness, fluid or electrolyte loss, impaired consciousness, low blood pressure, low blood sugar, nausea, shock, slow or rapid heartbeat, thirst, vomiting, weakness

Large overdoses may interfere with breathing or cause delirium, coma, or convulsions.

ZIAGEN

Pronounced: ZYE-a-jen
Generic name: Abacavir sulfate

Why is this drug prescribed?

Ziagen helps to halt the inroads of the human immunodeficiency virus (HIV). Without treatment, HIV gradually undermines the body's immune system, encouraging other infections to take hold until the body succumbs to full-blown acquired immune deficiency syndrome (AIDS).

Like other anti-HIV drugs, Ziagen holds back the advance of the virus by disrupting its reproductive cycle. This medication is used only as part of a drug regimen that attacks the virus on several fronts. It is not prescribed alone.

Most important fact about this drug

Ziagen is not a cure for HIV infection or AIDS. It does not completely eliminate HIV from the body or totally restore the immune system. You will continue to face the danger of serious opportunistic infections (unusual infections that develop only when the immune system falters). It's important, therefore, to continue seeing your doctor for regular blood counts and tests, and to notify him immediately of any changes in your general health.

How should you take this medication?

It is important to keep adequate levels of Ziagen in your bloodstream at all times, so be sure to keep a supply on hand at all times and take this drug exactly as prescribed, even when you're feeling better. Ziagen may be taken with or without food.

■ *If you miss a dose...*
 Take it as soon as you remember. If it is almost time for your next dose, skip the one you missed and go back to your regular schedule. Do not take 2 doses at once.

■ *Storage instructions...*
 Both the tablets and the oral solution may be stored at room temperature. The oral solution may also be refrigerated, but do not allow it to freeze.

What side effects may occur?

Side effects cannot be anticipated. If any develop or change in intensity, inform your doctor as soon as possible. Only your doctor can determine if it is safe for you to continue taking Ziagen.

■ *Side effects may include:*
 Abdominal pain, cough, diarrhea, fatigue, fever or chills, generally ill feeling, headache/migraine, joint pain, mouth ulcers, muscle aches or

weakness, nausea, rash, severe blisters in the mouth and eyes, severely peeling skin, shortness of breath, skin tingling or burning, sleep disorders, sore throat, swelling, tiredness, vomiting

Why should this drug not be prescribed?

If the active ingredient abacavir (found in Ziagen and Trizivir) gives you an allergic reaction, you must never take it again. If you've failed to get any benefit from HIV drugs that work the same way as Ziagen (Epivir, Videx, or Hivid), this drug probably won't work for you either. Make sure the doctor knows the results of all the drug treatments you've been given.

You will not be able to use Ziagen if you have moderate to severe liver disease.

Special warnings about this medication

Be alert for development of a skin rash, severe peeling skin, or two or more of the following sets of symptoms:

Fever
Nausea, vomiting, diarrhea, or abdominal pain
Severe tiredness, achiness, or a generally ill feeling
Sore throat, shortness of breath, or cough

If these symptoms appear, stop taking Ziagen and call your doctor immediately. You may be experiencing a potentially fatal allergic reaction. Once you've had such a reaction, never take Ziagen again. In fact, avoid Ziagen permanently if there's even a possibility that you've had an allergic reaction. Additional doses could trigger a dangerous drop in blood pressure and other life-threatening symptoms.

Keep in mind, too, that a severe and even fatal allergic reaction is possible when you resume taking Ziagen after an interruption in therapy—even if you've never experienced signs of an allergic reaction before. Resume Ziagen therapy only under your doctor's close supervision.

If you are overweight or have been taking HIV drugs similar to Ziagen (Epivir, Videx, or Hivid) for a long period of time, you are more likely to develop liver problems and a complication called lactic acidosis (a buildup of lactic acid in the body). If you develop either of these conditions, your doctor will take you off of Ziagen.

Like other HIV drugs, Ziagen sometimes causes a redistribution of body fat, resulting in added weight around the waist, a "buffalo hump" of fat on the upper back, breast enlargement, and wasting of the face, arms, and legs. It's not known why this occurs, or what long-term effects it might have.

Because Ziagen and other HIV medications do not completely eliminate the virus, it remains possible to infect others with HIV through sexual contact or blood contamination. Continue to practice safe sex while using Ziagen.

Possible food and drug interactions when taking this medication
If you are taking methadone, there is a slight chance that your dosage of methadone may need to be increased.

Special information if you are pregnant or breastfeeding
The effects of Ziagen during pregnancy have not been adequately studied. If you are pregnant or plan to become pregnant, tell your doctor immediately.

Since HIV infection can be passed to your baby through breast milk, you should avoid breastfeeding.

Recommended dosage

ADULTS

The recommended dose is 300 milligrams twice a day in combination with other anti-HIV drugs.

CHILDREN

The recommended dose for children and adolescents 3 months to 16 years of age is 8 milligrams per 2.2 pounds of body weight twice a day in combination with other anti-HIV drugs. Do not exceed 300 milligrams twice a day.

DOSAGE ADJUSTMENT

Ziagen oral solution is recommended for people with mild liver problems. The usual dose is 10 milliliters (200 milligrams) twice a day.

Overdosage
Any medication taken in excess can have serious consequences. If you suspect an overdose of Ziagen, seek medical attention immediately.

Zidovudine See Retrovir, page 1245.

Zileuton See Zyflo, page 1663.

Ziprasidone See Geodon, page 617.

ZITHROMAX
Pronounced: ZITH-roh-macks
Generic name: Azithromycin

Why is this drug prescribed?
Zithromax is an antibiotic related to erythromycin. It is prescribed for adults to treat certain mild to moderate skin infections; upper and lower respiratory tract infections, including pharyngitis (strep throat), tonsillitis, sinus infections, worsening of chronic obstructive pulmonary dis-

ease, and pneumonia; sexually transmitted infections of the cervix or urinary tract; and genital ulcer disease in men. In children, Zithromax is used to treat middle ear infection, pneumonia, tonsillitis, and strep throat.

Most important fact about this drug
There is a possibility of rare but very serious reactions to Zithromax, including angioedema (swelling of the face, lips, and neck that impedes speaking, swallowing, and breathing), anaphylaxis (a violent, even fatal allergic reaction), and serious skin diseases. If you develop these symptoms, stop taking Zithromax and call your doctor immediately.

How should you take this medication?
Take Zithromax capsules at least 1 hour before or 2 hours after a meal. Zithromax tablets and oral suspension can be taken with or without food. Do not take any form with an antacid that contains aluminum or magnesium, such as Di-Gel, Gelusil, Maalox, and others.

If you are using single-dose packets of Zithromax powder for oral suspension, mix the entire contents of each packet with 2 ounces of water, drink immediately, then add an additional 2 ounces of water, mix again, and drink to make sure you've taken the entire dose. When giving the pediatric suspension, shake the bottle thoroughly before each use and measure the dose with the supplied calibrated dropper. Use the pediatric suspension within 10 days and throw out any that remains.

Your doctor will prescribe Zithromax only to treat a bacterial infection; it will not cure a viral infection, such as the common cold. It's important to take the full dosage schedule of Zithromax, even if you're feeling better in a few days. Not completing the full dosage schedule may decrease the drug's effectiveness and increase the chances that the bacteria may become resistant to Zithromax and similar antibiotics.

■ *If you miss a dose...*
Take the forgotten dose as soon as you remember. If you don't remember until the next day, skip the dose and go back to your regular schedule. Never try to catch up by doubling the dose.
■ *Storage instructions...*
Zithromax should be stored at room temperature.

What side effects may occur?
Side effects cannot be anticipated. If any develop or change in intensity, inform your doctor as soon as possible. Only your doctor can determine if it is safe for you to continue taking Zithromax.

■ *Side effects may include:*
Abdominal pain, diarrhea or loose stools, nausea or vomiting

The single large dose of Zithromax that is prescribed to treat sexually transmitted infection of the cervix or urinary tract is more likely to cause stomach and bowel side effects than the smaller doses prescribed for a skin or respiratory tract infection.

Why should this drug not be prescribed?
Do not take Zithromax if you have ever had an allergic reaction to it or to similar antibiotics such as erythromycin (E.E.S., PCE, and others).

Special warnings about this medication
Like certain other antibiotics, Zithromax may cause a potentially life-threatening form of diarrhea called pseudomembranous colitis. Pseudomembranous colitis may clear up spontaneously when the drug is stopped; if it doesn't, hospital treatment may be required. If you develop diarrhea, check with your doctor immediately.

If you have a liver problem, your doctor should monitor you very carefully while you are taking Zithromax.

Possible food and drug interactions when taking this medication
Do not take Zithromax with antacids containing aluminum or magnesium, such as Maalox and Mylanta.

If Zithromax is taken with certain other drugs, the effects of either could be increased, decreased, or altered. It is especially important to check with your doctor before combining Zithromax with the following:

Cyclosporine (Neoral, Sandimmune)
Digoxin (Lanoxicaps, Lanoxin)
Ergot-containing drugs such as Cafergot and D.H.E.
Hexobarbital
Nelfinavir (Viracept)
Phenytoin (Dilantin)
Warfarin (Coumadin)

Special information if you are pregnant or breastfeeding
If you are pregnant or plan to become pregnant, inform your doctor immediately. You should take Zithromax during pregnancy only if it is clearly needed. It is not known whether Zithromax can make its way into breast milk. If the drug is essential to your health, your doctor may advise you to stop breastfeeding until your treatment is finished.

Recommended dosage

ADULTS

Pneumonia, Chronic Obstructive Pulmonary Disease, Tonsillitis, Strep Throat, and Skin Infections
The usual dose of Zithromax is 500 milligrams in a single dose the first day. This is followed by 250 milligrams once daily for the next 4 days. Alternatively, patients with chronic obstructive pulmonary disease may be prescribed 500 milligrams a day for 3 days.

Sinus Infection
The usual dose of Zithromax is 500 milligrams once a day for 3 days.

Genital Ulcer Disease
The usual dose is a single gram (1,000 milligrams) one time only.

Sexually Transmitted Diseases
The usual dose is a single 2-gram (2,000 milligrams) dose.

CHILDREN

Middle Ear Infection
For children aged 6 months and up, treatment may be given three ways. One option is a single dose of 30 milligrams per 2.2 pounds of body weight. Another option is a dose of 10 milligrams per 2.2 pounds given each day for 3 days. Zithromax can also be given over a period of 5 days, starting with a dose of 10 milligrams per 2.2 pounds on the first day and continuing with daily doses of 5 milligrams per 2.2 pounds for the next 4 days.

Sinus Infection
For children aged 6 months and up, the usual dose is 10 milligrams of Zithromax suspension per 2.2 pounds of body weight given once daily for 3 days.

Pneumonia
For children aged 6 months and up, the usual dose is 10 milligrams of Zithromax suspension per 2.2 pounds of body weight in a single dose the first day, followed by 5 milligrams per 2.2 pounds for the next 4 days.

Strep Throat and Tonsillitis
For children aged 2 years and up, the usual dose is 12 milligrams per 2.2 pounds of body weight once daily for 5 days.

Overdosage
Although no specific information on Zithromax overdose is available, any medication taken in excess can have serious consequences. If you suspect an overdose, seek medical attention immediately.

ZOCOR
Pronounced: ZOH-core
Generic name: Simvastatin

Why is this drug prescribed?
Zocor is a cholesterol-lowering drug. Your doctor may prescribe Zocor in addition to a cholesterol-lowering diet if your blood cholesterol level is too high, and if you have been unable to lower it by diet alone. For people at high risk of heart disease, current guidelines call for considering drug

therapy when LDL levels reach 130. For people at lower risk, the cutoff is 160. For those at little or no risk, it's 190.

In people with high cholesterol and heart disease, Zocor reduces the risk of heart attack, stroke, and mini-stroke (transient ischemic attack) and can stave off the need for bypass surgery or angioplasty to clear clogged arteries. Zocor can also reduce these risks in people with diabetes, peripheral vascular disease, and a history of stroke.

Most important fact about this drug

Zocor is usually prescribed only if diet, exercise, and weight loss fail to bring your cholesterol level under control. It's important to remember that Zocor is a supplement to—not a substitute for—those other measures. To get the full benefit of the medication, you need to stick to the diet and exercise program prescribed by your doctor. All these efforts to keep your cholesterol levels normal are important because together they may lower your risk of heart disease.

How should you take this medication?

Take Zocor exactly as prescribed.

■ *If you miss a dose...*
Take it as soon as you remember. If it is almost time for your next dose, skip the one you missed and go back to your regular schedule. Do not take 2 doses at once.

■ *Storage instructions...*
Store at room temperature.

What side effects may occur?

Side effects cannot be anticipated. If any develop or change in intensity, inform your doctor as soon as possible. Only your doctor can determine whether it is safe for you to continue taking Zocor.

■ *Side effects may include:*
Abdominal pain, headache

Why should this drug not be prescribed?

Do not take Zocor if you have ever had an allergic reaction to it or are sensitive to it.

Do not take Zocor if you have active liver disease.

Do not take Zocor if you are pregnant or plan to become pregnant.

Special warnings about this medication

Because Zocor may damage the liver, your doctor may order a blood test to check your liver enzyme levels before you start taking the drug. Blood tests will probably be done before your treatment is started and at periodic intervals for a year after your final dosage increase. If your liver enzyme levels rise too high, your doctor may tell you to stop taking Zocor.

Since Zocor may cause damage to muscle tissue, be sure to tell your doctor of any unexplained muscle tenderness, weakness, or pain right away, especially if you also have a fever or feel sick. Your doctor may want to do a blood test to check for signs of muscle damage.

If you are scheduled for major surgery, your doctor will have you stop taking Zocor a few days before the operation.

Possible food and drug interactions when taking this medication

Zocor tends to enhance the effects of the blood-thinning drug Coumadin and the heart medication Lanoxin. Combining it with the following drugs increases the chance of muscle damage:

Amiodarone (Cordarone)
Clarithromycin (Biaxin)
Clofibrate (Atromid-S)
Cyclosporine (Sandimmune, Neoral)
Erythromycin (PCE and others)
Fenofibrate (Tricor)
Gemfibrozil (Lopid)
Itraconazole (Sporanox)
Ketoconazole (Nizoral)
Nefazodone (Serzone)
Nicotinic acid or niacin (Niaspan)
Protease inhibitors (used in the treatment of HIV), including
    Agenerase, Crixivan, Fortovase, Invirase, Norvir, and Viracept
Verapamil (Calan)

If you are taking Zocor with any of these drugs (or with large quantities of grapefruit juice) alert your doctor immediately at the first sign of muscle pain or weakness. If you need to take erythromycin, Biaxin, Nizoral, or Sporanox, the doctor may temporarily take you off Zocor.

Special information if you are pregnant or breastfeeding

You must not become pregnant while taking Zocor. This drug lowers cholesterol, and cholesterol is needed for a baby to develop properly. If you do become pregnant while taking Zocor, notify your doctor right away. Based on studies of other cholesterol-lowering drugs, it is assumed that Zocor could appear in breast milk and could cause severe adverse effects in a nursing baby. Do not take Zocor while breastfeeding your baby.

Recommended dosage

You will have to follow a standard cholesterol-lowering diet before starting treatment with Zocor and continue this diet while using Zocor.

All doses should be adjusted to your individual needs.

ADULTS

The usual starting dose is 20 to 40 milligrams once a day in the evening. If your cholesterol level or heart attack risk is especially high, the doctor may start with a dose of 40 milligrams. The dosage can be adjusted every 4 weeks. Some people with severe, hereditary high cholesterol may be prescribed as much as 80 milligrams a day, taken in doses of 20, 20, and 40 milligrams, along with other treatments.

Those who have severe kidney disease should use Zocor with caution. The recommended starting dose is 5 milligrams per day.

When combined with cyclosporine, niacin, Atromid-S, Lopid, or Tricor, the dosage of Zocor should not exceed 10 milligrams a day. When combined with Calan or Cordarone, the dosage of Zocor should not exceed 20 milligrams a day.

CHILDREN 10 TO 17 YEARS OLD

The recommended starting dose is 10 milligrams once a day in the evening. The dosage may be increased every 4 weeks, as determined by the doctor, up to a maximum of 40 milligrams a day. Girls must have been menstruating for at least 1 year before starting therapy with Zocor.

The safety and effectiveness of Zocor in children under 10 years old or in doses greater than 40 milligrams a day have not been studied.

Overdosage

Although no specific information about Zocor overdose is available, any medication taken in excess can have serious consequences. If you suspect an overdose of Zocor, seek medical attention immediately.

ZOFRAN

Pronounced: ZOH-fran
Generic name: Ondansetron hydrochloride
Other brand name: Zofran ODT

Why is this drug prescribed?

Zofran is used for the prevention of nausea and vomiting caused by radiation therapy and chemotherapy for cancer, and, in some cases, to prevent these problems following surgery.

Most important fact about this drug

To ensure the maximum effect, it is important to take all doses of Zofran exactly as prescribed by your doctor.

How should you take this medication?

Your doctor will tell you how much drug to take and how often, depending on the type of therapy you will be having.

Zofran is available in three forms: an oral solution, tablets that you swallow with water, and orally disintegrating tablets that can be swallowed with saliva alone (Zofran ODT). If you're taking the orally disintegrating tablets, don't remove them from the blister pack until it's time for a dose. Then peel off the foil backing with dry hands, gently remove the tablet, and immediately place it on your tongue. Do not attempt to push the tablets through the foil.

■ *If you miss a dose...*
Take the forgotten dose as soon as you remember.
■ *Storage instructions...*
Store Zofran at room temperature. Protect from light. Keep the drug in the carton it came in. Store oral solution bottles upright.

What side effects may occur?
Side effects cannot be anticipated. If any develop or change in intensity, inform your doctor as soon as possible. Only your doctor can determine if it is safe for you to continue taking Zofran.

■ *Side effects may include:*
Constipation, diarrhea, dizziness, fatigue, headache
■ *When Zofran is used to prevent nausea and vomiting after surgery, the following side effects may occur:*
Anxiety, difficulty breathing, difficulty urinating, dizziness, drowsiness, female reproductive disorders, fever, headache, itching, low blood pressure, shivers, slow heartbeat

Why should this drug not be prescribed?
If you are sensitive to or have ever had an allergic reaction to ondansetron hydrochloride, you should not take this medication. Make sure that your doctor is aware of any drug reactions that you have experienced.

Special warnings about this medication
If drugs similar to Zofran (for instance, Anzemet or Kytril) have given you a reaction, Zofran may cause one too.

If you suffer from phenylketonuria (an excess of the amino acid phenylalanine) remember that Zofran contains this substance.

Possible food and drug interactions when taking this medication
No interactions with Zofran have been reported.

Special information if you are pregnant or breastfeeding
The effects of Zofran during pregnancy have not been adequately studied. If you are pregnant or plan to become pregnant, inform your doctor immediately. Zofran may appear in breast milk and could affect a nursing infant. If this medication is essential to your health, your doctor may advise you to discontinue breastfeeding until your treatment with this medication is finished.

Recommended dosage

Dosage is the same for both regular and orally disintegrating tablets. If you have poor liver function, you should take no more than 8 milligrams of Zofran per day.

PREVENTION OF NAUSEA AND VOMITING DUE TO CHEMOTHERAPY

Adults and Children 12 Years of Age and Older

The recommended dose of Zofran is one 8-milligram tablet or 2 teaspoonfuls of oral solution taken twice a day. The first dose should be taken 30 minutes before the start of treatment. The other dose should be taken 8 hours after the first dose. One 8-milligram tablet or 2 teaspoonfuls should be taken twice a day (every 12 hours) for 1 to 2 days after completing chemotherapy.

If the chemotherapy is especially likely to cause nausea and vomiting, the recommended dosage is one 24-milligram tablet taken 30 minutes before the treatment.

Children 4 through 11 Years of Age

The recommended dose of Zofran is one 4-milligram tablet or 1 teaspoonful of oral solution taken 3 times a day. The first dose should be taken 30 minutes before the start of chemotherapy. The other 2 doses should be taken 4 and 8 hours after the first dose. One 4-milligram tablet or 1 teaspoonful should be taken 3 times a day (every 8 hours) for 1 to 2 days after completing chemotherapy.

PREVENTION OF NAUSEA AND VOMITING DUE TO RADIATION THERAPY

Adults

The usual dosage is one 8-milligram tablet or 2 teaspoonfuls of oral solution taken 3 times a day. You will take the first dose 1 to 2 hours before therapy; the other intervals will depend on the type of radiation therapy you are receiving.

Children

Zofran has not been used for this purpose in children.

PREVENTION OF NAUSEA AND VOMITING AFTER SURGERY

Adults

The usual dose is two 8-milligram tablets or 4 teaspoonfuls of oral solution taken 1 hour before undergoing anesthesia.

Children

Zofran has not been used for this purpose in children.

Overdosage

Any medication taken in excess can have serious consequences. If you suspect an overdose, seek medical attention immediately.

■ *Symptoms of Zofran overdose may include:*
Low blood pressure and fainting, severe constipation, sudden blindness

ZOLADEX

Pronounced: ZO-luh-dex
Generic name: Goserelin acetate

Why is this drug prescribed?

Zoladex relieves the symptoms of advanced prostate cancer in men and advanced breast cancer in premenopausal women. In combination with other forms of therapy, it is also prescribed during treatment of early prostate cancer.

In addition, it can be used in the treatment of endometriosis, a condition in which tissue from the lining of the uterus invades the abdomen. If you are scheduled for surgical removal of the lining, the drug may be used to thin the lining prior to the operation.

Zoladex works by reducing levels of testosterone in men and estrogen in women. These hormones can encourage the growth of certain cancers.

Most important fact about this drug

Symptoms may actually get worse during the first few weeks of therapy. However, as hormone levels subside, you should begin to feel an improvement.

How should you take this medication?

Doses are implanted under the skin of the upper abdomen every 4 or 12 weeks by your physician or a nurse.

■ *If you miss a dose...*
Make an appointment as soon as possible.

What side effects may occur?

Side effects cannot be anticipated. If any develop or change in intensity, tell your doctor as soon as possible. Only your doctor can determine if it is safe for you to continue using Zoladex.

■ *Side effects may include:*
Acne, application site reactions, breast development in men or enlargement in women, breast tenderness or pain, change in sex drive, depression, dizziness, emotional problems, flu-like symptoms, fluid retention and swelling, hair growth in women, headache, hot flashes,

infection, insomnia, lethargy, loss of appetite, loss of breast tissue in women, lung problems, nausea, nervousness, pain, rash, sexual impairment, sore throat, sweating, urinary problems, vaginal dryness, vaginal inflammation, voice changes, weak heart, weakness, weight gain

Why should this drug not be prescribed?

If Zoladex gives you an allergic reaction, it cannot be used. It should also be avoided during pregnancy and breastfeeding, and if you have unexplained abnormal vaginal bleeding. Women of childbearing age should use nonhormonal contraceptive measures while taking Zoladex.

Special warnings about this medication

Zoladex therapy can weaken the bones and cause bone pain. In men under treatment for prostate cancer, it has been known to cause osteoporosis and fractures. If you are a heavy drinker, smoke a lot, have family members with brittle bones, or take anticonvulsant drugs (such as Dilantin) or steroids (such as prednisone), make sure your doctor is aware of the situation.

Men with a blockage in the tube from the kidney to the bladder (the ureter) or a case of spinal cord compression should get treatment for these conditions before beginning Zoladex therapy.

Severe allergic reactions, including hives and swelling of the lips and throat, have been reported with drugs similar to Zoladex. If these symptoms occur, call your doctor immediately.

When given with sex hormones, Zoladex may lead to overstimulation of the ovaries. It has also been known to cause ovarian cysts.

Women should remember that even though Zoladex stops menstruation, it is possible to become pregnant if you miss a dose. Since Zoladex could harm the developing baby, it's important to observe strict contraceptive precautions throughout Zoladex therapy.

If you are taking Zoladex to relieve endometriosis, your doctor may recommend hormone-replacement therapy to limit the effects of the reduced estrogen levels that result from Zoladex therapy.

Possible food and drug interactions when taking this medication

No interactions have been reported.

Special information if you are pregnant or breastfeeding

Zoladex can harm developing babies and newborn infants. It must not be used during pregnancy or breastfeeding.

Recommended dosage

Typically, the doctor will implant a dose of 3.6 milligrams every 4 weeks. Treatment for endometriosis lasts no longer than 6 months. Cancer therapy generally continues for a longer term.

For prostate cancer, the doctor can administer a longer-lasting implant of 10.8 milligrams every 12 weeks. When the drug is given with Flutamide, the treatment is one 3.6-millgram implant followed by one 10.8-milligram implant 4 weeks later.

If the drug is being used in preparation for endometrial surgery, you'll receive 1 or 2 implants before the operation.

Overdosage

An overdose of Zoladex is highly unlikely, and if one were to occur, it would not cause any harm.

Zolmitriptan See Zomig, page 1650.

ZOLOFT

Pronounced: ZOE-loft
Generic name: Sertraline

Why is this drug prescribed?

Zoloft is prescribed for major depression—a persistently low mood that interferes with everyday living. Symptoms may include loss of interest in your usual activities, disturbed sleep, change in appetite, constant fidgeting or lethargic movement, fatigue, feelings of worthlessness or guilt, difficulty thinking or concentrating, and recurrent thoughts of suicide.

Zoloft is also used to treat the following:

Premenstrual dysphoric disorder (PMDD), a condition marked by a depressed mood, anxiety or tension, emotional instability, and anger or irritability in the two weeks preceding menstruation.

Obsessive-compulsive disorder (unwanted thoughts that won't go away and an irresistible urge to keep repeating certain actions, such as hand washing or counting).

Panic disorder (unexpected attacks of overwhelming anxiety, accompanied by fear of their return).

Social anxiety disorder (extreme shyness in social situations that interferes with an individual's work and social life).

Post-traumatic stress disorder (re-experiencing a dangerous or life-threatening event through intrusive thoughts, flashbacks, and intense psychological distress).

Zoloft belongs to a class of drugs called selective serotonin re-uptake inhibitors (SSRIs). Serotonin is one of the chemical messengers believed to govern moods. Ordinarily, it is quickly reabsorbed after its release at the junctures between nerves. Re-uptake inhibitors such as Zoloft slow this process, thereby boosting the levels of serotonin available in the brain.

Most important fact about this drug

Do not take Zoloft within 2 weeks of taking any drug classified as an MAO inhibitor. Drugs in this category include the antidepressants Marplan, Nardil, and Parnate. When serotonin boosters such as Zoloft are combined with MAO inhibitors, serious and sometimes fatal reactions can occur. In addition, you should not combine Zoloft with the drug pimozide (Orap).

How should you take this medication?

Take Zoloft exactly as prescribed: once a day, in either the morning or the evening.

Zoloft is available in capsule and oral concentrate forms. To prepare Zoloft oral concentrate, use the dropper provided. Measure out the amount of concentrate prescribed by your doctor and mix it with 4 ounces of water, ginger ale, lemon/lime soda, lemonade, or orange juice. (Do not mix the concentrate with any other type of beverage.) Drink the mixture immediately; do not prepare it in advance for later use. At times, a slight haze may appear after mixing, but this is normal.

Improvement with Zoloft may not be seen for several days to a few weeks. You should expect to keep taking it for at least several months.

Zoloft may make your mouth dry. For temporary relief, suck a hard candy, chew gum, or melt bits of ice in your mouth.

■ *If you miss a dose...*
Take the forgotten dose as soon as you remember. If several hours have passed, skip the dose. Never try to catch up by doubling the dose.

■ *Storage instructions...*
Store at room temperature.

What side effects may occur?

Side effects cannot be anticipated. If any develop or change in intensity, inform your doctor as soon as possible. Only your doctor can determine if it is safe for you to continue taking Zoloft.

■ *Side effects may include:*
Abdominal pain, agitation, anxiety, constipation, decreased appetite, decreased sex drive, diarrhea or loose stools, difficulty with ejaculation, dizziness, dry mouth, fatigue, gas, headache, increased sweating, indigestion, insomnia, nausea, nervousness, pain, rash, sleepiness, sore throat, tingling or pins and needles, tremor, vision problems, vomiting

Many people lose a pound or two of body weight while taking Zoloft. This usually poses no problem but may be a concern if your depression has already caused you to lose a great deal of weight.

In a few people, Zoloft may trigger the grandiose, inappropriate, out-of-control behavior called mania or the similar, but less dramatic, state called hypomania.

Why should this drug not be prescribed?

Do not use this drug while taking an MAO inhibitor or the drug pimozide (Orap) (see *Most important fact about this drug*). Avoid Zoloft if it causes an allergic-type reaction.

Special warnings about this medication

In clinical studies, antidepressants increased the risk of suicidal thinking and behavior in children and adolescents with depression and other psychiatric disorders. Anyone considering the use of Zoloft or any other antidepressant in a child or adolescent must balance this risk with the clinical need. Zoloft is approved for treating obsessive-compulsive disorder only in children 6 years and older.

Additionally, the progression of major depression is associated with a worsening of symptoms and/or the emergence of suicidal thinking or behavior in both adults and children, whether or not they are taking antidepressants. Individuals being treated with Zoloft and their caregivers should watch for any change in symptoms or any new symptoms that appear suddenly—especially agitation, anxiety, hostility, panic, restlessness, extreme hyperactivity, and suicidal thinking or behavior—and report them to the doctor immediately. Be especially observant at the beginning of treatment or whenever there is a change in dose.

Use Zoloft cautiously and under close medical supervision if you have a history of kidney or liver disorders, heart disease, seizures, or bleeding problems. Your doctor may limit your dosage if you have one of these conditions.

Zoloft could cause weight loss in children. The manufacturer recommends regular monitoring of weight and growth during long-term treatment in children.

SSRI antidepressants could potentially cause stomach bleeding, especially when combined with nonsteroidal anti-inflammatory drugs (NSAIDs) such as aspirin, ibuprofen (Advil, Motrin), naproxen (Aleve), and ketoprofen (Orudis KT). Consult your doctor before combining Zoloft with NSAIDs or blood-thinning medications.

Like all antidepressants, Zoloft could trigger a manic episode. Let the doctor know if you've ever had this problem.

Zoloft has not been found to impair the ability to drive or operate machinery. Nevertheless, the manufacturer recommends caution until you know how the drug affects you.

If you are sensitive to latex, use caution when handling the dropper provided with the oral concentrate.

Possible food and drug interactions when taking this medication
Remember that Zoloft must never be combined with pimozide (Orap) or an MAO inhibitor (see *Most important fact about this drug*).

You should not drink alcoholic beverages while taking Zoloft. Use over-the-counter remedies with caution. Although none is known to interact with Zoloft, interactions remain a possibility.

If Zoloft is taken with certain other drugs, the effects of either could be increased, decreased, or altered. It is especially important to check with your doctor before combining Zoloft with the following:

Antidepressants that boost serotonin, such as Paxil and Prozac
Other antidepressants, including tricyclics such as Elavil and
    Pamelor
Cimetidine (Tagamet)
Diazepam (Valium)
Digitoxin (Crystodigin)
Flecainide (Tambocor)
Lithium (Eskalith, Lithobid)
Over-the-counter drugs such as cold remedies
Propafenone (Rythmol)
Sumatriptan (Imitrex)
Tolbutamide (Orinase)
Warfarin (Coumadin)

If you are using the oral concentrate form of Zoloft, do not take disulfiram (Antabuse)

Special information if you are pregnant or breastfeeding
The effects of Zoloft during pregnancy have not been adequately studied. If you are pregnant or plan to become pregnant, inform your doctor immediately. Zoloft should be taken during pregnancy only if it is clearly needed. It is not known whether Zoloft appears in breast milk. Caution is advised when using Zoloft during breastfeeding.

Recommended dosage

ADULTS

Depression or Obsessive-Compulsive Disorder
The usual starting dose is 50 milligrams once a day, taken either in the morning or in the evening. Your doctor may increase your dose depending upon your response. The maximum dose is 200 milligrams in a day.

Premenstrual Dysphoric Disorder
Doses may be prescribed throughout the menstrual cycle or limited to the 2 weeks preceding menstruation. The starting dose is 50 milligrams a day. If this proves insufficient, your doctor will increase the dose in 50-milligram steps at the start of each new menstrual cycle up to a maximum

of 100 milligrams per day in the 2-week regimen or 150 milligrams per day in the full-cycle regimen. (During the first 3 days of the 2-week regimen, doses are always limited to 50 milligrams.)

Panic Disorder, Post-Traumatic Stress Disorder, and Social Anxiety Disorder

During the first week, the usual dose is 25 milligrams once a day. After that, the dose increases to 50 milligrams once a day. Depending on your response, you're the doctor may continue to increase your dose up to a maximum of 200 milligrams a day.

CHILDREN 6 TO 17 YEARS OLD

Obsessive-Compulsive Disorder

The starting dose for children aged 6 to 12 is 25 milligrams and for adolescents aged 13 to 17, 50 milligrams. The doctor will adjust the dose as necessary.

Safety and effectiveness have not been established for children under 6.

DOSAGE ADJUSTMENT

The doctor will need to reduce the dosage if you have liver disease.

Overdosage

Any medication taken in excess can have serious consequences. An overdose of Zoloft can be fatal. If you suspect an overdose, seek medical attention immediately.

■ *Common symptoms of Zoloft overdose include:*
Agitation, dizziness, nausea, rapid heartbeat, sleepiness, tremor, vomiting

Other possible symptoms include coma, stupor, fainting, convulsions, delirium, hallucinations, mania, high or low blood pressure, and slow, rapid, or irregular heartbeat

Zolpidem See Ambien, page 89.

ZOMIG

Pronounced: ZOE-mig
Generic name: Zolmitriptan

Why is this drug prescribed?

Zomig relieves migraine headaches. It's effective whether or not the headache is preceded by an aura (visual disturbances such as halos and flickering lights). For most people Zomig provides relief within 2 hours, but it will not abort an attack or reduce the number of headaches you experience.

Migraines are thought to be caused by expansion and inflammation of blood vessels in the head. Zomig ends a migraine attack by constricting these blood vessels and reducing inflammation.

Most important fact about this drug

Zomig is for use only on common and classic migraine headaches. It should not be used for other types of headache, including certain unusual types of migraine. It has not been tested for cluster headaches, a type of severe headache more common among men.

How should you take this medication?

Take Zomig as soon as your first symptoms appear. If the headache comes back after your first dose, you may take a second one 2 hours later. However, if the first dose has no effect at all, do not take a second one unless your doctor advises it, and never take more than 10 milligrams in a day. If taking an orally disintegrating Zomig ZMT tablet, do not remove it from the blister pack until just before use, then immediately place it on your tongue, where it will dissolve in the saliva. Do not break the tablet. Throw away any unused tablets already removed from the blister packaging.

■ *If you miss a dose...*
Zomig is not for regular use. Take it only when you are having a migraine attack.

■ *Storage instructions...*
Store Zomig at room temperature, away from heat, light, and moisture. Throw away any remaining tablets after the expiration date printed on the package. Also discard any leftover medicine if your doctor decides to stop treatment with Zomig.

What side effects may occur?

Side effects cannot be anticipated. If any develop or change in intensity, inform your doctor as soon as possible. Only your doctor can determine if it is safe for you to continue taking Zomig.

■ *Side effects may include:*
Chest pain or tightness, cold sensation, dizziness, drowsiness, dry mouth, feeling of heaviness in the chest or elsewhere, indigestion, jaw pain or tightness, nausea, neck pain or tightness, pain, skin tingling, sweating, throat pain or tightness, warm sensation, weakness

Why should this drug not be prescribed?

You should not take Zomig if you have certain types of heart disease, including angina (chest pain), a history of heart attack, and certain heart irregularities. Also avoid the drug if you have uncontrolled high blood pressure.

Do not use Zomig within 24 hours of taking an ergotamine-based migraine medication such as Cafergot, Ergostat, or Sansert, or a drug in the same class as Zomig, such as Imitrex.

Avoid using Zomig within 2 weeks of taking a drug classified as an MAO inhibitor, such as the antidepressants Nardil and Parnate.

If Zomig gives you an allergic reaction, do not take it again.

Special warnings about this medication

If the first dose of Zomig does not relieve your symptoms, ask your doctor to reevaluate you; migraine may not be the problem.

Although the danger is very remote, this type of medication has been known to trigger serious and even life-threatening heart problems in people with heart disease. If you have a heart disorder, make sure the doctor knows about it. Do not take Zomig if you suffer from irregular heartbeat.

Very rarely, Zomig has caused serious intestinal problems. See your doctor immediately if you have bloody diarrhea or stomach pain.

If you have risk factors for heart disease, your doctor may ask you to take your first dose of Zomig in the office, and may want to monitor you carefully thereafter. Risk factors that signal the need for caution include high blood pressure, high cholesterol, smoking, excess weight, diabetes, and a strong family history of heart disease or hardening of the arteries. Heart disease is also more likely in postmenopausal women and men over 40.

Use Zomig with caution if you have liver or kidney disease. These conditions could alter the effect of the drug. If you have a history of seizures, make sure the doctor is aware of it. Also, if you develop any trouble with your eyes, alert your doctor. There is a possibility the problem could be related to Zomig.

If you experience pain or tightness in your chest or throat when using Zomig, tell your doctor. If the chest pain is severe or does not go away, seek medical attention immediately. These pains could be symptoms of a previously undetected heart condition.

If you develop shortness of breath, wheezing, a throbbing heartbeat, swelling of the eyelids, face, or lips, or a skin rash, skin lumps, or hives after taking Zomig, call your doctor immediately, and do not take any more of the drug without your doctor's approval.

If a headache feels different from your usual migraine, check with your doctor before using Zomig.

If you must avoid phenylalanine, do not use the orally disintegrating Zomig ZMT tablets, which contain this substance.

Possible food and drug interactions when taking this medication

Remember that Zomig should never be combined with the following drugs (see *Why should this drug not be prescribed?*):

MAO inhibitors such as the antidepressant drugs Nardil and Parnate
Ergotamine-type drugs such as Cafergot, D.H.E. 45 Injection,
    Ergostat, and Sansert
Sumatriptan (Imitrex)

If Zomig is taken with certain other drugs, the effects of either may be increased, decreased, or altered. It is especially important to check with your doctor before combining Zomig with the following:

Acetaminophen (Tylenol)
Cimetidine (Tagamet)
Fluoxetine (Prozac)
Fluvoxamine (Luvox)
Oral contraceptives
Paroxetine (Paxil)
Propranolol (Inderal)
Sertraline (Zoloft)

Special information if you are pregnant or breastfeeding

The effects of Zomig during pregnancy have not been adequately studied. If you are pregnant or plan to become pregnant, inform your doctor immediately. Although researchers have not confirmed it, Zomig may appear in breast milk and could affect a nursing infant. Check with your doctor before using Zomig while breastfeeding.

Recommended dosage

ADULTS

The recommended starting dose is no more than 2.5 milligrams. Higher doses have little additional effect, but tend to cause more side effects. If the headache returns, the dose may be repeated after 2 hours. Do not exceed 10 milligrams in a day.

If you have liver disease, your doctor will prescribe a lower dose and closely monitor your blood pressure.

CHILDREN AND OLDER ADULTS

The safety and effectiveness of Zomig have not been established in children and adults over 65.

Overdosage

The only known symptom of Zomig overdose is drowsiness. However, any medication taken in excess can have serious consequences. If you suspect an overdose, seek medical attention immediately.

ZONEGRAN

Pronounced: ZAH-nah-gran
Generic name: Zonisamide

Why is this drug prescribed?

Zonegran helps reduce the frequency of partial epileptic seizures, a form of epilepsy in which neural disturbances are limited to a specific region of the brain and the victim remains conscious throughout the attack. The drug is used in combination with other antiseizure medications, not by itself.

Most important fact about this drug

Do not stop taking this drug on your own. If the doctor decides to discontinue Zonegran, he will tell you how to taper off slowly. Abrupt discontinuation of Zonegran can cause seizures.

How should you take this medication?

Zonegran capsules should be swallowed whole and can be taken with or without food.

■ *If you miss a dose...*
Take it as soon as you remember. If it is almost time for your next dose, skip the one you missed and go back to your regular schedule. Never take 2 doses at the same time.

■ *Storage instructions...*
Store at room temperature in a dry place. Protect from light.

What side effects may occur?

Side effects cannot be anticipated. If any develop or change in intensity, inform your doctor as soon as possible. Only your doctor can determine if it is safe for you to continue taking Zonegran.

■ *Side effects may include:*
Abdominal pain, agitation, confusion, depression, diarrhea, difficulty concentrating, difficulty with memory, dizziness, double vision and other visual disturbances, drowsiness, fatigue, flu syndrome, headache, insomnia, irritability, loss of appetite, loss of muscle coordination, mental slowing, nausea, prickling or burning skin, rash, speech abnormalities, tiredness

Why should this drug not be prescribed?

Do not take Zonegran if you are allergic to sulfa drugs such as Bactrim.

Special warnings about this medication

If you develop a rash while taking Zonegran, call your physician immediately. It could be a sign of an allergic reaction.

Zonegran may cause drowsiness. Do not drive a car or operate dangerous machinery until you know how the drug affects you.

People who take Zonegran are prone to develop kidney stones. To reduce the risk of stone formation, be sure to drink plenty of fluids. Call your doctor immediately if you develop symptoms of kidney stones such as back pain, abdominal pain, painful urination, or blood in the urine.

Call your doctor if you start to bruise easily or develop a fever, a sore throat, or blisters in the mouth. These could be signs of anemia or other blood problems that Zonegran has been known to trigger in very rare cases.

Contact your doctor immediately if you develop severe muscle pain or weakness.

Contact your doctor immediately if your seizures worsen.

Zonegran may interfere with a child's ability to perspire and control body temperature, leading to a medical emergency. Zonegran is not approved for use in children under 16.

Possible food and drug interactions when taking this medication

If Zonegran is taken with certain other drugs, the effects if either could be increased, decreased, or altered. It is especially important to check with your doctor before combining Zonegran with the following:

Carbamazepine (Tegretol)
Phenobarbital
Phenytoin (Dilantin)
Valproate (Depakote)

Special information if you are pregnant or breastfeeding

In most cases, Zonegran should not be taken by pregnant women because there is a chance that it could harm the developing baby. If you are pregnant or plan to become pregnant, tell your doctor immediately.

It is not known whether Zonegran appears in breast milk, but because it could cause a serious reaction if it did, you'll probably need to make a choice between breastfeeding and continuing your Zonegran therapy. Be sure to discuss the question with your doctor.

Recommended dosage

ADULTS

The recommended starting dose for adults over the age of 16 is 100 milligrams daily as your doctor directs.

Your physician may wish to increase the dose by 100 milligrams every 2 weeks to a maximum of 600 milligrams per day. Larger doses can be divided into 2 smaller doses taken twice a day.

Overdosage

Any medication taken in excess can have serious consequences. If you suspect an overdose, seek medical attention immediately.

■ *Symptoms of Zonegran overdose may include:*
Diminished breathing, loss of consciousness, low blood pressure, slow heartbeat

Zonisamide *See Zonegran, page 1654.*

Zovia *See Oral Contraceptives, page 1000.*

ZOVIRAX

Pronounced: zoh-VIGH-racks
Generic name: Acyclovir

Why is this drug prescribed?

Zovirax liquid, capsules, and tablets are used in the treatment of certain infections with herpes viruses. These include genital herpes, shingles, and chickenpox. This drug may not be appropriate for everyone, and its use should be thoroughly discussed with your doctor. Zovirax ointment is used to treat initial episodes of genital herpes and certain herpes simplex infections of the skin and mucous membranes. Zovirax cream is used for herpes cold sores on the lips and face only.

Some doctors use Zovirax, along with other drugs, in the treatment of AIDS, and for unusual herpes infections such as those following kidney and bone marrow transplants.

Most important fact about this drug

Zovirax does not cure herpes. However, it does reduce pain and may help the sores caused by herpes to heal faster. Genital herpes is a sexually transmitted disease. To reduce the chance of infecting your partner, forgo intercourse and other sexual contact while you have sores or any other symptom.

How should you take this medication?

Your medication should not be shared with others, and the prescribed dose should not be exceeded. You can take Zovirax with or without food.

Zovirax ointment should not be used in or near the eyes. To reduce the risk of spreading the infection, use a rubber glove to apply the ointment.

Zovirax cream should not be used in or near the eyes, or inside the nose or mouth. The medication can, however, be applied on the outside of the lips. Apply the cream with your fingers to clean, dry skin. Be sure to wash your hands before and after applying Zovirax cream, and avoid bathing or swimming afterward to prevent it from washing off. Do not cover the cold sore with a bandage or makeup unless your doctor approves.

■ *If you miss a dose...*
Take it as soon as you remember. If it is almost time for your next dose, skip the one you missed and go back to your regular schedule. Never take 2 doses at the same time.

If you are using the ointment, apply it as soon as you remember and continue your regular schedule.

■ *Storage instructions...*
Store Zovirax at room temperature in a dry place.

What side effects may occur?
Side effects cannot be anticipated. If any develop or change in intensity, inform your doctor as soon as possible. Only your doctor can determine if it is safe for you to continue taking Zovirax.

■ *Side effects may include:*
Diarrhea, general feeling of bodily discomfort, nausea, vomiting

■ *Side effects of Zovirax ointment may include:*
Burning, itching, mild pain, skin rash, stinging, vaginal inflammation

■ *Side effects of Zovirax cream may include:*
Allergic reactions, burning, dry or cracked lips, dry or flaky skin, eczema (inflamed, irritated patches of skin), hives, inflammation, itchy spots, stinging

Why should this drug not be prescribed?
If you are sensitive to or have ever had an allergic reaction to Zovirax or similar drugs, you should not take this medication. Make sure that your doctor is aware of any drug reactions that you have experienced.

Special warnings about this medication
If you are being treated for a kidney disorder, consult your doctor before taking Zovirax. The drug has been known to cause kidney failure.

If you develop unusual bruising or bleeding under the skin, be sure to alert your doctor. It could signal a dangerous blood disorder.

Possible food and drug interactions when taking this medication
If Zovirax is taken with certain other drugs, the effects of either could be increased, decreased, or altered. It is especially important to check with your doctor before combining Zovirax with the following:

Cyclosporine (Neoral, Sandimmune)
Interferon (Roferon-A)
Probenecid (Benemid)
Zidovudine (Retrovir)

Special information if you are pregnant or breastfeeding

Zovirax seems relatively safe during pregnancy. Nevertheless, it should be used only if its benefits outweigh the potential risk to the baby. If you are pregnant or plan to become pregnant, inform your doctor immediately. Zovirax appears in breast milk and could affect a nursing infant. If this medication is essential to your health, your doctor may advise you to discontinue breastfeeding your baby until your treatment with Zovirax is finished.

Recommended dosage

ADULTS

Genital Herpes

The usual dose is one 200-milligram capsule or 1 teaspoonful of liquid every 4 hours, 5 times daily for 10 days. If the herpes is recurrent, the usual adult dose is 400 milligrams (two 200-milligram capsules, one 400-milligram tablet or 2 teaspoonfuls) 2 times daily for up to 12 months.

If genital herpes is intermittent, the usual adult dose is one 200-milligram capsule or 1 teaspoon of liquid every 4 hours, 5 times a day for 5 days. Therapy should be started at the earliest sign or symptom.

Ointment: Apply ointment to affected area every 3 hours, 6 times per day, for 7 days. Use enough ointment (approximately one-half inch ribbon of ointment per 4 square inches of surface area) to cover the affected area.

Herpes Cold Sores

Apply Zovirax cream to the affected area 5 times a day for 4 days. Therapy should begin as soon as possible after the first sign of a cold sore such as a bump, tingling, redness, or itchiness.

Herpes Zoster (Shingles)

The usual adult dose is 800 milligrams (one 800-milligram tablet or 4 teaspoonfuls of liquid) every 4 hours, 5 times daily for 7 to 10 days.

Chickenpox

The usual adult dose is 800 milligrams 4 times a day for 5 days.

If you have a kidney disorder, the dose will need to be adjusted by your doctor.

CHILDREN

The usual dose for chickenpox in children 2 years of age and older is 20 milligrams per 2.2 pounds of body weight taken orally 4 times daily, for a total of 80 milligrams per 2.2 pounds, for 5 days. A child weighing more than 88 pounds should take the adult dose.

The safety and effectiveness of oral Zovirax have not been established in children under 2 years of age. However, your doctor may decide that the benefits of this medication outweigh the potential risks. The safety and effectiveness of Zovirax ointment in children have not been established. Zovirax cream has not been studied in children less than 12 years old.

OLDER ADULTS

Your doctor will start you at the low end of the dosage range, since older adults are more apt to have kidney problems or other disease, or to be taking other medications.

Overdosage

Zovirax is generally safe. However, any medication taken in excess can have serious consequences. If you suspect an overdose, seek medical attention immediately.

■ *Symptoms of Zovirax overdose may include:*
Agitation, coma, kidney failure, lethargy, seizures

ZYBAN

Pronounced: ZIGH-ban
Generic name: Bupropion hydrochloride

Why is this drug prescribed?

Zyban is a nicotine-free quit-smoking aid. Instead of nicotine, it contains the same active ingredient as the antidepressant medication Wellbutrin. It works by boosting the levels of several chemical messengers in the brain. With more of these chemicals at work, you experience a reduction in nicotine withdrawal symptoms and a weakening of the urge to smoke. More than a third of the people who take Zyban while participating in a support program are able to quit smoking for at least 1 month. Zyban can also prove helpful when people with conditions such as chronic bronchitis and emphysema decide it's time to quit.

Most important fact about this drug

About 1 person in 1,000 suffers a seizure while taking Zyban. For this reason, people with epilepsy and certain other disorders should never take the drug. Don't share Zyban with friends. Only a doctor can decide whether it's safe for a particular individual.

How should you take this medication?

Treatment with this drug begins while you are still smoking. Zyban needs about a week to reach an effective level in your body; so to improve your chance of success, you should not attempt to quit until the second week of treatment. Set a firm date for quitting. If you are still smoking after that date, your odds of breaking the habit will be worse. You should keep taking Zyban for 7 to 12 weeks.

You can use nicotine patches along with Zyban. However, combining the two treatments can raise your blood pressure, so it's important to tell your doctor if you plan to use both. Do not smoke while using a patch, because too much nicotine can cause serious side effects.

Participating in a counseling or support program will make success more likely. Your doctor can recommend a local program for you.

Swallow Zyban tablets whole. Do not chew, divide, or crush them. Take them exactly as prescribed.

■ *If you miss a dose...*
Do not take an extra tablet to catch up on the missed dose. Skip the dose and take your next tablet at the regularly scheduled time.

■ *Storage instructions...*
Store at room temperature in a tightly closed container. Keep out of direct sunlight.

What side effects may occur?
Side effects cannot be anticipated. If any develop or change in intensity, inform your doctor as soon as possible. Only your doctor can determine if it is safe for you to continue taking Zyban.

■ *Side effects may include:*
Dry mouth, sleeplessness

These are generally mild and usually disappear after a few weeks. If you have difficulty sleeping, avoid taking Zyban close to bedtime and ask your doctor about reducing your dosage.

Why should this drug not be prescribed?
Because Zyban has been known to trigger convulsions, no one with a seizure disorder should take this drug. Also avoid Zyban if you are taking Wellbutrin or any other drug that contains bupropion, Zyban's active ingredient. The more bupropion you take, the more likely you are to have a seizure.

Zyban's seizure-triggering potential is greater in people with an eating disorder such as bulimia or anorexia, and in those undergoing abrupt withdrawal from alcohol, sedatives, and tranquilizers such as Librium and Valium. If you suffer from one of these problems, never take Zyban. Avoid it, too, if you are taking a drug classified as an MAO inhibitor, such as the antidepressants Nardil and Parnate. Allow at least 14 days to pass between taking one of these drugs and starting your Zyban therapy.

If bupropion or any other ingredient in Zyban has ever given you an allergic reaction, the drug is not for you.

Special warnings about this medication
In clinical studies, antidepressants increased the risk of suicidal thinking and behavior in children and adolescents with depression and other psychiatric disorders. Because Zyban contains the same ingredient as the antidepressant Wellbutrin, anyone considering the use of Zyban or any other antidepressant in a child or adolescent must balance this risk with

the clinical need. Zyban has not been studied in children or adolescents and is not approved for treating anyone less than 18 years old.

Additionally, the progression of major depression is associated with a worsening of symptoms and/or the emergence of suicidal thinking or behavior in both adults and children, whether or not they are taking antidepressants. Individuals being treated with Zyban and their caregivers should watch for any change in symptoms or any new symptoms that appear suddenly—especially agitation, anxiety, hostility, panic, restlessness, extreme hyperactivity, and suicidal thinking or behavior—and report them to the doctor immediately. Be especially observant at the beginning of treatment or whenever there is a change in dose.

Because the chance of a seizure from Zyban rises with the amount in your system, never take more than one 150-milligram tablet at a time, and limit your total daily intake to 2 doses (300 milligrams).

A variety of conditions can predispose you to seizures, including:

Prior head injuries
Prior seizures
Central nervous system tumors
Cirrhosis of the liver
Too much alcohol
Abrupt withdrawal from alcohol, tranquilizers, or sedatives
Addiction to narcotics or cocaine
Use of over-the-counter stimulants or diet pills
Use of diabetes medications
Use of antidepressants, major tranquilizers, steroids, or theophylline

If any of these apply to you, use Zyban with care. If you do have a seizure while taking Zyban, stop taking the drug and never take it again.

Stop taking Zyban and call your doctor immediately if you have difficulty breathing or swallowing; notice swelling in your face, lips, tongue, or throat; develop swollen arms and legs; or break out with itchy eruptions. These are warning signs of a potentially severe allergic reaction.

If you have a liver or kidney condition, make sure the doctor is aware of it. Your dosage may need to be reduced. (If you have severe cirrhosis of the liver, your dosage *must* be reduced.) Also make certain the doctor knows about any heart condition you may have.

Zyban can interfere with your driving ability. Don't drive or operate dangerous machinery until you are certain of the drug's effect on you.

Possible food and drug interactions when taking this medication
If Zyban is used with certain other drugs, the effects of either could be increased, decreased, or altered. It is especially important to check with your doctor before combining Zyban with the following:

Alcohol
Amantadine (Symmetrel)

Antidepressants such as Norpramin, Pamelor, Paxil, Prozac, Tofranil, and Zoloft

Beta-blockers (heart and blood pressure medications) such as Inderal, Lopressor, and Tenormin

Carbamazepine (Tegretol)

Cimetidine (Tagamet)

Cyclophosphamide (Cytoxan)

Heart-stabilizing drugs such as Rythmol and Tambocor

Levodopa (Dopar, Larodopa, Sinemet)

Major tranquilizers such as Haldol, Risperdal, and Thorazine

MAO inhibitors such as the antidepressants Nardil and Parnate

Orphenadrine (Norflex)

Phenobarbital

Phenytoin (Dilantin)

Steroids such as hydrocortisone and prednisone

Theophylline (Theo-Dur, Theolair)

Warfarin (Coumadin)

Quitting smoking, with or without Zyban treatment, could change the way your body metabolizes certain drugs, for example, theophylline and warfarin. Make sure your doctor knows all the prescription and over-the-counter medicines you're taking.

Special information if you are pregnant or breastfeeding

Zyban has not been tested in pregnant women. If you are pregnant or plan to become pregnant, do your best to quit smoking with the aid of counseling and support before turning to drug therapy. For the sake of the baby, you should avoid smoking or taking nicotine in any other form while pregnant.

Zyban appears in breast milk and could affect a nursing infant. Ask your doctor whether it will be better to discontinue the medication or to stop breastfeeding.

Recommended dosage

ADULTS

The usual starting dose is one 150-milligram tablet in the morning for the first 3 days. After that, take one 150-milligram tablet in the morning and another in the early evening. Keep doses at least 8 hours apart. The maximum recommended dose is 300 milligrams daily.

Continue taking Zyban for 7 to 12 weeks. Your doctor may recommend continuing treatment for up to 6 months.

Kidney and Liver Disease

Your doctor may reduce the frequency of your doses to avoid high blood levels of Zyban. If you have severe cirrhosis of the liver, you should take no more than 150 milligrams every *other* day.

CHILDREN

The safety and efficacy of Zyban have not been established in children under 18.

Overdosage

Information on Zyban overdose is limited. However, any medication taken in excess can have serious consequences. If you suspect an overdose, seek medical attention immediately.

■ *Symptoms of Zyban overdose may include:*
Blurred vision, confusion, grogginess, jitteriness, light-headedness, nausea, seizure, sluggishness, visual hallucinations

Zydone *See Vicodin, page 1557.*

ZYFLO

Pronounced: ZIGH-flow
Generic name: Zileuton

Why is this drug prescribed?

Zyflo tablets prevent and relieve the symptoms of chronic asthma. The drug works by relaxing the muscles in the walls of your airways, allowing them to open wider, and by reducing inflammation, swelling, and mucus secretion in the lungs.

Most important fact about this drug

Zyflo has been known to cause liver damage. Be sure to see your doctor every few months for liver function tests.

How should you take this medication?

Zyflo should be taken 4 times a day. Although you can take it with or without meals, it may be easier to remember if you take it with meals and at bedtime. Take Zyflo exactly as prescribed, even when symptoms subside.

While taking Zyflo, you should continue taking all other asthma medications your doctor has prescribed, unless directed otherwise. Do not decrease the dose or stop taking any of these drugs.

■ *If you miss a dose...*
Take the forgotten dose as soon as you remember. If it is almost time for your next dose, skip the one you missed and go back to your regular schedule. Never take 2 doses at the same time.

■ *Storage instructions...*
Store at room temperature, away from light.

What side effects may occur?

Side effects cannot be anticipated. If any develop or change in intensity, inform your doctor as soon as possible. Only your doctor can determine if it is safe for you to continue taking Zyflo.

■ *Side effects may include:*
Abdominal pain, headache, indigestion, loss of strength, muscle aches, nausea, pain

Why should this drug not be prescribed?

If you have liver disease, you should not take this medication. You should also avoid Zyflo if you have ever had an allergic reaction to it or its ingredients.

Special warnings about this medication

Zyflo will not help an acute asthma attack in which immediate opening of the airways is needed.

If you find that you have to use your other asthma medications—such as an inhaler—more often, report this to your doctor.

Because Zyflo can affect the liver, make sure your doctor is aware of any problems you've had in the past. Warn the doctor, too, if you're a heavy drinker. Your liver function will be tested before you start Zyflo, and regularly thereafter. Be sure to go in for these tests. If they reveal liver damage, you'll have to stop taking Zyflo. Also be sure to tell your doctor immediately if you develop any symptoms of liver disease. These include pain in the upper right abdomen, nausea, fatigue, lethargy, itching, general discomfort, and jaundice (yellowing of the skin and eyes).

Possible food and drug interactions when taking this medication

If Zyflo is taken with certain other drugs, the effects of either could be increased, decreased, or altered. You should check with your doctor before stopping or starting any prescription or nonprescription medicine. This is especially important with the following:

Astemizole (Hismanal)
Beta-blockers (a type of heart and blood pressure medication) such as Inderal, Sectral, and Tenormin
Calcium channel blockers (another type of heart and blood pressure medication) such as Calan, Cardizem, and Procardia
Cisapride (Propulsid)
Cyclosporine (Sandimmune, Neoral)
Terfenadine (Seldane)
Theophylline (Theo-Dur)
Warfarin (Coumadin)

While you are taking Zyflo, your theophylline dosage may need to be lowered, and your theophylline levels will have to be carefully watched.

Dosages of Inderal may also need reduction, and warfarin dosages may need adjustment as well.

Special information if you are pregnant or breastfeeding

The effects of Zyflo in pregnancy have not been adequately studied. If you are pregnant or plan to become pregnant, ask your doctor whether you should continue taking Zyflo. It is not certain that the drug appears in breast milk, but taking Zyflo while nursing is not recommended. Discuss with your doctor whether it's best to stop taking the drug or to give up breastfeeding.

Recommended dosage

ADULTS

The recommended dosage is one 600-milligram tablet 4 times a day.

CHILDREN

The safety and effectiveness of Zyflo in children under 12 years of age have not been established.

Overdosage

Because Zyflo is a relatively new drug, little is known about overdosage. However, any medication taken in excess can have serious consequences. If you suspect an overdose, seek medical treatment immediately.

ZYLOPRIM

Pronounced: ZYE-loe-prim
Generic name: Allopurinol

Why is this drug prescribed?

Zyloprim is used in the treatment of many symptoms of gout, including acute attacks, tophi (collection of uric acid crystals in the tissues, especially around joints), joint destruction, and uric acid stones. Gout is a form of arthritis characterized by increased blood levels of uric acid. Zyloprim works by reducing uric acid production in the body, thus preventing crystals from forming.

Zyloprim is also used to manage the increased uric acid levels in the blood of people with certain cancers, such as leukemia. It is also prescribed to manage some types of kidney stones.

Most important fact about this drug

Zyloprim will not stop a gout attack that is already under way. However, when taken over a period of several months, this drug will begin to reduce your symptoms. It's important to keep taking it regularly, even if it seems to have no immediate effect.

How should you take this medication?

Take Zyloprim exactly as prescribed. Your doctor will probably start you on a low dosage, increasing it gradually each week until you reach the dosage that is best for you.

A typical starting dose is one 100-milligram tablet per day. You may want to take Zyloprim immediately after a meal to minimize the risk of stomach irritation.

You should avoid taking large doses of vitamin C because of the increased possibility of kidney stone formation.

While taking Zyloprim you should drink plenty of liquids—10 to 12 glasses (8 ounces each) per day—unless otherwise prescribed by your doctor.

To help prevent attacks of gout, you should also avoid beer, wine, and purine-rich foods such as anchovies, sardines, liver, kidneys, lentils, and sweetbreads.

If you have been taking colchicine and/or an anti-inflammatory drug, such as Anaprox, Indocin, and others, to relieve your gout, your doctor will probably want you to continue taking this medication while your Zyloprim dosage is being adjusted. Later, when you have had no attacks of gout for several months, you may be able to stop taking these other medications.

If you have been taking a drug that promotes the excretion of uric acid in the urine, such as probenecid (Benemid) or sulfinpyrazone (Anturane), to try to prevent attacks of gout, your doctor will probably want to reduce or stop your dosage of this drug while increasing your dosage of Zyloprim.

■ *If you miss a dose...*
Take it as soon as you remember. If it is almost time for your next dose, skip the one you missed and go back to your regular schedule. Do not take 2 doses at once.

■ *Storage instructions...*
Store at room temperature in a cool, dry place, away from light.

What side effects may occur?

Side effects cannot be anticipated. If any develop or change in intensity, inform your doctor as soon as possible. Only your doctor can determine if it is safe for you to continue taking Zyloprim.

Because a skin reaction, the most common side effect of Zyloprim, may occasionally become severe or even fatal, you should stop taking Zyloprim if you notice even the beginnings of a rash. Such a rash may be itchy or scaly or may make your skin peel off in sheets; it may be accompanied by chills and fever, aching joints, or jaundice.

■ *Side effects may include:*
Acute attack of gout, diarrhea, nausea, rash

Why should this drug not be prescribed?

Do not take Zyloprim if you have ever had a severe reaction to it in the past.

Special warnings about this medication

If you notice a rash or other signs of an allergic reaction, stop taking Zyloprim immediately and consult your doctor. In some people, a Zyloprim-induced rash may lead to a serious skin disease, generalized inflammation of a blood or lymph vessel, irreversible liver damage, or even death.

You may experience acute attacks of gout more often in the early stages of Zyloprim therapy, even when normal uric acid levels have been attained. These attacks will become shorter and less severe after several months of therapy.

A kidney problem may turn a normal dose of Zyloprim into an overdose. If you have a kidney disease, or a condition such as diabetes or high blood pressure that may affect your kidneys, your doctor should prescribe Zyloprim cautiously and order periodic blood and urine tests to assess your kidney function.

Because Zyloprim may make you drowsy, do not drive or perform hazardous tasks until you know how the medication affects you.

It may be 2 to 6 weeks before you see any results from this medication.

Possible food and drug interactions when taking this medication

If Zyloprim is taken with certain other drugs, the effects of either could be increased, decreased, or altered. It is especially important to check with your doctor before combining Zyloprim with the following:

Amoxicillin (Amoxil, Trimox, Wymox)
Ampicillin (Omnipen, Principen)
Azathioprine (Imuran)
Blood thinners such as Coumadin
Cyclosporine (Sandimmune, Neoral)
Drugs for diabetes, such as Diabinese and Orinase
Mercaptopurine (Purinethol)
Probenecid (Benemid, ColBENEMID)
Sulfinpyrazone (Anturane)
Theophylline (Theo-Dur, Slo-Phyllin, and others)
Thiazide diuretics such as Diuril, HydroDIURIL, and others
Vitamin C

Special information if you are pregnant or breastfeeding

The effects of Zyloprim during pregnancy have not been adequately studied. If you are pregnant or plan to become pregnant, notify your doctor immediately. Zyloprim should be taken during pregnancy only if it is clearly needed.

Zyloprim appears in breast milk; what effect it may have on a nursing baby is unknown. Caution is advised when Zyloprim is taken during breastfeeding.

Recommended dosage

ADULTS

Your doctor will tailor your dosage of Zyloprim individually to control the severity of symptoms and to bring the uric acid levels to normal or near normal.

Gout

The usual starting dose is 100 milligrams once daily. Your doctor may increase your dose by 100 milligrams per day at 1-week intervals until desired results are attained. The average dose is 200 to 300 milligrams per day for mild gout and 400 to 600 milligrams daily for moderate to severe gout. The most you should take in a day is 800 milligrams.

Recurrent Kidney Stones

The usual dose is 200 to 300 milligrams daily, divided into smaller doses or taken as one dose.

Management of Uric Acid Levels in Certain Cancers

The usual dose is 600 to 800 milligrams daily for 2 to 3 days, together with a high fluid intake.

CHILDREN

The usual recommended dose for children 6 to 10 years of age is 300 milligrams daily for the management of uric acid levels in certain types of cancer. Children under 6 years of age are generally given 150 milligrams daily.

Overdosage

Although no specific information is available regarding Zyloprim overdosage, any medication taken in excess can have serious consequences. If you suspect an overdose of Zyloprim, seek medical attention immediately.

ZYMAR

Pronounced: ZIE-mar
Generic name: Gatifloxacin

Why is this drug prescribed?

Zymar is an antibiotic used in the treatment of eye infections such as conjunctivitis (pinkeye) and other bacterial infections. Gatifloxacin, the active ingredient, is a member of the quinolone family of antibiotics.

Most important fact about this drug

Other forms of gatifloxacin have been known to cause allergic reactions in a few patients. These reactions can be extremely serious, leading to loss of consciousness and cardiovascular collapse. Early warning signs include a skin rash, hives, and itching. Other symptoms may include swelling of the face or throat, shortness of breath, and being unable to breathe. If you develop any of these symptoms, seek emergency help immediately.

How should you take this medication?

Zymar solution is administered with an eyedropper. To avoid contaminating the solution, do not touch the tip of the dropper to your eye, finger, or any other surface.

■ *If you miss a dose…*
Take it as soon as you remember. If it is almost time for your next dose, skip the one you missed and go back to your regular schedule. Do not take 2 doses at once.

■ *Storage instructions…*
Store at room temperature; do not freeze.

What side effects may occur?

Side effects cannot be anticipated. If any develop or change in intensity, tell your doctor as soon as possible. Only your doctor can determine if it is safe to continue using Zymar.

■ *Side effects may include:*
Eye irritation, increased tearing, inflammation of the cornea or other parts of the eye

Why should this drug not be prescribed?

Do not use Zymar if you've ever had an allergic reaction to the drug or to other quinolone antibiotics such as Cipro, Floxin, Levaquin, Noroxin, Avelox, or Tequin.

Special warnings about this medication

Long-term use of Zymar could promote the growth of germs that are resistant to the medication. The doctor will examine your eyes as needed to watch for signs of this development.

Be sure to tell the doctor if you wear contact lenses. People with eye infections generally should not wear contact lenses.

Zymar has not been studied in infants less than 1 year old.

Possible food and drug interactions when taking this medication

There is no information on interactions with Zymar. When taken internally, however, gatifloxacin is known to interact with the following:

Caffeine
Cyclosporine (Neoral, Sandimmune)
Theophylline (Theo-Dur)
Warfarin (Coumadin)

Special information if you are pregnant or breastfeeding

Zymar has not been adequately studied in pregnant women. If you are pregnant or plan to become pregnant, alert your doctor immediately.

Researchers do not know whether Zymar can be passed to a breastfeeding infant. However, animal studies indicate that it could appear in breast milk. If you plan to breastfeed, discuss your medication options with your doctor.

Recommended dosage

For days 1 and 2, insert one drop in each affected eye every 2 hours, up to a maximum of eight times a day. For days 3 through 7, insert one drop up to a maximum of four times a day. Zymar should be used during your normal waking hours. You do not have to wake up from sleeping to take the medication.

Overdosage

There is no information on Zymar overdose. However, any medication taken in excess can have serious consequences. If you suspect an overdose, seek medical attention immediately.

ZYPREXA

Pronounced: Zye-PRECKS-ah
Generic name: Olanzapine

Why is this drug prescribed?

Zyprexa helps manage symptoms of schizophrenia, the manic phase of bipolar disorder, and other psychotic disorders. It is thought to work by opposing the action of serotonin and dopamine, two of the brain's major chemical messengers. The drug is available as Zyprexa tablets and Zyprexa Zydis, which dissolves rapidly with or without liquid.

Most important fact about this drug

At the start of Zyprexa therapy, the drug can cause extreme low blood pressure, increased heart rate, dizziness, and, in rare cases, a tendency to faint when first standing up. These problems are more likely if you are dehydrated, have heart disease, or take blood pressure medicine. To avoid such problems, your doctor may start with a low dose of Zyprexa and increase the dosage gradually.

Drugs such as Zyprexa may increase the risk of death in elderly people with dementia-related psychosis. Zyprexa is not approved for use in such patients.

How should you take this medication?

Zyprexa should be taken once a day with or without food. To use Zyprexa Zydis, open the sachet, peel back the foil on the blister pack, remove the tablet, and place the entire tablet in the mouth. Do not push the tablet through the foil. The medication can be taken with or without water; the saliva in your mouth will cause the tablet to dissolve.

■ *If you miss a dose...*
Take it as soon as you remember. If it is almost time for your next dose, skip the one you missed and go back to your regular schedule. Do not take 2 doses at once.

■ *Storage instructions...*
Store at room temperature away from light and moisture.

What side effects may occur?

Side effects cannot be anticipated. If any develop or change in intensity, inform your doctor as soon as possible. Only your doctor can determine if it is safe for you to continue taking Zyprexa.

■ *Side effects may include:*
Agitation, change in personality, constipation, dizziness, dry mouth, increased appetite, indigestion, low blood pressure upon standing, sleepiness, tremor, weakness, weight gain

Why should this drug not be prescribed?

If Zyprexa gives you an allergic reaction, you cannot take the drug.

Special warnings about this drug

Certain antipsychotic drugs, including Zyprexa, are associated with an increased risk of developing high blood sugar, which on rare occasions has led to coma or death. See your doctor right away if you develop signs of high blood sugar, including dry mouth, unusual thirst, increased urination, and tiredness. If you have diabetes or have a high risk of developing it, see your doctor regularly for blood sugar testing.

Use Zyprexa with caution if you have any of the following conditions: Alzheimer's disease, Parkinson's disease, trouble swallowing, narrow angle glaucoma (high pressure in the eye), an enlarged prostate, heart irregularities, heart disease, heart failure, liver disease, or a history of heart attack, seizures, or intestinal blockage.

Drugs such as Zyprexa sometimes cause a condition called Neuroleptic Malignant Syndrome (NMS). Symptoms include high fever, muscle rigidity, irregular pulse or blood pressure, rapid heartbeat, excessive sweating, and changes in heart rhythm. If these symptoms appear, contact your doctor right away. You'll have to discontinue using Zyprexa while the condition is under treatment.

There is also a risk of developing tardive dyskinesia, a condition marked by slow, rhythmical, involuntary movements. This problem is more likely to surface in older adults, especially elderly women. When it does, use of Zyprexa is usually stopped.

Animal studies suggest that Zyprexa may increase the risk of breast cancer, although human studies have not confirmed such a risk. If you have a history of breast cancer, see your doctor regularly for checkups.

People at high risk of suicide attempts should be prescribed the lowest dose possible to reduce the risk of intentional overdose.

Zyprexa sometimes causes drowsiness and can impair your judgment, thinking, and motor skills. Use caution while driving and don't operate dangerous machinery until you know how the drug affects you.

Medicines such as Zyprexa can interfere with regulation of the body's temperature. Do not get overheated or become dehydrated while taking Zyprexa. Avoid extreme heat and drink plenty of fluids.

Zyprexa can cause low blood pressure upon standing, resulting in dizziness, rapid heartbeat, and fainting, especially at the start of therapy. Let the doctor know if you develop this problem; your dosage can be adjusted to reduce the symptoms.

If you have phenylketonuria and must avoid the amino acid phenylalanine, you should not take Zyprexa Zydis, which contains this substance.

The safety and effectiveness of Zyprexa have not been studied in children.

Possible food and drug interactions when taking this medication
Avoid alcohol while taking Zyprexa. The combination can cause a sudden drop in blood pressure.

If Zyprexa is taken with certain other drugs, the effects of either can be increased, decreased, or altered. Ask your doctor before taking any prescription or over-the-counter drugs. It is especially important to check before combining Zyprexa with the following:

Blood pressure medications
Carbamazepine (Tegretol)
Diazepam (Valium)
Drugs that boost the effect of dopamine, such as the Parkinson's
     medications Mirapex, Parlodel, Permax, and Requip
Fluvoxamine
Levodopa (Larodopa)
Omeprazole (Prilosec)
Rifampin (Rifadin, Rimactane)

Special information if you are pregnant or breastfeeding

If you are pregnant or plan to become pregnant, inform your doctor immediately. Zyprexa should be used during pregnancy only if absolutely necessary. The drug may appear in breast milk; do not breastfeed while on Zyprexa therapy.

Recommended dosage

ADULTS

Schizophrenia

The usual starting dose is 5 to 10 milligrams once a day. If you start at the lower dose, after a few days the doctor will increase it to 10. After that, the dosage will be increased no more than once a week, 5 milligrams at a time, up to a maximum of 20 milligrams a day.

Those most likely to start at 5 milligrams are people who are weak, people prone to low blood pressure, and nonsmoking women over 65 (because they tend to have a slow metabolism).

Manic Episodes in Bipolar Disorder

The usual starting dose is 10 to 15 milligrams once a day. If needed, the dose can be increased every 24 hours by 5 milligrams a day, up to a maximum daily dose of 20 milligrams. After the person is stabilized, the doctor may continue maintenance therapy at a dosage range of 5 to 20 milligrams a day. If Zyprexa is being combined with lithium or valproate (Depakene, Depakote), the usual starting dose is 10 milligrams once a day.

Overdosage

An overdose of Zyprexa is usually not life-threatening, but fatalities have been reported. If you suspect an overdose, seek medical attention immediately.

■ *Symptoms of Zyprexa overdose may include:*
   Agitation, drowsiness, rapid or irregular heartbeat, slurred or disrupted speech, stupor

Overdoses of Zyprexa have also led to breathing difficulties, changes in blood pressure, excessive perspiration, fever, muscle rigidity, cardiac arrest, coma, and convulsions.

ZYRTEC

Pronounced: ZEER-tek
Generic name: Cetirizine hydrochloride

Why is this drug prescribed?

Zyrtec is an antihistamine. It is prescribed to treat the sneezing; itchy, runny nose; and itchy, red, watery eyes caused by seasonal allergies such as hay fever. Zyrtec also relieves the symptoms of year-round allergies due to dust, mold, and animal dander. This medication is also used in the treatment of chronic itchy skin and hives.

Most important fact about this drug

Zyrtec may cause drowsiness. Be especially careful driving or operating dangerous machinery or participating in any hazardous activity that requires full mental alertness until you know how you react to this medication.

How should you take this medication?

Take Zyrtec once a day, exactly as prescribed. This medication can be taken with or without food.

Zyrtec may make your mouth dry. Sucking hard candy, chewing a stick of gum, or melting bits of ice in your mouth can provide relief.

- *If you miss a dose...*
  If you are taking this medication on a regular schedule, take the forgotten dose as soon as you remember. If it is almost time for your next dose, skip the one you missed and go back to your regular schedule. Do not take 2 doses at once.
- *Storage instructions...*
  Store the tablets and syrup at room temperature. The syrup may be refrigerated.

What side effects may occur?

Side effects cannot be anticipated. If any develop or change in intensity, tell your doctor as soon as possible. Only your doctor can determine if it is safe for you to continue taking Zyrtec.

- *Side effects in adults may include:*
  Drowsiness, dry mouth, fatigue
- *Side effects in children aged 6 to 11 may include:*
  Abdominal pain, coughing, diarrhea, headache, nosebleed, sleepiness, sore throat, wheezing

Why should this drug not be prescribed?

Avoid Zyrtec if it causes a reaction, or if you have ever had a reaction to the similar drug Atarax.

Special warnings about this medication

If you have kidney or liver disease, be sure to tell your doctor. Your dose of this medication may have to be reduced.

Possible food and drug interactions when taking this medication

You should avoid drinking alcohol or taking sedatives, tranquilizers, sleeping pills, or muscle relaxants while using Zyrtec. They can lead to increased drowsiness and reduced mental alertness. Among the products to avoid are the following:

Antidepressants such as Anafranil, Elavil, Ludiomil, and Tofranil
Muscle relaxants such as Soma and Valium
Pain-relieving narcotics such as codeine, Demerol, and Percocet
Sedatives such as Nembutal, phenobarbital, and Seconal
Sleeping pills such as Ambien, Halcion, and Restoril
High doses of theophylline (Theo-Dur)

Special information if you are pregnant or breastfeeding

The effects of Zyrtec during pregnancy have not been adequately studied. If you are pregnant or plan to become pregnant, tell your doctor immediately. Zyrtec appears in breast milk and should not be used if you are breastfeeding.

Recommended dosage

ADULTS AND CHILDREN 12 YEARS AND OLDER

The usual starting dose is 5 or 10 milligrams once a day, depending on the severity of your symptoms. If you have a kidney or liver condition, the doctor will probably prescribe 5 milligrams daily.

CHILDREN 6 TO 11 YEARS

The usual starting dose is 5 or 10 milligrams (1 or 2 teaspoonfuls of syrup) once a day. If your child has a kidney or liver condition, the doctor will probably prescribe the lower dose.

CHILDREN 2 TO 5 YEARS

The usual starting dose is 2.5 milligrams (one-half teaspoonful) once a day. Dosage may be increased to a maximum of 5 milligrams (1 teaspoonful) once daily or 2.5 milligrams (one-half teaspoonful) every 12 hours. If the child has a kidney or liver condition, Zyrtec should not be given.

CHILDREN 6 TO 23 MONTHS

The usual starting dose is 2.5 milligrams (one-half teaspoonful) once a day. In children 12 to 23 months old, the dose can be increased to a maximum of 5 milligrams a day, given as 2.5 milligrams (one-half teaspoonful) every 12 hours. Zyrtec should not be used if your child has kidney or liver problems.

Overdosage

Any medication taken in excess can have serious consequences. In adults, the primary symptom of a Zyrtec overdose is extreme sleepiness. In children, restlessness and irritability may precede drowsiness. If you suspect an overdose, seek medical treatment immediately.

ZYRTEC-D

Pronounced: ZEER-tek
Generic ingredients: Cetirizine hydrochloride,
  Pseudoephedrine hydrochloride

Why is this drug prescribed?

Zyrtec-D contains the same antihistamine found in regular Zyrtec, plus the decongestant pseudoephedrine. The drug is prescribed to relieve the symptoms of hay fever and similar allergies, whether seasonal or year-round.

Most important fact about this drug

Unlike regular Zyrtec, this drug should be avoided by anyone with severe heart or blood pressure problems.

How should you take this medication?

Zyrtec-D comes in 12-hour extended release tablets, and should be taken no more than twice a day. The tablet may be taken with or without food, but should be swallowed whole, without breaking or chewing.

■ *If you miss a dose...*
  Take it as soon as you remember. If it is almost time for your next dose, skip the one you missed and go back to your regular schedule. Do not take 2 doses at once.
■ *Storage instructions...*
  Store at room temperature.

What side effects may occur?

■ *Side effects may include:*
  Dry mouth, fatigue, insomnia, sleepiness

Why should this drug not be prescribed?

If you are allergic to any of Zyrtec-D's ingredients, to the similar drug Atarax, or to certain drugs that tend to raise blood pressure (adrenergic agents), do not take Zyrtec-D. Symptoms that indicate a sensitivity to adrenergic agents include insomnia, dizziness, weakness, tremor, or irregular heartbeat.

You should also avoid Zyrtec-D if you have severely high blood pressure, severe heart disease, high pressure in the eye (glaucoma), or difficulty urinating. Never combine Zyrtec-D with a drug classified as an MAO inhibitor, such as the antidepressants Nardil and Parnate.

Special warnings about this medication

If you have a mild case of high blood pressure or heart disease, use Zyrtec-D sparingly. Be cautious, too, if you have diabetes, a tendency to increased pressure in the eye (glaucoma), an overactive thyroid gland, or an enlarged prostate gland. If you have kidney or liver problems, make sure your doctor is aware of it. Your dosage may have to be reduced.

Zyrtec-D makes some people sleepy. Exercise caution when driving a car or operating potentially dangerous machinery after taking this drug.

This drug is not recommended for children under 12 years of age.

Possible food and drug interactions when taking this medication

Avoid Zyrtec-D if you've taken an MAO inhibitor such as Nardil or Parnate anytime within the preceding 14 days. Also avoid combining Zyrtec-D with alcohol, antidepressants, muscle relaxants, tranquilizers, sedatives, sleeping pills, or pain-relieving narcotics; they increase the likelihood of drowsiness.

If Zyrtec-D is taken with certain other drugs, the effects of either could be increased, decreased, or altered. It is especially important to check with your doctor before combining Zyrtec-D with the following:

Certain drugs used to treat high blood pressure, including Aldomet, Inversine, and reserpine
Digitalis
Drugs that tend to raise blood pressure
High doses of theophylline (Theo-Dur)

Special information if you are pregnant or breastfeeding

If you are pregnant or plan to become pregnant, check with your doctor before taking Zyrtec-D. The possibility of harm to the developing baby has not be ruled out.

Both of the active agents in Zyrtec-D make their way into human breast milk. It is not recommended for nursing mothers.

Recommended dosage

ADULTS

The recommended dose for adults and children 12 years of age and older is 1 tablet twice daily. If you have kidney or liver problems, your doctor may recommend only 1 dose per day.

Overdosage

An overdose of Zyrtec-D can have serious consequences. If you suspect an overdose, seek medical care immediately.

■ *Symptoms of Zyrtec-D overdose may include:*
Chest pain, coma, convulsions, delusions, drowsiness, giddiness, hallucinations, headache, insomnia, irregular heartbeat, irritability, muscle weakness, nausea, palpitations, respiratory failure, restlessness, sweating, thirst, urination problems, vomiting

ZYVOX

Pronounced: ZIGH-vox
Generic name: Linezolid

Why is this drug prescribed?

Zyvox is a member of the class of antibiotics called oxazolidinones. It is used to treat certain types of pneumonia, some forms of skin infection, and infections involving certain strains of a germ called *Enterococcus faecium*.

Most important fact about this drug

Antibiotic treatment can cause a type of diarrhea that, in rare cases, becomes extremely severe. If you develop diarrhea after starting Zyvox, be sure to notify your doctor immediately.

If you need to take Zyvox for more than two weeks, your doctor will perform blood tests to check for blood abnormalities. Blood tests are also needed if you tend to bleed easily or are taking medications that increase your chance of bleeding.

Zyvox could cause a very rare—but potentially fatal—side effect known as lactic acidosis, especially if the treatment lasts longer than the recommended 28 days. It is caused by a buildup of lactic acid in the blood. Lactic acidosis is a medical emergency that must be treated in a hospital. Notify your doctor immediately if you experience repeated nausea and vomiting or any of the following:

- *Symptoms of lactic acidosis may include:*
  Dizziness, extreme weakness or tiredness, light-headedness, low body temperature, rapid breathing or trouble breathing, sleepiness, slow or irregular heartbeat, unexpected or unusual stomach discomfort, unusual muscle pain

How should you take this medication?

Zyvox should be taken twice a day, every 12 hours, until the prescription is finished. Do not stop taking the medicine when you start to feel better. If you discontinue it too soon, surviving germs may cause a relapse. Zyvox may be taken with or without food.

If you are taking the liquid formulation of Zyvox, gently mix it before each use by turning the bottle upside down and upright 3 to 5 times. Do not shake the bottle.

Your doctor will prescribe Zyvox only to treat a bacterial infection; it will not cure a viral infection, such as the common cold. It's important to take the full dosage schedule of this medication, even if you're feeling better in a few days. Not completing the full dosage schedule may decrease the drug's effectiveness and increase the chances that the bacteria may become resistant to Zyvox and similar antibiotics.

■ *If you miss a dose...*
Take it as soon as you remember. If it is almost time for your next dose, skip the one you missed and go back to your regular schedule. Never take 2 doses at the same time.

■ *Storage instructions...*
Both Zyvox tablets and Zyvox liquid can be stored at room temperature. Keep the bottles tightly closed and protect from light and moisture. The liquid formulation should be used within 21 days.

What side effects may occur?
Side effects cannot be anticipated. If any develop or change in intensity, inform your doctor as soon as possible. Only your doctor can determine if it is safe for you to continue taking Zyvox.

■ *Side effects reported in adults may include:*
Diarrhea, headache, nausea, vomiting

■ *Side effects reported in children may include:*
Anemia, blood infection, diarrhea, fever, rash, upper respiratory infection, vomiting

Why should this drug not be prescribed?
If Zyvox gives you an allergic reaction, you won't be able to use it.

Special warnings about this medication
Let the doctor know if you have high blood pressure. Zyvox has not been tested under these conditions.

If you have a condition called phenylketonuria and must avoid the amino acid phenylalanine, it's important to know that the liquid formulation of Zyvox contains this substance.

Possible food and drug interactions when taking this medication
If Zyvox is taken with certain other drugs, the effects of either could be increased, decreased, or altered. It is especially important to check with your doctor before combining Zyvox with the following:

Decongestants such as Entex and Sudafed
Over-the-counter cold medicines and cough syrups that contain
  pseudoephedrine
Serotonin-boosting antidepressants such as Paxil, Prozac, and
  Zoloft, as well as other antidepressants such as Elavil and
  Tofranil

While taking Zyvox, it's important to avoid eating large amounts of foods that contain a chemical called tyramine. Food products high in tyramine include aged cheese, fermented or air-dried meats such as dry sausage, sauerkraut, soy sauce, red wine, tap beers, and any protein-rich food that has been improperly refrigerated.

Special information if you are pregnant or breastfeeding

Zyvox has not been studied in pregnant women or nursing mothers. Because the possibility of harm to the developing baby has not been ruled out, Zyvox should be used during pregnancy only if the potential benefit outweighs the possible risk. If you wish to breastfeed your infant, discuss your treatment options with your doctor.

Recommended dosage

ADULTS AND ADOLESCENTS 12 AND OLDER

Pneumonia and Complicated Skin Infections
The usual dosage is 600 milligrams every 12 hours for 10 to 14 days.

Uncomplicated Skin Infections
Adults: The usual dosage is 400 milligrams every 12 hours for 10 to 14 days.
   Adolescents 12 years and older: The usual dosage is 600 milligrams every 12 hours for 10 to 14 days.

Enterococcus faecium *Infections*
The usual dosage is 600 milligrams every 12 hours for 14 to 28 days.

CHILDREN (BIRTH TO 11 YEARS OLD)

Pneumonia and Complicated Skin Infections
The usual dosage is 10 milligrams for every 2.2 pounds of body weight taken every 8 hours for 10 to 14 days.

Uncomplicated Skin Infections
Children under 5 years old: The usual dosage is 10 milligrams for every 2.2 pounds of body weight taken every 8 hours for 10 to 14 days.
   Children 5 to 11 years old: The usual dosage is 10 milligrams for every 2.2 pounds of body weight taken every 12 hours for 10 to 14 days.

Enterococcus faecium *Infections*
The usual dosage is 10 milligrams for every 2.2 pounds of body weight taken every 8 hours for 14 to 28 days.

Overdosage

Little is known about the effects of a Zyvox overdose. However, any medication taken in excess can have serious consequences, so if you suspect an overdose, seek medical attention immediately.

Disease & Disorder Index

Appendices

Disease & Disorder Index

Use this index to find out which drugs are available for a specific medical problem. Both brand and generic names are listed: the generic names are shown in italics. Only brands covered in the drug profiles are included.

Inderal, 676
*Isometheptene, Dichloral-
    phenazone, and Acetaminophen.
    See* Midrin
Maxalt, 812
Midrin, 858
Migranal, 859
Naratriptan. See Amerge
Propranolol. See Inderal
Relpax, 1229
Rizatriptan. See Maxalt
Sumatriptan. See Imitrex
Topamax, 1461
Topiramate. See Topamax
Zolmitriptan. See Zomig
Zomig, 1650

Headache, simple
See Pain

Headache, tension
Anolor 300. *See* Fioricet
*Butalbital, Acetaminophen and
    Caffeine. See* Fioricet
*Butalbital, Aspirin, and Caffeine.
    See* Fiorinal
*Butalbital, Codeine, Aspirin, and
    Caffeine. See* Fiorinal with
    Codeine
Esgic. *See* Fioricet
Fioricet, 565
Fiorinal, 568
Fiorinal with Codeine, 571

Heart attack, risk reduction
Altace, 77
Aspirin, 132
Atorvastatin. See Lipitor
Clopidogrel. See Plavix
Ecotrin. See Aspirin
Empirin. See Aspirin
Genuine Bayer. *See* Aspirin
Lipitor, 764
Lovastatin. See Mevacor
Mevacor, 839
Plavix, 1108
Pravachol, 1120
Pravastatin. See Pravachol

Pravastatin with Aspirin. See
    Pravigard PAC
Pravigard PAC, 1123
Ramipril. See Altace
Simvastatin. *See* Zocor
Zocor, 1638

Heart attack, treatment of
Atenolol. See Tenormin
Coreg, 335
Carvedilol. See Coreg
Inderal, 676
Lisinopril. See Zestril
Lopressor, 775
Mavik, 809
Metoprolol. See Lopressor
Prinivil. *See* Zestril
Propranolol. See Inderal
Tenormin, 1405
Trandolapril. See Mavik
Zestril, 1624

**Heartburn and related stomach
    problems**
AcipHex, 19
Cimetidine. See Tagamet
Esomeprazole. See Nexium
Famotidine. *See* Pepcid
Lansoprazole. See Prevacid
Metoclopramide. See Reglan
Nexium, 934
Omeprazole. See Prilosec
Pantoprazole. See Protonix
Pepcid, 1070
Prevacid, 1143
Prilosec, 1155
Protonix, 1182
Rabeprazole. See AcipHex
Reglan, 1222
Tagamet, 1378

Heart failure, congestive
See also Fluid retention
Accupril, 6
Acetazolamide. See Diamox
Altace, 77
*Amiloride with Hydrochlorothiazide.
    See* Moduretic

Ampicillin, 98
Augmentin, 150
Bactrim, 188
Ceclor, 261
Cefaclor. See Ceclor
Cefadroxil. See Duricef
Ceftin, 266
Cefuroxime. See Ceftin
Cephalexin. See Keflex
Cipro, 289
Ciprofloxacin. See Cipro
Doryx, 474
Doxycycline. See Doryx
Duricef, 483
Dynacin. See Minocin
E.E.S. *See* Erythromycin, Oral
E-Mycin. *See* Erythromycin, Oral
ERYC. *See* Erythromycin, Oral
Ery-Tab. *See* Erythromycin, Oral
Erythrocin. *See* Erythromycin,
    Oral
Erythromycin, Oral, 520
Flagyl, 574
Floxin, 581
Fosfomycin. See Monurol
Gantrisin, 612
Gatifloxacin. See Tequin
Keflex, 703
Keftab. *See* Keflex
Levaquin, 735
Levofloxacin. See Levaquin
Lomefloxacin. See Maxaquin
Lorabid, 781
Loracarbef. See Lorabid
Macrobid. See Macrodantin
Macrodantin, 806
Maxaquin, 814
Methenamine. See Urised
Metronidazole. See Flagyl
Minocin, 867
Minocycline. See Minocin
Monurol, 893
Nitrofurantoin. See Macrodantin
Norfloxacin. See Noroxin
Noroxin, 966
Ofloxacin. See Floxin
PCE. *See* Erythromycin, Oral
Principen. See Ampicillin

Septra. *See* Bactrim
Sulfisoxazole. See Gantrisin
Sumycin. See Tetracycline
Tequin, 1410
Tetracycline, 1422
*Trimethoprim with
    Sulfamethoxazole. See*
    Bactrim
Urised, 1532
Vibramycin. See Doryx
Vibra-Tabs. See Doryx

Infertility, female
Clomid. *See* Clomiphene Citrate
Clomiphene Citrate, 307
Prochieve, 1165
Progesterone gel. See Prochieve
Serophene. *See* Clomiphene
    Citrate

Inflammation, rectal
Canasa. *See* Rowasa
Mesalamine. See Rowasa
Rowasa, 1280

Inflammatory diseases
Anaprox, 105
Decadron Tablets, 394
Dexamethasone. See Decadron
    Tablets
Medrol, 817
Methylprednisolone. See Medrol
Naprelan. *See* Anaprox
Naproxen sodium. See Anaprox
Pediapred, 1048
*Prednisolone Sodium Phosphate.
    See* Pediapred
Prednisone, 1132

Inflammatory diseases of the eye
Alamast, 59
Ciloxan, 287
Ciprofloxacin, ocular. See Ciloxan
Crolom, 365
Cromolyn, ocular. See Crolom
Fluorometholone. See FML
FML, 594

NicoDerm CQ. *See* Nicotine
  Patches
Nicotine Patches, 939
Nicotrol. *See* Nicotine Patches
Nicotrol Inhaler, 944
Nicotrol NS, 946
Zyban, 1659

Social anxiety disorder
Effexor XR. *See* Effexor
Paroxetine. See Paxil
Paxil, 1042
Sertraline. See Zoloft
Zoloft, 1646

Sore throat symptoms
See Coughs and colds

Sore throat treatment
*See Infections, upper respiratory
  tract*

Spastic colon
Anaspaz. *See* Levsin
Bellatal. *See* Donnatal
Bentyl, 201
*Chlordiazepoxide with Clidinium.
  See* Librax
Dicyclomine. See Bentyl
Donnatal, 469
Hyoscyamine. See Levsin
Levbid. *See* Levsin
Levsin, 742
Levsinex. *See* Levsin
Librax, 756
NuLev. *See* Levsin
*Phenobarbital, Hyoscyamine,
  Atropine, and Scopolamine. See*
  Donnatal

Spasticity
Tizanidine. See Zanaflex
Zanaflex, 1607

Stroke, risk reduction
Aggrenox, 57
Altace, 77
Aspirin, 132

*Aspirin with Extended-release
  dipyridamole. See* Aggrenox
Clopidogrel. See Plavix
Ecotrin. *See* Aspirin
Empirin. *See* Aspirin
Genuine Bayer. *See* Aspirin
Plavix, 1108
Pravastatin with Aspirin. See
  Pravigard PAC
Pravigard PAC, 1123
Ramipril. See Altace
Simvastatin. See Zocor
Zocor, 1638

Syphilis
See Sexually transmitted diseases

Testosterone deficiency
Androderm. *See* Testosterone
  Patches
AndroGel, 109
Striant, 1351
Testim. *See* AndroGel
Testoderm. *See* Testosterone
  Patches
Testopel, 1417
*Testosterone buccal system, oral.
  See* Striant
Testosterone gel. See AndroGel
Testosterone Patches, 1420
Testosterone pellets. See
  Testopel

Thyroid hormone deficiency
Armour Thyroid, 127
Levothroid. See Synthroid
Levothyroxine. See Synthroid
Levoxyl. *See* Synthroid
Synthroid, 1375
Unithroid. *See* Synthroid

Tick fevers
See Infections, rickettsiae

Tics
Haldol, 646
Haloperidol. See Haldol

APPENDIX 1
Safe Medication Use

Using medications safely is largely a matter of common sense and caution. The following are general guidelines to keep in mind:

You and your doctor

- Tell your doctor everything about your medical history, including reactions to medications you've used in the past.
- Tell the doctor about any medications you are using now, even if they are over-the-counter drugs, dietary supplements (such as glucosamine), or herbal medicines (such as St. John's wort).
- Keep track of your reactions to a medication and report them to your doctor.
- Ask your doctor what you can do when given a new drug. For example, are there any foods to avoid when taking the drug? Should you avoid alcohol? Should you avoid driving?
- Never change your dose schedule unless your doctor tells you to do so—and always finish all the medication unless instructed otherwise.

You and your pharmacist

- See if there are any written instructions that you can take with you.
- Ask the pharmacist to explain clearly when and how to take the drug.
- Ask about any possible interactions between the new prescription and any other drugs, dietary supplements, or herbals that you might be taking.
- Ask how long the medication remains effective. Don't take it after its expiration date.
- If you are going on a vacation, make sure your drug can be used in different climates—and make sure you have enough to get you through your trip.

You and your medications

- Never take someone else's medication; and don't share your own medicines.
- Check the label each time you take a drug. Don't take—or dispense—a drug in the dark.
- Keep your medications in a dry, safe spot.

- Keep each medicine in the bottle from the drug store. Don't mix medicines together in a single bottle.
- If you think you are pregnant, consult with your doctor before using any medication.
- Destroy any unused portions of a drug and dispose of the bottle.
- Periodically check your medicine cabinet for expired medications. Toss them if they've expired.
- If you need a certain medicine (for instance, insulin) in case of emergency, carry the information with you.

Your medicines and your children

- Keep all medications in a locked cabinet or in a spot well out of the reach of children.
- Ask for child-proof safety bottles.
- Be alert and awake when giving a child medication.
- Make sure that children know medications can be dangerous if misused.
- Keep antidotes such as syrup of ipecac (which induces vomiting) on hand.
- Keep the numbers of your EMS and poison control centers handy.

APPENDIX 2
Poison Control Centers

The American Association of Poison Control Centers (AAPCC) uses a single, nationwide emergency number to automatically link callers with their regional poison center. This toll-free number, **800-222-1222**, also works for teletype lines (TTY) for the hearing-impaired and telecommunication devices (TTD) for individuals who are deaf. However, a few local poison centers and the ASPCA/Animal Poison Control Center are not part of this nationwide system and continue to use separate numbers.

Most of the centers listed below are certified by the AAPCC. **Certified centers are marked by an asterisk after the name.** Each has to meet certain criteria. It must, for example, serve a large geographic area; it must be open 24 hours a day and provide direct-dial or toll-free access; it must be supervised by a medical director; and it must have registered pharmacists or nurses available to answer questions from the public. Within each state, centers are listed alphabetically by city. Some state poison centers also list their original emergency numbers (including TTY/TDD) that only work within that state. For these listings, callers may use either the state number or the nationwide 800 number.

ALABAMA

BIRMINGHAM
Regional Poison Control Center, The Children's Hospital of Alabama (*)
1600 7th Ave. South
Birmingham, AL 35233-1711
Business: 205-939-9201
Emergency: 800-222-1222
                 800-292-6678 (AL)
www.chsys.org

TUSCALOOSA
Alabama Poison Center (*)
2503 Phoenix Dr.
Tuscaloosa, AL 35405
Business: 205-345-0600
Emergency: 800-222-1222
                 800-462-0800 (AL)
www.alapoisoncenter.org

ALASKA

JUNEAU
Alaska Poison Control System
Section of Community Health and EMS
410 Willoughby Ave.,
Room 109
Box 110616
Juneau, AK 99811-0616
Business: 907-465-3027
Emergency: 800-222-1222
www.chems.alaska.gov

(PORTLAND, OR)
Oregon Poison Center (*)
Oregon Health Sciences University
3181 SW Sam Jackson Park Rd.
CB550
Portland, OR 97239
Business: 503-494-8600
Emergency: 800-222-1222
www.oregonpoison.com

ARIZONA

PHOENIX
Banner Poison Control Center (*)
Banner Good Samaritan Medical Center
901 E. Willetta St.
Room 2701
Phoenix, AZ 85006
Business: 602-495-6360
Emergency: 800-222-1222
              800-362-0101 (AZ)
              602-253-3334 (AZ)
www.bannerpoisoncontrol.com

TUCSON
Arizona Poison and Drug Information Center (*)
Arizona Health Sciences Center
1501 N. Campbell Ave.
Room 1156
Tucson, AZ 85724
Business: 520-626-7899
Emergency: 800-222-1222

ARKANSAS

LITTLE ROCK
Arkansas Poison and Drug Information Center
College of Pharmacy—UAMS
4301 West Markham St.
Mail Slot 522-2
Little Rock, AR 72205-7122
Business: 501-686-5540
Emergency: 800-222-1222
              800-376-4766 (AR)
TDD/TTY: 800-641-3805

ASPCA/ANIMAL POISON CONTROL CENTER

1717 South Philo Rd.
Suite 36
Urbana, IL 61802
Business: 217-337-5030
Emergency: 888-426-4435
              800-548-2423
www.napcc.aspca.org

CALIFORNIA

FRESNO/MADERA
California Poison Control System-Fresno/Madera Div.(*)
Children's Hospital of Central California
9300 Valley Children's Place
MB 15
Madera, CA 93638-8762
Business: 559-622-2300
Emergency: 800-222-1222
              800-876-4766 (CA)
TDD/TTY: 800-972-3323
www.calpoison.org

SACRAMENTO
California Poison Control System-Sacramento Div.(*)
UC Davis Medical Center
Room HSF 1024
2315 Stockton Blvd.
Sacramento, CA 95817
Business: 916-227-1400
Emergency: 800-222-1222
              800-876-4766 (CA)
TDD/TTY: 800-972-3323
www.calpoison.org

SAN DIEGO
California Poison Control
System-San Diego Div. (*)
UC San Diego Medical Center
200 West Arbor Dr.
San Diego, CA 92103-8925
Business: 858-715-6300
Emergency: 800-222-1222
800-876-4766 (CA)
TDD/TTY: 800-972-3323
www.calpoison.org

SAN FRANCISCO
California Poison Control
System-San Francisco Div.(*)
San Francisco General Hospital
University of California San
Francisco
Box 1369
San Francisco, CA 94143-1369
Business: 415-502-6000
Emergency: 800-222-1222
800-876-4766 (CA)
TDD/TTY: 800-972-3323
www.calpoison.org

COLORADO

DENVER
Rocky Mountain Poison
and Drug Center (*)
777 Bannock St.
Mail Code 0180
Denver CO 80204-4507
Business: 303-739-1100
Emergency: 800-222-1222
TDD/TTY: 303-739-1127 (CO)
www.RMPDC.org

CONNECTICUT

FARMINGTON
Connecticut Regional
Poison Control Center (*)
University of Connecticut Health
Center
263 Farmington Ave.
Farmington, CT 06030-5365
Business: 860-679-4540
Emergency: 800-222-1222
TDD/TTY: 866-218-5372
http://poisoncontrol.uchc.edu

DELAWARE

(PHILADELPHIA, PA)
The Poison Control Center (*)
Children's Hospital of Philadelphia
34th St. & Civic Center Blvd.
Philadelphia, PA 19104-4303
Business: 215-590-2003
Emergency: 800-222-1222
800-722-7112 (DE)
TDD/TTY: 215-590-8789
www.poisoncontrol.chop.edu

DISTRICT OF COLUMBIA

WASHINGTON, DC
National Capital Poison Center (*)
3201 New Mexico Ave., NW
Suite 310
Washington, DC 20016
Business: 202-362-3867
Emergency: 800-222-1222
TDD/TTY: 202-362-8563
www.poison.org

FLORIDA

JACKSONVILLE
Florida Poison Information
Center-Jacksonville (*)
SHANDS Hospital
655 West 8th St.
Jacksonville, FL 32209
Business: 904-244-4465
Emergency: 800-222-1222
http://fpicjax.org

MIAMI
Florida Poison Information
Center-Miami (*)
University of Miami–
Department of Pediatrics
P.O. Box 016960 (R-131)
Miami, FL 33101
Business: 305-585-5250
Emergency: 800-222-1222
www.miami.edu/poison-center

TAMPA
Florida Poison
Information Center-Tampa (*)
Tampa General Hospital
P.O. Box 1289
Tampa, FL 33601-1289
Business: 813-844-7044
Emergency: 800-222-1222
www.poisoncentertampa.org

GEORGIA

ATLANTA
Georgia Poison Center (*)
Hughes Spalding Children's
Hospital, Grady Health System
80 Jesse Hill Jr. Dr., SE
P.O. Box 26066
Atlanta, GA 30303-3050
Business: 404-616-9237
Emergency: 800-222-1222
            404-616-9000
            (Atlanta)
TDD: 404-616-9287
www.georgiapoisoncenter.org

HAWAII

(DENVER, CO)
Rocky Mountain Poison
and Drug Center (*)
777 Bannock St.
Mail Code 0180
Denver CO 80204-4507
Business: 303-739-1100
Emergency: 800-222-1222
www.RMPDC.org

IDAHO

(DENVER, CO)
Rocky Mountain Poison
& Drug Center (*)
777 Bannock St.
Mail Code 0180
Denver CO 80204-4507
Business: 303-739-1100
Emergency: 800-222-1222
www.RMPDC.org

ILLINOIS

CHICAGO
Illinois Poison Center (*)
222 South Riverside Plaza
Suite 1900
Chicago, IL 60606
Business: 312-906-6136
Emergency: 800-222-1222
TDD/TTY: 312-906-6185
www.illinoispoisoncenter.org

INDIANA

INDIANAPOLIS
Indiana Poison Control Center (*)
Clarian Health Partners Methodist Hospital
I-65 at 21st St.
Indianapolis, IN 46206-1367
Business: 317-962-2335
Emergency: 800-222-1222
            800-382-9097
            317-962-2323
            (Indianapolis)
TTY: 317-962-2336
www.clarian.org/clinical/poisoncontrol

IOWA

SIOUX CITY
Iowa Statewide Poison Control Center
Iowa Health System and the University of Iowa Hospitals and Clinics
2910 Hamilton Blvd., Suite 101
Sioux City, IA 51104
Business: 712-279-3710
Emergency: 800-222-1222
          712-277-2222 (IA)
www.iowapoison.org

KANSAS

KANSAS CITY
Mid-America Poison Control Center
University of Kansas Medical Center
3901 Rainbow Blvd.
Room B-400
Kansas City, KS 66160-7231
Business   913-588-6638
Emergency: 800-222-1222
          800-332-6633 (KS)
TDD: 913-588-6639
www.kumc.edu/poison

KENTUCKY

LOUISVILLE
Kentucky Regional Poison Center (*)
PO Box 35070
Louisville, KY 40232-5070
Business: 502-629-7264
Emergency: 800-222-1222
          502-589-8222
          (Louisville)
www.krpc.com

LOUISIANA

MONROE
Louisiana Drug and Poison Information Center (*)
University of Louisiana at Monroe
700 University Ave.
Monroe, LA 71209-6430
Business: 318-342-3648
Emergency: 800-222-1222
www.lapcc.org

MAINE

PORTLAND
Northern New England Poison Center
Maine Medical Center
22 Bramhall St.
Portland, ME 04102
Business: 207-842-7220
Emergency: 800-222-1222
          207-871-2879 (ME)
TDD/TTY: 877-299-4447 (ME)
          207-871-2879 (ME)

MARYLAND

BALTIMORE
Maryland Poison Center (*)
University of Maryland at Baltimore
School of Pharmacy
20 North Pine St., PH 772
Baltimore, MD 21201
Business: 410-706-7604
Emergency: 800-222-1222
TDD: 410-706-1858
www.mdpoison.com

(WASHINGTON, DC)
National Capital
Poison Center (*)
3201 New Mexico Ave., NW
Suite 310
Washington DC 20016
Business: 202-362-3867
Emergency: 800-222-1222
TDD/TTY: 202-362-8563 (MD)
www.poison.org

MASSACHUSETTS

BOSTON
Regional Center for Poison Control and Prevention (*)
(Serving Massachusetts and Rhode Island)
300 Longwood Ave.
Boston, MA 02115
Business: 617-355-6609
Emergency: 800-222-1222
TDD/TTY: 888-244-5313
www.maripoisoncenter.com

MICHIGAN

DETROIT
Regional Poison
Control Center (*)
Children's Hospital of Michigan
4160 John R. Harper
Professional Office Bldg.
Suite 616
Detroit, MI 48201
Business: 313-745-5335
Emergency: 800-222-1222
TDD/TTY: 800-356-3232
www.mitoxic.org/pcc

GRAND RAPIDS
DeVos Children's Hospital
Regional Poison Center (*)
100 Michigan St., NE
Grand Rapids, MI 49503
Business: 616-391-3690
Emergency: 800-222-1222
http://poisoncenter.devoschildrens.org

MINNESOTA

MINNEAPOLIS
Minnesota Poison Control System (*) Hennepin County Medical Center
701 Park Ave.
Mail Code 820
Minneapolis, MN 55415
Business: 612-873-6000
Emergency: 800-222-1222
TTY: 612-904-4691
www.mnpoison.org

MISSISSIPPI

JACKSON
Mississippi Regional Poison Control Center, University of Mississippi Medical Center
2500 North State St.
Jackson, MS 39216
Business: 601-984-1675
Emergency: 800-222-1222

MISSOURI

ST. LOUIS
Missouri Regional Poison Center (*)
Cardinal Glennon Children's Hospital
7980 Clayton Rd.
Suite 200
St. Louis, MO 63117
Business: 314-772-5200
Emergency: 800-222-1222
TDD/TTY: 314-612-5705
www.cardinalglennon.com

MONTANA

(DENVER, CO)
Rocky Mountain Poison and Drug Center (*)
777 Bannock St.
Mail Code 0180
Denver CO 80204-4507
Business: 303-739-1100
Emergency: 800-222-1222
TDD/TTY: 303-739-1127
www.RMPDC.org

NEBRASKA

OMAHA
The Poison Center (*)
Children's Hospital
8200 Dodge St.
Omaha, NE 68114
Business: 402-955-5555
Emergency: 800-222-1222
www.poison-center.com

NEVADA

(DENVER, CO)
Rocky Mountain Poison and Drug Center (*)
777 Bannock St.
Mail Code 0180
Denver CO 80204-4507
Business: 303-739-1100
Emergency: 800-222-1222
www.RMPDC.org

(PORTLAND, OR)
Oregon Poison Center (*)
Oregon Health Sciences University
3181 SW Sam Jackson Park Rd.
Portland, OR 97201
Business: 503-494-8600
Emergency: 800-222-1222
www.oregonpoison.com

NEW HAMPSHIRE

(PORTLAND, ME)
Northern New England Poison Center
Maine Medical Center
22 Bramhall St.
Portland, ME 04102
Business: 207-842-7220
Emergency: 800-222-1222

NEW JERSEY

NEWARK
New Jersey Poison Information and Education System (*)
UMDNJ
65 Bergen St.
Newark, NJ 07101
Business: 973-972-9280
Emergency: 800-222-1222
TDD/TTY: 973-926-8008
www.njpies.org

NEW MEXICO

ALBUQUERQUE
**New Mexico Poison and
Drug Information Center (*)**
MSC09-5080
1 University of New Mexico
Albuquerque, NM 87131-0001
Business: 505-272-4261
Emergency: 800-222-1222
http://HSC.UNM.edu/pharmacy/poison

NEW YORK

BUFFALO
**Western New York Regional
Poison Control Center (*)**
Children's Hospital of Buffalo
219 Bryant St.
Buffalo, NY 14222
Business: 716-878-7654
Emergency: 800-222-1222
www.fingerlakespoison.org

MINEOLA
**Long Island Regional Poison
and Drug Information Center (*)**
Winthrop University Hospital
259 First St.
Mineola, NY 11501
Business: 516-663-2650
Emergency: 800-222-1222
TDD: 516-747-3323
              (Nassau)
              516-924-8811
              (Suffolk)
www.lirpdic.org

NEW YORK CITY
**New York City
Poison Control Center (*)**
NYC Dept. of Health
455 First Ave., Room 123
New York, NY 10016
Business: 212-447-8152
Emergency: 800-222-1222
(English)   212-340-4494
              212-POISONS
              (212-764-7667)
Emergency: 212-VENENOS
(Spanish)   (212-836-3667)
TDD: 212-689-9014

ROCHESTER
**Finger Lakes Regional Poison
and Drug Information Center (*)**
**University of Rochester
Medical Center**
601 Elmwood Ave.
Box 321
Rochester, NY 14642
Business: 585-273-4155
Emergency: 800-222-1222
TTY: 585-273-3854

SYRACUSE
**Central New York
Poison Center (*)**
SUNY Upstate Medical University
750 East Adams St.
Syracuse, NY 13210
Business: 315-464-7078
Emergency: 800-222-1222
www.cnypoison.org

NORTH CAROLINA

CHARLOTTE
Carolinas Poison Center (*)
Carolinas Medical Center
PO Box 32861
Charlotte, NC 28232
Business: 704-395-3795
Emergency: 800-222-1222
TDD: 800-735-8262
TTY: 800-735-2962
www.ncpoisoncenter.org

NORTH DAKOTA

(MINNEAPOLIS, MN)
Minnesota Poison Control
System (*) Hennepin County
Medical Center
701 Park Ave.
Mail Code 820
Minneapolis, MN 55415
Business: 612-873-3144
Emergency: 800-222-1222
www.ndpoison.org

OHIO

CINCINNATI
Cincinnati Drug and Poison
Information Center (*)
Regional Poison Control System
3333 Burnet Ave.
Vernon Place, 3rd Floor
Cincinnati, OH 45229
Business: 513-636-5111
Emergency: 800-222-1222
TDD/TTY: 800-253-7955
www.cincinnatichildrens.org/dpic

CLEVELAND
Greater Cleveland
Poison Control Center
11100 Euclid Ave.
MP 6007
Cleveland, OH 44106-6007
Business: 216-844-1573
Emergency: 800-222-1222
                216-231-4455 (OH)

COLUMBUS
Central Ohio Poison Center (*)
700 Children's Dr.
Room L032
Columbus, OH 43205-2696
Business: 614-722-2635
Emergency: 614-228-1323
                800-222-1222
                937-222-2227
                (Dayton region)
TTY: 614-228-2272
www.bepoisonsmart.com

OKLAHOMA

OKLAHOMA CITY
Oklahoma Poison
Control Center (*)
Children's Hospital at
OU Medical Center
940 Northeast 13th St.
Room 3510
Oklahoma City, OK 73104
Business: 405-271-5062
Emergency: 800-222-1222
www.oklahomapoison.org

OREGON

PORTLAND
Oregon Poison Center (*)
Oregon Health Sciences University
3181 S.W. Sam Jackson Park Rd.,
CB550
Portland, OR 97239
Business: 503-494-8600
Emergency: 800-222-1222
www.oregonpoison.com

PENNSYLVANIA

PHILADELPHIA
The Poison Control Center (*)
Children's Hospital of Philadelphia
34th Street & Civic Center Blvd.
Philadelphia, PA 19104-4399
Business: 215-590-2003
Emergency: 800-222-1222
                215-386-2100 (PA)
TDD/TTY: 215-590-8789
www.poisoncontrol.chop.edu

PITTSBURGH
Pittsburgh Poison Center (*)
Children's Hospital of Pittsburgh
3705 Fifth Ave.
Pittsburgh, PA 15213
Business: 412-390-3300
Emergency: 800-222-1222
                412-681-6669
www.chp.edu/clinical/03a_poison.php

PUERTO RICO

SANTURCE
San Jorge Children's Hospital
Poison Center
258 San Jorge St.
Santurce, PR 00912
Business: 787-726-5660
Emergency: 800-222-1222
TTY: 787-641-1934
www.poisoncenter.net

RHODE ISLAND

(BOSTON, MA)
Regional Center for Poison Control
and Prevention (*)
(Serving Massachusetts and
Rhode Island)
300 Longwood Ave.
Boston, MA 02115
Business: 617-355-6609
Emergency: 800-222-1222
TDD/TTY: 888-244-5313
www.maripoisoncenter.com

SOUTH CAROLINA

COLUMBIA
Palmetto Poison Center (*)
College of Pharmacy
University of South Carolina
Columbia, SC 29208
Business: 803-777-7909
Drug Info: 800-777-7804
Emergency: 800-222-1222
              803-777-1117 (SC)
www.pharm.sc.edu/PPS/pps.htm

SOUTH DAKOTA

(MINNEAPOLIS, MN)
Hennepin Regional Poison
Center (*) Hennepin County
Medical Center
701 Park Ave.
Minneapolis, MN 55415
Business: 612-873-6000
Emergency: 800-222-1222
TTY: 612-904-4691
www.mnpoison.org

SIOUX FALLS
Provides education only—
Does not manage exposure cases.
Sioux Valley Poison Control
Center (*)
1305 W. 18th St.
Box 5039
Sioux Falls, SD 57117-5039
Business: 605-333-6638
www.sdpoison.org

TENNESSEE

NASHVILLE
Tennessee Poison Center (*)
1161 21st Ave. South
501 Oxford House
Nashville, TN 37232-4632
Business: 615-936-0760
Emergency: 800-222-1222
www.poisonlifeline.org

TEXAS

AMARILLO
Texas Panhandle
Poison Center (*)
Northwest Texas Hospital
1501 S. Coulter Dr.
Amarillo, TX 79106
Business: 806-354-1630
Emergency: 800-222-1222
www.poisoncontrol.org

DALLAS
North Texas Poison Center (*)
Texas Poison Center Network
Parkland Health and Hospital
System
5201 Harry Hines Blvd.
Dallas, TX 75235
Business: 214-589-0911
Emergency: 800-222-1222
www.poisoncontrol.org

EL PASO
West Texas Regional
Poison Center (*)
Thomason Hospital
4815 Alameda Ave.
El Paso, TX 79905
Business   915-534-3800
Emergency: 800-222-1222
www.poisoncontrol.org

GALVESTON
Southeast Texas
Poison Center (*)
The University of Texas
Medical Branch
3.112 Trauma Bldg.
301 University Ave.
Galveston, TX 77555-1175
Business: 409-766-4403
Emergency: 800-222-1222
www.poisoncontrol.org

SAN ANTONIO
South Texas
Poison Center (*)
The University of Texas Health
Science Center–San Antonio
7703 Floyd Curl Dr., MC 7849
San Antonio, TX 78229-3900
Business: 210-567-5762
Emergency: 800-222-1222
www.poisoncontrol.org

TEMPLE
Central Texas Poison Center (*)
Scott & White Memorial Hospital
2401 South 31st St.
Temple, TX 76508
Business: 254-724-7401
Emergency: 800-222-1222
www.poisoncontrol.org

UTAH

SALT LAKE CITY
Utah Poison Control Center (*)
585 Komas Dr.
Suite 200
Salt Lake City, UT 84108
Business: 801-581-7504
Emergency: 800-222-1222
                801-587-0600 (UT)
http://uuhsc.utah.edu/poison

VERMONT

(PORTLAND, ME)
Northern New England
Poison Center
Maine Medical Center
22 Bramhall St.
Portland, ME 04102
Business: 207-842-7220
Emergency: 800-222-1222

VIRGINIA

CHARLOTTESVILLE
Blue Ridge Poison Center (*)
University of Virginia Health
System
PO Box 800774
Charlottesville, VA 22908-0774
Business: 434-924-0347
Emergency: 800-222-1222
                800-451-1428 (VA)
www.healthsystem.virginia.edu.brpc

RICHMOND
Virginia Poison Center (*)
Virginia Commonwealth University
P.O. Box 980522
Richmond, VA 23298-0522
Business: 804-828-4780
Emergency: 800-222-1222
              804-828-9123
TDD/TTY: 804-828-9123

WASHINGTON

SEATTLE
Washington Poison Center (*)
155 NE 100th St.
Suite 400
Seattle, WA 98125-8011
Business: 206-517-2351
Emergency: 800-222-1222
              206-526-2121 (WA)
TDD: 800-572-0638 (WA)
              206-517-2394
              (Seattle)
www.wapc.org

WEST VIRGINIA

CHARLESTON
West Virginia Poison Center (*)
3110 MacCorkle Ave. SE
Charleston, WV 25304
Business: 304-347-1212
Emergency: 800-222-1222
www.wvpoisoncontrol.org

WISCONSIN

MILWAUKEE
Children's Hospital
of Wisconsin Statewide
Poison Center
9000 W. Wisconsin Ave.
P.O. Box 1997, Mail Station 677A
Milwaukee, WI 53226
Business: 414-266-2000
Emergency: 800-222-1222
TDD/TTY: 414-964-3497
www.chw.org

WYOMING

(OMAHA, NE)
The Poison Center (*)
Children's Hospital
8200 Dodge St.
Omaha, NE 68114
Business: 402-955-5555
Emergency: 800-222-1222
www.poison-center.com

APPENDIX 3

Top 200 Brand-Name Drugs

The following list contains the top-selling brands prescribed during 2004, measured by the total number of prescriptions filled. The information was compiled by the market research group Verispan, based in Yardley, Pennsylvania.

Rank	Product	Rank	Product
1.	Lipitor	34.	Celexa
2.	Synthroid	35.	Ortho Evra
3.	Norvasc	36.	Diovan HCT
4.	Toprol XL	37.	Accupril
5.	Zoloft	38.	Paxil CR
6.	Zocor	39.	Actonel
7.	Zithromax Z-Pak	40.	Actos
8.	Ambien	41.	Wellbutrin XL
9.	Lexapro	42.	Cozaar
10.	Prevacid	43.	Zetia
11.	Nexium	44.	Yasmin 28
12.	Singulair	45.	Avandia
13.	Levoxyl	46.	Aciphex
14.	Celebrex	47.	Zithromax
15.	Fosamax	48.	Adderall XR
16.	Effexor XR	49.	Concerta
17.	Premarin	50.	Flomax
18.	Allegra	51.	Risperdal
19.	Plavix	52.	Digitek
20.	Protonix	53.	Tricor
21.	Zyrtec	54.	Seroquel
22.	Advair Diskus	55.	Nasonex
23.	Neurontin	56.	Clarinex
24.	Flonase	57.	Xalatan
25.	Viagra	58.	Diflucan
26.	Levaquin	59.	Coumadin
27.	Pravachol	60.	Lantus
28.	Lotrel	61.	Amaryl
29.	Diovan	62.	Hyzaar
30.	Vioxx	63.	Combivent
31.	Altace	64.	Valtrex
32.	Klor-Con	65.	Crestor
33.	Bextra	66.	Ortho Tri-Cyclen

Rank	Product	Rank	Product
67.	Coreg	111.	Prempro
68.	Evista	112.	Ditropan XL
69.	OxyContin	113.	Glucovance
70.	Zithromax	114.	Inderal LA
71.	Allegra-D	115.	Apri
72.	Metformin HCl ER	116.	Trivora-28
73.	Ortho Tri-Cyclen Lo	117.	Biaxin XL
74.	Zyprexa	118.	Lescol XL
75.	Trinessa	119.	Low-Ogestrel
76.	Strattera	120.	Amoxil
77.	Avapro	121.	Avelox
78.	Topamax	122.	Cefzil
79.	Endocet	123.	Humulin 70/30
80.	Ultracet	124.	Augmentin XR
81.	Omnicef	125.	Tussionex
82.	Flovent	126.	Necon 1/35
83.	Zyrtec	127.	Trileptal
84.	Detrol LA	128.	Alphagan P
85.	Lanoxin	129.	Atacand
86.	Depakote	130.	Proscar
87.	Nasacort AQ	131.	Avandamet
88.	Imitrex Oral	132.	Budeprion SR
89.	Rhinocort Aqua	133.	Thyroid, Armour
90.	Wellbutrin SR	134.	Depakote ER
91.	Skelaxin	135.	Tobradex
92.	Levothroid	136.	Miacalcin Nasal
93.	Duragesic	137.	Cialis
94.	Aviane	138.	Cosopt
95.	Mobic	139.	Lamisil Oral
96.	Aricept	140.	Pulmicort Respules
97.	Niaspan	141.	Bactroban
98.	Elidel	142.	Plendil
99.	Humulin N	143.	Vivelle-DOT
100.	Humalog	144.	Abilify
101.	Benicar	145.	Vigamox
102.	Patanol	146.	Serevent Diskus
103.	Lamictal	147.	Xopenex
104.	Tri-Sprintec	148.	Biaxin
105.	Miralax	149.	Prometrium
106.	Zyrtec-D	150.	BenzaClin
107.	Avalide	151.	Cipro
108.	Dilantin	152.	Benicar HCT
109.	Augmentin ES-600	153.	Astelin
110.	Kariva	154.	Sprintec

Rank	Product	Rank	Product
155.	Orapred	178.	Zantac
156.	Ovcon-35	179.	Provigil
157.	Levitra	180.	Methadose
158.	Glucotrol XL	181.	Mavik
159.	Cipro XR	182.	Glucophage XR
160.	Lescol	183.	Femhrt
161.	Lotensin	184.	Depo-Provera
162.	Flexeril	185.	Elocon
163.	NuvaRing	186.	Zymar
164.	Roxicet	187.	Catapres-TTS
165.	MetroGel-Vaginal	188.	Micardis
166.	Paxil	189.	Keppra
167.	Asacol	190.	Humulin R
168.	Differin	191.	Prilosec
169.	Lidoderm	192.	Macrobid
170.	Zelnorm	193.	Sonata
171.	Atrovent	194.	Necon 0.5/35E
172.	Climara	195.	Premarin Vaginal
173.	Lumigan	196.	Zovia 1/35
174.	Glycolax	197.	Activella
175.	Tequin	198.	Humalog Mix 75/25
176.	Levora	199.	Mircette
177.	Estrostep Fe	200.	Taztia XT